Trauma: A Comprehensive Emergency Medicine Approach

Trauma: A Comprehensive Emergency Medicine Approach

Edited by

Eric Legome

Kings County Hospital Center and SUNY Downstate Medical School Brooklyn, New York

Lee W. Shockley

Denver Health Medical Center and University of Colorado School of Medicine Denver, Colorado

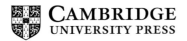
CAMBRIDGE
UNIVERSITY PRESS

CAMBRIDGE UNIVERSITY PRESS
Cambridge, New York, Melbourne, Madrid, Cape Town,
Singapore, São Paulo, Delhi, Tokyo, Mexico City

Cambridge University Press
The Edinburgh Building, Cambridge CB2 8RU, UK

Published in the United States of America by
Cambridge University Press, New York

www.cambridge.org
Information on this title: www.cambridge.org/9780521870573

First published 2011

Printed in the United Kingdom at the University Press, Cambridge

A catalogue record for this publication is available from the British Library

Library of Congress Cataloging-in-Publication Data

Trauma : a comprehensive emergency medicine approach / edited by
Eric Legome, Kings County Hospital, and Lee W. Shockley, University
of Colorado and Denver Health Sciences Center.
       p. ; cm.
     Includes bibliographical references and index.
     ISBN 978-0-521-87057-3 (Hardback)
1. Traumatology.   2. Wounds and injuries.   I. Legome, Eric, editor.
II. Shockley, Lee W., editor.   III. Title.
     [DNLM: 1. Wounds and Injuries–therapy.   2. Critical Care–methods.
3. Emergencies.   4. Emergency Medical Services–methods.
5. Emergency Treatment–methods.   6. Wounds and
Injuries–diagnosis. WO 700]
     RD93.T673 2011
     617.1–dc22
                                                                    2010046403

ISBN 978-0-521-87057-3 Hardback

We would like to dedicate this book to all the front line emergency physicians, nurses, and providers who work each day in difficult circumstances to provide the best trauma care possible.

Contents

Contributors

Giustino Albanese MD
Radiology Residency
University of Colorado School of Medicine
Aurora, Colorado

Andrew Amaranto MD
Instructor in Medicine, Division of Emergency
Medicine
Weill Cornell Medical School
New York–Presbyterian Hospital
New York, New York

Brandon H. Backlund MD, FACEP
Assistant Professor, Department of Emergency
Medicine
University of Colorado School of Medicine
Staff Physician, Denver Health Medical Center
Denver, Colorado

Alexander Baxter MD
Assistant Professor, Department of Radiology
NYU School of Medicine
Emergency Radiology
New York University Langone Medical Center
Bellevue Hospital Center
New York, New York

Abraham Berger MD
Assistant Professor in Emergency Medicine
Albert Einstein College of Medicine
Department of Emergency Medicine
Beth Israel Medical Center
New York, New York

Mark Bernstein MD
Assistant Professor, Department of Radiology
NYU School of Medicine
Emergency Radiology
New York University Langone Medical Center
Bellevue Hospital Center
New York, New York

Marian E. Betz MD, MPH
Instructor, Department of Emergency
Medicine
University of Colorado School of Medicine
Attending Physician, University of Colorado
Denver School of Medicine
Anschutz Medical Campus
Denver, Colorado

Omar Bholat MD
Assistant Professor, Department of Surgery
Division of Trauma and Critical Care
New York University School of Medicine
New York University Langone Medical Center
Bellevue Hospital Center
New York, New York

Suzanne Bigelow MD
Attending Physician, Providence Regional
Medical Center Everett Washington
Clinical Instructor, Division of Emergency
Medicine
University of Washington
Seattle, Washington

Carl Bonnett MD
Staff Physician
Littleton Adventist Hospital
Littleton, Colorado

Elizabeth Borock MD
Assistant Professor, University of Washington
School of Medicine
Attending Physician, University of Washington
Medical Center
Seattle, Washington

Christopher B. Colwell MD
Associate Professor, University of Colorado
School of Medicine
Director, Emergency Medical Services

Medical Director, Paramedic Division
Medical Director, Denver Fire Department
Staff Physician, Denver Health Medical Center
Denver, Colorado

Alasdair Conn MD
Associate Professor of Surgery, Department
of Surgery
Harvard Medical School
Chief, Emergency Medical Services
Massachusetts General Hospital
Boston, Massachusetts

Moira Davenport MD
Assistant Professor of Emergency Medicine
Drexel University College of Medicine
Associate Program Director, Allegheny General
Hospital Emergency
Medicine Residency
Attending Physician, Departments of Emergency
Medicine and Orthopedic Surgery
Allegheny General Hospital
Pittsburgh, Pennsylvania

David Dreitlein MD
Staff Physician
Montrose Memorial Hospital
Montrose, Colorado

Aaron Eberhardt MD
Staff Physician
Denver Health Medical Center
Denver, Colorado

Ugo A. Ezenkwele MD, MPH
Assistant Professor, Department of Emergency
Medicine
New York University School of Medicine
New York University Langone Medical Center
Bellevue Hospital Center
New York, New York

Diana Felton MD
Staff Physician
Whidden Memorial Hospital
Cambridge Health Alliance
Everett, Massachusetts

Spiros G. Frangos MD, MPH
Assistant Professor, Department of Surgery
Division of Trauma and Critical Care

New York University School of Medicine
New York University Langone Medical Center
Bellevue Hospital Center
New York, New York

John E. Frank MD
Director, ENT
Manhattan's Physicians Group
New York, New York

Jonathan S. Gates MD
Assistant Professor, Department of Surgery
Harvard Medical School
Medical Director, Trauma Services
Division of Trauma, Burns, and Critical Care
Brigham and Women's Hospital
Boston, Massachusetts

Lewis Goldfrank MD
Professor and Chair, Department of Emergency
Medicine
NYU School of Medicine
Director, NewYork Poison Control Center
Bellevue Hospital Center
New York, New York

Pinchas Halpern MD
Chair, Emergency Department
Tel Aviv Medical Center,
Tel Aviv, Israel

Jean Hammel MD
Assistant Professor, Division of Emergency
Medicine
Yale University School of Medicine
Staff Physician, Norwalk Hospital
Norwalk, Connecticut

Kristin E. Harkin MD FACEP
Assistant Professor of Emergency Medicine
Albert Einstein College of Medicine
Jacobi Medical Center
New York, New York

Jason S. Haukoos MD, MSc
Associate Professor, University of Colorado
School of Medicine
Department of Emergency Medicine, School
of Medicine in Denver
Department of Preventive Medicine and Biometrics,
School of Medicine in Denver

Denver, Colorado
Department of Integrative Physiology, University
of Colorado
Boulder, Colorado
Staff Physician, Department of Emergency Medicine
Denver Health Medical Center
Denver, Colorado
Research Director, Department of Emergency
Medicine
Denver Health Medical Center
Denver, Colorado

E. Parker Hays, Jr. MD, FACEP
Department of Emergency Medicine
Carolinas Medical Center
Charlotte, North Carolina
Adjunct Professor of Emergency Medicine
University of North Carolina School of Medicine
Chapel Hill, North Carolina

Aaron Hexdall MD
Assistant Professor of Emergency Medicine
Tufts University School of Medicine
Baystate Medical Center
Springfield, Massachusetts

James F. Holmes MD, MPH
Professor, Department of Emergency Medicine
Department of Emergency Medicine
UC Davis School of Medicine
Sacramento, California

Debra Houry MD, MPH
Assistant Professor, Vice Chair for Research,
Department of Emergency Medicine
Emory University School of Medicine and
Department of Behavioral Science and Health
Education at the Rollins School of Public Health
Director, Center for Injury Control, Rollins
School of Public Health
Emory University
Atlanta, Georgia

Jennifer Isenhour MD
Department of Emergency Medicine
Carolinas Medical Center
Charlotte, North Carolina
Assistant Professor of Emergency Medicine
University of North Carolina School of Medicine
Chapel Hill, North Carolina

Andy Jagoda MD
Professor and Chair, Department of Emergency
Medicine
Mt. Sinai School of Medicine
Medical Director, Department of Emergency
Medicine
Mt. Sinai Medical Center
New York, New York

John L. Kendall MD, FACEP
Associate Professor, Department of Emergency
Medicine
University of Colorado School of Medicine
Director, Emergency Ultrasound
Denver Health Medical Center
Denver, Colorado

Erica Kreisman MD
Assistant Professor, Department of Emergency
Medicine
NYU School of Medicine
North Shore University Hospital
Assistant Residency Director, North Shore
University Hospital Emergency Medicine
Residency
New York, New York

Nancy Kwon MD
Assistant Professor, Department of Emergency
Medicine
NYU School of Medicine
New York University Langone Medical Center
Bellevue Hospital Center
New York, New York

Eric Legome MD FACEP
Visiting Associate Professor of Emergency
Medicine
State University New York Downstate Medical School
Associate Professor of Emergency Medicine
New York Medical College
Chief of Service, Kings County Medical Center
Brooklyn, New York

Matthew R. Levine MD
Assistant Professor and Director, Trauma Services
Department of Emergency Medicine
Northwestern University, Feinberg School of
Medicine
Chicago, Illinois

Phillip D. Levy MD, MPH
Assistant Professor, Wayne State University
School of Medicine
Associate Director of Clinical Research
Director of Resident Research
Detroit Receiving Hospital
Department of Emergency Medicine
Detroit, Michigan

Charles Little DO
Associate Professor of Surgery, Department
of Emergency Medicine
University of Colorado Denver School
of Medicine
Univeristy of Colorado Hospital
Denver, Colorado

Marion Machado RN
Head Nurse, Bellevue Emergency Ward
Bellevue Hospital
New York, New York

Heather Mahoney MA, MD
Assistant Professor, Department of Emergency
Medicine
NYU School of Medicine
Assistant Residency Director, NYU/Bellevue
Emergency Medicine Residency
New York University Langone Medical
Center
Bellevue Hospital Center
New York, New York

Vincent J. Markovchick MD
Staff Physician, Denver Health Medical
Center
Professor, University of Colorado Denver
School of Medicine
Denver, Colorado

Nancy Martin RN, ACNP
Trauma Program Director
Virginia Commonwealth University
Richmond, Virginia

John Marx MD
Chair and Chief of the Department of Emergency
Medicine
Carolinas Medical Center
Adjunct Professor of Emergency
Medicine
University of North Carolina, Chapel Hill
Charlotte, North Carolina

Julie Mayglothling MD
Assistant Professor, Department of Emergency
Medicine
Department of Surgery, Division of Trauma
Critical Care
Virginia Commonwealth University
Richmond, Virginia

Ron Medzon MD
Associate Professor, Department of Emergency
Medicine
Boston University School of Medicine
Medical Director, Clinical Training Center
Director for Medical Simulation
Boston Medical Center
Boston, Massachusetts

Maurizio A. Miglietta DO, FACOS
Assistant Professor, Department of Surgery
Columbia University College of Physicians and
Surgeons
Chief, Division of Acute Care Surgery
Trauma and Emergency Surgery
Columbia University College of Physicians and
Surgeons
NewYork-Presbyterian Hospital
New York, New York

Elizabeth L. Mitchell MD
Associate Professor, Department of Emergency
Medicine
Boston University School of Medicine
Attending Physician, Boston Medical
Center
Boston, Massachusetts

Ernest Moore MD
Chief of Surgery and Trauma Services, Denver
Health Medical Center
Professor and Vice Chair of Research, University
of Colorado Denver
Denver, Colorado

Maria E. Moreira MD
Director, Residency in Emergency Medicine
Staff Physician, Denver Health Medical
Center
Assistant Professor, University of Colorado

School of Medicine
Denver, Colorado

Sassan Naderi MD
Director, International Emergency Medicine
Fellowship
North Shore – LIJ Health System
Assistant Professor of Emergency Medicine
Albert Einstein College of Medicine
New York, New York

Salvatore Pardo MD
Associate Chairman, Department of Emergency
Medicine
Long Island Jewish Medical Center
Assistant Professor of Emergency Medicine
Albert Einstein College of Medicine
New York, New York

Sajan Patel MS
New York University School of Medicine
New York, New York

David Peak MD
Instructor in Medicine, Division of Emergency
Medicine
Harvard Medical School
Assistant Program Director, Harvard Affiliated
Residency in Emergency Medicine
Attending Physician, Massachusetts General
Hospital
Boston, Massachusetts

Christine Preblick MD
Assistant Professor, Emergency Medicine
Department of Emergency Medicine
Beth Israel Medical Center
New York, New York

Niels K. Rathlev MD
Professor and Chair, Department of Emergency
Medicine
Tufts University School of Medicine
Department of Emergency Medicine
Baystate Medical Center
Springfield, Massachusetts

Charles Ray Jr. MD
Professor of Radiology
Faculty, Interventional Radiology
Department of Radiology

University of Colorado at Denver
Denver, Colorado

Phillip L. Rice, Jr. MD
Instructor in Medicine, Division of Emergency Medicine
Harvard Medical School
Attending Physician
North Shore Medical Center
Salem, Massachusetts

Carlo L. Rosen MD
Assistant Professor, Medicine
Harvard Medical School
Director, Emergency Medicine Residency
Beth Israel Deaconess Medical Center
Harvard Affiliated Emergency Medicine Residency
Department of Emergency Medicine
Beth Israel Deaconess Medical Center
Boston, Massachusetts

Peter Rosen MD
Senior Lecturer on Medicine
Harvard Medical School
Department of Emergency Medicine
Beth Israel Deaconess Medical Center
Boston, Massachusetts

Livia Santiago-Rosado MDD
Assistant Professor, Emergency Medicine
Mt. Sinai School of Medicine
Associate Director, Department of Emergency Medicine
Queens Hospital Center
Jamaica, New York

Tamara A. Scerpella MD
Professor, Department of Orthopedics and
Rehabilitation
University of Wisconsin-Madison
Madison, Wisconsin

David T. Schwartz MD
Clinical Associate Professor
Department of Emergency Medicine
NYU School of Medicine
NewYork University Langone Medical Center
Bellevue Hospital Center
New York, New York

Fred Severyn MD
Associate Professor of Surgery
Department of Emergency Medicine

University of Colorado, School of Medicine
University of Colorado Hospital
Denver, Colorado

Kaushal Shah MD

Assistant Professor, Emergency Medicine
Mt. Sinai School of Medicine
Site Residency Director
Mt. Sinai Emergency Medicine Residency
Elmhurst Hospital
Queens, New York

Lee W. Shockley MD, MBA, FACEP, FAAEM, CPE

Medical Director, Emergency Department
Associate Director of Emergency Medical Services
Denver Health Medical Center
Professor, Department of Emergency Medicine
University of Colorado School of Medicine
Denver, Colorado

Mari Siegel MD

Clinical Instructor, Division of Emergency Medicine
Stanford University
Stanford, California

Matthew Simons MD

Assistant Professor of Emergency Medicine
Mt. Sinai School of Medicine
Assistant Director of Emergency Medicine
Queens Hospital Center
Jamaica, New York

Michael Stern MD

Assistant Professor, Weill Medical College of Cornell University
Director of Geriatric Emergency Medicine
NewYork Presbyterian Hospital
New York, New York

D. Matthew Sullivan MD

Associate Director of Emergency Department Operations
Director of Observational Medicine
Attending Physician, Carolinas Medical Center
Charlotte, North Carolina

Carrie D. Tibbles MD

Assistant Professor, Harvard Medical School
Associate Residency Director
Beth Israel Deaconess Medical Center
Harvard/BIDMC Affiliated Emergency Medicine Residency
Boston, Massachusetts

Knox H. Todd MD, MPH

Professor and Chair
Department of Emergency Medicine
MD Anderson
Cancer Center
Houston, Texas

Shawn Ulrich RN, NPM

Department of Emergency Medicine
Denver Health Medical Center
Denver, Colorado

Neil Waldman MD

Emergency Physician
Montrose Memorial Hospital
Montrose, Colorado

Kurt Whitaker MD

Staff Physician
Department of Emergency Medicine
Intermountain Medical Center
Murray, Utah

Stephen J. Wolf MD, FACEP

Associate Dean, University of Colorado
Denver School of Medicine
Staff Physician, Denver Health Medicial Center
Associate Professor, University of Colorado
School of Medicine
Denver, Colorado

Daniel Zlogar MD

Attending Physician
Kalispell Regional Medical Center,
Kalispell, Montana

Preface

Traumatic injuries, both intentionally inflicted and unintentional, have major health consequences worldwide. Although primarily a disease of younger adults, its morbidity and mortality are increasingly severe at the extremes of age. Expert multidisciplinary trauma care is recognized as the most important determinant of survival. This concept has far reaching implications for medical education, public health, public policy, economics, and research.

There are a number of very fine textbooks on trauma that the student and experienced clinician can reference. However, the overwhelming majority of those texts are written primarily from a surgical perspective; they detail the resuscitation, operative management, and intensive care of trauma patients. Emergency physicians with proficiency in trauma management are crucial elements in initial approach to these trauma patients. Furthermore, there are many traumatic injuries treated in the emergency department by emergency physicians and nurses; outpatient follow up may be performed by a variety of specialists after the initial visit. Less tends to be written about these patients yet they consume the majority of trauma care provided in emergency departments.

We have assembled over eighty authorities in emergency trauma care to craft a comprehensive reference for all practitioners called upon to provide care for patients with emergency presentations of traumatic injuries. While specifically targeted at practicing emergency physicians, emergency medicine residents in training, physician assistants, nurse practitioners, and emergency nurses will find that this text provides insights and assistance for their trauma management. In addition, the surgical trauma specialist will glean insights that are topical and useful about care in the emergency department. The internist and family practitioner who may evaluate minor trauma in the office will benefit from discussions on ways to manage minor trauma, expedite care of their patients, and understand which patients may require more emergent care and the resources available in emergency departments. Although primarily authored by emergency physicians, multiple consultants and subspecialists lent their expertise to this book, affirming that trauma is truly a "team sport" that often requires efforts of multiple specialties to attain optimal outcomes.

This text covers aspects of trauma care from resuscitation procedures to implications for rural settings, from disaster preparedness to trauma in special populations, from medical concerns in the trauma patient to professionalism, communications, and interpersonal issues. The authors in this book are clinicians, teachers, writers, researchers, and administrators renowned as the experts in modern trauma care in the emergency department.

Acknowledgments

To my wife, Ann, and my daughters, Dorian and Darby, for your love and understanding. To my mother, Doris, for your guidance and strength. To my father, Orville, for your inspiration and example; I wish you were here to receive a signed first edition. To my in-laws, Ann and Bill, for your encouragement. To my teachers for giving me the benefit of your knowledge and wisdom. For my residents and students for keeping me sharp and excited about emergency medicine. For the nurses, technicians, clerks, and colleagues for keeping me out of trouble. And for my patients who have allowed me to serve them when they needed it the most.

LS

To my family, which doubled in size during the development of this book. My wife Lisa and my children Giselle and Jack provided me with the love, energy, and time necessary to complete this project. To my parents for their support throughout the years. To all my mentors, colleagues and residents that have taught me over the years and continue to do so on a daily basis. For all the daily support I receive from the nurses, technicians, clerks, and administrative assistants that help me care for our patients and department; I appreciate it every day. To the consultants who provide insight and knowledge to help us care for our patients. To all my wonderful colleagues at the former St. Vincent's Hospital, Manhattan. For all injured patients, whom this book is really for.

EL

A special thanks to all the people that helped us with this project, especially Mark Strauss, Katherine Tengco, Katie James, and Alice Nelson from the publishing end, Mark Bernstein, MD for his tremendous assistance with radiographs, the NYU Anatomy department, Sajan Patel MS, Taku Taira, MD for his photography skills and Nick Setty for his legal skills.

EL and LS

Decision making in trauma

Julie Mayglothling, Peter Rosen, and Ernest Moore

Introduction

With the development of trauma systems in the 1970s, the care of the injured trauma patient has become more organized, specialized, evidence based, and of improved quality. Organized trauma systems have improved mortality by providing expert care to trauma patients.[1–3] The goal of trauma systems is to match the severity of injury and resources required for optimal care with the appropriate trauma facility and personnel. On a theoretical basis, all patients with significant traumatic injuries and mechanisms of trauma would ideally be brought to a trauma center. This is not possible in the United States, due to funding, the geographic size of the country, the dispersal of the population, and the lack of a financial means of supporting those physicians who would confine their practice to trauma. Proficient trauma care is accomplished by not only having appropriate resources and specialists available in special trauma centers, but by having practitioners well educated and trained in the sophisticated care of the injured patient, even in the institutions that rarely manage trauma. A challenge is how to maintain trauma skills in the physicians and nurses who practice in institutions that rarely care for traumatic injuries, but may need to during a disaster or other critical situation.

It is difficult to predict in advance what specific needs an injured patient will require. Therefore, clinical decisions are made both in the prehospital setting, as well as on patient arrival to the emergency department (ED), based on a consistent and compulsive evaluation of each patient, rather than trying to guess what is the most likely extent of injury that is present. A routine and complete evaluation of the patient will avoid missing significant pathology. For this reason, adequate information about the mechanism of injury and the magnitude of the trauma sustained is an important part of the evaluation of each patient, and requires detailed communication and trust between the prehospital providers and the in-house trauma team.

The trauma team

An efficiently functioning trauma team is integral to the successful care of the severely injured patient. The team may range from a single emergency physician and emergency nurse at a small rural hospital, to a large, multiperson team at an urban Level I trauma center. Each member of the team should have an understood and well-defined role in the resuscitation and evaluation of the patient. Routine tasks must be performed simultaneously, in a coordinated manner, to identify and treat life-threatening injuries as early as possible.[4] Frequently, in rural institutions with a paucity of manpower, tasks that can be performed in parallel by the team in the trauma center will have to be performed serially. It may be useful to have assistance from the prehospital personnel, if they can stay at the ED to assist. The trauma captain is responsible for the overall management of the trauma resuscitation. He or she designates team members' responsibilities prior to the patient's arrival and ensures that all members of the team perform their duties. The captain is responsible for the overall assessment of the patient, and should not become involved in the performance of procedures unless there is no other choice. All roles on the team can be interchanged for educational variety, but this should be established in advance rather than during the resuscitation. For example, in an academic institution, the team captain may be surgical resident one day or emergency medicine resident another. At smaller hospitals, an

Trauma: A Comprehensive Emergency Medicine Approach, eds. Eric Legome and Lee W. Shockley. Published by Cambridge University Press. © Cambridge University Press 2011.

emergency physician may be the only physician available in house, and assumes responsibility for whatever comes through the door. When there are multiple physicians present, it is imperative that there is a chain of command which works through the trauma captain. If the trauma captain becomes involved in a difficult procedure such as an intubation or central line placement, the overall responsibility of being captain must be handed off to another physician who is not involved in the procedure. In institutions with housestaff, the emergency medicine attending physician is responsible for the patient until the trauma attending physician is physically present and a transfer of care has occurred.

At designated American College of Surgeons (ACS) certified trauma centers, the ACS mandates that a surgeon must be present on arrival of all severely injured patients and that he or she act as the trauma team leader.[5] This tenet initially was put into practice when a high percentage of trauma patients required operative intervention and many EDs were staffed with non-emergency medicine trained physicians with little or no trauma training. However, with increasing numbers of EDs staffed by residency trained emergency physicians and lower rates of exploratory laparotomy, this tenet is being re-evaluated and challenged.[6,7] Currently, the debate surrounds what is meant by severely injured. There is no question as to the need for a trauma surgeon's presence in a patient with penetrating trauma to the torso and hypotension. A more reasonable goal may be to have a trauma surgeon present on patient arrival when there is a high likelihood of a patient requiring urgent operative intervention. Many hospitals have developed a multitiered trauma activation system to more efficiently utilize the attending trauma surgeon's expertise. These systems spare the trauma surgeon from being present for all trauma team alerts and reserve their efforts for those patients that have high likelihood of requiring operative intervention.[8] The reality of trauma practice is that few institutions can meet the mandate of the ACS. What is most important is that there is an emergency physician present who has trauma expertise and that there is an orderly transition of responsibility between the emergency physician and the trauma surgeon. If there are no institutional surgeons with trauma expertise, there needs to be a system to transfer the patient to a trauma center that has those capabilities.

Prehospital personnel are important to the success of any trauma resuscitation. They provide a unique perspective as to the changing condition of the patient, from injury to hospital presentation. They communicate important information regarding mechanism of injury, initial presentation, and changes in clinical condition. Many times, the history obtained from the field personnel is the only source available. In addition, prehospital personnel often initiate life-saving therapy such as airway control, needle decompression for pneumothorax, and fluid resuscitation.

An experienced trauma nurse is a valuable asset to a severely injured patient. A nurse familiar with trauma resuscitation is able to anticipate the needs of the trauma captain, and has medications or supplies ready even before they are needed. In most cases, the trauma nurses are the personnel who spend the most time with the patient, from initial presentation to disposition, and are therefore more likely to notice subtle changes in vital signs or other signs of deterioration, and can notify the captain in a timely manner. The trauma nurse maintains records of intravenous (IV) fluids and blood products administered, medications given, and procedures performed.

The trauma team may also include physician assistants, emergency medics, or medical technicians whose responsibilities may include obtaining IV access, attaining adequate exposure of the patient, and assisting in rolling and transporting the patient in a safe and expeditious manner. The level of responsibility is often dependent upon training and the center where they practice.

The appropriate and timely evaluation of the trauma patient is also dependent on other support personnel, such as radiology and computed tomography (CT) technicians. The accuracy of radiographs is imperative to the appropriate workup of a trauma patient. A knowledgeable radiology technician can safely and quickly obtain needed films with minimal disruption of the evaluation. An experienced CT technician can have a large impact on the timeliness of a trauma evaluation. They can rapidly obtain multiple scans and promptly get patients back to the resuscitation area.

Additional surgical subspecialists, such as neurosurgeons and orthopedic surgeons, may be members of the trauma team and provide a unique set of skills and knowledge. Neurologic trauma, including head injury and spinal cord injury, is common in trauma patients. Traumatic brain injury accounts for 40% of all deaths from acute trauma. The availability of neurosurgeons to provide neurotrauma care promptly and continuously is a prerequisite for a level I trauma center. However, access to neurosurgical care remains a problem, most acutely in rural communities. For those trauma centers and community hospitals that do not provide routine neurosurgeon coverage, it may be important to transfer patients with spinal cord injury or moderate to severe traumatic brain injury to a higher level of care as soon as possible where these patients can receive care by neurotrauma specialists. However, this should be done with consideration of the full range of injuries, with life-threatening hemorrhage control taking precedence.

More than half of all hospitalized trauma patients have one or more musculoskeletal injuries that could be life or limb threatening or that might result in significant functional impairment. Patients with isolated simple fractures with low-grade soft tissue injuries are appropriately treated in any well-equipped hospital by orthopedic surgeons. Patients who have multiple fractures, complex fractures (including pelvic, acetabular, intra-articular, and spinal column), or high-grade soft tissue injuries are appropriate candidates for musculoskeletal trauma care at a Level I or II trauma center. The multiple trauma patient is best served by being admitted to the trauma service with subspecialty consultation rather than admitting such patients to one or other of the subspecialty services. This may allow for better overall coordination of care and diagnosis of occult internal injuries.

Box 1.1   Trauma team essentials

- An efficiently functioning trauma team is integral to the successful care of the severely injured patient. The team may range from a single emergency physician and emergency nurse at a small rural hospital to a large, multiperson team at an urban level I trauma center.
- Each member of the team should have an understood and well-defined role in the resuscitation and evaluation of the patient.
- When there are multiple physicians present, it is imperative that there is a chain of command that works through the trauma captain.
- The multiple trauma patient is best served by being admitted to the trauma service with subspecialty consultation rather than admitting

---

such patients to one or other of the subspecialty services. This may allow for better overall coordination of care and diagnosis of occult internal injuries.

Prehospital

The initial challenge in the prehospital management of trauma is finding and gaining access to the trauma victim. This can be difficult due to problems with communication (e.g., inadequate phone coverage in rural areas), dispatch (lack of clear jurisdictional authority), and access (e.g., traffic congestion, lack of roads, or weather). The major forms of prehospital transport are by ambulance, helicopter, or, rarely, fixed-wing. The goal of prehospital trauma triage is to identify and provide rapid treatment for the most severely injured trauma patients and to transport them to the most appropriate center able to manage their injuries.

There is no national consensus on trauma triage criteria and many trauma systems have adopted their own guidelines. Most systems use some variation of the field triage scheme outlined by the ACS Committee on Trauma (Figure 1.1). These guidelines have been shown to have > 95% sensitivity for identification of severely injured trauma patients.[9,10] Multiple variables are included, such as physiologic, anatomic, and mechanistic criteria, as well as patient age and comorbidities. Physiologic criteria, such as systolic blood pressure (SBP), Glasgow Coma Scale (GCS), or Revised Trauma Score (RTS) have been shown to have the highest sensitivity (56–65%) in predicting severe injury when used alone. The sensitivity of physiologic criteria is increased even more when used in combination with anatomic or mechanistic criteria. An SBP < 90 mmHg, a mechanism of gunshot wounds (GSWs), and endotracheal intubation (ETI) predicts the need for intensive care unit (ICU) admission and operative intervention; a GCS < 8, SBP < 90 mmHg and ETI are associated with mortality.[11]

Anatomic criteria used for field triage include penetrating injuries to the head, neck, torso, and proximal extremity; two or more proximal long bone fractures; crushed or mangled extremity; pelvic fractures; open or depressed skull fractures; and paralysis. The Injury Severity Score (ISS) is an anatomic scoring system that is used to assess the extent of injury and has been found to correlate with morbidity and

3

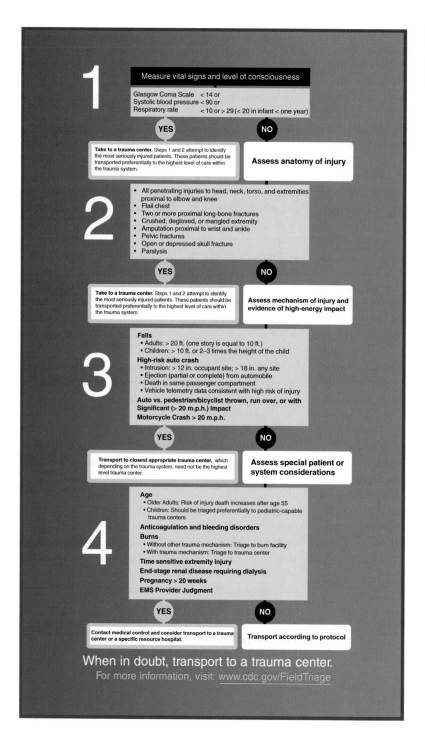

Figure 1.1 Field triage decision scheme: The National Trauma Triage Protocol. (Courtesy of the US Department of Health and Human Services Centers for Disease Control and Prevention.)

mortality. Patients with an ISS score > 15 have been shown to benefit from transport to a trauma center.[12] However, the ISS is calculated at discharge, and is difficult, if not impossible, to accurately calculate in the field. In fact, trauma scores have generally not worked prospectively in large part because they can only be derived from data that is not available until late in the trauma patient's course. However, the use of any anatomic criteria alone to triage patients has a lower sensitivity (45%) in predicting severe injury.[9] Certain anatomic criteria, such as paraplegia or a mangled extremity, may alert the trauma team to a significant mechanism possibly causing other injuries or the need for subspecialists, such as orthopedic surgeons or neurosurgeons.

Mechanistic criteria, such as pedestrian stuck by a vehicle, motor vehicle collision (MVC) with prolonged extrication, vehicle damage, or intrusion, and death of another vehicle occupant have had mixed results; however, when used alone have generally been shown to be poorly predictive of severe injury or need for trauma team activation.[13-17] When used in combination with anatomic or physiologic criteria, the sensitivity increases. Multiple studies have attempted to identify which mechanistic criteria are more sensitive for the risk of severe injury; however, there is no consensus. Many trauma systems tailor their own triage guidelines depending on which mechanistic criteria appear to be the most sensitive for their unique patient populations.[8,18] Like any screening test, field triage will have a level of sensitivity and specificity. A gain in one will lead to a loss in others. Generally it is felt that overtriage, or loss of specificity and gain of sensitivity, is preferable to undertriage. The ACS uses a number of > 25% overtriage as acceptable to achieve < 5% undertriage.

Geriatric trauma patients present a difficult challenge in the evaluation of injury. Patients > 65 years old have higher mortality and complication rates and longer hospital stays than younger patients with similar injury severity.[19] Several prehospital trauma triage guidelines that do not contain criteria to include elderly trauma patients have found that it results in unacceptable levels of undertriage in patients > 65 years old with potentially life-threatening injuries.[20,21]

Box 1.2 Prehospital essentials

- The goal of prehospital trauma triage is to identify and provide rapid treatment for the most severely injured trauma patients and transport them to the most appropriate center able to manage their injuries.
- There is no national consensus on trauma triage criteria and many trauma systems have adopted their own guidelines.
- Generally it is felt that overtriage to trauma centers, or loss of specificity and gain of sensitivity, is preferable to undertriage.

Hospital presentation

Patient management must consist of rapid primary survey, resuscitation of vital functions, a more detailed secondary assessment, and, finally, the initiation of definitive care. The goals of the primary survey are to identify and target potentially life-threatening causes of injury on patient presentation. The primary survey is the same regardless of whether the injured patient is delivered to a small community hospital or a level I trauma center. Trauma surveys must be performed compulsively on each patient.

The ultimate goal of resuscitation is to restore organ perfusion. This is accomplished by controlling hemorrhage as much as is possible, administering isotonic fluids to replace lost intravascular volume, infusing packed red blood cells to avoid critical anemia, and monitoring the patient response to intervention in order to tailor further resuscitative efforts. In attempting to restore organ perfusion, there are multiple criteria clinicians use to assess patients' response: blood pressure, heart rate, mental status, and urine output are the most commonly used endpoints of resuscitation in the ED. Serum lactate and base deficit values may be helpful because they may alert the physician to organ hypoperfusion in the setting of apparently normal vital signs, particularly in the elderly. One of the recent controversies in the patient with ongoing bleeding is the concept of "permissive hypotension," where the goal of organ perfusion is balanced with the risks of rebleeding by accepting a lower than normal blood pressure. For decades the standard approach to the trauma victim who is hypotensive from presumed hemorrhage has been to infuse isotonic fluid as early and rapidly as possible, with the goal of restoration of intravascular volume and vitals signs to normal. Multiple studies, mostly in animal models of uncontrolled hemorrhage, have suggested that this practice may be harmful and increase mortality by accelerating hemorrhage through increasing hydrostatic pressure at the hemorrhage site, breaking clots, and dilution of clotting factors.[22-24] However, this is countered by concerns that delayed resuscitation may lead to tissue hypoperfusion, organ failure, and subsequent death. Special consideration should be taken with patients with traumatic brain injury, where avoiding a SBP < 90 mmHg is important. Currently there is no universal consensus pertaining to the optimal resuscitation strategy in trauma patients. However, a policy of

5

judicious fluid administration to maintain a mean arterial pressure (MAP) > 65 mmHg is advisable once the patient is in the hospital. The most important early step in actively hemorrhaging patients is control of the bleeding. In these cases, early involvement of a trauma surgeon is appropriate.

Imaging

One of the decisions a clinician needs to make in the setting of significant trauma is what imaging to obtain. With the availability and diagnostic capability of the CT scan and the emergence of ultrasonography in the ED, imaging in trauma has changed significantly in the past several years. Various factors influence the decision of what imaging to obtain. A combination of mechanism of injury, vital signs, reliability and findings of the physical examination, clinical appearance of the patient, age, and existing comorbidities all contribute to the extent of imaging required.

The screening anteroposterior (AP) chest radiograph remains routine for patients sustaining significant blunt or penetrating trauma to the head, chest, or abdomen. This can often identify potential life-threatening injuries, such as pneumothorax or hemothorax, which may need to be addressed before transport to the CT scan, the operating room, or transfer to another facility. In addition, plain chest radiographs may identify free intra-abdominal air, mediastinal hematomas, or mediastinal air that may mandate additional imaging.

The single-view pelvis radiograph has traditionally been one of the screening radiographs obtained during initial trauma resuscitation. However, the utility of obtaining this film has been questioned.[25–27] The main goal for the screening pelvis radiograph is to identify unstable pelvic fractures or hip dislocations that need emergent intervention. In patients who are hemodynamically stable and have no clinical suggestion of an unstable pelvis fracture or hip dislocation, and who will undergo abdominal and pelvic imaging with the CT scan, it appears safe, cost effective, and appropriate to forgo pelvic radiographs. The CT scan is virtually 100% sensitive in diagnosing significant pelvic fractures.[28] On the other hand, patients who have an unstable pelvis on physical examination or evidence of hypotension should have a pelvis film in the trauma bay. These patients may have suffered an unstable pelvic fracture that needs to

be urgently stabilized or a posterior hip dislocation that warrants prompt reduction.

Historically, lateral view cervical spine radiographs were standard in initial trauma evaluation. Previously, it was deemed essential to clear the cervical spine radiographically before undertaking any active airway management. When it was decided that not all uncleared airway patients required a surgical airway as opposed to being safely intubated orally, the need for immediate imaging clearance of the spine became less time constrained. However, the inefficiency of plain radiographs and the use of CT imaging have made cervical spine radiographs much less common. So long as the stabilization of the cervical spine is maintained, the trauma team can now wait until more critical injuries have been identified and managed. Films can then be obtained according to which modality is the most accurate.[29] Plain radiographs of the cervical spine have reported sensitivity as low as 31% for identification of cervical spine injury.[30,31] Not only are radiographs not sensitive for detection of cervical spine injury, 72–79% of films are inadequate.[30,32] Many radiographs need to be repeated to get adequate views and the time it takes to obtain adequate views can average up to 22 minutes, more than double the time for cervical spine CT.[32] The atlanto-occipital and lower cervical areas are most difficult to evaluate on cervical spine radiographs and are the ones most likely to be repeated.

Box 1.3 Initial imaging essentials

- The screening AP chest radiograph in the trauma bay generally remains routine for patients sustaining significant blunt or penetrating trauma to the head, chest, or abdomen.
- In major patients who are hemodynamically stable and have no clinical suggestion of an unstable pelvic fracture or hip dislocation, and who will undergo abdominal and pelvic imaging with CT scan, it appears safe, cost effective, and appropriate to forgo pelvic radiograph in the trauma bay.
- The CT scan is virtually 100% sensitive in diagnosing significant pelvic fractures.
- In the neurologically intact patient, if stabilization of the cervical spine is maintained, the lateral cervical spine film may be withheld in the trauma bay while more critical injuries are identified and managed.
- Radiographs can then be obtained according to which modality (CT or plain film) is the most appropriate for the situation.

The cost-effectiveness of cervical spine CT relative to cervical spine radiographs has been studied. For example, Grogan et al. found that it was more cost effective to obtain cervical spine CT scans rather than plain radiographs for patients with any of the following criteria: age over 50 years; a high injury mechanism; any patient with focal neurologic deficit; or evidence of head injury.[33] Most patients requiring trauma team activation likely meet at least one of these criteria. The difficult decision arises when a patient presents with low to moderate risk of injury and any indication for imaging by either the National Emergency X-Radiography Utilization Study (NEXUS) Criteria or the Canadian Cervical Spine Rule. For moderate risk of injury, cervical spine CT is preferred, but controversial. The benefits have to be balanced with the low yield of positive scans as well as the additional cost and radiation exposure. For low-risk patients, those patients under 50 years of age with low to moderate mechanism for injury, cervical spine CT has not been shown to be cost effective.[34,35] The exception may be the patients with a large body habitus in whom it is unlikely to achieve adequate radiographs and multiple plain films are anticipated. Regardless of the modality used, the clinician needs to take into consideration the potentially devastating consequences of missed cervical spine injury and use clinical decision rules and imaging appropriately.

Evaluation for potential intra-abdominal injury is where many evaluation errors were made historically. Today, there is more acceptance of a need for objective evaluation of the abdomen in patients with blunt abdominal injury, especially if there are concomitant injuries, intoxication with drugs or alcohol, extremes of age, and where there has been a significant mechanism of injury. Patients suffering from MVCs, pedestrians struck by vehicles, patients with significant falls, or patients with penetrating trauma to the torso are at high risk for abdominal injuries. One of the complicating factors in the evaluation of these patients is the difficulty of clinical assessment, especially in the multiply injured patient. The sensitivity of physical examination alone in blunt abdominal trauma, even with serial examinations, has been well studied and is accepted as being relatively inaccurate with sensitivities of detecting intra-abdominal injury of only 65%.[36]

Determining the need for emergent operative care is the top priority in the evaluation of patients sustaining abdominal trauma. Patients who are hemodynamically unstable need to have intra-abdominal hemorrhage identified and controlled expeditiously. Time spent in the ED and severity of hypotension increases risk of death in patients with isolated operative blunt abdominal trauma.[37] In patients with penetrating trauma, hypotension is an indication for immediate operative intervention. Historically, bedside diagnostic peritoneal lavage (DPL) was the diagnostic modality of choice to rule out intra-abdominal hemorrhage or injury in unstable patients suffering from blunt abdominal trauma. The emergence of ultrasonography in trauma, specifically the focused abdominal sonography in trauma (FAST) exam, has markedly reduced the need for DPL. Reported sensitivity of FAST in detecting hemoperitoneum varies from 65% to 95%,[38,39] but in the hypotensive patient the sensitivity is thought to increase to close to 97% in patients requiring surgical intervention.[40] Given this relatively high detection of hemoperitoneum, most trauma centers employ FAST early on in evaluation of hypotensive patients with blunt trauma. The FAST exam needs to be interpreted in light of the patient's condition. It is dangerous to rely solely on a single study without context. As with a DPL, a positive FAST examination only tells you there is blood present in the abdomen. It does not identify the source, nor the magnitude of injury, and thus there is still place for the trauma team to use judgment about which patient must go directly to the operating room for management. This is more true of blunt rather than penetrating trauma.

For hemodynamically stable patients, the introduction of the CT scan in the mid-1980s has fundamentally changed the evaluation and treatment of the multisystem trauma patient, especially in evaluation of abdominal trauma. The emergence of non-operative management for many abdominal injuries and the decreased need for exploratory laparotomy is in large part due to the availability, speed, and accuracy of the CT scan. The CT scan has improved the diagnosis of both solid and hollow viscous injury after blunt abdominal trauma. Only CT scans with IV contrast are likely to be adequate for the evaluation of abdominal trauma.[41] Clinicians must balance the risks of giving IV contrast to high-risk patients with decreased glomerular filtration rate (GFR), diabetes, or history of allergic reactions to contrast medium with the risk of missed injury. However, a non-IV contrast abdominal CT should not give the clinician a false sense of security that there is no injury because this study is inadequate to fully rule out intra-abdominal injury.

There has been some controversy regarding ultrasonography vs. CT in the evaluation of hemodynamically stable patients with blunt abdominal trauma. Ultrasound is fast and allows other evaluations to proceed while the patient is being scanned. It also avoids exposure of the patient to ionizing radiation and IV contrast medium. But the sensitivity of ultrasound in diagnosing intra-abdominal injury is lower than the CT scan. Significant abdominal injury has been reported in one third of patients without hemoperitoneum.[38] These results indicate the lesser or absent ability of ultrasound to detect organ injury in the absence of free fluid. In the unstable patient who should not be placed in a CT scanner, a FAST examination or a DPL should be performed for the detection of intra-abdominal fluid. However, in the stable multisystem trauma patient, given the greater diagnostic capability and accuracy of the CT scan and the relatively low sensitivity of physical exam, clinicians should have a low threshold for evaluation with abdominal CT scan. Patients with tenderness on abdominal exam or evidence of abdominal wall trauma, such as contusion or a seat belt sign, also warrant evaluation with CT. If the physician elects not to obtain a CT scan and monitor the patient with serial abdominal exams, a CT can be subsequently obtained if the physical exam changes. A benefit of abdominal CT scan is the safe, expeditious disposition of patients. Patients with a negative abdominal CT scan may be safely discharged with a high degree of certainty from the hospital without admission or observation for occult intra-abdominal injury.[42] This decision is also dependent upon concomitant injuries, diseases, the examination, and social circumstances of the patient, as well as the mechanism of injury. There are patients who will benefit from a period of observation even if the initial studies are negative.

Box 1.4   Essentials of CT in decision making

- The emergence of non-operative management for many abdominal injuries and the decreased need for exploratory laparotomy is in large part due to the availability, speed, and accuracy of CT scan.
- CT scans with IV contrast only are likely adequate for the evaluation of abdominal trauma.
- Clinicians must balance the risks of giving IV contrast to high-risk patients with decreased GFR, diabetes, or history of allergic reactions to contrast medium with the risk of missed injury.

- However, a non-IV contrast abdominal CT should not give the clinician a false sense of security that there is no injury because this study is inadequate to fully rule out intra-abdominal injury.
- In the stable multisystem trauma patient, given the greater diagnostic capability and accuracy of the CT scan and the relatively low sensitivity of a physical exam, clinicians should have a low threshold for evaluation with abdominal CT scan.
- A benefit of abdominal CT scan is the safe, expeditious disposition of patients.

Rural and non-trauma centers

Although algorithms are in place for Emergency Medical Services (EMS) personnel to bypass community hospitals in favor of trauma centers for patients meeting selected criteria, often there is no trauma center in the vicinity. Furthermore, there are patients who arrive at the community or rural hospital with seemingly mild trauma and are found to have more extensive injury upon diagnostic review than what was apparent upon initial assessment by the EMS providers in the field. Therefore, protocols must be in place to transfer patients to appropriate facilities to manage their injuries.

The decision to transfer a patient depends on the extent of injury as well as the capabilities of the local hospital. Patients with certain injuries, combinations of injuries, or who have findings indicating high energy mechanisms may be at risk for severe injury and they are candidates for early transfer to a trauma center.[43] For example, patients who present with decreased GCS and evidence of closed head injury, obtaining CT scans or other diagnostic studies should not unduly delay transfer to a higher level of care. On the other hand, for patients who are hemodynamically stable, it may be more prudent to obtain the appropriate workup at the local hospital in order to rule out any injury requiring a trauma center. Therefore, if the studies are negative, the transfer can be avoided. If there is an injury diagnosed and the patient requires further care, transfer to a higher level facility may occur at that time.

There should be in place an easy to arrange transfer mechanism. It is far safer to accept the transfer that turns out to be a patient without significant injury than to prevent transfer of the patient with significant injuries. Prior to transfer of a critically injured patient to a higher level of care, the patient should be resuscitated and attempts should be made to stabilize the patient's condition. Interventions such as definitive airway control if indicated, chest tube placement or mechanical ventilation if appropriate, sufficient IV access, and control of external bleeding as much as possible should occur before the patient leaves the initial hospital. The receiving hospital must not demand performance of tasks that are beyond the capacity of the transferring hospital, such as difficult airway management or central line placement. The personnel in the transferring hospital may not have the necessary experience and expertise to perform them safely.

Conclusions

The care of the severely injured trauma patient is complex. A multidisciplinary team made up of individuals familiar with the care of trauma patients is essential to promptly evaluate and treat these patients. Injury assessment is based on prehospital data, vital signs, clinical presentation, and imaging studies. Trauma patients may have suffered significant injuries despite normal vital signs and an initially benign physical examination. The appropriate use of imaging studies can promptly diagnose occult injuries and help to make quick and safe dispositions. The placement of patients where they can receive definitive care, whether in the operating room, the ICU, or another facility, is a high priority in trauma care.

References

1. West JG, Cales RH, Gazanigga AB. Impact of regionalization: the Orange County experience. *Archiv Surg* 1983;**118**(6):740–4.

2. Kilberg L, Clemmer TP, Clawson J, et al. Effectiveness of implementing a trauma triage system on outcome: a prospective evaluation. *J Trauma* 1988;**28**(10): 1493–8.

3. Celso B, Tepas B, Langland-Orbon B, et al. A systematic review and meta-analysis comparing outcome of severely injured patients treated in trauma centers following the establishment of trauma systems. *J Trauma* 2006;**60**:371–8.

4. Driscoll PA, Vincent CA. Organizing an efficient trauma team. *Injury* 1992;**23**:107–10.

5. American College of Surgeons Committee on Trauma. *American College of Surgeons Resources for Optimal Care of the Injured Patient.* Chicago, IL: American College of Surgeons, 2006.

6. Green SM. Is there evidence to support the need for routine surgeon presence on trauma patient arrival? *Ann Emerg Med* 2006;**47**(5):405–11.

7. Ciesla DJ, Moore EE, Moore JB, Johnson JL, Cothren CC. Intubation alone does not mandate trauma surgeon presence on patient arrival to the emergency department. *J Trauma* 2004;**56**:937–42.

8. Markovchick VJ, Moore EE. Optimal trauma outcome: trauma system design and the trauma team. *Emerg Med Clin N Am* 2007;**25**:643–54.

9. Norcross ED, Ford DW, Cooper ME, et al. Application of American College of Surgeons field triage guidelines by pre-hospital personnel. *J Am Coll Surg* 1995;**181**:539–44.

10. Lerner EB. Studies evaluating current field triage: 1966–2005. *Prehosp Emerg Care* 2006;**10**(3):303–6.

11. Tinkoff GH, O'Connor RE. Validation of new trauma triage rules for trauma attending response to the emergency department. *J Trauma* 2002;**52**(6):1153–8.

12. Nirula R, Brasel K. Do trauma centers improve functional outcomes: A National Trauma Data Bank analysis. *J Trauma* 2006;**61**(2):268–71.

13. Lowe DK, Oh GR, Neely KW, Peterson CG. Evaluation of injury mechanism as a criterion in trauma triage. *Amer J Surg* 1986;**152**(1):6–10.

14. Hunt RC. Is mechanism of injury dead? *Preshosp Emerg Care* 1999;**3**(1):70–3.

15. Velmahos GC, Jindal A, Chan LS, et al. "Insignificant" mechanism of injury: not to be taken lightly. *J Amer Coll Surg* 2001;**192**(2):147–52.

16. Boyle MJ. Is mechanism of injury alone in the prehospital setting a predictor of major trauma – a review of the literature. *J Trauma Manage Outcomes* 2007;**26**(1):1–4.

17. Lehmann RK, Arthurs ZM, Cuadrado DG, et al. Trauma team activation: simplified criteria safely reduces overtriage. *Am J Surg* 2007;**193**:630–5.

18. Kohn, MA, Hammel JM, Bretz SW, Tangby A. Trauma team activation criteria as predictors of patient disposition from the emergency department. *Acad Emerg Med* 2004;**11**(1):1–9.

19. Champion HR, Copes WS, Buyer D, et al. Major trauma in geriatric patients. *Am J Public Health* 1989;**79**(9):1278–82.

20. Phillips S, Rond PC, Kelly SM, Swartz PD. The failure of triage guidelines to identify geriatric patients with trauma: results from the Florida Trauma Triage Study. *J Trauma* 1996;**40**(2):278–83.

21. Chang DC, Bass RR, Cornwell EE, Mackenzie EJ. Undertriage of elderly trauma patients to state-designated trauma centers. *Archiv Surg* 2008;**143**(8):776–81.

22. Stern SA, Dronen SC, Birrer P, Wang X. Effect of blood pressure on hemorrhage volume and survival in a near-fatal hemorrhage model incorporating a vascular injury. *Ann Emerg Med* 1993;**22**:155–63.

23. Burris D, Rhee P, Kaufmann C, et al. Controlled resuscitation for uncontrolled hemorrhagic shock. *J Trauma* 1999;**46**:216–23.

24. Dutton RP, Mackenzie CF, Scalea TM. Hypotensive resuscitation during active hemorrhage: impact on in-hospital mortality. *J Trauma* 2002;**52**(6):1141–6.

25. Guillamondequi OD, Pryor JP, Gracias VH, et al. Pelvic radiography in blunt trauma resuscitation: a diminishing role. *J Trauma* 2002; **53**(6):1043–7.

26. Obaid AK, Barleben A, Porral D, Lush S, Cinat M. Utility of plain pelvic radiographs in blunt trauma patients in the emergency department. *Amer Surg* 2006;**72**(10):951–4.

27. Duane TM, Dechert T, Wolfe LG, et al. Clinical examination is superior to plain films to diagnose pelvic fractures compared to CT. *Amer Surg* 2008;**74**(6):476–9.

28. Herzog C, Ahle H, Mack MG, et al. Traumatic injuries of the pelvis and thoracic and lumbar spine: does thin slice multi-detector-row CT increase diagnostic accuracy? *Eur Radiol* 2004;**14**(10):1751–60.

29. Rosen P, Wolfe RE. Therapeutic legends of emergency medicine. *J Emerg Med* 1989;**7**(4):387–9.

30. Griffen MM. Radiographic clearance of blunt cervical spine injury: Plain radiograph or computed tomography scan? *J Trauma* 2003;**55**:222–7.

31. Gale SC, Garcias VH, Reilly PM, et al. The inefficiency of plain radiography to evaluate the cervical spine after blunt trauma. *J Trauma* 2005;**59**:1121–5.

32. Daffner RH. Helical CT of the cervical spine for trauma: a time study. *AJR Am J Roentgenol* 2001;**177**(3):677–9.

33. Grogan EL, Morris JA, Jr., Dittus RS, et al. Cervical spine evaluation in urban trauma center: lowering

institutional costs and complications through helical CT scan. *J Am Coll Surg* 2005;**200**:160–5.

34. Blackmore CC, Ramsey SD, Mann FA, et al. Cervical spine screening with CT in trauma patients: a cost effectiveness analysis. *Radiology* 1999;**212**:117–25.

35. Hunink MG. Decision making in the face of uncertainty and resource constraints: examples from trauma imaging. *Radiology* 205;**235**(2):375–83.

36. Schurink GW, Bode PJ, van Lujit PA, van Vugt AB. The value of physical exam in the diagnosis of patients with blunt abdominal trauma: a retrospective study. *Injury* 1997;**28**(4)261–5.

37. Clarke JR, Trooskin SZ, Doshi PJ, Greenwald L, Mode CJ. Time to laparotomy for intra-abdominal bleeding from trauma does affect survival for delays up to 90 minutes. *J Trauma* 2002;**52**(3):420–5.

38. Chiu WC, Cushing BM, Rodriguez A, et al. Abdominal injuries without hemoperitoneum; a potential limitation of focused abdominal sonography for trauma (FAST). *J Trauma* 1997;**42**:617–25.

39. Dolich MO, McKenney MG, Varela JE, et al. 2576 ultrasounds for blunt abdominal trauma. *J Trauma* 2001;**50**(1):108–12.

40. Farahmand N, Sirlin CB, Brown MA, et al. Hypotensive patients with blunt abdominal trauma: performance of screening US. *Radiology* 2005;**235**:436–43.

41. Stuhlfaut JW, Soto JA, Lucey BC, et al. Blunt abdominal trauma: performance of CT without oral contrast material. *Radiology* 2004;**233**(3):689–94.

42. Livingston DH, Lavery RF, Passannante MR, et al. Admission or observation is not necessary after a negative abdominal computed tomographic scan in patients with suspected blunt abdominal trauma: results of a prospective, multi-institutional trial. *J Trauma* 1998;**44**(2):273–80.

43. American College of Surgeons Committee on Trauma. *Advanced Trauma Life (ATLS®), Support Program for Doctors*, 7th edn. Chicago, IL: American College of Surgeons, 2004.

Chapter

2

Initial approach to trauma

Marian E. Betz, Carrie D. Tibbles, and Carlo L. Rosen

Introduction

Injuries remain the leading cause of death in the United States from age 1 to 34. Optimal initial management of the trauma patient during the first several hours after injury offers the best chance of a good outcome.[1] The establishment of trauma center designation has lowered overall trauma mortality by approximately 15%.[2] The resuscitation begins with appropriate prehospital triage and field care and continues in the emergency department (ED). The ABCs remain the foundation of the initial evaluation of the trauma patient, with rapid but thorough assessment of the patient's airway, breathing, circulation, and potential disabilities. The early recognition and aggressive treatment of hemorrhagic shock in trauma patients has advanced in recent years. The use of bedside ultrasound allows for the rapid detection of intraperitoneal or pericardial fluid. Additionally, a better understanding of shock physiology has led to the use of metabolic markers, such as base deficit and lactate, to detect occult hypoperfusion. As emergency medicine continues to mature as a specialty, the ability of the emergency physician to provide optimal initial care for the major trauma patient continues to grow.

Box 2.1   Essential concepts in trauma care

- Prehospital care and triage
- ABCs of primary survey
- Secondary survey
- Use of radiologic studies and bedside ultrasound
- Use of laboratory tests
- Consultation with specialists
- Patient disposition

Prehospital care

Rapid prehospital transport is an integral part of the optimal management of trauma patients. Regional organization of trauma systems, with hospital designations based on capability to care for the complex trauma patient, has been shown to improve patient outcomes,[2–5] but appropriate field triage of patients remains difficult. Various criteria have been used, including anatomic (e.g., type of injury), physiologic (e.g., vital signs), and mechanism of injury, modified by the presence of comorbid conditions such as the extremes of age and third trimester pregnancy. Most trauma centers have two levels of trauma activation (with additional personnel reporting to severe traumas) and use similar criteria. The criteria recommended by the American College of Surgeons (ACS) for the activation of the expanded trauma team for a major trauma include physiologic criteria (traumatic arrest, heart rate below 50 or over 120, systolic blood pressure below 90 mmHg, a Glasgow Coma Scale [GCS] score below 10, paralysis, and age over 65) as well as two mechanistic criteria (gunshot wound to torso, head, or neck, or burn over 20% of body surface area). The criteria for a minor trauma activation are all based on mechanism (gunshot wound to an extremity; fall over 20 ft; motor vehicle collision [MVC] with ejection, rollover or occupant death; pedestrian struck by car; crush or degloving to extremity; or stab wound to torso, head, neck, or thigh).[6,7] Physiologic criteria have a higher specificity for major trauma (defined as the need for emergent surgery or intensive care unit [ICU] admission, or death in the ED) but the use of mechanistic criteria can add sensitivity and decrease the rate of undertriage, since some patients may initially maintain

---

Trauma: A Comprehensive Emergency Medicine Approach, eds. Eric Legome and Lee W. Shockley. Published by Cambridge University Press. © Cambridge University Press 2011.

Table 2.1 Trauma mechanism and suspected injuries

Mechanism	Injury
MVC (broken windshield or steering wheel damage)	• Closed head injury
	• Chest: myocardial contusion, aortic injury, pulmonary contusion, flail chest
	• Abdomen: diaphragm rupture, liver and spleen injuries
	• Hip dislocation
MVC (ejection)	• Head injury
	• Aortic injury
	• Renal pedicle injury
Falls (deceleration)	• Aortic injury
	• Renal pedicle injury
	• Calcaneal fracture, lumbar fractures
Bicycle handlebar	• Duodenal hematoma
	• Pancreatic injury

MVC, motor vehicle collision.

hemodynamic stability in the face of significant injury.[6] Of the mechanistic criteria most frequently used in triage, the four least predictive of surgery, ICU admission, or death are: (1) pedestrian struck by car; (2) motorcycle crash with separation of rider; (3) MVC with rollover; (4) and MVC with occupant death.[6] In children with blunt trauma, the mechanism most associated with immediate or delayed need for surgical management is falls from playground equipment.[8] Certain mechanisms are more likely to cause severe injuries; gunshot wounds and MVCs combined are responsible for one half of all injury deaths in the United States.[8,9] However, the ability of any particular injury mechanism to predict severity of injury and ultimate outcome depends on multiple other factors, including mechanism details (e.g., speed of crash, type of bullet), exact location of injury (e.g., damage to major vessels or organs), and patient factors (e.g., age and comorbidities). Although mechanism of injury is still often a part of triage criteria, it is clear that serious mechanisms may result in minimal injury and, conversely, apparently benign mechanisms may cause significant injuries (Table 2.1).[8,10,11]

The ACS guidelines for Level I trauma centers require the presence of the attending trauma surgeon at the ED arrival of trauma patients requiring *major resuscitation*, or within 15 minutes in cases of short advance notification. The minimum criteria for a *major resuscitation* as defined by the ACS are: hypotension (confirmed blood pressure below 90 for adults or age-appropriate level for children); intubation or respiratory obstruction or compromise; gunshot wounds to neck, chest, or abdomen; a GCS < 8 (attributed to trauma); transfer patients receiving blood transfusions for hemodynamic stability; and ED physician discretion.[12] Although research has shown that these criteria are associated with increased mortality, more severe injuries, and longer ICU and hospital stays,[7] whether the physical presence of a trauma surgeon in the initial resuscitation influences outcomes is debated.[7,13–15] The use of intubation or airway compromise as the sole reason for trauma surgeon presence upon arrival of the trauma patient has been studied. Of these patients only 2% require emergent operation for hemorrhage control. Patients who arrive intubated and otherwise stable are actually more likely to require neurosurgical or orthopedic intervention than trauma surgeon intervention.[14]

Regardless of trauma severity, certain information from prehospital providers is useful in guiding ED approach and management. Basic patient background, including details such as age, past medical history, medications and allergies, and medications given en route, remains important. Additional helpful information concerns patient injuries (including prehospital treatment such as splinting or needle decompression), patient hemodynamics en route, and mechanism of injury.[1] A study from 2003 showed that isolated prehospital hypotension – with normal blood pressure on presentation at the ED – was associated with an increased mortality and need for operative intervention.[16] For MVCs, useful mechanistic information includes estimated speed, patient position in car, use of restraints or airbags, patient ejection from vehicle, time of extrication, fatalities in crash, vehicle condition after crash (e.g., windshield or intrusion damage), and explosion or fire. For trauma from falls, the height of fall is important, as is the surface upon which the body lands and the orientation of the body. For stab or gunshot wounds, description of the weapon (length or caliber), number of shots heard, and a rough estimate of the wound path are important. For any trauma, additional useful prehospital information is the reason for injury (e.g., suspected electrocution or syncope), ambient temperature, and alcohol or drug use. It is important to consider medical causes for trauma, such as hypoglycemia, anaphylaxis, and myocardial infarction, especially in single car crashes.

Protocols for field care vary somewhat by region, and physicians should be aware of guidelines in their system. Certain field interventions will influence ED management. For example, prehospital needle decompression of the chest will necessitate tube thoracostomy in the ED. For patients intubated by Emergency Medical Services (EMS), endotracheal tube placement should be verified upon arrival in the ED by some combination of auscultation, end tidal carbon dioxide monitoring, chest radiography, and direct visualization. Extremities splinted in the field should be examined to ensure splints are not compromising vascular flow. Appropriate prehospital care of amputated parts will also affect the possibility of replantation.

Emergency department evaluation and treatment

Identification of life-threatening injuries is the priority in the initial evaluation of a trauma patient and is generally accomplished through the step-wise approach established by the ACS as described in the Advanced Trauma Life Support® (ATLS®) course.[17] However, with an efficient and well-staffed trauma team, multiple steps occur simultaneously. As the physician assesses the airway, other providers are establishing intravenous (IV) access and exposing the patient. Furthermore, this standard algorithm is illogical for certain mechanisms or particular situations. For instance, a patient with a single stab wound to the left chest likely needs a focused abdominal sonography in trauma (FAST) exam to evaluate a potential pericardial effusion prior to a full extremity examination. All trauma patients need a thorough evaluation to avoid missing injuries overshadowed by the life threat(s), but the order of evaluation may differ depending on the specific case.

Primary survey

The initial approach to the trauma patient begins with the primary survey. This is a rapid assessment for immediate life-threatening conditions. As in other types of ED patients, the airway, breathing, and circulation evaluation comes first. As injuries are identified, they are treated rapidly before the rest of the primary survey is completed. This systematic approach avoids missing life-threatening injuries. The speed of this initial assessment depends on the clinical stability of the patient. The goal is to address the airway, treat any major chest injuries, treat shock, and then identify any injuries that require immediate operative repair.

Airway management

Airway assessment and management is the first step in the care of an injured patient because inadequate oxygenation or ventilation presents an immediate life threat that may be easily reversible. This assessment may be as simple as establishing that a patient is awake and speaking normally without facial trauma, but may be much more challenging in cases of significant facial or neck trauma. Multiple modalities are available for intubation, including rapid sequence with in-line manual cervical immobilization, blind nasotracheal, oral awake, cricothyrotomy, bougie, fiberoptic, and lighted stylet. Factors affecting the choice of method include the presence of obvious or possible facial, anterior neck, intracranial, or cervical spine injuries. In trauma, rapid establishment of the airway is critical. Due to the presence of life-threatening injuries that require immediate operative management, there may not be time to attempt difficult airway techniques, and the physician must be prepared to perform a surgical airway when oral intubation fails or is contraindicated. New wire-guided (Seldinger technique) or catheter-over-needle kits for cricothyrotomy may be superior to traditional surgical approaches. In one study, procedure duration and complication rates were similar for wire-guided and surgical approaches but physicians preferred the wire-guided approach, which also required smaller skin incisions.[18] In children under 8 years of age a needle cricothyrotomy is preferred to a surgical cricothyrotomy.

Box 2.2 Indications for intubation

- Airway obstruction
- Airway protection
- GCS < 8
- Inadequate ventilation
- Head injury requiring hyperventilation
- Persistent hypotension
- Anticipated future course (e.g., need for multiple radiologic studies or operating room)

Breathing: ventilation and oxygenation

This step of the primary survey focuses on identification of chest injuries that may impair ventilation. The emergency physician should inspect for chest wounds, listen for breath sounds, and palpate for subcutaneous air or flail chest. Physical exam findings consistent with a tension pneumothorax are indications for immediate chest decompression with a needle or chest tube prior to a chest radiograph. These include hypotension in addition to subcutaneous air, or decreased breath sounds in blunt trauma and hypotension in addition to decreased breath sounds in penetrating trauma. A chest radiograph can aid in the diagnosis of chest injury but should not delay resuscitation of an unstable patient. However, in stable patients with suspected chest trauma it may be reasonable to obtain a chest radiograph prior to placing a chest tube. All major trauma patients should receive supplemental oxygen, especially if room-air saturations are abnormally low or for preoxygenation if intubation is imminent.

Bedside ultrasound may be useful in detecting pneumothorax, as it is faster and more sensitive than portable chest radiography and can identify small pneumothoraces that would be otherwise seen only on computed tomography (CT); some advocate for including the lungs in an extended FAST exam.[19] For diagnosis of pneumothorax (with CT as the gold standard), ultrasound has a sensitivity of 92–100% and a specificity of 94–100%.[20-22]

Box 2.3 Chest injuries that impair ventilation

- Tension pneumothorax
- Flail chest
- Open pneumothorax
- Hemothorax

Circulation

The primary circulation survey of the trauma patient includes establishment of vascular access, assessment and control of hemorrhage (internal or external), fluid resuscitation with crystalloid or blood, and assessment of shock. Major trauma patients need at least two large-bore (14 or 16 gauge) peripheral IVs. Physician judgment may be used for stable patients with lesser mechanisms, some of whom may require only one IV. If peripheral IV placement is difficult or impossible, the patient will require a saphenous vein cut down, central access (subclavian, internal jugular, or femoral) or an intraosseous line (IO). A single-lumen, large-bore central line should be used rather than a multilumen line to ensure rapid delivery of fluids and medications. In children, an IO line should be attempted prior to a central line. This technique has also been studied recently for use in adult patients.[23]

The primary circulation survey should address possible external or internal hemorrhage, including assessment of blood pressure, pulse, and skin perfusion. Compressive dressings should be applied to sites of obvious external hemorrhage. In stable patients with bleeding head wounds, rapid closure in the trauma bay may be advisable prior to radiologic studies given the potential for ongoing hemorrhage. Raney clips may be useful for temporarily closing scalp wounds to control hemorrhage. Given the concern over possible scatter artifact from scalp staples, it is ideal to obtain the head CT prior to wound closure with staples, but wounds with ongoing hemorrhage need to be controlled if they interfere with or hinder resuscitation. Significant internal bleeding may be from intra-abdominal or intrathoracic injuries, pelvic or femur fractures, or from arterial or venous involvement of penetrating injuries.[24] Intracranial hemorrhage will not cause hypotension from hemorrhage, although it may cause neurologic disability and hypertension with bradycardia (Cushing reflex).

Fluid resuscitation should begin with 2–3 L of isotonic fluid, either normal saline (NS) or lactated Ringer's (LR). Although both fluid types are good choices for initial resuscitation, NS can cause hypercloremic acidosis when given in large volumes, especially in a patient with impaired renal function.[17] Pediatric resuscitation is based on weight, with an initial one or two 20 ml/kg crystalloid boluses followed by 10 ml/kg of blood as indicated. Fluids should be warmed to minimize hypothermia, although it should be noted that by the time warm fluids reach the patient via IV tubing they may have cooled to room temperature unless administered via a rapid infuser.[25] Blood transfusion is indicated for patients who remain hemodynamically unstable after 2–3 L or have ongoing blood loss (e.g., open-book pelvic fracture). Patients with life-threatening hemorrhage should receive O-negative blood, which should be immediately available in all EDs; O-positive blood can be used instead in males and females past child-bearing age. Patients with transient response to crystalloid should receive type-specific blood, which is compatible with ABO and Rh blood types and requires 10–30 minutes for matching. For all patients, fully cross-matched blood is preferable, but the time required for matching (1 hour) should not delay care.

Any patient with major pelvic trauma should receive blood immediately in anticipation of major blood loss, even before hematocrit results are available. Patients with major open-book or other pelvic fractures that are associated with significant bleeding may also be temporally stabilized by the application of a commercially available pelvic stabilization binder. Alternatively, the emergency physician can tightly wrap a sheet around the pelvis.

Conventional protocols, including ATLS®, recommend resuscitation of hemorrhaging patients with the goal of maintaining a normal blood pressure. This approach has been questioned, with the rationale that fluid administration may actually increase bleeding because of increased vessel wall pressure and dilution of coagulation factors. Multiple animal studies have supported this hypothesis, and research is ongoing to examine the effects of permissive hypotension on the outcome of hemorrhaging trauma patients.[26–28] While certain trauma patients may benefit from smaller volumes of fluid replacement, those with head injuries need resuscitation. In those with head injuries, hypotension results in increased mortality rates, and aggressive fluid resuscitation improves outcomes, decreases the risk of secondary brain injury, and lowers the relative risk of death or vegetative state.[28–30] In multiply injured patients, hypertonic saline dextran (HSD) may be useful, as it decreases intracranial pressure and increases cerebral compliance without having detrimental systemic hemodynamic effects.[29,31,32]

Patients receiving large volumes of fluid or blood may need replacement of other blood components, including fresh frozen plasma (FFP), platelets, and cryoprecipitate.[24] The use of recombinant factor VIIa for coagulation factor replacement in trauma is an area of great current interest, as several case series and retrospective studies have demonstrated decreased transfusion requirements and perhaps decreased mortality.[33] Although initial reports are hopeful, additional studies concerning safety, timing of dosage, and indications and contraindications are needed before recombinant factor VIIa becomes standard practice for treating hemorrhage due to trauma.[33]

While hemorrhage is the most common etiology of shock in the trauma patient, other clinical entities should be considered. Non-hemorrhagic etiologies of shock include cardiogenic, tension pneumothorax, and neurogenic. Cardiac contusion and rupture after blunt trauma and cardiac tamponade after penetrating trauma can acutely decrease cardiac output and blood pressure. Tension pneumothorax and cardiac tamponade obstruct cardiac outflow and may present with muffled heart sounds, tachycardia, jugular venous distention (JVD), and hypotension. Physical exam findings consistent with a tension pneumothorax, such as subcutaneous air, tracheal shift, and the absence of breath sounds, will help differentiate between the two diagnoses. As mentioned above, ultrasound is useful in detecting a pneumothorax, and it can also be used to diagnose a hemothorax or a pericardial effusion. Bedside ultrasound is 96% sensitive and 100% specific for hemothorax,[34] and 95% sensitive and 100% specific for tamponade.[35] Rapid treatment of pneumothorax or tamponade with chest decompression or pericardiocentesis, respectively, is critical to management. Pericardiocentesis is indicated in hypotensive patients with a pericardial effusion. Emergency department thoracotomy is indicated in penetrating trauma patients who had vital signs in the field or on arrival but lose them in the ED, or in blunt trauma patients who had vital signs on arrival but lose them in the ED.

Neurogenic shock causes hypotension through peripheral vascular relaxation due to the loss of sympathetic tone. Cardiac output is not obstructed, and tachycardia is usually absent. Treatment of spinal shock is IV crystalloid, followed by vasopressors if needed.[22]

Box 2.4 Circulatory assessment and management (for major trauma)

Component	Comments
Vascular access	Minimum of two large-bore peripheral IVs, with central access or IO line if IVs are unobtainable
Hemorrhage control	Sources include extremities, intra-abdominal, intrathoracic, pelvis, or femur fracture, and arterial or venous involvement of penetrating injuries

Box 2.4 *(cont.)*

Fluid resuscitation	Begin with 2–3 L of warmed crystalloid (NS or Ringer's lactate), then transfuse type-specific or type-O blood if patient still unstable or bleeding. (Other acceptable options include limited resuscitation, although this remains controversial)
Assessment of shock	Types of shock include hemorrhagic, cardiogenic (myocardial contusion, tamponade), tension pneumothorax, and neurogenic (spinal shock)

Disability

The primary survey also includes a brief global assessment of neurologic disabilities. Providers should calculate a GCS, with pediatric modifications as appropriate. Eye, verbal, and motor responses are totaled for the final GCS scale, ranging from 3 (comatose) to 15 (normal). Intubation will make assessment of the verbal component impossible, and the total score should be annotated to identify the patient as being intubated. The initial GCS scale can give providers a marker of injury severity and can guide treatment priorities. For example, a GCS of < 8 in a trauma patient is a criterion for activation of the first-tier (expanded) trauma team and is an indication for intubation. Although intoxication with alcohol or other drugs may alter a patient's sensorium, there is evidence that it does not significantly alter the GCS in patients with head injuries, suggesting that a lower than normal GCS should be assumed to be due to the brain injury rather than the intoxication.[36] Providers should also consider whether an alteration in mental status is the etiology, rather than the result, of the injury and evaluate for hypoglycemia, seizure, stroke, ingestions, or other entities as indicated.

The primary neurologic survey should include assessment of pupil size and reactivity as well, as this can provide clues to possible intracranial injury. In addition, a quick determination of gross motor function should be performed. The secondary survey and more complete exams should include a more thorough neurologic assessment, including detailed motor and sensory exams in any injured extremity.

Box 2.5 Glasgow Coma Scale (with pediatric modifications)

Score	Best eye response	Best verbal response	Best motor response
1	No eye opening	No verbal response	No motor response
2	Eye opening to pain	Incomprehensible sounds (inconsolable, agitated)	Extension to pain
3	Eye opening to verbal command	Inappropriate words (inconsistently consolable, moaning)	Flexion to pain
4	Eyes open spontaneously	Confused (cries but is consolable, inappropriate interactions)	Withdrawal from pain
5	–	Oriented (smiles, oriented to sounds, follows objects, interacts)	Localizing pain
6	–	–	Obeys commands

Exposure

All trauma patients should be undressed to facilitate a complete exam to assess for injuries. The removal of clothing can be performed by assistants while the physician assesses the airway, breathing, and circulation. Part of exposing a patient's injuries involves rolling the patient (using in-line cervical spine immobilization) to examine the back for wounds or evidence of injury.

The exposure component of the primary survey also reminds the physician to assess patient exposure to the elements prior to arrival and in the resuscitation room. Hypo- or hyperthermia should be addressed rapidly. Once undressed, patients should be covered with warm blankets to avoid iatrogenic hypothermia.

Secondary survey and ancillary studies

Once the primary survey is complete, the goal is to perform a complete search to diagnose injuries and to identify indications for further imaging or operative intervention. The secondary survey begins with a more thorough physical examination to diagnose potential injuries. This exam should include assessment of the face, oropharynx, and dentition, the extremities, and general motor and sensory function. Imaging of potential fractures is indicated, and injuries such as facial fractures or complex wounds may require consultation with specialists.

A main focus of the secondary survey is the abdominal exam. In blunt trauma, abdominal injuries may present with frank hypovolemic shock but can also have a more insidious presentation. Up to 25% of major trauma patients will require an exploratory laparotomy,[37,38] and approximately 1% of all trauma patients have an abdominal injury.[39] Certain mechanisms raise the likelihood of intra-abdominal trauma, including MVCs with steering wheel deformity (when the patient is the front-seat passenger) and impact against bicycle handlebars.[38,40,41] The trauma abdominal exam in the resuscitation bay should begin with observation and inspection for ecchymoses, abrasions, distension, or penetrating wounds. An important physical exam finding is the "seat belt sign," bruising, or other markings in the seat belt region. This finding has been associated with hollow viscous, pancreatic, and mesenteric injuries,[38,42–45] and should prompt physicians to obtain diagnostic imaging.

Palpation for abdominal tenderness or peritonitis remains an important part of the trauma exam, and the presence of abdominal pain or tenderness should not be ignored. However, a normal examination may be falsely reassuring in patients who are intoxicated or distracted by other injuries. The abdominal exam has a sensitivity of 82% for intra-abdominal injury. Therefore, the absence of pain or tenderness does not rule out significant injury.[38,46] Certain injuries should alert the physician to possible intra-abdominal injuries even in the absence of abdominal pain or tenderness, including pelvic fractures, chest injuries, and significant (and multiple) extremity fractures.[46] Thoracolumbar flexion–distraction ("Chance") fractures, often from lap seat belt use, are associated with intra-abdominal injuries, especially to the small bowel.[38,47,48] Lower rib fractures should raise concern for injury to the liver, spleen, or kidneys, even in the absence of abdominal pain.[38,46,47,49]

The difficult part of the secondary survey is deciding which patients require workup with CT for abdominal injuries. This has not been well studied.

It is clear that the physical examination is not a perfect test and that up to 19% of patients with positive abdominal CT have no abdominal tenderness.[50] In stable patients who are awake and without a distracting injury that would prevent them from feeling the pain of an abdominal injury, the decision to scan or not is largely based on physician judgment and experience. The mechanism of injury should also be considered. A high-speed mechanism or other high-velocity trauma to the abdomen may be associated with an injury that would not be detected by physical examination. Given the high rate of normal examinations in patients with abnormal CT scans, one could make an argument to scan patients with a high-velocity mechanism. Prehospital hypotension should also be used as an indication for abdominal CT scanning. Many patients who are not intoxicated and have no other significant injuries can be safely observed in the ED for a short period of time (4 hours) and then discharged with careful discharge instructions.[51] Other high-risk findings that might be considered indications for CT scanning include the following: GCS < 14; abdominal or costal margin tenderness; a "seat belt sign"; femur fractures; hematuria (> 25 red blood cells per high powered field [RBC/hpf]); and rib fractures or pneumothorax on chest radiography. The absence of any of these findings is associated with a 99% negative predictive value for abdominal injury.[52]

The FAST examination has become routine in trauma resuscitations. The timing varies, but usually it is performed late in the primary survey or early in the secondary survey. The FAST exam is both sensitive and specific (range: 87–100%) for the identification of free fluid in the abdomen of the blunt trauma patient,[24,53] even when performed by non-radiologists. The FAST exam may also be useful during the primary survey for assessment of hypovolemia and cardiac tamponade. The main benefit of the FAST exam is the rapid detection of intraperitoneal blood in the hypotensive blunt trauma patient. It is also very useful to detect pericardial blood after penetrating chest trauma. As with many aspects of trauma care, there are various algorithms for the use of FAST results in determining patient care.[53]

Even in stable blunt trauma patient, a FAST exam should be performed as part of the secondary survey. This allows faster triage to CT if the ultrasound is positive. If the patient becomes unstable, it also helps the clinicians make rapid decisions about the need for operative management and the cause of the instability. Furthermore, serial ultrasound exams can be performed if the initial FAST is negative and there is any change in clinical status. This will increase the sensitivity for detecting hemoperitoneum.

Foley catheter placement is necessary in patients who are unstable in order to monitor urine output. For those unable to stand up or use a bedpan to urinate, a Foley catheter placement may also be required to obtain a sample for urinalysis, in order to evaluate for hematuria as evidence for bladder or kidney injury. Gross hematuria is an indication for further workup with a CT cystogram. Contraindications to a Foley placement are signs of urethral injury, such as blood from the meatus, hemoscrotum, and inability to palpate the prostate. Finally, in patients undergoing diagnostic peritoneal lavage (DPL), a Foley catheter should be placed to avoid penetrating a distended bladder with the DPL trocar or needle.

Nasogastric (NG) tube placement is also recommended in patients undergoing a DPL to avoid gastric penetration. Patients who are intubated should also have decompression of their stomachs with an oro-gastric or NG tube. For the awake patient, NG tube placement should be avoided as it may induce vomiting and cause the patient to move his or her head excessively in the presence of a potential cervical spine injury.

If not already provided by prehospital providers, the secondary survey should include a focused patient history. Patients should be questioned concerning allergies, medications, past medical history, and the time of last oral intake. As discussed above, questions concerning the event can give insight to possible injuries and predisposing medical conditions, such as syncope leading to an MVC. Certain injury mechanisms suggest possible injuries and can help guide the workup.

Initial radiography

A chest radiograph is still recommended for patients with blunt trauma or penetrating trauma to the chest or abdomen, since it is a rapid and safe way to identify a pneumo- or hemothorax, a widened mediastinum or other signs of traumatic aortic injury, or intra-peritoneal free air. However, patients who are asymptomatic with minimal mechanisms of injury may not require a chest radiograph. Although most trauma anteroposterior (AP) chest radiographs are obtained in the supine position because of spinal precautions, an upright posteroanterior (PA) chest radiograph is ideal because it limits the impression of a widened mediastinum due to the supine technique.

A pelvis radiograph, also traditionally a part of the standard trauma resuscitation, may not be necessary for every patient. A pelvis film taken in the resuscitation bay may be helpful in identifying an unstable pelvic fracture as a source of bleeding in the unstable patient, and it may also identify hip dislocations. However, in the awake and sober patient without symptoms, physical exam findings, or distracting injuries, imaging of the pelvis may not be necessary. For the trauma patient who is hemodynamically stable and who will have a CT scan of the abdomen and pelvis, pelvis radiography in the resuscitation bay is not needed. Computed tomography identifies more pelvis fractures and provides far more information about fracture patterns. Compared to CT, pelvis radiography is 68% sensitive and 98% specific for pelvic fractures.[54] The three main indications for obtaining a plain radiograph of the pelvis in the resuscitation bay are: (1) hemodynamic instability; (2) suspicion (by exam or mechanism) of a hip dislocation that should be reduced emergently; and (3) the emergent need for a procedure outside of the ED (e.g., operating room or angiography) without time for CT scans.[54,55]

Box 2.6 Main indications for trauma room pelvic radiography in patients undergoing CT of the abdomen and pelvis[54,55]

- Hemodynamic instability
- Suspicion (by exam or mechanism) of a hip dislocation that should be reduced emergently
- Emergent need for a procedure outside of the ED (e.g., operating room or angiography) without time for CT scans

---

Cervical spine radiographs were also traditionally part of the initial evaluation of the trauma patient, starting with a lateral radiograph taken in the resuscitation room. If all 7 vertebrae are visualized, a lateral radiograph detects 90% of fractures, with the yield increasing to 100% when anteroposterior and odontoid radiographs are included. Although plain cervical radiographs are still used, there is a growing reliance on CT scans for diagnosing cervical spine injuries. Helical CT scans have a sensitivity of 98.1% and a negative predictive value of 99.7% for cervical spine injuries,[56] and they can save time since plain radiographs are often inadequate and require additional images. In patients undergoing other CT scans, it is cost effective to perform cervical CT. With the advent of new helical CT scanners, there is some evidence that even ligamentous injury may be ruled out and thus the spine cleared in obtunded patients.[56–58]

Commonly used guidelines for cervical spine imaging include the National Emergency X-Radiography Utilization Study (NEXUS) Criteria and the Canadian Cervical Spine Rule. Under the NEXUS Criteria, patients are at low risk of cervical injury and do not need cervical spine imaging if they meet all five of the following criteria: (1) a normal level of alertness and (2) no evidence of intoxication; (3) no posterior midline cervical spine tenderness (4) no focal neurologic deficits on exam; and (5) no painful distracting injury.[59] The Canadian Cervical Spine Rules applies to alert, stable trauma patients with a GCS of 15. These patients are at low risk of cervical injury and do not need injury if they meet all of the following criteria: (1) no high-risk factors (age over 65, certain dangerous mechanisms, or extremity paresthesias); (2) have at least one low-risk factor allowing range of motion assessment (simple rear-end MVC, sitting up in ED, ambulatory after crash, delayed onset of neck pain, or lack of midline cervical spine tenderness); and (3) are able to actively rotate the neck 45° right and left.[60]

Guidelines for imaging of the thoracolumbar spine are similar to the cervical spine. Imaging is generally indicated for any patient with a high energy mechanism plus the presence of at least one of the following: (1) back pain or tenderness on palpation; (2) focal sign of injury on the back; (3) neurologic deficit; (4) cervical spine fracture; (5) GCS lower than 15; (6) painful distracting injury; or (7) intoxication with alcohol or other substances.[61,62] As with clearance of the cervical spine, even a slight alteration in mental status (from intoxication, brain injury, or other etiology) makes the physical exam of the thoracolumbar spine inaccurate.[62–64] Computed tomography is more sensitive than conventional radiography for spine fractures,[65] and trauma CT scans of the chest, abdomen, and pelvis are adequate for identification of thoracolumbar injuries without the need for additional dedicated imaging.[65–67]

Patients who present with obvious major joint dislocations, such as hip deformities or knee dislocations, should undergo radiographs of the joint in the trauma room with subsequent reduction prior to being moved to the CT scanner. This will depend on the stability of the patient and concern for more life-threatening injuries.

Complicating factors

Up to 70% of trauma patients are intoxicated with alcohol or other substances,[68] making the initial history and physical examination difficult to interpret. Similarly, patients with a "distracting" injury may not notice pain elsewhere in their body – such as the cervical spine or abdomen – and thereby complicate the physician's task. The guidelines developed by NEXUS discuss the need for cervical spine imaging when a "distracting injury" prevents accurate physical examination, and define a distracting painful injury as: "(a) a long bone fracture; (b) a visceral injury requiring surgical consultation; (c) a large laceration, degloving injury, or crush injury; (d) large burns; or (e) any other injury producing acute functional impairment."[69] Studies have attempted to narrow the definition of a painful distracting injury,[70] but there still is no precise definition and the principle typically is applied to any injury that is thought to cloud the rest of the evaluation.[64,70] Hypoxia, head injuries, or metabolic derangements may also alter a patient's perception and expression of pain. Evaluation of such patients must rely on a combination of objective clinical signs – such as vital signs and physical findings – and mechanistic details of the trauma. Thus, for an intoxicated patient who was the unrestrained, ejected driver in a high-speed rollover MVC, it may be prudent to obtain diagnostic imaging even in the absence of pain or tenderness. Conversely, for an intoxicated patient who fell from standing, it may be appropriate to observe the patient with repeated exams but no imaging until clinically sober.[71,72]

> **Box 2.7 Potential distracting injuries in cervical spine evaluation**[70]
>
> - Long bone fracture
> - Visceral injury requiring surgical consultation
> - Large laceration, degloving injury or crush injury
> - Large burns
> - Any other injury producing acute functional impairment

Laboratory studies

Most hospitals obtain a standard panel of labs in every trauma patient, although in many cases these have little impact on the initial management. This panel includes chemistries, blood counts, toxicological screens, pregnancy test, and coagulation factors. Critical labs in patients with major trauma include a baseline hematocrit, platelet count, blood clot for typing, pregnancy test, and coagulation panel. A baseline hematocrit is useful for subsequent management of the patient. However, it takes time for equilibration to occur, so a normal initial hematocrit should not be reassuring. An initially low hematocrit is worrisome for significant bleeding. In certain patients other useful labs may include a blood glucose fingerstick, creatinine (for the stable patient in whom IV contrast may pose a risk) and a toxicological screen.

Serum lactate levels and base excess measurements have recently emerged as useful metabolic markers to guide the initial resuscitation of the trauma patient. Elevated lactate levels suggest tissue hypoperfusion, even with normal vital signs, and studies have shown an association between clearance of lactate and trauma mortality.[24,73–75] The association is not perfect, as some patients with hypoperfusion have normal lactate levels and some patients without hypoperfusion (but with other conditions such as seizures or with certain medications) have elevated lactate levels. Lactate may not perfectly predict mortality,[76] especially in patients with minor trauma, but it may be useful in identifying early shock and in directing care over the first 24–48 hours when followed as a trend. It may be especially helpful in elderly trauma patients, in whom elevated lactate in normotensive patients reflects occult hypoperfusion and a higher mortality.[77] Similarly, base excess may also provide insight into tissue hypoperfusion, though it is also not a perfect marker.

Other diagnostic studies

Patients with external evidence of chest trauma or who are complaining of chest pain should have an electrocardiogram (ECG) to evaluate for potential blunt cardiac injury. Additionally, an ECG should also be obtained in a patient at risk for myocardial infarction, particularly those in a single car accident, as it may reveal myocardial ischemia as the precipitating cause of the trauma.

Consultation of specialists

Certain findings during the initial evaluation of the trauma exam mandate a specialist consultation or (after stabilization) transfer to a higher level facility where a specialist is available. Open fractures or unstable pelvic fractures will need orthopedic intervention. Patients with intracranial injuries should be evaluated by a neurosurgeon, ideally prior to sedation, paralysis, and intubation, but consultation should not delay resuscitation or imaging. Although they should not distract from resuscitation and management of potential life threats, serious injuries such as globe rupture, orbital fracture with entrapment, facial trauma, degloving, compartment syndrome, and extremity crush injuries need consultation with an ophthalmologist, plastic surgeon, microvascular surgeon, or other appropriate specialist.

Disposition

The majority of patients will be admitted to the hospital following major trauma for the management of their injuries. In patients with significant high-speed blunt mechanisms without obvious injuries, a period of observation is recommended. This should be at least 4 hours and may be longer if the patient is intoxicated. Repeat examinations and serial ultrasound examinations can be used to detect evolving intraperitoneal bleeding or other injuries.

Patients with less significant mechanisms of injury, who remain hemodynamically stable and have benign physical examinations may not require a full trauma workup as described above. There are few rules or studies that assist the clinician and these decisions are based largely on judgment and experience. The negative predictive value of a negative abdominal CT scan in blunt trauma patients is 99%. Thus, patients can usually be sent home from the ED after a negative CT and do not require admission for observation.[50] Similarly, patients with minimal head injury (GCS of 14 or 15) and a normal head CT without other body system injuries who have a normal neurologic examination can generally be discharged. In these patients, the negative predictive value of CT is 99.7%.[50]

References

1. Legome EL, Rosen P. General principles of trauma. In Wolfson AB (ed.), *Harwood-Nuss' Clinical Practice of Emergency Medicine*, 4th edn. Philadelphia, PA: Lippincott, Williams and Wilkins, 2005: pp. 890–8.

2. Celso B, Tepas J, Langland-Orban B, et al. A systematic review and meta-analysis comparing outcome of severely injured patients treated in trauma centers following the establishment of trauma systems. *J Trauma* 2006;**60**(2):371–8; discussion 8.

3. Mann NC, Mullins RJ, MacKenzie EJ, et al. Systematic review of published evidence regarding trauma system effectiveness. *J Trauma* 1999;**47**(3 Suppl.): S25–33.

4. Clancy TV, Gary Maxwell J, Covington DL, et al. A statewide analysis of Level I and II trauma centers for patients with major injuries. *J Trauma* 2001; **51**(2):346–51.

5. Chiara O, Cimbanassi S. Organized trauma care: does volume matter and do trauma centers save lives? *Curr Opin Crit Care* 2003;**9**(6):510–14.

6. Kohn MA, Hammel JM, Bretz SW, et al. Trauma team activation criteria as predictors of patient disposition from the emergency department. *Acad Emerg Med* 2004;**11**(1):1–9.

7. Tinkoff GH, O'Connor RE. Validation of new trauma triage rules for trauma attending response to the emergency department. *J Trauma* 2002;**52**(6):1153–8; discussion 8–9.

8. Burd RS, Jang TS, Nair SS. Evaluation of the relationship between mechanism of injury and outcome in pediatric trauma. *J Trauma* 2007; **62**(4):1004–14.

9. Mackenzie EJ, Fowler C. Epidemiology of trauma. In Mattox KJ, Feliciano DV, Moore EE (eds.), *Trauma*, 5th edn. Stamford, CT: Appleton and Lange, 2004: pp. 21–39.

10. Santaniello JM, Esposito TJ, Luchette FA, et al. Mechanism of injury does not predict acuity or level of service need: field triage criteria revisited. *Surgery* 2003;**134**(4):698–703; discussion 4.

11. Velmahos GC, Jindal A, Chan LS, et al. "Insignificant" mechanism of injury: not to be taken lightly. *J Am Coll Surg* 2001;**192**(2):147–52.

12. American College of Surgeons Committee on Trauma. *American College of Surgeons Resources for Optimal Care of the Injured Patient*. Chicago, IL: American College of Surgeons, 2006.

13. Green SM. Is there evidence to support the need for routine surgeon presence on trauma patient arrival? *Ann Emerg Med* 2006;**47**(5):405–11.

14. Steele R, Gill M, Green SM, et al. Do the American College of Surgeons' "Major Resuscitation" trauma triage criteria predict emergency operative management? *Ann Emerg Med* 2007;**50**(1):15–17.

15. Ciesla DJ, Moore EE, Moore JB, et al. Intubation alone does not mandate trauma surgeon presence on patient arrival to the emergency department. *J Trauma* 2004;**56**(5):937–41; discussion 41–2.

16. Shapiro NI, Kociszewski C, Harrison T, et al. Isolated prehospital hypotension after traumatic injuries: a predictor of mortality? *J Emerg Med* 2003;**25**(2):175–9.

17. American College of Surgeons Committee on Trauma. *Advanced Trauma Life (ATLS®), Support Program for Doctors*, 7th edn. Chicago, IL: American College of Surgeons, 2004.

18. Chan TC, Vilke GM, Bramwell KJ, et al. Comparison of wire-guided cricothyrotomy versus standard surgical cricothyrotomy technique. *J Emerg Med* 1999;**17**(6):957–62.

19. Kirkpatrick AW, Sirois M, Laupland KB, et al. Hand-held thoracic sonography for detecting post-traumatic pneumothoraces: The Extended Focused Assessment with Sonography for Trauma (EFAST). *J Trauma* 2004;**57**(2):288–95.

20. Rowan KR, Kirkpatrick AW, Liu D, et al. Traumatic pneumothorax detection with thoracic US: correlation with chest radiography and CT – initial experience. *Radiology* 2002;**225**(1):210–14.

21. Knudtson JL, Dort JM, Helmer SD, et al. Surgeon-performed ultrasound for pneumothorax in the trauma suite. *J Trauma* 2004;**56**(3):527–30.

22. Mandavia DP, Joseph A. Bedside echocardiography in chest trauma. *Emerg Med Clin North Am* 2004; **22**(3):601–19.

23. Macnab A, Christenson J, Findlay J, et al. A new system for sternal intraosseous infusion in adults. *Prehosp Emerg Care* 2000;**4**(2):173–7.

24. Cocchi M, Kimlin E, Walsh M, et al. Identification and resuscitation of the trauma patient in shock. *Emerg Med Clin N Am* 2007;**25**(3):623–42, vii.

25. Handrigan MT, Wright RO, Becker BM, et al. Factors and methodology in achieving ideal delivery temperatures for intravenous and lavage fluid in hypothermia. *Am J Emerg Med* 1997;**15**(4):350–3.

26. Bickell WH, Wall MJ, Jr., Pepe PE, et al. Immediate versus delayed fluid resuscitation for hypotensive patients with penetrating torso injuries. *N Engl J Med* 1994;**331**(17):1105–9.

27. Dutton RP, Mackenzie CF, Scalea TM. Hypotensive resuscitation during active hemorrhage: impact on in-hospital mortality. *J Trauma* 2002;**52**(6):1141–6.

28. Fowler R, Pepe PE. Fluid resuscitation of the patient with major trauma. *Curr Opin Anaesthesiol* 2002; **15**(2):173–8.

29. Dutton RP, McCunn M. Traumatic brain injury. *Curr Opin Crit Care* 2003;**9**(6):503–9.

30. Pepe PE, Mosesso VN, Jr., Falk JL. Prehospital fluid resuscitation of the patient with major trauma. *Prehosp Emerg Care* 2002;**6**(1):81–91.

31. Vassar MJ, Perry CA, Holcroft JW. Prehospital resuscitation of hypotensive trauma patients with 7.5% NaCl vs. 7.5% NaCl with added dextran: a controlled trial. *J Trauma* 1993;**34**(5):622–32; discussion 32–3.

32. Vassar MJ, Perry CA, Gannaway WL, et al. Seven point five percent sodium chloride/dextran for resuscitation of trauma patients undergoing helicopter transport. *Arch Surg* 1991;**126**(9):1065–72.

33. Mohr AM, Holcomb JB, Dutton RP, et al. Recombinant activated factor VIIa and hemostasis in critical care: a focus on trauma. *Crit Care* 2005; **9**(Suppl. 5):S37–42.

34. Ma OJ, Mateer JR, Ogata M, et al. Prospective analysis of a rapid trauma ultrasound examination performed by emergency physicians. *J Trauma* 1995; **38**(6):879–85.

35. Plummer D. The sensitivity, specificity, and accuracy of ED echocardiography.Abstract. *Acad Emerg Med* 1995;**2**:339.

36. Sperry JL, Gentilello LM, Minei JP, et al. Waiting for the patient to "sober up": effect of alcohol intoxication on Glasgow Coma Scale score of brain injured patients. *J Trauma* 2006;**61**(6):1305–11.

37. Hoyt DB, Coimbra R, Potenza B. Management of acute trauma. In Townsend CM, Beauchamp RD, Evers BM, et al. (eds.), *Sabiston Textbook of Surgery*, 17th edn. Philadelphia, PA: WB Saunders, 2004: pp. 311–44.

38. Rosen C, Legome EL, Wolfe RE. Blunt abdominal trauma. In Adams J (ed.), *Emergency Medicine*. Philadelphia, PA: WB Saunders, 2008: pp. 827–40.

39. Rutledge R, Hunt JP, Lentz CW, et al. A statewide, population-based time-series analysis of the increasing frequency of nonoperative management of abdominal solid organ injury. *Ann Surg* 1995;**222**(3):311–22; discussion 22–6.

40. Newgard CD, Lewis RJ, Kraus JF. Steering wheel deformity and serious thoracic or abdominal injury among drivers and passengers involved in motor vehicle crashes. *Ann Emerg Med* 2005;**45**(1):43–50.

41. Nadler EP, Potoka DA, Shultz BL, et al. The high morbidity associated with handlebar injuries in children. *J Trauma* 2005;**58**(6):1171–4.

42. Chandler CF, Lane JS, Waxman KS. Seatbelt sign following blunt trauma is associated with increased incidence of abdominal injury. *Am Surg* 1997; **63**(10):885–8.

43. Velmahos GC, Tatevossian R, Demetriades D. The "seat belt mark" sign: a call for increased vigilance among physicians treating victims of motor vehicle accidents. *Am Surg* 1999;**65**(2):181–5.

44. Wotherspoon S, Chu K, Brown AF. Abdominal injury and the seat-belt sign. *Emerg Med (Fremantle)* 2001; **13**(1):61–5.

45. Sokolove PE, Kuppermann N, Holmes JF. Association between the "seat belt sign" and intra-abdominal injury in children with blunt torso trauma. *Acad Emerg Med* 2005;**12**(9):808–13.

46. Ferrera PC, Verdile VP, Bartfield JM, et al. Injuries distracting from intraabdominal injuries after blunt trauma. *Am J Emerg Med* 1998;**16**(2):145–9.

47. Tyroch AH, McGuire EL, McLean SF, et al. The association between chance fractures and intra-abdominal injuries revisited: a multicenter review. *Am Surg* 2005;**71**(5):434–8.

48. Bernstein MP, Mirvis SE, Shanmuganathan K. Chance-type fractures of the thoracolumbar spine: imaging analysis in 53 patients. *AJR Am J Roentgenol* 2006;**187**(4):859–68.

49. Holmes JF, Offerman SR, Chang CH, et al. Performance of helical computed tomography without oral contrast for the detection of gastrointestinal injuries. *Ann Emerg Med* 2004;**43**(1):120–8.

50. Livingston DH, Lavery RF, Passannante MR, et al. Admission or observation is not necessary after a negative abdominal computed tomographic scan in patients with suspected blunt abdominal trauma: results of a prospective, multi-institutional trial. *J Trauma* 1998;**44**(2):273–80; discussion 80–2.

51. Branney SW, Moore EE, Cantrill SV, et al. Ultrasound based key clinical pathway reduces the use of hospital resources for the evaluation of blunt abdominal trauma. *J Trauma* 1997;**42**(6): 1086–90.

52. Holmes J, Wisner D, McGahan J, et al. A clinical prediction instrument for the abdominal evaluation of adult blunt trauma patients: abstract. *Acad Emerg Med* 2007;**14**(5):S62.

53. Rose JS. Ultrasound in abdominal trauma. *Emerg Med Clin North Am* 2004;**22**(3):581–99, vii.

54. Guillamondegui OD, Pryor JP, Gracias VH, et al. Pelvic radiography in blunt trauma resuscitation: a diminishing role. *J Trauma* 2002;**53**(6):1043–7.

55. Kessel B, Sevi R, Jeroukhimov I, et al. Is routine portable pelvic X-ray in stable multiple trauma patients always justified in a high technology era? *Injury* 2007;**38**:559–63.

56. Brohi K, Healy M, Fotheringham T, et al. Helical computed tomographic scanning for the evaluation of the cervical spine in the unconscious, intubated trauma patient. *J Trauma* 2005;**58**(5):897–901.

57. Schuster R, Waxman K, Sanchez B, et al. Magnetic resonance imaging is not needed to clear cervical spines in blunt trauma patients with normal computed tomographic results and no motor deficits. *Arch Surg* 2005;**140**(8):762–6.

58. Hogan GJ, Mirvis SE, Shanmuganathan K, et al. Exclusion of unstable cervical spine injury in obtunded patients with blunt trauma: is MR imaging needed when multi-detector row CT findings are normal? *Radiology* 2005;**237**(1):106–13.

59. Hoffman JR, Mower WR, Wolfson AB, et al. Validity of a set of clinical criteria to rule out injury to the cervical spine in patients with blunt trauma. National

Emergency X-Radiography Utilization Study Group. *N Engl J Med* 2000;**343**(2):94–9.

60. Stiell IG, Clement CM, McKnight RD, et al. The Canadian C-spine Rule versus the NEXUS Low-risk Criteria in patients with trauma. *N Engl J Med* 2003;**349**(26):2510–18.

61. Hsu JM, Joseph T, Ellis AM. Thoracolumbar fracture in blunt trauma patients: guidelines for diagnosis and imaging. *Injury* 2003;**34**(6):426–33.

62. Terregino CA, Ross SE, Lipinski MF, et al. Selective indications for thoracic and lumbar radiography in blunt trauma. *Ann Emerg Med* 1995; **26**(2):126–9.

63. Sava J, Williams MD, Kennedy S, et al. Thoracolumbar fracture in blunt trauma: is clinical exam enough for awake patients? *J Trauma* 2006;**61**(1):168–71.

64. Chang CH, Holmes JF, Mower WR, et al. Distracting injuries in patients with vertebral injuries. *J Emerg Med* 2005;**28**(2):147–52.

65. Antevil JL, Sise MJ, Sack DI, et al. Spiral computed tomography for the initial evaluation of spine trauma: a new standard of care? *J Trauma* 2006;**61**(2):382–7.

66. Hauser CJ, Visvikis G, Hinrichs C, et al. Prospective validation of computed tomographic screening of the thoracolumbar spine in trauma. *J Trauma* 2003; **55**(2):228–34; discussion 34–5.

67. Berry GE, Adams S, Harris MB, et al. Are plain radiographs of the spine necessary during evaluation after blunt trauma? Accuracy of screening torso computed tomography in thoracic/lumbar spine fracture diagnosis. *J Trauma* 2005;**59**(6):1410–13; discussion 13.

68. Rootman DB, Mustard R, Kalia V, et al. Increased incidence of complications in trauma patients cointoxicated with alcohol and other drugs. *J Trauma* 2007;**62**(3):755–8.

69. Hoffman JR, Wolfson AB, Todd K, et al. Selective cervical spine radiography in blunt trauma: methodology of the National Emergency X-Radiography Utilization Study (NEXUS). *Ann Emerg Med* 1998;**32**(4):461–9.

70. Heffernan DS, Schermer CR, Lu SW. What defines a distracting injury in cervical spine assessment? *J Trauma* 2005;**59**(6):1396–9.

71. American Association of Neurological Surgeons and the Congress of Neurological Surgeons. Radiographic assessment of the cervical spine in asymptomatic trauma patients. *Neurosurgery* 2002; **50**(Suppl. 3):S30–5.

72. Marion D, Domeier R, Dunham CM, et al. *Determination of Cervical Spine Stability in Trauma Patients. Update of the 1997 EAST Cervical Spine Clearance Document*. Chicago, IL: Eastern Association for the Surgery of Trauma, 2000: pp. 1–9.

73. Abramson D, Scalea TM, Hitchcock R, et al. Lactate clearance and survival following injury. *J Trauma* 1993;**35**(4):584–8; discussion 8–9.

74. Lavery RF, Livingston DH, Tortella BJ, et al. The utility of venous lactate to triage injured patients in the trauma center. *J Am Coll Surg* 2000;**190**(6): 656–64.

75. Bilkovski RN, Rivers EP, Horst HM. Targeted resuscitation strategies after injury. *Curr Opin Crit Care* 2004;**10**(6):529–38.

76. Pal JD, Victorino GP, Twomey P, et al. Admission serum lactate levels do not predict mortality in the acutely injured patient. *J Trauma* 2006;**60**(3):583–7; discussion 7–9.

77. Callaway D, Rosen C, Baker C, et al. Lactic acidosis predicts mortality in normotensive elderly patients with traumatic injury: abstract. *Acad Emerg Med* 2007;**145**(5):S152.

Mechanism of injury

Aaron Hexdall and Maurizio A. Miglietta

Introduction

Traumatic injuries are the most common cause of death in people between the ages of 1 and 44 years of age in the United States and the 5th most common cause of death overall.[1] In 2004 there were 167 184 traumatic deaths, yielding a mortality rate of 56.2 per 100 000 people. Motor vehicle collisions (MVCs) account for the largest number of traumatic deaths each year, 43 432 in 2004. The 10 most common mechanisms of traumatic death are listed by age group in Figure 3.1. (Unintentional injuries are highlighted, as many non-traumatic mechanisms such as self-poisoning are also considered injury deaths for statistical purposes.) A systematically organized approach to trauma evaluation and management has been shown to reduce mortality, morbidity, and length of hospital stay.[2–4] The severity of initial injuries and outcomes in trauma are determined by two principal non-modifiable factors: the mechanism of injury and patient-related physiological factors, such as age and comorbid illness. Traditionally the mechanism of injury has been used in the prehospital setting to triage the patient to the appropriate level of care (i.e., a Level I, II, or III trauma center) and often helps to anticipate common injury patterns.

It is intuitive that higher energy mechanisms will result in more severe injuries. Yet experience has proven that trauma is a complex multisystem disease and even apparently innocuous mechanisms can result in severe injuries, and severe mechanism may not. One study that examined "insignificant" mechanisms, primarily low level falls and unconscious patients without external signs of trauma, reported a 37% incidence of severe injuries.[5] Thus, while the mechanism of injury has been traditionally held as the main predictor of injury, recent advances in diagnostic systems and algorithms have emphasized objective physiologic factors.

In the future, more precise descriptions of a traumatic event, such as prehospital telemedicine systems, and more precise physiologic assessment tools may enhance our ability to perform early trauma triage.

Numerous scoring systems have been developed for trauma. Trauma scoring tools include anatomically-based systems, physiologic-based systems, and combined anatomic- and physiologic-based scoring systems. Some of the more familiar trauma scoring tools are listed in Box 3.1. Research has shown that many of these tools assist with resource utilization and help predict mortality, although the authors' experience is that, outside of the Glasgow Coma Scale (GCS), they are rarely used in clinical triage practice. While scoring systems are unlikely to trump the clinical acumen of experienced providers, the utility of such systems is to produce a uniform descriptive vocabulary that will allow for comparative research and facilitate rapid communication.[6–8]

Box 3.1 Trauma scoring systems

Anatomical trauma scores
- Injury Severity Score (ISS)[9]
- New Injury Severity Score (NISS)[10]
- Abbreviated Injury Score (AIS)[8,11]
- Anatomic Profile[8]

Physiological trauma scores
- Glasgow Coma Scale (GCS)[12]
- Acute Physiology and Chronic Health Evaluation II (APACHE II)[13]
- Revised Trauma Score (RTS)[14]

Combined trauma scores
- Trauma and Injury Severity Score (TRISS)[15]
- International Classification of Disease-based ISS (ICDISS)[8]

Rank	<1	1–4	5–9	10–14	15–24	25–34	35–44	45–54	55–64	65+	Total
	Age groups										
1	Congenital anomalies 5622	Unintentional injury 1641	Unintentional injury 1126	Unintentional injury 1540	Unintentional injury 15449	Unintentional injury 13032	Unintentional injury 16471	Malignant neoplasms 49520	Malignant neoplasms 96956	Heart disease 533302	Heart disease 652486
2	Short gestation 4642	Congenital anomalies 569	Malignant neoplasms 526	Malignant neoplasms 493	Homicide 5085	Suicide 5074	Malignant neoplasms 14723	Heart disease 37556	Heart disease 63613	Malignant neoplasms 385847	Malignant neoplasms 553888
3	SIDS 2246	Malignant neoplasms 399	Congenital anomalies 205	Suicide 283	Suicide 4316	Homicide 4495	Heart disease 12925	Unintentional injury 16942	Chronic low. respiratory disease 11754	Cerebro-vascular 130538	Cerebro-vascular 150074
4	Maternal pregnancy comp. 1715	Homicide 377	Homicide 122	Homicide 207	Malignant neoplasms 1709	Malignant neoplasms 3633	Suicide 6638	Liver disease 7496	Diabetes mellitus 10780	Chronic low. respiratory disease 105197	Chronic low. respiratory disease 121987
5	Unintentional injury 1052	Heart disease 187	Heart disease 83	Congenital anomalies 184	Heart disease 1038	Heart disease 3163	HIV 4826	Suicide 6906	Cerebro-vascular 9966	Alzheimer's disease 65313	Unintentional injury 112012
6	Placenta Cord membranes 1042	Influenza and pneumonia 119	Chronic low. respiratory disease 46	Heart disease 162	Congenital anomalies 483	HIV 1468	Homicide 2984	Cerebro-vascular 6181	Unintentional injury 9651	Diabetes mellitus 53956	Diabetes mellitus 73138
7	Respiratory distress 875	Septicemia 84	Benign neoplasms 41	Chronic low. respiratory disease 74	Cerebro-vascular 211	Diabetes mellitus 599	Liver disease 2799	Diabetes mellitus 5567	Liver disease 6569	Influenza and pneumonia 52760	Alzheimer's disease 65965
8	Bacterial sepsis 827	Perinatal period 61	Septicemia 38	Influenza and pneumonia 49	HIV 191	Cerebro-vascular 567	Cerebro-vascular 2361	HIV 4422	Suicide 4011	Nephritis 35105	Influenza and pneumonia 59664
9	Neonatal hemorrhage 616	Benign neoplasms 53	Cerebro-vascular 34	Benign neoplasms 43	Influenza and pneumonia 185	Congenital anomalies 420	Diabetes mellitus 2026	Chronic low. respiratory disease 3511	Nephritis 3963	Unintentional injury 35020	Nephritis 42480
10	Circulatory system disease 593	Chronic low. respiratory disease 48	Influenza and pneumonia 33	Cerebro-vascular 43	Chronic low. Respiratory Disease 179	Septicemia 328	Influenza and pneumonia 891	Septicemia 2251	Septicemia 3745	Septicemia 25644	Septicemia 33373

Figure 3.1 The 10 leading causes of injury death by age group in the United States, 2004. (Courtesy of the National Vital Statistics System, National Center for Health Statistics, CDC.)

The Injury Severity Score (ISS), for example, is one of the more common and simplest scores to calculate. An ordinal Abbreviated Injury Score (AIS) value from 1 (minor injury) to 6 (fatal injury) is assigned to the most severe injury in each of six body areas. The square of the AIS in the three most severely injured areas is summed to calculate the ISS. The ISS ranges from 0 to 75, and an AIS of 6 in any one area automatically gives an ISS of 75.[16] Severe injury is routinely defined as an ISS > 15. Amongst many shortcomings of the ISS is that it underestimates the impact of severe isolated head injury and the severity of penetrating trauma and it is not a linear scale – many scores simply cannot occur because of the mathematical formula used to derive it. It is rarely useful early on as the information needed to calculate the score cannot be obtained until all the injuries are known, sometimes at surgery or autopsy. The ISS treats the six AIS body areas as being equal with the same severity; this may not be true. It may also underestimate severity at the extremes of age, i.e., the elderly and young children. In addition, the ISS is a poor indicator of severity and survival with multiple injuries in one body region. Nonetheless, it is a widely recognized descriptive tool. A modification to the ISS focusing on the three most severe injuries regardless of body area is more accurate and easier to calculate (called the New Injury Severity Score [NISS]).[10] As a general rule, trauma scoring systems with more data-points provide a more accurate description but are likewise more complicated to calculate.

Many of the most common and severe injuries are caused by mixed mechanisms, polytrauma. For example, high-speed motor vehicle crashes often combine deceleration, blunt, and penetrating injuries and are the single most common cause of death in young people. Thus, polytrauma is the norm rather than the exception in high mortality injuries. Many Level I trauma centers use mechanism of injury to trigger trauma team activation, although this routine practice is controversial and less widely accepted.[17,18] Current recommendations are that individual centers decide their own criteria for trauma team activation. Some commonly accepted mechanisms are listed in Box 3.2 below.[19] The presence of emergency physicians who can receive and resuscitate the patient has impacted the need for immediate surgical evaluation in trauma centers of all levels. Whether major mechanisms of injury alone should automatically activate the trauma team will be hotly debated in the coming years as economic pressures on hospitals and providers mount.[18]

Box 3.2 Common indications for trauma team activation

- Motor vehicle crash with death of another passenger or ejection
- Motor vehicle crash at speed > 40 mph, deceleration > 20 mph
- Rollover MVC
- Motorcycle crash > 20 mph or separation of the rider from the bike
- Pedestrian or bicyclist struck by automobile
- Major vehicle damage: intrusion of > 12 inches into passenger compartment or vehicle deformity > 20 inches
- Penetrating trauma to the head, neck, torso, or abdomen
- Fall from height, generally > 10 ft
- Closed head trauma with loss of consciousness and/or GCS < 14
- Amputation proximal to the ankles or wrists
- Discretion of the receiving physician

Blunt and penetrating trauma mechanisms

Blunt trauma results from energy transfer through intact skin to vital organs and anatomic structures. Common blunt trauma mechanisms are MVCs, falls, and interpersonal violence. Often, blunt trauma is more complex than penetrating trauma in that more energy is dispersed over a larger area rather than dispersed along the path of a penetrating injury. Penetrating trauma is usually caused by gunshot wounds (GSWs) and stab wounds (SWs), although virtually any object can cause a penetrating injury if it has adequate force. Stab wounds are low energy and the nature of the injury is determined by the size of

the sharp object and its trajectory of penetration and path. Both blunt and penetrating traumas are divided into high-energy and low-energy mechanisms.

Blunt trauma: Kinematics of acceleration and deceleration as it relates to motor vehicle crashes:

Acceleration is defined as a change in velocity over time ($\Delta v/t$). Acceleration (a) or deceleration (–a) exerts force on a body. This force can be expressed in terms of G force or the acceleration due to the earth's gravitational field (1 G = a/g, where a is acceleration and g is the gravitational constant of the earth, 32 ft/s^2 or 9.8 m/s^2).

$$Gs = \frac{a}{-g} = \frac{V_0^2}{\Delta d \times 32.2\, \text{ft/s}^2}.^{[20]}$$

If one assumes that the final velocity is zero, this formula can easily be reworked for MVCs to reveal that stopping distance is inversely proportional to G force.

$$Gs = \frac{(\text{Velocity change}[\text{ft/s}])^2}{30 \times \text{Stopping distance}(\text{ft})}^{[20,]}$$

in this formula 30 approximates the gravitational constant, g.

The shorter the stopping distance, the greater the G forces exerted will be. Thus doubling the stopping distance will result in half the G force being applied. While a healthy person can withstand brief forces ("jolt force") of 30–40 Gs in the anterior posterior direction, abrupt acceleration or deceleration can result in extreme G force stress. Human tolerance to G forces is significantly less in a cephalad caudad or in a side-to-side direction. Instantaneous changes in velocity, deceleration of > 40 km/hour (25 mph) have been associated with more severe injuries.[21]

In the case of MVCs, the vehicle and safety devices such as airbags and seat belts may absorb much of the energy that is generated, thus protecting the passengers. The first impact is that of the vehicle, which may absorb a substantial amount of energy through crumple zones or other deformities of the vehicle structure. The second impact is the person against any interior structure, such as an airbag, steering wheel, or car surfaces. The third impact is that of the person's internal organs against their bony skeleton. Lastly, there may be unrestrained objects, including passengers or cargo, which result in additional impacts.[20] In cases of ejection, little or no protection exists and the entire G force of deceleration may be absorbed by the patient.

Common blunt trauma-related injury patterns

Non-fatal blunt trauma results in more than 14 million emergency department (ED) visits per year, with falls accounting for approximately half of the visits. The next most common causes of blunt trauma are MVCs, assault, and pedestrian crashes.[22] Some common injury patterns associated with blunt trauma are described below.

Motor vehicle crashes

In the United States, across all ages below 65 years, MVCs represent the leading cause of death. In 2005, there were more than 6 million MVCs, which resulted in 39 189 deaths. The majority of MVCs result in property damage only (69.9%), injury occurs in 1 in 3 incidents (29.5%), and fatalities are rare, occurring in only 0.6% of incidents. Since 1966, the fatality rate in MVCs has declined from 25.89 to 14.66 per 100 000 people. More notable is that while driving (mileage) has more than tripled since 1966, the fatality rate has dropped from 5.50 to 1.45 deaths per 1 million miles driven.[23] This trend is graphically illustrated over 20 years in Figure 3.2.

Safety belts reduce MVC mortality by nearly half; unfortunately more than half of MVC fatalities (55%) occur in unrestrained occupants.[21,23] Alcohol intoxication was implicated in 39% of fatal MVCs in 2005, which remained consistent over the prior decade after 3 decades of significant reductions in alcohol-related fatalities. Saturdays and Sundays from midnight to 3 am are the deadliest hours, and alcohol is implicated in 75% of fatalities during these hours.[21]

Hallmarks of more severe MVCs are vehicle damage findings such as vehicle crush, intrusion into the passenger compartment, and "spidering" or "helmeting" of the windshield. Vehicle rollover may be a harbinger of more serious injuries: rollover is associated with fatal MVCs (21.1%) more than MVCs which result in injury (5.3%), or in MVCs that result in property damage only (1.3%). A recent analysis of MVC mechanism also identified lateral impact crashes ("T-bone crashes") as having a higher mortality than front impact incidents (17% vs. 11%).[21] Lateral impact MVCs are associated with a higher ISS than other impacts (mean ISS 25 for lateral impacts vs. 20 for others), and are associated with more severe chest and abdominal injuries. Frontal impacts are associated with more severe facial injuries.[24] These results are likely because of the increased protection provided by crumple zones and airbags in front impact crashes, and the fact that three-point restraints (i.e., seat belts) are less effective in lateral impacts.

Seat belt sign and steering wheel marks

A seat belt sign is an area of erythema or ecchymosis located over the abdomen, chest, or neck where a seat belt was placed. It has been associated with more severe injuries. An erythematous or ecchymotic imprint of the steering wheel raises suspicion for deceleration injuries to the thoracic aorta and other blunt trauma to the chest (95% of blunt aortic injuries will be to the thoracic aorta, and > 80% result from MVCs).[25,26] Reports of aortic dissection or rupture, vertebral fractures and spinal cord injury, and gastrointestinal injuries associated with a seat belt sign are

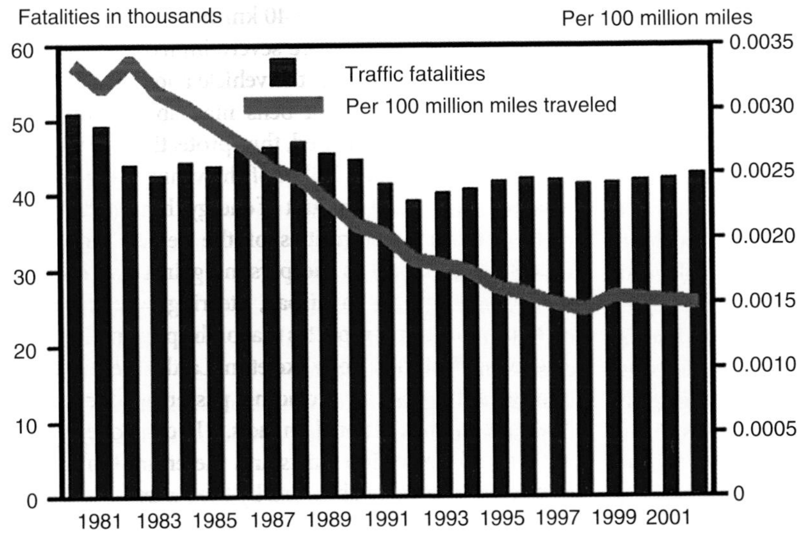

Fatalities in thousands   Per 100 million miles

Traffic fatalities

Per 100 million miles traveled

Figure 3.2 Traffic fatalities per miles traveled. (Courtesy of the US National Highway Traffic Safety Administration.)

frequent, especially in head-on type MVCs in which the primary vector of force is perpendicular to the seat belt restraint. In one study of children, an abdominal seat belt sign was associated with gastrointestinal and pancreatic injuries, but not with solid organ injuries.[27] A prospective study of the 131 patients with either cervical or thoracic seat belt sign showed a 3% incidence of significant vascular trauma (carotid artery injuries), and half of these patients died. Another study that looked at a cervical seat belt sign, but did not correlate it with physical exam, failed to show it to be an independent predictor of carotid or cervical spine injury.[28] Thus, a clinical algorithm such as the one developed by Rozycki et al. may be useful in detecting these otherwise occult and devastating injuries: all patients presenting with a thoracic or cervical seat belt sign were evaluated for possible vascular injury: patients with abnormal mental status (GCS < 14) or an abnormal neurovascular exam received immediate imaging (usually CT angiogram).[29] Those with a cervical seat belt sign and normal exam received vascular evaluation within 24 hours.[29] While an isolated seat belt sign in the absence of pain or other abnormalities on physical exam has no predictive value, the inappropriate application of seat belts, especially in children, has been associated with severe injuries.[30]

Airbag injuries

Airbags are reported to reduce fatalities by about 30% in purely frontal MVCs, and by 11% in all MVCs. Airbags are designed to protect an unrestrained occupant by deploying within 50 ms of impact; a pyrotechnic oxidation reaction of sodium azide and other oxides produces nitrogen gas and sodium hydroxide.[31] Not long after the mandatory introduction of airbags in 1995, serious injuries associated with their deployment were noted, especially in children.[32] Common injuries are hearing loss and tinnitus, chemical burns to the face and eyes, irritant induced asthma, and forearm trauma such as fractures. In those of short stature and children, more serious injuries include cervical fractures and dislocations with spinal cord injury and suffocation. It is recommended that children under the age of 12 and rear-facing child seats should not be in the front passenger seat. Side airbags have been shown to decrease the AIS score in the head, chest, and extremity by 2, compared with similar crashes without these bags. However, in another study, there was an increased risk of moderate to serious

upper extremity injuries with side airbags as well as an increase in upper extremity orthopedic dislocations.[33,34] There was no increase in fractures.

Pedestrian crashes

Pedestrian crashes results in a disproportionate amount of MVC-related death and disability; 4482 deaths were reported in 2005 (mortality rate 6.6% for pedestrians struck, as opposed to 1.3% for vehicle-only MVCs).[23] Most pedestrian crash events that arrive to the hospital occur at relatively lower speeds of 5–50 km/hour (3–30 mph). In experimental models the sequence of impact is usually lateral to the pedestrian's tibia or fibula by the vehicle bumper, followed by roll-up trajectory of the victim onto the vehicle hood with impacts to the chest and abdomen, and finally impact to the windshield by the victim's head.[35] This pattern is greatly influenced by vehicle geometry and pedestrian size. For example, larger vehicles such as SUVs may initially impact the pedestrian's femur or hip and throw the victim downward rather than the roll-up trajectory described for passenger cars. Injury patterns in pedestrians struck include fractures (77%), followed by head (34%), abdomen (21%), and chest injuries (15%). While the triad of lower extremity fracture, abdominal injury, and head injury was first described by Waddell in 1971 is intuitively appealing for its simplicity, its true usefulness is questionable because few patients have all three injuries.[36]

Falls from height

Falls are the most common trauma, accounting for nearly 8 million ED visits annually. Falls from standing height are common in the elderly and others with gait or balance disturbances. Hip, rib, spine, long bone fractures and closed head trauma are commonly associated injuries. Although long-term sequelea can be substantial, these injuries are generally low energy and have a consequently low acute mortality.[37,38]

Falls from height are higher energy injuries and have an acute mortality that may reach 35%.[39] Three meters (∼ 10 ft) is a commonly accepted height at which serious injuries should be suspected, although there is not a linear relationship between the distance of fall and mortality in patients that survive to ED admission.[40] Intuitively, however, the height of the fall is an appealing predictor of outcome, as the velocity of impact is described by the Newtonian formula,

$$V = \sqrt{2}\,gh$$

(velocity equals the square root of 2 × gravitational constant [9.8 m/s] × height [m]).

When prehospital deaths are included in the analysis, the factors predicting mortality after a fall from height are the distance fallen (in floors, more than two floors), patient age, the surface on which the patient lands (hard or soft), and the part of the body that first impacts (landing on feet was associated with lower mortality than landing on the chest, head, or lateral body). The circumstances of the fall (suicide vs. accidental) and intervening impacts during the fall do not predict mortality.[39] The mortality ranges from 6% to 20% in patients that survive to ED admission.[41] The injury patterns associated with falls from height have been extensively investigated. The most common site of impact is the feet. Energy is transferred through the bony skeleton to the spine leading to a high incidence of occult vertebral fractures, especially in the region of the thoraco-lumbar junction. A high index of suspicion for vertebral fracture is warranted in all falls from height; because distracting injuries such as long bone fractures are common, one quarter of patients with spinal injury may not complain of back pain or be tender on exam. A recent retrospective analysis of 414 falls from height found vertebral fractures in 31% of patients, half of whom had multiple vertebral fractures (15% were at non-contiguous levels).[42]

Box 3.3 Factors predicting mortality in falls from height[39]

Factors predicting mortality in falls from height	Comment/risk stratification	OR of death
Patient age	> 40 (42 ± 17 years vs. 36 ± 15 years)	1.05
Height fallen in floors	> 2 floors (5 floors vs. 2 floors)	1.24
Impact surface	Hard (39% mortality) vs. soft (22% mortality)	2.7
Body part impacting first	Head, anterior face, or lateral body high mortality vs. feet (lower mortality)	10.6–16.7

OR, odds ratio.

Penetrating trauma: ballistics

Gunshot wounds are the leading cause of homicidal death in the United States, accounting for about 30 000 deaths annually.[43,44] The case fatality rate in GSWs is 30%, substantially higher than the case fatality rate for all other injuries combined (< 1%).[45]

Gunshot wounds are potentially complex injuries and at least a minimal understanding of ballistics is useful in evaluating these injuries. Several factors determine the severity of a GSW (Box 3.5). The kinetic energy imparted from a projectile is described by the equation $KE = \frac{1}{2}MV^2$ (kinetic energy equals one-half the mass times the velocity squared). This formula predicts that heavier and higher velocity projectiles will have greater energy. While this is true, it does not always follow that higher velocity projectiles will lead to more severe injuries. The behavior of the bullet within the tissue has been recognized as the major determinant of injury severity. Bullet deformation, fragmentation, and yaw result in more energy being deposited in the surrounding tissue. Bullet yaw refers to the tendency of the bullet to tumble in tissue.

Bullet design is also a major determinant of injury: the size, shape, and behavior of the bullet at impact determines how much kinetic energy is transferred to the tissue and over what area. Bullets passing through the body intact, transferring relatively little energy, may result in less severe injury. If the bullet fragments, transferring more of its energy into the surrounding tissues, the injury will be more severe. In particular, soft-tipped and hollow-point bullets (which were banned by the articles of the Hague Convention in 1899 for military use) are more likely to cause severe injury and are more common in civilian GSWs. These bullets expand at impact to 2–3 times their original diameter, thus causing significantly more tissue damage. Shotgun shells are also worth mentioning because while the projectile velocity is low, the blast area and the volume of pellets (i.e., mass) are large (Figure 3.3).

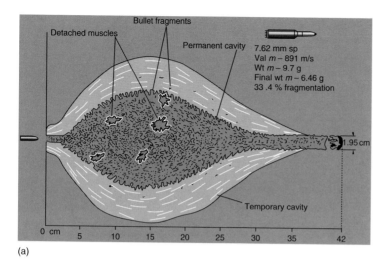

(a)

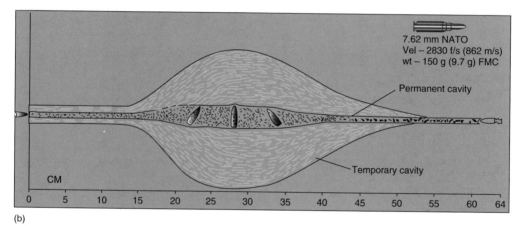

(b)

Figure 3.3 (a) Effect of North Atlantic Treaty Organization (NATO) 7.62 high-speed projectile when fired through ballistic gelatin when unjacketed (non-military) round is used. Note the bullet tendency to fragment and, thus, convert most of its velocity into wounding energy. Resultant permanent cavity is much larger than that of similar jacketed round. Vel, velocity; m/s, meters per second. (b) Effect of NATO 7.62 high-speed projectile in ballistic gelatin when jacketed (military) round is used. Note the bullet tendency to remain intact with resulting small conversion of velocity into wounding potential and relatively small permanent cavity. Also note that bullet takes single tumble at 30 cm and continues to travel backwards, which is a common characteristic of military rifle rounds also seen with Russian AK-47. 41Vel, velocity. (From NATO. *Emergency War Surgery: NATO Handbook, US revision 2*. Washington, DC: US Government Printing Office, 1988.)

Box 3.4   Factors determining the severity of injury in GSWs

Factor	Comment
Bullet trajectory and path	Vital structures impacted
Velocity	High, medium, low
Mass	Bullet caliber
Bullet design	Jacketed (military) vs. non-jacketed (hunting) rounds, and the likelihood of bullet deformity or fragmentation: Dum Dum rounds, hollow-tipped rounds
Yaw	Increase in forward cross-sectional area
Number of bullet wounds received	–

Blast injuries

Blast injuries are uncommon causes of traumatic injury in US civilian medical practice; much of what we know has been gleaned from military experiences and terrorist mass casualty events.[46] Blast injuries are complex. These events are caused by the detonation of explosive devices and are categorized into high-energy and low-energy ordinance. High-energy explosives include TNT (trinitrotoluene), Semtex, nitroglycerine, C-4 (cyclotrimethylene trinitramine) and ammonium nitrate fuel oils (ANFO). Low-energy ordinance include gunpowder, most pipe bombs, petroleum-based incendiary devices, and most improvised explosive devices (IEDs) which do not produce an over-pressurized energy wave. The determinants of the severity of blast injuries are listed in Table 3.1.

The hallmark of high-energy explosions is an over-pressurized pulse of energy that is referred to as a "blast wave" and is different from the "blast wind," which refers to the accelerated super-heated air that can be produced by both high- and low-energy devices. When high-energy explosives are detonated, a solid or a liquid is converted into a highly pressurized gas: this gas expands from the blast epicenter, compressing the surrounding air to create the blast wave. The over-pressurized blast wave creates primary blast injuries that are characteristic of high-energy explosions: C4, for example, can produce pressures of 4 million pounds per square inch.[47] Secondary injuries are caused by blunt and penetrating trauma from flying debris and bomb fragments. Shrapnel injuries are the most common cause of immediate death in blast injuries. Injury patterns are similar to those seen in conventional polytrauma, although shrapnel deposition may occur in unexpected locations such as the eyes. Tertiary injuries occur when the victim is thrown by the blast wind and are largely blunt trauma injury patterns similar to falls from height. Lastly, quaternary injuries represent the thermal injuries, toxic inhalation, and radiation exposure. Burns may occur from the blast itself or subsequent super-heated blast wind (Figure 3.4).[48]

Over-pressurization in high-energy explosions produces injuries that may not have obvious external signs of trauma: air containing structures such as the lungs, the gastrointestinal tract, and the middle ear are at highest risk for such injuries due to rapid changes in velocity of the blast wave at air–tissue interfaces. Blast lung, which is the most common

Table 3.1 Severity of blast injuries

Nature of the device	High- or low-energy material, and the amount of material
Method of delivery	Explosive or incendiary
Nature of the blast environment	Open space or closed space
Distance from the device to the victim	–
Intervening protective barriers and personal protective equipment	–
Projectiles	Flying debris and bomb fragments

cause of early death in initial survivors, is a direct result of barotrauma (air expansion) and sheer stress at the air–tissue interface causing alveolar-venous tearing.[47] Clinically blast lung may appear similar to pulmonary contusion as the patient may complain of dyspnea, cough, chest pain, or have hemoptysis. The triad of apnea, bradycardia, and hypotension seen in blast lung is likely vagally mediated and differentiates this process from conventional blunt trauma. Hypoxia and butterfly or bat-wing appearance seen on initial chest X-ray is *sine qua non* for blast lung. In patients with isolated pulmonary injury, early airway management and mechanical ventilation improves outcomes. Because of the high incidence of air embolism and occult gas trapping, prophylactic chest tube insertion is recommended prior to positive pressure ventilation (e.g., anesthesia) or air transport.[49]

The intestine is also at high risk for primary blast injury because it is air containing. Sheer stress may produce intestinal perforations, rupture, contusions, hemorrhages, mesenteric injury, and air embolic phenomena similar to blast lung. Early and late tension pneumoperitoneum or intestinal perforations have also been reported.[50,51] External signs of trauma may be absent, but these injuries should be suspected if abdominal complaints or unexplained hypovolemia are present. The presence of tympanic membrane rupture is common and indicates exposure to over-pressurization, although it has not been shown to be an indicator of more serious occult injuries such as blast lung.[52] The sensitivity of this is unknown; that is, the absence of this may not rule out a significant injury. Other important primary blast injuries related

31

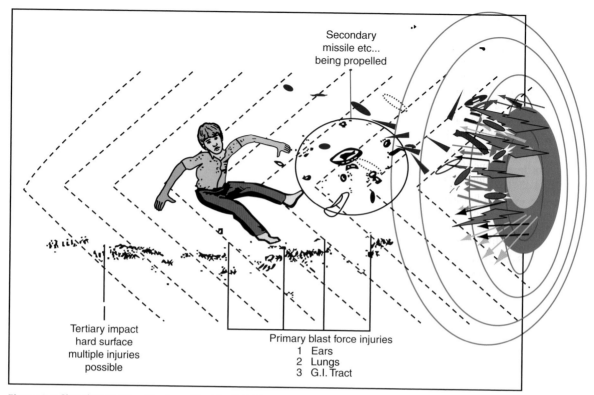

Secondary
missile etc...
being propelled

Tertiary impact
hard surface
multiple injuries
possible

Primary blast force injuries
1 Ears
2 Lungs
3 G.I. Tract

Figure 3.4 Blast characteristics. (Courtesy of Lt. John T. McManus, US Army.)

to over-pressurization include traumatic brain injuries without signs of external trauma (Table 3.1).

Box 3.5 Primary blast injuries

- Injury from blast wave impacting the body surface
- Tympanic membrane (TM) rupture
- Pulmonary damage and air embolization
- Hollow viscus injury

Conclusions

The mechanism of injury can provide important information and aid clinicians in anticipating injury patterns, most importantly, life-threatening injuries which require immediate attention. Some mechanisms of injury are strongly associated with severe injuries and may warrant activation of the trauma team or a similar response. An optimal approach to prehospital or ED triage incorporates the mechanism of injury along with the objective physiological assessment of the patient's condition.

References

1. National Center for Injury Prevention and Control, Centers for Disease Contral and Prevention. *Ten Leading Causes of Death, United States, 2004, All Races, Both Sexes.* Washington, DC: Office of Statistics and Programming and National Vital Statistics, 2004.

2. Nathens AB, Jurkovich GJ, Maier RV, et al. Relationship between trauma center volume and outcomes. *JAMA* 2001;**285**(9):1164–71.

3. MacKenzie EJ, Rivara FP, Jurkovich GJ, et al. A national evaluation of the effect of trauma-center care on mortality. *N Engl J Med* 2006;**354**(4):366–78.

4. Celso B, Tepas J, Langland-Orban B, et al. A systematic review and meta-analysis comparing outcome of severely injured patients treated in trauma centers following the establishment of trauma systems. *J Trauma* 2006;**60**(2):371–8; discussion 8.

5. Velmahos GC, Jindal A, Chan LS, et al. "Insignificant" mechanism of injury: not to be taken lightly. *J Am Coll Surg* 2001;**192**(2):147–52.

6. Foreman BP, Caesar RR, Parks J, et al. Usefulness of the Abbreviated Injury Score and the Injury Severity Score in comparison to the Glasgow Coma Scale in predicting

outcome after traumatic brain injury. *J Trauma* 2007; **62**(4):946–50.

7. Rutledge R, Osler T, Emery S, et al. The end of the Injury Severity Score (ISS) and the Trauma and Injury Severity Score (TRISS): ICISS, an International Classification of Diseases, ninth revision-based prediction tool, outperforms both ISS and TRISS as predictors of trauma patient survival, hospital charges, and hospital length of stay. *J Trauma* 1998;**44**(1): 41–9.

8. Chawda MN, Hildebrandb F, Pape HC, et al. Predicting outcome after multiple trauma: which scoring system? *Injury* 2004;**35**(4):347–58.

9. Baker SP, O'Neill B, Haddon W, Jr., et al. The injury severity score: a method for describing patients with multiple injuries and evaluating emergency care. *J Trauma* 1974;**14**(3):187–96.

10. Osler T, Baker SP, Long W. A modification of the injury severity score that both improves accuracy and simplifies scoring. *J Trauma* 1997;**43**(6):922–5; discussion 5–6.

11. Committee on Medical Aspects of Automotive Safety. Rating the severity of tissue damage. *JAMA* 1971; **215**:277–80.

12. Healey C, Osler T, Rogers F, et al. Improving the Glasgow Coma Scale score: motor score alone is a better predictor. *J Trauma* 2003;**54**(4):671–8; discussion 78–80.

13. Knaus WA, Draper EA, Wagner DP, et al. APACHE II: a severity of disease classification system. *Crit Care Med* 1985;**13**(10):818–29.

14. Champion HR, Sacco WJ, Copes WS. A revision of the Trauma Score. *J Trauma* 1989;**29**(5):623–9.

15. Boyd CR, Tolson MA, Copes WS. Evaluating trauma care: the TRISS method, Trauma Score and the Injury Severity Score. *J Trauma* 1987;**27**(4):370–8.

16. Baker SP, O'Neill B. The Injury Severity Score: an update. *J Trauma* 1976;**16**(11):882–5.

17. Burd RS, Jang TS, Nair SS. Evaluation of the relationship between mechanism of injury and outcome in pediatric trauma. *J Trauma* 2007;**62**(4):1004–14.

18. Shatney CH, Sensaki K. Trauma team activation for "mechanism of injury" blunt trauma victims: time for a change? *J Trauma* 1994;**37**(2):275–81; discussion 81–2.

19. American College of Surgeons Committee on Trauma. *Resources for Optimal Care of the Injured Patient, 1999.* Chicago, IL: American College of Surgeons, 1999.

20. Peterson TD, Jolly BT, Runge JW, et al. Motor vehicle safety: current concepts and challenges for emergency physicians. *Ann Emerg Med* 1999;**34**(3):384–93.

21. Ryb GE, Dischinger PC, Ku fera JA, et al. Delta V, principal direction of force, and restraint use

contributions to motor vehicle crash mortality. *J Trauma* 2007;**63**(5):1000–5.

22. National Electronic Injury Surveillance System, US Consumer Product Safety Commission. *National Estimates of the 10 Leading Causes of Nonfatal injuries Treated in Hospital Emergency Departments, United States, 2006.* Washington, DC: Office of Statistics and Programming, National Center for Injury Prevention and Control, 2006.

23. National Highway Traffic Safety Administration. *Traffic Safety Facts 2006: A Compilation of Motor Vehicle Crash Data from the Fatality Analysis Reporting System and the General Estimates.* Washington, DC: National Center for Statistics and Analysis, US Department of Transportation, 2006.

24. McLellan BA, Rizoli SB, Brenneman FD, et al. Injury pattern and severity in lateral motor vehicle collisions: a Canadian experience. *J Trauma* 1996;**41**(4):708–13.

25. Fabian TC, Davis KA, Gavant ML, et al. Prospective study of blunt aortic injury: Multicenter Trial of the American Association for the Surgery of Trauma. *J Trauma* 1997;**42**(3):374–80; discussion 80–3.

26. Roth SM, Wheeler MD, Jr., Gregory RT, et al. Blunt injury of the abdominal aorta: a review. *J Trauma* 1997;**42**(4):748–55.

27. Sokolove PE, Kuppermann N, Holmes JF. Association between the "seat belt sign" and intra-abdominal injury in children with blunt torso trauma. *Acad Emerg Med* 2005;**12**(9):808–13.

28. DiPerna CA, Rowe VL, Terramani TT, et al. Clinical importance of the "seat belt sign" in blunt trauma to the neck. *Am Surg* 2002;**68**(5):441–5.

29. Rozycki GS, Tremblay L, Feliciano DV, et al. A prospective study for the detection of vascular injury in adult and pediatric patients with cervicothoracic seat belt signs. *J Trauma* 2002;**52**(4):618–23; discussion 23–4.

30. Shweiki E, Klena JW, Halm KA, et al. Seat belt injury to the abdominal aorta. *Am J Emerg Med* 2000;**18**(2):236–7.

31. Schreck RM, Rouhana SW, Santrock J, et al. Physical and chemical characterization of airbag effluents. *J Trauma* 1995;**38**(4):528–32.

32. Centers for Disease Control and Prevention. Update: fatal air bag-related injuries to children – United States, 1993–1996. *JAMA* 1997;**277**(1):11–12. Erratum appears in *JAMA* 1997;**277**(5):372.

33. Yoganandan N, Pintar FA, Zhang J, et al. Lateral impact injuries with side airbag deployments–a descriptive study. *Accid Anal Prev* 2007;**39**(1):22–7.

34. McGwin G, Jr., Metzger J, Alonso JE, et al. Association between upper extremity injuries and side airbag availability. *J Trauma* 2008;**64**(5):1297–301.

35. Thollon L, Jammes C, Behr M, et al. How to decrease pedestrian injuries: conceptual evolutions starting from 137 crash tests. *J Trauma* 2007;**62**(2):512–19; discussion 9.

36. Orsborn R, Haley K, Hammond S, et al. Pediatric pedestrian versus motor vehicle patterns of injury: debunking the myth. *Air Med J* 1999;**18**(3):107–10.

37. Chang JT, Morton SC, Rubenstein LZ, et al. Interventions for the prevention of falls in older adults: systematic review and meta-analysis of randomised clinical trials. *BMJ* 2004;**328**(7441):680.

38. Woolf AD, Akesson K. Preventing fractures in elderly people. *BMJ*, 2003;**327**(7406):89–95. Erratum appears in *BMJ* 2003;**327**(7416):663.

39. Lapostolle F, Gere C, Borron SW, et al. Prognostic factors in victims of falls from height. *Crit Care Med* 2005;**33**(6):1239–42.

40. Goodacre S, Than M, Goyder EC, et al. Can the distance fallen predict serious injury after a fall from a height? *J Trauma* 1999;**46**(6):1055–8.

41. Lallier M, Bouchard S, St-Vil D, et al. Falls from heights among children: a retrospective review. *J Pediatr Surg* 1999;**34**(7):1060–3.

42. Velmahos GC, Spaniolas K, Alam HB, et al. Falls from height: spine, spine, spine! *J Am Coll Surg* 2006;**203**(5):605–11.

43. NEISS All Injury Program operated by the Consumer Product Safety Commission (CPSC). *Ten Leading Causes of Nonfatal Unintentional Injury, United States 2005, All Races, Males, Disposition: All Cases.* Atlanta, GA: Office of Statistics and Programming, National Center for Injury Prevention and Control, Centers for Disease Control, 2005.

44. Denton JS, Segovia A, Filkins JA. Practical pathology of gunshot wounds. *Arch Pathol Lab Med* 2006;**130**(9):1283–9.

45. Gotsch KEA, Mercy JL, Ryan JA, George W. Surveillance for fatal and nonfatal firearm-related injuries – United States, 1993–1998. *MMWR Morb Mortal Wkly Rep* 2001;**50**(SS02):1–32.

46. Mallonee S, Shariat S, Stennies G, et al. Physical injuries and fatalities resulting from the Oklahoma City bombing. *JAMA* 1996;**276**(5):382–7.

47. Wightman JM, Gladish SL. Explosions and blast injuries. *Ann Emerg Med* 2001;**37**(6):664–78.

48. National Center for Injury Prevention and Control (NCIPC), Office of Noncommunicable Diseases, Injury and Environmental Health. *Explosions and Blast Injuries: A Primer for Clinicians.* Atlanta, GA: Centers for Disease Control and Prevention, 2006.

49. Avidan V, Hersch M, Armon Y, et al. Blast lung injury: clinical manifestations, treatment, and outcome. *Am J Surg* 2005;**190**(6):927–31.

50. Oppenheim A, Pizov R, Pikarsky A, et al. Tension pneumoperitoneum after blast injury: dramatic improvement in ventilatory and hemodynamic parameters after surgical decompression. *J Trauma* 1998;**44**(5):915–17.

51. Paran H, Neufeld D, Shwartz I, et al. Perforation of the terminal ileum induced by blast injury: delayed diagnosis or delayed perforation? *J Trauma* 1996;**40**(3):472–5.

52. Leibovici D, Gofrit ON, Shapira SC. Eardrum perforation in explosion survivors: is it a marker of pulmonary blast injury? *Ann Emerg Med* 1999;**34**(2):168–72.

Chapter

4
Multiple casualties and disaster preparedness

Carl Bonnett, Shawn Ulrich, Charles Little, and Fred Severyn

Introduction

A disaster is an event that generates a group of patients overwhelming an emergency department (ED), either by virtue of the numbers of patients or their unique pathology. The net result of such an incident will be to cause an ED to change its normal operations, sometimes dramatically. Any number of man-made or natural disasters can strike a community and potentially send a flood of casualties to local EDs. In addition, the same event may damage the hospital itself and compromise its ability to respond to the disaster. Because disasters are relatively rare events with the potential for significant casualties and disruption of hospital operations, it is critical for EDs to develop and practice a response plan before an actual event. Unfortunately, the same characteristics that make disasters disruptive also create disincentives for preparation. Unlike almost any other activity that the hospital engages in, disaster preparedness involves investing time and money into preparing for an event that may never happen. Therefore, from a business viewpoint, any activity which does not lead to increased profits for an organization will naturally meet some resistance.[1] Additionally, on an individual level, personnel within a healthcare organization are busy with projects and deadlines relating to problems that are more tangible and immediate. This creates a situation where disaster preparedness constantly keeps getting pushed aside "until we have more time."[2]

Emergency department administrators and providers should consider giving a higher priority to disaster preparedness for several reasons. The primary reason is that a failure to adequately prepare may lead to increased death and morbidity among initial survivors. Making the assumption that the local trauma center will handle most of the casualties from a disaster is inappropriate and not supported by the literature. Numerous disasters including the bombing of the Alfred P. Murrah Federal Building in Oklahoma City in 1995, the Rhode Island nightclub fire in 2003, and the Madrid, Spain train bombings in 2004 have shown that the majority of patients present to the nearest available facility; many of these after bypassing the formal on-scene triage system.[3–8] Those events demonstrate the potential for any ED to become overwhelmed by patients. After the Rhode Island nightclub fire for instance, a local hospital received 67 patients in the first hour; 22 of these required endotracheal intubation.[5,6] A second reason to prepare for disasters is that it is required by the Joint Commission for hospital accreditation. Under the new standards establishing emergency management as a separate independent chapter, hospitals are under increased scrutiny for disaster management. Preparedness now encompasses two categories: leadership standards and environment of care. Under the leadership category there should be a disaster plan in place and resources should be available in the event of a disaster. Under the environment of care standard, everyone in the institution should know his or her role during a disaster. Disaster drills should also be carried out in the hospital per the hospital's policy.

Finally, disasters generate a tremendous amount of media attention. Hospital administrators should realize that their success or failure in managing a disaster will be seen as a public relations benefit or downfall for their institution.

The framework for thinking about disasters divides the process into those activities that are performed *before* an event (mitigation and preparation) from those which are done *after* an event (response and recovery).

Trauma: A Comprehensive Emergency Medicine Approach, eds. Eric Legome and Lee W. Shockley. Published by Cambridge University Press. © Cambridge University Press 2011.

> **Box 4.1** Basic processes that encompass disaster planning
> - **Before event:**
>   Mitigation and preparation
> - **After event:**
>   Response and recovery

Mitigation

Mitigation involves actions that can be taken prior to a disaster in order to prevent or reduce the damage and injuries. A simple analogy is the wearing of a seat belt while driving a car; its use mitigates the risk of serious injury to the driver involved in a crash.[9]

Before mitigation strategies can be implemented; however, one must determine what risks and hazards may exist. To do this, emergency planners conduct a hazard vulnerability analysis. This is a comprehensive look at what situations can occur in and around the hospital that could create a large increase in the number of patients. The hazards faced will be unique to each hospital. For instance, a hospital in Des Moines, Iowa will not have to worry about hurricanes; one in Miami, Florida will. Both hospitals, however, will have to consider airplane crashes, pandemic influenza, and acts of terrorism.

Specifically hospitals need to evaluate three issues of a potential event; the human impact, the property impact, and the business impact. The human impact will be the most immediately pressing if the hospital is near an industrial site, for instance, then it may face a higher likelihood of having to respond to chemically contaminated patients.

When looking at the property impact it is important for planners to determine if the hospital itself is likely to incur damage. One useful tool is a geographical informational system (GIS) maintained by many states and some municipal emergency management offices.[9,10] A GIS is a sophisticated computerized tool that combines multiple types of information into one map and can gives planners a comprehensive picture of the threats a locality may face. For example, a road map can be overlaid on maps showing flood planes and demographic information to determine if low-income residents with poor access to transportation may be trapped by floodwaters. At minimum, hospital planners should examine street maps and drive around the neighborhoods surrounding the hospital to identify risks.

Once planners determine what risks and hazards exist, there are two broad categories of mitigation to be used: structural and procedural. Structural mitigation is ideally done during the design phase of a new facility; it can also be accomplished by retrofitting existing facilities. An example of a structural mitigation strategy is ensuring a redundant power supply (e.g., generators) that is not vulnerable to flooding. During Tropical Storm Allison, a Houston hospital had its basement flooded, causing a short circuit in the electrical switching gear.[11] Another consideration with generators would be their fuel and the need for resupply trucks to be able to get to the hospital.

In addition to mitigating the effects of natural disasters, planners should take into account the potential for violent crime and terrorism. Hospitals should consider deploying physical barriers that prevent unauthorized people from entering EDs, screening devices for weapons, and physical objects to prevent vehicles from being driven into an ED, e.g., large concrete planters.[12]

Preparation

Preparation involves those activities that can be done before an event to facilitate an effective response after it occurs. To expand the earlier analogy further, this could be carrying a fire extinguisher in one's automobile. In this case the driver has not only mitigated his risk by wearing a seat belt but he is now prepared to respond to a fire that may result from a crash.

Preparation consists of two broad categories; planning and equipment acquisition. The end result of the planning process is the disaster plan; however, viewing this document as an end in itself is a mistake. The plan should be thought of as a process with continual drills and exercises being conducted to refine it. The economic considerations of exercises and drills must be considered. For example, if an exercise is to be conducted with employees who are off duty, are they going to be paid for their participation or will it be voluntary?

In general the hospital disaster plan should address how to take care of the patients and families that are expected to arrive and also how to care for the staff members that will be taking care of this influx.[13,14]

A disaster plan has three fundamental components: it should define what activates the plan, who gets notified, and what happens in response to the event. These three components of the plan are known as the initiation criteria, notification requirements, and operational responses.

The initiation criteria are the list of events that would trigger the activation of the plan. It is the point at which the volume and/or pathology of patients arriving exceeds the resources which would be available under normal operations. This point demands a fundamental shift in operations. This may or may not be a dramatic shift. The absolute number of patients that triggers this shift may vary greatly between institutions and at different times of the day. Events that might overwhelm an ED on an overnight shift with limited staff coverage may cause no difficulties in the middle of the afternoon. It might be prudent for the plan to suggest a number of patients for initiating the disaster plan but to ultimately leave it up to the ED physician and charge nurse to assess the situation and activate it as needed.

Other reasons to initiate the disaster plan would include events that are far outside of ordinary operations. One example could be an act of terrorism that might be a diversionary attack in preparation for larger attacks to follow. In such a situation, healthcare facilities may be targeted. Another example might be multiple patients with chemical or radiological contamination from an industrial accident. Any events like this are rare but have the potential for significant disruption of operations. Therefore they should garner a more aggressive response from the hospital.

The second component of the plan is the notification requirements. This is the list of people to be notified when the disaster plan is activated. A tool known as an activation matrix often describes the initial steps in making notifications of a event that will impact the hospital. This may be done in a two-tiered fashion. First, there are certain people who should be notified regardless of the nature of the event. This may include a hospital administrator, the hospital nursing supervisor, the director of security personnel, and an in-house hospitalist or intensivist. The second tier would include individuals who would be notified for specific types of events. For example, the trauma surgeon on-call would be notified for an explosion; a toxicologist would be notified for a chemical release; a radiation safety officer would be notified for a radiation contamination event. Inherent in this part of the plan is the requirement for an effective call-down list that is updated and tested regularly.

The final component of the disaster plan defines the operational responses. This would be the heart of the plan; it describes the actual response to an event. Generally, emergency managers create plans with an "all-hazards" approach rather than have multiple plans for each potential event. In such a plan, the operational response section should begin with a list of actions that are accomplished for any event. Following that section, it is appropriate to have supplemental sections describing additional actions to be taken for specific events. One example may be a requirement that on-call staff members are to be called to establish contact even if they are not actually needed to come in. An event-specific action may be to move any stable or boarding patients in the ED to the inpatient units to be boarded in the hallway or discharged in order to open beds in the ED to enhance surge capacity.

It is important to have the buy-in of all interested parties as the plan is developed. Failure to do so will almost ensure that the response to an event will not be optimal. If the plan calls for certain individuals to be called and for them to perform certain duties, it would be prudent for these individuals to be aware of this and agree to it ahead of time. Additionally, regularly exercising the plan is important because if it sits on the shelf long enough the people who fill key roles may have left. Just because the person who filled a role in the past agreed to perform a certain task in the disaster plan does not mean that the person who now holds that position can be counted on.

Event

There are numerous types of events that may create a disaster. These may appear to be very different but they share an ability to overload a healthcare system's resources and capabilities. Emergency planners must understand disasters from a "big-picture" conceptual level. The lack of universally accepted definitions has led to the use of a number of terms and categories of disasters in the medical literature. Some authors have described static and dynamic events as the first decision point.[15] This describes whether the event was a discrete event ("static") that has done all the damage that it will do (e.g., an isolated bombing in a shopping mall) or is the "disaster" an unfolding event ("dynamic") expected to keep causing problems and generating new casualties (e.g., widespread civil disturbance in a metropolitan area). Other authors have used the terms "contained" or "population-based" disasters.[16] A contained event is one that is limited to a defined geographic area. Conceivably it could be static or dynamic, but it effects only one location. This could range anywhere from an isolated bombing to a riot but it is localized to one metropolitan area (e.g., the Los Angeles riots of April 1992). A population-based event would be one that has poorly defined boundaries. This may include events such as a spreading pandemic or concurrent civil disturbances in multiple cities after an economic or political crisis. It is difficult to devise a system of terminology that can accurately describe all kinds of crises without being so overly complicated as to limit its usefulness. One of the important aspects of these differentiations is the ability to determine what outside resources are available. For example, in a contained event such as Hurricane Katrina of 2005, the infrastructure of the rest of the United States was unaffected making it possible for unaffected areas to send personnel and resources to assist. If there was an influenza pandemic, however, conceivably all municipalities in the United States could be affected, thereby limiting the possibility of outside help.

Response

The response phase involves those actions that occur immediately after the event has transpired; these actions attempt to contain the event, treat casualties, and prevent further damage and injuries. To revisit the earlier analogy, the response is like a motorist using that fire extinguisher that was carried in the car for such an event. Incident response can be a complex and intricate system. Some of the critical components that form the foundation of a response operation include the Incident Command System, triage, surge capacity, decontamination, and communications.

National Incident Management System and Incident Command System

The Incident Command System (ICS) is a flexible system that standardizes the command structure for an incident response.[9] The model grew out of the work of the US Forest Service and the fire-fighting community that battled wildfires in California in the early 1970s. It is based on a very simple yet powerful framework that centers on an Incident Commander

(IC). That person then has four subordinate Section Chiefs that oversee the Planning, Operations, Logistics, and Finance/Administration Sections. The IC also has a Command Staff consisting of Information, Safety, and Liaison Officers who assist with their respective roles. Each section may have subordinate groups, sections, and resources. The ICS uses a system of common terminology and standardized structure which allows various agencies and responders to integrate their efforts on short notice and work effectively to respond to a crisis. After the Department of Homeland Security was created in the aftermath of the September 11th, 2001 attacks, the National Incident Management System (NIMS) was created by the Homeland Security Presidential Directive 5. Its purpose was to guide government agencies and non-governmental organizations in their prevention, preparation, response, and recovery from disasters of any type and scope. While the NIMS covers a large number of issues, the ICS is its foundation. Information about the Federal Emergency Management Agency (FEMA), various resources, and free training materials related to NIMS and ICS are available from http://www.fema.gov/emergency/nims/ (Figures 4.1 and 4.2).

Triage

In order to do the most good for the greatest number of victims, emergency providers must have a means to categorize patients into those who need the most immediate help and those who can wait. Traditionally, victims have been sorted into one of four categories that are represented by colors. The exact terms and colors vary somewhat by organizations. As an example, the US military uses the the categories listed in Table 4.1.

The colors traditionally assigned to these categories are red, yellow, green, and black, respectively. There is some debate in the medical literature as to what the best method is to triage casualties.[17–20] All studies on triage methodology are retrospective and somewhat anecdotal. Further, a variety of commercially developed triage systems are available, each using its own proprietary educational materials and patient-tracking cards. Examples of these systems include Simple Triage and Rapid Treatment (START), JumpSTART (for kids), Homebush, Triage Sieve, Pediatric Triage Tape, CareFlite, Sacco Triage Method, Military Triage, and CESIRA. Information

Table 4.1 US military triage criteria

Immediate	Patients with life-threatening injuries that require immediate treatment
Delayed	Patients that can wait 6–8 hours before definitive treatment
Minor	Patients that can wait indefinitely for further treatment
Expectant	Patients who are dead or who will die despite aggressive treatment

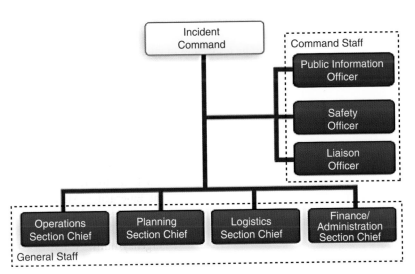

Figure 4.1 Incident command leadership table of organization. (Courtesy of FEMA Resource Center, Homeland Security National Incident Command System, 2008.)

Figure 4.2 National Incident Management System (NIMS) overview. (Courtesy of FEMA Resource Center, Homeland Security National Incident Command System, 2008.)

What NIMS Is:	What NIMS Is NOT:
• A comprehensive, nationwide, systematic approach to incident management, including the Incident Command System. Multiagency Coordination Systems, and Public Information • A set of preparedness concepts and principles for all hazards • Essential principles for a common operating picture and interoperability of communications and information management • Standardized resource management procedures that enable coordination among different jurisdictions or organizations • Scalable, so it may be used for all incidents (from day-to-day to large-scale) • A dynamic system that promotes ongoing management and maintenance	• A response plan • Only used during large-scale incidents • A communications plan • Only applicable to certain emergency management/incident response personnel • Only the Incident Command System or an organization chart • A static system

Box 4.2   Triage systems

Homebush

- http://www.ema.gov.au/agd/EMA/rwpattach.nsf/viewasattachmentpersonal/(C86520E41F5EA5C8AAB6E66B851038D8)~An_Australian_mass_casualty_incident_triage_system.pdf/$file/An_Australian_mass_casualty_incident_triage_system.pdf

Triage seive

- http://www.triagesystems.co.uk/cwctriage.html

Sacco triage method

- http://www.sharpthinkers.com/STM_Site/stm_home.htm

on several of the methods can be obtained from the websites listed in Box 4.2.

Regardless of the triage system chosen, it is important to pick one, plan for its implementation, and train with it.

Surge capacity

A surge capacity plan defines how the facility will alter its structure and protocols to accommodate a large influx of patients. It should be in place before a disaster occurs or may be expected.[16,21] One of the first priorities of a surge capacity plan is to empty or "decompress" the ED as quickly as practical prior to the arrival of the majority of the disaster patients. Frequently, there is some advance notice of multiple casualties arriving: the surge plan should be activated when this information is appropriately confirmed. Prior agreements should be in place for inpatient units to accept patients that may be boarding in the ED or are in the midst of an evaluation. This requires agreements among physician, nursing, and admission leaders. There should be a clear understanding and agreement of when and who activates the surge capacity plan.

The inpatient physician groups should have a standing agreement with the ED leaders to continue workups, or open alternate care sites outside of the ED. The agreement should have outlined how and when patients are accepted from the ED when the surge capacity plan is activated. These agreements should include the department of surgery. Operating rooms (ORs) can easily become overwhelmed in a mass casualty situation: it is important to have prior

agreements in place to efficiently maximize the use of OR space. Depending on the event, it may be appropriate to have a surgeon in the ED working with the emergency physician to prioritize surgical triage; however, they may be required in the OR. Junior residents are not appropriate substitutes, however. Communication between the OR and the ED is essential; it should be consistent and uniform in the institution. Since telephones in the ED and the OR can become overwhelmed in a disaster, radios may be used to facilitate real-time communication. Radios should be tested and maintained. A supply of replacement batteries is necessary. Standard phraseology and assigned frequencies are critical to limit communication errors.

Prior to a disaster, emergency nursing leaders and the inpatient nursing leaders should have agreements about how to accept more than the normal capacity on the inpatient units. Nursing leaders on the inpatient floors must convey to inpatient staff that the normal patient ratios do not apply during a surge capacity activation. Nursing inpatient leaders should also have a call-down list for their staff to accept the influx of patients. There should be a plan to bed these patients either in disaster cots or alternate arrangements.

Admissions personnel should understand the surge capacity plan. Tracking of patients after they have been "surged" to the inpatient floor can be challenging. If the facility uses an electronic tracking system it should be reviewed prior to a disaster to determine whether the potential to add "surge" beds within the system architecture exists. If that is possible, a solution to add these beds or have a "toggle" to increase the capacity of the electronic tracking system should be implemented. In addition, it is important to have a back-up paper tracking process in preparation for potential system failures.

Hospital decontamination

In an incident involving potential contamination with chemical, biologic, or radioactive agents, hospitals should be prepared to perform patient decontamination.[22] Each hospital must have this capability regardless of regional capability. The hospital plan cannot rely on all patients being decontaminated at the scene. All hospitals are required by national standards to maintain a decontamination team. These teams are required to meet the Occupational Safety and Health Administration (OSHA) standards for equipment and training. In addition to a team, it may be useful to set up specific areas or transport corridors so, if a hospital does experience contamination, the contamination is limited to a confined or small area. This may also include closing off ventilation to the rest of the hospital and laying floor covering.

The process of decontamination is straightforward. Staff and patient safety is paramount. Decontamination teams need initial and ongoing training. Decontamination gear is categorized by levels of protection as A, B, C, or D. Level A suits are heavy duty chemically resistant material, vapor sealed with a self-contained breathing apparatus (SCBA) within the suit. These are generally used by field HazMat teams. The training, cost, and physical requirements to use these suits are typically prohibitive for hospitals. Level B is a lighter protective suit with chemically resistant gloves and boots. Level B maintains high respiratory protection with an SCBA external to the suit. Level B suits are less effective against chemicals than Level A suits. Level C protection uses a protective suit similar to Level B coupled with a respirator (face mask) fitted with chemical filters. A common type of respirator used by hospitals is a powered air purified respirator (PAPR). The PAPR draws air though the filter system to a loose fitting hood that does not require the individual to be fitted with a face mask.

Level D protection is a particulate-resistant suit with gloves, boots, eye protection, and masks. The use of surgical gowns, boots, and double gloves is field-expedient protective gear that would be adequate for simple particulate protection such as for radiation or anthrax contamination.

Box 4.3   Decontamination suits

Level	Suit characteristics
A	Heavy duty chemically resistant material, vapor sealed with a SCBA Generally used by field HazMat
B	Maintains high respiratory protection with a SCBA external to the suit
C	Protective suit similar to Level B coupled with a respirator (face mask) fitted with chemical filters
D	Particulate-resistant suit with gloves, boots, eye protection, and mask

More information about protective suits can be obtained at: http://www.osha.gov/pls/oshaweb/owadisp.show_document?p_table=STANDARDS&p_id=9767 and http://www.au.af.mil/au/awc/awcgate/army/sbccom_decon.pdf.

The approach to decontamination depends on the suspected agent. It is important to quickly determine if any contamination is present even if it appears that the event was caused by a conventional explosive. It is prudent to assume that all explosions may be terrorist attacks until proven otherwise. In especially large or unusual explosions, hospital personnel would be wise to survey the first arriving patients with a radiation detector to detect any radiation contamination (e.g., from a "dirty bomb"). The goal is to prevent hospital contamination, which may not cause immediate problems but would be detrimental to the longer-term health of hospital employees.

Decontamination can be either "hasty" (e.g., with fire hoses) or deliberate. With overwhelming numbers of patients, hasty decontamination may be all that is practical. More thorough decontamination is preferable, particularly with patients suffering the effects of a chemical exposure. Chemical decontamination should ideally be performed in a specially built hospital shower (with exterior exhaust) or in a tent outside the hospital. The layout is divided into zones called "hot," "warm," and "cold." No one will move from hot to cold zones without decontamination. Healthcare providers in the hot and warm zones should have at least Level C protection.

Patients in the "hot zone" are instructed to bag their belongings and enter the showers ("warm zone"). Non-ambulatory patients enter on stretchers and have their clothing cut off. The majority of contamination (up to 90%) on patients is removed by removing the clothing. Soap and water is used to wash the patient head to toe. With radiation contamination a survey meter is used to monitor the process. After completion of decontamination the patient enters the cold zone. They will then require fresh clothing and medical treatment.

Non-critical patients contaminated with radiation should be decontaminated before treatment. Radiation is easily detected with counters and is generally a minimal risk to medical personnel. Patients with life-threatening injuries should be treated as trauma patients with hospital contamination limited as much as is practical. The hospital facilities can be decontaminated later as needed.

41

Chemical contamination

Patients contaminated with dangerous chemicals should be decontaminated prior to entry to the hospital, regardless of condition, to prevent injury to individuals in the facility. Scene information as to chemical types is very helpful and should be actively sought.

Biologic exposures

Patients contaminated with biologic agents (i.e., anthrax spores) should be decontaminated in the same fashion as with chemicals exposures. Biologic agents may cause contamination (the agent existing on the patient) or infection (the agent causing illness); the infected patient may also be contagious. After initial exposure, an infected patient may require isolation but will generally not require decontamination days later.

Emergency workers in protective gear doing decontamination need frequent rest breaks. A substitution plan to rotate workers in and out of the decontamination area is necessary. The run off from showers should ideally be contained to prevent environmental contamination. In a terrorist (criminal) event clothing and material should be saved for forensic evaluation.

Crisis communication

Consideration of the manner in which information is released to the media and the public is important. After taking care of the victims themselves it is important to address the needs of the families and friends of those victims. A well-run communication plan will get families the information they need, facilitate an orderly response to the event, and maintain a co-operative relationship between a healthcare facility and the community. A poorly run communications plan could lead to undue emotional upset amongst relatives of the victims, significant animosity directed towards the healthcare facility, panic in the community, and negative treatment in the press.[23–25] There are a few key principles in crisis communication. First, it is best to have one person serving as the spokesperson for the organization; contradictory statements from different people are counterproductive. Second, the spokesperson should have some training in crisis communication. This person should give facts clearly and succinctly; speculation should be

> **Box 4.4 Essentials of crisis communication**
>
> - A well-run communication plan will get families the information they need, facilitate an orderly response to the event, and maintain a co-operative relationship between a healthcare facility and the community.
> - It is best to have one person serving as the spokesperson for the organization; contradictory statements from different people are counterproductive.
> - The spokesperson should have some training in crisis communication.
> - If the answer is not known the speaker should say so and offer to make the information available as soon as possible.
> - It is prudent to give people something tangible that they can do to help.

avoided. If the answer is not known the speaker should say so and offer to make the information available as soon as possible. Any attempt to lie, cover up, or otherwise gloss over the facts may be exposed and could create a public relations problem for the institution as well as lead to loss of credibility when it is needed. Lastly, it is prudent to give people something tangible that they can do to help. For example, families can be told to assemble at a given hotel where they all will be given updates on a situation. Alternatively, people can be instructed to go and donate blood if that is required. Disasters can be psychologically overwhelming: it can be helpful to restore a sense of control for people by giving them something that they can do to assist.

Recovery

The recovery phase involves repairing and rebuilding the infrastructure that was damaged during the event as well as replenishing medical supplies and equipment. It also involves transitioning from disaster operations back to normal operations. Depending on the nature of the incident there may have been a suspension of the usual course of care. If so, then patients should be re-evaluated, charting updated, and efforts made to ensure that nothing has "slipped through the cracks."

It will also be essential to address the physical and mental health of care providers. For many staff, the event will have been the most horrific experience of their careers. By virtue of the fact that the healthcare system was overwhelmed, it is quite possible that some number of patients experience morbidity or mortality which, under normal circumstances, would not have occurred. This situation can lead healthcare providers to feel that they failed or were in some way inadequate. In light of this it may be helpful for ED and hospital administration to address these concerns and arrange for debriefing, such as a critical incident stress debriefing (CISD).[2]

Finally, because no disaster will ever go "as planned," it is important for hospitals to conduct an after action review (AAR) to take a critical look at what went well and what needs to be improved upon. It is important for a person of authority to take charge of this meeting and keep it focused: there can be a tendency for participants in these reviews to avoid personal blame and assign fault for deficiencies during the planning and response.[26]

Conclusion

Planning for a disaster can be one of the most challenging tasks that healthcare providers will face. As disasters can occur in a multitude of forms and in a wide range of scales, trying to adequately plan and prepare for an event can be a daunting task. In addition to the potential human suffering that may unfold, emergency planners must take into account the scrutiny they will face in the political, legal, and media arenas. Anyone who occupies an administrative role should consider themselves obliged to educate themselves about disaster planning and make it a priority to make the appropriate preparations in their healthcare facilities and systems.

References

1. Rodriguez H, Aguirre BE. Hurricane Katrina and the healthcare infrastructure: a focus on disaster preparedness, response, and resiliency. *Front Health Serv Manage* 2006;**23**(1):13–23.

2. Auf der Heide E. Disaster planning, Part II. Disaster problems, issues, and challenges identified in the research literature. *Emerg Med Clin North Am* 1996;**14**(2):453–80.

3. Hogan DE, Waeckerle JF, Dire DJ, Lillibridge SR. Emergency department impact of the Oklahoma City terrorist bombing. *Ann Emerg Med* 1999;**34**(2):160–7.

4. Gutierrez de Ceballos JP, Turegano FF, Perez DD et al. Casualties treated at the closest hospital in the Madrid, March 11, terrorist bombings. *Crit Care Med* 2005;**33**(1 Suppl.):S107–12.

5. Dunbar JA. The Rhode Island nightclub fire: the story from the perspective of an on-duty ED nurse. *J Emerg Nurs* 2004;**30**(5):464–6.

6. Dacey MJ. Tragedy and response – the Rhode Island nightclub fire. *N Engl J Med* 2003;**349**(21):1990–2.

7. Tokuda Y, Kikuchi M, Takahashi O, Stein GH. Prehospital management of sarin nerve gas terrorism in urban settings: 10 years of progress after the Tokyo subway sarin attack. *Resuscitation* 2006;**68**(2):193–202.

8. Auf der Heide E. The importance of evidence-based disaster planning. *Ann Emerg Med* 2006;**47**(1):34–49.

9. Haddow GD, Bullock JA, Coppola DP. *Introduction to Emergency Management*, 2nd edn. Burlington, MA: Elsevier Butterworth-Heinemann; 2006.

10. Boulos MN, Honda K. Web GIS in practice IV: publishing your health maps and connecting to remote WMS sources using the Open Source UMN MapServer and DM Solutions MapLab. *Int J Health Geogr* 2006;**5**:6.

11. Cocanour CS, Allen SJ, Mazabob J, et al. Lessons learned from the evacuation of an urban teaching hospital. *Arch Surg* 2002;**137**(10):1141–5.

12. Bullard TB, Strack G, Scharoun K. Emergency department security: a call for reassessment. *Health Care Manag (Frederick)* 2002;**21**(1):65–73.

13. Bonnet C, Ullruch S, Shockley L, et al. *Writing Cell Emergency Department Disaster Plan*, 2007 edn. Denver, CO: Denver Health Medical Center, 2008.

14. Van Dyke S. *Surge Capacity Plan*. Denver, CO: Denver Health Medical Center, 2008.

15. Koenig K, Dinerman N, Kuehl AE. Disaster nomenclature – a functional impact approach: the PICE system. *Acad Emerg Med* 1996;**3**:723–7.

16. Bonnett CJ, Peery BN, Cantrill SV, et al. Surge capacity: a proposed conceptual framework. *Am J Emerg Med* 2007;**25**(3):297–306.

17. Gebhart ME, Pence R. START triage: does it work? *Disaster Manag Response* 2007;**5**(3):68–73.

18. Asaeda G. The day that the START triage system came to a STOP: observations from the World Trade Center disaster. *Acad Emerg Med* 2002;**9**(3):255–6.

19. Zoraster RM, Chidester C, Koenig W. Field triage and patient maldistribution in a mass-casualty incident. *Prehosp Disaster Med* 2007;**22**(3):224–9.

20. Lerner EB, Schwartz RB, Coule PL, et al. Mass casualty triage: an evaluation of the data and development of a proposed national guideline. *Disaster Med Public Health Prep* 2008;**2**(Suppl. 1):S25–34.

21. Hick JL, Hanfling D, Burstein JL, et al. Health care facility and community strategies for patient care surge capacity. *Ann Emerg Med* 2004;**44**(3):253–61.

22. Currance PL. *Medical Response to Weapons of Mass Destruction*. St. Louis, MO: Elsevier Mosby; 2005.

23. Levi L, Michaelson M, Admi H, Bregman D, Bar-Nahor R. National strategy for mass casualty situations and its effects on the hospital. *Prehosp Disaster Med* 2002;**17**(1): 12–16.

24. Lynn M, Gurr D, Memon A, Kaliff J. Management of conventional mass casualty incidents: 10 commandments for hospital planning. *J Burn Care Res* 2006;**27**(5):649–58.

25. Partington AJ, Savage PE. Disaster planning: managing the media. *Br Med J (Clin Res Ed)* 1985; **291**(6495):590–2.

26. Hoffman B. The capability of emergency departments and emergency medical systems in the US to respond to mass casualty events resulting from terrorist attacks. Written testimony submitted to website: http://oversight.house.gov/documents/20080505103219.pdf.

Chapter 5

Trauma airway

Abraham Berger, Christine Preblick, and Pinchas Halpern

Introduction

Control of the airway in a major trauma patient may be the most important contributor to survival. The emergency physician must be facile in emergent airway management. Timely recognition of the need to secure an airway, identification of the potentially difficult airway, and an awareness of the resources available (equipment and medications) are necessary.

The initial evaluation

The initial assessment of the airway can be very brief and basic; however, a more thorough assessment is eventually required based on patient factors and findings. Just speaking with the patient and having them answer appropriately in a full sentence gives the clinician some measure of comfort that immediate aggressive management may not be required. An intoxicated patient with minor trauma may just require a chin thrust and observation, while a severely head-injured unconscious patient needs early intubation.

The initial point of assessment in the trauma patient and the decision to intubate is a clinical one made at the bedside. If the physician feels that the airway is threatened then it should be secured with intubation. To aid in this decision, the physician may use a four-question assessment tool:

1. Is there failure of airway maintenance or protection?
2. Is there failure of oxygenation?
3. Is there failure of ventilation?
4. Is there an anticipated need for intubation?

Having the patient speak often assesses a failure of airway maintenance or protection. Patients who are able to speak clearly and control and swallow their secretions are generally able to protect their airways. Many clinicians rely upon the lack of a gag reflex as an indication for intubation. However, the gag reflex is a poor discriminator for the need for intubation.[1–4] By eliciting the gag reflex, one runs the risk of causing a patient to vomit and aspirate.

An airway should also be considered threatened if it is anatomically distorted (as in the case of maxillofacial trauma) or if the patient's consciousness is altered (as in intoxication or brain injury). On the other hand, experience and clinical judgment can and should take into account other factors before a patient is reflexively intubated. For example, the patient with head trauma after a relatively minor mechanism and with a computed tomography (CT) scan readily available may be a better candidate for sedation rather than intubation. If there is a severe mechanism, however, with a high potential for intracranial injury, early intubation may be more appropriate, even if the patient is most likely just intoxicated. If intubation is deferred, however, close monitoring is necessary with the ability to rapidly secure an airway if needed. One commonly accepted scoring system that serves to guide the decision to intubate is the Glasgow Coma Scale (GCS). A GCS < 8 in a trauma patient warrants intubation.

Failure of oxygenation can be assessed by several means. Patients who are quite hypoxic may appear cyanotic. However, this is an insensitive sign for moderate degrees of hypoxia. Non-invasive pulse-oximetry devices have become commonplace in nearly all emergency departments (EDs) and most ambulances. Pulse oximetry is as sensitive as 92% and as specific as 90% for the detection of hypoxia in normal individuals.[5] However, pulse oximetry accuracy can be affected by motion, hypotension, vasoconstriction, hypothermia anemia, hemoglobinopathies, certain dyes (such as methylene blue, indocyanine green, and indigo carmine), nail polish, ambient light, and skin pigmentation. Lastly, arterial blood gas determination can demonstrate hypoxia. However, this takes time to obtain the sample and run the test and it is rarely necessary when used solely as a means of making intubation decisions.

Failure of ventilation is most often determined by the clinical examination. Patients with inadequate chest rise and fall, with poor air movement on auscultation, or low respiratory rates may be candidates for emergent intubation. The exception may be the patient with an expected short-term impairment of ventilation, such as that caused by over-sedation. In such a situation, assisting the patient's ventilations with a bag-valve-mask (BVM) device or administering a reversal agent may be more prudent than proceeding to endotracheal intubation. End-tidal carbon dioxide (ETCO$_2$) monitors may also help in the recognition of a hypoventilating patient. However, ETCO$_2$ monitors are prone to sampling errors (e.g., poor cardiac output, rapid respiratory rates, low tidal volumes, hypothermia, and malpositioning of the sampling instrument).[6,7] Similarly, arterial blood gases can demonstrate hypercapnea. However, as in determining hypoxia, the test takes time to obtain the sample and run the test and it is rarely necessary when used solely as a means of making intubation decisions.

The ability to anticipate a need for intubation is one mark of a thoughtful clinician exercising sound judgment. Some cases are very straightforward. For example, the patient with penetrating neck trauma with an expanding hematoma that is compressing the airway should be intubated expeditiously. However, an inexperienced clinician may not recognize the potential for rapid airway deterioration in the same patient who presents moments after the injury before the hematoma has developed. In such a circumstance, the risks and benefits of performing the procedure early must be weighed carefully against the risks and benefits of performing the procedure later, when it may be considerably more difficult or impossible. In making the intubation decision, the clinician should consider:

- What is the likelihood of significant deterioration that will require emergent intubation?
- If deterioration is a reasonable possibility, how much time will I likely have to respond? Will this be a "crash" situation?
- What resources are available to handle the situation now and in the future (including airway options, personnel, and medications)?
- Where could this patient be if and when he or she deteriorates (CT scan, elevator, exam room, helicopter)?

Even though a patient may have one or more of the four assessment tool conditions, endotracheal intubation may not always be the most appropriate response. For example, a patient who is hypoxic because of a pneumothorax would benefit more from a chest tube thoracostomy than intubation (which may be harmful instead).

It is important to consider intracranial injury or intoxication that can also compromise ventilation. High level cervical spine injury may also compromise ventilation via respiratory muscle paralysis. Patients with significant chest trauma may need intubation. Lung contusions may cause respiratory failure and may progress rapidly from minor to severe symptoms. It is important to monitor these patients closely for the need for intubation and following intubation for hypoxia and hypotension which may be a result of their lung injury. Direct facial trauma may also compromise the airway. Evidence of burn injury in the form of soot or singed facial hair may also be an indicator of injury to the lungs or trachea which may cause airway compromise.

Finally, the decision to secure an airway may also be directed by the anticipated clinical course for the patient. Injuries to the neck, trachea, or larynx should alert the physician to potential airway compromise and warrant early establishment of an artificial airway. Patients who will require multiple procedures including CT scans, chest tubes, fixation of broken bones, or eventually will go to the operating room (OR) or intensive care unit (ICU) setting should also be considered for early intubation. Patients who are being transported out of the security of the ED, e.g., CT scanner or transfer to another institution, should also be considered for intubation.

Box 5.1 **High-risk situations often requiring advanced airway management**

- Head-injured patients
- Burn injury
- Direct airway injury (trachea, neck, larynx)
- Need for multiple procedures
- Need for transport out of ED
- Multiple injuries
- Significant chest trauma

Predicting the difficult airway

The difficult airway can be defined as the clinical situation in which adequate face mask ventilation of the upper airway or tracheal intubation is challenging.[8] The airway may be made difficult by the interactions of patient factors, the clinical setting, and the skills of the physician. A patient with a history of prior airway difficulties should alert the physician to potential problems with intubation. However, this information is rarely available in the acute trauma setting. A quick, focused examination of the airway anatomy can help the physician assess the potential risk of encountering difficulties (Table 5.1[8]).

The Mallampati classification compares tongue size to pharyngeal size.[9,10] As originally described, the test is performed with the patient seated. The patient's head is held in a neutral position with the mouth wide open and the tongue protruding. The extent of the visibility of the pharyngeal structures determines the classification (Figure 5.1):

Class I: Visualization of the soft palate, uvula, anterior and the posterior pillars.

Class II: Visualization of the soft palate and uvula.

Class III: Visualization of soft palate and base of uvula.

Class IV: Only hard palate is visible.

An airway assessment mnemonic, LEMON, takes into account many of the anatomic factors in a scoring system.[11–13] LEMON is a 10-point scale (up to 1 point for each factor) (Table 5.2). Although never validated, in general, patients with higher LEMON scores are more likely to have difficult intubations.

Assessment of most of these physical examination findings require either a cooperative, awake patient or require the ability to safely extend the neck. In many circumstances the ability to predict difficulty is not readily apparent. Unless obvious by external findings,

Table 5.1 Components of the preintubation airway physical examination – concerning factors[8]

Anatomic factor	Predictor of potential difficulty
Length of upper incisors	Relatively long
Relation of maxillary and mandibular incisors during normal jaw closure	Prominent "overbite" (maxillary incisors anterior to mandibular incisors)
Relation of maxillary and mandibular incisors during voluntary protrusion of mandible	Patient cannot bring mandibular incisors anterior to (in mandible front of) maxillary incisors
Interincisor distance	< 3 cm
Visibility of uvula	Not visible when tongue is protruded with patient in sitting position (e.g., Mallampati class > II)
Shape of palate	Highly arched or very narrow
Compliance of mandibular space	Stiff, indurated, occupied by mass, or non-resilient
Thyromental distance	< 3 Ordinary finger breadths
Length of neck	Short
Thickness of neck	Thick
Range of motion of head and neck	Patient cannot touch tip of chin to chest or cannot extend neck

Table 5.2 The LEMON Scale

Variable	Factors/points
L = Look externally	Facial trauma = 1, large incisors = 1, beard or moustache = 1, and large tongue = 1
E = Evaluate the 3–3–2 rule	Mouth opening distance < 3 fingerbreadths = 1, hyoid/mental distance < 3 fingerbreadths = 1, thyroid-to-mouth distance < 2 fingerbreadths = 1
M = Mallampati	Mallampati score 3 or greater = 1
O = Obstruction	Presence of any condition that could cause an obstructed airway = 1
N = Neck mobility	Limited neck mobility = 1

47

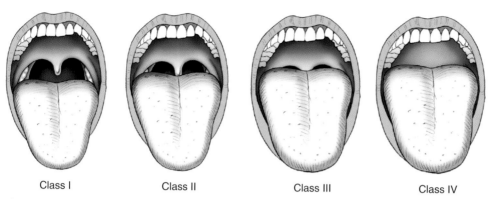

Class I   Class II   Class III   Class IV

Figure 5.1 Mallampati classification. The classification of tongue size relative to the size of the oral cavity as described by Mallampati and colleagues. Class I: faucial pillars, soft palate, and uvula visualized. Class II: faucial pillars and soft palate visualized, but the uvula is masked by the base of the tongue. Class III: only the base of the uvula can be visualized. Class IV: none of the three structures can be visualized. (From Mahadevan S, Garmel G. *An Introduction to Clinical Emergency Medicine.* Cambridge: Cambridge University Press, 2005.)

difficulty can be very hard to predict; the laryngoscopic view will ultimately indicate the severity of the difficulty. Faced with this situation, the prudent physician should have access to multiple rescue techniques and a "Plan B" if airway problems are encountered.

Options for intubation

Rapid sequence inbutation: theory and practice

Rapid sequence intubation (RSI) is the technique most often utilized for trauma intubations.[14] It involves the use of a paralytic agent along with a sedative to ease intubation and reduce the risk of gastric aspiration as well as a spike in intracranial pressure. The use of paralytic agents poses a risk of hypoventilation and hypoxia in the difficult airway. Some have argued that paralytics should be avoided in patients who may be difficult to ventilate or in situations where one anticipates a difficult airway, although this is generally outweighed by the benefits and is generally considered the standard of care in the ED.[15] Certain circumstances, e.g., penetrating neck trauma with hematoma, may warrant careful consideration of alternative approaches.

Rapid sequence intubation has been broken into seven steps, the seven Ps. These are described below.

Preparation

All resources and the patient should be prepared for intubation. The patient should be placed on a cardiac monitor, and a pulse oximeter with blood

pressure measurements. An intravenous (IV) line should be placed and the patient assessed for a possible difficult airway. Equipment should be prepared at the bedside, including bag valve mask connected to oxygen, a Yankauer suction, $ETCO_2$ detector (or continuous CO_2 monitor), laryngoscopes (with functioning light source), and endotracheal tubes. The endotracheal tube should be prepped with a stylet in place and a 10 ml syringe attached to the balloon port. The balloon should be inflated and then deflated to test for leaks. All RSI medications should be drawn and ready for administration.

Preoxygenation

Because RSI patients are rendered apneic during the procedure, they should be adequately preoxygenated prior to administration of medications. Patients are given at least 3 minutes of normal tidal volume breathing or 8 vital capacity breaths with as close to 100% oxygen as practical. A well-fitting non-rebreathing face mask at 15+ L of oxygen per minute may be used; if necessary, a BVM device may also be used. However, this technique risks forcing air down the esophagus, inflating the stomach, and potentially precipitating aspiration.

Pretreatment

Pretreatment medications are used by many clinicians to attempt to blunt the parasympathetic and sympathetic stimulation caused by direct laryngoscopy and intubation for specific patients. These medications include lidocaine (1.5 mg/kg IV) and fentanyl (1–3 mcg/kg IV) for patients with suspected intracranial injuries. If used, they should be given 3 minutes prior to paralysis. The benefits from these drugs have never been quantified and intubations in trauma without them are acceptable, especially when time is a factor.

Paralysis of anesthesia

Induction agents may include narcotics, short-acting barbiturates, benzodiazepines, ketamine, etomidate, propofol, and others. Because of its cardiovascular neutrality (not causing hypotension, hypertension, bradycardia, or tachycardia) many clinicians prefer etomidate (0.3 mg/kg IV). Simultaneous administration of a paralytic accompanies the sedative/induction agent. Paralytics should not be used without adequate sedation. Commonly used paralytics include succinylcholine (1.5 mg/kg IV), a depolarizing agent, and rocuronium (1 mg/kg IV), a non-depolarizing agent.

Protection

If the patient was being ventilated with a BVM device, this is suspended after the paralytic is given. It should not be necessary to continue if the patient was adequately preoxygenated and the risk of instilling air down the esophagus rises while the patient is becoming paralyzed.

Many practitioners advocate applying the Sellick maneuver once the patient becomes unconscious in an effort to prevent gastric regurgitation. The Sellick maneuver involves an assistant applying firm pressure on the cricoid cartilage in an attempt to close the esophagus. If the patient begins to vomit then pressure should be released. The utility of the Sellick maneuver, however, has not been proven and may make intubation more difficult by partially collapsing the upper trachea. One modification of this maneuver has been shown to increase the chances of success, the BURP maneuver. This maneuver involves placing the larynx into a position that optimizes the view for an intubator holding a laryngoscope in the left hand by applying *Backward* (towards the spine), *Upward* (towards the mouth), *Rightward Pressure*. Excessive pressure may, however, make the view worse.[16,17] Concern for cervical spine injury should lead to in-line traction by an assistant to prevent neck hyperextension during laryngoscopy.

Placement

Confirmation of paralysis can be made in a number of ways (loss of body movements, loss of chest rise and fall, loss of corneal reflexes); the most germane, however, may be the laxity of the mandible to upward

and downward movement by the intubator. An endotracheal tube is then inserted under direct laryngoscopy with visualization of the vocal cords. The cuff is then inflated, the stylette is removed, and tracheal placement is confirmed by color change with an $ETCO_2$ detector or capnograph, condensation within the tube on exhalation, the observation of chest rise and fall, and auscultation over the stomach and both axilla. Other additional confirmatory techniques may include the passage of a lighted stylette, fiberoptic bronchoscopy through the endotracheal tube, ultrasonography, the use of a pneumatic esophageal detector device (EDD), or chest radiography. Care must be taken to always guard the endotracheal tube's position by grasping it close to the teeth until it can be secured with tape or string.

Post-intubation management

The endotracheal tube is connected to a mechanical ventilation device (a ventilator or a BVM). Additional sedation, with or without longer acting paralytic agents, is administered and restraints are applied to prevent self-extubation (Figure 5.2).

Other options besides standard RSI

The prudent emergency physician should acquire skills in using adjuncts to assist RSI, as well as develop familiarity with other airway techniques that may be used in place of RSI, or as rescue techniques in the case of the failure of RSI:

- awake intubation
- retrograde intubation
- laryngeal mask airways (LMA)
- combitube and laryngeal tube
- lighted stylet intubation
- semi-rigid fiberoptic stylets
- nasal and orotracheal intubation over a flexible fiberoptic
- rigid fiberoptic laryngoscopy
- video-assisted laryngoscopy
- blind nasotracheal intubation
- transtracheal jet ventilation
- surgical airways (cricothyroidotomy)
- bougie assisted intubation.

Post-intubation care

Once the airway is established and the patient is intubated it is important to maintain adequate sedation for both patient comfort and safety. Depending on the

Typical RSI time

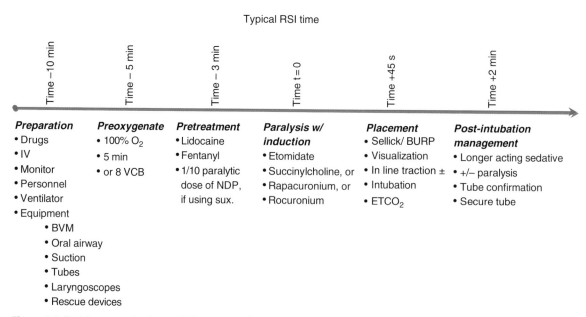

| Time −10 min | Time − 5 min | Time − 3 min | Time t = 0 | Time +45 s | Time +2 min |

Preparation
- Drugs
- IV
- Monitor
- Personnel
- Ventilator
- Equipment
  - BVM
  - Oral airway
  - Suction
  - Tubes
  - Laryngoscopes
  - Rescue devices

Preoxygenate
- 100% O_2
- 5 min
- or 8 VCB

Pretreatment
- Lidocaine
- Fentanyl
- 1/10 paralytic dose of NDP, if using sux.

Paralysis w/ induction
- Etomidate
- Succinylcholine, or
- Rapacuronium, or
- Rocuronium

Placement
- Sellick/ BURP
- Visualization
- In line traction ±
- Intubation
- $ETCO_2$

Post-intubation management
- Longer acting sedative
- +/− paralysis
- Tube confirmation
- Secure tube

Figure 5.2 Rapid sequence intubation (RSI): sequence of events. BVM, bag-valve-mask; $ETCO_2$, end-tidal carbon dioxide; IV, intravenous; NPD, ethosuximide; VCB, vital capacity breaths.

clinical scenario, sedative induction medications can be continued to maintain sedation. These medications are titrated to sedation and the Richmond Agitation Sedation Score can be utilized to help ensure patient comfort post-intubation (Table 5.3[18,19]).

Proper sedation requires frequent clinical monitoring and observation for agitation and hypotension (common post-intubation). In addition, the use of two-point wrist restraints should be considered to prevent self-extubation.

Prehospital intubation

In the prehospital setting the same basic principles for securing the airway are applied. The techniques available are determined by the training of the provider, the equipment available, and the agency's policies and procedures, as determined by the medical director. Supplemental oxygen and the chin lift maneuver may be adequate in some trauma patients; others may require ventilation with a BVM device. Many prehospital systems provide the option for unmedicated endotracheal intubation in the field; some provide RSI. Other airway options may be chosen from the list above. The decision to intubate a trauma patient in the field, especially if that procedure will delay transportation, is a controversial one. In many cases a stable patient can safely be transported with a non-rebreather or BVM device, deferring the intubation to the more controlled setting of the ED where a wider array of procedures and personnel are available.

An Ontario Prehospital Advanced Life Support (OPALS) study examined the question of whether invasive airway management should be done in the field and whether this would change the survival of patients with traumatic injuries.[20] Other authors have investigated this topic and discovered that there is an increase in mortality in severe head-injury patients when intubated vs. receiving BVM ventilation. Placement of the endotracheal tube can increase the risk of aspiration and also lead to a rise in intracranial pressure furthering the neurologic insult. Another factor contributing to potential risks from early intubation is inappropriate ventilation. Studies have found that once intubation is accomplished, prehospital personel commonly hyperventilate head-injured patients, even when protocols are set otherwise.[21–24]

In the prehospital arena patients with suspected blunt neck injuries should be transported in a supine position, with a cervical collar and oxygen. Bleeding should be controlled with direct pressure. Blind intubations are not recommended because of the risk of creating a false route or completely transecting a partially damaged airway. Laryngeal mask and RSI are relatively contraindicated in patients with laryngotracheal disruption.

Table 5.3 Richmond Agitation Sedation Scale[18,19]

Score	Term	Description	
+4	Combative	Overtly combative, violent, immediate danger to staff	
+3	Very agitated	Pulls or removes tube(s) or catheter(s); aggressive	
+2	Agitated	Frequent non-purposeful movement, fights ventilator	
+1	Restless	Anxious but movements not vigorously aggressive	
0	Alert and calm	–	
−1	Drowsy	Not fully alert, but has sustained awakening (eye-opening/eye contact) to voice (> 10 s)	Verbal stimulation
−2	Light sedation	Briefly awakens with eye contact to voice (< 10 s)	
−3	Moderate sedation	Movement or eye opening to voice (but no eye contact)	
−4	Deep sedation	No response to voice, but movement or eye opening to physical stimulation	Physical stimulation
−5	Unarousable	No response to voice or physical stimulation	

Box 5.2 Key concepts in the trauma airway

- The four-question assessment tool is a valuable aid in assessing the need for intubating a trauma patient:
  1. Is there failure of airway maintenance or protection?
  2. Is there failure of oxygenation?
  3. Is there failure of ventilation?
  4. Is there an anticipated need for intubation?
- Difficult airway management can often be predicted by the airway assessment mnemonic, LEMON:
  L = Look externally
  E = Evaluate the 3–3–2 rule
  M = Mallampati
  O = Obstruction
  N = Neck mobility
- While RSI is generally considered the standard in the emergency management of the airway, it is prudent to consider other options with a very high-risk airway and always have a "Plan B" rescue option, including the ability to create a surgical airway by cricothyroidotomy.

References

1. Kulig K, Rumack BH, Rosen P. Gag reflex in assessing level of consciousness. *Lancet* 1982;**1**(8271):565.

2. Chan B, Gaudry P, Grattan-Smith TM, et al. The use of Glasgow Coma Scale in poisoning. *J Emerg Med* 1993;**11**(5):579–82.

3. Davies AE, Kidd D, Stone SP, et al. Pharyngeal sensation and gag reflex in healthy subjects. *Lancet* 1995;**345** (8948):487–8.

4. Leder SB. Gag reflex and dysphagia. *Head Neck* 1996;**18** (2):138–41.

5. Lee WW, Mayberry K, Crapo R, et al. The accuracy of pulse oximetry in the emergency department. *Am J Emerg Med* 2000;**18**(4):427–31.

6. Fukuda K, Ichinohe T, Kaneko Y. Is measurement of end-tidal CO2 through a nasal cannula reliable? *Anesth Prog* 1997;**44**(1):23–6.

7. Ornato JP, Shipley JB, Racht EM, et al. Multicenter study of a portable, hand-size, colorimetric end-tidal carbon dioxide detection device. *Ann Emerg Med* 1992;**21**(5):518–23.

8. Caplan R, Benumof JL, Berry FA, Blitt CD. Practice guidelines for management of the difficult airway: an updated report by the American Society of Anesthesiologists Task Force on Management of the Difficult Airway. *Anesthesiology* 2003;**98**(5):1269–77.

9. Mallampati SR, Gatt SP, Giigino LD, et al. A clinical sign to predict difficult tracheal intubation: a prospective study. *Can Anaesth Soc J* 1985;**32**(4):429–34.

10. Samsoon GL, Young JR. Difficult tracheal intubation: a retrospective study. *Anaesthesia* 1987;**42**(5):487–90.

11. Murphy MF. The difficult and failed airway. Walls RM (ed.), *Manual of Emergency Airway Management*. Chicago, IL: Lipincott, Williams and Wilkins, 2000: pp. 31–9.

12. Reed MJ, Dunn MJ, McKeown DW. Can an airway assessment score predict difficulty at intubation in the emergency department? *Emerg Med J* 2005;**22**(2):99–102.

13. Sunanda G, Sharma R, Jain D. Airway assesment: predictors of difficult airway. *Indian J Anaesth* 2005;**49**(4):257–62.

14. Sagarin MJ, Barton ED, Chng YM, et al. Airway management by US and Canadian emergency medicine residents: a multicenter analysis of more than 6000 endotracheal intubation attempts. *Ann Emerg Med* 2005;**46**(4):328–36.

15. Mace SE. Challenges and advances in intubation: rapid sequence intubation. *Emerg Med Clin North Am* 2008;**26**(4):1043–68.

16. Snider DD, Clarke D, Finucane BT. The "BURP" maneuver worsens the glottic view when applied in combination with cricoid pressure. *Can J Anaesth* 2005;**52**(1):100–4.

17. Takahata O, Kubota M, Mamiya K, et al. The efficacy of the "BURP" maneuver during a difficult laryngoscopy. *Anesth Analg* 1997;**84**(2):419–21.

18. Ely EW, Truman B, Shintani A, et al. Monitoring sedation status over time in ICU patients: reliability and validity of the Richmond Agitation-Sedation Scale (RASS). *JAMA* 2003;**289**(22):2983–91.

19. Sessler CN, Gosnell MS, Grap MJ, et al. The Richmond Agitation-Sedation Scale: validity and reliability in adult intensive care unit patients. *Am J Respir Crit Care Med* 2002;**166**(10):1338–44.

20. Stiell IG, Nesbitt L, Pickett W, et al. The OPALS Major Trauma Study: impact of advanced life-support on survival and morbidity. *CMAJ* 2008;**178**(9):1141–52.

21. Bernard SA. Paramedic intubation of patients with severe head injury: a review of current Australian practice and recommendations for change. *Emerg Med Australas* 2006;**18**(3):221–8.

22. Davis DP, Douglas DJ, Koenig W, et al. Hyperventilation following aero-medical rapid sequence intubation may be a deliberate response to hypoxemia. *Resuscitation* 2007;**73**(3):354–61.

23. Davis DP, Fakhry SM, Wang HE, et al. Paramedic rapid sequence intubation for severe traumatic brain injury: perspectives from an expert panel. *Prehosp Emerg Care* 2007;**11**(1):1–8.

24. Davis DP, Peay J, Sise MJ, et al. The impact of prehospital endotracheal intubation on outcome in moderate to severe traumatic brain injury. *J Trauma* 2005;**58**(5):933–9.

Head trauma

Livia Santiago-Rosado, Matthew Simons, and Andy Jagoda

Definitions

Head trauma (*or head injury*) includes the full spectrum of injury to the head, from superficial contusions, abrasions, and lacerations of the soft tissues that overlie the cranium, to injuries deep within the skull. The vast majority of patients who present to the emergency department (ED) with head trauma have blunt trauma or closed head injury, which is the focus of this chapter.

A *traumatic brain injury* (TBI) implies disruption of brain tissue as a result of a blunt directional or rotational shearing force on the brain. Although the presence of obvious signs of trauma above the clavicles may be associated with intracranial injury, patients who sustain a TBI may not have external signs of trauma.[1] In addition, while some patients with severe TBI have a depressed mental status, the majority of patients with TBI have less severe injuries with an intact or minimally altered mental status and no neurologic deficit.

In 1974, Teasdale and Jennett developed the Glasgow Coma Scale (GCS) as a surrogate measurement of mental status.[2] The original score was developed for use in adults, but was subsequently amended to include children and infants (Table 6.1).[2–4] The main utility of the GCS lies in its application over time, as it helps to document improvement or deterioration. A key concept is that a single GCS score in the field or in the ED has limited diagnostic or prognostic value.

The vast majority of injured patients fall into the *mild traumatic brain injury* (MTBI) category, i.e., a GCS score of 13–15. Patients with MTBI at increased risk for sequelae include the elderly, as well as any patient having had blunt head injury resulting in either loss of consciousness (LOC) < 30 minutes, post-traumatic amnesia (PTA) lasting < 24 hours,

or confusion. However, these characteristics fail to identify all patients at risk for significant acute injury or for developing sequelae.

Epidemiology

An estimated 1.5 million people seek medical care for TBI annually in the United States. Approximately 1.6% of ED visits are for a head injury; up to 90% of these are for MTBI.[5,6] Traumatic brain injury is responsible for up to 235 000 hospital admissions and 50 000 deaths per year, totaling one third to one half of all trauma-related deaths.[7] Risk factors for intracranial injury include male sex, increasing age, and alcohol intoxication.[8] There is a 2 : 1 male to female preponderance; in elderly patients and infants, the difference is slightly less marked, presumably because the factors that influence head trauma in those populations affect both sexes equally.[9]

The most common causes of head trauma in the United States are motor vehicle collisions, falls, and assaults. The relative incidence of specific causes varies according to geographic setting – urban vs. rural – and population issues, including age and socioeconomic status. Children and the elderly are more frequently victims of falls, whereas assault is a common cause of head trauma among males in urban environments. The rate of hospitalization according to age has a trimodal distribution: children under 4 years of age; young adults aged 15–24 (strongly male predominant); and elderly patients aged over 75.[9]

Approximately 5–10% of patients with MTBI will have an abnormal head computed tomography (CT) scan, but only 0.5–1.0% will require acute neurosurgical intervention for intracranial injury.[5] Head injured patients with an abnormal GCS score, even mildly abnormal, have significantly higher rates of

Trauma: A Comprehensive Emergency Medicine Approach, eds. Eric Legome and Lee W. Shockley. Published by Cambridge University Press. © Cambridge University Press 2011.

Table 6.1 The Glasgow Coma Scale (GCS)[2,3]

Score*	Adult	Children aged 1–5	Infants
Best eye response			
1	No eye opening	No eye opening	No eye opening
2	Eye opening to pain	Eye opening to pain	Eye opening to pain
3	Eye opening to voice	Eye opening to voice	Eye opening to voice
4	Eyes open spontaneously	Eyes open spontaneously	Eyes open spontaneously
Best verbal response[†4]			
1	No response	No response	No response
2	Incomprehensible sounds	Incomprehensible, restless, unaware	Moans to pain
3	Inappropriate words	Inappropriate words, inconsolable, unaware	Cries to pain
4	Confused	Disoriented, consolable, aware	Irritable cry
5	Oriented	Oriented, social, interactive	Coos, babbles
Best motor response			
1	No response	No response	No response
2	Decerebrate posturing	Decerebrate posturing	Decerebrate posturing
3	Decorticate posturing	Decorticate posturing	Decorticate posturing
4	Withdraws from pain	Withdraws from pain	Withdraws from pain
5	Localizes pain	Localizes pain	Withdraws to touch
6	Follows commands	Normal spontaneous movement	Normal spontaneous movement

*Note that lowest possible combined score is 3; highest is 15.
†Since intubated patients cannot be evaluated for the verbal component, a "Derived Verbal Score" was elucidated via linear regression analysis using the motor and eye components.[4]
Derived Verbal Score = $-0.3756 + [\text{Motor Score} \times (0.5713)] + [\text{Eye Score} \times (0.4233)]$.
By definition: mild traumatic brain injury (TBI) = GCS score 13–15; moderate TBI = GCS score 9–12; severe TBI = GCS score 3–8.

intracranial injury than patients with a GCS of 15.[10] In one illustrative study, the rate of neurosurgical intervention among patients with a GCS of 13 was 1.3%, and the rate of positive CT findings about 20%. In contrast, in patients with a normal GCS score of 15 the rates were 0.4% and 5.5%, respectively.[6] In another review, the respective percentages of CT abnormalities were 38%, 24%, and 13% for GCS scores of 13, 14, and 15, respectively.[11]

Between 1980 and 1995, there was a 50% reduction in hospitalization and a 22% decline in the number of deaths secondary to TBI. During that same period, there was a 29% reduction in hospitalization for all causes. It is plausible that the proportionally greater reduction in TBI may be due to the success of preventive measures as well as to the increase in use of CT brain imaging to exclude significant intracranial injury, thus obviating the need to admit these patients for observation.[12] While injury to the central nervous system (CNS) is a common cause of death and disability, injuries to the head often do not occur in isolation; cervical spine injuries are the most significant associated injuries, while extremity injuries are the most common.[13]

Anatomy

The scalp is composed of five layers: skin, subcutaneous tissue, galea, areolar tissue, and pericranium. The dermis of the scalp contains a rich blood supply, which if disrupted can result in large hemorrhage as the blood vessels there are unable to fully constrict in response to laceration. The galea is the tough fascial layer which contains the occipitofrontalis and temporoparietalis muscles. The areolar tissue lies under the galea, and it is comprised of loose tissue

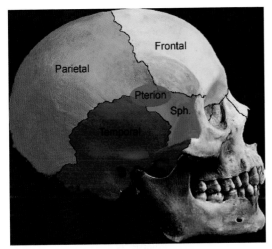

Figure 6.1 The weakest part of the skull, the pterion lies at the junction of the multiple bones and overlies the middle meningeal artery. Injury to this area may cause epidural hematomas. Sph., sphenoid.

attachments, allowing for the formation and spread of large hematomas, as well as tissue avulsion. The areolar tissue lies above the pericranium, which adheres to the skull.

The skull is comprised of eight fused bones which are composed of solid inner and outer layers surrounding a layer of cancellous bone. This structure lends added rigidity and strength to the bone. The thinnest areas of the skull are at the pterions, where the temporal, parietal, sphenoid, and frontal bones join (Figure 6.1). Fractures in this area may result in epidural hematoma by laceration of the underlying middle meningeal artery.

The brain occupies 80% of the volume of the skull, and is divided by the *dura mater*, which adheres to the inner lining of the skull, and its intracranial reflections. The *falx cerebri* separates the two cerebral hemispheres sagittally, and the *tentorium cerebelli* transversely separates the cerebellum and brainstem from the cerebrum. Both of the attachments are fixed, and herniation most frequently occurs when the uncus herniates along the inner edge of the *tentorium cerebelli*. The dura also separates into two layers to form the dural venous sinuses which drain blood and cerebrospinal fluid (CSF) from the brain. The *arachnoid mater* lies underneath the dura, and perforates the dura at the venous sinuses to filter and drain CSF through the arachnoid granulations. The *pia mater* is a thin innermost layer that lies on the surface of the brain.

Between the arachnoid mater and the pia mater is the *subarachnoid space*, in which circulates the CSF. Cerebrospinal fluid is produced by the choroid plexuses located in the lateral ventricles. Approximately 500 ml of CSF is produced per 24 hours. The four ventricles within the brain are the two lateral ventricles, and the midline third and fourth ventricles. The CSF drains from the lateral ventricles to the third ventricle via the foramen of Monroe, and from the third ventricle to the fourth ventricle via the aqueduct of Sylvius. The CSF exits the fourth ventricle into the subarachnoid space via the foramina of Luschka and Magendie.

Pathophysiology

Primary head injuries refer to the damage directly related to a traumatic event, such as fractures, lacerations, or hematomas. *Secondary injury* refers to the damage incurred as a result of subsequent ischemia, edema, or inflammation. Secondary injury contributes greatly to overall morbidity and mortality in TBI, and ED management of these patients is aimed at mitigating these events.

Injury to the brain parenchyma occurs when sudden deceleration or rotational forces cause shearing of small blood vessels and axons. Injuries to the blood vessels cause the development of hematomas. Small intraparenchymal vessel damage results in petechial bleeds. Disruption of bridging veins or arterial injury results in subdural or epidural hematomas, respectively.

Diffuse axonal injury (DAI) refers to a pattern of injury associated with disruption of axonal transport, which results in swelling and Wallerian degeneration. Subsequent release of excitatory amino acids and generation of oxygen radicals then perpetuate secondary neuronal injury.

Epidural hematomas (Figure 6.2) are the result of arterial injury, commonly to the middle meningeal artery, as a result of direct compressive forces. Since they involve arterial disruption, these can bleed rapidly and may result in a rapid deterioration of the patient's neurological status, classically following a "lucid interval." Epidural bleeds can precipitate herniation, and emergent evacuation of the hematoma is frequently indicated, either in the operating room (OR) by neurosurgery or by burr hole in the ED if the OR is unavailable. Injuries due to direct force, including epidural hematomas and skull fractures,

55

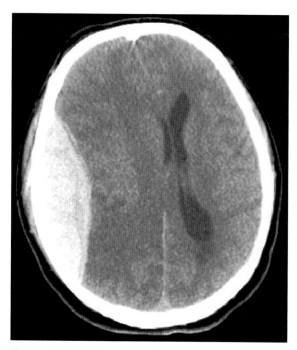

Figure 6.2 Epidural hematomas form as a result of trauma to an artery, commonly the middle meningeal artery, and thus can expand rapidly. Classically, the hyperdense acute blood appears as a lens-shaped or lenticular lesion adjacent to the cranium, with associated brain edema.

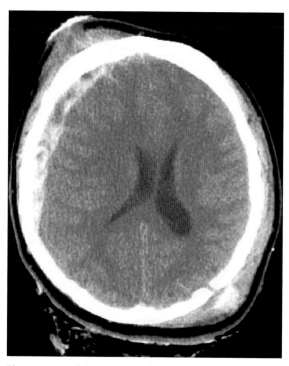

Figure 6.3 A subdural hematoma may result when bridging veins between the cerebral cortex and dural sinuses are stretched and torn. The hematoma is a crescent-shaped hyperdense lesion adjacent to the cortex, with varying degrees of edema in the surrounding brain tissue.

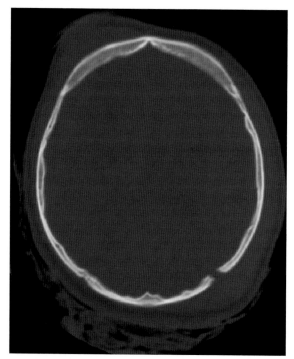

Figure 6.4 Bone windows are useful for highlighting skull fractures that may occur with concomitant brain injury.

are sometimes referred to as "coup" injuries. These are in contrast to "contracoup" injuries, which occur when the brain is set in motion and strikes the opposite inner surface of the skull, causing rapid deceleration.

Subdural hematomas (Figure 6.3) occur when the bridging veins from the cortex to the dura become disrupted. Typically, these venous bleeds progress more slowly than epidural bleeds, which are arterial. Large subdural hematomas can still produce severe neurological deterioration and may require emergent neurosurgical intervention. Figure 6.4 highlights an associated skull fracture.

Subarachnoid hemorrhage, or SAH, consists of bleeding in the subarachnoid space and can occur either in isolation or in combination with other intra-cranial bleeds.

Intracerebral hematomas are caused by disruption of the small intraparenchymal vessels secondary to shearing forces (Figure 6.5). Like patients presenting with subdural hematomas, these patients may exhibit a slow decline in neurologic state, or possibly

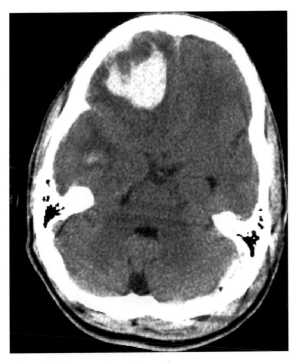

Figure 6.5 Intraparenchymal hemorrhage.

Table 6.2 Common intracranial injuries

Structure	Common injury
Scalp	Lacerations, contusions
Skull	Fractures: linear, depressed
Dura	Epidural hematoma
Bridging veins	Subdural hematoma
Subarachnoid space	Subarachnoid hemorrhage
Brain parenchyma	Parenchymal bleed, herniation
White matter	Diffuse axonal injury (DAI)
Gray matter	Diffuse axonal injury (DAI)

no focal neurological signs whatsoever. Management of these bleeds depends on their location and size, as well as on the patient's clinical neurological status.

Cerebral herniation occurs as the result of critical elevations of intracranial pressure (ICP), either due to cerebral swelling or mass effect secondary to hematoma formation. Signs of herniation include fixation or dilation of one or both pupils, rapid deterioration in GCS, and decerebrate (extensor) posturing. The classic sign of a unilateral fixed, dilated pupil (Hutchinson's pupil) occurs when herniation of the uncus of the hippocampal gyrus compresses the outer parasympathetic fibers of the ipsilateral third cranial nerve, and may be associated with a contralateral hemiparesis. Kernohan's phenomenon occurs in a small percentage of patients, in which a notch on the contralateral cerebral peduncle (Kernohan's notch) is formed when the peduncle is pressed against the tentorium, resulting in a hemiparesis ipsilateral to the dilated pupil. Bilaterally fixed and dilated pupils are suggestive of brainstem injury. It should be noted, however, that hypotension or hypoxia may also produce the same finding and thus the patient should be aggressively resuscitated.

The *Cushing reflex* is defined as systemic hypertension and bradycardia that occurs as a reflex in response to increased ICP. It is generally regarded as a sign that the ICP has risen to a critical level.

Common types of intracranial injuries and affected structures are summarized in Table 6.2.

Cerebral hemodynamics

Cerebral blood flow (CBF) is maintained by cerebral autoregulation in response to physiologic conditions and metabolic rate. Regional CBF is held constant when the mean arterial pressure (MAP) is between 60 and 150 mmHg. Cerebral arteries constrict in response to hypocapnia, hypertension, and alkalosis and dilate from the opposite conditions.

Vascular response in relation to carbon dioxide is linear between PCO_2 levels of 20–60 mmHg.[14] Below 20 mmHg, vasoconstriction may accelerate and contribute to cerebral hypoxia or ischemia.[15] Vasoconstriction in response to hypocapnia is also subject to desensitization over time, and in the setting of prolonged hyperventilation-induced hypocapnia, injured vessels may become dilated, increasing swelling and ICP.[16]

Cerebral perfusion pressure (CPP) is defined as MAP minus ICP (Box 6.1). It is this pressure gradient that drives CBF, and is therefore the integral variable related to cerebral ischemia. In the setting of acute TBI, CBF is often decreased as a result of cerebral vasospasm and possibly lower perfusion pressures as a result of systemic hypotension. For this reason, clinical interventions after TBI are aimed at enhancing CPP to avoid cerebral ischemia. A CPP of 50 mmHg or lower has been associated with cerebral hypoxia and increased morbidity and mortality. Current guidelines suggest that maintenance of CPP above 60 mmHg is associated with improved outcomes in the TBI patient.[17]

Box 6.1 Essentials of cerebral hemodynamics
- $CPP = MAP - ICP$
- Goal $SBP > 90$
- Goal $ICP < 20$; mental status changes occur with $ICP \geq 20$
- Goal $CPP > 60$

Prehospital

Prehospital providers are often the vital link between the injury and definitive care. They are responsible for initiating interventions which can minimize mortality and morbidity. In a study from Colorado, the incidence of TBI was higher in rural than in urban populations and the mortality of rural patients was higher.[18] These findings are supported by similar results in an Australian study.[19] The mortality associated with TBI sustained in rural settings is partially due to delayed access to definitive care, but also emphasizes the pivotal role prehospital providers play.

Recognizing the importance of prehospital care of TBI patients, the US government provided a grant to the Brain Trauma Foundation (BTF) to develop guidelines to assist prehospital care providers in assessing and managing the TBI patient (Figure 6.6). First published in 1998 and disseminated through a national education initiative, the guidelines were revised in 2007.[17]

Prehospital assessment

On the initial encounter, it is seldom possible to accurately determine the degree of brain injury. In patients who appear to have sustained a minor blunt head injury, the only historical parameters proven useful in identifying patients with lesions requiring neurosurgical intervention are LOC and amnesia.[20] The presence of either of these findings prompts the need for careful serial examinations and consideration for transport to a hospital with neurosurgical capabilities. Although the mechanism of injury may direct additional inquiries, there is no evidence that mechanism alone is predictive of an intracranial injury in blunt head trauma.[21] Patients with a history of a penetrating injury, or the potential for a penetrating injury such as a gunshot to the scalp, deserve special attention and should be transported directly to a trauma center even if the injury appears inconsequential.[22] A history of alcohol use, anticoagulant therapy, hemophilia, or age over 60 years should prompt consideration of transport to a trauma center.

The patient should be examined for open wounds, blood from the external auditory canal, and clear or bloody nasal or ear drainage, concerning for CSF rhinorrhea and otorrhea. All patients require a minimum assessment of: (1) blood pressure; (2) oxygenation; (3) pupils; and (4) GCS score.

The Traumatic Data Coma Bank (TDCB) provides the best scientific evidence in which hypotension was defined as a single observation of a systolic blood pressure (SBP) < 90 mmHg, and hypoxemia defined as apnea, cyanosis, or a hemoglobin oxygen saturation $< 90\%$ in the field.[23] The TDCB found that hypotension and hypoxemia were predictors of a poor outcome independent of other major predictors, such as age, GCS score, intracranial diagnosis, and pupillary status. A single episode of hypotension was associated with a doubling of mortality and an increased morbidity when compared with a matched group of patients without hypotension.

The pupillary examination consists of determining pupil size, symmetry, and reactivity to light. Hypoxemia, hypotension, and hypothermia may cause dilated pupil size and abnormal reactivity, making it necessary to resuscitate and stabilize the patient before accurate pupillary assessment can occur.[24] Serial evaluation of the pupils during transport remains a standard, although unproven, assessment parameter in that signs of intracranial hypertension may prompt temporizing interventions to lower ICP.

The key to employing the GCS is in serial determinations. In one of the original multicenter studies validating the scale, approximately 13% of patients who ultimately were in coma had an initial GCS of 15.[25] A single GCS determination is of little utility.

Box 6.2 Essentials of the prehospital management of head injured patients
- Hypoxemia and hypotension are predictors of outcome in TBI patients and thus should be carefully monitored and treated appropriately.
- A single GCS score determination has low predictive value and thus the GCS must be repeated serially.
- Clinical signs of increased ICP include dilated fixed pupil(s) or posturing.
- Patients with moderate or severe TBI should be transported to a hospital with neurosurgical monitoring capabilities.

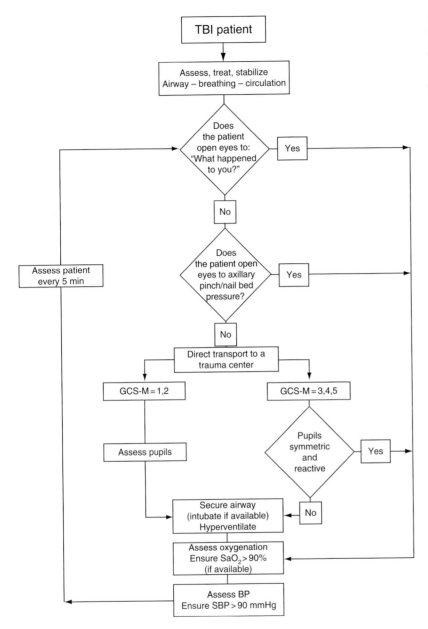

Figure 6.6 Algorithm for the prehospital management of traumatic brain injury (TBI). BP, blood pressure; GCS-M, Glasgow Coma Scale Motor Score; SBP, systolic blood pressure; M, molar score. (Courtesy of the Brain Trauma Foundation.)

Prehospital management

The prehospital management of the TBI patient focuses on stabilizing and maintaining oxygenation and blood pressure. All head injured patients have potential cervical injury and should be immobilized if there is cervical tenderness or pain, a neurologic deficit, altered mental status, or distracting injuries.[26] Anticipate and prepare for potential eventualities such as vomiting, seizures, and aberrations of blood pressure or oxygenation. Consideration should be given to intravenous (IV) access, and to pulse oximetry, blood pressure, and cardiac monitoring.

Indications for a field intubation include failure to protect the airway, failure to ventilate, or failure to oxygenate despite supplemental oxygen administration. It is reasonable to consider proactively securing the airway if it is anticipated that one of the above may occur during transport. In one retrospective case-controlled study of 1092 patients with severe TBI, the outcome of patients endotracheally intubated in the field was compared to patients who were not intubated.[27] Paramedics intubated only if patients were apneic, unconscious with ineffective ventilation, and had no gag reflex. The study suggested that prehospital endotracheal intubation significantly improved survival in select patients. More controversial is the question whether paramedics should use rapid sequence intubation (RSI) for securing the airway in TBI patients who are able to oxygenate but who either have a decreased gag or who have the potential for deterioration during transport. Investigators in San Diego conducted a prospective observational case controlled study involving 209 suspected TBI patients and 627 matched controls.[28] The authors found that the patients who underwent RSI had a higher mortality rate and worse neurologic outcomes than patients who did not undergo intubation. A subsequent study by the same investigators on 59 intubated TBI patients found that low end-tidal carbon dioxide ($ETCO_2$) in intubated patients (inadvertent hyperventilation) was correlated with increased mortality.[29] In addition to hyperventilation, studies have found a not insignificant rate of inadvertent esophageal intubation in the prehospital setting, with concomitant worse outcomes.[30] Based on these findings, current prehospital airway recommendations caution against RSI in the field (Box 6.3).

Box 6.3 **Recommendations for the prehospital airway management[17]**

- An airway should be established in patients who have severe TBI, the inability to maintain an adequate airway, or hypoxemia not corrected by supplemental oxygen by the most appropriate means available.
- Emergency medical service systems implementing endotracheal intubation protocols including the use of RSI should monitor blood pressure, oxygenation, and $ETCO_2$.
- In ground-transported patients in urban environments, the routine use of paralytics to assist endotracheal intubation in patients who are spontaneously breathing and maintaining oxygen saturation above 90% on supplemental oxygen is not recommended.
- Hyperventilation ($ETCO_2$ < 30–35) should be avoided unless the patient shows signs of herniation and corrected immediately when identified.*

*While not required, $ETCO_2$ is the preferred method of monitoring CO_2 in the field.

Hypotension is another critical factor associated with an increased morbidity and mortality in head injured patients. Generally, isotonic IV crystalloid administration has been the mainstay of prehospital treatment of hypotension. Vassar et al.[31] reported that the prehospital administration of hypertonic (7.5%) saline to a subgroup of severely head injured patients resulted in improved outcomes. However, a well-designed randomized double-blind prehospital study comparing hypertonic saline to lactated Ringer's found no survival benefit in severely head injured patients.[32] At the present time whether there is a role for hypertonic saline is unclear and in need of additional study.

The signs of cerebral herniation include a dilated, fixed pupil(s), posturing, or a decrease in the GCS score by two or more points. Hyperventilation can decrease ICP by inducing vasoconstriction and is the recommended first-line intervention for the field management of patients demonstrating signs of intracranial hypertension. Since capnography is generally unavailable in the prehospital setting, a rough guideline is to give 18–20 breaths/min when the patient shows any of the above signs. Hyperventilation is discontinued when the signs of herniation resolve or when other ICP treatment modalities are available.

Mannitol does not have a role in the field management of patients with brain injury and increased ICP. While concern exists that it may cause hypovolemic hypotension, one pilot study demonstrated that mannitol does not cause hypotension when given in the field.[33] However, with no outcome data and theoretical harm, its use is not recommended.

A potential pitfall in the management of the head injury patient is to assume that trauma is entirely responsible for altered mental status. Consideration must be given to the reversible causes of altered mental status that include hypoglycemia, hypoxemia, hypotension, hypothermia, infection, and drug toxicity. At least one case series highlighted problems of unrecognized hypoglycemia in trauma patients and emphasized the importance of a comprehensive approach to patient care.[34]

Severely head injured patients can experience episodes of agitation and combativeness, both of which tend to increase ICP. Therefore, as first line treatment for these patients, analgesics and sedatives should be considered. These medications should have a short duration of action. Narcotic analgesics, such as fentanyl, or a benzodiazepine, such as midazolam, are typically used. The GCS score should be determined before these agents are given. Although haloperidol is commonly used to control agitation in ED patients, in the head injured population there are arguments, based on theory, against it. However, there are no conclusive data to argue for or against its use.

Box 6.4 Essentials of the prehospital management of head injured patients

- Hypoxemia and hypotension are predictors of poor outcome in TBI patients and thus should be carefully monitored and treated appropriately.
- A single GCS score determination has low predictive value and thus the GCS must be repeated serially.
- Clinical signs of increased ICP include dilated fixed pupil(s) or posturing.
- Patients with moderate or severe TBI should be transported to a hospital with neurosurgical monitoring capabilities.

Emergency department evaluation and management

The first few minutes

The initial evaluation of the head injured patient is the same as for all trauma patients. Evaluate and stabilize with particular attention to the ABCs and cervical spine. Because the consequences of ventilatory and circulatory failure are dismal in the setting of TBI, early intervention to ensure adequate oxygenation and perfusion are crucial.[35] In cases of altered mental status, it is imperative to maintain a broad differential diagnosis so as to avoid missing concomitant medical issues, including intoxication and hypoglycemia. Patients presenting with altered mental status require a stat serum glucose determination, core temperature, and oxygen saturation determination. In select patients where an opioid toxidrome is suspected, judicious naloxone administration may be considered as a diagnostic agent.

If endotracheal intubation is necessary by traditional parameters or due to an inability to control a combative patient with a high suspicion of intracranial injury, the principles of RSI apply. Preoxygenation minimizes the risk of hypoxia during intubation while pretreatment medications minimize changes in ICP during the procedure. Patients may be pretreated with fentanyl and lidocaine in order to blunt the ICP response to laryngoscopy; a non-depolarizing paralytic can also be used adjunctively. Given the lack of proven clear benefit, however, this should be considered an option only when time is available. Following pretreatment, induction and paralysis are performed. Ideally, patients should have continuous capnography post-intubation to prevent inadvertent hyper- or hypoventilation. Cervical spine precautions should be maintained at all times.

Ventilatory support in the intubated patient should be dictated by the clinical condition. Typically, all patients should be placed on a ventilator that delivers 100% oxygen in a tidal volume approximately 5–7 cc/kg of ideal patient weight. The respiratory rate is typically set at 14–16 breaths/min. There is evidence that hyperventilation may be deleterious and, if used at all, should be reserved as a temporizing measure for patients exhibiting acute signs of increased ICP.[17]

Cerebral ischemia is likely the most important predictor of poor outcomes following TBI.[36–38] An adequate CPP is critical to minimize the incidence and severity of ischemic events and should be maintained above 60 mmHg.[17] Given that ICP measurements are frequently not available in the ED, steps directed at maintaining an adequate systemic blood pressure (and MAP) are crucial in preventing reductions in CPP. Even a single episode of hypotension results in a 150% relative increase in mortality.[23] The most likely causes of hypotension in the patient with TBI are due to extracranial trauma.[39] Less likely, hypotension and shock may be neurogenic secondary to concomitant spinal cord injury.

Patients at risk of compromised perfusion will require IV access and monitoring. Intravenous fluid, either normal saline or lactated Ringer's, is used for the resuscitation of head injured patients. Studies have suggested that a 250 ml bolus of hypertonic saline (HTS) as an initial resuscitation fluid is more effective in raising blood pressure when compared to normal saline and may reduce overall fluid requirements.[40] In cases of hypotension refractory to fluid resuscitation, pressors may be indicated to maintain adequate CPP. If pressors are required, limited data suggest that norepinephrine may be more predictable in maintaining an adequate CPP than dopamine.[41] Since the ICP is seldom known in the ED, one reasonable option is to use a SBP of > 90–100 mmHg as a target. While never specifically studied, keeping the systemic pressure low in cases of "hypotensive resuscitation" or "permissive hypotension" may potentially result in detriment to the injured brain.

Once the ABCs have been addressed, the patient is assessed for gross neurologic disability including mental status, pupillary response, motor function, and GCS. Pupil size and response should be assessed and followed; a unilateral fixed and dilated pupil in an obtunded patient should prompt identification and aggressive management of a presumed brain herniation. Bilateral fixed, dilated pupils may indicate brainstem injury. Motor response should be evaluated in all four extremities; look for evidence of decreased response or asymmetry in the setting of noxious stimuli. Decorticate posturing involves abnormal flexion of the upper extremities associated with extension of the lower extremities. It is present when there is damage to the corticospinal tracts but implies an intact brainstem. Decerebrate posturing is more ominous, and involves extension of the upper and lower extremities as well as arching of the neck. Decerebrate posturing is frequently a sign of intracranial hypertension and portends a poor prognosis, as it is often caused by acute uncal herniation compressing the brainstem.

The history

History-taking should never preclude or delay active stabilization, but should occur concurrently. Evidence of amnesia and LOC should be queried. One difficulty with this question is that it is frequently unwitnessed, poorly defined, and defined differently in relevant literature depending on the study. Corroboration and additional history may be obtained from witnesses, relatives, and paramedics. While mechanism is poorly predictive of injury, trauma sustained from greater force or deceleration should raise more suspicion for significant injury and deterioration than low-velocity, low-impact trauma.

Age is an important factor in head trauma. The extremes of age are particularly worrisome, as they are at higher risk for significant injury. Elderly patients are at risk for significant TBI because the age-related atrophy of their brains results in the stretching and possible rupture of bridging with subsequent subdural hematomas. Infants, on the other hand, are at risk for significant TBI due to a thinner skull and open cranial fontanelles.

It is helpful to find out about the patient's medical history and medications. Medical conditions, such as seizure disorder or heart disease, may predispose patients to traumatic events. In addition, conditions associated with impaired coagulation, including hemophilia, advanced liver disease, and anticoagulant use, require special consideration. Due to their coagulopathy, these patients are at risk of significant morbidity from what may otherwise be a relatively harmless minor trauma. Certain medications may predispose patients to trauma. Elderly patients are particularly susceptible to the effects of medications that may cause dizziness or sedation. Polypharmacy creates additional risk due to medication interactions and synergistic effects.

Where obtainable, a social history should be sought. Ingestion of intoxicants, both acutely and chronically, may predispose the patient to injury, and may be contributing to an altered mental status. Interpersonal violence including domestic violence, elder and child abuse may be difficult to elicit without specific questioning. A history in which the mechanism seems inconsistent with the observed injuries should raise suspicion of the possibility of abuse.

Physical exam

An effort should be made to identify concomitant trauma and evidence of underlying predisposing medical conditions, such as medical alert bracelets, surgical scars, or implanted devices. Any external sign of head trauma should be noted, including hematomas, lacerations, and contusions (Box 6.5). Pupils should be checked for size, shape, symmetry, and reactivity. If feasible, funduscopy should be performed to assess for intraocular pathology, including post-traumatic retinal hemorrhage or detachment. Cranial nerve assessment is performed, paying special attention to extraocular muscle (EOM) function. It is important to note that in studies predicting risk in head injured patients with LOC and MTBI, no specific physical sign has been associated with need for intervention; any sign of "trauma above the clavicles" was an independent risk factor in these patients.[10]

Battle's sign and raccoon eyes are infrequently seen early in the course of the injury, but when present

> **Box 6.5 Signs of skull fracture**
> - Skull depression/step-off
> - Hemotympanum
> - Raccoon eyes (periorbital ecchymosis)
> - Battle's sign (postauricular ecchymosis)
> - Cerebrospinal fluid leak
> - Rhinorrhea
> - Otorrhea
> - Scalp hematoma (especially infants)

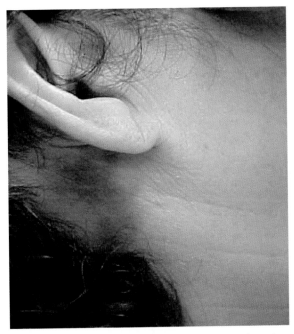

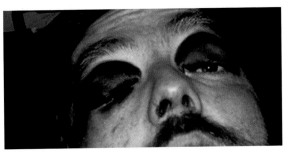

Figure 6.8 Raccoon eyes. Periorbital ecchymosis, unilateral or bilateral, may follow direct trauma to the orbits or basilar skull fracture. (with permission from eMedicine.com, 2007. Available from http://www.emedicine.com/med/topic3221.htm.)

Figure 6.7 Battle's sign. Retroauricular ecchymosis may be a sign of basilar skull fracture. (Courtesy of Immediate Action Services.)

Management: general principles

The initial assessment of the patient and GCS score determination will dictate further testing. The evaluation and management will largely depend on the severity of the injury. An outline of general treatment goals in TBI is given in Box 6.6.

Box 6.6 Basic treatment goals in TBI

- Secure airway
- Prevent ICP rise
- Lower elevated ICP
- Maintain
  - O_2 saturation $> 90\%$
  - SBP > 90 mmHg
  - ICP ≤ 20 mmHg
- Correct hypoglycemia
- Avoid hyperglycemia
- Avoid hyperthermia
- Analgesia
- Wound care
- Prevent seizures

---

should raise suspicion for a basilar fracture (Figures 6.7 and 6.8). The external auditory canals should be examined with an otoscope to look for lacerations, tympanic membrane (TM) rupture, or evidence of CSF otorrhea and hemotympanum. Cerebrospinal fluid otorrhea is a CSF leak due to skull fracture with associated TM rupture. Cerebrospinal fluid rhinorrhea, or nasal leak, may be present if there is violation of the cribriform plate with associated dural disruption. The diagnosis of CSF otorrhea and rhinorrhea may be elusive, as blood and other secretions, including mucus, may mimic CSF. Testing the fluid for glucose may be a way to differentiate CSF from other secretions; normal CSF has a glucose concentration equal to two thirds that of the serum glucose, whereas nasal secretions are essentially glucose-free. The test can be done using a dextrose stick and glucometer. The historical "target sign" elicited by dripping the leaking fluid onto a sheet or other absorbent material, and observing color separation of dark blood in the center and clearer fluid peripherally, is inaccurate.

Finally, a focused neurologic evaluation of the patient should be performed including motor function and gross cerebellar function. The remainder of the clinical evaluation should be directed towards identifying concomitant injuries.

Sedation

Many patients with TBI will have alterations in mental status and violent behavior. Agitated patients are at increased risk for self harm or harm to care providers. In many cases, sedation is indicated to allow for evaluation, stabilization, and diagnostic testing. Sedation is preferentially accomplished via the use of a benzodiazepine or antipsychotic.[42] Etomidate or propofol in low doses may also be used. Ketamine should probably be avoided, as it may cause increased ICP. Many sedative agents, including barbiturates, may cause systemic hypotension, respiratory depression, and airway compromise. The clinician should thus have a low threshold to intubate and take over the airway in patients with head trauma who require sedation. This must be balanced with appropriate clinical decision making, i.e., an agitated or belligerent patient with a low likelihood of intracranial injury should not be subjected to the risks of intubation if not required.

Analgesia

There has been considerable discussion in the literature regarding inadequate analgesia in patients presenting with a complaint of pain.[43] The same appears to hold true in TBI. Bazarian et al. found that only 46% of TBI patients with documented pain received analgesia.[44] As with any painful condition, pain following head trauma should be treated. Acetaminophen may be useful in the treatment of mild headache due to head trauma. There is some theoretical concern regarding treatment with aspirin and non-steroidal anti-inflammatory drugs (NSAIDs) given their propensity to cause bleeding via platelet inhibition. Opioids should be reserved for the treatment of moderate to severe pain. These medications, particularly when administered parenterally, may cause hypotension, respiratory depression, or alteration in mental status. If used, judicious aliquots of parenteral medication with close monitoring is the safest course.

There is no answer or research on the use of oral opioids, e.g., hydrocodone, on the patient who has been clinically or radiographically cleared of intracranial injury. Clinical judgment and local customs tend to predominate.

Glucose control

Data have identified hyperglycemia as a significant secondary insult, portending a poor prognosis. It is unclear if hyperglycemia is more prevalent in patients who have had more severe injuries and is a marker of a severe stress response, or whether the high levels of glucose are causative of increased morbidity.[45] Since hypoglycemia may further complicate the management of the head injured patient, glucose control with a goal of englycemia should be an objective of early stabilization.

Seizure prophylaxis

The incidence of post-traumatic seizure (PTS) following severe TBI is relatively high, ranging between 5 and 35%.[46,47] In general, a higher severity injury increases the chance of developing PTS. Post-traumatic seizure is categorized as occurring early,

within 7 days of head injury, or late, after the 7-day period. Most instances of PTS will occur in the first 24 hours after injury. Both phenytoin and valproate have been found to be comparably effective in reducing the incidence of early PTS, but not late PTS.[46,48–50] While there are insufficient data to show that the prevention of early PTS improves overall outcomes, it is reasonable to assume that seizures may result in immediate adverse effects, which have the potential to exacerbate secondary brain injury.

For most patients, seizure prophylaxis is unnecessary. However, injuries involving the dura and intracranial hemorrhages are considered high risk for developing PTS. Penetrating head injuries carry particular risk. It is recommended that either phenytoin or valproate be used prophylactically for the first week following a high-risk TBI. There is no indication to continue seizure prophylaxis beyond the first 7 days, unless the patient has recurrent late seizures.[17]

Blood pressure management

There is a significant body of literature delineating the risks of hypotension in head trauma. There is also some evidence that there may be a role in controlling hypertension in the management of spontaneous intracranial hemorrhage.[51] In the setting of traumatic intracranial hemorrhage, on the other hand, there is no benefit to aggressive management of hypertension. In fact, because the autoregulatory mechanisms that maintain cerebral blood flow are altered in head trauma, lowering the blood pressure may cause acute decreases in CPP. Thus, hypertension in the head injured patient should not be acutely lowered. When systemic hypertension is associated with bradycardia, the cause may be intracranial hypertension, via Cushing's reflex; the ICP should be aggressively treated, not the systemic pressure.[52]

Wound care

General wound care principles apply in the TBI population. Any bleeding should be controlled; direct pressure will suffice in most cases. Since larger scalp vessels do not retract after being lacerated, blood loss may be significant.[53] Occasionally, injuries to these vessels require surgical intervention, such as deep sutures or ligation, to halt bleeding. Abrasions, lacerations, and avulsions should be examined for the presence of foreign bodies. External wounds should be debrided, cleaned, and, if contaminated, irrigated copiously. Following cleansing and irrigation, abrasions can be dressed with sterile gauze following application of a topical antibiotic ointment. Lacerations and avulsions may lend themselves to closure, discussed below. Some patients will present with hematomas and ecchymoses without associated skin breaks. These resolve spontaneously via resorption. Ice may be useful in decreasing associated swelling. Tetanus status should be checked and immunization provided when indicated.

Laceration repair

Patients with head trauma may sustain avulsions and lacerations to the scalp or face. As always, care of these injuries starts with meticulous cleansing. A local anesthetic such as lidocaine should be used to allow for a careful deep examination, debridement, and closure, if appropriate. Preparations containing epinephrine are useful in the well-vascularized scalp and face and are recommended if no contraindications to their use exist. Routine shaving prior to closure is not recommended; eyebrows should never be shaved. When a scalp laceration is present, it should be carefully examined for violation of the galea, the layer of fibrous tissue surrounding the skull. If the galea is torn, it should be repaired using non-absorbable sutures to prevent the formation of a subgaleal hematoma, which can in turn become infected. The scalp can then be closed using sutures or staples. It should be noted that staples, due to their metallic composition, may create artifact on CT. If a patient is to undergo CT scanning, it may be advisable to delay staple closure until the initial CT has been performed. Staples should never be used on the face. Simple interrupted sutures using a thin nylon suture (preferably 6–0) is preferred for facial lacerations. Deep sutures may also be placed if necessary to better appose deeper tissues. Synthetic absorbable sutures made primarily of polyglycolic acid (e.g., Vicryl® or Dexon®) and catgut sutures are both acceptable for this purpose. Additionally, some evidence supports the use of rapidly absorbable external sutures for the face. Finally, superficial, linear lacerations on the face and scalp may be appropriate for closure with a cyanoacrylate adhesive.

Antibiotics

Due to the vascularity of the scalp and face, superficial injuries to these areas infrequently become infected and generally do not benefit from prophylactic antibiotics. However, some patients may benefit from antibiotic prophylaxis following head trauma. Blunt trauma to the skin or scalp resulting in significant tissue maceration or contamination may warrant antibiotic administration. More importantly, violation of the dura mater with subsequent exposure of intracranial contents to pathogens may predispose the patient to developing meningitis, encephalitis, brain abscess, and other dangerous and potentially lethal infections. When imaging reveals an open skull fracture or fracture into a sinus cavity (e.g., orbital floor fracture with maxillary sinus involvement), especially when there is a CSF leak or penetrating injury, antibiotics are sometimes recommended. There have been no randomized controlled trials to determine when antibiotic prophylaxis is indicated, nor any proof that it is effective.[54] First-generation cephalosporins are the first-line agents used for skin and scalp wound prophylaxis. A broader-spectrum agent such as amoxicillin–clavulanate may be used when the injury causes communication with the sinuses or respiratory passages. Changing bacteriology in the patient population, such as community acquired Methicillin-resistant *Staphylococcus aureus*, may require a different spectrum of antibiotic.

Penetrating injury

Though much less common than blunt head trauma, penetrating trauma to the head, whether caused by projectiles or direct penetration from a stab wound, can have devastating effects. It is almost always associated with intracranial hemorrhage and swelling, as well as intracranial hypertension. Patients with this type of injury should have emergent imaging with non-contrast CT. Some penetrating injuries occur in the context of blunt trauma, such as impaled skull fragments. When any impaled foreign body protrudes from the head it should never be removed in the ED. The effect of the indwelling foreign body may be to tamponade bleeding, and removal outside the controlled environment of the operating room may cause uncontrolled bleeding and rapid deterioration. These injuries are particularly prone to subsequent complications, including infection and seizures. Prophylaxis with antiepileptic medications and antibiotics is recommended in cases of penetrating TBI.[55]

Severe TBI

Patients with a GCS score of 8 or less will invariably require stabilization, including intubation. Prevention of acute increases in ICP is of particular importance. Non-contrast CT of the brain and neurosurgical consultation should be obtained promptly. If the patient presents to a facility without neurosurgical backup, early initiation of patient transfer to a trauma center is advisable. In general, transfer should not be delayed for the purpose of imaging.

Initial stabilization and resuscitation are directed at mitigating hypotension and hypoxemia and managing increased ICP. Intracranial pressure monitoring requires the placement of an invasive catheter into either the patient's brain parenchyma or a lateral ventricle.[17] While it is recommended to guide the care of all salvageable severe TBI patients, ICP monitoring is generally reserved for the intensive care unit (ICU) setting, as it is often not available during ED management. When ICP cannot be directly monitored, therapeutic interventions are based on the presence of clinical signs of increased ICP (Box 6.7).

Box 6.7 Clinical signs of increased ICP

- Unilateral fixed, dilated pupil
- Decrease in GCS greater or equal to 2 points in a patient with severe TBI
- Posturing
- Cushing reflex

One small study suggested that the measurement of intraocular pressure (IOP) with a handheld tonometer accurately detected or ruled out elevated ICP 100% of the time when using a cut-off of 20 cmH$_2$O.[56] Intraocular pressure measurements using handheld tonometry may prove be a useful adjunct to early detection of ICP elevation in these patients when invasive monitoring is not available.

Increased ICP

The early detection and management of increased ICP has been the cornerstone of stabilization of TBI patients. The techniques used to decrease ICP have traditionally included hyperventilation, osmotic agents, barbiturates, and surgical decompression. These modalities have at times been overused, or applied in settings when there is no evidence of increased ICP, possibly with deleterious effects.

Hyperventilation

For many years, hyperventilation was widely used in the management of patients with severe TBI; at times

it was instituted prophylactically without clear signs of increased ICP. Hyperventilation causes a reduction in ICP by lowering PCO_2, which induces cerebral vasoconstriction and results in decreased cerebral blood volume.[57] However, in addition to lowering ICP, vasoconstriction also causes a decreased CBF and therefore carries a high risk of contributing significantly to brain ischemia. For this reason, the use of hyperventilation as a mainstay of treatment is no longer recommended.

Hyperventilation is recommended only as a temporizing measure in the setting of elevated ICP. The BTF[17] recommends that hyperventilation be avoided in the first 24 hours following acute injury, as this is the time period when cerebral perfusion may be critically reduced, and vasoconstriction induced by hyperventilation may worsen cerebral ischemia. Prophylactic hyperventilation in the absence of signs of increased ICP should be avoided.

Osmotic agents

Hyperosmolar agents increase CBF and reduce ICP through both hemodynamic and osmotic mechanisms. First, hyperosmolar fluid administration draws water in from tissues and red blood cells into the plasma, causing plasma expansion and reduced volume and rigidity of red blood cells.[58] This decreases blood viscosity, and though a rheologic effect, results in reduced vascular resistance and increased CBF. The osmotic effect occurs partially through the direct removal of water from the brain parenchyma. This is a delayed effect that depends on the development of an osmotic gradient between the plasma and tissue, and it may take up to 30 minutes to develop.[59] The more immediate rheological effects of these agents may be the primary cause of ICP reduction.

The main osmotherapeutic agent used today is mannitol. Unfortunately, while there are numerous studies that demonstrate beneficial physiologic effects, there is a paucity of clinical studies to show a correlation between the use of mannitol and improved clinical outcomes. It is also worth noting that a rebound phenomenon causing a paradoxical increase of ICP has been associated with the use of osmotic agents, including mannitol.[60]

Despite the widespread use of mannitol as a therapeutic agent in the management of patients with severe TBI, there have been no studies comparing mannitol to placebo in a clinical trial. While many studies have shown that mannitol decreases ICP and increases CBF, the lack of clinical trials makes definitive recommendations on its use and dosage difficult.[61] The BTF recommends the use of mannitol in patients with severe TBI and "signs of transtentorial herniation or progressive neurological deterioration not attributable to extracranial explanations."[17] The BTF guidelines recommend a dose of mannitol ranging from 0.25 to 1.0 g/kg of body weight. However, there have been three recent studies, by the same investigators, that have shown improved neurological outcomes with the use of early, high dose (1.4 g/kg) mannitol in severe TBI when compared with conventional dose mannitol.[62–64] Mannitol boluses should be administered over 15–30 minutes to avoid hypotension, and euvolemia should be maintained by concomitant isotonic fluid replacement.[65] Hypotension (SBP < 90 mmHg) is a relative contraindication to mannitol use.

Hypertonic saline has been shown to reduce ICP in patients with severe TBI, including cases that were refractory to mannitol.[66–69] Like mannitol, it appears to lower ICP through both hemodynamic and osmotic mechanisms. However, HTS is less likely to cross the blood–brain barrier and therefore less likely to result in rebound increases in cerebral edema and ICP.[70] Two studies have suggested that HTS may be superior to mannitol for reducing ICP.[68,69] As with mannitol, however, there is a potential for adverse effects. Infusions of HTS may result in central pontine myelinolysis when administered to patients with pre-existing chronic hyponatremia, and should not be initiated until hyponatremia has been excluded. Hypertonic saline may also precipitate renal failure in hypovolemic patients and pulmonary edema in patients with underlying cardiac or pulmonary problems.[71,72] Hypertonic saline may be used independently or as an adjunct to mannitol to lower ICP.

Barbiturates

High-dose barbiturates have been used to manage elevated ICP in patients with severe TBI. They have several protective mechanisms of action. First, they cause a dose-dependent depression on cerebral metabolism, which via auto-regulation leads to a decreased CBF, thereby reducing cerebral blood volume and ICP. Second, barbiturates increase cerebrovascular tone. Finally, they inhibit free radical mediated lipid peroxidation and inhibit excitotoxicity.[73,74]

Barbiturates also have well-described side effects, the most significant of which is systemic hypotension due to decreased systemic vascular resistance and myocardial depression. The Cochrane Injuries Group released a meta-analysis of three barbiturate trials in 2005 and concluded there was no definitive evidence that barbiturate therapy improves outcome in patients with severe head injury, and that its hypotensive effects negate the benefit of its ICP-lowering properties.[75] Therefore, the use of high-dose barbiturates should only be considered in patients who have refractory elevated ICP despite maximal medical and surgical therapy, and should not be used prophylactically. If barbiturate therapy is initiated, close hemodynamic monitoring, preferably in an ICU setting, is recommended.

Neurosurgical intervention

Some patients with severe TBI will need emergent neurosurgical procedures; involving a neurosurgeon early is prudent. Patients with mild or moderate TBI, but worsening or lateralizing neurologic examinations should receive early consultation. Neurosurgical interventions include ICP monitoring, craniotomy (Figure 6.9), and ventriculostomy. Recent guidelines outline the indications for operative management of specific injuries (Table 6.3).[76]

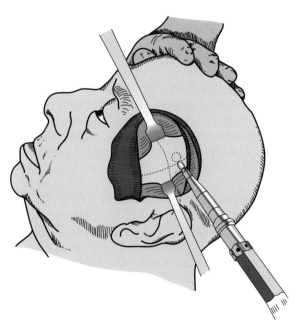

Figure 6.9 Craniotomy. A temporal burr hole is placed two finger breadths anterior to the external auditory meatus and two finger breadths above the zygomatic arch.

Table 6.3 Guidelines for neurosurgical intervention[76]

	Surgical intervention	Non-operative management
Epidural hematoma (EDH)	EDH > 30 cm³ regardless of GCS	EDH < 30 cm³ and < 15 mm thick and < 5 mm shift and GCS > 8 without focal deficit
Subdural hematoma (SDH)	SDH > 10 mm thick or > 5 mm shift	SDH < 10 mm thick and < 5 mm shift; monitor ICP if GCS < 9
Parenchymal lesions	Progressive neurologic deterioration Medically refractory ↑ICP Signs of mass effect on CT	Absence of specific indication for surgery
Cranial fractures	Open fractures Fractures depressed beyond thickness of cranium	Linear, mildly depressed skull fractures

CT, computed tomography; GCS, Glasgow Coma Scale; ICP, intracranial pressure.

Burr holes

In cases where maximal medical management is ineffective and the patient is exhibiting signs of acute uncal herniation, burr-hole placement may be considered. Ideally, this procedure should be performed by a neurosurgeon but, in the case that one is unavailable, the emergency physician may perform the procedure in a life-saving effort. Given the availability of rapid CT scans throughout EDs in the United States, exploratory burr holes are generally not indicated, and placement should be guided by findings on the scan. However, in the case that CT is not available, it should be noted that abnormal pupillary changes occur ipsilateral to hematoma formation in 85% of cases and epidural hematomas occur in the area of the pterion in about 70% of patients.[77]

Three major anatomical areas for burr-hole placement are frontal, temporal, and parietal. The frontal burr hole is made immediately anterior to the coronal suture, 3 cm lateral from the midline, or in the mid-pupillary line. It can also be used for the placement of

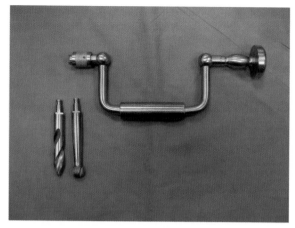

Figure 6.10 Photograph of the Hudson brace drill with perforator and burr bits.

a ventriculostomy catheter. A temporal burr hole is placed two finger breadths anterior to the external auditory meatus and two finger breadths above the zygomatic arch. The parietal burr hole is placed two finger breadths behind the external auditory meatus and three finger breadths above the mastoid process.

Before initiating the procedure, the patient's airway should be secured by endotracheal intubation. After choosing the appropriate location for burr-hole procedure, the scalp should be shaved and prepped. A Hudson brace drill is typically used for burr-hole placement (Figure 6.10).

Moderate TBI

There is a general lack of consensus as to the management of moderate TBI. These patients have a GCS score that ranges from 9 to 12. Clinical presentation and CT findings are varied in this population, as are prognosis and long-term outcomes.[78] In most cases, moderate TBI is treated like severe TBI, as this is a patient population at risk for rapid and severe deterioration. Patients in the moderate TBI category will often require intubation for airway protection and must be imaged with CT scanning as soon as possible. Since neurosurgical intervention may be required, early neurosurgical consultation is optimal. When there is evidence of increased ICP, it must be managed expeditiously to prevent deterioration.

Mild TBI

Patients with MTBI and GCS scores 13–15, are the most diverse and in some ways the most challenging to manage. The vast majority of these patients do well, even those in whom there is evidence of intracranial injury on CT. A significant minority of MTBI patients go on to have neurospsychiatric sequelae, known as the postconcussive syndrome, which may affect their functioning for months or years. It is unclear which MTBI patients will go on to develop these symptoms.

There are a myriad of studies addressing the approach to the MTBI patient, including clinical decision instruments attempting to discern who needs CT, who needs admission, and what follow-up is required.[1,20,79,80] In addition, guidelines have been developed to address concussion in the setting of sport-related injuries, given that these patients tend to have recurrent insults.[11]

Imaging in MTBI

While the history and physical exam are important in the patient presenting with head trauma, they are relatively insensitive in the diagnosis of MTBI. Thus, the emergency physician often must rely on ancillary studies to help guide the treatment. Ideally clinical decision making is geared towards obtaining the highest sensitivity possible, while understanding the cost and risks of obtaining brain CTs.

Skull radiography

Historically plain films of the skull were the cornerstone of imaging prior to wide CT availability. However they are insensitive for intracranial lesions, as the majority of TBI occurs in the absence of skull fractures. Computed tomography has supplanted skull radiographs almost entirely (Figure 6.11). Some authors have touted the use of skull films in the evaluation of pediatric patients, but there seems to be little or no role for this study in adults (see Pediatric considerations, below.) The American College of Emergency Physicians (ACEP) guideline regarding decision making in MTBI concludes that plain skull radiographs in head injured adults are not sufficiently sensitive to be a useful screening test and are therefore not recommended.[81]

Computed head tomography

Non-contrast CT is the modality of choice for imaging the brain after head trauma. Much of the recent literature on MTBI has revolved around the appropriate use of CT in head injured patients. There are two competing goals: to identify all clinically

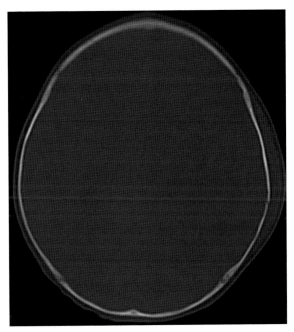

Figure 6.11 Skull fracture CT is the preferred study to identify skull fractures, especially when bone windows are viewed.

significant injuries, and to reduce the number of unnecessary studies. While some authors have argued for liberal CT scanning in MTBI, others have advocated a more selective approach, attempting to derive prediction rules that identify patients in whom CT may be safely obviated.[1,82]

Beginning in the early 1990s, research focused on early CT scanning of all MTBI patients with a history of LOC or PTA. Because they included patients with a GCS of 13–15, based on the definition of MTBI, those studies found a positive CT rate in the range of 13–17%. It has been shown that patients with a GCS score of 13, despite being classified as mild, have a prognosis similar to those with moderate head injury and a GCS of 9–12.[36] In addition, while patients with a GCS of 14 typically do significantly better than those who score 13, they have a much higher rate of positive CT results than those with a GCS of 15. Thus, most authors recommend imaging all patients with an abnormal GCS. The question still remains as to the optimal management of the largest subset of MTBI patients: those presenting with a normal GCS and no focal neurologic signs.

Stiell et al.[1] developed the Canadian CT Head Rule (CCHR) and Haydel et al.[20] published a decision instrument referred to as the New Orleans Criteria

69

(NOC). They both were developed to identify which patients have such a low risk of significant injury that they can safely forgo CT scanning. Table 6.4 compares the NOC and CCHR.

A subgroup analysis was performed by the Canadian group to exclusively study those patients with a GCS of 15. They found that neurosurgical intervention was rare in this group (0.2%) but that potential warning signs included any vomiting, any GCS score decrease within 6 hours of arrival in the hospital, and the presence of severe headache, focal temporal blow, restlessness, or confusion.[83]

In 2002, ACEP published guidelines that address the issue of neuroimaging in MTBI.[81] Because the literature is unclear on which patients deteriorate or are at risk for developing sequelae including the post-concussive syndrome, they chose "presence of acute intracranial injury" as their primary outcome. The conclusion was that head CT is not indicated in the absence of headache, vomiting, age > 60 years, drug or alcohol intoxication, deficits in short-term memory, physical evidence of trauma above the clavicle, and seizure. The absence of all seven risk factors had a negative predictive value of 100%.

In 2005, two studies were published comparing the performance of the CCHR and NOC criteria. Stiell et al.[84] (who had developed the CCHR) performed a prospective cohort study of both rules on patients presenting with a GCS of 15. Both rules had a sensitivity of 100% for the need for neurosurgical intervention and for clinically important brain injury, and the sensitivity for all cases of brain injury, including those termed clinically "unimportant," was 93.1% for CCHR and 98.6% for NOC. They found that the NOC had much lower specificity than CCHR, necessitating a CT rate of 88%, vs. 52% if the CCHR rule was followed.

The second study, by Smits et al.[85] in the Netherlands, found both rules to have a sensitivity of 100% for neurosurgical intervention. However, while the NOC identified 98–99% of any positive finding on CT, the CCHR was 83–87% sensitive. The Dutch group included patients without LOC in their sample; of note, 30% of the patients that required neurosurgical intervention did not report LOC.

Given these results, Smits et al.[6] have gone on to develop their own decision rule. The CT in Head Injury Patients (CHIP) prediction rule was developed for the selective use of CT scanning in a more undifferentiated population. Patients with a GCS of 15 were included if they had *any* of several risk factors

(LOC, PTA, seizure, vomiting, severe headache, evidence of intoxication, coagulopathy, external evidence of trauma above the clavicles, or neurologic deficit) in combination with predictive criteria (Table 6.5).[6] The CHIP rule results in 100% sensitivity for neurosurgical intervention, with a sensitivity of 94–96% for all intracranial positive findings on CT. However, the specificity in the 25–32% range is not much better than the other decision rules.

Prior studies involving MTBI patients had incorporated LOC and PTA into their inclusion criteria, leading to a practice where patients without these symptoms were commonly discharged without imaging or observation. Among the most salient features of the CHIP rule is that LOC and PTA are removed from the inclusion criteria and instead become independent risk factors for intracranial injury. This shift was further explored in a recent publication by the same group which found that patients *without* LOC and PTA required neurosurgical intervention at the same rate as patients *with* these findings.[86] The common approach of discharging patients with a normal mental status who have not had LOC or PTA without imaging or observation may thus not be justified, particularly if other known risk factors are present.

The clinical bottom line to all of the studies is that the ACEP guidelines propose a reasonable and effective strategy to diminish CT usage without missing major injury. However, these guidelines, although based on good evidence, cannot fit every clinical situation. If the clinical picture is highly worrisome due to underlying patient morbidity, symptomatology, or mechanism, it may be fully appropriate to perform a non-contrast CT to exclude intracranial bleeding. On the other hand, CT scans are somewhat costly, use limited resources, and deliver ionizing radiation to the brain. Therefore indiscriminate use for every minor head injury is neither medically appropriate nor effective.

Magnetic resonance imaging

While CT scanning is the gold standard in neuroimaging after head trauma, there is some utility to alternate imaging studies, particularly magnetic resonance imaging (MRI). It is more sensitive than CT in detecting DAI and small intraparenchymal hemorrhages, particularly in the brainstem. On the other hand, CT is clearly superior at detecting subarachnoid hemorrhages and skull fractures. When compared

Table 6.4 Comparison of Canadian CT Head Rule (CCHR) and the New Orleans Criteria (NOC)

	CCHR	NOC
Objective	Identify patients who need CT	Identify patients who can safely forgo CT
Inclusion	Age ≥ 16 years	Age > 3 years
	GCS 13–15 with LOC/PTA	GCS 15 with LOC/PTA
	Head injury within 24 hours	Head injury within 24 hours
Risk factors identified	**High-risk** Failure to reach GCS of 15 within 2 hours	Headache Vomiting
	Suspected open skull fracture	Age > 60 years
	Sign of basilar skull fracture	Drug or alcohol intoxication
	Vomiting ≥ 2 episodes	Short-term memory deficits
	Age ≥ 65 years	Physical evidence of trauma above clavicles
	Medium-risk	
	Amnesia before impact > 30 minutes	Seizure
	Dangerous mechanism of injury (pedestrian struck, ejection from motor vehicle, fall from height > 3 ft or 5 stairs)	
Exclusion criteria	No LOC or PTA	No LOC or PTA
	Penetrating skull injuries	Patient declined CT
	Unstable vital signs associated with major trauma	Concurrent injuries precluding CT
	Seizure before assessment in the ED	
	Bleeding disorder or oral anticoagulants	
	Returned for reassessment of the same injury	
	Pregnant	
Outcome measures	Neurosurgical intervention; and "clinically important" brain injury on CT	Neurosurgical injury and any positive finding on CT (any hematoma or hemorrhage, contusion or depressed skull fracture)
	"Unimportant" findings included: solitary contusion < 5 mm in diameter, localized subarachnoid blood < 1 mm thick, smear subdural hematoma < 4 mm thick, isolated pneumocephaly or closed depressed skull fracture not through the inner table	
Sensitivity for injuries requiring neurosurgical intervention	100%	100%
Main limitation	Only two thirds of patients received CT	Low specificity does not greatly decrease number of CTs

CT, computed tomography; ED, emergency department; GCS, Glasgow Coma Scale; LOC, loss of consciousness; PTA, post-traumatic amnesia.

Table 6.5 CHIP Rule: simple prediction model[6]

CT is indicated in the presence of one major criterion	CT is indicated in the presence of at least two minor criteria
Pedestrian or cyclist vs. vehicle	Fall from any elevation
Ejected from vehicle	Persistent anterograde amnesia
Vomiting	PTA of 2–4 hours
PTA $\geq$ 4 hours	Contusion of the skull
Clinical signs of skull fracture	Neurologic deficit
GCS score < 15	Loss of consciousness
GCS deterioration $\geq$ 2 points (1 hour after presentation)	GCS deterioration of 1 point (1 hour after presentation)
Use of anticoagulant therapy	Age 40–60 years
Post-traumatic seizure	
Age > 60 years	

CHIP, CT in Head Injury Patients; CT, computed tomography; GCS, Glasgow Coma Scale; PTA, post-traumatic amnesia.

Table 6.6 The Glasgow Outcome Scale (GOS)[88]

Score	Description
1	**Death**
2	**Persistent vegetative state**
	Patient exhibits no obvious cortical function
3	**Severe disability**
	(Conscious but disabled.) Patient depends upon others for daily support due to mental or physical disability or both
4	**Moderate disability**
	(Disabled but independent.) Patient is independent as far as daily life is concerned. The disabilities found include varying degrees of dysphasia, hemiparesis, or ataxia, as well as intellectual and memory deficits and personality changes
5	**Good recovery**
	Resumption of normal activities even though there may be minor neurological or psychological deficits

with CT in the setting of intracerebral hemorrhage, MRI was superior at detecting a subset of small acute hemorrhages and chronic bleeds.[87] This advantage has limited utility in the trauma patient, however. In contrast, MRI has several disadvantages, including increased study duration (thus increasing the time during which the patient is out of the ED), increased cost, and myriad contraindications, including the introduction of magnetic objects into the room. At this time, MRI is not recommended as part of the initial evaluation of the head injured patient in the ED.

Complications of TBI

Predictably, the most common short- and long-term complications of TBI are neurologic. In the majority of cases, the frequency, degree, and duration of these complications are related to the severity of the initial injury. Both focal and global neurologic deficits may persist and result in long-term disability. The range of such sequelae is broad, from mild paresis of an extremity to persistent unconsciousness to death. The Glasgow Outcome Scale (GOS) was developed in order to classify functional neurologic outcomes

in patients with TBI.[88] This is a useful tool for population studies of TBI patients (Table 6.6).[88]

Seizures are a potential complication of TBI, most commonly within the first 24 hours to 1 week. On occasion, TBI leads to a post-traumatic seizure disorder or epilepsy. Infection may also complicate TBI. Most commonly, local infections occur, particularly in the setting of penetrating trauma or dural tears. These range from cellulitis and soft tissue infections to meningitis and brain abscess. In TBI patients, systemic infections may also ensue; mental status changes and vomiting in the setting of TBI predispose patients to aspiration pneumonia. Moreover, since many patients with significant brain injuries are admitted to the hospital, and frequently to the ICU, they may contract a spectrum of infections.

While complication rates tend to be lower among patients with milder injuries, there are distinct phenomena that may follow MTBI, namely the postconcussive syndrome and the second-impact syndrome.

Postconcussive syndrome

The postconcussive syndrome includes neurologic and psychological manifestations such as chronic headaches, visual changes, depression, irritability, decreased concentration, and memory impairment. Postconcussive syndrome has been reported in up to 80% of patients with MTBI. While in most patients these symptoms usually resolve spontaneously within the first 3 months, they may persist. Approximately 30% of patients will have symptoms at 3 months, and half of those will have persistent symptoms at one year.[14] Initially thought to be primarily due to psychological mechanisms, recent advances in brain imaging with MRI and positron emission tomography (PET) have correlated the clinical findings to subtle changes in brain structure and physiology.[80,89] However, there is a body of evidence which suggests that the patient's psychosocial situation influences the incidence of these symptoms and the timing of their resolution.[80]

There is some evidence that early follow up of patients at risk for developing postconcussive syndrome may decrease the incidence of these symptoms 6 months after the injury. Wade et al.[80] found that interventions including counseling and neuropsychological assessment and treatment decreased patients' social disability and the rate of postconcussive symptoms.

Sports-related injuries and the second impact syndrome

A significant proportion of TBI cases are sports related. Often referred to as "concussion" in sports-related literature, MTBI carries significant morbidity in this setting. Because these patients are exposed to repeated insults, they are at risk for developing second impact syndrome. This syndrome occurs when the brain is traumatized a second time prior to fully recovering from a first impact. The already injured brain may suffer additive damage and has a diminished capability to recover. Significant disability and even deaths have been reported as a result of this syndrome. Patients who practice contact sports, such as boxing and football, are at particular risk. Concussions vary in grade, from mild insults resulting in confusion to those leading to LOC. The risk of developing second impact syndrome rises as the grade of the concussion increases. Practical management guidelines, based mainly on consensus opinion rather than robust literature, have been developed for this group of patients (Table 6.7).[11]

Table 6.7 Management of patients with sports-related concussion[11]

Grade I	Confusion but no LOC/PTA	• Remove from activity and observe
		• After return to baseline, return to full activity if patient is asymptomatic with exertion
Grade II	Confusion and PTA, but no LOC	• Remove from activity for the rest of the day
		• Reassess in 24 hours
		• Return to activity after 1 week if patient remains asymptomatic
		• After two grade II concussions, no activity that places patient at risk for 3 months
Grade III	LOC	• Transport to ED for evaluation and CT
		• Return to activity after 1 month and asymptomatic for 2 weeks
		• After two grade III concussions, terminate season and consider terminating high-risk activity indefinitely

CT, computed tomography; ED, emergency department; LOC, loss of consciousness; PTA, post-traumatic amnesia.

Pediatric considerations

Trauma is the leading cause of death among children, and head injury is responsible for up to 3000 annual deaths in children. Infants under 1 year of age have a worse prognosis after trauma to the head, with a high incidence of brain injury.[90] Unfortunately, clinical signs have limited predictive value in children, and the majority of patients with headache, vomiting, and lethargy have no demonstrable injury on CT. To complicate matters, infants often lack physical signs, including LOC, mental status changes, and vomiting even when significant TBI is present.

Infants to 2 years

Because they are preverbal and have a limited behavioral range at baseline, young infants are most at risk for having a missed intracranial injury, as "common" signs of TBI are frequently absent.[91] Thus, current clinical decision rules developed for adults are inadequate for evaluating children, particularly preverbal ones. Even LOC, a variable that has been used in risk stratifying adult patients with head trauma, is highly insensitive as a marker in these children, with a sensitivity as low as 3%.[92] In their study on intracranial injury in infants, Greenes and Schutzman found that among infants with documented intracranial injury (ICI), 27% of those younger than 6 months, and 15% of those between 6 months and 1 year of age, had no symptoms.[93] However, the vast majority of those with significant ICI had a scalp hematoma. Thus, the clinician should have a low threshold to image infants, especially those with scalp hematomas.

Children 2 years and older

In older children, LOC acquires greater sensitivity, as do other clinical risk factors. Much like in the adult patient, the question then becomes which children need neuroimaging. In addition to cost considerations, increased lengths of stay in the ED, and the concern regarding transferring a patient out of the ED for imaging, there are several disadvantages to routine CT scanning in children. Radiation exposure is a concern in the pediatric patient, due to children's increased susceptibility to the effects of radiation. In addition, many children require sedation in order to undergo CT scanning, and sedation places the patient at risk for complications including respiratory depression and aspiration.

In 1999, the American Academy of Pediatrics published a guideline for the management of MTBI in children, addressing patients aged 2–20 with isolated closed head trauma.[93] In patients who present with normal mental status, non-focal neurologic exams and no clinical evidence of skull fracture, CT is not indicated if there was no LOC. In patients with brief LOC (defined by the authors as < 1 minute), either CT scanning or observation are appropriate. Palchak and colleagues at UC Davis found that the

Table 6.8 Pediatric high-risk[94,95]

UC Davis Rule	NEXUS II
Clinical signs of skull fracture	Evidence of skull fracture
Abnormal mental status	Altered level of consciousness
High-risk vomiting	Neurologic deficit
Scalp hematoma age < 2 years	Persistent vomiting
Severe headache	Scalp hematoma
	Abnormal behavior
	Coagulopathy

NEXUS, National Emergency X-Radiography Utilization Study.

presence of high-risk clinical signs had a sensitivity of 100% for TBI requiring acute intervention.[94] Their decision rule, which has yet to be validated, also had a negative predictive value of 100% when all high risk variables were absent. Oman and the NEXUS II investigators evaluated a decision rule to reduce unnecessary CT scanning in young children.[95] They concluded that ICI is extremely unlikely in any child who does not exhibit any of the defined high-risk criteria (Table 6.8).[94,95]

There has been a paucity of data on the rates of TBI among undifferentiated pediatric head injury patients. Some research suggests that among neurologically intact children with MTBI, the rate of radiographically evident injury is as high as 3–6%. However, the clinical significance of these data is unknown. The majority of children who have had MTBI will experience a full recovery. Children have lower complication rates than adults following head trauma, and the postconcussive syndrome described in adult patients does not appear to affect most children.[96]

Another source of controversy has been the use of skull radiography in the evaluation of pediatric TBI patients. In children, skull fractures are not uncommon and are more predictive of intracranial injury than in adults.[90] Moreover, skull fractures have important sequelae in children given their potential to develop leptomeningeal cysts and fracture non-union. Finally, unlike in CT scanning, sedation is typically not required in patients undergoing skull plain films so these are used by some

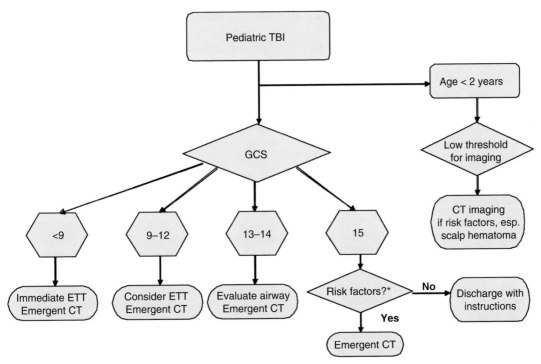

Figure 6.12 Approach to pediatric head trauma. CT, computed tomography; ETT, endotracheal tube; GCS, Glasgow Coma Scale; TBI, traumatic brain injury. *Risk factors include evidence of skull fracture, altered level of consciousness, neurologic deficit, persistent vomiting, scalp hematoma, abnormal behavior, and coagulopathy.

practitioners to screen for skull fractures. If a skull fracture is identified on plain film radiography, a CT should be performed to assess for intracranial pathology. A normal radiograph, however, cannot rule out, but can diminish the likelihood of intracranial pathology.

Child abuse is frequently manifested by head trauma. The stated mechanism of injury must be consistent with the child's developmental maturity and with the presenting signs of injury, if any. When the history is suspect, inconsistent, or repeatedly changing, abuse should be entertained. In suspected cases of child abuse, a full radiologic survey is indicated ("baby-gram") to identify evidence of previous or concomitant injuries.

The optimal management of the pediatric head trauma patient remains controversial. We outline a reasonable approach in Figure 6.12.

Considerations in the elderly

While trauma is the leading cause of death among young people, it is also a significant cause of death among the elderly. It is, in fact, the seventh leading cause of death among patients over age 65. In this population, falls are the primary cause of TBI.

The elderly are prone to falls due to polypharmacy and the pathophysiology of aging. Their balance and proprioception may be impaired. Slower reflexes may prevent them from stopping a fall, or from protecting their heads when they do. They may also have comorbid conditions that predispose them to increased morbidity and mortality, including coagulopathy and osteopenia. Mosenthal et al. studied patients with isolated TBI and found that increasing age predicted increasing mortality in these patients regardless of initial injury severity.[9] Moreover, for patients who survived their injury, age predicted an increased rate of poor functional outcome.

Donohue et al. studied patients aged 65 and over and found that the relative risk of death in this population remains elevated for at least 2 years following the injury.[97] With the exception of the most severely injured patients, overall mortality following head injury was dependent on general health as much as on injury severity. Poorer outcomes may be related to the elderly patient's decrease in "physiologic reserve," increased post-injury complications, and delay in onset of neurologic findings, perhaps delaying diagnosis and aggressive treatment.

These findings may be partially explained by the increased risk of elderly patients of sustaining subdural hematoma after head trauma. Brain atrophy due to normal aging causes increased tension on bridging veins within the subdural space and places them at risk of rupture following head trauma. Because brain atrophy results in increased potential intracranial space, mass effect and shift may not occur early on, even in the setting of a major intracranial lesion. Thus, the elderly are less likely to have early changes in GCS or focal neurologic signs, and clinical assessment is less useful in stratifying head trauma among the elderly. Some of these are the often described "talk and die" patients.[98] Thus CT scanning should be performed on elderly patients who have sustained MTBI. Emergency physicians should also have a low threshold to image elderly patients with minimal head injury without neurologic signs or symptoms, particularly if they take anticoagulants.

Anticoagulation

It is intuitive that patients with congenital and acquired coagulopathies, including therapeutic anticoagulation, are at increased risk for intracranial pathology in the setting of head injury. One small study showed a probability of intracranial hemorrhage of up to 25% even in patients presenting without apparent neurologic abnormalities.[99] A protocol with rapid reversal of anticoagulation in these patients with CT findings has been shown to significantly decrease mortality.[100] These patients are at high risk and generally should be prioritized for a rapid brain CT. An abnormal one should be followed by immediate reversal of anticoagulation and a normal one should also be followed by consideration for reversal if the International Normalized Ratio (INR) is significantly out of range. Reversal is generally accomplished by using fresh frozen plasma (FFP). In cases where reversal is high risk, e.g., mechanical valves, lowering the INR to the low range of therapeutic, and observation, may be the safest course.

With the widespread use of antiplatelet agents, including aspirin and clopidogrel, there is a potential for similar complications in patients with head trauma. A retrospective review of trauma patients taking clopidogrel found an increase in morbidity, including the need for surgical intervention.[101] Another study compared a cohort of patients aged over 50 taking aspirin or clopidogrel with a control group and found a significant increase in mortality in the antiplatelet group.[102] Reversal of antiplatelet agents with platelets or FFP has not been studied, but should be considered particularly in patients who require operative intervention.

Disposition

Patient disposition following TBI varies according to injury severity. Patients with severe head trauma need close monitoring and ventilatory support. Many of them will require neurosurgical intervention, and while some may be managed expectantly, all will require admission to an ICU. Similarly, patients with moderate head trauma (GCS of 9–12) may require ICU admission and airway management. At a minimum, patients with moderate TBI require admission and frequent neurologic checks, as they are at risk for rapid deterioration. In cases of MTBI, disposition is again a source of controversy. Patients who have undergone CT imaging should be admitted if there is evidence of intracranial hemorrhage or depressed skull fracture. Some studies have used the term "clinically important" to refer to CT findings that would require the patient to be admitted, while clinically unimportant findings would not warrant admission. Others have postulated that any CT finding is clinically important enough to admit the patient for further observation. Because there is a paucity of data elucidating the incidence of deterioration and long-term prognosis of patients following these "unimportant" injuries, it is generally recommended that all patients with intracranial findings on CT be admitted for observation.

The disposition of MTBI patients with a normal head CT has been debated in the literature. It would be prudent to adopt a conservative approach where patients with abnormal GCS scores (13–14) are admitted for observation even when CT results are normal. After reviewing the literature, the ACEP guidelines concluded that a patient with a GCS score of 15 and a negative CT can safely be discharged after a period of observation of 6 hours from the time of injury.[103] The observation period may be shorter if the patient is discharged in the care of a responsible third party. While the risk of delayed deterioration in discharged patients is low, it is not zero. On the other hand, the negative predictive value of a negative CT scan for any intervention is close to 99%, and if the patient is otherwise stable, admission probably offers little.[99] The major, although rare, concern is in a patient on whom a CT scan is not performed. Any patient in whom discharge is considered must have clear instructions as to important reasons to return for re-evaluation. These patients should only be discharged if there is reasonable proximity and access to re-evaluation in case of worsening condition. It is preferable that a responsible adult is able to check on the patient repeatedly and has the ability to transport the patient back to an acute care facility quickly if the patient deteriorates. Patients and their relatives or caretakers should be encouraged to return to the ED immediately for any deterioration of mental status, worsening of headache, vomiting, or evolving neurologic deficit.

Transfer criteria

Patients who present to hospitals and other settings that are not equipped or able to deliver specialized care often need to be transferred from one institution to another.[104] The circumstances and timing surrounding such transfers need careful evaluation by the transferring physician in order to prevent deterioration. As discussed previously, patients at risk for decompensation during transfer may need to be intubated for airway protection. Measures should be taken to avoid hypoxia and hypotension, common causes of secondary injury. Once the decision has been made to transfer the patient, transfer proceedings should begin as soon as practical. Transfer criteria vary based on the type of injury and the potential benefits. The general principles are that the patient should be transferred if there is an injury that may require specialized care that is unavailable at the transferring institution, but can be provided at the receiving center, and that the patient has been reasonably stabilized to allow for a safe transfer.

Future research directions

Neuroimaging

Non-contrast CT of the brain is the test of choice in identifying and excluding intracranial hemorrhage. However, significant symptoms and sequelae may manifest themselves in patients with negative head CT. It is becoming increasingly clear that other modalities may aid in the diagnosis of subtle findings associated with DAI and other mild derangements in brain structure and physiologic function, including those that predispose patients to postconcussive symptoms. Belanger et al. reviewed some of the promising techniques in neuroimaging for TBI.[89] Magnetic resonance imaging

has already been used to image evidence of DAI, which is typically not captured on CT. Diffusion tensor imaging (DTI) measures the directional diffusion of water molecules as a marker of structural integrity in the brain. It may be used in the future to predict recovery in patients with TBI. Magnetic resonance spectroscopy (MRS) yields *in vivo* neurochemical information about the brain by measuring specific metabolites in brain tissue. Functional MRI (fMRI) is also being studied to observe "real-time" brain functioning. Positron emission tomography (PET) and single photon emission computed tomography (SPECT) are techniques for imaging regional brain metabolism via regional cerebral blood flow. Like fMRI, PET specifically provides a "real-time" measurement. All of these imaging techniques are currently being studied, and the structural and physiologic abnormalities being identified correlate with clinical outcomes. The eventual application of these techniques will likely be outside the realm of the ED, but future research into the use of these modalities may reveal optimal strategies for the initial management of patients in the ED.

Therapeutic hypothermia

In recent years, hypothermia has been considered to be an attractive treatment adjunct in trauma patients. Several studies have suggested better neurological outcomes in patients treated with systemic cooling when compared to normothermic controls. However, the largest randomized study did not support this theory. A recent meta-analysis published by the BTF found that the use of therapeutic hypothermia in patients with severe TBI resulted in significantly higher Glasgow Outcome Scale (GOS) scores.[17] There was no difference in overall mortality, but data suggested improved mortality rates when hypothermia was used for more than 48 hours.[17] Some investigators have also examined selective head and neck cooling as an alternative.[105]

Research suggests that hypothermia may be most beneficial among severe TBI patients with increased ICP not controlled by conventional means; the optimal timing of onset and cessation is controversial. There are significant difficulties with inducing and maintaining hypothermia along with detrimental side effects such as systemic coagulopathy. A randomized prospective study was terminated prematurely due to lack of effect of therapeutic hypothermia vs. normothermia.[106] The lack of effect may be due to a missed therapeutic window; patients who are hypothermic on arrival in the ED –from ambient causes, for instance – and are kept hypothermic, did better than patients in whom hypothermia was induced after arrival.[107] In addition, when patients who arrive hypothermic are actively rewarmed to achieve normothermia, they have worse outcomes than if they are allowed to remain hypothermic. It may be that the rebound effects of rewarming, rather than the hypothermia itself, adversely affect outcomes.[108] We also may not be maintaining hypothermia long enough to observe neuroprotective effects, as cerebral edema is often greatest more than 48 hours after traumatic insults. A recent study by Inamasu et al. suggests that patients with isolated subdural hematoma have decreased mortality and improved outcomes when hypothermia is employed; this effect was not seen in patients who had concomitant cerebral contusion or other injuries.[109]

In sum, therapeutic hypothermia, while initially promising, may not have utility. It may be that patients already hypothermic with severe TBI benefit from maintaining hypothermia. However, inducing hypothermia, at least in the short term, does not appear to confer a major clinical benefit on these patients.

Factor VIIa

Recombinant factor VIIa (rFVIIa) is a hemostatic agent approved by the US Food and Drug Administration (FDA) for the treatment of bleeding in hemophiliacs who have circulating inhibitors to factor VIII or IX. Over the last few years, additional "off-label" uses have been studied, including reversal of coagulopathy in non-hemophiliacs and treatment of traumatic hemorrhage. Even a small dose of rFVIIa will normalize an elevated INR, and its mechanism of action suggests that hemostatic activity is limited to the site of injury without systemic activation of the coagulation cascade.[110] However, while thromboembolic complications are rare among hemophiliacs, these events may pose particular risk to non-hemophiliac patients, possibly increasing mortality, as was shown in atraumatic intracranial hemorrhage. Recent studies have examined both the use of rFVIIa in trauma and its complications, and point to the importance of weighing the risk of thromboembolic event vs. the possible benefit of hemostasis.[111,112] Of note, the high cost of the agent would dictate that alternative treatments be given if available, and that its use be reserved for patients who stand to benefit the most from its administration. This subset of patients is yet to be firmly identified, but it likely includes coagulopathic TBI patients.

Summary

Head trauma, and specifically TBI, is a leading cause of morbidity and mortality. It is incumbent upon the emergency physician to understand its pathophysiology and treatment. In addition to the damage caused by the initial traumatic event, secondary injury may occur due to hypoxia, hypotension, and other metabolic insults. Traumatic brain injury is classified into severe, moderate, and mild: the management, disposition, and prognosis of each varies. Because the clinical evaluation is insufficiently sensitive to identify all TBI among head injured patients, CT scanning has emerged as an integral imaging modality. Epidural hematomas, subdural hematomas, subarachnoid hemorrhage, and intraparenchymal bleeds are the main CT-apparent injuries in TBI. The treatment for TBI revolves around preventing complications, especially intracranial hypertension. Some patient populations, such as children, the elderly, coagulopathic patients, and those with penetrating trauma, require special consideration. Long-term complications of TBI include neuropsychiatric sequelae that may persist, even after mild injury. Future research promises to further elucidate the optimal management of these patients and may uncover new treatment strategies.

Box 6.8   Clinical pearls in head trauma

- Traumatic brain injury is classified as severe, moderate, or mild depending on presentation.
- Primary injury refers to damage due to direct compressive forces; secondary injury includes subsequent damage due to insults at the cellular level.
- The clinical evaluation may be insufficient to diagnose significant injuries in the head-injured patient.
- Head CT is the preferred imaging modality following head trauma and detects intracranial injury requiring intervention.
- Poor outcomes are associated with increasing injury severity.
- There is no specific treatment for primary injury in head trauma; treatment strategies are directed towards minimizing secondary injury and preventing complications, principally intracranial hypertension.
- Management of severe head injury should be directed to the prevention of hypotension and hypoxia, both of which are clearly associated with increased morbidity and mortality.

References

1. Stiell IG, Wells GA, Vandemheen K, et al. The Canadian CT Head Rule for patients with minor head injury. *Lancet* 2001;**357**:1391–6.

2. Teasdale G, Jennett BA. Assessment of coma and impaired consciousness: a practical scale. *Lancet* 2;1974:81–4.

3. Reilly PL, Simpson DA, Sprod R, et al. Assessing the conscious level in infants and young children: a paediatric version of the Glasgow Coma Scale. *Childs Nerv Syst* 1988;**4**:30–3.

4. Meredith W, Rutledge R, Fakhry SM, et al. The conundrum of the Glasgow Coma Scale in intubated patients: a linear regression prediction of the Glasgow verbal score from the Glasgow Eye and Motor Scores. *J Trauma Injury Infect Crit Care* 1998;**44**:839–45.

5. Bazarian JJ, Pope C, McClung J, et al. Ethinic and racial disparities in emergency department care for mild traumatic brain injury. *Acad Emerg Med* 2003;**10**:1209–17.

6. Smits M, Dippel DWJ, Steyerberg EW, et al. Predicting intracranial traumatic findings on computed tomography in patients with minor head injury: the CHIP prediction rule. *Ann Intern Med* 2007;**146**:397–405.

7. Centers for Disease Control. Rates of hospitalization related to traumatic brain injury: nine states, 2003. *MMWR* 2007;**56**:167.

8. Yates PJ, Williams WH, Harris A, et al. An epidemiological study of head injuries in a UK population attending an emergency department. *J Neurol Neurosurg Psychiatry* 2006;**77**:699–701.

9. Mosenthal AC, Lavery RF, Addis M, et al. Isolated traumatic brain injury: age is an independent predictor of mortality and early outcome. *J Trauma* 2002;**52**:907–11.

10. Haydel MJ. Clinical decision instruments for CT scanning in minor head injury. *JAMA* 2005;**294**:1551–3.

11. Cushman JG, Agarwal N, Fabian TC, et al. Practice management guidelines for the management of mild traumatic brain injury. *J Trauma* 2001;**51**:1016–26.

12. Thurman D, Guerrero J Trends in hospitalization associated with traumatic brain injury. *JAMA* 1999;**282**:954–7.

13. Henry GL, Jagoda A, Little N, Pellegrino TR. *Neurologic Emergencies: A Symptom-Oriented Approach*, 2nd edn. New York: McGraw-Hill, 2003.

14. Reivech M. Arterial PCO_2 and cerebral hemodynamics. *Am J Physiol* 1964;**206**:25.

15. Stringer WA, Hasso AN, Thompson JR, et al. Hyperventilation induced cerebral ischemia in patients with acute brain lesions: demonstration by xenon enhanced CT. *Am J Neuroradiol* 1993;**14**:475.

16. Marion DW, Darby J, Yonas H. Acute regional/cerebral blood flow changes caused by severe head injuries. *J Neurosurg* 1991;**74**:407–14.

17. Brain Trauma Foundation. *Guidelines for the Management of Severe Traumatic Brain Injury*, 3rd edn. New York: Brain Trauma Foundation Press, 2007.

18. Gabella B, Hoffman R, Marine W, Stallones L. Urban and rural traumatic brain injuries in Colorado. *Ann Epidemiol* 1997;**7**:207–12.

19. Woodward A, Dorsch M, Simpson D. Head injuries in country and city: a study of hospital separations in South Australia. *Med J Australia* 1984;**141**:13–17.

20. Haydel MJ, Preston CA, Mills TJ, et al. Indications for computed tomography in patients with minor head injury. *N Engl J Med* 200;**343**:100–5.

21. Jeret JS, Mandell M, Anziska B, et al. Clinical predictors of abnormality disclosed by computed tomography after mild head trauma. *Neurosurg* 1993;**32**:9–15.

22. Anglin D, Hutson H, Luftman J, et al. Intracranial hemorrhage associated with tangential gunshot wounds to the head. *Acad Emerg Med* 1998;**5**:672–8.

23. Chestnut RM, Marshall LF, Klauber MR, et al. The role of secondary brain injury in determining outcome from severe head injury. *J Trauma* 1993;**34**:216–22.

24. Meyer S, Gibb T, Jurkovich G. Evaluation and significance of the pupillary light reflex in trauma patients. *Ann Emerg Med* 1993;**22**:1052–7.

25. Jennett B, Teasdale G, Galbraith S, et al. Severe head injuries in three countries. *J Neurol Neurosurg Psych* 1977;**40**:291–8.

26. Hoffman JR, Mower WR, Wolfson AB, et al. Validity of a set of clinical criteria to rule out injury to the cervical spine in patients with blunt trauma. *N Engl J Med* 2000;**343**:94–9.

27. Winchell RJ, Hoyt DB. Endotracheal intubation in the field improves survival in patients with severe head injury. *Arch Surg* 1997;**132**:592–7.

28. Davis D, Hoyt D, Ochs M, et al. The effect of paramedic rapid sequence intubation on outcome in patients with severe traumatic brain injury. *J Trauma* 2003;**54**:444–53.

29. Davis D, Dunford J, Poste J, et al. The impact of hypoxia and hyperventilation on outcome after paramedic rapid sequence intubation of severely head injured patients. *J Trauma* 2004;**57**:1–10.

30. Wirtz DD, Ortiz C, Newman DH, et al. Unrecognized misplacement of endotracheal tubes by ground prehospital providers. *Prehosp Emerg Care* 2007;**11**:213–18.

31. Vassar MJ, Perry CA, Holcroft JW. Prehospital resuscitation of hypotensive trauma patients with 7.5% NaCl versus 7.5% NaCl with added dextran: a controlled trial. *J Trauma* 1993;**34**:622–32.

32. Cooper J, Myles P, McDermott F, et al. Prehospital hypertonic saline resuscitation of patients with hypotension and severe traumatic brain injury. *JAMA* 2004;**291**:1350–7.

33. Sayre M, Daily S, Stern S, et al. Out-of-hospital administration of mannitol to head-injured patients does not change systolic blood pressure. *Acad Emerg Med* 1996;**3**:840–8.

34. Luber S, Brady W, Brand A, et al. Acute hypoglycemia masquerading as head trauma: a report of four cases. *Am J Emerg Med* 1996;**14**:543–7.

35. McHugh GS, Engel DC, Butcher I, et al. Prognostic value of secondary insults in traumatic brain injury: results from the IMPACT study. *J Neurotrauma* 2007;**24**:287–93.

36. Miller JD. Head injury and brain ischemia – implications for threrapy. *Br J Anaesth* 1985;**57**:120–30.

37. Changaris DG, McGraw CP, Richardson JD, et al. Correlation of cerebral perfusion pressure and Glasgow Coma Scale to outcome. *J Trauma* 1987;**27**:1007–13.

38. Cruz J. The first decade of continuous monitoring of jugular bulb oxyhemoglobin saturation: management strategies and clinical outcome. *Crit Care Med* 1998;**26**:344–51.

39. Siegel JH. The effect of associated injuries, blood loss, and oxygen debt on death and disability in blunt traumatic brain injury: the need for early physiologic predictors of severity. *J Neurotrauma* 1995;**12**:579–90.

40. Vassar MJ, Perry CA, Gannaway WL, et al. 7.5% sodium chloride/dextran for resuscitation of trauma patients undergoing helicopter transport. *Arch Surg* 1991;**126**:1065–72.

41. Steiner LA, Johnston AJ, Czosnyka M, et al. Direct comparison of cerebrovascular effects of norepinephrine and dopamine in head-injured patients. *Crit Care Med* 2004;**32**:1049–54.

42. Rund D, Ewing J, Mitzel K, et al. The use of intramuscular benzodiazepines and antipsychotic agents in the treatment of acute agitation or violence in the emergency department. *J Emerg Med* 2006;**31**:317–24.

43. Todd KH, Ducharme J, Choiniere M, et al. Pain in the emergency department: results of the Pain and Emergency Medicine Initiative (PEMI) Multicenter Study. *J Pain* 2007;**8**:460–6.

44. Bazarian JJ, McClung J, Cheng YT, et al. Emergency department management of mild traumatic brain injury in the USA. *Emerg Med J* 2005;**22**:473–7.

45. Walia S, Sutcliffe AJ. The relationship between blood glucose, mean arterial blood pressure and outcome after severe head injury: an observational study. *Injury, Int J Care Injured* 2002;**33**:339–44.

46. Temkin NR, Dikmen SS, Wilensky AJ, et al. A randomized, double-blind study of phenytoin for the prevention of post-traumatic seizures. *N Engl J Med* 1990;**323**:497–502.

47. Yablon SA. Posttraumatic seizures. *Arch Phys Med Rehabil* 1993;**74**:983–1001.

48. Manaka S. Cooperative prospective study on posttraumatic epilepsy: risk factors and the effect of prophylactic anticonvulsant. *Jpn J Psychiatry Neurol* 1992;**46**:311–15.

49. Temkin NR, Dikmen SS, Anderson GD, et al. Valproate therapy for prevention of posttraumatic seizures: a randomized trial. *J Neurosurg* 1999;**91**:593–600.

50. Young B, Rapp RP, Nortan JA, et al. Failure of prophylactically administered phenytoin to prevent late posttraumatic seizures. *J Neurosurg* 1983;**58**:236–41.

51. Pancioli AM. Hypertension management in neurologic emergencies. *Ann Emerg Med* 2008;**51**:S24–7.

52. Shutter LA, Narayan RK. Blood pressure management in traumatic brain injury. *Ann Emerg Med* 2008;**51**:S37–8.

53. Lemos MJ, Clark DE. Scalp lacerations resulting in hemorrhagic shock: case reports and recommended management. *J Emerg Med* 1988;**6**:377–9.

54. Villalobos T, Arango C, Kubilis P, et al. Antibiotic prophylaxis after basilar skull fractures: a meta-analysis. *Clin Infect Dis* 1998;**27**:364–9.

55. Bayston R, de Louvois J, Brown EM, et al. Use of antibiotics in penetrating craniocerebral injuries "Infection in Neurosurgery" Working Party of British Society for Antimicrobial Chemotherapy. *Lancet* 2000;**355**:1813–17.

56. Lashutka MK, Chandra A, Murray HN, et al. The relationship of intraocular pressure to intracranial pressure. *Ann Emerg Med* 2004;**43**:585–91.

57. Raichle ME, Plum F. Hyperventilation and cerebral blood flow. *Stroke* 1972;**3**:566–75.

58. Burke AM, Quest DO, Chien S, Cerri C. The effects of mannitol on blood viscosity. *J Neurosurg* 1981;**55**:550–3.

59. Barry KG, Berman AR. Mannitol infusion: the acute effect of the intravenous infusion of mannitol on blood and plasma volumes. *N Engl J Med* 1961;**264**:1085–8.

60. Javid M, Gilboe D, Cesario T. The rebound phenomenon and hypertonic solutions. *J Neurosurg* 1964;**21**:1059–66.

61. Wakai A, Roberts I, Schierhout G. Mannitol for acute traumatic brain injury. *Cochrane Database Syst Rev* 2007;**1**:CD001049.

62. Cruz J, Minoja G, Okuchi K. Improving clinical outcomes from acute subdural hematomas with the emergency preoperative administration of high doses of mannitol: a randomized trial. *Neurosurgery* 2001;**49**:864–71.

63. Cruz J, Minoja G, Okuchi K. Major clinical and physiological benefits of early high doses of mannitol for intraparenchymal temporal lobe hemorrhages with abnormal papillary widening: a randomized trial. *Neurosurgery* 2002;**51**:628–37.

64. Cruz J, Minoja G, Okuchi K, Facco E. Successful use of the new high-dose mannitol treatment in patients with Glasgow Coma Scale scores of 3 and bilateral abnormal papillary widening: a randomized trial. *J Neurosurg* 2004;**100**:376–83.

65. Paczynski RP. Osmotherapy. Basic concepts and controversies. *Crit Care Clin* 1997;**13**:105–29.

66. Härtl R, Medary M, Ruge M, et al. Hypertonic/hyperoncotic saline attenuates microcirculatory disturbances after traumatic brain injury. *J Trauma* 1977;**42**:S41–7.

67. Horn P, Munch E, Vajkoczy P, et al. Hypertonic saline solution for control of elevated intracranial pressure in patients with exhausted response to mannitol and barbiturates. *Neurol Res* 1999;**21**:758–64.

68. Battison C, Andrews PJ, Graham C, Petty T. Randomized, controlled trial on the effect of a 20% mannitol solution and a 7.5% saline/6% dextran solution on increased intracranial pressure after brain injury. *Crit Care Med* 2005;**33**:196–202.

69. Vialet R, Albanese J, Thomachot L, et al. Isovolume hypertonic solutes (sodium chloride or mannitol) in the treatment of refractory posttraumatic intracranial hypertension: 2 ml/kg 7.5% saline is more effective than 2 ml/kg 20% mannitol. *Crit Care Med* 2003;**31**:1683–7.

70. Bhardwaj A, Ulatowski JA. Hypertonic saline solutions in brain injury. *Curr Opin Crit Care* 2004;**10**:126–31.

71. Khanna S, Davis D, Peterson B, et al. Use of hypertonic saline in the treatment of severe refractory posttraumatic intracranial hypertension in pediatric traumatic brain injury. *Crit Care Med* 2000;**28**:1144–51.

72. Qureshi AI, Suarez JI, Castro A, Bhardwaj A. Use of hypertonic saline/acetate infusion in treatment of cerebral edema in patients with head trauma: experience at a single center. *J Trauma* 1999;**47**:659–65.

73. Demopoulous HB, Flamm ES, Pietronigro DD, et al. The free radical pathology and the microcirculation in the major central nervous system trauma. *Acta Physiol Scand Suppl* 1980;**492**:91–119.

74. Kassell NF, Hitchon PW, Gerk MK, et al. Alterations in cerebral blood flow, oxygen metabolism, and electrical activity produced by high-dose thiopental. *Neurosurgery* 1980;**7**:598–603.

75. Roberts I, Sydenham E. Barbiturates for acute traumatic brain injury. *Cochrane Database Syst Rev* 1999;**3**:CD000033.

76. Bullock MR, Chesnut R, Ghajar J, et al. Guidelines for the surgical management of traumatic brain injury. *Neurosurgery* 2006;**58**(S2):1–60.

77. Ghandi Y, Penny DW. Burr holes. In Reichman EF, Simon RR (eds), *Emergency Medicine Procedures*. New York: McGraw-Hill, 2004: pp. 881–9.

78. Rimel RW, Giordani B, Barth JT, et al. Moderate head injury: completing the clinical spectrum of brain trauma. *Neurosurgery* 1982;**11**:344–51.

79. Servadei F, Teasdale G, Merry G, et al. Defining acute mild head injury in adults: a proposal based on prognostic factors, diagnosis and management. *J Neurotrauma* 2001;**18**:657–64.

80. Wade DT, King NS, Wenden FJ, et al. Routine follow up after head injury: a second randomized trial. *J Neurol Neurosurg Psychiatry* 1998;**65**:177–83.

81. Jagoda AS, Cantrill SV, Wears RL, et al. Clinical policy: neuroimaging and decisionmaking in adult mild traumatic brain injury in the acute setting. *Ann Emerg Med* 2002;**40**:231–49.

82. Stein SC, Ross SE. Mild head injury: a plea for routine early CT scanning. *J Trauma* 1992;**33**:11–13.

83. Clement CM, Stiell IG, Schull MJ, et al. Clinical features of head injury patients presenting with a Glasgow Coma Scale score of 15 and who require neurosurgical intervention. *Ann Emerg Med* 2006;**48**:245–51.

84. Stiell IG, Clement CM, Rowe BH, et al. Comparison of the Canadian CT Head Rule and the New Orleans Criteria in patients with minor head injury. *JAMA* 2005;**294**:1511–18.

85. Smits M, Dippel DWJ, de Haan GG, et al. External validation of the Canadian CT Head Rule and the New

Orleans Criteria for CT scanning in patients with minor head injury. *JAMA* 2005;**294**:1519–25.

86. Smits M, Hunink M, Nederkoorn PJ, et al. A history of loss of consciousness or post-traumatic amnesia in minor head injury: "condition sine qua non" or one of the risk factors? *J Neurol Neurosurg Psychiatry* 2007;**78**:1359–64.

87. Kidwell CS, Chalela JA, Saver JL, et al. Comparison of MRI and CT for detection of acute intracerebral hemorrhage. *JAMA* 2004;**292**:1823–30.

88. Jennett B, Bond M. Assessment of outcome after severe brain damage. *Lancet* 1975;**1**(7905):480–4.

89. Belanger HG, Vanderploeg RD, Curtiss G, et al. Recent neuroimaging techniques in mild traumatic brain injury. *J Neuropsych Clin Neurosci* 2007;**19**:5–20.

90. American Academy of Pediatrics, Committee on Quality Improvement. The management of minor closed head injury in children. *Pediatrics* 1999;**104**:1407–15.

91. Schutzman SA, Barnes P, Duhaime AC, et al. Evaluation and management of children younger than two years old with apparently minor head trauma: proposed guidelines. *Pediatrics* 2001;**107**:983–93.

92. Greenes DS. Decision making in pediatric minor head trauma. *Ann Emerg Med* 2003;**42**:515–18.

93. Greenes DS, Schutzman SA. Occult intracranial injury in infants. *Ann Emerg Med* 1998;**32**:680–6.

94. Palchak MJ, Holmes JF, Vance CW, et al. A decision rule for identifying children at low risk for brain injuries after blunt head trauma. *Ann Emerg Med* 2003;**42**:492–506.

95. Oman JA, Cooper RJ, Holmes JF, et al. Performance of a decision rule to predict need for computed tomography among children with blunt head trauma. *Pediatrics* 2006;**117**: e238–46.

96. Savitsky EA, Votey SR. Current controversies in the management of minor head injuries. *Am J Emerg Med* 2000;**18**:96–101.

97. Donohue JT, Clark DE, DeLorenzo MA. Longterm survival of Medicare patients with head injury. *J Trauma* 2007;**62**:419–23.

98. Goldschlager T, Rosenfeld JV, Winter CD. 'Talk and Die' patients presenting to a major trauma centre over a 10 year period: a critical review. *J Clin Neurosci* 2007;**14**:618–23.

99. Reynolds FD, Dietz PA, Higgins D, et al. Time to deterioration of the elderly, anticoagulated, minor head injury patient who presents without evidence of neurologic abnormality. *J Trauma* 2003;**54**:492–6.

100. Ivascu FA, Howells GA, Junn FS, et al. Rapid warfarin reversal in anticoagulated patients with traumatic intracranial hemorrhage reduces hemorrhage progression and mortality. *J Trauma* 2005;**59**:1131–7.

101. Jones K, Sharp C, Mangram A, et al. The effects of preinjury clopidogrel use on older trauma patients with head injuries. *Am J Surg* 2006; **192**:743–5.

102. Ohm C, Mina A, Howells G, et al. Effects of antiplatelet agents of outcomes for elderly patients with traumatic intracranial hemorrhage. *J Trauma* 2005;**58**:518–22.

103. Livingston DH, Lavery RF, Passannante MR, et al. Emergency department discharge of patients with a negative cranial computed tomography scan after minimal head injury. *Ann Surg* 2000;**232**:126–32.

104. McConnell K, Newgard C, Mullins R, et al. (2005). Mortality benefit of transfer to Level I versus Level II trauma centers for head injured patients. *Health Serv Res* 2005;**40**:435–57.

105. Qiu W, Shen H, Zhang Y, et al. Noninvasive selective brain cooling by head and neck cooling is protective in severe traumatic brain injury. *J Clin Neurosci* 2006;**13**:995–1000.

106. Clifton GL, Miller ER, Choi SC, et al. Lack of effect of induction of hypothermia after acute brain injury. *N Engl J Med* 2001;**344**:556–63.

107. Clifton GL. Is keeping cool still hot? An update on hypothermia in brain injury. *Curr Opin Crit Care* 2004;**10**:116–19.

108. Jiang J, Yang X. Current status of cerebral protection with mild-to-moderate hypothermia after traumatic brain injury. *Curr Opin Crit Care* 2007;**13**:153–5.

109. Inamasu J, Saito R, Nakamura Y, et al. Therapeutic hypothermia for severely head-injured patients with acute subdural hematoma. *J Clin Neurosci* 2006;**13**:733–7.

110. White CE, Schrank AE, Baskin TW, et al. Effects of recombinant activated factor VII in traumatic nonsurgical intracranial hemorrhage. *Curr Surg* 2006;**63**:310–17.

111. Yusim Y, Perel A, Berkenstadt H, et al. The use of recombinant factor VIIa (NovoSeven) for treatment of active or impending bleeding in brain injury: broadening the indications. *J Clin Anesth* 2006;**18**:545–51.

112. Rhys Thomas GO, Dutton RP, Hemlock B, et al. Thromboembolic complications associated with factor VIIa administration. *J Trauma* 2007;**62**:564–9.

7

Oral and maxillofacial trauma

Kurt Whitaker and John E. Frank

Introduction

The spectrum of facial trauma varies by age and mechanism. The most common causes of minor trauma are household injuries, sports, violence, traffic accidents, and workplace accidents. The most common cause of more severe injuries, such as facial fractures, is automobile collisions.[1] Older patients are prone to fractures (increase of 4.4% per year of age) while younger patients are more susceptible to dentoalveolar trauma (decrease of 4.5% per year of age).[2]

Concomitant injuries are common in facial trauma. In patients with facial fractures, up to 6% also have cervical spine injury,[3,4] and up to 45% have brain injury or skull fracture.[5] Laryngo-tracheal injuries and pulmonary injuries are also common. The hospital complication rate in patients with multisystem trauma and facial injuries is high and may be related to missed injuries, including vascular injuries and ocular injuries.

The percentage of patients reporting significant post-traumatic complaints, such as visual problems, anosmia, difficulty masticating or breathing, and epiphora (overflow of tears), increases with the severity of injury.[6] It is also this severely injured population that reports the greatest percentage of injury-related disability, hindering employment at long-term follow up.

Box 7.1 Essentials of facial trauma

- Focus on the ABCs – Do not be distracted by the impressive visual nature of facial trauma.
- Orally intubate early if oropharyngeal deformity or bleeding threatens the airway.
- Have a surgical airway kit ready and the neck prepped before attempting intubation.

- Computed tomography (CT) scan is the most important diagnostic test.
- No medications in the acute setting have been proven to reduce the mortality or morbidity of facial trauma.

Clinical anatomy and pathophysiology

The face encompasses a complex region of sensory and motor neural systems. The protective bony framework facilitates integrated functions such as vision, olfaction, and mastication yet also maintains a very important protective role during trauma. While the thick maxillary, orbital, frontal, zygomatic, pterygoid, and sphenoid bones comprise both a vertical and horizontal buttress system, the thinner maxillary, ethmoid, sphenoid, and frontal sinuses absorb considerable force when crushed. For instance, the anterior wall of the frontal sinus (frontal bone) may easily be depressed into the sinus, while the extremely thick posterior wall resists fracturing and the brain is well protected. The globe, which is housed in its rigid bony framework, is also protected. The thin orbital walls and floor will fracture and collapse, thereby absorbing the impact of trauma to the globe, protecting the globe from rupture (Figure 7.1).

The skin of the face is durable because of its high collagen content. The musculature and subcutaneous fat protect underlying structures. Lacerations heal quickly because the face is well vascularized. This is generally an advantage; however bleeding from facial trauma can be severe if not controlled expeditiously.

For the purpose of fracture management, the face is divided into the lower face or mandible, midface (maxillae, zygomata, nasal bones, and orbits), and

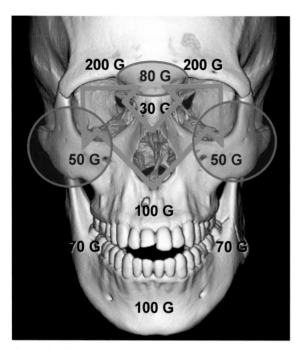

Figure 7.1 Force required to fracture. (Low G forces: nasal bones < zygoma < nasal bridge. High G forces: maxilla < supraorbital. Low and high G forces: frontal bone.)

the upper face or frontal bone. The likelihood of death from neurologic injury is lowest for mandible fractures and highest for frontal fractures.[7]

Prehospital

Most serious injuries to the face are associated with concomitant trauma to other organ systems. The trauma to the face may be immediately evident and may be quite distracting secondary to impressive bleeding or the disfiguring nature of the injury. Facial trauma, however, is rarely an immediate threat to life unless airway compromise occurs. If significant facial deformities endanger the airway (e.g., segmental mandible fracture with the tongue and soft tissues falling posteriorly into the hypopharynx and obstructing the airway), early intubation is strongly recommended. If intubation is not in the local emergency medical services protocol, then an oral airway, bag-valve-mask (BVM), laryngeal mask airway, or combination tube may be acceptable alternatives. Though cervical spine precautions must be maintained, there is no contraindication to performing jaw thrust or applying a BVM with pressure on a patient with presumed facial fractures. There is, however, a relative contraindication to nasal intubation in patients with significant trauma to

the head and face. Because skull base fractures may be present, a nasal trumpet or endotracheal tube passed through the nose could potentially pass into the cranial vault and penetrate the meninges and brain. Due to this extremely rare but reported complication, it is generally advised to avoid placing a nasal airway in patients with significant facial trauma in the prehospital setting.

If significant intraoral or nasal hemorrhage is present, placing the patient in a cervical collar on a backboard may endanger the airway by funneling bleeding down the airway. A patient with a gunshot wound or major blunt trauma to the mouth or midface can have copious bleeding from the lingual artery, facial artery, branches of the maxillary artery, or the internal carotid. In a supine patient, this bleeding will cause airway compromise or disordered oxygenation before hemorrhagic shock develops. Orotracheal intubation should be performed early if possible. Packing the oropharynx following intubation may decrease bleeding. Penetrating trauma to the face with a no spinal neurologic finding has an extremely low incidence of an unstable cervical spine. It may be necessary and appropriate to forgo spinal immobilization in order to allow for easier airway control.

In some instances, massive bleeding or disfiguring injury to the structures of the oropharynx and larynx will make intubation through the oro- or nasopharynx impossible. Unfortunately, these are the same patients in which oxygenation with a BVM device will be equally challenging. This situation may necessitate a field cricothyrotomy, which may be performed by trained personnel as a salvage procedure.

As with all trauma patients, the critical aspect of the prehospital management is rapid transport. As little time as possible should be spent at the scene, and the patient should be rapidly transported to the closest appropriate trauma center.

> **Box 7.2 Essential interventions**
>
> - Evidence of airway compromise; orally intubate (if in protocol).
> - Oxygenate all patients, oxygen (O_2) saturation should remain > 90%.
> - Obtain large-bore peripheral intravenous (IV) access.
> - Presume concomitant injuries to brain, spine, chest, and abdomen based on reasonable mechanism.
> - Board and collar.
> - Use direct pressure to control sources of significant hemorrhage.

Emergency department evaluation and management

Presentation

Severe

The patient with life-threatening facial fractures generally has a threat to the airway. A common cause would be a crush injury or blast injury to the mandible, resulting in loss of bony support for the tongue in a supine patient. Loss of the suspension support of the mandible allows the tongue to sag back into the posterior pharynx and obstruct the airway. Profuse bleeding from the oropharynx can result in airway compromise as well, particularly in open fractures with lacerations and gunshot wounds that transect a major artery, such as the facial artery or lingual artery. Bleeding directly from the well-vascularized face, if left unstaunched, may occasionally result in hemorrhagic shock. Dislocated teeth may be aspirated and cause airway obstruction at the level of the bronchial tree. Injuries directly to the eye can result in loss of vision. Secondary injuries to the eye – such as increased intraocular pressure and traction on the optic nerve – can result from facial trauma and may be a severe threat to vision.

Moderate

Facial fractures and severe lacerations can cause loss of normal facial contour and aesthetics, loss of function of the facial nerve or one of its branches, transection of the parotid duct, long-term loss or derangement of the nasal airway, and other morbidity.

Minor

The majority of injuries to the face are not life threatening and result in little morbidity. An avulsed tooth, an eyebrow laceration, or a nasal fracture will cause pain, inconvenience, and may have a negative impact on cosmesis. This may be lessened by expert closure of wounds and referral as necessary to facial plastics specialists.

Occult facial trauma is uncommon, though occult injuries may lie beneath seemingly routine trauma such as lacerations. Intoxicated or head injured patients may under-report their pain or may not be able to detect malocclusion of their teeth. Patients with serious injuries to the eye may have swelling impairing eye opening and examination, resulting in lack of recognition of a vision threatening injury. Another category of what might be considered "occult" in the setting of facial trauma is the true cause: the clinician should maintain a high index of suspicion for domestic violence in patients with facial trauma, particularly women, children, and the elderly.

Initial evaluation

Physical examination

The primary and secondary surveys should be performed. After threats to life have been addressed, particular attention should be paid to pupil reactivity, the intraoral examination including the teeth, the tympanic membranes, facial stability, and any significant sources of bleeding. Significant bleeding in the posterior pharynx may be present without any external evidence. A thorough neurologic evaluation of the face and eyes should be performed. A facial nerve injury may result in significant long-term morbidity. Failure to document facial nerve function prior to the debridement and closure of a complex facial laceration could contribute to significant medicolegal liability. The parotid duct should be identified and examined in the event of any severe cheek laceration. If a deep wound crosses the duct, consultation with facial plastics should be obtained to rule out ductal laceration or transection.

Studies

There are no emergent trauma room studies necessary for screening patients with isolated facial trauma. If the cervical spine cannot be clinically cleared, the patient should remain in a hard collar.

Acute interventions

Trauma patients frequently have altered mentation secondary to concomitant head injury or intoxication, so oro-pharyngeal bleeding may cause airway compromise as well as significant blood loss. Although the airway should be addressed by this point, continued suspicion, vigilance, and early intervention will prevent airway catastrophes. External bleeding should be controlled with pressure. Any posterior pharyngeal or oral bleeding should be addressed immediately as well. This may be achieved by direct pressure as an initial step. Endotracheal intubation followed by oro- and/or naso-pharyngeal packing, or emergent interventional radiology for embolization or surgery to stop the bleeding may be neccesary.

Table 7.1 Focused history in facial trauma

Questions to ask victims of facial trauma	Screening for what injury?
Have you had any change in vision? Is there any change in your color vision?	Retrobulbar hematoma, hyphema, perforated globe, retinal detachment, optic nerve injury
Does it hurt when you move your eyes? Do you see double?	Orbital wall fractures, extraocular muscle entrapment, retrobulbar hematoma
Can you breathe, speak, and swallow normally?	Laryngeal injuries, tracheal injuries, blood, teeth or foreign bodies in the airway
Can you open your jaw all the way?	Mandible fractures
Is anywhere on your face feeling numb?	Peripheral nerve injuries
Do your teeth come together okay?	Mandible, maxilla, or alveolar ridge fracture
Are any teeth you had when you woke up this morning missing now?	Missing teeth, possibly aspirated
How is your hearing?	Traumatic ear injury or basilar skull fracture

Secondary evaluation

History

For all facial trauma other than superficial lacerations or contusions, a focused history should be obtained. Careful questioning can be used to identify any functional derangement.

This history is intended to be highly sensitive, rather than specific, for detecting facial injuries that may require intervention. For example, many patients without mandible fracture will have masseter spasm that causes trismus. Patients with simple periorbital hematomas may report blurred vision. The goal is to identify areas to focus on in the physical exam for further clinical and radiographic evaluation.

Physical exam

Inspection

The clinician should visually inspect the face, making note of lacerations, areas of asymmetry, dislodged teeth, and foreign bodies. Pay particular attention to the eyes and the oropharynx. Use the history to focus your exam (Table 7.1). If the injury is the result of an impact with glass, or a retained foreign body, duct or nerve laceration may exist. If the patient reports a loss of vision in the one eye, the majority of the exam should be focused on detailing the nature of the injury e.g., floaters, field cut, etc.

Palpation

Palpate the bony protuberances of the forehead, the orbital rims, the zygomata, the maxillae, the mandible (including the temporamandibular joints), and the teeth. Note areas of tenderness, crepitus, and bony deformity. Contusions will often result in significant hematoma and swelling because the tissues are well-vascularized. Patients tend to report tenderness at any area of swelling or bruising. The clinician should make an attempt to palpate the underlying bones *without* palpating the tender area of skin over it where possible. For example, a patient with a swollen, tender superior orbital rim might respond to palpation of the area with significant pain. Apply upward traction to the skin of the forehead, drawing the tender area superiorly off of the orbital rim. The rim may be palpated from below – essentially palpating through the tissue of the superior eyelid – without the confounder of whether the tenderness is secondary to the soft tissue injury or an underlying bony injury. A similar approach may be used for the anterior maxillary wall and anterior aspect of the zygoma by palpating the bones through the oral cavity rather than through facial edema.

Soft tissue edema may obscure exam of nasal bones, frontal bones, maxilla, and orbits.

Neurologic exam of the face

Perform a motor exam of cranial nerves 3, 4, 5, 6, and 7. Evaluate for conjugate eye movements in all cardinal directions and check sensory function by using a cotton swab lightly brushed on the forehead, cheek, and jaw on both sides of the face. Compare the strength of the injured side to the uninjured side, understanding however that asymmetry may exist

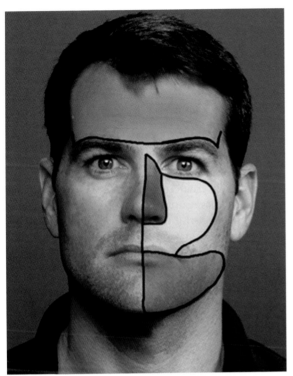

Figure 7.2 Distribution of the infraorbital nerve (yellow), supraorbital nerve (red), anterior ethmoidal nerve (brown), and mental nerve (blue). (From Burton J, Miner J. *Emergency Sedation and Pain Management.* Cambridge: Cambridge University Press, 2008.)

simply because of swelling rather than nerve injury. Certain tasks, such as pursing the lips and puffing out the cheeks, may be impossible secondary to lacerations, pain, or edema. Perform a sensory exam on the three branches of the trigeminal nerve. Next, evaluate the sensation of the distribution of the infraorbital nerve, supraorbital nerve, and inferior alveolar nerve (cranial nerve 5). Injuries to these nerves may occur in direct trauma as well as secondary to nerve compression in the setting of fractures to the inferior orbital rim, superior orbital rim, or mandible respectively (Figure 7.2).

Midface stability

Assess the midface by palpation. Note any crepitus or deformity. Grasp the nasal bone between the thumb and index finger of one hand while grasping the hard palate between the thumb and index finger of the other hand. The patient may have pain or palpable laxity to anterior and posterior and lateral movement if Le Fort type fractures are present.

Oral exam

Have the patient open his mouth as far as possible. The clinician will need to seek an explanation for the cause of any patient who can not open his mouth to three finger breadths. A cervical collar may impede jaw opening, so testing may need to be performed with the collar briefly opened and the cervical spine manually stabilized, or when the spine has been cleared. Ask the patient to bite down firmly and assess for malocclusion. Open the mouth again and inspect the oral cavity with adequate, focal lighting. An operating room light in a trauma bay, an otoscope without a speculum, headlight, or a flashlight may be used for lighting. Evaluate for dislodged or missing teeth. If a tooth has been avulsed and remains in the oro- or hypo-pharynx, it should be removed with forceps and the socket should be identified. Even if the tooth has been avulsed for up to an hour, it may still remain viable because saliva is an excellent medium for the preservation of avulsed teeth. Place the tooth into milk or Hanks balanced salt solution (HBSS) until it can be reimplanted. Grasp or tap each tooth individually to check for tenderness or laxity within the socket.

Evaluate for lacerations of the tongue or oral mucosa. Use suction to facilitate the exam if bleeding obstructs the view. Perform a full sweep of the buccal mucosa, gingival mucosa, and all sides of the tongue searching for abraded tissue and lacerations. Some lacerations of the buccal mucosa will essentially fall back together and appear as if they are only superficial abrasions or avulsions of the mucosa. Place traction on the wound edges to evaluate for a true laceration. If there is an external facial laceration lying over an abraded or lacerated area inside the mouth, a cotton swab or the tip of a hemostat can be passed through the external portion after the wound is anesthetized. If the swab or clamp enters the oral cavity, a through-and-through laceration is present. A significant error in the management of peri-oral lacerations is the failure to recognize that they communicate intraorally. A through-and-through laceration of the lip or cheek that is treated as a superficial laceration with a one layer closure is a higher risk for infection. Poor cosmetic outcome or functional deficit such as prolonged drooling or altered speech may be a consequence.

Mandibular exam

Again, evaluate for trismus. Palpate the jaw from the temporomandibular joint to the chin. Place a finger in the external canal of the ear and palpate anteriorly as the patient opens and closes his jaw, checking for instability or tenderness of the mandibular condyle. Stress the jaw by manipulating with both hands and applying traction. In a patient with jaw pain and no evidence of instability or malocclusion, perform the tongue-blade test to evaluate for fracture. The tongue blade is inserted lengthwise into the mouth between the upper and lower molars on one side of the mouth. The patient then bites down on the tongue blade forcefully. The patient then twists the tongue blade until it breaks and comes apart. If pain or malocclusion prevents the patient from successfully gripping of the tongue blade on both sides, then further evaluation of the mandible with radiologic studies is required. This test has high, but not perfect reported sensitivity, so if there is a high clinical suspicion with a negative test, further imaging is appropriate.[8] Low suspicion can probably rule out a mandible fracture with a normal test. It may not be appropriate in intoxicated or altered patients. Clinical judgment must be used.

Test for numbness of the lips or gums to evaluate for injury to the inferior alveolar nerve.

Orbital and eye exam

Examine the eye without placing any pressure on the globe itself. If significant periorbital swelling exists, the clinician must gently open the eyelids using eyelid retractors without applying pressure to the eye. These retractors are comprised of a loop of smooth material, such as plastic or aluminum, with eyelid restraining blades positioned on opposite sides. A common quick substitute may be a bent paperclip, although this is not optimal if a formal retractor is available. The metal in the clip can flake off into the eye and cause an abrasion, so care must be taken when bending. Evaluate for ex- or enophtholmos. Perform visual acuity testing. Test each eye individually and both eyes together. This can be performed with a handheld Snellen eye chart in a supine trauma patient in a cervical collar. Test the extraocular muscle function to evaluate for cranial nerve 3, 4, or 6 injury or extra-ocular muscle entrapment. Test sensation around the eye to assess the infraorbital and supraorbital nerves. Palpate the bones about the eye and along the medial canthus. Lacerations over the medial canthus or between the medial canthus and the nasal bone may cause injury to the nasolacrimal duct, so explore these injuries thoroughly and evaluate the duct. In the setting of blunt trauma, tenderness over the medial canthus, or excessive epiphora may indicate medial orbital wall fracture or duct injury. Fluoroscein staining, intraocular pressure testing, and slit-lamp exam should be performed when practical. Perform a visual field exam to evaluate for traumatic retinal tears. Ophthalmologic consultation is required for full fundoscopic examination if retinal detachment is suspected.

Ear exam

Inspect the entire external ear including auricle, pinna, and external auditory canal. Lacerations and avulsions of tissue are common on the ear, and they may go undetected if they are on the posterior aspect of the pinna. Evaluate the architecture of the ear and compare it to the contralateral side. If it is focally swollen, if it has purple discoloration, or the ridges of underlying cartilage are indistinct, a subperichondral hematoma may be present. These subperichondral fluid collections will be tender on palpation and may feel either tense or fluctuant. Evaluate the tympanic membrane for laceration, rupture, or hemotympanum, which may be present in basilar skull fractures.

Diagnostic studies
Labs

Laboratory values are not useful in the evaluation of facial trauma, with the exception of screening for blood loss or concomitant illness or injury. The clinician should order appropriate laboratory studies based on the suspicion for multisystem trauma or need for urgent operative repair. In a patient with facial injuries in whom significant bleeding is suspected, a complete blood count may be sufficient.

Plain films

Historically, plain films of the face were the initial radiographic modality. With the increased availability of CT scanning, however, plain films are much less commonly used.

Computed tomography

The discussion regarding CT in facial trauma has evolved from the question of whether CT scanning or plain films of the face should be ordered to what kind of CT is required and on whom (Figure 7.3).

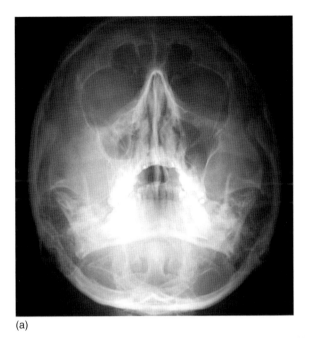

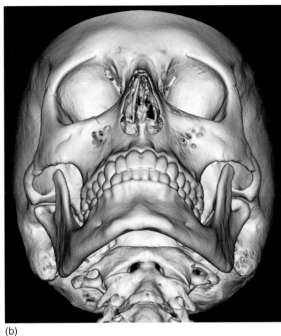

(a) (b)

Figure 7.3 (a) Radiograph of facial bones and (b) reconstruction of facial bones (with permission).

Computed tomography scanning is the test of choice in facial trauma. It has both superior sensitivity and specificity over plain films, and it allows better preoperative planning. There are two challenges for the clinician, however, regarding CT scans in facial trauma. The first is deciding which minimally injured facial trauma victims need CT scanning of the face. The second is deciding if a non-contrast head CT alone, rather than dedicated thin-slice facial CT, is sufficient in patients suspected of having multisystem trauma. A non-contrast CT is a relatively quick and simple way to screen for fractures, whereas contrast CT is preferred for more complete and detailed examination assessing soft tissue, blood vessels, and other fluid collections such as an abscess.

For many years, panoramic views (Panorex®) of the mandible were considered the best modality for the evaluation for mandible fractures.[9] More recently, coronal CT has been found to have superior accuracy in the evaluation of mandible fractures over panoramic plain films, mandible series, and axial CT.[10] Coronal CT has improved sensitivity over plain films for fractures of the mandibular condyle.[11] In one recent study, the sensitivity of helical CT was 100% in diagnosing mandibular fractures; this compared with 86% for panoramic tomography, in which significantly more fractures were missed.[12] Helical CT has also been found to have enhanced imaging quality, excellent sensitivity in identification of fractures, decreased interpretation error, and greater interphysician agreement in the identification of mandible fractures.[13]

A recent study found 100% sensitivity and negative predictive values of a negative non-enhanced head CT scan when screening for fractures. The authors found a negative non-enhanced head CT scan precludes the need for a dedicated facial bone or orbital CT scan in the evaluation for orbital, maxillary, or zygomatic fractures.[14] Contradicting this result is a more recent study that showed that 12% of trauma patients requiring head CT had facial fractures, and that orbital fractures may be missed on the screening head CT. Most of these missed fractures however were nasal fractures. Significant facial trauma seemed to be an indicator of underlying facial fractures.[15] For that reason, many clinicians opt for dedicated facial CT in addition to a non-contrast head CT in obtunded or multiply injured trauma patients.

Some research has been done regarding using the physical exam to guide whether dedicated facial CT scanning is required in trauma patients already receiving a head CT. Lacerations occurring in areas of the lips, nose, and intraorally, as well as wounds leading to periorbital contusion and subconjunctival hemorrhage, have been found to increase the odds of finding underlying fracture.[16] Conversely, scalp lacerations and scalp contusions were significantly higher in the non-fracture group.

Magnetic resonance imaging

Recently, magnetic resonance imaging (MRI) has begun to take on a role in the grading of severity of dento-alveolar trauma, particularly for preoperative planning.[17] The MRI may be used in a severe condylar fracture to evaluate for hemarthrosis and capsular tear.[17,18] However, because MRI does not image bone as well as CT, it plays a minor role in the evaluation of acute facial trauma. In addition, the practicality of obtaining MRI may also be challenging. Computed tomography of the face has better sensitivity and is superior in identifying and grading facial fractures[19]; therefore, MRI is rarely pertinent to the emergency department (ED) management of facial trauma.

Angiography

Life-threatening hemorrhage from facial trauma is rare. The initial approach to these injuries should be pressure, packing, volume replacement, and correction of coagulopathy. If bleeding continues, angiography is the best approach to both characterize and treat severe bleeding from facial trauma.[20,21] Once the interventionalist has identified the source of bleeding, selective embolization may be performed in an attempt to control it (Figure 7.4).

Regardless of the imaging modality chosen, maintain a high degree of suspicion for airway obstruction in order to avoid disastrous consequences which can occur while the patient is being scanned.

Specific injuries

Lacerations

Face

The face presents some unique challenges because of the intricate musculature and the dense vascularization and innervation. Pay particular attention to the identification of injuries to underlying structures, such as the parotid duct or facial nerve. Debride any small areas of devitalized tissue and remove all foreign bodies. Irrigate the wound. Close any lacerations through the facial musculature with deep sutures to repair the defect. If this is not done, poor cosmesis results for two reasons. First, a depressed, elevated or even pigmented scar may appear at the site of the wound; second, active facial expressions will exacerbate the defect with further dimpling. Facial lacerations may be closed up to 24 hours after the event, if an acceptable level of wound cleanliness can be achieved. Extremely dirty wounds and wounds left open for > 24 hours generally require delayed primary closure, healing by secondary intent, or other facial plastic management.

Peri-oral

The key to insuring a good cosmetic outcome in peri-oral lacerations, as with any facial laceration, is to restore the tissue architecture working from the "bottom of the hole" up to the skin. If the underlying muscle, such as the orbicularis oris is lacerated, close it tightly with 5–0 Vicryl® or similar absorbable suture. Take tension off of the skin edges by placing an intermediate depth or subcuticular layer of sutures, making sure to close any potential space that would remain. At this point of the closure, the wound should be well aligned without any significant gaping at the edges. Then the skin may be closed with small bites of a non-absorbable monofilament suture, such as 6–0 nylon or a synthetic non-absorbable polypropylene suture, to essentially fine-tune the horizontal and vertical alignment of the wound and slightly evert the edges.

Consider all lacerations to the lips or cheeks to have a high likelihood of communicating with the oral cavity. Conduct a thorough search of the oral cavity to insure that the laceration is not through and through. If a laceration is present on the cheek and another laceration is present in the same vicinity inside the mouth, use traction to investigate for a communicating tract. The clinician can also pass a cotton swab or hemostat through the laceration to see if it enters the mouth. If the instrument does not enter the oral cavity, ask the patient to keep their lips tightly sealed while the wound is irrigated with normal saline. If the patient detects a salty taste in the mouth during irrigation, then the wound communicates with the oral cavity. After ample anesthesia is achieved, through-and-through lacerations should be closed as described in Box 7.3.

These wounds are at risk of infection. The goal in using this method is to avoid contamination of the wound with intraoral contents. Through-and-through lacerations may require either a three layer (buccal mucosa, deep, and skin) or a four-layer (buccal

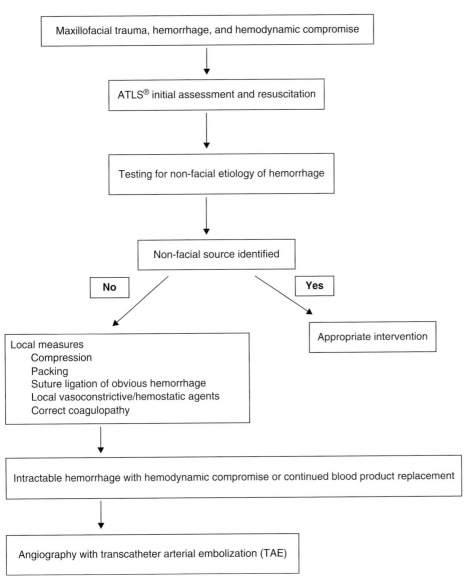

Figure 7.4 Algorithm for management of life-threatening bleeding from facial trauma (From Bynoe RP, Kerwin AJ, Parker HH, et al. Maxillofacial injuries and life-threatening hemorrhage: treatment with transcatheter arterial embolization. *J Trauma* 2003;**55**(1):77.)

Box 7.3   Closure of through-and-through facial lacerations

1. Place traction on the cheek or lip to expose the intraoral wound.
2. Irrigate the wound from first the buccal surface and then the skin surface.
3. If exposure is inadequate a rolled sterile 4 × 4 between the gingival surface and the area to be sewn may improve the view.
4. Close the intraoral portion with assistant providing proper exposure. Use 5–0 Vicryl® sutures and make the closure water tight. Burying the knot may allow for a more comfortable closure.
5. Change to a new suture kit and new sterile gloves.
6. Reirrigate the wound.
7. Close the wound from the outside in as you would any other non-through-and-through facial laceration, i.e., closing the muscle then skin.

mucosa, muscle layer, dermal, and skin) closure. Though it is controversial, many specialists will place the patient on a prophylactic three day course of antibiotics, such as penicillin or clindamycin, to reduce the risk of infection. A recent analyses looking at this question found few investigations adequately studied the question. Generally, it was felt that for through-and-through wounds there may be a benefit, but the number needed to treat is considerable. The downsides of antibiotics were not adequately studied. There is no absolute answer, and clinical judgment as well as patient and provider preference must be used.[22]

Lacerations of the lips require special attention. The lip itself is composed of an epidermal layer, fatty soft tissue, small salivary glands, the labial artery, the orbicularis oris muscle, and the inner labial mucosa. Close them as described above for through-and-through facial lacerations, with a couple of adjustments in technique. If the lip is "split," i.e., cut through the labial epidermis, muscle, and labial mucosa, the muscle layer should be closed first, then the labial mucosa, followed by the labial epidermis. The orbicularis oris is the sphincter muscle of the mouth. Failure to correct defects in it will result in asymmetry in the shape of the mouth. If the laceration passes through the epidermis of the face and the lip, crossing the vermillion border, realign the vermillion border with the first stitch placed. Then the lip mucosa should be closed with interrupted 5–0 or 6–0 Vicryl® with the knot buried. If nylon or synthetic polypropelene (e.g., Prolene) is used on the lip mucosa, the cut ends of the knot will irritate the tongue and the lips. If simple, rather than buried, knots are employed, the patient will worry the exposed knot with their tongue or habitually nibble on it until it loosens or unties. Complete the closure by suturing the facial skin portion with a non-absorbable suture as one would close any facial wound. Misalignment of important lip structures such as the oral commissure, vermilion borders, or nearby structures such the philtral columns may result in readily visible defects.

Parotid gland, parotid duct, and facial nerve

Injuries to the cheek cause damage to the skin and soft tissue; the deeper, functional structures are also at risk. The parotid gland and duct may be injured. The best time to evaluate is prior to repair of the open wound. The duct follows a line from the tragus to the corner of the mouth and any deep injury crossing this line is suspicious for causing damage to the parotid duct. One way to look for an injured duct is massaging the parotid gland while evaluating for saliva spilling from the severed proximal end of the duct. Cannulating Stenson's duct and papilla in the buccal mucosa opposite the second molar to look for the distal end in the wound is a more involved, definitive procedure, typically performed by facial plastic specialists. If possible, the duct can be anastamosed end-to-end over a stent by an otolaryngologist or facial plastic surgeon. Alternatively, the proximal end can be sutured directly to the papilla and stented open for several weeks. A surgeon may also repair the gland parenchyma as well as the capsule in order to prevent delayed sialocele. However, with any work in and around the parotid gland and duct one must be very careful not to damage the branches of the facial nerve; indiscriminate suturing, cautery, traction, and clamping should be avoided. For the facial nerve, proximal damage creates significant functional loss. For example, lacerations medial to the lateral canthus of the eye may damage the distal branches, whose fine threads are typically unrepairable. However, the functional deficit is minimal. Damage lateral to the lateral canthus can damage the main trunk of the facial nerve, creating motor loss in several branches. This causes a large functional deficit. Primary anastamosis or nerve cable grafting would be required to re-establish continuity. For facial nerve injury as well as parotid gland and duct injury, the best time to explore is through the open wound and therefore, consultation with a facial plastic specialist should not be delayed. This is especially true for facial nerve injury as significant neuromuscular damage may begin within three days.

Ear, including canal

Lacerations to the ear frequently pass through the cartilage. Keep in mind three goals in closing these lacerations. First, the cartilage must be completely covered with skin; if necessary, trim back up to 3–4 mm of cartilage to guarantee that there is none exposed. Second, the perichondrium must be aligned on both sides of the cartilage for its blood supply to aid healing of the avascular cartilage. This can be effected either by taking full three-layer bites (skin, cartilage, skin) with a non-absorbable suture on both sides of the laceration, or by suturing the cartilage independently with absorbable suture and then closing both skin layers separately with non-absorbable skin sutures

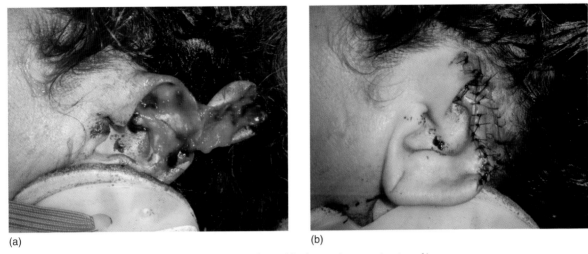

Figure 7.5 (a and b) Severely lacerated ear requiring significant debriding and reapproximation of layers.

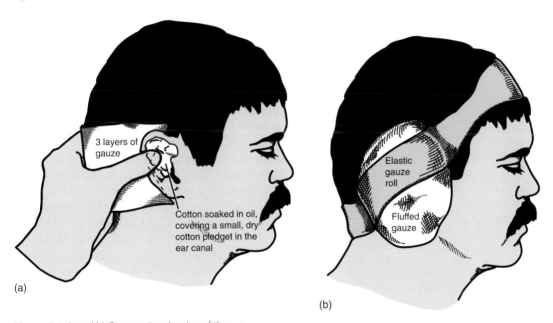

Figure 7.6 (a and b) Compression dressing of the ear.

(Figure 7.5). Third, a subperichondral hematoma must not be allowed to form. Place a compressive dressing over the ear as shown in Figure 7.6. Lacerations of the external canal should prompt a search for serious underlying causes. If they are the result of blunt trauma to the head, computed tomography should be performed to evaluate for basilar skull fracture. If lacerations to the canal are the result of direct trauma with an implement into the ear and are superficial, they may be treated conservatively with irrigation and updating tetanus vaccine without attempting closure. A small expandable cotton "wick" may be placed in the canal and antibiotic

drops applied to minimize the risk of otitis externa. Follow up with an otolaryngologist should be arranged to minimize the risk of canal stenosis.

Tongue

The tongue is composed primarily of muscle tissue that is extremely well vascularized, so lacerations may bleed profusely. Anesthetize the tongue initially by placing a 2 × 2 gauze soaked in 4% lidocaine with epinephrine over the wound for 5 minutes with the patient applying pressure. If inadequate anesthesia is achieved, then anesthesia may be injected directly

93

through the already partially anesthetized wound edge to achieve sufficient pain control. Do not exceed the recommended 5–7 mg/kg dosing for lidocaine with epinephrine, including the amount used in the initial topical stage. Injecting anesthetic directly into the tongue is extremely painful. Consider procedural sedation (especially in children) or a lingual nerve block for large lacerations requiring lengthy closure. Ketamine may be an excellent choice for procedural sedation. Through and through lacerations, lacerations > 1 cm involving the muscle, flaps, or deep lacerations involving the tongue edge (e.g., resulting in a forked tongue) require closure. If bleeding is the only indication for closure, superficial lidocaine with epinephrine and pressure may be sufficient. If bleeding continues, inject buffered lidocaine with epinephrine at the site. If the bleeding still does not resolve, silver nitrate sticks applied briefly to a small localized area may staunch it. If not, closure is indicated. Exposure of the wound is challenging. If the patient is sedated or the tip of the tongue is anesthetized, a towel clip or a 1–0 Prolene stitch may be used through the tip of the tongue to place traction on it for improved exposure. An assistant may be helpful, but neither the caregiver nor the assistant should place their fingers between the patients teeth until a bite block, such as a large roll of gauze between the maxillary and mandibular teeth on one side of the mouth, is in place. Close lacerations to the tongue with 3–0 or 4–0 absorbable suture and large bites of tissue. Start with the inferior mucosa and muscle layer, proceed to the superior mucosa and muscle layer, and finally, close the tip or edge with large bites as well. A buried knot may improve patient comfort.

Dental injuries

With sufficient traumatic forces applied, the teeth may be subluxed, avulsed, or fractured. Associated injuries may include alveolar ridge fracture, mandible, or maxillary fracture, as well as facial or oral laceration.

Concussion or minor subluxation (loosening) of the teeth does not require specific treatment. Concussion is characterized by tenderness to tap but no laxity. If a tooth has a minor amount of laxity in its socket on exam, soft foods, pain control, gentle chewing, and referral to a dentist are sufficient treatment. Splinting or extraction is not necessary. Depending on the findings, the dentist may place a mechanical block on neighboring teeth to prevent occlusion directly on the injured tooth.

Significant subluxation indicates tears to the attachment apparatus and carries a significant risk of pulp and tooth necrosis. Subluxations are described by the direction in which they occur: intrusive, extrusive, or lateral. Fractures either of the base of the tooth or the alveolar bone at the point of attachment are relatively common. There are two options for management: (1) a dentist or oral surgeon may be consulted to see the patient in the ED; or (2) the clinician caring for the patient may reposition the tooth in anatomic alignment and splint the tooth using common periodontal dressing, such as Coe-Pak.

Reimplantation needs to occur rapidly to be successful. Decidual or "baby teeth" do not require reimplantation. The likelihood of successful reimplantation degrades significantly with time. If a tooth has been dislodged (or partially dislodged) from its socket for more than 6 hours, even if it has been properly stored, successful implantation is extremely unlikely. The goal is to maintain the viability of the periodontal ligament in avulsed teeth. They should be stored either in the patient's mouth (held under the tongue), in Hanks' solution, or in milk until they can be reimplanted. Manipulate them as little as possible. Rinse them gently with saline. Do not scrub or mechanically attempt to debride them if soiled. After performing a dental block, rinse out the socket gently to remove clot and debris. Be cognizant not to disrupt the remaining periodontal ligament. The tooth or teeth are repositioned into proper anatomic position and then a rapidly curing periodontal dressing, such as Coe-Pak or other commercially available products, is applied. The periodontal dressing is rolled into a malleable cylinder long enough to extend two teeth in each direction beyond the affected tooth or teeth. It is then molded over the top of the teeth down, including both the internal and external surfaces of the teeth, even extending down over the gingiva to provide stability. It is allowed to harden with the patient's mouth open. This approach will temporarily stabilize the teeth until dental or oral surgery consultation can be obtained.

Dental fractures are a common occurrence. Up until recently, emergency medicine textbooks commonly referred to the Ellis classification for tooth fractures. This simple system is divided by what layers of tooth are involved. An Ellis I fracture goes through the enamel only. An Ellis II fracture goes through enamel and dentin. An Ellis III fracture is characterized by pulp involvement. Unfortunately, dentists and oral surgeons may be unfamiliar with the Ellis classification system and generally use a different system.[23]

Table 7.2 Overview of dental fractures[24]

Category	Description	Management
Enamel infraction	Incomplete fracture of the enamel without loss of tooth substance	Routine dental follow up.
Enamel fracture	Fracture with loss of tooth substance confined to the enamel	Routine dental follow up.
Enamel–dentin fracture (also called uncomplicated crown fracture)	Fracture including enamel and dentin but not pulp	Cover with calcium hydroxide or glass ionomer cement. Dental follow up within 24 hours.*
Complicated crown fracture	Fracture involving enamel, dentin, and pulp	Cover with calcium hydroxide or glass ionomer cement. Same day or within 8–12 hours dental follow up.*
Uncomplicated crown–root fracture	Fracture involving enamel, dentin, and cementum, but not the pulp	Cover with calcium hydroxide or glass ionomer cement. Dental follow up within 24 hours.*
Complicated crown–root fracture	Fracture involving enamel, dentin, cementum, and pulp	Cover with calcium hydroxide or glass ionomer cement. Same day or within 8–12 hours dental follow up.*
Root fracture	Fracture involving dentin, cementum, and pulp	Cover with calcium hydroxide or glass ionomer cement. Same day or within 8–12 hours dental follow up.*

*Note. A dentist or oral surgeon may be consulted to see the patient at the emergency department clinician's discretion, or if urgent follow up is unavailable.

Use this terminology to facilitate communication with consultants (Table 7.2).[24]

The clinician should manage fractures to the teeth based on whether dentin or pulp is exposed. If the fracture goes through only the smooth, white enamel, then no treatment is necessary in the ED. Refer the patient to a dentist for smoothing of any sharp or unsightly edges as needed. If the dentin – the yellow-tinged, porous material which contributes most of the volume of the tooth – is exposed, then place a commercially available calcium hydroxide coating over the cleaned and dried fracture surface. Exposed pulp, which is made up of the tooth's nerve and blood supply, appears pink or bloody at the fracture surface. This is extremely painful and usually requires anesthesia prior to any further manipulation. It must be covered with a calcium hydroxide coating after cleaning and drying it well. The porous dentin and the pulp are subject to inflammation and infection if exposed to saliva and oral flora. Frequently, tooth necrosis occurs as a result of these injuries and

extraction or root canal is necessary. Follow up within 24 hours with a dentist or oral surgeon is required.

If it appears that teeth in series are dislodged, then examine gingiva and alveolar ridge at the base of the teeth closely. If the teeth appear to be in their sockets, but they move as a set when grasped and gently shaken, then an alveolar ridge fracture is present. Alveolar ridge fractures often result in tooth necrosis or ankylosis. Consult an oral surgeon to evaluate the patient in the ED.

Facial fractures
Nasal fractures

Nasal bone fracture is the most common facial fracture. The nasal bones project out from the surface of the maxillae and therefore often receive direct, isolated trauma. The skin overlying the bones is thin and has no underlying musculature. Forces are transmitted efficiently to the relatively thin and weak nasal bone. Associated injuries may include maxillary or orbital fractures, dental fractures, or septal hematoma.

Table 7.3 Reduction of a nasal fracture

1. Instill 3–5 cc of viscous lidocaine gel into each nare, being careful not to exceed the patient's weight-based lidocaine dosing

2. Give the patient an appropriate dose of a short-acting parenteral pain medication, such as fentanyl. Perform a nasal block with lidocaine from the nasion running a wheal inferolaterally toward the nasolabial fold on each side

3. Wrap 2 needle drivers in kerlex or 4 × 4 gauze (may also use scalpel handles)

4. Gently introduce the wrapped needle drivers or scalpel handles into the nares and slide them up until they gently rest against the internal mucosa underlying the nasal bones

5. Briefly apply upward and/or lateral pressure to the depressed or deviated area. This should be performed rapidly (2–3 s) because it is a profound noxious stimulus

Patients present with nose pain and may have swelling, inability to breathe through the nose, and epistaxis. Exam findings include swelling, deviation, tenderness, and crepitus. Always check inside the nose and the oropharynx in a patient with suspected nasal fracture. Introduce a nasal speculum gently into both nares (Table 7.3). Evaluate the patient for a septal hematoma, which is a subperichondral blood collection that appears as a purple lump or deviation of the septum. This fluid must be drained or the patient is at risk for either seeding of the hemotoma and bacterial infection, or avascular necrosis of the nasal septum from loss of the perichondral blood supply. Saddle nose deformity may result.

To drain the nasal septal hematoma, incise the perichondrium over the blood collection. If the hematoma is acute, it will drain as soon as it is incised. Suction may be required. If the hematoma is more than 6–8 hours old, it may be coagulated. The clinician should gently milk the clot out. After evacuating the blood, irrigate gently with saline. The nare should then be packed to prevent reaccumulation of blood and to maintain the perichondrium in close proximity to the septum and facilitate healing. The patient should be placed on prophylactic antibiotics, such as amoxicillin or trimethoprim–sulfamethoxazole to cover routine sinus flora, for 48 hours. After 48 hours, the patient should return to the ED or an otolaryngologist for packing removal and re-examination.

Most isolated nasal fractures may be diagnosed clinically. Plain radiographs are unlikely to add clinically useful information. If there is suspected concomitant midface and orbital fractures, CT scanning is the test of choice (Figure 7.7).

Reduction of the nasal fracture is possible in the ED, but the clinician may decide to defer reduction

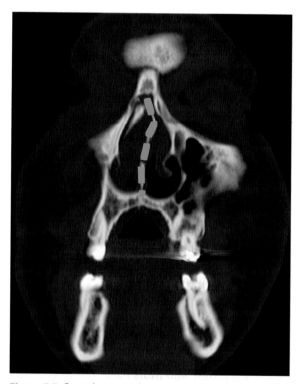

Figure 7.7 Coronal computed tomography (CT) showing nasal bone fracture.

until the patient is seen by an otolaryngologist. Edema of the nasal soft tissues may increase over the first 48 hours and thereby limit the ability to accurately reduce the fracture. Waiting up to several weeks until the edema has resolved is an acceptable plan for reducing nasal fractures.

Mandible fractures

Almost 50% of patients with facial fractures have fractures of the mandible,[22,25] making it the second

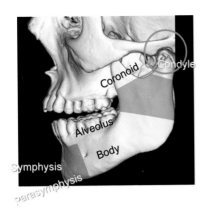

Figure 7.8
Mandible anatomy.

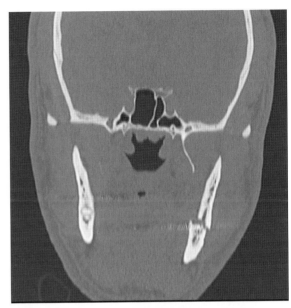

Figure 7.9 Fracture of left ascending ramus of mandible.

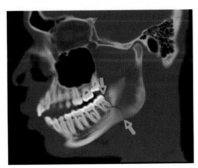

Figure 7.10 Open mandible fracture.

most common facial bone to be fractured. In decreasing order of frequency, fractures occur at the angle, body, condyle, symphysis, and ramus (Figure 7.8). Assault is the most common mechanism, followed by motor vehicle collisions, falls, and sporting accidents. Patients may complain of pain, malocclusion, inability to fully open the mouth, blood in the mouth, or even inability to breathe. Patients with altered mental status secondary to head trauma or intoxication may not report complaints localized to the jaw; a repeat exam when sober or stable is warranted.

The tongue-blade test is an excellent screening tool for mandibular fracture, and it has higher sensitivity than plain film series of the mandible. In the authors' opinion, a sober patient with a normal mental status exam who passes the tongue-blade test does not require imaging to evaluate for jaw fracture. Research has shown a very high sensitivity for the test and a normal test should only be followed by imaging with a high suspicion or severe pain (Figure 7.9).

If jaw fracture is diagnosed, the patient must be seen by a specialist who treats these fractures. This is commonly an oral-maxillofacial surgeon, otolaryngologist, or plastic surgeon. A dilemma in the ED is the timing of the consultation. If the patient can not maintain his or her airway when lying flat, cannot handle his or her own secretions, cannot handle oral intake of liquids or medications, or has inadequate pain control with oral medications, he or she must be admitted to the hospital for further treatment. Patients may also require admission if they have a poor social situation making follow-up treatment impossible. Many fractures are treated with immobilization by wiring the teeth of the maxilla to the teeth of the mandible. Open reduction and internal fixation is another common approach, depending on the location and type of fracture(s). A short-term (48 hour) course of antibiotics should be prescribed for open mandibular fracture (Figure 7.10) to prevent infections; however, this is not indicated for closed condylar fracture.[26]

Orbital fractures

Orbital wall fractures occur commonly in facial trauma. Fractures occur most often to the medial wall, followed by the orbital floor.[27] Serious injuries to the globe itself in blunt facial trauma causing orbital fractures occur commonly. In one recent study, the most common positive ocular finding in the presence of orbital wall fracture was *commotio retinae* (9%). This was followed in frequency by traumatic mydriasis (8%), and traumatic iritis (6%).[28] Other associated

97

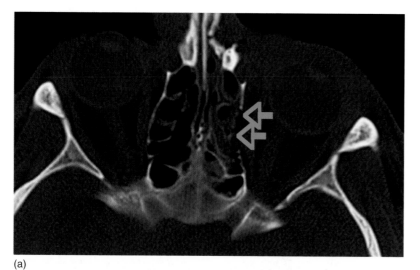

(a)

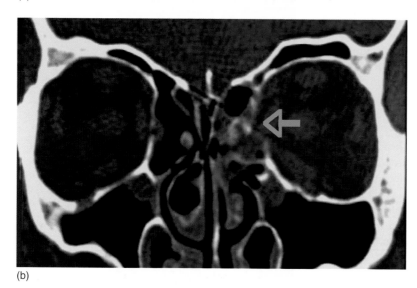

(b)

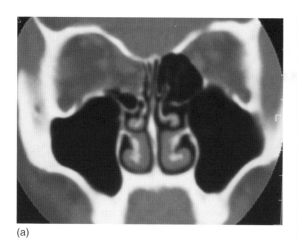

(a)

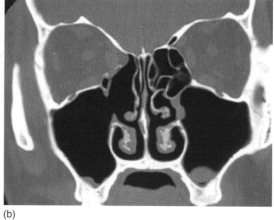

(b)

Figure 7.12 (a) Preoperative CT scan shows a large blowout fracture of the right medial orbital wall with herniation of orbital tissue. (b) CT scan taken at 8 weeks after surgery shows a well-reduced medial orbital wall. *Otolaryngol Head Neck Surg* 2007;**136**(1):38–44, with permission.

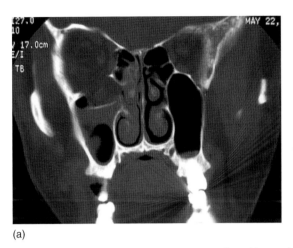 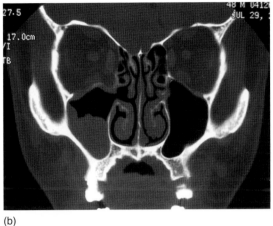

(a)   (b)

Figure 7.13 (a) Preoperative CT scan shows an inferior blowout fracture of the right orbit. (b) CT scan taken at two months after surgery shows a well-reduced orbital floor. *Otolaryngol Head Neck Surg* 2007;**136**(1):38–44, with permission.

injuries include ruptured globe, hyphema, and corneal abrasions and lacerations. Severe ocular injuries are associated with orbital apex fractures, lateral wall fractures, and Le Fort type III fractures.[29]

Patients may complain of diplopia or eye pain. On exam, the clinician may note enophthalmos, exophthalmos, tenderness over the medial canthus, or upward gaze palsy secondary to inferior rectus entrapment. These findings should prompt the order of a thin slice facial CT with reconstructions to characterize the fractures present and appropriately refer the patient for specialty follow up. Orbital wall fractures, even with inferior rectus muscle entrapment, rarely need emergent evaluation by an ophthalmologist or facial surgeon in the ED. Next day follow up is sufficient, unless there are other factors – such as concomitant ocular injury or inability to follow up for social or economic reasons – which mandate emergent management. For this reason, the emergency physician should perform a thorough eye exam, including papillary reactivity, visual acuity, visual fields, fluoroscein, and slit-lamp exam, on patients with orbital wall fractures. If a visual field defect is present, suspect a retinal detachment and consult ophthalmology to see the patient in the ED.

In follow up, visual acuity, ocular motility, exophthalmometry, and forced duction is evaluated. Persistent diplopia, restriction of eye movement with CT evidence of extra-ocular muscle entrapment, or an enophtalmos of > 2 mm may be considered indications for surgery (Figures 7.11–7.14).[30]

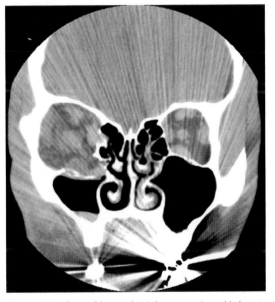

Figure 7.14 Severe blow to the right eye causing orbital contents to extrude into maxillary and ethmoid sinuses.

A special condition that requires immediate care is retrobulbar hematoma, which is the accumulation of blood behind the globe causing increased pressure and traction on the optic nerve. Symptoms may include eye pain, double vision, and blurred or obscured vision. Suspicious findings include exophthalmos, a sluggish or non-reactive pupil, decreased visual acuity, and increased intra-ocular pressure. Untreated, retrobulbar hematoma will lead

99

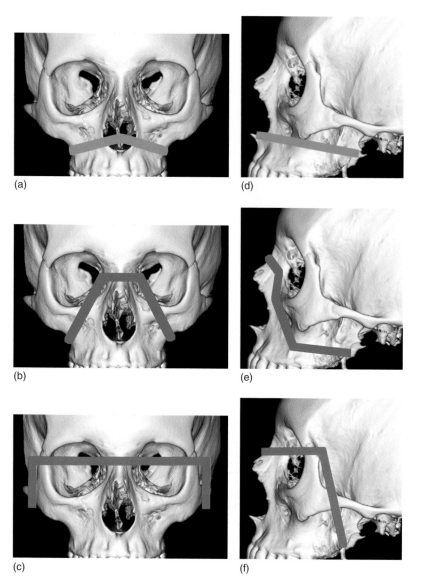

Figure 7.15 (a) Le Fort I fracture pattern. (b) Le Fort II fracture pattern. (c) Le Fort III fracture pattern. (d) Le Fort I lateral view. (e) Le Fort II lateral view. (f) Le Fort III lateral view.

to permanent vision loss in the affected eye. If this condition is suspected, the emergency physician should emergently consult ophthalmology and if not immediately available, perform a lateral canthotomy.

Midface fractures

Depending upon the direction of the trauma as well as the force applied, any of the bones of the midface may fracture causing functional and cosmetic defects. Anterior trauma may result in frontal, nasal, and maxillary fractures, including dental-alveoloar and the spectrum of Le Fort fractures. Lateral trauma may injure the zygomatic arch or temporal bone.

Maxillary and Le Fort fractures

Maxillary wall fracture is the most common midface fracture. The anterior, posterior, medial, and lateral maxillary walls may fracture. Fractures are usually detected on CT scan and findings may include directly visualized fractures or simply fluid in the maxillary sinus, possibly indicating bleeding from a non-visualized fracture. The absence of free paranasal sinus fluid after facial trauma is a highly reliable criterion to exclude fractures involving the paranasal sinus walls.[31] Maxillary fractures may disrupt innervation to the teeth or skin of the cheek, resulting in anesthesia. This may be temporary or permanent depending on type of injury to the nerve, but generally acute treatment is not performed. The clinician should evaluate for and document these deficits at the time of initial evaluation.

More extensive injuries are classified through the continuum of Le Fort I, II, and III injuries depending upon the level of the fracture line and the extent of injury.[32] Le Fort I fractures may result in a "floating palate," more extensive Le Fort II injuries usually run through parts of the orbit, whereas with the extensive Le Fort III injury, the entire facial skeleton may become detached from the cranial base (Figure 7.15).

Should the cribiform plate and dura mater become injured, then cerebrospinal fluid (CSF) rhinorrhea may be noted and must be treated accordingly. Similarly, longitudinal and transverse temporal bone fractures may also damage the dura of the middle or posterior cranial fossa resulting in CSF otorrhea. Research to date has not shown antibiotic prophylaxis to be effective with basilar skull fracture and its use cannot be supported nor completely refuted. It has not been conclusively shown to prevent meningitis and it may select more resistant organisms. Isolated maxillary sinus fractures likewise have no evidence for the need or exclusion of antibiotics and local custom is usually followed.[33]

A *tripod fracture* is essentially a "floating cheekbone." The anterior wall of the maxilla is fractured in conjuction with the zygoma and the lateral orbital wall.

The zygoma comprises the underlying bony architecture for the upper cheek and lateral eye. Because of its superolateral positioning in the face, it is both extremely important to facial symmetry and commonly fractured. The zygoma may be fractured as part of a complex facial fracture or it may be an isolated fracture. Sixty percent of isolated zygomatic arch fractures are displaced or comminuted.[34] The minority of patients with non-displaced fractures may be managed conservatively without operative repair. Zygomatic arch fractures, which are part of a complex fracture pattern involving the bones to which it attaches, generally require operative repair, as do displaced or comminuted fractures. Patients with any zygomatic fracture other than an isolated linear non-displaced fracture must be referred to an otolaryngologist or facial plastic surgeon for evaluation and treatment. Without operative intervention, these fractures typically result in poor cosmetic outcomes. Paresis of the orbicularis oculi and zygomaticus muscles may occur as a result of fracture or operative repair. Also, injury to the zygomaticofacial branch

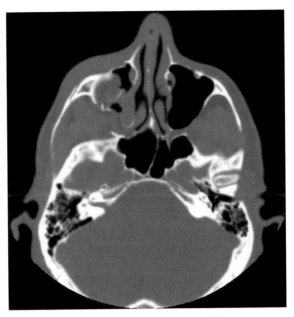

Figure 7.16 Maxillary computed tomography (CT) showing injury to right zygomatic arch (as well as fractures of right maxilla).

of the trigeminal nerve may result in sensory deficit over the prominence of the cheek (Figure 7.16).

A frequent fracture pattern is the tetrapod fracture. This fracture was formerly referred to as a tripod fracture, but it is better described as a tetrapod: the fracture involves the frontal, maxillary, and temporal articulation of the zygoma along with an orbital extension of the fracture pattern into the greater wing of the sphenoid (Figures 7.17 and 7.18).[31,32] This fracture requires operative treatment.

Frontal fractures

The frontal bone is thick and resistant to fracture. An impact of 200 times the force of gravity is required for fracture. Ten percent of patients with facial fractures have frontal bone fracture.[31,35] The clinician should consider any frontal bone fracture, excepting those that only involve the anterior wall of the frontal sinus, as a skull fracture and treat it as such. Evaluate the patient for intracranial and cervical spine injuries. Frontal bone fractures are associated with skull base fractures as well, and cerebrospinal fluid leak may complicate these injuries. Non-displaced fractures to the anterior wall of the frontal bone may be managed non-operatively, though management by an otolaryngologist or a facial plastic surgeon is optimal. If the fracture is significantly displaced or the frontal sinus is obliterated, the likelihood of complication

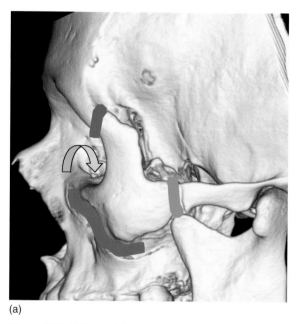

(a)

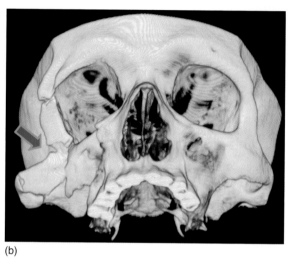

(b)

Figure 7.17 (a) Tetrapod fracture anatomy. Pink = maxilla; blue = frontal bone; green = arch of temporal bone; yellow = greater wing of sphenoid. (b) Zymagoticomaxillary fracture.

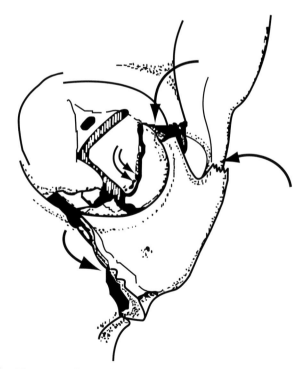

Figure 7.18 Zygoma-lateral orbital complex fracture. (From Zingg M, Laedrach K, Chen J, et al. Classification and treatment of zygomatic fractures. *J Oral Maxillofac Surg* 1992;**50**(8):79, with permission.)

Table 7.4 Overview of documentation in facial trauma

History: AMPLE (Allergies, medications, past medical history, last meal, and events leading up to the injury). Include any drug or alcohol abuse, as well as functional deficits

Physical: Include all cosmetic defects and functional deficits

Workup: Include all laboratory testing and radiographic studies

Therapies: Include intravenous fluids and medications given, as well as procedural sedation

Procedures: Include indication, timing, consent, and technical steps

Consultations: Include all services consulted, along with timing

Medical decision making: Include differential diagnosis and interpretation of results of history, physical, testing, and consultations

Patient instructions: Include what you told the patient to expect regarding functional and cosmetic outcomes, as well as medications prescribed and timing and service of follow up

Table 7.5 Disposition and transfer criteria

Consider admission*	Admission necessary
Open mandible fracture	Mandible fracture with inadequate pain control, difficulty breathing, or inability to manage secretions
Frontal bone or sinus fracture	Depressed frontal bone fracture or fracture through posterior wall of frontal sinus
Tetrapod or midface fractures requiring surgery	Midface crunch or multiple displaced fractures
Retrobulbar hematoma status post-drainage	Open globe
Extra-ocular muscle entrapment with double vision	–
Transfer criteria	
Concomitant injuries requiring trauma center management	–
Admission criteria above and no qualified surgeon available	–

*Please note possible admission and discharge criteria are usually based on the patient's characteristics, including comorbidities, ability to be observed, access to rapid follow-up, and symptomology.

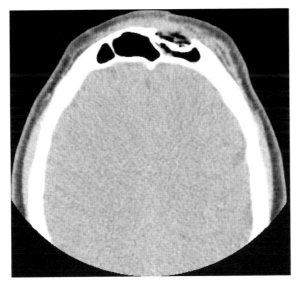

Figure 7.19 Depressed fracture of the anterior wall of frontal sinus caused by severe blow to forehead. Note the integrity of the posterior wall.

such as brain abscess, contour deformity, osteomyelitis, hematoma, meningitis, and mucocele increases (Tables 7.4 and 7.5; Figure 7.19).

> **Box 7.4 Essential ED interventions: facial fractures**
> - Intubation for altered mental status, airway collapse, or uncontrolled hemorrhage
> - General trauma management for possible multi-system trauma
> - Spinal immobilization
> - CT scan as diagnostic test of choice
> - Evaluate for concomitant injuries (especially intracranial, ocular, cervical, pulmonary)
> - Closure of lacerations

References

1. Alvi A, Doherty T, Lewen G. Facial fractures and concomitant injuries in trauma patients. *Laryngoscope* 2003;**113**(1):102–6.

2. Gassner R, Tuli T, Hächl O, et al. Cranio-maxillofacial trauma: a 10 year review of 9543 cases with 21067 injuries. *J Craniomaxillofac Surg* 2003;**31**(1):51–61.

3. Lalani Z, Bonanthaya KM. Cervical spine injury in maxillofacial trauma. *Br J Oral Maxillofac Surg* 1997;**35**(4):243–5.

4. Hackl W, Hausberger K and Sailer R, et al. Prevalence of cervical spine injuries in patients with facial trauma. *Oral Surg Oral Med Oral Pathol Oral Radiol Endod* 2001;**92**(4):370–6.

5. Pappachan B, Alexander M. Correlating facial fractures and cranial injuries. *J Oral Maxillofac Surg* 2006;**64**(7):1023–9.

6. Girotto JA, Mackenzie F, Fowler C, et al. Long-term physical impairment and functional outcomes after complex facial fractures. *Plast Reconstr Surg* 2001;**108**(2):312–27.

7. Plaisier BR, Punjabi AP, Super DM, et al. The relationship between facial fractures and death from neurologic injury. *J Oral Maxillofac Surg* 2000;**58**(7):708–12; discussion 12–13.

8. Malhotra R, Dunning J. The utility of the tongue blade test for the diagnosis of mandibular fracture. *Emerg Med J* 2003;**20**(6):552–3.

9. Moilanen A. Primary radiographic diagnosis of fractures in the mandible. *Int J Oral Surg* 1982;**11**(5):299–303.

10. Markowitz BL, Sinow JD, Kawamoto HK, Jr., et al. Prospective comparison of axial computed tomography and standard and panoramic radiographs in the diagnosis of mandibular fractures. *Ann Plast Surg* 1999;**42**(2):163–9.

11. Chacon GE, Dawson KH, Myall R, et al. A comparative study of 2 imaging techniques for the diagnosis of

103

condylar fractures in children. *J Oral Maxillofac Surg* 2003;**61**(6):668–72; discussion 73.

12. Wilson IF, Lokeh A, Benjamin CI, et al. Prospective comparison of panoramic tomography (zonography) and helical computed tomography in the diagnosis and operative management of mandibular fractures. *Plast Reconstr Surg* 2001;**107**(6):1369–75.

13. Roth FS, Kokoska MS, Awwad EE, et al. The identification of mandible fractures by helical computed tomography and panorex tomography. *J Craniofac Surg*, 2005;**16**(3):394–9.

14. Lewandowski RJ, Rhodes CA, McCarroll K, et al. Role of routine nonenhanced head computed tomography scan in excluding orbital, maxillary, or zygomatic fractures secondary to blunt head trauma. *Emerg Radiol* 2004;**10**(4):173–5.

15. Holmgren EP, Dierks EJ, Homer LD, et al. Facial computed tomography use in trauma patients who require a head computed tomogram. *J Oral Maxillofac Surg* 2004;**62**(8):913–18.

16. Holmgren EP, Dierks EJ, Assael LA, et al. Facial soft tissue injuries as an aid to ordering a combination head and facial computed tomography in trauma patients. *J Oral Maxillofac Surg* 2005;**63**(5):651–4.

17. Cohenca N, Simon JH, Roges R, et al. Clinical indications for digital imaging in dento-alveolar trauma. Part 1: traumatic injuries. *Dent Traumatol* 2007;**23**(2):95–104.

18. Gerhard S, Ennemoser T, Rudisch A, et al. Condylar injury: magnetic resonance imaging findings of temporomandibular joint soft-tissue changes. *Int J Oral Maxillofac Surg* 2007;**36**(3):214–18.

19. Sun JK, LeMay DR. Imaging of facial trauma. *Neuroimaging Clin N Am* 2002;**12**(2):295–309.

20. Ho K, Hutterb JJ, Eskridgec J, et al. The management of life-threatening haemorrhage following blunt facial trauma. *J Plast Reconstr Aesthet Surg* 2006;**59**(12):1257–62.

21. Bynoe RP, Kerwin AJ, Parker HH, 3rd, et al. Maxillofacial injuries and life-threatening hemorrhage: treatment with transcatheter arterial embolization. *J Trauma* 2003;**55**(1):74–9.

22. Mark DG, Granquist EJ. Are prophylactic oral antibiotics indicated for the treatment of intraoral wounds? *Ann Emerg Med* 2008;**52**(4):368–72.

23. Vinson DR. The Ellis fracture: an anachronistic eponym in dentistry. *Ann Emerg Med* 1999;**33**(5):599–600.

24. Andreasen JO, Andreasen FM. *Textbook and Color Atlas of Traumatic Injuries to the Teeth*, 3rd edn. St Louis: Mosby, 1994: pp. 151–5.

25. Ellis, E, 3rd. Treatment methods for fractures of the mandibular angle. *Int J Oral Maxillofac Surg* 1999;**28**(4):243–52.

26. Andreasen JO, Jensen SS, Schwartz O, et al. A systematic review of prophylactic antibiotics in the surgical treatment of maxillofacial fractures. *J Oral Maxillofac Surg* 2006;**64**(11):1664–8.

27. Burm JS, Chung CH, Oh SJ. Pure orbital blowout fracture: new concepts and importance of medial orbital blowout fracture. *Plast Reconstr Surg* 1999;**103**(7):1839–49.

28. He D, Blomquist PH, Ellis E, 3rd. Association between ocular injuries and internal orbital fractures. *J Oral Maxillofac Surg* 2007;**65**(4):713–20.

29. Read RW, Sires BS. Association between orbital fracture location and ocular injury: a retrospective study. *J Craniomaxillofac Trauma* 1998;**4**(3):10–15.

30. Jin HR, Shin SO, Choo MJ, et al. Endoscopic versus external repair of orbital blowout fractures. *Otolaryngol Head Neck Surg* 2007;**136**(1):38–44.

31. Lambert DM, Mirvis SE, Shanmuganathan K, et al. Computed tomography exclusion of osseous paranasal sinus injury in blunt trauma patients: the "clear sinus" sign. *J Oral Maxillofac Surg* 1997;**55**(11):1207–10; discussion 10–11.

32. Zingg M, Chowdhury K, Vuillemin T, et al. Treatment of 813 zygoma-lateral orbital complex fractures. New aspects. *Arch Otolaryngol Head Neck Surg* 1991;**117**(6):611–20; discussion 21–2.

33. Martin B, Ghosh A. Antibiotics in orbital floor fractures. *Emerg Med J* 2003;**20**(1):66.

34. Covington DS, Wainwright DJ, Teichgraeber JF, et al. Changing patterns in the epidemiology and treatment of zygoma fractures: 10-year review. *J Trauma* 1994;**37**(2):243–8.

35. Bell RB, Dierks EJ, Brar P, et al. A protocol for the management of frontal sinus fractures emphasizing sinus preservation. *J Oral Maxillofac Surg* 2007;**65**(5):825–39.

Chapter

8

Ocular trauma

Heather Mahoney

Introduction

Traumatic injuries to the eye may result in severe disability. After initial stabilization, a rapid eye evaluation can be performed to identify immediate threats to vision. A more thorough evaluation can be done after definitive management of other serious injuries.

The incidence in ocular injury has decreased in the past years due to intense focus on prevention including changes in the break patterns of windshields and requiring protective eye wear in the workplace. In 2005 6.98 per 1000 of the population experienced an eye injury in the United States requiring treatment. Rates were highest in white males in their twenties.[1,2]

A retrospective analysis done in the United Kingdom found a significant association between facial factures and ocular injury. In patients with major trauma, 2.3% of patients had associated ocular injury and 10.4% had a facial fracture. More importantly, the odds ratio of an eye injury in patients with facial fractures is 6.7. Almost 60% of ocular injuries were associated with motor vehicle collisions.[3]

> **Box 8.1 Essential information/highlights of ocular trauma**
>
> - Ocular injuries can lead to vision loss and should be considered in all major trauma, especially when the patient is unable to describe injuries.
> - Major trauma has been associated with ocular injury of 2.3%.
> - Ocular injuries are common and more prevalent in young white males.
> - Facial fractures significantly raise the likelihood of an ocular injury.

Relevant anatomy

The eye is a complex structure consisting of the globe and its accessory organs. Understanding the anatomy allows one to predict patterns of injury. The functions of the eyelids are: (1) to protect the anterior surface of the globe from local injury; (2) to assist with regulation of light reaching the eye; (3) to maintain tear film maintenance; and (4) to adjust tear flow by their pumping action on the conjunctival sac and lacrimal sac. The layers of the eyelids are composed of a thin skin outer layer (< 1 mm), eyelashes at the palpebral junction in rows of 2–3 follicles, orbicularis oculi skeletal muscle, tarsal plate, and the inner layer of palpebral conjunctiva contiguous with the fornix and bulbar conjunctiva (Figure 8.1). On the palpebral edge of the eyelid the tarsal plate extends beneath the orbicularis oculi muscles. The tarsal plate consists of a fibrous band of tissue about 29 mm long and about 1 mm thick which connects to the orbital septum. The orbital septum creates the anterior border of the intraorbital space. This septum has connection with the lid retractors (including the levator aponeurosis) and with the periosteum of the orbital rim superiorly and inferiorly. The medial and lateral canthus, two fibrous structures at the creases of the eyes, connect to the orbital septum. This fibrous meshwork maintains the intraorbital contents in position (Figure 8.2). With intraorbital bleeding this layer can be cut to release the pressure on the optic nerve. Posterior to the orbital septum there are fat pads in both eyelids and the lacrimal system in the lateral aspect of the upper eyelid. Disruption of the orbital septum and intraorbital penetration may be noted by visualization of the yellow fatty tissue in this layer or the pinkish tissue of the lacrimal system. The nasolacrimal ducts are in the medial palpebral crease of the eye and

Trauma: A Comprehensive Emergency Medicine Approach, eds. Eric Legome and Lee W. Shockley. Published by Cambridge University Press. © Cambridge University Press 2011.

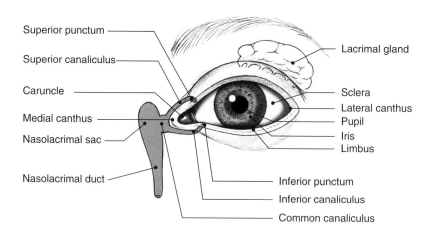

Superior punctum

Superior canaliculus

Caruncle

Medial canthus

Nasolacrimal sac

Nasolacrimal duct

Lacrimal gland

Sclera

Lateral canthus

Pupil

Iris

Limbus

Inferior punctum

Inferior canaliculus

Common canaliculus

Figure 8.1 Anterior view of the eye and adnexal structures. Lacrimal gland is situated superotemporally. The superior and inferior puncta drain into the canalicular system, which eventually empties into the nasal cavity. (From Mahadevan S, Garmel G. *An Introduction to Clinical Emergency Medicine.* Cambridge: Cambridge University Press, 2005.)

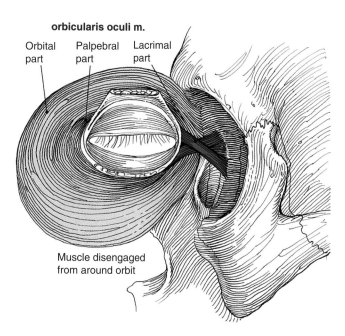

orbicularis oculi m.

Orbital part

Palpebral part

Lacrimal part

Muscle disengaged from around orbit

Figure 8.2 On the palpebral edge of the eyelid the tarsal plate extends beneath the orbicularis oculi muscles. (From Melloni J, Dox I, Melloni H, Melloni B. *Attorney's Reference on Human Anatomy.* Cambridge: Cambridge University Press, 2008.)

any injury in this area should alert the physician to potential disruption of this duct.

The orbital structures consist of the extraocular muscles, the globe, nerves, and vessels (Figure 8.3). Awareness of the attachments and identification of disruption can help predict injuries unable to be directly visualized. Any fractures of the orbit or increased pressure in the orbit can restrict the function of these muscles. The most commonly entrapped muscles in the orbit are the inferior rectus or inferior oblique after a "blowout" fracture. The outer cover of the eye consists of a fibrous layer in two parts: (1) the cornea (transparent layer for vision); and (2) the sclera. The cornea is a structure that is part of the visual pathway. It covers the anterior chamber, iris, and pupil. The surface of the globe that communicates with the outside environment and lids is covered with an epithelial layer called the ocular or bulbar conjunctiva. The globe is divided into the anterior and posterior segments. The anterior chamber consists of the cornea, iris, ciliary body, and lens. The posterior segment includes the vitreous, choroid, retina, macula, optic nerve, and central retinal artery and vein. Both segments are fluid-filled chambers, the anterior filled with aqueous humor and the posterior filled with vitreous humor. The choroid is the vascular layer between the retina and the sclera. The junction of the optic nerve to the globe marks the end of

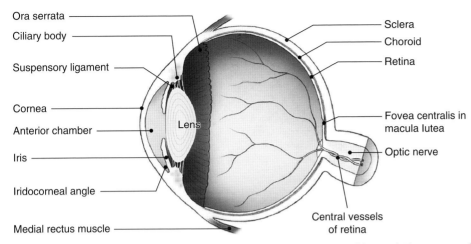

Ora serrata
Ciliary body
Suspensory ligament
Cornea
Anterior chamber
Lens
Iris
Iridocorneal angle
Medial rectus muscle

Sclera
Choroid
Retina
Fovea centralis in macula lutea
Optic nerve
Central vessels of retina

Figure 8.3 The globe in cross section. The iris diaphragm outlines the margins of the pupil. The anterior surface of the lens abuts the posterior surface of the iris. Zonular suspensory fibers are seen emanating from the ciliary body, adjacent to the iris root. (From Mahadevan S, Garmel G. *An Introduction to Clinical Emergency Medicine*. Cambridge: Cambridge University Press, 2005.)

the retina and choroids. As the optic nerve exits the globe, it is covered by all three meningeal layers of the brain. In addition, the optic nerve encases the central retinal artery and vein that supply the blood flow to the retina.

Prehospital management

Prehospital care for a patient with obvious ocular injury consists of application of an eye shield to prevent further damage. In the cases of chemical exposures without foreign body projectile injury, copious saline (normal saline or lactated Ringer's) irrigation should be initiated. Penetrating objects should be left in place and stabilized if necessary. Since the eyes track together, the contralateral uninjured eye benefits from patching also. If possible, pain control and antiemetics should be administered to prevent an increase in intraocular pressure (IOP) from vomiting.

Emergency department evaluation and management

Ocular exam in trauma

In the trauma patient who requires airway intervention, the initial choice of intubation medications may be important in the setting of an intraocular injury. Studies have suggested an increase in IOP with succinylcholine that is significantly higher than with other agents, such as rocuronium.[4,5] The clinical

significance of this increase is unknown; the use of non-depolarizing paralytic agents such as rocuronium may be an advantage in patients with suspected ocular injury. The use of premedication with lidocaine 1.5 mg/kg intravenously (IV) 2 minutes prior to intubation to blunt the increase in IOP can also be considered, however, with the caveat there remains no known outcome benefit from this.[6,7]

Secondary survey includes head, eye, ear, nose and throat (HEENT) examination to assess for both ocular injury as well as any damage along the visual pathway suggesting intracranial pathology. A quick assessment for immediate threats to a patient's vision (e.g., retrobulbar hematoma, globe rupture, or retinal detachment) should be performed in order to initiate prevention of further injury and arrange for coordinated repair along with life-saving measures. Ideally this examination should be completed early in the evaluation as development of periorbital edema may obscure a full evaluation later. The eye should be examined in a systematic fashion from external to internal structures. Any unnecessary pressure on the globe should be avoided. If chemical exposure has occurred, irrigation should be initiated unless globe rupture is suspected. In the event of globe rupture the necessity for removal of any further exposure to a chemical an especially, alkaline substance, should be discussed with an ophthalmologist. At any point a globe rupture is suspected or discovered, the exam should be stopped, an eye shield placed, and ophthalmology expeditiously consulted.

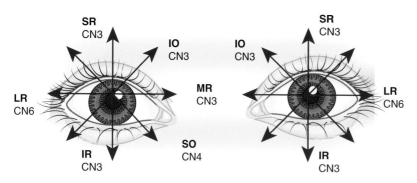

Figure 8.4 Depiction of extraocular muscle innervation by cranial nerves III, IV, VI, and the direction of eye movements that result with contraction of the different extraocular muscles. CN, cranial nerve; IO, inferior oblique; IR, inferior rectus; LR, lateral rectus; MR, medial rectus; SO, superior oblique; SR, superior rectus. (From Shah SM, Kelly KM. *Principles and Practice of Emergency Neurology.* Cambridge: Cambridge University Press, 1999: p. 199.)

In an alert patient, first ask questions relating to visual acuity: light perception, finger counting, Snellen eye chart at bedside, visual fields, and floaters. Pain in the eye indicates injuries to the portions of the globe with sensory innervation including the periorbital and retrobulbar structures, bulbar conjunctiva, and anterior chamber structures. Change in vision indicates any injury that affects the visual pathways of the eye. Patients should be checked not only for pupillary reflex but also for afferent pupillary defect. The afferent pupillary defect in an indication of decreased light perception. It is assessed by using the swinging light test. The usual pupillary response to direct light is that both pupils contract equally if there is nothing wrong with either pupil. If you move the light rapidly from one eye to the other, both pupils remain contracted. To perform the test on an afferent pupillary defect, one shines a light directly in one eye observing for pupillary constriction in both eyes. The examiner then swings the light to the other eye. When there is an injury to the optic nerve, the nerve will also transmit light but to a lesser and slower degree. Consequently, when the light is moved from the good to the injured eye the brain interprets this as receiving less light, or less light coming into the eye. The response is to cause both pupils to dilate to allow more light in to the eye. This is a bilateral response, although only one eye is affected. After this test, note the red light reflex in all patients to detect possible blood or other injury to the posterior chamber. If any defect is found on this exam, a more detailed exam should be performed to identify the cause and help indicate how quickly an intervention is needed. Next assess extraocular movements in the alert patient. A defect here will require a computed tomography (CT) scan of the head and orbit to further assess. An ophthalmology consultation may be valuable at any point in the examination if one is unable to fully

Table 8.1 Highlights of the examination

Structure	Notable findings
Face	Bony deformity, crepitus, loss of sensation
General	Proptosis, endopthalmos/ enophthalmos, loss of extraocular movements, decreased vision, RAPD, diplopia, increased intraocular pressure
Eyelids	Laceration, edema, hematoma
Sclera/ conjunctiva	Laceration or subconjunctival hemorrhage, foreign body
Cornea	Laceration, abrasion, foreign body
Anterior chamber	Hyphema, pupillary irregularities
Posterior chamber and retina	Hemorrhage, detachment, papilledema

RAPD, relative afferent pupillary defect.

assess and the history is concerning, or there are abnormal findings consistent with serious injury, or if there is rapid edema that may obscure further ocular evaluation (Figure 8.4). Highlights of the examination are shown in Table 8.1.

In the case of a patient with a negative exam and no obvious facial trauma, the likelihood of a vision-threatening injury is extremely low. However, even if the exam is negative but the patient has significant facial trauma in the extraocular area, a complete slit-lamp examination and possible ophthalmology follow up within 48 hours for repeat exam is appropriate.

The slit lamp can be utilized in the mobile patient with minimal trauma or isolated facial injury. The high magnification of the slit lamp can help identify injuries not seen with gross external inspection, such as occult globe rupture, hyphema, foreign objects, or small lacerations. Using fluorescein (which binds to the amine group on proteins inside cells) with ultraviolet light identifies defects in the epithelial surface of the eye such as corneal abrasions, conjunctival lacerations, or globe rupture. Globe rupture is noted by fluorescein streaming from the site of rupture, and this is called a positive Seidel test (Figure 8.5). A positive test is indicated when the fluorescein streams down the eye and is taken up by the extruding vitreous humor and turns bright green under Cobalt blue light. In bedbound patients, a portable blue Cobalt light can be used for a beside fluorescein exam. If no globe rupture has been detected at this point, but the patient has persistent pain, IOP should be measured. Normal ranges are 10–20 mmHg with an acceptable difference between eyes of 3–6 mmHg. Most commonly this is measured in the ED with an applanation tonometer, e.g., Tono-Pen®.

The history of injury is a valuable asset in predicting findings. For example, in cases of projectiles, intraocular or intraorbital foreign objects should be investigated. Certain chemical exposures require emergency treatment even without obvious early signs of damage. In cases of blunt trauma, there is a well-recognized pattern of injury due to the transmission of force placed on the globe and the weakest points that rupture (Figure 8.6). This means that physical examination, while essential, needs to be interpreted in the light of clinical suspicion. Even with minimal findings, the examination may need to be supplanted with diagnostic testing.

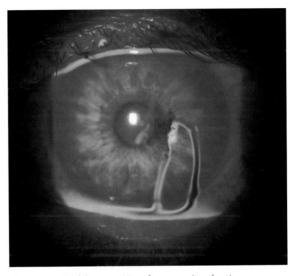

Figure 8.5 Seidel test positive after corneal perforation.

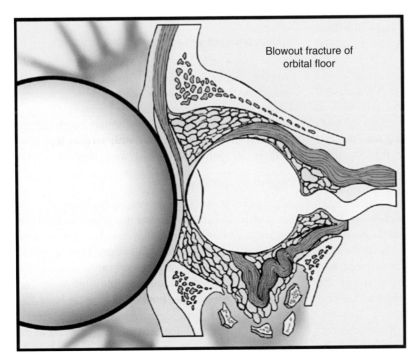

Blowout fracture of orbital floor

Figure 8.6 Illustration showing typical mechanism of injury that produces an orbital blowout fracture. (From Mandavia D, Newton E, Demetriades D. *Colour Atlas of Emergency Trauma*. Cambridge: Cambridge University Press, 2003.)

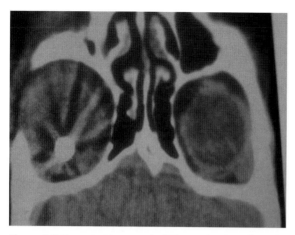

Figure 8.7 Computed tomography (CT) scan showing orbit with intraocular foreign object. (Courtesy of Lawrence Jacobson, MD.)

Imaging in ocular trauma

When imaging to evaluate ocular trauma, three modalities are now utilized: computed tomography (CT), magnetic resonance imaging (MRI), and ultrasound. Magnetic resonance imaging is limited by availability, cost, transportation logistics (patient stability), and fear of complications, e.g., damage caused by undiagnosed metallic foreign objects. With significant facial trauma, edema, and pain, most patients require imaging. Determining which imaging studies are adequate is not always clear. Computed tomography scanning is most useful for evaluating orbital pathology including retrobulbar hematoma, orbital fractures, and intraocular foreign objects (Figure 8.7). However, certain materials such as vegetable and organic matter may not be visualized on CT scan and should be suspected by the history of injury. If high suspicion exists and a metallic foreign object has been ruled out in hemodynamically stable patients, an MRI can evaluate for these substances.[8]

Ultrasound has also been used in ocular trauma and is better at evaluating intraocular pathology, especially when periorbital trauma obscures a direct ophthalmoscope exam. However, in order to perform ultrasonography, external pressure has to be placed on the globe, which is contraindicated in globe rupture. Only when and if rupture has been ruled out, ultrasonography may be used to further image the globe including intraocular foreign objects (radiolucent or opaque), choroidal/scleral rupture, lens dislocation, vitreous hemorrhage, retinal detachment, retrobulbar hematoma, and IOP. Although it has not reached widespread use, in some academic centers it has been shown to provide additional information. There are few prospective randomized trials to evaluate the role of ultrasound in the emergency department (ED), but one study revealed it to have a sensitivity of 100% and specificity of 97.2% evaluating ocular pathology when performed by emergency physicians.[9] This included lens dislocation, retrobulbar hemorrhage, intraocular foreign object, and retinal detachment. This may be useful as a rapid screening test, but is unlikely to supplant CT scan. Plain films are rarely indicated. They may be used to screen for metal prior to MRI or when CT is unavailable.

General principles: key points
Anesthesia

Anesthesia of the cornea and conjunctiva is best accomplished with topical agents. Most common is the use of proparacaine or tetracaine. If the adnexal or deep structures of the eye are involved then parenteral or oral pain control is also necessary. Globe ruptures should avoid topical medications. Occasionally topical non-steroidal anti-inflammatory drugs (NSAIDs) are effective for pain relief;[10,11] however, this should be limited to cases of severe pain not relieved with oral analgesics. Topical NSAIDs have been associated with corneal toxicity including keratitis, ulceration, and perforation in limited case reports.[12–14]

Irrigation/wound preparation

In the event of a chemical exposure without globe rupture, copious irrigation of the ocular surface should be initiated as soon as possible with lactated Ringer's or normal saline. There is limited evidence to suggest one ocular irrigation solution over another; however, lactated Ringer's and normal saline are considered safe and readily available in the ED.

Prophylactic antibiotics

All open injuries require tetanus immunization if not up to date. Topical antibiotics recommended for the eye should be broad spectrum antibiotics to prevent secondary infection when the globe surface is disrupted. Sulfacetamide, erythromycin, tobramycin, or a fluoroquinolone are the most commonly prescribed prophylactic topical medications. Neomycin has fallen out of favor due to its significant incidence of hypersensitivity reactions. Bacitracin ointment applied to the eye nightly is also recommended as a prophylactic agent. Contact wearers are commonly prescribed fluoroquinolones topically due to the higher risk of pseudomonal infection. If the globe is ruptured, a systemic antibiotic regimen is recommended within 6 hours of injury.

Dressing and shielding

Eye patching is no longer considered a treatment in corneal abrasions since it has not been shown to promote re-epithelization nor decrease discomfort. However, if there is a globe rupture or hyphema, a hard shield should be placed over the eye until evaluated by ophthalmology.

Pupil dilation to facilitate exam

Topical drops with tropicamide 1% one drop or phenylephrine 2.5% one drop can be used to facilitate direct ophthalmoscopy and evaluation of the posterior chamber in select patients. However, they should only be used in select cases taking into account the possibility of precipitating an acute attack of narrow-angle closure glaucoma and the possible systemic affects of topical medications.

Common traumatic ocular injuries

Periorbital contusions

This is the most common presentation of direct blunt injury to the orbit. As swelling and edema can make the exam challenging, an early examination is best. A Desmarres retractor (or bent paper clip) can be used to retract the swollen lids, but it must be used with caution so as not to apply additional external pressure on the globe. One challenge in the ED is determining which patients require further imaging to exclude underlying orbital fractures. Some studies have reported 58.3% incidence of orbital fractures with isolated blepharohematoma.[15] However, the significance or necessity for emergent intervention for these fractures was not discussed. Depending on the severity of the mechanism and extent of periorbital trauma, it is up to the emergency physician's judgment when to order an orbital CT with isolated periorbital contusions. Any ocular injury, crepitus, decreased periorbital sensation, or limited examination secondary to edema warrants orbital CT to evaluate for fracture. Treatment of contusions consists simply of ice and head elevation, and should resolve in 2–3 weeks. All patients with significant contusion and an inability to fully visualize the globe

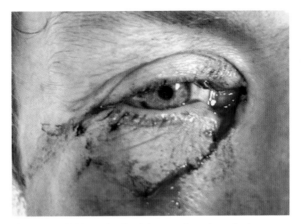

Figure 8.8 Lid laceration involving margin and canaliculus. (Courtesy of Andrew Doan, MD.)

and fundi should be given early ophthalmology follow up for a comprehensive examination of the posterior chamber and retina. Any loss of vision, floaters, or severe pain should prompt ED consultation.

Eyelid lacerations

Many eyelid lacerations require ophthalmology or plastic surgery consultation for repair due to the very thin, complex structure of the eyelid. The job of the emergency physician is to fully evaluate the depth of laceration, assess for penetration into the globe, and identify any foreign objects. Careful evaluation consists of examining and everting the lid without applying external pressure onto the globe. Important structures to examine include tarsal plate, lacrimal gland, or canalicular system. The tarsal plate, thin muscle layers of the orbicularis oculi, and canalicular system require separate layers of closure and alignment (Figure 8.8). Specialized stenting of the canalicular system may be required if there is duct involvement. This will prevent loss of function and cosmetic appearance and the collapse of ducts and epiphora (excessive tearing of the eye). The emergency physician should be concerned about this when the wound is in the medial corner of the eye. Examine the globe surface beneath the lid in the full range of motion. Note if there is penetration into the orbit. Also note injury to the extraocular muscles. Following this, evaluate with fluorescein and the slit lamp or a handheld Wood's lamp of the eye surface to identify any disruptions in the epithelial layer of the eye, corneoscleral lacerations, foreign objects, or globe rupture. If the wound involves the canicular structures, fluorescein placed in the eye may be taken up and leak

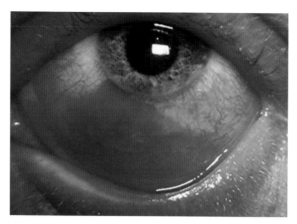

Figure 8.9 Subconjunctival hemorrhage from foreign body found under lid. (Courtesy of William Caccamise Sr, MD.)

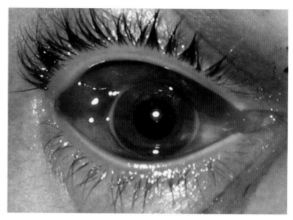

Figure 8.10 Bullous subconjunctival hemorrhage from fist blow. (Courtesy of Jordan M. Graff, MD.)

out of the wound. Superficial (partial thickness) eyelid lacerations without involvement of the lid margin or the above mentioned structures can be repaired primarily by the emergency physician. Repair can be done under local anesthetic. Supraorbital or infraorbital blocks may not be adequate for complete eyelid anesthesia because parts of the eyelid are innervated by branches of the supratrochlear, infratrochlear, and lacrimal nerves. Suture the laceration with 6–0 or 7–0 non-absorbable sutures. Sutures should be removed in 3–5 days. Any laceration that is unable to be sutured primarily by the emergency physician in the ED may be treated with cold compress and antibiotics and referred to an ophthalmologist to see the next day in their office, although follow up must be assured.

Subconjunctival hemorrhage

These are hemorrhages visualized on the surface of the eye contained underneath the conjunctival layer due to rupture of small blood vessels (Figure 8.9). This can occur due to simple blunt trauma, scratching, with forceful valsalva actions such as vomiting, or spontaneously. Most patients have no symptoms, so if a patient describes pain, photophobia, or decreased vision, a more serious injury such as penetrating injury or post-traumatic iritis must be considered. Evaluation consists of a thorough eye exam under the slit lamp to rule out any lacerations or globe rupture. Subconjunctival hemorrhages appear flat on exam. If the hematoma is raised, one should consider the diagnosis of bloody chemosis, a more serious condition. Large circumferential hematomas around the cornea can be associated with occult globe rupture. Therefore, a

detailed exam with fluorescein is indicated; even if normal, these large injuries should have a re-evaluation with ophthalmology within 24–48 hours. Treatment of isolated subconjunctival hemorrhage can be cold compresses for 24 hours, although it is not clear if this is better that watchful waiting. They should resolve spontaneously in 2–3 weeks. Warning the patient that color changes, such as seen with any resolution of a contusion, may be seen and are not concerning.

Bloody chemosis or bullous subconjunctival hemorrhage

This injury is due to bleeding within the conjunctival tissues and edema (Figure 8.10). This is suggestive of more serious injury such as scleral or globe rupture, foreign objects, chemical or thermal injuries, or infection. Treatment is based upon the cause.

Conjunctival lacerations

Conjunctival lacerations cause pain, conjunctival injection, and bloody chemosis (Figure 8.11).

The conjunctiva is less innervated than the cornea; therefore, conjunctival lacerations may not produce the same level of pain as corneal injuries. The conjunctiva will appear injected, patients may complain of pain and foreign object sensation, tearing may occur, and there may be bleeding seen in addition to subconjunctival hemorrhage or chemosis. The main concerns are retained foreign body, scleral involvement, or globe penetration. If the Seidel test is negative, a careful exam under topical anesthesia using a saline-moistened

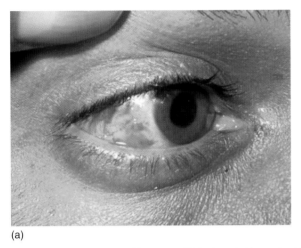

(a)

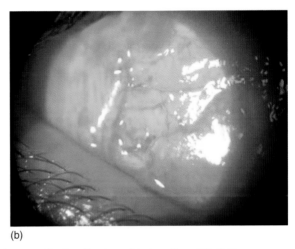

(b)

Figure 8.11 (a) Conjunctival laceration. (b) Conjunctival laceration higher magnification. (Courtesy of Andrew Doan, MD, PhD.)

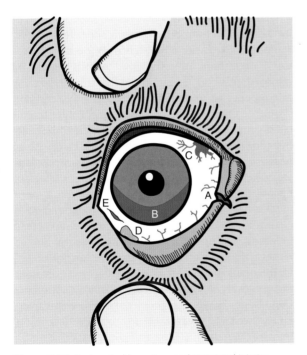

Figure 8.12 Conjunctival lacerations and associated injuries. A: Marginal laceration. B: Hyphema. C: Subconjunctival hemorrhage. D. Globe rupture with leakage. E. Conjunctival laceration.

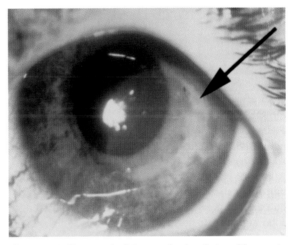

Figure 8.13 Photograph of the eye after installation of fluorescein dye showing bright yellow-green uptake of dye lateral to the pupil (arrow). (From Mandavia D, Newton E, Demetriades D. *Colour Atlas of Emergency Trauma*. Cambridge: Cambridge University Press, 2003.)

cotton-tip applicator can manipulate the laceration to evaluate the depth and extent. Conjunctival lacerations < 1 cm in size are generally left to heal without suturing. Applying topical antibiotic ointment until fully healed within a few days is appropriate. Lacerations > 1 cm and some smaller lacerations that have tissue avulsion or gaping or poor appositional closure involving the plica, semilunar fold, or caruncle, warrant closure to prevent scarring and poor cosmesis (Figure 8.12). Referral to an ophthalmologist within 24 hours for primary closure in these cases is necessary. A perforated eye shield may be applied on discharge.

Corneal abrasions

A corneal abrasion is a disruption in the outer epithelial layer of the cornea (Figure 8.13). This can be caused by blunt trauma, penetration trauma, foreign objects, and chemical/environmental exposures. They can cause pain, blurry vision, conjunctival injection, tearing, and a foreign object sensation. The abrasion can sometimes be seen during general inspection of the eye but is clearly delineated under fluorescein exam. Linear abrasions may suggest a foreign object under the eyelid (ice rink sign) and should be fully investigated. Streaming of fluorescein may suggest penetration into the anterior chamber, consistent with a globe rupture; an eye shield should be placed and emergent ophthalmology consultation obtained. A simple abrasion can be treated with topical broad spectrum antibiotics and lubricating drops. In the past, cycloplegics or mydriatics were suggested in treatment to reduce ciliary spasm and pain. While there is limited data on this subject, a literature review has failed to show any benefit compared to lubricating drops.[16] The only randomized control study on the subject found no benefit in comparison to lubrication.[17] Therefore, unnecessary pharmacologic treatment may increase risk of unwarranted side effects, and their routine use is not encouraged. Eye patching is probably unnecessary; it does not seem to increase comfort and may delay re-epithelization.[18,19] Topical anesthetics should never be prescribed or dispensed to go with the patients: repetitive use impedes healing and may mask development of more serious injury. As discussed previously, topical NSAIDs for short periods may provide additional pain relief, although different case studies have shown concern for corneal toxicity without a clear dose–toxicity relationship. Cautious use for only a few days is recommended, and NSAIDS should generally not be used in conjunction with steroids.[10–14] Most corneal abrasions heal within 1–3 days. It is prudent to follow up the patient with a repeat examination in 24–48 hours. Large defects or those in the central visual axis, i.e., passing though the middle of the pupil, require 24 hour referral to an ophthalmologist.

Corneal foreign objects

Foreign body sensation or irritation and conjunctival injection or corneal infiltration may suggest a corneal foreign body (Figure 8.14). Evaluation should be done under slit lamp with high magnification (if possible) using fluorescein to evaluate for rupture and corneal abrasion. In addition, certain materials such as plaster, cement, mortar, and whitewash may also cause an alkali injury as these substances contain lime. Ocular pH (normal 7.0–7.5) should be checked and irrigation may need to be initiated. Any burning or pain, or abnormal pH requires immediate copious irrigation with reassessment of pain and ocular pH every 1 L of

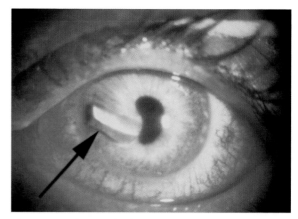

Figure 8.14 Photograph of the eye showing a metallic foreign body on the cornea that is deforming the iris and pupil (arrow). (From Mandavia D, Newton E, Demetriades D. *Colour Atlas of Emergency Trauma*. Cambridge: Cambridge University Press, 2003.)

irrigation. Multiple liters may be required to normalize the pH. After topical anesthesia, superficial objects can be removed with a moistened cotton-tip applicator or irrigation. Any visualized objects should be removed prior to irrigation, and any irrigation for microscopic or unvisualized foreign body sensation should be done without a Morgan lens. Under the slit lamp, high magnification lens, small, minimally imbedded objects can be removed with a 18–25-gauge needle or eye spud held parallel to the corneal plane and used to lift the object gently off the surface. If unable to easily remove with this technique, or if there is deep penetration, referral to an ophthalmologist within 24 hours is necessary. Ferrous objects tend to leave a rust ring that may require a corneal burr to remove the ring after removal of the metal object. Ophthalmology referral within 24 hours can be done for removal of the rust ring. Topical antibiotics should be prescribed as prophylaxis. Emergent referral is needed in cases of any corneal laceration, positive Seidel test, evidence of corneal ulcer or infiltrate, deeply imbedded foreign object, hypopyon, or significant anterior chamber reaction such as iritis.

Corneoscleral lacerations

Disruption of the corneal or scleral layers can be deep enough to disrupt the integrity of the globe (Figure 8.15). For this reason, any corneoscleral laceration requires immediate eye shield and emergent ophthalmologic evaluation. Most patients report pain or decreased visual acuity. Even without globe rupture, all patients require their tetanus immunization

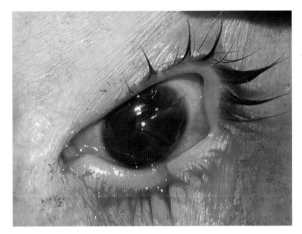

Figure 8.15 Open globe with corneal laceration due to bungee cord injury. (Courtesy of James Howard, MD.)

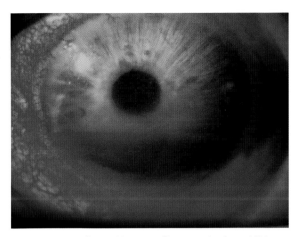

Figure 8.16 Hyphema. (Courtesy of Lawence Jacobson, MD.)

updated and broad spectrum parenteral antibiotics for prevention of post-traumatic endophthalmitis. Most of these patients are admitted to the hospital.

Hyphema

A hyphema is a collection of blood in the anterior chamber of the eye (Figure 8.16). The etiologies include blunt trauma from small tears in the ciliary muscle or iris or from penetrating trauma. Hyphemas are classified by Grade 0–4:

Grade 0: Microscopic can only be detected on slit-lamp examination.

Grade 1: Layered blood occupying less than one third of the anterior chamber.

Grade 2: Blood filling one third to one half of the anterior chamber.

Grade 3: Layered blood filling one half to less than total of the anterior chamber.

Grade 4: Total clotted blood, often referred to as blackball or eight-ball hyphema.

Hyphemas are measured in millimeters of height from the inferior edge of the anterior chamber and as a percentage of the anterior chamber filled. Examination must include patient history of any blood dyscrasias or treatment with anticoagulants, visual acuity, fluorescein exam with slit lamp, retinal exam, and IOP measurements. Management is dependent on the etiology. With penetrating trauma, it is considered an open globe; an eye shield is placed and emergent ophthalmology consultation is required. In the setting of closed globe trauma, the managment is more varied. In

general, consultation with an ophalmologist is preferred in the ED for all hyphemas. The main treatment goals are to prevent rebleeding, and increased IOP in order to prevent corneal bloodstaining and optic atrophy and promote the best visual outcome. Patients should be placed in a bed with head elevated to 30°. An eye shield may be placed although the science behind it is not conclusive. In a prospective randomized double-blind study, bilateral patching, unilateral patching, and no patching appear to be associated with the same visual outcome.[20] However, some recommend a perforated (to protect binocular vision) eye shield to prevent further trauma to the eye and a non-perforated eye shield to reduce light exposure for reducing corneal bloodstaining in select patients. The decision should be made in consultation with an ophthalmologist. Bed rest used to be the mainstay of treatment; however, limited studies have suggested no increase in rebleeding rates in patients placed on bed rest vs. quiet ambulation (no strenuous activity).[21] Surgery is usually reserved for patients with delayed complications but it may be performed early in patients with sickle cell or total hyphema. Medical management is also focused on healing and preventing rebleeding. Rebleeding is the most common complication and occurs 2–5 days after injury, when the clot retracts and loosens, and has an incidence of 3.5–38.0% depending on numerous patient factors. A series of topical and systemic medications, administered in coordination with an ophthalmologist, may be used. These include cycloplegics, such as atropine 1% daily, although numerous retrospective studies have found no effect on outcome.[22–24] However, consensus opinion still recommends their use for patient comfort, prevention of formation of posterior synechiae, and to decrease rebleed in patients on aspirin.[25] A topical corticosteroid (prednisolone acetate 1% QID) is also recommended to reduce intraocular inflammation, the risk of anterior or posterior synechiae, and rebleeding. While numerous studies on topical steroids have been performed, the data has varied based upon the severity of the hyphema, patient population, and dosage of corticosteroid. A full evaluation of the literature still provides inconclusive evidence but suggests that even systemic corticosteroids may be beneficial in preventing rebleeding in select high-risk patients. Systemic antifibrinolytic agents (i.e., tranexamic acid and aminocaproic acid) significantly lower the rate of rebleeding after traumatic hyphema and also may delay clot resorption, based on numerous studies since 1966, but they have not been proven to statistically improve visual outcome in traumatic hyphema.[26] Due to this reason and the large number of adverse side effects they are much less commonly used. In the event of elevated IOP, agents that decrease IOP (see section on glaucoma, below) such as timolol eye drops and acetazolamide (except in sickle cell patients) should be initiated. In limited cases the patient can be discharged home with daily ophthalmology evaluation for rebleeding and IOP monitoring. A recent review discusses the limited evidence on outpatient management of traumatic hyphema stressing the lack of prospective randomized studies and limited patient populations.[21] Their recommendations consist of considering outpatient management for patients without associated ocular injury requiring admission, over 12 years of age, with hyphema less than half of anterior chamber volume, with satisfactory IOP < 24 mmHg, no blood dyscrasia, and compliant.[21] Complications of hyphema include traumatic or future angle-recession glaucoma and rebleeding, synechiae formation, optic atrophy, and corneal staining from blood. Visual prognosis is substantially worse for total hyphema than subtotal hyphema, with studies showing a recovery of good visual acuity (> 20/50) occurring in 76% of patients with a subtotal hyphema but in only 35% of patients with a total hyphema.[27] Depending on the extent, hyphemas should resolve in about a week. Patients should avoid aspirin or non-steroidal medications.

Traumatic glaucoma

This can either be an immediate sequelae or delayed complication of trauma. Blood, particles released from the iris or lens, direct contusion to the trabecular meshwork, or lens dislocation into the anterior chamber may block aqueous flow out of the anterior chamber. Patients may present with pain, blurred vision, colored halos around lights, frontal headache, nausea, and vomiting. On exam, conjunctival injection will be noted and in severe cases a fixed, middilated pupil, and corneal edema. The hallmark is an acute increase in IOP > 20 mmHg or a difference > 3–6 mmHg between eyes. Treatment consists of medications to decrease the IOP immediately. Consult ophthalmology immediately but do not delay treatment. Start a beta-blocker topically (Timoptic® 0.5%, one drop every 30 minutes for two doses) and an alpha-agonist topically (Alphagan® one drop TID or apraclonidine one drop every 30 minutes for two doses). Patients may also require pain medications and antiemetics to prevent increases in IOP due to vomiting. If pressure is not decreasing after an hour of topical drops, systemic medications such as carbonic anhydrase inhibitors or hyperosmotic agents may be started if the patient is hemodynamically stable. If the angle is mechanically obstructed, surgery is required. Delayed glaucoma can occur 1–3 weeks post-injury and may be from scarring to the trabecular meshwork or angle recession or hemosiderin deposits in the anterior chamber. Treatment is medical but may require surgery. An expedited ED ophthalmology consultation should occur with cases of elevated IOP.

Iris sphincter tears/traumatic mydriasis

The etiology of sphincter tears and traumatic mydriasis is from blunt trauma to the eye with the transmission of forces through the globe. Complaints usually include pain and photophobia. Examination finding is an irregular and often dilated pupil with a possible associated hyphema. In addition, IOP must be measured as these can have an association with glaucoma, more likely in a delayed presentation. Smaller tears are best left alone and followed for healing. Larger sphincter tears with resultant mydriasis and photophobia may be managed pharmacologically with topically miotic agents or by the use of a tinted contact lens or sunglasses. Some may require surgery. If isolated injury has occurred without other injuries immediately threatening vision, the patient can be re-evaluated by ophthalmology within 24 hours. Although mydriasis can also be caused by intracranial injury and damage to the third cranial nerve, the

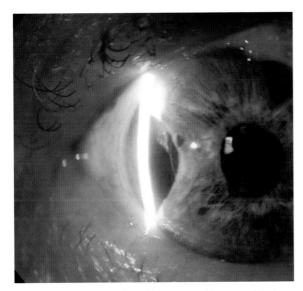

Figure 8.17 Iridodialysis from blunt trauma. (Courtesy of Andrew Doan, MD, PhD.)

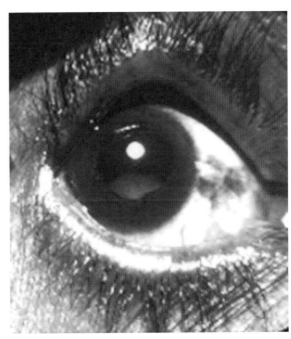

Figure 8.18 Subluxed lens. (Courtesy of William Caccamise Sr, MD.)

history and mental status examination should be able to distinguish between them.

Iridodialysis

This is a localized traumatic separation of the iris root from the ciliary body seen in trauma due to blunt force to the eye (Figure 8.17). An associated hyphema may be present in addition to other more serious injuries. Symptoms include monocular diplopia, pain, and photophobia. The examination will show appearance of polycoria (multiple pupils, see Figure 8.17). Treatment is generally urgent surgical repair if anything other than minimal. High suspicion for other injuries should exist due to the amount of force required to cause this injury. This finding requires an ophthalmology consult within 24 hours if an isolated injury, normal IOP, and no concern for globe rupture or other sight-threatening injuries exist.

Subluxation/dislocation of the lens (ecoptia lentis)

This may result from either blunt or penetrating trauma. In subluxation, the lens is partially decentered but will remain visible through the pupillary aperture, a crescent-shaped defect may be noted (Figure 8.18). In dislocation, the lens may be fully displaced from the pupillary aperture. Symptoms consist of diplopia or decreased vision and pain.

Exam shows a crescent-shaped red reflex or defect in addition to possible increased IOP. An open globe should be suspected until proven otherwise. Measurement of IOP after fluorescein exam is required. Surgical correction is necessary and ophthalmology should be immediately involved especially due to the possibility of the lens subluxing to create secondary acute angle closure glaucoma at any time.

Post-traumatic cataract formation

The stretching and pulling forces exerted on the lens during blunt trauma can cause edema and scarring and eventual cataract formation. Penetrating trauma causes direct injury as it passes through the lens. Both mechanisms are commonly associated with lens subluxation or dislocation as well as associated glaucoma, uveitis, and globe rupture. Acute cases will present immediately or within a day of injury. Delayed cataract formation normally occurs weeks to months following the injury. Patients may complain of diplopia or decreased vision, and cataracts are detected by a cloudy appearance or opacification of the lens on exam (Figure 8.19). Treatment requires surgery when vision is impaired and necessitates IOP monitoring. Ophthalmology should be consulted in the ED if the lens is subluxed/dislocated or other

117

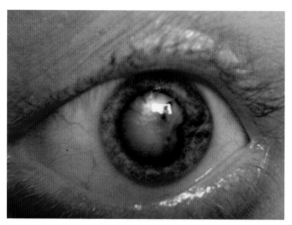

Figure 8.19 Post-traumatic cataract and synechie formation. (Courtesy of William Caccamise Sr, MD.)

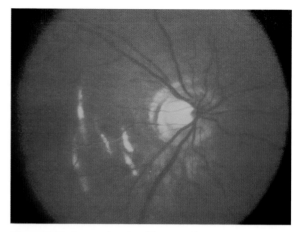

Figure 8.20 Commotio retina. (Courtesy of Lawrence Jacobson, MD.)

associated injuries are noted in acute presentations. Isolated delayed cataract formation can be re-evaluated by ophthalmology within 24 hours if IOP is normal.

Vitreous hemorrhage

This is blood in the posterior chamber. Symptoms include loss of vision or small bleeds described as floaters, shadows, or haziness. On ophthalmoscopic examination, the hemorrhage may be visible in the posterior chamber or the red reflex may be decreased or absent. Blood in the posterior chamber should alert the emergency physician to potential retinal detachment. Studies show 11–44% of traumatic vitreous hemorrhages are associated with retinal tears.[28] Additionally, vitreous hemorrhage can be associated with subarachnoid hemorrhage (Terson syndrome) and indicates a poorer prognosis in subarachnoid hemorrhage. Vitreous or retinal hemorrhage in any child < 3 years old should prompt a high index of suspicion for child abuse. In the event of penetrating injuries, this indicates globe penetration and possible intraocular foreign object necessitating a CT scan of the orbit. The patient's head should be kept elevated at 30° and emergent ophthalmology consult should be obtained. If rupture is suspected, place a shield over the eye. When the exam is limited by periobital contusion and rupture is not suspected, ultrasound may be helpful in detecting retinal detachment; however, it can miss a substantial number of retinal tears (50%).[29] If the ophthalmologist has excluded other pathology, patients with isolated vitreous hemorrhages can be discharged with strict instructions for head elevation,

avoiding aspirin and non-steroidal medications, and limited physical activity. These hemorrhages usually resolve spontaneously in a few weeks to months.

Retinal detachment

These injuries cause complete or partial peripheral loss of vision. There may be a history of progressive visual field loss as the detachment advances. The same symptoms as in vitreous hemorrhage may be described; in addition flashing lights from stimulated retinal neurons may occur. This is painless by itself, unless there are other associated injuries. These can also have a delayed presentation, up to months after the initial injury. Sometimes the hazy, gray membrane of the retina billowing forward can be seen on direct ophthalmoscopy; however, smaller and more peripheral tears may not be seen and any patient suspected of this should be examined under indirect ophthalmoscopy by the ophthalmologist emergently. These patients require emergent surgery within 24 hours.

Commotio retina

Blunt trauma can contuse the retina. *Commotio retina* consists of disruption of the retinal photoreceptors and normally occurs as a contracoup injury in the traumatized eye. Patients are asymptomatic or complain of decreased visual acuity if the macula is involved (called Berlin's edema). On exam, a patchy gray–white opacification of the retina is seen within a few hours of injury (Figure 8.20). While this condition resolves spontaneously, concurrent retinal hemorrhages, tears, or detachment may be present.

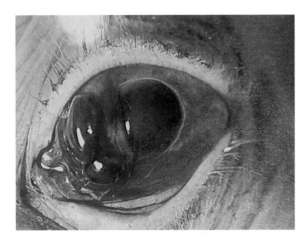

Figure 8.21 Scleral rupture and protruding vitreous. (Courtesy of Lawrence Jacobson, MD.)

Long-term visual loss may also be found when the injury results in macular scarring, reactive pigment hyperplasia or atrophy, or macular holes. This may lead to central visual loss. As the differential diagnosis includes other injuries, ED evaluation by ophthalmology is indicated when visual acuity or peripheral fields are affected; however, asymptomatic patients with this found incidentally on exam can follow up with ophthalmology within 24 hours.

Traumatic optic neuropathy

This is an injury to the optic nerve due to trauma. It can be by indirect or shearing forces in head trauma or due to direct compression of the nerve from bony fragments or other injuries. Patients may complain of various degrees of vision loss (decreased visual acuity, visual field abnormalities, or loss of color vision especially red desaturation). There will be an afferent pupillary defect that can not be accounted for by other injuries. In most cases the optic nerve appears normal on funduscopic exam during the acute phase. Atrophy may be seen 3–4 weeks post-injury. There is a high association with concurrent head trauma in these patients. A head and orbital CT scan should be done to evaluate for intracranial injury or optic nerve compression. Treatment consists of systemic corticosteroids alone or in conjunction with optic nerve decompression. Ophthamology consultation is emergently indicated.

Globe rupture

Globe rupture is a major cause of monocular blindness and should always be suspected in any blunt

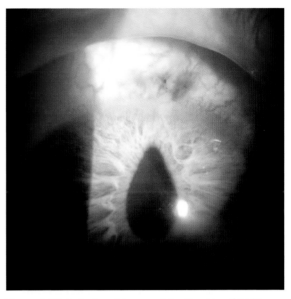

Figure 8.22 Peaked pupil in open globe. (Courtesy of Andrew Doan, MD, PhD.)

or penetrating trauma to the eye. Sometimes this can be an obvious diagnosis (Figure 8.21), but occult globe rupture can be difficult to diagnose and must be suspected by noting associated findings (Figure 8.21). These include decreased visual acuity, severe subconjunctival hemorrhage (> 50%), bloody chemosis, a peaked pupil (Figure 8.22), a deep or shallow anterior chamber, limitation of extraocular motion, and an afferent pupillary defect. In the event that none of these signs are present, continue examination as described earlier including a fluorescein exam looking particularly for the Seidel sign (see Figure 8.5). The locations to search for occult globe rupture in blunt trauma are at the points of attachment to the globe by accessory organs, insertion of the extraocular muscles, or by the corneal limbus where the sclera is the thinnest. Treatment consists of eye shield placement and emergent ophthalmologic consultation. Administer IV antibiotics and tetanus immunization. In adults, antibiotic regimens may include a combination of cefazolin and ciprofloxacin. In pediatrics, fluoroquinolones should not be used and gentamicin is recommended instead. In some regions with a high methicillin-resistant *Staphylococcus aureus* incidence, vancomycin may be added. In addition, anti-emetics to prevent increased IOP from vomiting may be given.

119

Globe luxation

This is a rare condition in which the globe is displaced out of the orbit. It may result from penetrating trauma, severe blunt trauma, or rare spontaneous cases. If awake, patients will have severe pain and decreased vision, exam will show proptosis with lid retraction behind the globe sometimes suspended by the optic nerve. The emergent treatment is to reduce traction on the optic nerve if possible until surgical correction. This is usually possible in spontaneous cases, while most traumatic cases will have obstruction posterior to the luxed globe preventing reduction. Although the treatment for a spontaneous luxation is as follows, it is not fully clear if this can be effective in traumatic luxation and should be done with great caution. Use a saline-moistened gauze pad, apply small pressure to the superior scleral region as the patient looks downward, if possible, to slowly reduce the globe towards or into the orbit only enough to reduce traction on the optic nerve. Then, leave the saline gauze cover and apply a hard protective eye shield over the entire area. If no reduction is possible or necessary, cover the area including the globe with a hard protective shield. Emergent ophthalmology consultation and surgery is indicated.

Penetrating foreign objects: intraocular and intraorbital

Penetrating objects can reside in the intraorbital or intraocular region. Sometimes the presentation is obvious with a foreign object protruding. Foreign objects should be suspected by the mechanism of injury, pain, vision loss, globe rupture, corneoscleral lacerations, or pupillary irregularity. Unless going emergently to the operating room, in these cases orbital CT scanning is essential. Organic material may not be noted on CT scan and further evaluation with ultrasound or MRI is warranted based on clinical circumstance. The material of the foreign object predicts the inflammation reaction and likely endophthalmitis that may help the decision to remove. Generally, the only foreign bodies left intraorbitally are small metallic fragments, except iron, lead, and copper which are highly inflammatory. All cases warrant emergent ophthalmologic consult.

Retrobulbar hematoma

This is a serious and uncommon complication of blunt trauma to the orbit. It is similar in pathophysiology to compartment syndrome. Bleeding accumulates behind the orbit, creating pressure behind the globe, pushing it forward and creating traction on the optic nerve. If there isn't an associated and displaced orbital wall fracture, this pressure may continue until patient loses vision. The damage can quickly become irreversible in as little as 90–120 minutes.[30–32] Signs and symptoms of a retrobulbar hematoma are proptosis, severe eye pain, periorbital edema, ophthalmoplegia, afferent pupillary defect, and vision loss (Figure 8.23). The IOP is increased, and palpation of the orbit will generally find a hard globe. Ophthalmoscopic findings include cherry red macula, absent pulsations of the central retinal artery, or choroidal folds. The emergent treatment is a lateral canthotomy. Absolute indications for lateral canthotomy include retrobulbar hemorrhage resulting in acute loss of visual acuity, afferent pupillary defect, increased IOP, and proptosis. An IOP > 40 mmHg in this clinical situation is an indication for lateral canthotomy (normal IOP is 10–21 mmHg). Medical treatments that decrease IOP can also be used but are never a replacement for surgical decompression and should not delay intervention. Ophthalmology should be involved in treatment emergently, but the lateral canthotomy should be performed by the emergency physician if they are not immediately available.

Orbital fractures and entrapment

Orbital trauma may result in entrapment of the extraocular muscles. This may be due to fracture requiring surgical decompression. Edema may also cause a global decrease of extraocular movements and diplopia, which resolves as the edema resolves. Entrapment is more likely if movement is restricted in only one or two directions. The most common muscle involved in entrapment is the inferior rectus due to fracture of the inferior wall of the orbit, resulting in diplopia on upward gaze (Figure 8.24). Generally, CT scanning is the test of choice to evaluate. Opthalmology consultation is indicated. In some centers, otolaryngology or plastic surgery may be the primary consulting service.

Chemical burns

Acid or alkali exposures can cause substantial damage and potential blindness. Immediate copious irrigation should begin when a patient arrives. Alkali substances cause more severe damage since they are lipophilic

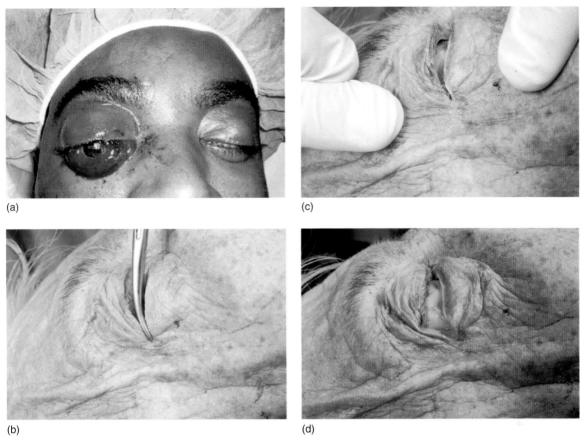

Figure 8.23 (a) Proptosis and periobital edema. (Courtesy of Lawrence Jacobson, MD.) (b–d) Lateral canthotomy performed on cadaver. (b) Cadaver undergoing lateral canthotomy with compression of lateral canthal fold. (c) Photograph shows all tissues layers cut along lateral canthal fold up to orbital rim. (d) Photograph shows cadaver after all tissue layers of canthal fold and lateral canthal membrane incised. (b–d, Courtesy of Taku Taira, MD and New York University School of Medicine.)

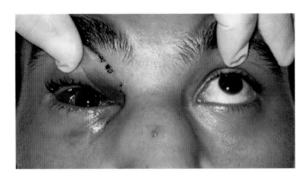

Figure 8.24 Blowout fracture with entrapment and upgaze restriction. (Courtesy of Jordan M. Graff, MD.)

and hydrophilic and can penetrate the cell membrane rapidly, within 5–15 minutes, and damage the anterior structures. Alkali substances include oven and drain cleaners (potassium hydroxide), lime in plaster (calcium hydroxide), fertilizers and sparklers (ammonium hydroxide), high concentration bleach (sodium hypochlorite), and sodium hydroxide from an air bag. Acidic agents may be less deeply penetrating due to the action of corneal proteins which act as a buffer and form a precipitate on the surface. Normal ocular pH is neutral, approximately 7.0–7.5 on litmus paper. Ocular pH can be measured after initial copious irrigation using a Morgan lens (if no particulate matter is present) and a topical anesthetic such as tetracaine. After each liter of irrigation, measure the pH and, if not neutral, continue irrigation. It is best not to complete a full and comprehensive examination until a neutral pH is established, which can take many liters. If an abnormal pH persists after 2 L of irrigation, a search for particulate matter in the folds of the eye should be done rapidly, with irrigation then continued. Once the pH is neutral, a more thorough eye exam can be done. This optimally includes a

121

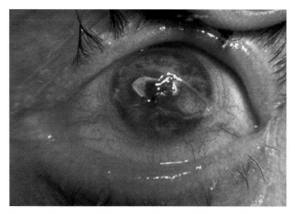

Figure 8.25 Burn of lid margin and cornea. (Courtesy of William Caccamise Sr, MD.)

slit-lamp, fluorescein exam, and measurement of IOP. Common findings with minor chemical burns include corneal abrasions or keratitis, conjunctival injection, or chemosis. Severe burns can cause corneal opacification (Figure 8.25), ulcers including perforation, and conjunctival ischemia. Ischemia is noted by the blanching of the conjunctival vessels (Figure 8.26). Eyelids may be edematous and periorbital skin may have first- or second-degree burns. Later the patient may develop glaucoma, cataracts, scarring of the cornea or conjunctiva, and problems associated with adnexa of the eye including the conjunctival cul-de-sac eyelid. Long-term disability is significant. In one study, one third of 131 patients with ocular burns were considered disabled; approximately 15% were considered blind. The success rate for transplants for this condition is < 50%.[33] Patients are treated with topical antibiotics and ophthalmology follow up within 24 hours with isolated corneal abrasions and skin involvement. Strict instructions to keep the eye moist with artificial tears or antibiotic ointment is important to prevent keratitis. Most alkali exposures and any other chemical injuries require emergent ophthalmologic evaluation and possible admission for corneal and IOP monitoring. Patients without a normal pH should not be discharged.

Thermal burns

Thermal burns can be caused by contact with any hot substance. Most injuries are superficial but thermal necrosis and penetration can occur. Burns that damage the periorbital structures such as the eyelids can cause contractures. Irrigation helps to clear debris and cool the ocular surface. The ocular exam should

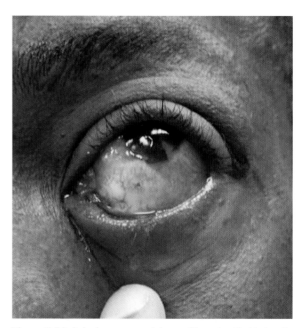

Figure 8.26 Anhydrous ammonia burn with conjunctival ischemia. (Courtesy of Andrew Doan, MD, PhD.)

evaluate for corneal abrasions, intraocular inflammation (uveitis, glaucoma), and globe penetration. The most common injury is corneal abrasion. Patients with isolated corneal abrasions and minor periorbital burns can be discharged to follow up with an ophthalmologist within 24 hours. Ointments should be used on the eye to ensure adequate lubrication and prevent keratitis especially if the eyelid is involved. More severe injuries require ophthalmology consult emergently.

Delayed complications

Traumatic iridiocyclitis (uveitis)

Iridiocyclitis or inflammation of the iris occurs when iris particles are released into the anterior chamber and cause a transient irritation that may be accompanied by an increase in IOP. This may be seen within 3 days after blunt trauma to the eye. Symptoms include photophobia even with the consensual light response, blurred vision, and eye pain. If the uveitis is severe enough, a small poorly dilating pupil may be seen. Signs include cells and flare in the anterior chamber on slit-lamp exam, which confirm this diagnosis. The differential includes the more concerning entity endopthalmitis and should be considered in patients with severe pain and chemosis and any patient with a hypopyon. Cycloplegics (homotropine

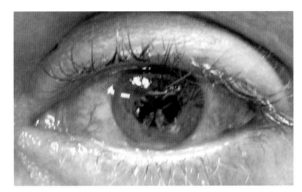

Figure 8.27 Traumatic endophthalmitis with small hypopyon. (Courtesy of Andrew Doan, MD, PhD.)

5%) can be prescribed for comfort and prevention of synechiae. In rare cases, topical corticosteroids (prednisolone acetate 1%) may be prescribed if inflammation has not resolved in 7 days and the patient does not have a corneal abrasion or dendritic fluorescein staining suggest herpes simplex virus (HSV). Most will spontaneously resolve within a week. Patients warrant follow up in 24–48 hours with an ophthalmologist.

Endophthalmitis

Inflammation of the deep structures of the eye after open globe injury occurs in 1–6% of patients. Risk factors associated with an increased risk of post-traumatic endophthalmitis include delayed primary repair, dirty wound, breach of lens capsule, retained intraocular foreign body (IOFB), visual acuity 20/1000 to light perception, and rural setting.[34–36] Signs and symptoms consist of pain, photophobia, variable visual loss, extreme conjunctival injection, chemosis, hypopyon, uveitis, and lid swelling (Figure 8.27). Fluorescein exam and IOP readings should be taken (Figure 8.28).

The possibility of endophthalmitis should be suspected in any painful red eye post-trauma whether hours to months after the incident. A study of post-traumatic endophthalmitis by Al-Omran et al. showed a large variety in species but the majority were *Streptococcus* and *Staphylococcus epidermidis* (most common with retained foreign bodies).[34] Bacillus was only isolated in 3% but has been cultured in up to 25% in other studies, especially in rural areas or in cases of organic foreign objects. Based on clinical circumstances, CT scan or ultrasound to look for retained foreign objects is important. Combination

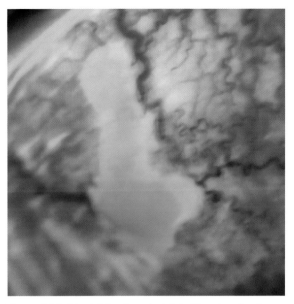

Figure 8.28 Scleral defect in endophthalmitis patient showing missed open globe. (Courtesy of Andrew Doan, MD, PhD.)

therapy of IV antibiotics is recommended such as vancomycin plus an aminoglycoside or a third-generation cephalosporin. Clindamycin should be considered to cover for Bacillus if soil contamination is suspected. Ophthalmology should be emergently contacted as patients require admission and may require surgery.

Sympathetic ophthalmia

Sympathetic ophthalmia is a granulomatous uveitis of both eyes following severe trauma to one eye. This is a rare but serious complication of unilateral severe eye injury, and it can cause blindness even in the uninjured eye. Floating spots and loss of accommodation are the earliest signs. Iridiocyclitis develops with pain and photophobia. This condition may develop from days to several years after eye injury but in 80% uveitis develops in 2–12 weeks following injury and 90% occur within a year.[37] The key to diagnosis is in the history of eye trauma and, especially penetrating, eye injury. Mild cases may respond to immunosuppressive therapy but many may require enucleation (removal of the globe) or evisceration (removal of the vitreous and aqueous humor, sclera is left) of the injured eye.[38] Preventing sympathetic ophthalmia is one reason enucleation or evisceration may be done immediately following severe trauma. All suspected cases require emergency ophthalmologic consultation.

Table 8.2 Ocular exam documentation

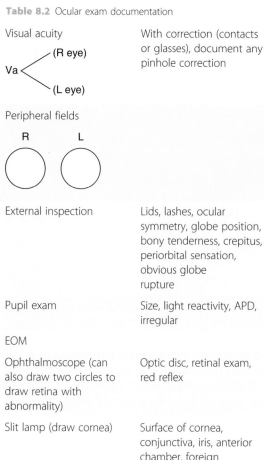

Visual acuity Va < (R eye) (L eye)	With correction (contacts or glasses), document any pinhole correction
Peripheral fields R L	
External inspection	Lids, lashes, ocular symmetry, globe position, bony tenderness, crepitus, periorbital sensation, obvious globe rupture
Pupil exam	Size, light reactivity, APD, irregular
EOM	
Ophthalmoscope (can also draw two circles to draw retina with abnormality)	Optic disc, retinal exam, red reflex
Slit lamp (draw cornea)	Surface of cornea, conjunctiva, iris, anterior chamber, foreign objects
Fluorescein (draw also)	Epithelial defects, Seidel test
Intraocular pressure	Normal < 20 mmHg or < 3–6 mmHg difference between eyes

APD, afferent pupillary defect; EOM, extraocular muscles.

Documentation

All patients should have ophthalmologic examination documented. Diagrams may aid in this (Table 8.2). This examination should include a visual acuity exam with spectacle correction when possible, peripheral fields, and extraocular movements. External lid and lash injuries should also be noted. Timing and response of consult with outpatient appointment should be in the chart.

Disposition

The role of the emergency physician in ocular trauma is to do a thorough evaluation, establish a provisional diagnosis, and treat an emergent condition when able. Minor injuries can be handled by the emergency physician as long as a high index of suspicion exists to rule out occult injuries that could threaten a patient's vision. Every patient with significant ocular injury should be reassessed by an ophthalmologist after discharge. Optometrists can follow up patients with superficial injuries such as corneal abrasions, conjunctival abrasions, and subconjunctival hemorrhages. The patient should be provided with clear discharge instructions to return if any signs of delayed complications develop.

References

1. McGwin G, Jr., Xie A, Owsley C. Rate of eye injury in the United States. *Arch Ophthalmol* 2005;**123**(7):970–6.

2. McGwin G, Jr., Owsley C. Incidence of emergency department-treated eye injury in the United States. *Arch Ophthalmol* 2005;**123**(5):662–6.

3. Guly CM, Guly HR, Bouamra O, et al. Ocular injuries in patients with major trauma. *Emerg Med J* 2006;**23**(12):915–17.

4. Vinik, HR. Intraocular pressure changes during rapid sequence induction and intubation: a comparison of rocuronium, atracurium, and succinylcholine. *J Clin Anesth* 1999;**11**(2):95–100.

5. Chiu CL, Jaais F, Wang CY. Effect of rocuronium compared with succinylcholine on intraocular pressure during rapid sequence induction of anaesthesia. *Br J Anaesth* 1999;**82**(5):757–60.

6. Lev R, Rosen P. Prophylactic lidocaine use preintubation: a review. *J Emerg Med* 1994;**12**(4):499–506.

7. Drenger B, Pe'er J, BenEzra D, et al. The effect of intravenous lidocaine on the increase in intraocular pressure induced by tracheal intubation. *Anesth Analg* 1985;**64**(12):1211–13.

8. Lakshmanan A, Bala S, Belfer KF. Intraorbital organic foreign body–a diagnostic challenge. *Orbit* 2008;**27**(2):131–3.

9. Blaivas M, Theodoro D, Sierzenski PR. A study of bedside ocular ultrasonography in the emergency department. *Acad Emerg Med* 2002;**9**(8):791–9.

10. Calder LA, Balasubramanian S, Fergusson D. Topical nonsteroidal anti-inflammatory drugs for corneal abrasions: meta-analysis of randomized trials. *Acad Emerg Med* 2005;**12**(5):467–73.

11. Weaver CS, Terrell KM. Evidence-based emergency medicine. Update: do ophthalmic nonsteroidal anti-inflammatory drugs reduce the pain associated with simple corneal abrasion without delaying healing? *Ann Emerg Med* 2003;**41**(1):134–40.

12. Guidera AC, Luchs JI, Udell IJ. Keratitis, ulceration, and perforation associated with topical nonsteroidal anti-inflammatory drugs. *Ophthalmology* 2001;**108**(5):936–44.

13. Flach AJ. Corneal melts associated with topically applied nonsteroidal anti-inflammatory drugs. *Trans Am Ophthalmol Soc* 2001;**99**:205–10; discussion 10–12.

14. Gaynes BI, Fiscella R. Topical nonsteroidal anti-inflammatory drugs for ophthalmic use: a safety review. *Drug Saf* 2002;**25**(4):233–50.

15. Exadaktylos AK, Sclabas GM, Smolka K, et al. The value of computed tomographic scanning in the diagnosis and management of orbital fractures associated with head trauma: a prospective, consecutive study at a Level I trauma center. *J Trauma* 2005;**58**(2):336–41.

16. Carley F, Carley S. Towards evidence based emergency medicine: best BETs from the Manchester Royal Infirmary. Mydriatics in corneal abrasion. *Emerg Med J* 2001;**18**(4):273.

17. Brahma AK, Shah S, Hillier VF, et al. Topical analgesia for superficial corneal injuries. *J Accid Emerg Med* 1996;**13**(3):186–8.

18. Arbour JD, Brunette I, Boisjoly HM, et al. Should we patch corneal erosions? *Arch Ophthalmol* 1997;**115**(3):313–17.

19. Kaiser PK, Pineda R, 2nd. A study of topical nonsteroidal anti-inflammatory drops and no pressure patching in the treatment of corneal abrasions. Corneal Abrasion Patching Study Group. *Ophthalmology* 1997;**104**(8):1353–9.

20. Rakusin W. Traumatic hyphema. *Am J Ophthalmol* 1972;**74**(2):284–92.

21. Walton W, Von Hagen S, Grigorian R, et al. Management of traumatic hyphema. *Surv Ophthalmol* 2002;**47**(4):297–334.

22. Coles WH. Traumatic hyphema: an analysis of 235 cases. *South Med J* 1968;**61**(8):813–16.

23. Fong LP. Secondary hemorrhage in traumatic hyphema. Predictive factors for selective prophylaxis. *Ophthalmology* 1994;**101**(9):1583–8.

24. Ng CS, Strong NP, Sparrow JM, et al. Factors related to the incidence of secondary haemorrhage in 462 patients with traumatic hyphema. *Eye* 1992;**6**(3):308–12.

25. Gorn RA. The detrimental effect of aspirin on hyphema rebleed. *Ann Ophthalmol* 1979;**11**(3):351–5.

26. Aylward GW, Dunlop IS, Little BC. Meta-analysis of systemic anti-fibrinolytics in traumatic hyphaema. *Eye* 1994;**8**(4):440–2.

27. Read J, Goldberg M. Comparison of medical treatment for traumatic hyphema. *Trans Am Acad Ophthalmol Otolaryngol* 1974;**78**:799.

28. Spraul CW, Grossniklaus, HE. Vitreous Hemorrhage. *Surv Ophthalmol* 1997;**42**(1):3–39.

29. Rabinowitz R, Yagev R, Shoham A, et al. Comparison between clinical and ultrasound findings in patients with vitreous hemorrhage. *Eye* 2004;**18**(3):253–6.

30. Larsen M, Wieslander, S. Acute orbital compartment syndrome after lateral blow-out fracture effectively relieved by lateral cantholysis. *Acta Ophthalmol Scand* 1999;**77**(2):232–3.

31. Popat H, Doyle PT, Davies SJ. Blindness following retrobulbar haemorrhage–it can be prevented. *Br J Oral Maxillofac Surg* 2007;**45**(2):163–4.

32. Hislop WS, Dutton GN. Retrobulbar haemorrhage: can blindness be prevented? *Injury* 1994;**25**(10):663–5.

33. Kuckelkorn R, Schrage N, Keller G, et al. Emergency treatment of chemical and thermal eye burns. *Acta Ophthalmol Scand* 2002;**80**(1):4–10.

34. Al-Omran AM, Abboud EB, Abu El-Asrar AM. Microbiologic spectrum and visual outcome of posttraumatic endophthalmitis. *Retina* 2007;**27**(2):236–42.

35. Essex RW, Yi Q, Charles PGP, et al. Post-traumatic endophthalmitis. *Ophthalmology* 2004;**111**(11):2015–22.

36. Thompson JT, Parver LM, Enger CL, et al. Infectious endophthalmitis after penetrating injuries with retained intraocular foreign bodies. National Eye Trauma System. *Ophthalmology* 1993;**100**(10):1468–74.

37. Zaharia MA, Lamarche J, Laurin M. Sympathetic uveitis 66 years after injury. *Can J Ophthalmol* 1984;**19**(5):240–3.

38. Damico FM, Kiss S, Young LH. Sympathetic ophthalmia. *Semin Ophthalmol* 2005;**20**(3):191–7.

Chapter

9

Neck trauma

Niels K. Rathlev

Introduction

Blunt and penetrating trauma to the neck results in a spectrum of injuries to vascular and aerodigestive structures that range from minor to life-threatening in severity. The injuries frequently demand immediate attention and intervention on the part of the emergency physician and trauma surgeon. The risk of devastating morbidity and mortality is significant because of the proximity of airway, neurological, digestive, and major vascular structures in closely confined fascial compartments.

Airway injuries challenge even the most skilled practitioners; familiarity with multiple approaches to securing a definitive airway is required to ensure successful management of patients with neck injuries; successful placement and maintenance of an appropriate airway is not assured with any single technique or modality. Ill-fated attempts at orotracheal intubation have resulted in the extension of partial airway lacerations and complete transaction of the trachea with disastrous consequences. Accordingly, intubation through an accessible neck wound and establishment of a surgical airway are procedural skills necessary for the successful management of victims of neck trauma. Arterial and spinal cord injuries cause significant morbidity and mortality in these patients. Major arterial structures such as the subclavian and internal, external, and common carotid arteries comprise critical vascular structures that may be involved in neck trauma. Injuries to these structures are a major source of morbidity because of exsanguinating hemorrhage, thrombosis, and distal embolus formation. They account for up to 50% of all deaths due to penetrating neck trauma.[1] Patients with esophageal injuries may demonstrate suggestive signs and symptoms initially; however, a significant

number present in subtle fashion. Aggressive initial evaluation is indicated since a more than 24-hour delay in diagnosis and definitive treatment of esophageal perforation is associated with a marked increase in mortality.

> **Box 9.1   Essential information**
> - Blunt and penetrating trauma to the neck can result in immediately life-threatening injuries due to airway, arterial, and spinal cord injuries.
> - The major role of the emergency physician is to protect the airway, manage hemorrhagic shock, and diagnose occult injuries that require intervention.
> - Diagnosis of laryngotracheal, esophageal, and major arterial injuries are a priority.
> - Providers must be skilled in several different approaches to airway management since no single method will be successful 100% of the time.
> - Thrombosis of the common and internal carotid arteries account for 50% of the deaths due to penetrating neck trauma.

Clinical anatomy and pathophysiology
Anatomy

For the purpose of describing wounds of the anterior neck, the surface anatomy is divided into three zones (Figure 9.1). Zone 1 comprises the thoracic outlet at the base of neck from the sternal notch to the cricoid cartilage. It contains the subclavian artery, the great vessels of the superior mediastinum, the trachea, and the esophagus. Zone 1 injuries are considered high risk because of concern for injury to critical thoracic and mediastinal structures. The area is not easily accessible to surgical exploration. Zone 2 is located between the cricoid cartilage and the angle of the

Trauma: A Comprehensive Emergency Medicine Approach, eds. Eric Legome and Lee W. Shockley. Published by Cambridge University Press. © Cambridge University Press 2011.

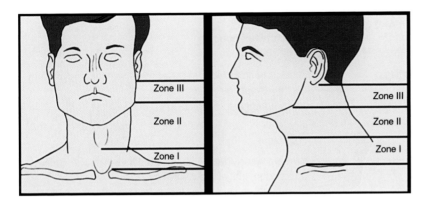

Figure 9.1 Zone I is confined between the clavicle and the cricoid cartilage, Zone II between the cricoid and the angle of the mandible, and Zone III between the angle of the mandible and the base of the skull. (From Mandavia D, Newton E, Demetriades D. Colour Atlas of Emergency Trauma. Cambridge: Cambridge University Press, 2003.)

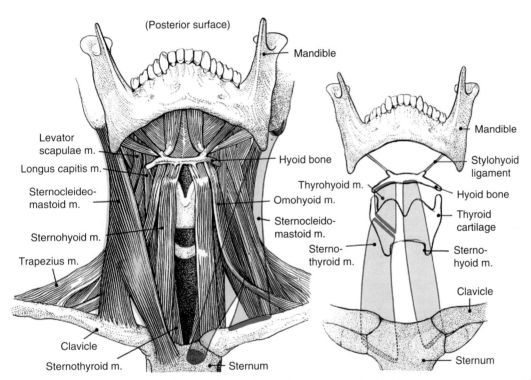

Figure 9.2 Drawing shows the sternocleidomastoid muscle with the anterior triangle highlighted. (From Melloni J, Dox I, Melloni H, Melloni B. Attorney's Reference on Human Anatomy. Cambridge: Cambridge University Press, 2008.)

mandible; the common and internal carotid arteries and the internal jugular vein are located close to the skin surface in this region and are easily accessible to surgical exposure and vascular control. The pharynx, larynx, and upper portions of the trachea and esophagus are also located in this zone. Zone 3 extends from the angle of the mandible to the base of the skull. It contains the vertebral and distal internal and external carotid arteries as well as the upper segments of the jugular veins. The internal carotid artery courses cephalad behind the body of the mandible which

obviously complicates efforts to achieve proximal and distal vascular control. For the purpose of surgical repair, part of the mandible may have to be partially dislocated and repositioned anteriorly in order to gain adequate exposure to the internal carotid artery above the level of C2.

The neck is also divided into the anterior and posterior triangles by the sternocleidomastoid muscle (Figure 9.2). The anterior triangle contains the carotid sheath which envelops important vascular structures such as the common and internal carotid arteries and

Table 9.1 Overview of surface anatomy of the neck

Surface anatomy		Structures of concern
Zone 1	Base of neck to cricoid cartilage	Subclavian artery, great vessels of the superior mediastinum, trachea, esophagus
Zone 2	Cricoid cartilage to the angle of the mandible	Common carotid and internal carotid arteries, internal jugular vein, pharynx, larynx, upper portions of trachea and esophagus
Zone 3	Above the angle of mandible	Vertebral artery, distal internal and external carotid arteries, upper segments of jugular veins
Anterior triangle	Anterior border of the sternocleidomastoid muscle to the midline	Common carotid and internal carotid arteries, internal jugular vein, vagus nerve, trachea, and esophagus
Posterior triangle	Posterior border of the sternocleidomastoid muscle to the trapezius muscle	Vertebral arteries

internal jugular vein; it extends from the midline to the anterior aspect of the sternocleidomastoid. The posterior triangle is located posterior to the sternocleidomastoid muscle extending to the anterior border of the trapezius muscle. The posterior triangle is considered a lower risk region of injury due to the paucity of critical vascular structures. The three zone nomenclature of anterior neck wounds does not apply to the posterior triangle. The vertebral arteries enter a bony canal known as the foramen tranversarium, created by the transverse processes of the vertebrae of the cervical spine, starting proximally at C6. The arteries continue cephalad within this well-protected bony canal until they exit from this foramen at C2 and enter the skull through the foramen magnum. Serious injuries to the vertebral arteries are rare because of this bony protection. Conversely, fractures involving the foramen tranversarium and facet joint dislocations due to either penetrating or blunt trauma should raise suspicion for vertebral artery injuries.[2] In the neck, vital structures are located in close proximity and are confined to compartments enclosed by relatively rigid and inflexible layers of fascia. The superficial and deep cervical fascial layers envelop these structures and offer protection vs. injury and excessive movement. The superficial fascia covers the platysma, a muscle that is only a couple of millimeters in width located just below the skin surface. The platysma is located between the superficial and deep cervical fascia and covers the entire anterolateral neck. It is an important landmark in the management of neck trauma because penetration of this muscle

should raise suspicion of injury to deeper structures. Historically, violation of the platysma was considered an indication for admission and observation or exploration in the absence of signs and symptoms of injury to vital structures.

The deep cervical fascia consists of several layers. The investing fascia surrounds the muscles of the neck circumferentially and envelops the sternocleidomastoid and trapezius. The pretracheal fascia adheres to the thyroid gland, cricoid and thyroid cartilages, trachea, and esophagus. It courses behind the sternum and inserts caudally into the pericardium. This fascial plane is clinically important because of its connection to the anterior mediastinum. Perforation of the esophagus, larynx, or trachea leads to spillage of luminal contents, including air and undigested food, into adjacent spaces. The anatomical connections of the deep fascial compartment allow these contents to enter the anterior mediastinum resulting in chemical, and eventually, infectious mediastinitis. Finally, the prevertebral fascia covers the muscles that stabilize the vertebrae and forms the axillary sheath that surrounds the subclavian artery. The carotid sheath envelops the common and internal carotid arteries, internal jugular vein, and vagus nerve (Table 9.1).

Case reports have documented, that in rare circumstances, the carotid sheath is able to deflect low-speed projectiles such as bullets from some handguns thereby preventing damage to critical vascular and neurological structures.[3] Because of the anatomic proximity of airway and major arterial structures, hemorrhage from a significant, adjacent vascular

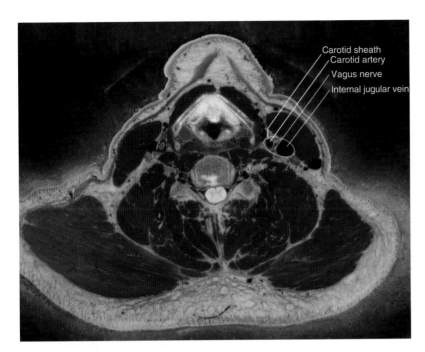

Carotid sheath
Carotid artery
Vagus nerve
Internal jugular vein

Figure 9.3 Transverse section of the neck at C7. (Courtesy of the Visible Human Project®, with permission.)

injury may externally compress and eventually distort the larynx and trachea (Figure 9.3). An expanding neck hematoma can quickly cause tracheal deviation and ultimately obstruct the airway. Accordingly, the size of a traumatic neck hematoma must be carefully assessed at regular intervals and a definitive airway should be established early if continued expansion is noted. This dramatic development can occur over a period of only minutes.

Pathophysiology

The majority of penetrating neck injuries is caused by knives and low-energy gunshot wounds. Fortunately, these weapons impart a lower level of kinetic energy to tissues in comparison with military rifles and shotguns. The current mortality rate from civilian penetrating injuries to the neck is approximately 3–6%.[4] This is in contrast to the military experience during the Korean and Vietnam conflicts when the mortality rates were significantly greater due to high-energy projectiles. The mortality rate in civilians has not changed appreciably in recent years, despite continued improvement in diagnostic and therapeutic techniques.[5] Unfortunately, this appears to reflect the fact that the prognosis for the subset of patients with spinal cord and major arterial injuries has not been appreciably altered despite advances in diagnostic imaging and interventions. Factors that

increase mortality include gunshot wounds, zone 1 entry or exit wounds, spinal cord injury, shock from uncontrolled hemorrhage and missed vascular injuries. In total, approximately 50% of all deaths are caused by arterial or venous injury. In addition, acute renal failure, stroke, air embolus, adult respiratory distress syndrome, severe brain injury, laryngo-tracheal trauma, and airway obstruction by hematoma also contribute as causes of death.[1] A missed esophageal perforation may occasionally result in mediastinitis, sepsis, and death. Fortunately, the mortality rate from perforation of the cervical esophagus due to a neck injury is lower than esophageal injuries caused by chest and abdominal wounds.

The demographic characteristics of the victims mirror the experience from penetrating trauma in general. Patients are primarily young men with injuries sustained as a result of interpersonal violence. Pooled data from civilian series published between 1963 and 1990, reported the frequency of these injuries among 2495 patients with penetrating neck trauma primarily caused by gunshot and stab wounds.[1] Approximately 51% of patients suffered significant injuries to vascular, airway, and digestive tract structures. The compiled data demonstrated that the common and internal carotid arteries were the most frequently involved structures accounting for almost 7% of all injuries. Nearly one third of these patients present with a concomitant neurological deficit due to thrombus formation and cerebrovascular ischemia. Hemispheric stroke and hemiplegia is an infrequent but devastating cause of long-term morbidity in survivors.[5] In descending order of frequency of injury, internal and common carotid artery injuries (6.7%) were followed by the subclavian (2%), external carotid (2%), and vertebral (1.3%) arteries. The internal jugular vein was the most frequently injured venous structure accounting for 9% of all victims.

Airway and digestive tract injuries are potentially life threatening and require a high index of suspicion in pursuit of the diagnosis. In the previously quoted pooled series of 2495 victims of penetrating neck trauma, laryngo-tracheal injuries occurred in 10% of the total number of victims. The pharynx and esophagus were damaged in 9% of patients.[1] Fortunately, injuries to these structures rarely require operative repair. Although complete airway occlusion is easily recognizable and rapidly fatal if not corrected immediately, other more insidious injuries to the airway and digestive tract prove no less fatal when the diagnosis is delayed. In a series of 12 789 consecutive trauma patients presenting over an 8-year period from 1988 to 1996, only 12 (0.09%) patients had airway or digestive tract injuries.[6] Other studies estimate the injury rate to be closer to 5%. Large randomized studies to determine optimal diagnostic and management decisions have not been published because of the infrequency of these injuries.

The most common mechanism causing blunt trauma to the neck are motor vehicle collisions.[7] These injuries typically result from rapid deceleration, or from direct blows to the anterior neck by the steering column, or dashboard crushing the trachea at the cricoid ring and compressing the esophagus against the cervical vertebrae. Injuries can also occur from increased intrathecal pressure against a closed glottis related to improper seat belt use.

Strangulation results from hangings, ligatures, manual choking, and excessive manipulation. The usual mechanism of death in hangings is compression of the jugular veins, preventing venous return and resulting in loss of consciousness from edema of the brain. Subsequently, the unconscious patient's body weight falls against the ligature, compressing the trachea and restricting airflow to the lungs. Irreversible asphyxiation follows in minutes.[8] Chokeholds typically generate even greater force and are no longer promoted in police training. While occasionally reported, carotid artery occlusion and dissection is

actually quite rare after strangulation injury.[9] Clothesline injuries occur in various contact sports such as football, as a result of tackling, and martial arts as well as in accidents involving all-terrain vehicles, motorcycles, and snowmobiles. Direct blows by fists, feet, and other blunt weapons and excessive cervical manipulation account for the remaining causes of blunt neck injury.[10,11]

Significant vascular injuries to the neck occur in approximately 1–3% of all major blunt trauma victims.[12–15] While high-speed motor vehicle accidents cause the majority of these injuries, other mechanisms include motorcycle crashes, pedestrians struck by motor vehicles, falls, and assaults with direct blows to the neck.[16,17] Intraoral trauma and basilar skull and cervical spine fractures are frequently associated injuries. Although vascular injuries are rare following blunt trauma, the morbidity and mortality rates are significantly higher than for penetrating trauma. The overall mortality related to blunt vascular injuries is 20–30%; in addition, 40–60% of the patients develop permanent neurologic deficits due to central nervous system ischemia.[18]

Both penetrating and blunt vascular trauma can result in the formation of pseudoaneurysms, arteriovenous fistulae, complete transections, and occlusions due to thrombus formation. In blunt trauma, injury to the cervical arteries is caused by rapid deceleration associated with distraction plus hyperextension or hyperflexion and rotation.[2] Vascular structures are stretched across bony prominences of the spine and the resulting shearing forces create intimal tears in the vessel wall.[19] With improved diagnostic imaging techniques, traumatic dissection is increasingly being recognized as the primary injury to the vessel wall. Hemispheric ischemic stroke and hemiplegia is a devastating consequence in these patients and is due to occlusive thrombus and embolus formation.[5]

Box 9.2 Pathophysiology of neck injuries

- Significant vascular injuries to the neck occur in approximately 1–3% of all major blunt trauma victims.
- Airway and digestive tract injuries are extremely rare.
- Motor vehicle collisions and strangulation are common mechanisms of blunt neck injuries.
- Knives and low-energy gunshot wounds cause most of the penetrating injuries.
- The mortality rate is 2–6% from penetrating trauma and 20–30% from blunt vascular injuries.

Prehospital care

Appropriate prehospital care of patients with potential airway and vascular injuries of the neck is crucial to patient outcomes. The natural inclination of prehospital providers is to immobilize the cervical spine for victims of both blunt and penetrating neck trauma. While evidence supports this practice in the former, immediate management of the airway and hemorrhage control of the victim of a penetrating neck wound should take precedence over cervical spine stabilization in alert patients with no neurological deficits.

There are no reports of unstable cervical spine injuries caused by penetrating neck trauma secondary to stab wounds. Conversely, these injuries are a recognized consequence of gunshot wounds to the neck. In order to create an unstable cervical spine fracture both anterior and posterior columns must be fractured. Consequently, the bullet must traverse the spinal cord to cause this injury, and the patient will invariably present with neurological signs and symptoms. A retrospective study of 19 patients sustaining gunshot wounds to the face and neck found that all patients with unstable cervical spine fractures also presented with neurological deficits; all were either comatose due to hemorrhagic shock or brain injury, or suffered para- or quadriplegia which was evident upon presentation to the emergency department (ED).[20] In this study, three awake and neurologically intact individuals presented with gunshot wounds to the face that resulted in stable cervical spine fractures. A previous series found no cervical spine injuries in 174 patients with gunshot wounds to the head.[21] Based on these results, emergent treatment, such as hemorrhage control or airway management, should take precedence over cervical spine stabilization in alert patients with no neurological deficits. This may involve removing the cervical collar to gain access to the injury. Once the immediate priorities have been addressed in the prehospital setting, the collar may be replaced during transport. In "non-judicial" hanging attempts, the risk of an unstable cervical spine fracture is extremely low. Moreover, the cervical collar may impede venous outflow from the head leading to an increased intracranial pressure.

Patients with progressive subcutaneous or mediastinal emphysema, uncontrolled hemorrhage, or an expanding hematoma require early airway intervention. This may be life saving for patients with severe airway compromise or vascular injuries because of potentially progressive distortion of normal, recognizable tissues and landmarks. In the care of experienced paramedics, it is far preferable to intubate a patient with relatively normal anatomy in the prehospital setting than waiting to perform a "crash" surgical airway in the ED or operating suite. Patients who require intubation for definitive airway control can be safely managed with in-line stabilization to minimize movement of the neck during the procedure. Standard procedure using direct laryngoscopy with a Macintosh or Miller laryngoscope blade causes minimal movement of the cervical spine, i.e., no more than 10–11° of extension in healthy patients positioned on a rigid board prior to intubation.[22]

Patients in hemorrhagic shock must be managed by stopping external bleeding and fluid resuscitation. External hemorrhage or a rapidly expanding hematoma of the neck must be controlled with uninterrupted, forceful, direct pressure. Intraoral bleeding may be controlled with gauze packing of the oropharynx once a definitive airway has been established. The strategy of accepting a lower than normal blood pressure while maintaining perfusion to vital organs is termed "controlled" or "permissive" resuscitation and remains controversial; it involves delaying aggressive fluid resuscitation until operative intervention. Favorable outcomes of delayed fluid resuscitation were obtained in patients with penetrating torso injuries but cannot yet be extrapolated to neck injuries.[23] Rapidly raising the blood pressure before the hemorrhage is controlled may theoretically promote further bleeding and increase mortality as evidenced by a transient or minimal response to resuscitation. Balancing the dual goals of maintaining organ perfusion and minimizing the risk of rebleeding can be difficult and requires constant monitoring of the victim.

Box 9.3 Essential rehospital interventions

- Oxygenate all patients, O_2 saturation should remain > 90%.
- Intravenous fluids to maintain perfusion to vital organs.
- Intubate early using standard protocols.
- Apply external pressure to stop hemorrhage.
- Board and collar all blunt trauma victims and patients who are comatose or demonstrate neurological deficits with penetrating trauma to the neck.

Emergency department evaluation and management

Patients who are awake and able to converse should be questioned about the timing and mechanism of injury. If the patient arrives via Emergency Medical Services, prehospital providers can provide further details, as may friends or family that accompany the patient. The initial clinical presentation ranges from patients who are entirely asymptomatic with no signs or symptoms of injury, to immediately life-threatening complications such as hemorrhagic shock, airway compromise, and coma.

The initial examination of any penetrating neck wound should determine the zone or zones of external wounds and the presence or absence of penetration of the platysma. It must be emphasized, that the zone of injury merely refers to the locations of wounds. Bullets notoriously travel in unpredictable directions once tissues are penetrated and bone is struck and redirects their course. The direction of stab wounds also cannot always be predicted. During the initial evaluation, injuries should therefore be sought in all zones of the neck as well as the head and chest. Patients commonly sustain significant injuries to vital organs that cannot be predicted based on the location of external wounds alone.

The airway must be secured when there is any question of compromise, and hemorrhage must be stopped with pressure and gauze packs. Direct pressure will usually successfully stop the bleeding while attempts to "blindly" clamp vascular structures under poor visualization are to be avoided. Other critical structures such as neurovascular bundles may be injured in the process; when managing zone 1 wounds, intravenous lines should be placed on the side opposite to the injury when possible. This is to avoid extravasation of fluids into the chest from a potential subclavian vein injury.

The pharynx must be examined by visual inspection when possible. Pharyngeal packing to tamponade severe oral bleeding will be necessary after a definite airway has been established. Patients with zone 1 injuries and refractory shock may require a thoracotomy for control of a suspected subclavian artery injury. A standard lateral thoracotomy may not allow proper exposure to the area of injury. In this instance, the help of a thoracic or trauma surgeon is required since a median sternotomy with extension to the involved side may be required for proximal control of the vessel.

The evaluation of blunt and penetrating neck trauma begins with the airway. Patients with airway injuries may present with abnormal respiratory patterns, stridor, dysphonia, tachypnea, cyanosis, progressive airway obstruction from an expanding hematoma that is compressing the airway, or cervical tenderness. Dyspnea, hoarseness, and cough also suggest the presence of an airway injury.[24] Bubbling of blood from a neck wound in synchrony with respirations is highly suggestive of a laryngeal or tracheal injury; however, hemoptysis may not be a reliable sign of serious injury to the airway. Kelly et al. published a 20-year study that examined 100 penetrating and 6 blunt neck trauma victims; all 80 patients with tracheal injuries had signs of airway compromise in the ED.[25] These signs included tachypnea, dyspnea, cyanosis, subcutaneous emphysema, and an abnormal respiratory pattern. Other investigators have found that breathing difficulties may not be present initially. Hemoptysis was an unreliable sign of serious injury and patients with major vascular or tracheal injuries rarely survived. Additional presenting features include voice alteration, stridor, drooling, cervical subcutaneous emphysema or crepitance, dyspnea, and distortion of the anatomy of anterior neck including loss of normal landmarks, asymmetry, flattened thyroid prominence, and tracheal deviation.[26]

Greene and Stark evaluated clinical signs of laryngeal fracture according to anatomic location.[24] Injuries above the glottis presented with cervical emphysema, progressive airway obstruction, palpable disruption of the thyroid cartilage, dysphagia, or hoarseness. Lesions located below the glottis presented with hemoptysis or a persistent air leak from the endotracheal tube in intubated patients but were not associated with swallowing difficulties and did not have early signs of airway compromise.

Under normal conditions, the esophagus is relatively mobile and collapsed, which partly explains why injuries to this organ are uncommon. Early detection of penetrating esophageal injuries remains difficult because clinical signs of injury are initially absent in 30% of patients.[27] In seriously injured patients, crepitance or subcutaneous emphysema may be found in the neck on physical exam and symptoms of dysphagia or hematemesis should raise suspicion of an acute esophageal injury. Unfortunately, clinical findings of odynophagia, drooling, and hematemesis are only approximately 80% sensitive for injury.[28] Blood in the saliva or nasogastric aspirate may be an early clue to esophageal damage. The average delay to diagnosis from the time of injury is usually many hours when using a selective approach to evaluation, and the resultant morbidity and mortality is significant.[29,30] While more than 90% of patients will survive if the injury is detected within 24 hours, the survival rate drops precipitously after this time, usually from infectious complications related to mediastinitis.[31]

Blunt esophageal injuries are equally uncommon. In subtle cases, there may be no initial signs of significant injury. Dysphagia, presence of a sucking neck wound, blood in oral gastric and nasogastric aspirate, and crepitance are all signs of esophageal rupture. The majority of injuries to the esophagus are associated with concomitant laryngotracheal trauma, which is to be expected given its posterior and protected location behind the airway structures.[28] Keogh et al. describe two cases in which minor neck trauma caused significant airway compromise from delayed neck hematomas.[32] Both patients were anticoagulated with warfarin.[32]

A careful physical examination is critical in stratifying vascular injuries that require further evaluation. Patients in extremis from hemorrhagic shock obviously require immediate transfer to the operating site. In terms of clinical decision making, the greater challenge rests in managing patients that do not have immediate indications for operative management. The presence of "hard" signs of vascular injury is useful in predicting injuries that require repair. They include: (1) a bruit or thrill which may be detected by palpation or auscultation in 45% of patients with a traumatic arteriovenous fistula; (2) active or pulsatile hemorrhage; (3) pulsatile or expanding hematoma.[30,33] The absence of "hard" signs reliably excludes significant zone 3 injuries that require intervention according to one series of 844 penetrating trauma patients.[34] "Soft" signs of vascular injury include: (1) hypotension and clinical shock; (2) stable or non-pulsatile hematoma; (3) proximity of the entry or exit wound to major vascular structures. In addition, neurological deficit due to ischemia is also considered a "soft" sign of vascular injury. Deficit due to a primary nerve injury occurs immediately whereas ischemic neuropathy is delayed and typically develops minutes to hours later.

Box 9.4 "Hard" and "soft" signs of vascular injury

Hard signs	Soft signs
Bruit or thrill	Hypotension and shock
	Central or peripheral nervous system ischemia
Expanding or pulsatile hematoma	Stable, non-pulsatile hematoma
Severe or pulsatile hemorrhage	Neurologic deficit from ischemia
Pulse deficit	

Diminished or absent pulses is not a sensitive finding; up to 25% of patients with major vascular injuries requiring surgical repair demonstrate normal pulses by physical exam.[35] Arterial flow may be maintained when these lesions are non-occlusive in nature. Fortunately, the majority of these non-occlusive injuries without "hard" signs resolve spontaneously over time.[36] The challenge, as always, is to detect subtle injuries that will eventually progress and require operative repair. A pseudoaneurysm, or false aneurysm, is a focal dilatation of the artery with disruption of one or more layers of the vessel wall. It is typically caused by leakage of blood into the surrounding tissues with persistent communication between the originating artery and the blood-filled cavity. Pseudoaneurysms of the neck may eventually present as a pulsatile mass if left untreated.

Blunt vascular injuries, involving the carotid or the vertebral arteries, are rare and the clinical presentation is often subtle and non-specific. McKevitt et al. documented that 60% of blunt cerebrovascular injuries were unsuspected at initial evaluation, and concomitant head or thoracic injuries frequently overshadowed the presenting symptoms.[37] When identified and treated early, the likelihood of permanent, devastating neurological dysfunction is reduced significantly. The diagnosis is often delayed because almost 25% of patients with injuries do not manifest signs and symptoms until 24 hours post-injury or later.

The classic presentation of a patient with a blunt vascular injury to the neck is a neurologically intact victim who subsequently develops hemiparesis after a high-speed motor vehicle crash. The vast majority of patients manifest neurological deficits at the time of diagnosis of blunt carotid injury.[12] Early signs and symptoms may include pain in the head and neck,

Table 9.2 High-risk criteria for blunt cerebrovascular injury[16]

- Glasgow Coma Scale score ≤ 6
- Petrous bone fracture
- Cervical spine fracture or subluxation especially involving C1–3 or the foramen tranversarium
- Diffuse axonal injury
- Le Fort II and III facial fracture

(NB. 20% of patients with lesions meet none of these criteria).

ptosis, and miosis; however, there are no reliable clinical means with which to diagnose blunt carotid injury prior to the development of neurological deficits or stroke.[38] Providers should screen for blunt cerebrovascular injury because significant lesions amenable to intervention are currently under-recognized and also because the typical latent period between initial presentation and onset of neurological deficits allows time for intervention. Finally, definitive treatment may improve patient outcomes. Based on a multiple logistic regression analysis, definitive diagnostic testing should be pursued for patients who demonstrate any of the high-risk features listed in Table 9.2.[16]

Since 20% of patients with blunt cerebrovascular injuries unfortunately meet none of these criteria, screening should be performed liberally, especially for survivors of near-hangings and severe hyperextension and hyperflexion injuries. With this approach, 72–80% of all blunt vascular injuries can be identified prior to the onset of neurologic deficits.[16,18,39] The presence of an ecchymosis on the neck caused by the shoulder portion of the seat belt is known as the "seat belt" sign. The risk of blunt carotid artery injury in patients with a neck "seat belt" sign is significantly higher when associated with an Injury Severity Score > 16, a Glasgow Coma Scale score < 14, or a clavicle or first rib fracture. Clearly, presence of this sign should raise suspicion of occult vascular injury and prompt further evaluation when accompanied by the previously stated criteria.[15]

Vertebral artery injuries are closely associated with cervical spine injuries. In one series, fully 33% of cervical spine fractures, excluding spinous process fractures, are associated with a vertebral artery injury.[14] Fractures involving the transverse foramen are present in 78% of patients while subluxation is associated with most of the remaining injuries; at least one of these bony injuries is present in 92% of

patients with vertebral artery injury. Bilateral injuries occur in approximately 15% of all patients.[12,18] Concurrent injuries to other organ systems are common; McKevitt et al. found that almost 95% of patients with blunt vascular injuries of the neck had a concomitant major thoracic injury or a Glasgow Coma Scale score < 8.[37]

Penetrating neck wounds should be examined with care to assess the depth of penetration by gently spreading the wound edges. The Trendelenburg position may be utilized if there is concern about an internal jugular vein injury and possible air embolus. Probing the wound is discouraged since it may inadvertently disrupt a thrombus or release a hematoma that was previously not actively bleeding. The wound should never be closed unless the depth is clearly visualized. Patients with progressive subcutaneous or mediastinal emphysema, severe dyspnea requiring intubation, difficulty in mechanical ventilation, uncontrolled hemorrhage, or patients with an air leak from their chest tubes should all be directed to the operating room for definitive surgical management.[40]

Box 9.5 Emergency department interventions for penetrating neck trauma

- Early intubation prior to airway compromise.
- Stop hemorrhage and resuscitate with blood products.
- Assess for "hard" and "soft" signs of vascular injury.
- Do not blindly probe wound.
- Patients with zone 1 injuries and refractory shock may require a thoracotomy for suspected subclavian artery injury.

Stable patients are approached from a selective set of criteria that are outlined in Figure 9.4 for penetrating trauma and Figure 9.5 for blunt injury.

Secondary evaluation

A lateral neck plain film and chest X-ray are useful as initial screening tests. The radiographs may reveal subcutaneous emphysema which is the most common presenting X-ray finding in patients with significant injuries to the airway and digestive tracts.[40] In patients with airway disruption, the surgical anatomy of the rupture creates patterns of air leak on plain films that may help predict the site of perforation. Patients with laryngeal transection tend to have gross,

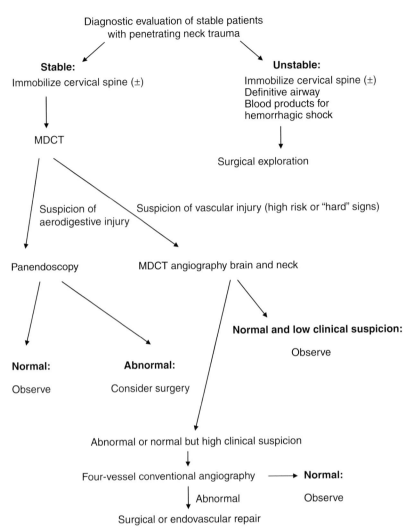

Diagnostic evaluation of stable patients
with penetrating neck trauma

Stable:
Immobilize cervical spine (±)

MDCT

Suspicion of
aerodigestive injury

Suspicion of vascular injury (high risk or "hard" signs)

Unstable:
Immobilize cervical spine (±)
Definitive airway
Blood products for
hemorrhagic shock

Surgical exploration

Panendoscopy

MDCT angiography brain and neck

Normal and low clinical suspicion:

Observe

Normal:

Observe

Abnormal:

Consider surgery

Abnormal or normal but high clinical suspicion

Four-vessel conventional angiography ⟶ **Normal:**

Abnormal

Observe

Surgical or endovascular repair

Figure 9.4 Diagnostic evaluation of stable patients with penetrating neck trauma. MDCT, multidetector computed tomography.

superficial, and deep emphysema of the face and neck, while patients with tracheal rupture often present with deep cervical and massive mediastinal emphysema without a pneumothorax (Figure 9.6).[41]

The improvement in speed and resolution of images by multidetector computed tomography (MDCT), including 64-row multiplanar reconstructions, has had a significant impact in facilitating widespread acceptance of the selective approach to evaluation of penetrating neck injuries. It has become clear that a normal MDCT may obviate surgical exploration in cases that previously would have gone directly to the operating room. Computed tomography can accurately identify extrapulmonary air, directly visualize tracheal wall disruption and signs of transtracheal balloon herniation in intubated patients, and locate extratracheal endotracheal tube position.[42] In intubations in cadavers with tracheal disruption, CT images closely match those obtained in live cases. Equally good results have been obtained when comparing CT to bronchoscopic images confirming the accuracy of CT.[43,44] Three-dimensional reconstructions also help the surgeon to choose the optimal surgical approach. Studies also note that it takes an extreme amount of pressure in order to rupture the tracheal rings in cadavers, suggesting it would be unusual for routine endotracheal tube balloon inflation during intubation to cause additional airway compromise in penetrating neck injuries.

Stable patients with suspected airway injuries should be evaluated with a combination of careful physical exam, plain films, MDCT, and bronchoscopy depending on the institutional resources and expertise. Three-dimensional reconstructive CT is

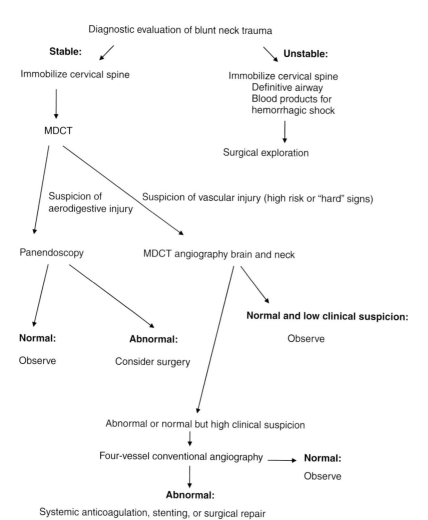

Diagnostic evaluation of blunt neck trauma

Stable:

Immobilize cervical spine

↓

MDCT

Suspicion of aerodigestive injury

Suspicion of vascular injury (high risk or "hard" signs)

Panendoscopy

MDCT angiography brain and neck

Normal:
Observe

Abnormal:
Consider surgery

Normal and low clinical suspicion:
Observe

Unstable:

Immobilize cervical spine
Definitive airway
Blood products for hemorrhagic shock

↓

Surgical exploration

Abnormal or normal but high clinical suspicion

↓

Four-vessel conventional angiography ⟶ **Normal:**
Observe

↓

Abnormal:
Systemic anticoagulation, stenting, or surgical repair

Figure 9.5 Diagnostic evaluation of blunt neck trauma. MDCT, multidetector computed tomography.

extremely sensitive in identifying and locating tracheal injuries. In the evaluation of esophageal injuries, barium swallow, flexible endoscopy, and rigid endoscopy all have sensitivities approaching 90%. In one study, the combination of rigid endoscope and barium swallow found 100% of esophageal injuries.[27] An MDCT scan may demonstrate free air in the neck adjacent to the esophagus suggesting perforation or rupture.

Imaging of the blunt trauma patient with a neck injury has also evolved with the advent of high resolution CT. Lateral soft tissue neck X-rays should never be used exclusively to rule out airway and digestive tract injuries, although significant injuries will typically reveal radiographic abnormalities.[41] The chest X-ray, however, remains an important element of the initial trauma workup to detect pneumothorax, hemothorax, and pneumomediastinum.

Computed tomography scanning is the initial imaging modality of choice in the hemodynamically stable blunt trauma patient and is used to guide selective operative management. As previously stated, Chen et al. found that CT accurately diagnosed tracheal rupture with deep cervical air in intubated cadavers,[42] and Moriwaki et al. found that three-dimensional CT accurately identified the site of injury, as confirmed by bronchoscopy.[43]

In conjunction with CT, panendoscopy ensures complete evaluation of the airway and digestive tracts. These procedures are recommended in the workup of all blunt and penetrating neck trauma patients with signs and symptoms of airway or digestive tract injury. Before embarking on this procedure, airway patency should be assessed and secured. Schaefer and Brown developed a classification system for laryngeal

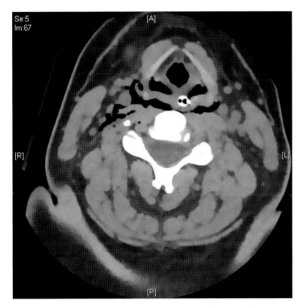

Figure 9.6 Multidetector computed tomography (MDCT) of the neck in a patient with tracheal disruption and deep tissue emphysema.

injuries based on a combination of CT scanning and endoscopy (Table 9.3).[45]

Fiberoptic nasopharyngoscopy is used to evaluate vocal cord function and to initially assess the extent of trauma of the glottis and above; direct laryngoscopy allows for a detailed view of the larynx and bronchoscopy is performed to examine the subglottic larynx. The combination of direct laryngoscopy and bronchoscopy appears to be highly sensitive for lesions of the larynx and trachea. Esophagoscopy allows detailed evaluation of esophageal mucosa. Additionally, barium swallow has been studied for esophageal injuries. It is commonly recognized that a swallow study alone does not rule out a pharyngeal or esophageal leak. Weigelt et al. examined 118 stable patients with cervical trauma and compared barium swallow with endoscopy.[27] All 10 esophageal injuries were identified when the 2 modalities were combined. Gastrograffin has currently replaced barium because of concern about chemical mediastinitis that may result from barium leakage through an esophageal perforation.

Conventional four-vessel cerebral angiography remains the "gold" standard for evaluating the carotid and the vertebral arteries with a sensitivity in excess of 99%. Very rarely do injuries missed by angiography require repair and a normal study is highly predictive of survival from vessel injury.[46]

Conversely, angiography is invasive, expensive, and resource intensive, and involves mobilizing interventional radiology. Complications usually involve the catheter insertion site or reactions to intravenous contrast. Biffl et al. developed a classification system for blunt carotid artery injuries based on angiographic findings that is utilized to guide further management (Table 9.4).[19] The lesions are categorized based on size, outcome, and treatment options.

In a series of penetrating neck injuries, MDCT angiography had a sensitivity of 90–100% compared with conventional angiography and surgical exploration.[47,48] High resolution CT angiography offers high diagnostic accuracy with minimal risk, making this the initial diagnostic study of choice when available. In addition, CT angiography can be used in lieu of conventional angiography to rule out an arterial injury in penetrating injuries to zone 2 of the neck.[49]

Most patients who meet screening criteria for blunt vascular injury of the neck undergo MDCT scanning for other injuries. Adding MDCT angiography of the neck to the clinical evaluation has increased the rate of identification of injuries by a factor of three, decreased the mean time to diagnosis and decreased the rate of permanent neurological sequelae from carotid arterial injuries.[18] In the evaluation of blunt injuries, MDCT angiography has a sensitivity of 68% and a specificity of 67%. In 2 series, it missed 55% of Grade I injuries, 14% of Grade II injuries, and 13% of Grade III injuries.[50,51] Approximately one third of the missed injuries were significant and resulted in stroke. Schneidereit et al. determined that the detection of blunt cerebrovascular injury increased from 0.17% to 1.40% after the implementation of screening with a protocol based on 8-slice MDCT angiography.[52] The protocol resulted in a decrease in the stroke rate from 67% to 0% ($P < 0.002$) and a decreased mortality from 38% to 0% ($P = 0.002$). Higher resolution, 64-slice technology will likely improve the sensitivity and specificity of MDCT angiography in blunt neck trauma. The modality is limited by artifacts from metallic fragments and occasionally by abundant soft tissue air.

Duplex ultrasonography is non-invasive, convenient, and low cost, but the technique remains highly operator-dependent. The technique relies on the detection of turbulent flow caused by vascular injuries. Consequently, duplex ultrasonography can miss non-occlusive injuries with preserved non-turbulent flow. Examples of such injuries include intimal flaps

Table 9.3 Treatment of laryngeal injury based on injury classification

Group	Symptoms	Signs	Management
I	Minor airway symptoms	Minor hematoma without laryngeal fracture	Observation and humidified oxygen
II	Airway compromise	Edema plus mucosal disruption	Tracheostomy followed by laryngoscopy and esophagoscopy
III	Airway compromise	Massive edema, exposed cartilage and vocal cord immobility	Tracheostomy followed by exploration and repair
IV	Airway compromise	Massive edema, exposed cartilage	Tracheostomy followed by exploration and repair Possible stent placement

Table 9.4 Grading scale for blunt carotid artery injury

Grade	Angiographic findings
1	Irregularity, < 25% narrowing of luminal diameter
2	Intimal flap, thrombus, > 25% narrowing of luminal diameter
3	Pseudoaneurysm
4	Total occlusion
5	Complete transaction

Box 9.6   Essentials of the secondary evaluation

- Conventional angiography remains the "gold" standard for vascular injuries.
- High resolution MDCT angiography defined as 64 slice or greater is the screening test of choice for patients without obvious indication for surgical intervention.
- Duplex ultrasonography is highly operator-dependent.
- Panendoscopy is required to rule out airway and digestive tract injuries.

---

and pseudoaneurysms that may require surgical repair. The technique is also limited by its ability to reliably evaluate only the extracranial arteries, i.e., the common and external carotid arteries. Unfortunately, most injuries involve the internal carotid artery, which is unfortunately not evaluated well by ultrasound. The technique is especially inaccurate in evaluating injuries at the base of the skull. When utilized by skilled, experienced operators, the sensitivity of duplex ultrasound vs. conventional angiography as the "gold" standard is reportedly 90–100% for injuries requiring intervention.[53] In spite of this and other favorable reports, duplex ultrasonography has largely been replaced by MDCT angiography in the assessment of patients without clear indications for surgical repair of vascular injuries.

Treatment

Early and rapid airway assessment, followed by definitive airway protection is critical to the management of both penetrating and blunt neck trauma. Most blunt neck trauma patients are placed in cervical spine collars that complicate the intubation. In-line cervical stabilization is a safe method for immobilizing the cervical spine during intubation. The optimal technique for intubating a patient with penetrating neck injuries is by direct laryngoscopy, though it has not been studied in detail in randomized trials. It remains a difficult decision when to expectantly observe a patient for signs of impending airway compromise, or to intubate the patient early before further distortion of the anatomy makes the procedure more difficult and possibly leads to an emergent surgical airway. Clearly any patient in shock, with hypoxia, or suspicion of airway compromise needs immediate intubation.

As described previously, immediate urgent treatment of the penetrating neck wound should take precedence over concerns for the cervical spine in awake and neurologically intact individuals. This includes removing the cervical collar to gain access to the injury or manage the airway, when necessary. However, a conservative but reasonable approach is that all patients with gunshot wounds to the neck and face should generally be immobilized in a cervical

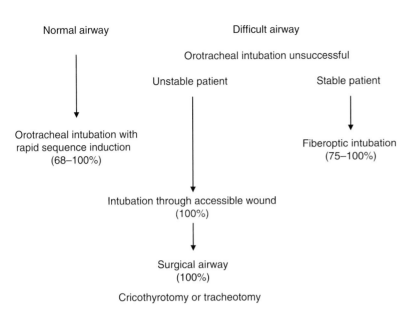

Normal airway

Difficult airway

Orotracheal intubation unsuccessful

Unstable patient

Stable patient

Orotracheal intubation with
rapid sequence induction
(68–100%)

Fiberoptic intubation
(75–100%)

Intubation through accessible wound
(100%)

Surgical airway
(100%)

Cricothyrotomy or tracheotomy

Figure 9.7 Airway techniques (success rates are listed in parentheses).

collar, understanding that the prevalence of unstable fracture is probably miniscule at most, until radiography definitively shows there is no fracture. Direct laryngoscopy using a Macintosh or Miller laryngoscope blade causes minimal movement of the cervical spine in healthy patients positioned on a spine board prior to intubation.[18] Patients who require intubation can be safely managed with in-line stabilization without a collar.

It is safe to use rapid sequence intubation using a short-acting paralytic along with an induction agent in these patients. In the most recent series in the literature, all of the 39 patients were successfully intubated using succinylcholine. In total, 12 patients underwent attempted fiberoptic intubation by otolaryngologists with three failures. Interestingly, those three patients were subsequently successfully intubated using rapid sequence intubation.[54] This series underscores the vital importance of using the technique with which the clinician is most comfortable during emergent airway management. If the airway can be directly visualized through the traumatic neck wound because of tracheal disruption, it may be possible to intubate the patient through the wound, but care must be exercised to stabilize the proximal end of the trachea. A single case report describes the use of the gum elastic bougie to facilitate the intubation of a patient with a self-induced deep slash wound to zone 2 and complete tracheal transection. When blind intubation failed, the bougie was

used to intubate the trachea. The tracheal rings caused a "clicking" sound to confirm the bougie's location, and the endotracheal tube was successfully placed into the trachea over the bougie.[55]

Numerous alternative intubation methods are available if direct laryngoscopy fails or cannot be used (Figure 9.7). Flexible fiberoptic endoscopes can be used both for orotracheal and nasotracheal intubations. These techniques require patient preparation with topical anesthetics, possible intravenous sedation, and are therefore time consuming and dependent upon the experience of the operator. Newer rigid fiberoptic endoscopes and video-laryngoscope blades may aid in visualizing the vocal cords for intubation, though all fiberoptic methods are difficult to use in the presence of bleeding or copious secretions.

Blind nasotracheal intubation historically has been discouraged due to a perceived high failure rate and potential for complications. A recent study of 40 patients intubated via the nasotracheal route in the prehospital setting demonstrated a 90% success rate with a similar mortality rate to matched patients who were orotracheally intubated.[56] It is reasonable to consider nasotracheal route as a viable alternative in the prehospital setting when emergency orotracheal intubation is not possible.

A surgical airway is used as a last resort. Cricothyrotomy or occasionally, tracheostomy, is the preferred procedure for securing the airway when other techniques have failed. There is a risk that the operator could open an otherwise stable hematoma while incising through fascial planes that have contained the bleeding. Significant hemorrhage may subsequently obscure the operative field and result in severe blood loss. There is also a risk of transforming a partial tracheal injury into a complete transection, which only further complicates the management of the patient.

In the past, controversy raged surrounding the choice between mandatory and selective evaluation of penetrating neck trauma. Selective surgical exploration has now become the standard of care for patients without obvious indications for surgical repair. This assumes that all necessary staffing, equipment, and radiographic and procedural expertise are available 24 hours a day for the management of these patients. In settings where these prerequisites are not available, exploration may be the safest course of action. This involves evaluation of vascular, airway, and digestive structures under direct visualization in the operating suite. The incision is made at the anterior border of the sternocleidomastoid, which is reflected posterior allowing easy access to zone 2 structures. Difficulty in exposure of critical structures renders exploration of zones 1 and 3 much more challenging. Mandatory exploration of zone 2 is a common therapeutic strategy in rural settings where transport to a level I trauma center is not an option and in developing countries. Non-operative techniques have proven to be sufficiently sensitive to safely rule out injuries to the airway, digestive tract, and vascular structures that require surgical intervention. Careful physical examination using protocols for serial examinations, including auscultation of the carotid arteries, is more than 95% sensitive for detecting arterial and aerodigestive tract injuries that require repair.[49] While esophageal and arterial injuries have reportedly been missed during selective evaluation, this has also been described during mandatory exploration. The selective approach is significantly more cost-effective than mandatory exploration because of a faster recovery period and a reduction in in-hospital days.[57]

The definitive treatment of penetrating and blunt cerebrovascular lesions is determined by the angiographic evaluation based on the proposed grading scale. In general, surgical repair is preferred for accessible Grade II–V lesions because the morbidity and mortality of these patients is significantly reduced compared with those who undergo simple ligation.

Adverse outcomes occur in 15% of individuals after repair vs. 50% after ligation. Consequently, ligation should be considered only for patients with coma and no antegrade flow in the internal carotid artery.[58] This unfortunate circumstance is thought to be associated with a high risk of converting an ischemic stroke into a hemorrhagic brain injury. Uncontrollable hemorrhage and inability to place a temporary shunt are also considered indications for ligation rather than primary repair. Fortunately, a shunt is rarely needed for repair of an internal or common carotid injury. A severe fixed neurological deficit related to either infarction or hemorrhage is considered a relative contraindication to definitive repair. On the other hand, primary repair is preferred over graft placement, when possible. Surgical intervention may also include resection or thrombectomy of lesions of the common or external carotid. Most blunt injuries involve the internal carotid artery, which is less accessible than the common and external carotid arteries. Complicating the approach to the internal carotid is the fact that subluxation and anterior repositioning of the mandible may be required for optimal surgical exposure of this vessel.

The surgical management of vertebral artery injuries should be guided by the results of four-vessel angiography. When conditions allow, vascular surgeons generally require this gold-standard study prior to definitive repair. The rate of detection of these lesions has increased dramatically since four-vessel angiography has been performed as a matter of routine. Vertebral artery injuries now comprise almost 20% of all cerebrovascular injuries, which is a much higher incidence than past experience had suggested.[59] The risks of adverse outcomes of vertebral artery lesions are low due to the presence of collateral flow through the Circle of Willis. Ligation is therefore more commonly performed than for carotid lesions. Brainstem ischemia occurs in 2–3% of patients following ligation and may be avoided by careful examination of a four-vessel angiogram.[60] Specifically, it is important to assess the vertebral artery on the opposite side of injury for evidence of anomaly or hypoplasia when deciding whether to perform primary repair vs. ligation. The presence of anatomic abnormalities will favor a decision to perform primary repair. In addition, angiography can help assess whether the posterior inferior cerebellar artery will remain adequately perfused after ligation. This is critical since lack of perfusion through this artery is likely to result in brainstem ischemia and a posterior circulation stroke. Consequently, primary repair is recommended if this concern is corroborated by angiographic findings.

While lesions of the external jugular veins can generally be managed with ligation, repair of internal jugular vein injuries is favored. This is especially true if bilateral internal jugular vein injuries are present. This approach also facilitates healing of the repair of a concomitant carotid artery lesion. Surgical repair of the vein may involve simple closure, resection, and reanastomosis or placement of an interposition graft.

The mural thrombus associated with traumatic dissection of the carotid and vertebral arteries may be a nidus for distal emboli. The potential development of cerebrovascular ischemia as a consequence, has prompted great interest in the prevention of this potentially devastating phenomenon. Anticoagulation and antiplatelet therapies have been recommended to reduce morbidity and mortality related to specific grades of injury to the carotid or vertebral arteries. Randomized trials have not been conducted on this topic; however, in case series, the rate of subsequent stroke in patients who are initially asymptomatic is decreased by 75% when systemic anticoagulation is instituted in comparison with historical controls. Heparin and antiplatelet drugs appear to be equivalent in promoting the healing of vascular injuries; however, heparin is more effective in improving neurologic outcome and in preventing stroke.[18] In asymptomatic patients studied by Biffl et al., the incidence of stroke was 1% with heparin, 9% with antiplatelet drugs, and 51% without any treatment.[19] A Cochrane review on the topic of cerebrovascular dissection documented a rate of subsequent stroke post-injury of 1.7% with anticoagulation, 3.3% without therapy, and 3.8% with antiplatelet therapy.[61] A statistically significant difference in patient outcomes between anticoagulation and antiplatelet therapy could not be demonstrated. Based on these results, anticoagulation therapy is therefore routinely administered, especially to blunt trauma patients with inaccessible Grade I–V lesions unless specifically contraindicated.[19] Antiplatelet therapy is employed when contraindications to systemic anticoagulation exist; e.g., in the presence of major, concurrent traumatic injuries. Routine follow-up angiography 7–10 days post-injury is recommended in order to plan further therapy.

Endovascular treatment by interventional radiologists is gaining popularity in the management of cerebrovascular injuries. The fact that definitive treatment potentially can be administered immediately following diagnostic angiography without moving the patient is a great advantage. Embolization of bleeding vessels by placement of coils has become the procedure of choice for vessels that are either expendable or difficult to access and expose in the operating suite. Branches of the external carotid artery are examples of the former and a classic example of the latter is the internal carotid artery at the base of the skull.[62] Complications of the procedure include thrombosis with distal embolus formation and pseudoaneurysms due to perforation of the vessel wall. Percutaneous angioplasty with stent placement after follow-up angiography has been used for the treatment of persistent blunt carotid injuries.[63,64] The intervention has raised concern regarding the danger of iatrogenic stroke and has yet to obtain wide acceptance.[65] In spite of this, it currently appears that the risks of the procedure outweigh the benefits, especially for carotid artery lesions.

Early detection of esophageal injuries allows a two-layer primary closure with wound irrigation, debridement, and drainage. Conversely, when the esophageal injury is diagnosed late, the tissue may not hold sutures because it is devitalized and frayed. In this case, several options exist including placement of a T-tube for drainage through a controlled fistula, and the injury site may be exteriorized in lower cervical esophageal perforations.[1] Optimal nutritional support and aggressive antibiotic treatment is imperative for healing. Moreover, it is important to maintain separation of the suture lines of the repairs if concomitant esophageal and tracheal lesions exist.

Approximately 10% of patients with injuries to the larynx or trachea require immediate surgery because of an unstable airway.[66] Severe hemorrhage, expanding neck hematoma that impinges on the airway, and an open wound into the airway are common indications for immediate surgical intervention. A tracheostomy must be performed if a definitive airway cannot be established by other means, or if a severe laryngeal injury is present. The procedure should not be placed through the repair since it may delay and complicate wound healing. Conversely, simple lacerations of the trachea can be closed primarily without tracheostomy. Closure is performed mucosa-to-mucosa and fractures are reduced and stabilized. Extensive disruption of tracheal cartilage may warrant placement of a soft laryngeal stent that remains in place for 4–6 weeks. Stent placement must be accompanied by a tracheostomy in order to insure proper healing.

Box 9.7 Essential treatments in ED for severe laryngeal or tracheal injuries

ED treatment	Definition and general indication
Establish definitive airway	Orotracheal intubation is the first choice
	Cricothyrotomy or tracheotomy
	Tracheal intubation through accessible wound
	Fiberoptic bronchoscopy in elective circumstances

Box 9.8 Common surgical interventions for penetrating neck trauma

Intervention	Definition and general indication
Mandatory exploration of zone 2 injuries	No longer recommended
Non-occlusive vascular injuries	Pseudoaneurysms and arteriovenous fistulae usually require surgical repair
Blunt vascular injuries	Accessible Grade 2–5 lesions require repair
	Non-accessible lesions are anticoagulated to prevent stroke
Endovascular techniques	Are gaining in acceptance and applicability

Documentation

The medical record is used as a communication tool with consultants and inpatient providers. As an effective instrument for hand-offs, it must reflect an accurate picture of the scenario leading up to the injury and include a detailed description of the mechanism and of the initial physical exam. The documentation must support the risk assessment of the emergency physician and justify further evaluation, definitive treatment, and the disposition of the patient. A secondary, but equally important goal is to provide a tool for risk management and medical–legal purposes.

Based on the ED record alone, the reader should be able to assess the presentation as either low risk in a patient that requires observation only, high risk in a patient that requires an aggressive evaluation including MDCT and panendoscopy, or life-threatening mandating immediate transport to the operating suite for definitive surgical intervention. In the case of interpersonal violence, the distance between the assailant and victim and the type of weapon must be established. As an example, it is critical to note whether a handgun, shotgun, or rifle was used by the assailant. The depth of penetration by a sharp object such as a knife or nail should be estimated and documented. In blunt trauma victims of motor vehicle crashes, the rate of speed prior to the accident and use of restraints are also important in terms of risk-stratifying the patient.

A carefully documented, detailed description of the primary survey and head-to-toe physical exam during the secondary survey is critical as it will serve as a basis for comparison for subsequent, serial evaluations. At minimum, a complete set of vital signs, detailed examination of the injured area with emphasis on evaluation of airway patency, pulses, and neurological function must be documented. The appearance and depth of any wounds and presence of foreign bodies or objects, crepitus, and subcutaneous emphysema should be noted. The presence of hematoma or ecchymosis on the skin surface of the neck and other areas of the body is of importance since follow-up examinations will use the initial exam as a baseline.

The record must justify the subsequent plan of action including notification of appropriate consultants. A brief, factual summary of the conversation with consulting physicians is mandatory, especially if the recommended course action is controversial or if transfer to another facility is planned. If discharge to home is contemplated for what is perceived to be very minor neck trauma, it is imperative that the ED record carefully describes in detail the benign nature of the injury. The record must clearly document the absence of previously described signs and symptoms of neurovascular, airway, and digestive tract injuries of the neck when further selective evaluation is not performed. In addition, it should be stated that no evidence of cardiac, pulmonary, abdominal, or neurological injuries are present. Appropriate, expeditious follow up with the surgical service must be documented when patients are discharged to home.

Disposition

The admission criteria for patients with blunt and penetrating neck trauma should be liberal. Any patient with signs or symptoms of organ damage to respiratory, digestive, or vascular structures, as described previously, should be transferred and admitted to a level I trauma center where constant observation by qualified surgeons can be undertaken. Only in this setting will interventional radiology, MDCT scanning, and panendoscopy be available 24 hours a day. In addition, patients with a wound that penetrates the platysma, which is only 2–3 mm in depth, should be admitted for observation. There is general agreement that this is a criterion for admission among trauma surgeons and emergency physicians alike. Even patients with apparently minor injuries may benefit from 24-hour observation in a hospital with appropriate staffing and resources, even when further evaluation is not planned initially. Practically speaking, "active" observation of the patient at regular intervals for signs and symptoms of significant organ injury are best provided in a level I trauma center.

Box 9.9 Consult, disposition, and transfer criteria

Admission criteria
1. Consider admission:
   - Penetration of the platysma (which is only 2–3 mm in depth).
2. Admission necessary:
   - Any signs or symptoms of injury to airway, digestive, or vascular structures.

Transfer criteria
Admission criteria above are indications for transfer to a level I trauma center.

Summary

Establishing a definitive airway early in the presentation is crucial to successful management of severe penetrating and blunt neck injuries. Orotracheal intubation is the initial method of choice; however,

no method will be successful 100% of the time. It is therefore crucial that practitioners are skilled in several different approaches to airway management including providing a surgical airway. In patients without obvious indications for operative intervention initially, evaluation for "hard" signs of vascular injury should be pursued. "Hard" signs include bruit, thrill, expanding or pulsatile hematoma, pulsatile or severe hemorrhage, pulse deficit, and central nervous system ischemia. The reference standard for vascular injury is conventional angiography. In addition, MDCT angiography is a non-invasive, less expensive, and more convenient alternative that is rapidly becoming the diagnostic tool of choice in the evaluation of cervical vascular injury due to both penetrating and blunt trauma. A high degree of suspicion should be maintained for neurological and esophageal injury. A careful, comprehensive neurological exam should be performed: MDCT is also a useful screening test for injuries to the airway and digestive structures. Unfortunately, radiographs do not exclude esophageal injury and panendoscopy is therefore the optimal diagnostic method for the evaluation of airway and digestive tract injuries. Diagnostic algorithms for the evaluation of penetrating and blunt trauma are provided in Figures 9.4 and 9.5 above.

References

1. McConnell DB, Trunkey DB. Management of penetrating trauma to the neck. *Adv Surg* 1994;**27**:97–127.

2. Inamasu J, Guiot BH. Vertebral artery injury after blunt cervical trauma: an update. *Surg Neurol* 2006;**65**(3):238–45.

3. May M, Tucker HM, Dillard BM. Penetrating wounds of the neck in civilians. *Otolaryngol Clin North Am* 1976;**9**(2):361–91

4. Carducci B, Lowe RA, Dalsey W. Penetrating neck trauma: consensus and controversies. *Ann Emerg Med* 1996;**15**(2):208–15.

5. Bell R, Osborn T, Dierks EJ, et al. Management of neck trauma: a new paradigm for civilian trauma. *J Oral and Maxillofacial Surg* 2007;**64**(4):691–704.

6. Huh J, Milliken JC, Chen JC. Management of tracheobronchial injuries following blunt and penetrating trauma. *Am Surg* 1997;**63**(10):896–9.

7. Levy D. *Neck Trauma*. Available from http://www.emedicine.com/emerg/topic331.htm, pp. 1–11. Last updated June 19, 2006.

8. Hawley D. Violence: recognition, management, and prevention. A review of 300 attempted strangulation

cases. Part III: Injuries in fatal cases. *J Emerg Med* 2001;**21**(3):317–22.

9. Clarot F, Vaz E, Papin F. Fatal and non-fatal carotid dissection after manual strangulation. *Forensic Sci* 2005;**149**(23):143–50.

10. Bernat RA. Combined laryngotracheal separation and esophageal injury following blunt neck trauma. *Facial Plastic Surg* 2005;**21**(3):187–90.

11. Shcweikh AM, Nadkarni AB. Laryngotracheal separation with pneumopericardium after blunt trauma to the neck. *Emerg Med J* 2001;**18**:410–11.

12. Fabian TC, Patton JH, Croce MA, et al. Blunt carotid injury: importance of early diagnosis and anticoagulant. *Ann Surg* 1996;**223**:513–25.

13. Kerwin AJ, Bynoe RP, Murray J, et al. Screening for blunt carotid and vertebral artery injuries is justified. *J Trauma* 2001;**51**:308–14.

14. Biffl. WL, Moore EE, Ryu RK, et al. The unrecognized epidemic of blunt carotid arterial injuries: early diagnosis improves neurologic outcome. *Ann Surg* 1998;**228**:462–70.

15. Rozycki GS, Tremblay L, Feliciano DV, et al. A prospective study for the detection of vascular injury in adult and pediatric patients with cervicothoracic seat belt signs. *J Trauma* 2002;**52**:618–24.

16. Biffl WL, Moore EE, Offner PJ, et al. Optimizing screening for blunt cerebrovascular injuries. *Am J Surg* 1999;**178**:517–22.

17. Biffl WL, Moore EE, Elliott JP, et al. The devastating potential of blunt vertebral artery injuries. *Ann Surg* 2000;**231**:672–81.

18. Miller PR, Fabian TC, Croce MA, et al. Screening for blunt cerebrovascular injuries: analysis of diagnostic modalities and outcomes. *Ann Surg* 2002;**236**: 386–95.

19. Biffl WL, Moore EE, Offner PJ, et al. Blunt carotid arterial injuries: implications of a new grading scale. *J Trauma* 1999;**47**:845–53.

20. Medzon R, Rothenhaus T, Bono CM, et al. Stability of the cervical spine after gunshot wounds to the head and neck. *Spine* 2005;**30**(20):2274–9.

21. Lanoix R, Gupta R, Leak L, et al. C-spine injury associated with gunshot wounds to the head: retrospective study and literature review. *J Trauma* 2000;**49**(5):860.

22. Hastings RH, Duong H, Burton DW, et al. Cervical spine movements during laryngoscopy with the Bullard, Macintosh, and Miller laryngoscopes. *Anesthesiology* 1995;**82**(4):859–69.

23. Bickell WH, Wall MJ, Jr., Pepe PE, et al. Immediate versus delayed fluid resuscitation for hypotensive patients with penetrating torso injuries. *NEJM* 1994;**331**(17):1105–9.

24. Greene R, Stark P. Trauma of the larynx and trachea. *Rad Clinics N Am* 1978;**16**(2):309.

25. Kelly JP, Webb WR, Moulder PV, et al. Management of airway trauma. I: tracheobronchial injuries. *Ann Thorac Surg* 1985;**40**(6):551–5.

26. Goudy SL, Miller FB, Bumpous JM. Neck crepitance: evaluation and management of suspected upper aerodigestive tract injury. *Laryngoscope* 2002;**112**:791–5.

27. Weigelt JA, Thal ER, Snyder WH, 3rd. Diagnosis of penetrating cervical esophageal injuries. *Am J Surg* 1987;**154**(6):619–22.

28. Sheely CH, Mattox KL, Beall AC, et al. Penetrating wounds of the cervical esophagus. *Am J Surg* 1975;**130**:707–11.

29. Arsensio JA, Berne J, Demetriades D, et al. Penetrating esophageal injuries: time interval of safety for preoperative evaluation-how long is safe? *J Trauma* 1997;**43**(2):319–24.

30. Demetriades D, Theodorou E, Cornwell E, et al. Evaluation of penetrating injuries of the neck: prospective study of 223 patients. *World J Surgery* 1997;**21**(1):41–8.

31. Sankaran S, Walt AJ. Penetrating wounds of the neck: principles and some controversies. *Surg Clin N Am* 1977;**57**:139–50.

32. Keogh IJ. Critical airway compromise caused by neck hematoma. *Clin Otolaryngol* 2002;**27**:244–5.

33. Rathlev NK. Penetrating neck trauma: mandatory versus selective exploration. *J Emerg Med* 1990;**8**:75–8.

34. Ferguson E, Dennis JW, Frykberg ER. Redefining the role of arterial imaging in the management of penetrating zone 3 neck injuries. *Vascular* 2005;**13** (3):158–63.

35. Hoffer EK, Sclafani SJ, Herskowitz MM, et al. Natural history of arterial injuries diagnosed with arteriography. *J Vasc Interv Radiol* 1997;**8**(1):43–53.

36. Dennis JW, Frykberg ER, Veldenz HC, et al: Validation of nonoperative management of occult vascular injuries and accuracy of physical examination alone in penetrating extremity trauma: 5- to 10-year follow-up. *J Trauma* 1998;**44**(2):243–52.

37. McKevitt EC, Kirkpatrick AW, Vertesi L, et al. Blunt vascular neck injuries: diagnosis and outcomes of extracranial vessel injury. *J Trauma* 2002;**53**:472–6.

38. Carrillo EH, Osborne DL, Spain DA, et al. Blunt carotid artery injuries: difficulties with the diagnosis prior to neurologic event. *J Trauma* 1999; **46**:1120–5.

39. Cothren CC, Moore EE, Biffl WL. Cervical spine fractures predictive of blunt vertebral artery injury. *J Trauma* 2003;**55**(5):811–13.

40. Gomez-Caro AA, Ausin HP, Moradiellos Diez FJ. Medical and surgical management of noniatrogenic traumatic tracheobronchial injuries. *Arch Bronconeumol* 2005;**41**(5):249–54.

41. Spencer JA, Rogers CE, Westaby S. Clinico-radiological correlates in rupture of the major airways. *Clin Radiol* 1991;**43**(6):371–6.

42. Chen JD, Shanmuganathan K, Mirvis SE, et al. Using CT to diagnose tracheal rupture. *AJR Am J Roentgenol* 2001;**176**(5):1273–80.

43. Moriwaki Y, Sugiyama M, Matsuda G, et al. Usefulness of the 3-dimensionally reconstructed computed tomography imaging for diagnosis of the site of tracheal injury (3D-tracheography). *World J Surg* 2005;**29**(1):102–5.

44. Scaglione M, Romano S, Pinto A. Acute tracheobronchial injuries: impact of imaging on diagnosis and management implications. *Eur J Radiol* 2006;**59**(3):336–43.

45. Schaefer SD, Brown OE. Selective application of CT in the management of laryngeal trauma. *Laryngoscope* 1983;**93**:1473–5.

46. Snyder WH, Thal ER, Bridges RA, et al. The validity of normal arteriograms in penetrating trauma. *Arch Surg* 1978;**113**:424.

47. Eastman A, Chason DP, Perez CL, et al. Computed tomographic angiography for the diagnosis of blunt cervical vascular injury: is it ready for primetime? *J Trauma* 2006;**60**(5):925–9.

48. Munera F, Soto JA, Palacio D, et al. Diagnosis of arterial injuries caused by penetrating trauma to the neck: comparison of helical CT angiography and conventional angiography. *Radiology* 2000;**216**:356–62.

49. Tisherman SA, Bokhari F, Collier B, et al. Clinical practice guideline: penetrating zone 2 neck trauma. *J Trauma* 2008;**64**(5):1392–1405.

50. Rogers FB, Baker EF, Osler TM, et al. Computed tomographic angiography as a screening modality for blunt cervical arterial injuries: preliminary results. *J Trauma* 1999;**46**:380–5.

51. Biffl WL, Ray CE, Moore EE, et al. Noninvasive diagnosis of blunt cerebrovascular injuries: a preliminary report. *J Trauma* 2002;**53**:850–6.

52. Schneidereit NP, Simons R, Nicolaou S, et al. Utility of screening for blunt vascular neck injuries with computed tomographic angiography. *J Trauma* 2006;**60**(1):209–15.

53. Kuzniec S, Kauffman P, Molnar LJ, et al. Diagnosis of limb and neck arterial trauma using duplex ultrasonography. *Cardiovasc Surg* 1998;**6**:358–64.

54. Mandavia D, Qualls S, Rokos I. Emergency airway management in penetrating neck injury. *Ann Emerg Med* 2000;**35**(3):221–5.

55. Scott JM, Lopez PP, Pierre E. Use of a gum elastic bougie (GEB) in a zone II penetrating neck trauma: a case report. *J of Emerg Med* 2004;**26**(3):353–4.

56. Weitzel N, Kendall J, Pons P. Blind nasotracheal intubation for patients with penetrating neck trauma. *J Trauma* 2004;**56**(5):1097–101.

57. Van As AB, Van Deurzen DF, Verleisdonk EJ, et al. Gunshots to the neck: selective angiography as part of conservative management. *Injury* 2002;**33**:453–6.

58. Weaver FA, Yellin AE, Wagner WH, et al. The role of arterial reconstruction in penetrating carotid injuries. *Arch Surg* 1988;**123**:1106–11.

59. Meier DE, Brink BE, Fry WJ. Vertebral artery trauma. *Arch Surg* 1981;**116**:236–9.

60. Thomas GI, Andersen KN, Hain RF. The significance of anomalous vertebral-basilar communications in operations on the heart and great vessels. *Surgery* 1959;**46**:747–57.

61. Lyrer P, Engelter S. Antithrombotic drugs for carotid artery dissection. *Cochrane Database Syst Rev* 2003;**3**: CD000255.

62. Mitchell WC, Whittaker DR, Martinez C, et al. Traumatic pseudoaneurysms of the head and neck: early endovascular intervention. *J Vasc Surg* 2007;**46**(6):1227–33.

63. Kerby JD, May AK, Gomez CR, et al. Treatment of bilateral blunt carotid injury using percutaneous angioplasty and stenting: case report and review of the literature. *J Trauma* 2000;**49**:784–7.

64. Shames ML, Davis JW, Evans AJ. Endoluminal stent placement for the treatment of traumatic carotid artery pseudoaneurysm: case report and review of the literature. *J Trauma* 1999;**46**:724–6.

65. Biffl WL, Moore EE, Ray C, et al. Emergent stenting of acute blunt carotid artery injuries: a cautionary note. *J Trauma* 2001;**50**:969–71.

66. Minard G, Kudak KA, Croce MA, et al. Laryngotracheal trauma. *Am Surg* 1992;**58**:181–7.

10

Injuries of the spine: musculoskeletal

Daniel Zlogar and Ron Medzon

Introduction

The spine is a complex bony structure providing stability and protection. The National Emergency X-Radiography Utilization Study (NEXUS) showed that 55% of all spine fractures were of the cervical spine.[1] Data from the Canadian Cervical Spine Study showed that in their country, like the United States, patients present much more often with neck injury that is non-bony. For example, in Canada, physicians treat 185 000 alert and stable trauma victims yearly who are at risk for cervical spine injury, but only 0.9% of these patients have suffered a cervical spine fracture.[2]

Injuries to the spine range from minor soft tissue contusions without structural abnormality, to bony fractures, severed ligaments, and nerve damage. Due to the potentially devastating morbidity, physicians are compelled to quickly and accurately identify serious injury. Recent research has provided guidelines to safely reduce the number of studies required to diagnose and treat bony spine fractures as well as choose the most efficient and cost-effective diagnostic test.

Box 10.1 Essentials of bony spinal trauma

- The NEXUS and the Canadian Cervical Spine Rule have reduced the number of cervical plain films in the evaluation of cervical spine fractures after blunt trauma.
- Computed tomography (CT) is becoming the study of choice for the evaluation of cervical spine fractures in moderate to high-risk trauma patients.

Clinical anatomy and pathophysiology

The spinal column is comprised of 33 vertebrae: 7 cervical, 12 thoracic, 5 lumbar, 5 sacral, and 4 coccygeal (Figures 10.1 and 10.2). The cervical, thoracic, and lumbar vertebrae are mobile, articulating via facet joints and intervertebral disks, and joined by multiple ligaments (Figure 10.3). The spine can be anatomically divided into upper cervical (C1–C2), lower cervical (C3–C7), and the remaining thoracic, lumbar, and sacral spine. The atlas (C1) articulates with the occipital condyles, the dens, and the facets of C2. The axis (C2) consists of the odontoid process that articulates with the anterior arch of C1 and the transverse ligament. The odontoid process is stabilized by the alar, transverse, and apical ligaments (Figures 10.4 and 10.5).

Stable vs. unstable fractures

Spinal instability causes abnormal or excessive spinal motion in response to normally tolerated physiologic loads, potentially injuring the spinal cord.

Historically, the bony cervical spine has been divided into three columns in order to describe its stability with different injury patterns. The theory is that if two contiguous columns are disrupted by trauma, the fracture is unstable. A recent study using a biomechanical trauma model validated the three-column theory of fractures by correlating multidirectional vertebral injuries to each of the three columns and subsequent instability. Sixteen fresh cadavers were subjected to bony spinal trauma. In addition to confirming the three-column theory, the results also demonstrate that the middle column is the primary determinant of mechanical stability of the lumbar spine.[3]

The anterior column consists of the anterior half of the vertebral body disc and annulus as well as the anterior longitudinal ligaments. The middle column is composed of the posterior half of the verterbral body disc and annulus, and the posterior longitudinal ligament. The posterior column is made up of the

Trauma: A Comprehensive Emergency Medicine Approach, eds. Eric Legome and Lee W. Shockley. Published by Cambridge University Press. © Cambridge University Press 2011.

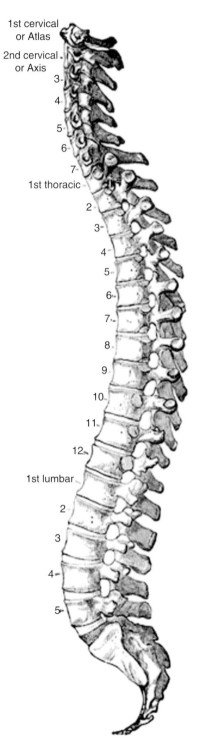

1st cervical
or Atlas

2nd cervical
or Axis

3

4

5

6

7

1st thoracic

2

3

4

5

6

7

8

9

10

11

12

1st lumbar

2

3

4

5

Figure 10.1
Vertebral columns.
(From *Gray's
Anatomy of the
Human Body*,
20th edn, in Public
Domain.)

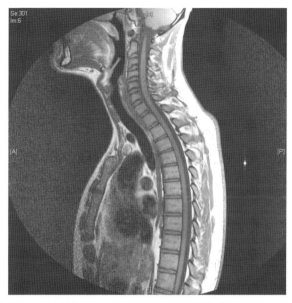

Figure 10.2 Magnetic resonance imaging (MRI) of spine.

interspinous, and infraspinous ligaments), the capsular ligaments and the ligamentum flavum. The thoracolumbar spine can be divided into three columns (anterior, middle, and posterior) similar to the cervical spine. Like the cervical spine, when at least two contiguous columns are injured there is biomechanical instability. Also, any spinal fracture with an associated neurological injury is unstable, except those injuries from penetrating trauma where the spinal column usually retains stability; the injury comes from direct cord trauma from the penetrating object.

Fracture patterns

Occipitocervical injuries consist of subluxations, dislocations, or condylar fractures and are extremely rare emergency department (ED) presentations and typically fatal.

C1 (atlas) injuries include five different types of fractures – posterior arch fracture, Jefferson burst fracture (Figure 10.6), lateral mass fracture, horizontal fracture of the anterior arch, and either a unilateral or bilateral transverse process fracture. Unstable fractures occur when the transverse ligament is disrupted. The Jefferson fracture describes a fracture of the anterior and posterior arches of C1 as well as the transverse ligament and is extremely unstable. On lateral plain film there will be a widening of the predental space between the anterior arch of C1 and the dens.

spinal canal, pedicles, transverse processes, articulating facets, laminae and spinous processes, and held stable by the nuchal ligament complex (supraspinous,

147

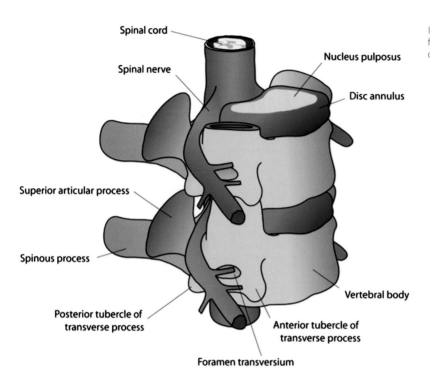

Spinal cord

Nucleus pulposus

Spinal nerve

Disc annulus

Superior articular process

Spinous process

Posterior tubercle of
transverse process

Anterior tubercle of
transverse process

Vertebral body

Foramen transversium

Figure 10.3 View of cervical vertebrae from an oblique viewpoint. (Courtesy of Creative Commons, Wikimedia.)

A space in excess of 3 mm in adults or 5 mm in children is abnormal (Figure 10.7).

Atlantoaxial joint injuries

Atlantoaxial joint injuries are subluxations which occur when the transverse ligament is disrupted and the ring of C1 remains intact. This is extremely unstable and has a high risk for neurological deficit. Rotary subluxations of C1–C2 clinically present with the patient's head in fixed rotation.

Odontoid fractures

Odontoid fractures are classified into three types. Type I fractures are through the apex of the dens and are very rare. Type 2 fractures are the most common and are transverse fractures at the junction of the dens and body of C2 These are unstable fractures and often result in non-union. Type 3 fractures extend into the body of C2 and are typically stable. Open mouth views are the best plain films to find these fractures, while CT can better define the extent of the fracture (Figure 10.8).

Clinical presentation will include pain and an inability to move the neck. A common complaint is the sensation of instability, as if the head is not being supported by the neck. Patients may hold their head with their hands to prevent any motion.

Traumatic spondylolisthesis of the axis (C2)

The so-called Hangman's fracture results from extreme hyperextension of the head and neck, such as the force of the hangman's noose as the victim's body is stopped short in free fall by the taut rope around his or her neck. The force is driven through C1 and C2, resulting in bilateral pedicle fractures of C2 and disruption of the anterior and middle columns. These injuries are very unstable; they should never be subjected to traction or distraction. Spinal cord injury is often minimal, as the fractured pedicles allow for cord decompression; the anteroposterior (AP) diameter of the spinal canal is greatest at C2. This injury pattern can be seen on lateral cervical plain film (Figure 10.9).

Subaxial cervical spine injuries (C3–C7)

Facet injuries include fractures, subluxations, and dislocations, and can be unilateral or involve both facets. Disruption of the facet joint initially leads to subluxation, then as either one or both of the facets shift superiorly over the inferior facet, can lead to a perched facet. With a more significant injury a perched facet can develop into a dislocation, with the superior facet lying in the intervertebral foramen (Figures 10.10–10.13).

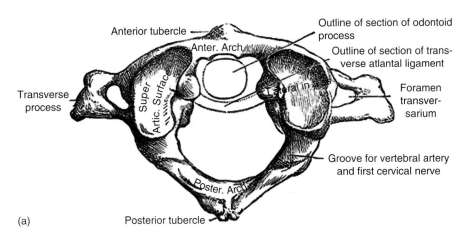

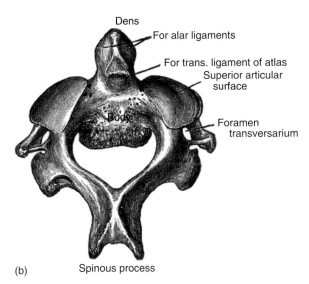

(a)

(b)

Figure 10.4 (a) First cervical vertebra, or atlas. (b) Second cervical vertebra from above. (From *Gray's Anatomy of the Human Body*, 20th edn, in Public Domain.)

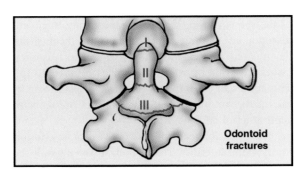

Figure 10.5 Schematic showing the ligamentous attachments of C1 and C2. (From Mandavia D, Newton E, Demetriades D. *Colour Atlas of Emergency Trauma*. Cambridge: Cambridge University Press, 2003.)

Unilateral facet dislocation occurs from flexion and rotation, and while this disrupts the posterior ligament, this essentially locks the facets and is considered a stable injury. Oblique plain films can be helpful in differentiating this from torticollis. In the thoracolumbar and lumbar areas, facet fracture is more common than dislocation, resulting in an unstable injury.

Subluxation

This injury involves ligamentous rupture without bony injury. It may be diagnosed on CT if there is significant soft tissue edema or bleeding. Magnetic resonance imaging (MRI) is the test of choice, however. Plain film

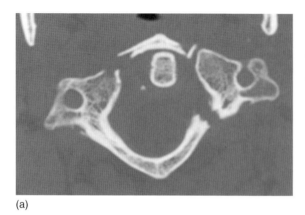
(a)

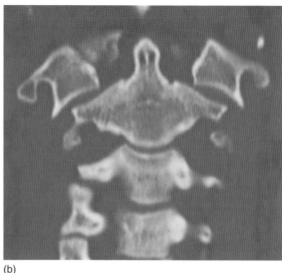
(b)

Figure 10.6 Transverse (a) and coronal (b) computed tomography (CT) view of Jefferson burst fracture.

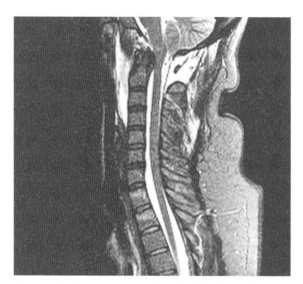

Figure 10.7 Magnetic resonance imaging (MRI) image of C1 compression fracture. Note the prevertebral soft tissue edema, which is white on this image.

may often miss this finding, and a delayed (after spasm has subsided) flexion–extension film may be necessary if this alone is the diagnostic choice.

Compression fractures

Simple wedge fractures are stable and occur as a result of flexion forces disrupting the anterior column, with the middle column intact. Neurological injury is rare. Severe wedge fractures include those in which over half of the vertebral body height is lost and posterior ligaments are disrupted or there are multiple adjacent wedge fractures present (Figure 10.14).

Burst fractures

Burst fractures occur most often in the cervical and lumbar regions of the spine and result from a large axial load (Figure 10.15). These fractures compromise the anterior and middle columns, with some protrusion into the neural canal. Unstable burst fractures have > 50% of body height loss, > 25° of angulation, > 50% of canal compromise, and/or present with neurological deficit.

Other fractures

The flexion teardrop fracture is an extremely unstable fracture and results from forceful flexion–compression of the spine, causing a wedge-shaped bony fragment, disruption of all three spinal columns, the ligamentum flavum, and anterior longitudinal ligament. It is often associated with neurological damage (Figure 10.16). This results in concomitant posterior displacement of the fracture into the spinal canal and can present with acute anterior cord syndrome.

The extension teardrop fracture is a stable avulsion injury of the anterior vertebral body, involving only the anterior spinal column. With forced extension, the anterior longitudinal ligament pulls the antero-inferior corner of the vertebral body away from the remainder of the vertebra – most commonly at C2.

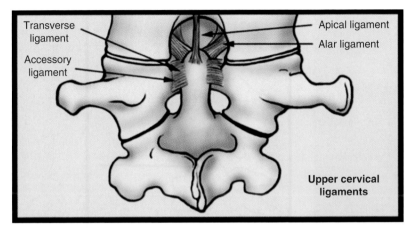

Transverse ligament

Accessory ligament

Apical ligament

Alar ligament

Upper cervical ligaments

(a)

Figure 10.8 (a) Schematic showing the three types of odontoid fracture. (From Mandavia D, Newton E, Demetriades D. *Colour Atlas of Emergency Trauma*. Cambridge: Cambridge University Press, 2003.) (b) Sagittal computed tomography (CT) of Type 2 dens fracture.(c) Sagittal CT of Type 3 dens fracture. (b and c: Courtesy of Mark Bernstein, MD.)

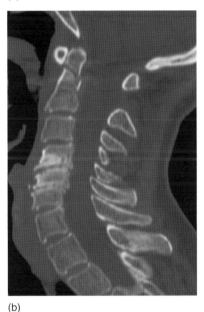

(b)

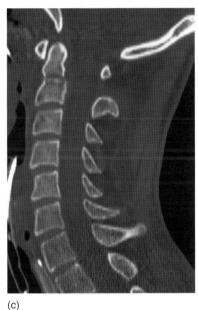

(c)

The so-called clay shoveler's fracture is a fracture of the base of the spinous process of one of the lower cervical vertebrae – most commonly at C7 (Figure 10.17). This injury results from direct trauma to the spinous process (e.g., from baseball bats) or sudden deceleration as in a motor vehicle collision (MVC) causing forceful flexion. A clay shoveler flexes his neck while placing his shovel into the clay. If his shovel becomes unexpectedly stuck in the clay as he exerts himself to lift the heavy load, he could experience a similar sudden deceleration and fracture, and hence the eponym "clay shoveler's fracture." Because this injury is isolated to the posterior column it is considered stable (Table 10.1).

Thoracic spine

A large amount of force is required to fracture the thoracic spine because of the added structural support offered by the ribs and sternum. This additional force often results in profound neurological deficits in patients (Figure 10.18).

Thoracolumbar spine

This area is highly susceptible to injury secondary to increased mobility and is only second to cervical spinal injuries in frequency of occurrence (Figure 10.19).

Compression fractures are the most common type of thoracolumbar fracture and present with a

151

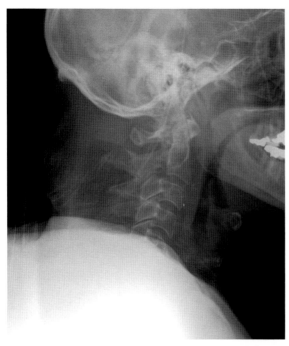

Figure 10.9 Lateral neck radiograph showing hangman's fracture at C2. (Courtesy of Mark Bernstein, MD.)

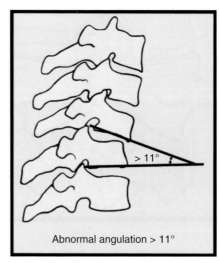

Abnormal angulation > 11°

Figure 10.10 Schematic illustrating abnormal angulation measurements with perched facets. (From Mandavia D, Newton E, Demetriades D. *Colour Atlas of Emergency Trauma*. Cambridge: Cambridge University Press, 2003.)

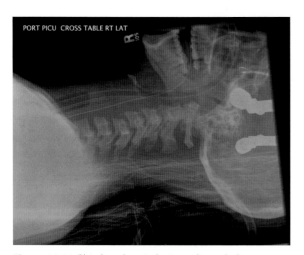

Figure 10.11 Plain lateral cervical spine radiograph shows a subluxation at C4–C5.

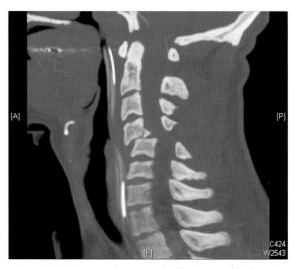

Figure 10.12 Computed tomography (CT) image of C4 fracture dislocation on C5.

decreased anterior vertebral body height without disruption of the posterior body or spinal cord.

Flexion–distraction/chance injuries

Chance fractures occur most commonly with high-speed frontal impact deceleration injuries when the patient is using the lap belt without the shoulder harness. This is a purely bony injury where the flexion and distraction in the lumbar region due to the lap belt causes a fracture beginning in the spinous process, progressing through the pedicles and the vertebral body. Chance fractures should be considered, especially in young patients found to have traumatic compression fracture following a MVC, and is diagnosed either by AP view (ruling out posterior injury) or CT scan. Devascularization or bowel rupture are also possible with this mechanism of injury. During

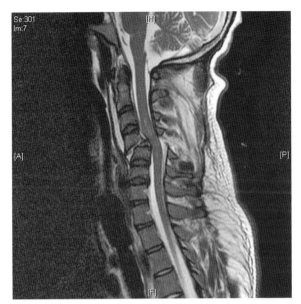

Figure 10.13 Magnetic resonance imaging (MRI) image of C4 fracture dislocation on C5. Note the different anatomical information provided between Figures 10.12 and 10.13.

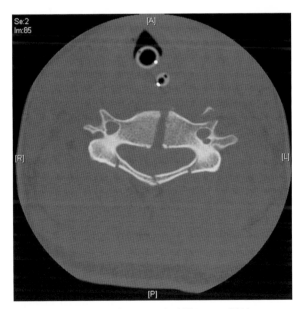

Figure 10.15 Computed tomography (CT) image of C4 burst fracture. The body of the vertebrae is fractured, as well as both laminae.

stabilization of this injury, all traction and distraction maneuvers should be avoided.

Fracture dislocations

Fracture dislocations are extremely unstable injuries caused by the spinal column being subjected to

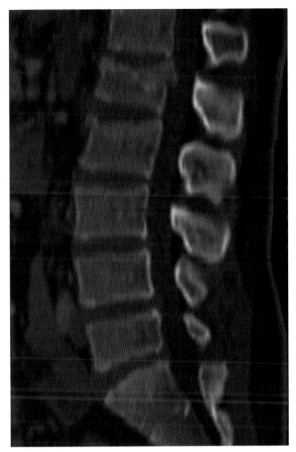

Figure 10.14 Sagittal computed tomography (CT) shows both simple compression fracture (L2) and burst fracture (L1). (Courtesy of Mark Bernstein, MD.)

various degrees of rotation, flexion, and translocation forces, causing all three columns to fail. Operative treatment is almost always needed. Neurologically incomplete injuries may benefit from early posterior reduction by surgical decompression and stabilization.

Isolated transverse process fractures are stable fractures.

Epidemiology of fractures

Fifty-five percent of all spine fractures are of the cervical spine. C2 fractures account for 24% of all fractures in the NEXUS, while fractures of C6 and C7 take up another 39.3%. C3 is the least fractured vertebrae of the cervical spine, and the vertebral body itself is the most common site of fracture. Dislocations occurred most frequently at the C5–C6 and C6–C7 interspaces.[4] The thoracolumbar spine is less

153

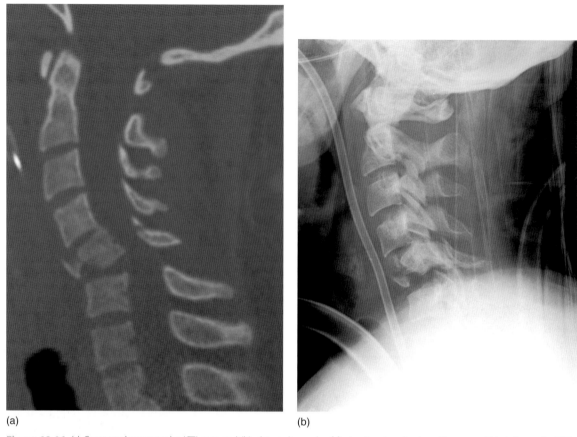

(a)   (b)

Figure 10.16 (a) Computed tomography (CT) scan and (b) plain radiograph of flexion teardrop fracture. (Courtesy of Mark Bernstein, MD.)

frequently injured than the cervical spine, with 8–15% of victims of blunt trauma suffering fractures.[5]

Studies looking at the most common contiguous fractures have pointed out a difference in fracture patterns between elderly and pediatric patients. C1–C2 contiguous fractures are more often found in the elderly, while C5–C6 fractures occur more commonly in children. Multiple regions of the vertebral column are involved in 7.8% of cervical spine injured patients.[6] A study from the United Kingdom shows that the most common spine injury in motorcyclists is forced hyperflexion and consequent thoracic spine injury, while car crash victims more commonly had cervical spine injuries.[7] Looking at injuries from falls, burst fractures at the thoracolumbar junction are the most common injuries.[8]

Prehospital

In the United States, spinal immobilization with a cervical collar and long board is currently considered the standard of care for hospital transport agencies such as Emergency Medical Services (EMS) systems, and by national guidelines like Advanced Trauma Life Support® (ATLS®), but the evidence supporting this is lacking.[9] The EMS system was instituted in 1971 and, after a decade, the number of patients presenting with complete spinal cord injuries dropped from 55% to 39%; however, there have been no randomized controlled studies showing the benefit of spinal immobilization in trauma patients. Indeed, a Cochrane database review concluded "the possibility that immobilization may increase mortality and morbidity cannot be excluded."[10] This concern is mainly due to airway issues in the immobilized patient.[10]

Interestingly, a study involving the University of Malaya (where none of the trauma patients were immobilized) and the University of New Mexico (where all of the transported trauma patients were immobilized) showed fewer injuries causing neurological disability in the non-immobilized patients.

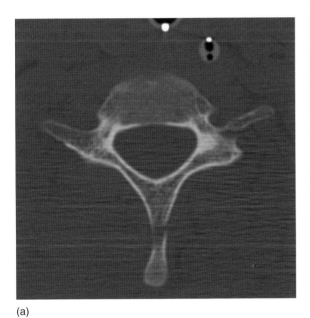

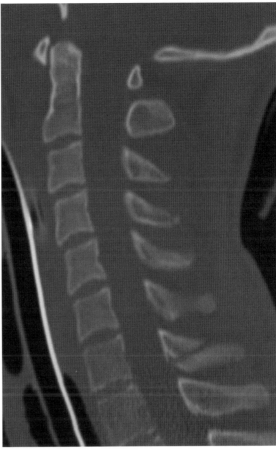

(a)   (b)

Figure 10.17 (a) Axial and (b) sagittal computed tomography (CT) of clay shoveler's fracture.

However, there were a larger percentage of motor vehicle accidents at the University of New Mexico, and the University of Malaya did not have any ambulances or EMS in place. The study authors hypothesized that cord damage occurs only at the time of initial trauma when high-energy forces are present, rather than during transport.[11]

It has been estimated that over 50% of immobilized trauma patients do not have neck or back pain prior to field immobilization,[12] while it should be noted that there are possible risks to patients by placing them on their backs in terms of airway compromise, aspiration, or pressure sores (prolonged immobilization with paralysis).

With these concerns over improper or unnecessary spinal immobilization, several studies have attempted to explore the possibility of prehospital spinal clearance. An observational study using modified NEXUS Low-risk Criteria to remove the cervical collar showed that EMS had approximately 95% sensitivity to clinically detect cervical spine fractures in the field.[13] This led to a follow-up prospective randomized study showing a 39% reduction in the number of patients immobilized. Unfortunately, 8% of patients with spine injuries (33/415) were not immobilized. None of the non-immobilized patients sustained cord injuries.[14] Maine also instituted a state-wide protocol for spinal immobilization that effectively reduced the number of immobilized trauma patients by over 50%; however, 13% of acute spinal fractures were not immobilized during the period of study.[15]

Also, transporting football, ice hockey, or lacrosse athletes with potential cervical spine injuries to the hospital can be accomplished with in-line stabilization with helmet and shoulder pads remaining in place.[16]

155

Table 10.1 Summary: common cervical spine fracture

Injury	Usual cause	Stability
Occipitocervical	Anterior, longitudinal or posterior displacement of occiput on atlas	All extremely unstable
Atlas (C1)		
Posterior arch (most common)	Extension	Potentially unstable
Jefferson	Compression	Extremely unstable
Atlantoaxial subluxation	Flexion	Extremely unstable
Odontoid (C2)	Flexion	Potentially unstable
Hangman's fracture (C2)	Extension	Unstable
Unilateral facet dislocation	Flexion–rotation	Stable
Bilateral facet dislocation	Flexion	Unstable
Wedge fracture	Compression	Stable
Burst fracture	Compression	Potentially unstable
Flexion teardrop fracture	Flexion	Extremely unstable
Extension teardrop fracture	Extension	Stable
Clay shoveler's fracture	Flexion	Stable
Chance fracture	Flexion–distraction	Unstable
Transverse process fracture	Flexion	Stable

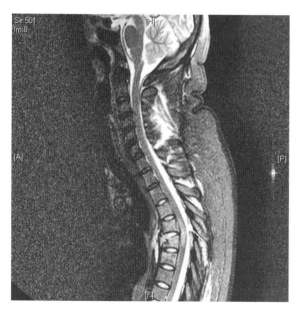

Figure 10.18 Magnetic resonance imaging (MRI) image of T4 fracture with spinal cord involvement.

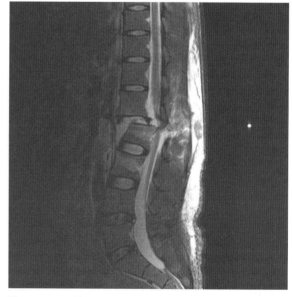

Figure 10.19 Magnetic resonance imaging (MRI) of L1–L2 dislocation with clinically devastating spinal cord compression and epidural hematoma.

To summarize, clearly a large number of trauma patients transported by EMS do not require spinal immobilization, but we do not yet have criteria that demonstrate high enough sensitivity and negative predictive value to change the current practice of immobilization. Further research may reveal a subset of patients where they can accurately be applied.

> **Box 10.2 Essentials of prehospital care in bony spinal trauma**
>
> - Immobilizing patients in a cervical collar and on a long board for transport is the current accepted practice.
> - There is no criteria sensitive enough to allow for cervical spine clearance in the prehospital setting.

Emergency department management and evaluation

Severe

While there is no standard definition of "severe" spinal injury, consider patients involved in high energy mechanisms or ones who have suffered multiple blunt trauma to have the potential for severe bony spine injury. High-risk factors include: fall $\geq$ 3 m, moderate velocity MVC or motorcycle crash, palpable step off, bruising, hematoma, pedestrian struck). Also, consider trauma patients presenting with a neurologic deficit as severe, as this suggests an unstable injury.

Moderate

Patients who are older, or have arthritic disease are at increased risk for spinal injury. Also, those patients with a history of malignancies which tend to metastasize to bone (prostate, breast, etc.) could suffer spinal trauma in the setting of an undiagnosed bony lesion. They should be viewed with closer attention even in lower mechanism traumas. The Canadian Cervical Spine Study recommends imaging patients over 65 years old, and an analysis of patients over the age of 64 in the NEXUS database found odontoid fractures four times more common in the elderly compared to the non-elderly population.[17]

One retrospective case-control study in 2005 evaluated blunt trauma patients 65 years and older with cervical spine fractures and compared them to randomly selected control subjects without fracture.[18] Composite predictors of fracture in the elderly included focal neurologic deficit (adjusted odds ratio [OR], 17.7; 95% clearance interval [CI]: 3.8–83.4), severe head injury (OR, 3.2; 95% CI 1.5–7.1), high energy mechanism (OR 6.7; 95% CI 3.1–14.8), and moderate energy mechanism (OR 3.3; 95% CI: 1.3–8.3).[18] While these factors may increase the odds of fracture, all except the moderate energy mechanism would have received a radiograph in NEXUS.

Minor

Minor spinal injury includes trauma that does not have any fracture or ligamentous injury. Because the cervical spine is the most vulnerable to injury, this section of the spine is the most filmed. In an attempt to reduce the number of needless plain films of the cervical spine, the Canadian Cervical Spine Rule and NEXUS Criteria were developed. Both allow the ordering clinician to categorize patients into a "minor" cervical spine injury not needing radiographic studies. Because the thoracic spine is inherently more stable with the additional support of the ribs and sternum, this area of the spinal column is less commonly injured. Currently, no criteria for thoracic and lumbar spinal injuries have been prospectively validated that allow the clinician to use certain patient factors to confidently exclude imaging in the at risk population.

Occult

The truly "occult" bony spinal has never been reported. There have been cases of delayed diagnosis due to altered mental status, painful distracting injuries, neurlogic impairments, etc. However, the patient with a cervical spine fracture who truly has no symptoms, but is otherwise intact, probably does not exist.

Initial evaluation

The initial physical exam for the severe, moderate, or minor trauma patient is the same as for any trauma patient, starting with the primary assessment of the airway, breathing, and circulation (ABCs).

The secondary survey should include carefully loosening the cervical collar (assuming the patient is cooperative) and checking for midline tenderness. Also the clinician should perform a detailed neurological exam. The extent of the exam depends on the clinical situation. A significantly injured patient should have an exam that includes sensation, reflexes, extremity movement, and rectal tone. Those patients, especially young, with minimal trauma and complaints may need a less thorough review.

With the help of several people, the patient should be log-rolled in order to remove the long board and examine the back. One person stands at the head of the bed to maintain in-line stabilization. It is easiest to keep the thumbs on the patient's clavicle, using the flat of the palm to cradle the head, then giving a three count to the rest of the team when the head and neck are stable to roll the patient. Another clinician examines the back for bruising, penetrating trauma, bony deformities, or bony step-offs (obvious interruptions in the otherwise linear position of the vertebrae).

Penetrating injury to the neck, via stab wound or gunshot, is approached in much the same way as any major trauma except that the cervical collar may be expendable. There are no reports in Western medical literature of an unstable cervical spine fracture resulting from a stabbing to the neck. The degree of force needed to fracture two columns of the cervical spine with a knife is considerable. Thus, any patient who requires emergent care of the neck wound, for example intubation because of an expanding hematoma, should have the collar removed for better access to the patient. Gunshot wounds to the head and neck present a problem in the patient with an acute airway emergency. The three-column theory of the bony spine would suggest that in order for a penetrating injury to create an unstable spine fracture, it would have to traverse the spinal cord to break at least two columns. It follows logically that a patient sustaining such an injury should have at minimum bony spine pain and tenderness, but more likely also neurological signs ranging from sensory changes to loss of motor function. Several studies confirm this thesis.[19–21] Some researchers have found no bony spine injury in alert patients with a normal neurological exam who have sustained gunshots to the neck or head and go so far as to recommend no need for a collar or further imaging.[22,23] However, one study noted that three patients who sustained gunshot wounds to the face were found to have cervical spine fractures, despite presenting as alert and oriented without pain or neurological signs on physical exam.[24] None of these fractures required surgical repair. Therefore a rational, although conservative, approach would recommend that the collar could be carefully removed during the physical exam of the neck and to perform any life-saving maneuvers but should be returned to the patient while awaiting radiographic studies.

Trauma room studies

No specific radiographic study of the spine are absolutely necessary in the trauma room. If the patient requires further imaging of the cervical, thoracic, or lumbar spine, they should proceed to the CT scanner or plain radiography suite once hemodynamically resuscitated. Some institutions still obtain lateral films in the trauma bay, although this has unclear utility.

Patients with a gunshot wound to the neck may benefit from plain films of the neck, head, and chest in the trauma room to localize the bullet and fragments.

Acute interventions

Managing the airway of a trauma patient with known or possible cervical spine injury can be challenging. Usually the cervical collar is removed and an assistant holds in-line stabilization with the clinician performing the intubation. New airway devices now rely on video camera assistance and specialized optics and allow for the cervical collar to remain in place during the entire process of intubation.

An unstable fracture at C3 or above can cause paralysis of the diaphragm. Pulmonary function testing, particularly the negative inspiratory pressures, can be evaluated if there is concern over a partially paralyzed or weakened diaphragm.

During in-line stabilization, the person responsible should be careful not to place any neck or head axial traction as this can cause unstable cervical spine injuries to distract or sublux.[25]

Any patient who is brought in on a long board in a cervical collar should be seen and evaluated in a timely manner by a clinician, as it is extremely uncomfortable for the patient, especially one who has sustained a significant injury. Patients who are paralyzed either by mechanism or chemically for intubation can develop decubitus ulcers if left on hard boards for prolonged periods of time. Any patient, even those with suspected thoracic or lumbar fracture, can be carefully removed from the long board. Those patients with suspected thoracic or lumbar fractures should remain supine, and be log-rolled whenever transfer is required. Patients presenting without prehospital care who have sustained a significant injury should have a cervical collar placed and be kept until further studies can be performed.

Pain control with parenteral medication can be very helpful.

Box 10.3   Initial interventions in spinal trauma

Acute interventions

- Stabilize ABCs
- Find and treat life-threatening injuries
- Oxygen
- Avoid hypotension (intravenous fluid/blood/pressors)
- Stop hemorrhage
- Maintain spinal immobilization

Most important evaluation in the first 10 minutes

- Assess and stabilize the ABCs
- Assess for vertebral body "step-offs"
- Assess lowest level of sensation/movement

Secondary evaluation

Minor

The cervical spine is the region of the neck most susceptible to injury and the most commonly filmed. In an effort to reduce unnecessary plain films (i.e., improve the specificity of radiography) but still maintain extremely high sensitivity, for diagnosing cervical spine injury, two separate and valid, decision rules – the NEXUS Low-risk Criteria (NLC) and the Canadian Cervical Spine Rule (CCR) (Figure 10.20) – have been developed.[1,2]

The NLC were based on a multicenter prospective observational study, in which 34 069 blunt trauma patients underwent either plain film or CT of the cervical

Canadian Cervical Spine Rule: (alert patients with a GCS score of 15)

Any high-risk factor that mandates radiography?

Age ≥ 65 years, or
Dangerous mechanism, or ·······················YES ·················→ Radiography
Paresthesias in extremities

Dangerous mechanism:

Fall ≥ 3 ft or 5 stairs
Axial load to head
NO   High-speed MVC (> 100 mph)
MVC with ejection, rollover
Collision of bike or motorized recreational vehicle

Any low-risk factor that allows safe assessment of range of motion?

Simple rear-end MVC, or
Patient in sitting position in ED, or
Patient ambulatory at any time, or
Delayed (not immediate) onset of neck pain, or ····· NO ·······→ Radiography
Absence of midline cervical-spine tenderness

"Simple rear-end MVC" excludes:

Being pushed into oncoming traffic
YES   Being hit by a bus or large truck or a high-speed vehicle
A rollover

Able to rotate neck actively? ············· UNABLE ···········→ Radiography

(45° to left and right)

YES

NO RADIOGRAPHY

Figure 10.20 Canadian Cervical Spine Rule. ED, emergency department; GCS, Glasgow Coma Scale; MVC, motor vehicle collision.

spine to identify significant spine injuries. The five questions that comprise the decision rule had a sensitivity of 99.6% (95% CI 98.6–99.6%), specificity of 12.9%, and a negative predictive value (NPV) of 99.9% (95% CI 99.6–100%) for the diagnosis of clinically important cervical spine injury.[1]

The NLC had no age criterion, although the CCR excluded patients younger than 16 years of age. One criticism of the NLC is that "no evidence of intoxication" and "no painful distracting injuries" were not well defined. One study attempted to narrow the definition of "distracting injury" to those only in the upper extremities.[26] Another study from Canada attempted to show that intoxicated blunt trauma patients may be able to have spine fractures requiring operative stabilization excluded using physical examination of the spine at presentation to the trauma center.[27] This study, however, only had a sensitivity of 60% for cervical spine abnormality on imaging.

Stiell et al. developed a decision rule that was prospectively evaluated against the NLC.[2] The CCR had a sensitivity of 99.4% and specificity of 45.1% in their study, compared to 90.7% and 36.8% (respectively) for the NLC.

Radiographs of the cervical spine should be obtained on patients who fail the low-risk criteria of either the CCR or NLC. For the low-risk patient with a good chance of obtaining a fully interpretable film, it is reasonable to use plain radiographs as a screening test. Plain films typically consist of the AP, lateral (including the top of T1), and open-mouth view. If plain films are inadequate, then CT is recommended. However, because in some studies, plain films miss up to 20% of cervical spine fractures (although usually have some abnormal findings), and many films need to be repeated or eventually require CT imaging, CT imaging has replaced plain radiographs as the first-line imaging modality in many centers (Figure 10.21).

On occasion there are plain films that on first look appear to be negative, but leave the clinician feeling that perhaps all is not quite right. Table 10.2 describes findings on plain films that are subtle but indicate vertebral instability.[28]

Table 10.2 Radiographic signs of vertebral instability[28]

Displacement implies injury to major ligamentous and articular structures

Wide interlaminar space implies injury to the posterior ligamentous structures and the facet joints

Wide facet joints imply injury to the posterior ligamentous structures

Disrupted posterior vertebral body line implies burst injury with disruption of anterior bony and posterior ligamentous structures

Wide vertebral canal implies injury to the entire vertebra in the sagittal plane

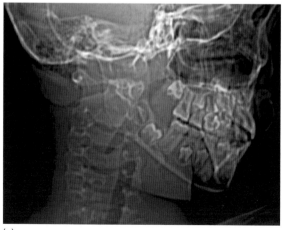

(a)

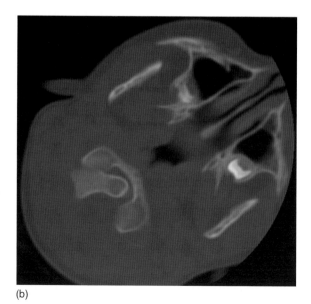

(b)

Figure 10.21 (a) Radiograph and (b) transaxial computed tomography (CT) of atlantoaxial rotary fixation.

CT scan

Imaging the spine with CT is becoming the preferred modality to evaluate for bony pathology after blunt trauma. The sensitivity of plain films for spinal fractures has been found to be as low as 32% for the cervical spine and 58% for thoracolumbar spine.[29–32] The greater radiation exposure with CT remains a concern due to the real but low risk of radiation-induced head and neck cancers. Other benefits include a more rapid removal of spine protection.[33] A CT scan can also help to identify foreign bodies, acute disk herniations, or extramedullary hematomas that can impinge on the spinal cord.[34]

For patients who suffer high-energy trauma or have a significantly depressed mental status, CT imaging is the study of choice to evaluate for bony fractures.[35] One decision analysis model found, using estimates and assumptions derived from the literature, that in moderate risk trauma patients CT is cost-effective and with low-risk patients CT may prevent rare cases of paralysis, but the incremental cost-effectiveness is low (about $80 000 per quality adjusted life year).[36] A recent meta-analysis concluded that there is insufficient evidence to state that CT of the cervical spine should replace plain films for initial screening for low-risk cervical spine injury.[35] However, others advocate for the use of CT imaging in the minor trauma patient if the cervical spine can not be cleared clinically.[37] The ultimate answer is dependent on the risk profile of the patient and the clinician's (and society's) tolerance for the risk of a serious adverse outcome, balanced with the increased cost, use of finite resources, and the radiation exposure that may cause ultimate harm.

Flexion–extension films

Most patient will have some discomfort or pain after their radiographs. When a patient continues to have persistent significant neck pain after negative plain films, CT should be the next imaging modality. If a patient continues to complain of significant cervical spine pain despite both negative plain films and CT imaging, there is still the rare possibility that a ligamentous injury could be present. Flexion–extension films of the cervical spine had been the next study to evaluate for ligamentous injury, but MRI is now preferred in the acute setting. Immediately following an injury, flexion–extension films are of limited use because up to 30% of films are limited by inadequate motion, most likely due to muscle spasms and pain.[38]

Flexion–extension films may be useful 7–10 days after injury when muscle spasm has abated. However, if flexion–extension films are negative and pain is severe and persistent, MRI should be used to evaluate for disc herniation or ligamentous injury. Flexion–extension films were never the only study to find cervical spine injury in the NEXUS study.[39]

Magnetic resonance imaging

The role of MRI in a blunt trauma patient is to identify ligamentous injury, the extent of spinal cord damage, and cases of spinal cord injury without radiographic abnormality (SCIWORA). An MRI may be superior to CT and plain film in identifying cervical spine ligamentous injury.[40,41] It is also helpful in identifying acute disk herniation, and in clearing the cervical spine in an obtunded or paralyzed trauma patient. However, recent studies have found that a normal motor exam and a negative cervical CT essentially negates the need for MRI in patients after blunt trauma.[42] Another retrospective review found CT imaging to have negative predicative value of 98.9% for ligamentous injury and those cases of ligamentous injury picked up by MRI were isolated to only one column. While controversial, these authors concluded that a normal CT of the cervical spine in obtunded or unreliable patients was sufficient to exclude unstable injuries.[28] A CT scan is still preferred to MRI for identifying osseous abnormalities, especially in the posterior column. In instances of penetrating trauma with a ferrous metal projectile, MRI is contraindicated because of potential bullet motion. Ultimately, CT may eventually be the single study to evaluate for both bony and ligamentous injury, but outside of some centers of expertise, it is more common at this time to obtain both when there is a significant concern or risk for ligamentous disruption and the CT scan is non-diagnostic.

Thoracolumbar spine

The thoracolumbar spine is structurally more stable, is less commonly injured, and is not imaged as frequently as the cervical spine. Most of the studies evaluating the thoracolumbar spine are retrospective reviews, and a prospectively validated decision rule has yet to be developed. However, certain risk factors have been associated with spinal fractures: Injury Severity Score (ISS) $\geq$ 15, positive clinical exam, fall $\geq$ 10 ft, ejection from motorcycle/MVC $\geq$ 50 mph, Glasgow Coma Scale (GCS) score $\leq$ 8, or neurologic deficit.[43,44] In one retrospective study, 40% of patients with spinal fracture had no documented complaints of pain at the fracture site, although many had distracting injuries.[44,45] Hsu et al. put forth guidelines for imaging the thoracolumbar spine if there is a high-energy traumatic mechanism and either back pain/midline tenderness, local signs of thoracolumbar injury, abnormal neurological signs, cervical spine fracture, GCS < 15, a major distracting injury, or alcohol/drug intoxication.[46] Following these guidelines, the majority of patients are filmed, but resulted in a sensitivity of 100%, specificity of 11.3%, and a NPV of 100%. This study also found that back pain/midline tenderness was the most sensitive finding at 62.1% and a palpable midline step had a specificity of 100%.[46] Interestingly, a retrospective review of patients involved in a MVC who then ambulated into the department complaining of back pain, showed that none of them had a fracture on plain film of the thoracic or lumbar spines.[47] If a patient has a high energy mechanism, has a known cervical spine fracture, or is obtunded, then CT imaging of the head or cervical spine is necessary, and CT imaging of the remaining spine is recommended.[48] Most times, however, this data can be reformatted from that obtained in trauma CT scans of the chest and abdomen performed with a multidetector CT scan (MDCT). One study showed CT sensitivity of 100% for thoracolumbar fracture and sensitivity of plain film of only 73%.[5]

Once a simple lumbar wedge-compression fracture has been identified, CT may help to determine if the fracture is stable.[49] The need may be based on the mechanism and suspicion.

Treatment

Most stable spinal fractures without neurological deficit are managed without surgical intervention, as most bony injuries can heal with proper orthotic immobilization. Ligamentous injuries require close follow up and will often require surgery.

Non-surgical options for treatment vary from cervical collars to halo rings. Cervical traction is often an option to reduce cervical spine deformity, via either placement of tongs or the halo apparatus. Braces can be used and include both cervical orthoses and high and low cervico-thoracic orthoses. The lumbar region is difficult to immobilize and often a brace extending 4–5 vertebra levels proximal and distal to unstable vertebrae is required. Thoracic bracing is also difficult because of inherent movement with respiration, however, with the sternum and ribs and shoulder, this area of the spine is inherently more stable.

Injuries that cause spinal instability, with or without neurological involvement, require surgery. Surgery allows for decompression of the neural canal, as well as restoration and maintenance of spinal stability and alignment. Immediate surgery is warranted when there is progressive neurological deterioration; early surgery is indicated in cases of impingement on the spinal cord caused by foreign bodies, herniated disks, bony fragments, or an epidural hematoma, although if the lesion is complete the prognosis is generally poor.[50,51] The extent of the injury (number of columns that are injured) may make an injury unstable, requiring stabilization with hardware (either anterior, posterior, or both). Fusion is the ultimate goal of these surgeries as the hardware will only provide short-term stability.

Numerous studies have questioned the need for surgical intervention for thoracolumbar burst fractures without neurological deficit.[52–54] A Cochrane review on the subject concluded that "there was no statistically significant difference on the functional outcome 2 years or more after therapy between operative and non-operative treatment for thoracolumbar burst fractures without neurological deficit."[55] However, proponents argue that surgery provides patients with a life with less pain and a greater chance of returning to work in their original jobs.[56,57]

Timing of surgery is also controversial, with some physicians advocating a waiting period to allow for reduction in tissue swelling, while others prefer earlier intervention. Some reports have shown that surgery results are best when performed within 4 days of injury and no later than 7–10 days (Table 10.3).[58–60]

Box 10.4   Essentials of spinal fracture treatment

- Stable spinal fractures can be often managed with proper orthotic immobilization.
- Unstable spinal fractures require surgical intervention.
- Emergent surgical intervention is warranted with progressive neurologic dysfunction or spinal impingement by bony fragment, hematoma, herniated disk, or foreign body.

Table 10.3 Common treatment patterns

Type	Treatment
Occipital cervical injuries	Fractures in which the transverse ligament is disrupted require traction initially to reduce the displaced lateral masses and then can be placed in a halo-vest
	Atlas fractures with significant displacement can require traction for up to 8 weeks before a halo-vest is subsequently worn. Surgery is usually not needed acutely
Atlantoaxial joint injuries	Patients are initially put in traction to achieve reduction. The definitive treatment is a posterior cervical fusion of C1–C2
	Rotary subluxations: These injuries usually reduce with traction and require only brace support
Burst fractures	Unstable injuries require surgery (anterior decompression and fusion) to realign and stabilize the fracture if reduction can't be achieved or maintained
	Stable burst fractures, can be treated with a halo-vest if there is no neurological deficit and alignment is acceptable, but require close follow up to insure that the spinal alignment is maintained. Surgery is warranted if both anterior and posterior longitudinal ligament injury occurs, surgical stabilization is required
Thoracic spine fractures	Stable fractures with intact neurological function (most often compression or burst fractures) can usually be treated with a brace. Unstable fractures either have associated neurological injury or excessive flexion, rotation, or translation
Flexion–distraction/ chance injuries	Closed reduction and bracing is appropriate in those injuries with < 30° of angulation of the bony spine at the site of injury. Surgical reduction and fixation are indicated for flexion–distraction injuries that involve primarily ligaments or disks that demonstrate more than 30° of angulation

Documentation

In spinal injury, a history of the trauma and examination, with details focusing on the CCR or NLC (if they are to be utilized) should be included, especially if the decision rules are being used to preclude imaging (Table 10.4). The physical exam should note any areas of bony tenderness, vertebral step-offs, decreased or limited extremity movement, and whether the patient presented boarded and collared. The chart should optimally include a thorough section on "medical decision making," explaining use of either the CCR or NEXUS to clear the cervical spine, and a re-evaluation of the patient after pain medication. With a spinal fracture, for persistent severe pain or pain out of proportion to expected despite negative plain films and CT, consultants should be contacted with proper documentation stating that the case was discussed and appropriate "hand-off" for follow-up care was put in place.

Disposition

Patients who are cleared either via the CCR or NRC may have their collars removed and do not require imaging. Soft cervical collars are often recommended;

Table 10.4 NEXUS Low-risk Criteria: cervical spine radiography is indicated unless patients meet all the following criteria[1]

1. No posterior midline cervical spine tenderness
2. No evidence of intoxication
3. A normal level of consciousness
4. No focal neurologic deficits
5. No painful distracting injuries

NEXUS, National Emergency X-Radiography Utilization Study.

however, the available data do not strongly support their use, and in some cases find it detrimental compared to active immobilization.[61–64] These patients may be discharged to home. Patients who do not meet criteria for either CCR or NLC, those who are obtunded, the elderly, or those with a higher-risk mechanism of energy should have imaging of the spine performed. An MDCT scan should be ordered if cervical spine films are inadequate, if there is a high suspicion of injury, or in those undergoing other MDCT imaging. Those patients who continue to have neurological symptoms (without demonstrable deficits), or persistent significant pain despite negative plain films or a negative MDCT should receive an MRI or be discharged with a cervical collar for delayed flexion–extension films or MRI, to evaluate for ligamentous injury. This should be a semi-rigid Philadelphia, Aspen, or Miami J collar. In patients with persistent pain, neurological symptoms, or concerning mechanism of injury, a discussion with the consulting service is appropriate. Once an unstable fracture is identified, the consulting service (trauma, neurosurgery, orthopedics) should be contacted and plans made for transfer or admission for definitive stabilizing therapy. Wedge fractures of the thoracic and lumbar spine may be best managed in the hospital (due to the need for parenteral narcotics, the usually large amount of force needed to cause the fracture and concern over internal organs, and because it is often associated with prolonged and occasionally delayed ileus).[47,65]

Some spinal fractures may be managed in the outpatient setting (isolated cervical vertebral body compression fractures or spinous process fractures) when the mechanism of injury and degree of patient distress are not significant and there is no evidence of neurologic impairment or associated ligamentous instability; in such a case orthopedic or neurosurgical consultation should first be made. Patients should be instructed to return immediately if they notice muscle weakness, increasing pain, numbness, or bowel or bladder incontinence.

Box 10.5 Essentials of disposition with spinal trauma

- Patients who have had their cervical spines cleared by either NLC or CCR, and whose pain is gone or mild, can be discharged.
- Consultation with the spinal service for treatment plan, disposition, and follow up should occur when a spinal injury (either bony or ligamentous) is identified.

References

1. Hoffman JR, Mower WR, Wolfson AB, Todd KH, Zucker MI. Validity of a set of clinical criteria to rule out injury to the cervical spine in patients with blunt trauma. National Emergency X-Radiography Utilization Study Group. *N Engl J Med* 2000;**343** (2):94–9.

2. Stiell IG, Grimshaw J, Wells GA, et al. A matched-pair cluster design study protocol to evaluate implementation of the Canadian C-spine Rule in hospital emergency departments: Phase III. *Implement Sci* 2007;**8**(2):4.

3. Panjabi MM, Oxland TR, Kifune M, et al. Validity of the three-column theory of thoracolumbar fractures. A biomechanic investigation. *Spine* 1995;**20** (10):1122–7.

4. Goldberg W, Mueller C, Panacek E, et al. Distribution and patterns of blunt traumatic cervical spine injury. *Ann Emerg Med* 2001;**38**(1):17–21.

5. Berry GE, Adams S, Harris MB, et al. Are plain radiographs of the spine necessary during evaluation after blunt trauma? Accuracy of screening torso computed tomography in thoracic/lumbar spine fracture diagnosis. *J Trauma* 2005;**59**(6):1410–13.

6. Sharma OP, Oswanski MF, Yazdi JS, Jindal S, Taylor M. Assessment for additional spinal trauma in patients with cervical spine injury. *Am Surg* 2007;**73**(1):70–4.

7. Robertson A, Branfoot T, Barlow IF, Giannoudis PV. Spinal injury patterns resulting from car and motorcycle accidents. *Spine* 2002;**27**(24):2825–30.

8. Bensch FV, Kiuru MJ, Koivikko MP, Koskinen SK. Spine fractures in falling accidents: analysis of multidetector CT findings. *Eur Radiol* 2004;**14** (4):618–24.

9. Baez AA, Schiebel N. Evidence-based emergency medicine/systematic review abstract. Is routine spinal immobilization an effective intervention for trauma patients? *Ann Emerg Med* 2006;**47**(1):110–12.

10. Kwan I, Bunn F, Roberts I. Spinal immobilization for trauma patients. *Cochrane Database Syst Rev* 2001;**2**: CD002803.

11. Hauswald M, Ong G, Tandberg D, Omar Z. Out-of-hospital spinal immobilization: its effect on neurological injury. *Acad Emerg Med* 1998;**5** (3):214–19.

12. McHugh TP, Taylor JP. Unnecessary out-of-hospital use of full spinal immobilization. *Acad Emerg Med* 1998;**5**(3):278–80.

13. Domeier RM, Swor RA, Evans RW, et al. Multicenter prospective validation of prehospital clinical spinal clearance criteria. *J Trauma* 2002;**53**(4):744–50.

14. Domeier RM, Frederiksen SM, Welch K. Prospective performance assessment of an out-of-hospital protocol for selective spine immobilization using clinical spine clearance criteria. *Ann Emerg Med* 2005;**46**(2):123–31.

15. Burton JH, Dunn MG, Harmon NR, Hermanson TA, Bradshaw JR. A statewide, prehospital emergency medical service selective patient spine immobilization protocol. *J Trauma* 2006;**61**(1):161–7.

16. Waninger KN, Richards JG, Pan WT, Shay AR, Shindle MK. An evaluation of head movement in

backboard-immobilized helmeted football, lacrosse and ice hockey players. *Clin J Sport Med* 2001;**11**(2):82–6.

17. Touger M, Gennis P, Nathanson N, et al. Validity of a decision rule to reduce cervical spine radiography in elderly patients with blunt trauma. *Ann Emerg Med* 2002;**40**(3):287–93.

18. Bub LD, Blackmore CC, Mann FA, Lomoschitz FM. Cervical spine fractures in patients 65 years and older: a clinical prediction rule for blunt trauma. *Radiology* 2005;**234**(1):143–9.

19. Rhee P, Kuncir EJ, Johnson L, et al. Cervical spine injury is highly dependent on the mechanism of injury following blunt and penetrating assault. *J Trauma* 2006;**61**(5):1166–70.

20. Barkana Y, Stein M, Scope A, et al. Prehospital stabilization of the cervical spine for penetrating injuries of the neck – is it necessary? *Injury* 2000;**31**(5):305–9.

21. Waters RL, Hu SS. Penetrating injuries of the spinal canal. Stab and gunshot injuries. In Frymoyer JW (ed.), *The Adult Spine*. New York:Raven Press, 1991: vol. 1, pp. 815–26.

22. Connell RA, Graham CA, Munro PT. Is spinal immobilisation necessary for all patients sustaining isolated penetrating trauma? *Injury* 2003;**34**(12):912–23.

23. Kaups KL, Davis JW. Patients with gunshot wounds to the head do not require cervical spine immobilization and evaluation. *J Trauma* 1998;**44**(5):865–7.

24. Medzon R, Rothenhaus T, Bono CM, Grindlinger G, Rathlev NK. Stability of cervical spine fractures after gunshot wounds to the head and neck. *Spine* 2005;**30**(20):2274–9.

25. Bivins HG, Ford S, Bezmalinovic Z, Price HM, Williams JL. The effect of axial traction during orotracheal intubation of the trauma victim with an unstable cervical spine. *Ann Emerg Med* 1988;**17**(1):25–9.

26. Heffernan DS, Schermer CR, Lu SW. What defines a distracting injury in cervical spine assessment? *J Trauma* 2005;**59**(6):1396–9.

27. Liberman M, Farooki N, Lavoie A, Mulder DS, Sampalis JS. Clinical evaluation of the spine in the intoxicated blunt trauma patient. *Injury* 2005;**36**(4):519–25.

28. Hogan GJ, Mirvis SE, Shanmuganathan K, Scalea TM. Exclusion of unstable cervical spine injury in obtunded patients with blunt trauma: is MR imaging needed when multi-detector row CT findings are normal? *Radiology* 2005;**237**(1):106–13.

29. Brohi K, Healy M, Fotheringham T, et al. Helical computed tomographic scanning for the evaluation of the cervical spine in the unconscious, intubated trauma patient. *J Trauma* 2005;**58**(5):897–901.

30. Gale SC, Gracias VH, Reilly PM, Schwab CW. The inefficiency of plain radiography to evaluate the cervical spine after blunt trauma. *J Trauma* 2005;**59**(5):1121–5.

31. Diaz JJ, Jr., Gillman C, Morris JA, Jr., et al. Are five-view plain films of the cervical spine unreliable? A prospective evaluation in blunt trauma patients with altered mental status. *J Trauma* 2003;**55**(4):658–63.

32. Brown CV, Antevil JL, Sise MJ, Sack DI. Spiral computed tomography for the diagnosis of cervical, thoracic, and lumbar spine fractures: its time has come. *J Trauma* 2005;**58**(5):890–5.

33. Hauser CJ, Visvikis G, Hinrichs C, et al. Prospective validation of computed tomographic screening of the thoracolumbar spine in trauma. *J Trauma* 2003;**55**(2):228–34.

34. Hockberger RS, Kirshenbaum KJ. Spine. In Marx JA, Hockberger RS, Walls RM (eds), *Rosen's Emergency Medicine: Concepts and Clinical Practice*. St. Louis, MO: Mosby, 2002: vol. 1, pp. 329–70.

35. Holmes JF, Akkinepalli R. Computed tomography versus plain radiography to screen for cervical spine injury: a meta-analysis. *J Trauma* 2005;**58**(5):902–5.

36. Blackmore CC, Ramsey SD, Mann FA, Deyo RA. Cervical spine screening with CT in trauma patients: a cost-effectiveness analysis. *Radiology* 1999;**212**(1):117–25.

37. Sanchez B, Waxman K, Jones T, et al. Cervical spine clearance in blunt trauma: evaluation of a computed tomography-based protocol. *J Trauma* 2005;**59**(1):179–83.

38. Insko EK, Gracias VH, Gupta R, et al. Utility of flexion and extension radiographs of the cervical spine in the acute evaluation of blunt trauma. *J Trauma* 2002;**53**(3):426–9.

39. Pollack CV, Jr., Hendey GW, Martin DR, et al. Use of flexion–extension radiographs of the cervical spine in blunt trauma. *Ann Emerg Med* 2001;**38**(1):8–11.

40. Diaz JJ, Jr., Aulino JM, Collier B, et al. The early work-up for isolated ligamentous injury of the cervical spine: does computed tomography scan have a role? *J Trauma* 2005;**59**(4):897–903.

41. Stassen NA, Williams VA, Gestring ML, Cheng JD, Bankey PE. Magnetic resonance imaging in combination with helical computed tomography provides a safe and efficient method of cervical spine clearance in the obtunded trauma patient. *J Trauma* 2006;**60**(1):171–7.

42. Schuster R, Waxman K, Sanchez B, et al. Magnetic resonance imaging is not needed to clear cervical

spines in blunt trauma patients with normal computed tomographic results and no motor deficits. *Arch Surg* 2005;**140**(8):762–6.

43. Durham RM, Luchtefeld WB, Wibbenmeyer L, et al. Evaluation of the thoracic and lumbar spine after blunt trauma. *Am J Surg* 1995;**170**(6):681–4.

44. Frankel HL, Rozycki GS, Ochsner MG, Harviel JD, Champion HR. Indications for obtaining surveillance thoracic and lumbar spine radiographs. *J Trauma* 1994;**37**(4):673–6.

45. D'Costa H, George G, Parry M, et al. Pitfalls in the clinical diagnosis of vertebral fractures: a case series in which posterior midline tenderness was absent. *Emerg Med J* 2005;**22**(5):330–2.

46. Hsu JM, Joseph T, Ellis AM. Thoracolumbar fracture in blunt trauma patients: guidelines for diagnosis and imaging. *Injury* 2003;**34**(6):426–33.

47. Tamir E, Anekstein Y, Mirovsky Y, Heim M, Dudkiewicz I. Thoracic and lumbar spine radiographs for walking trauma patients–is it necessary? *J Emerg Med* 2006;**31**(4):403–5.

48. Winslow JE, Hensberry R, Bozeman WP, Hill KD, Miller PR. Risk of thoracolumbar fractures doubled in victims of motor vehicle collisions with cervical spine fractures. *J Trauma* 2006;**61**(3):686–7.

49. Campbell SE, Phillips CD, Dubovsky E, Cail WS, Omary RA. The value of CT in determining potential instability of simple wedge-compression fractures of the lumbar spine. *AJNR Am J Neuroradiol* 1995;**16**(7):1385–92.

50. Vaccaro AR, Daugherty RJ, Sheehan TP, et al. Neurological outcome of early versus late surgery for cervical spinal cord injury. *Spine* 1997;**22**(22):2609–13.

51. Mirza SK, Krengel WF, 3rd, Chapman JR, et al. Early versus delayed surgery for acute cervical spinal cord injury. *Clin Orthop Relat Res* 1999;(**359**):104–14.

52. Wood K, Buttermann G, Mehbod A, et al. Operative compared with nonoperative treatment of a thoracolumbar burst fracture without neurological deficit. A prospective, randomized study. *J Bone Joint Surg Am* 2003;**85**A(5):773–81.

53. James KS, Wenger KH, Schlegel JD, Dunn HK. Biomechanical evaluation of the stability of thoracolumbar burst fractures. *Spine* 1994;**19**(15):1731–40.

54. Knight RQ, Stornelli DP, Chan DP, Devanny JR, Jackson KV. Comparison of operative versus nonoperative treatment of lumbar burst fractures. *Clin Orthop Relat Res* 1993;(293):112–21.

55. Yi L, Jingping B, Gele J, Baoleri X, Taixiang W. Operative versus non-operative treatment for thoracolumbar burst fractures without neurological deficit. *Cochrane Database Syst Rev* 2006;**4**:CD005079.

56. Siebenga J, Leferink VJ, Segers MJ, et al. Treatment of traumatic thoracolumbar spine fractures: a multicenter prospective randomized study of operative versus nonsurgical treatment. *Spine* 2006;**31**(25):2881–90.

57. Dai LD. Low lumbar spinal fractures: management options. *Injury* 2002;**33**(7):579–82.

58. Croce MA, Bee TK, Pritchard E, Miller PR, Fabian TC. Does optimal timing for spine fracture fixation exist? *Ann Surg* 2001;**233**(6):851–8.

59. Arnold PM, Malone DG, Han PP. Bilateral locked facets of the lumbosacral spine: treatment with open reduction and transpedicular fixation. *J Spinal Cord Med* 2004;**27**(3):269–72.

60. Albert TJ, Kim DH. Timing of surgical stabilization after cervical and thoracic trauma. Invited submission from the Joint Section Meeting on Disorders of the Spine and Peripheral Nerves, March 2004. *J Neurosurg Spine* 2005;**3**(3):182–90.

61. Schnabel M, Ferrari R, Vassiliou T, Kaluza G. Randomised, controlled outcome study of active mobilisation compared with collar therapy for whiplash injury. *Emerg Med J* 2004;**21**(3):306–10.

62. Kongsted A, Qerama E, Kasch H, et al. Neck collar, "act-as-usual" or active mobilization for whiplash injury? A randomized parallel-group trial. *Spine* 2007;**32**(6):618–26.

63. Crawford JR, Khan RJ, Varley GW. Early management and outcome following soft tissue injuries of the neck-a randomised controlled trial. *Injury* 2004;**35**(9):891–5.

64. Gennis P, Miller L, Gallagher EJ, et al. The effect of soft cervical collars on persistent neck pain in patients with whiplash injury. *Acad Emerg Med* 1996;**3**(6):568–73.

65. Ong AW, Rodriguez A, Kelly R, et al. Detection of cervical spine injuries in alert, asymptomatic geriatric blunt trauma patients: who benefits from radiologic imaging? *Am Surg* 2006;**72**(9):773–6.

Injuries of the spine: Nerve

Suzanne Bigelow and Ron Medzon

Introduction

A spinal cord injury (SCI) is a sudden, life-altering event. Damage to the spinal cord results in a disruption, either temporary or permanent, of the normal motor, sensory, or autonomic function of the spinal cord. The annual incidence is estimated to range between 15 and 40 cases per million.[1,2] In the United States, 12 000 new cases occur yearly.[3] The good news is that survival amongst patients with SCI has improved.[2] In the United States an estimated 177 000 persons were living with SCI in 1988, compared to an estimated 255 700–300 000 persons in 2008.[3,4] Spinal cord injury impacts society strongly, in medical expenses/use of resources, loss of productivity, and income. The estimated lifetime costs for someone with a high cervical spine injury (C1–C4) at the age of 25 years is > 3 million dollars. This figure does not include losses in wages, benefits, and productivity.[3] Missed SCI not only has litigious implications for the physician, but can be devastating for the patient in terms of complications, neurological abilities, and familial emotions.

Epidemiology

In 2005, the National Spinal Cord Injury Statistical Center released facts and figures regarding SCI from 2000 to 2005. They have recorded data on 13% of new SCIs (annually). There appear to be changes in the epidemiology, risk factors, and demographics of spinal cord injured patients when compared to data from the previous several decades. Average age of the SCI patient has increased from 28.7 years to 37.6 years (attributed to the overall aging of the general population).[3] African-Americans now comprise a larger percentage of the total population with SCI (an increase from 14% to 22%).[3,5] Men suffer a

sobering 80% of all SCI, with Caucasians topping the list with 63% of total cases. Conversely, being female, Hispanic, African-American, or < 18 years of age carries a reduced risk of cervical spine injury. In the United States, motor vehicle crashes account for 47.5% of SCI cases, followed by falls (22.9%), violence (13.8%), and sports/recreational activities.[3,5]

Box 11.1 Summary of spinal cord injury epidemiology

Risk factors for SCI	Causes of SCI	Reduced risk of SCI
Male (4 : 1 male : female)	Motor vehicle crash (47.5%)	Female
Caucasian	Falls (22.9%)	Hispanic or African-American
Young age (over 18 years)	Violence (13.8%)	Age younger than 18 years
Motor vehicle crash	Sports/ recreational activities	

The annual incidence of SCI ranges from 15 to 40 cases per million.[1,2,6,7] A majority (55–60%) of SCI occurs in the cervical spine region (C1–T1). The location of SCI is spread evenly between the remainder of the spinal areas (15% thoracic, T1–T11; 15% thoracolumbar, T11/12–L1/2; 15% lumbar and sacral areas).[7,8] In one retrospective review of patients presenting with new SCI, associated spinal fracture was seen in 56% of patients with cervical SCI, 100% of thoracic SCI, and 85% of lumbar SCI.[9]

Spinal cord injury carries a high mortality. It is estimated that 4000 patients with acute SCI die before

---

Trauma: A Comprehensive Emergency Medicine Approach, eds. Eric Legome and Lee W. Shockley. Published by Cambridge University Press. © Cambridge University Press 2011.

reaching the hospital. This number is extrapolated, as solid data on prehospital deaths do not exist. Out of 12 000 annual estimated new cases of SCI (paraplegia and tetraplegia), 1000 people die during their acute hospitalization.[10-12] Cervical spine injury carries the highest mortality.[9] In the thoracolumbar region, L1 is the most commonly injured level (16%), with L2 second (15%), L3 third (11%), followed by T12 (10%).[13] The most common neurologic diagnosis at discharge from the hospital after the initial admission was incomplete tetraplegia.[3] In one Canadian study, falls were responsible for 63% of SCI in patients 65 years or older.[9]

Recent major changes in evaluation and management

Over the past 40 years, roughly 66% of patients presenting with SCI had complete cord injury. Recent numbers show a decrease to 41%.[3] A limited number of preventive, diagnostic, and therapeutic improvements have been made in the past 20 years: improved prehospital care and retrieval systems, increased awareness of the need for spinal immobilization after an accident, introduction of airbags and restraint devices in motor vehicles, and hospital-based interventions (including avoidance of hypotension, hypoxia, and careful manipulation of the patient). Multislice computed tomography (CT) and magnetic resonance imaging (MRI) are now widely available for evaluating spine injuries.[14] Although steroids have become more commonly used in management, evolving treatments are now trending away from their use as standard in all cases.[14,15]

Box 11.2 Essentials of spinal cord injury epidemiology

- The annual incidence estimated to range between 15 and 40 cases per million.[1,2] In the United States, 12 000 new cases occur yearly.
- The estimated lifetime costs for someone with a high cervical spine injury (C1–C4) at the age of 25 years is > 3 million dollars (exclusive of losses in wages, benefits, and productivity).
- Men suffer 80% of all SCI.
- A majority (55–60%) of SCI occurs in the cervical spine region (C1–T1).
- The rest is spread evenly between the remainder of the spinal areas.
- A limited number of preventive, diagnostic, and therapeutic improvements have been made in

---

the past 20 years: improved prehospital care and retrieval systems, increased awareness of the need for spinal immobilization after an accident, introduction of airbags and restraint devices in motor vehicles, and hospital-based interventions (including avoidance of hypotension, hypoxia, and careful manipulation of the patient).

Clinical anatomy/pathophysiology

The bony spinal column encases and protects the spinal cord. The spinal cord is 40–45 cm in length, cylindrical in shape, starts at the base of the brain, exiting through the foramen magnum, and terminates in the conus medullaris at roughly L1–L2, although this can range from T12 to L3. The cauda equina emanate from the cona medullaris. The spinal cord is divided into neurological units, labeled after vertebral levels, i.e., C1, C2, etc. However, within the spinal cord, a C8 neurological level exists. This is not true of the bony spine.[16]

The spinal cord gives off 31 spinal nerves, (8 cervical, 12 thoracic, 5 lumbar, 5 sacral, 1 coccygeal). Spinal nerves consist of anterior (ventral) and posterior (dorsal) nerves, containing efferent and afferent axons, respectively. These nerves exit the spinal column through bony foramina. From C1 to C7, the nerve roots exit the spinal column above the corresponding vertebra. At the C7 vertebra, C8 roots exit below the vertebra. All roots caudal to C7 exit inferior to the vertebra.[16]

Fusiform enlargements of the spinal cord exist in the cervical as well as the lower thoracic/upper lumbar regions. The enlargements give rise to the brachial and lumbo-sacral plexuses that innervate the arms and legs respectively. The amount of space not occupied by the cord is reduced at these levels. Consequently, the cord is more easily compressed in these locations.[17,18] The most commonly injured spinal cord level is C5, whereas the thoracolumbar junction (T12–L1) is the most frequent lumbar level.[19] Transection of the cord above C5 causes tetraplegia. Respiratory failure may occur if the transection is superior to C4 (Figure 11.1).[16]

Mirroring the brain, the cord is covered by three meningeal layers, the pia, arachnoid, and dura maters.

Vascular system

Vascular supply of the spinal cord is divided into anterior and posterior vessels.

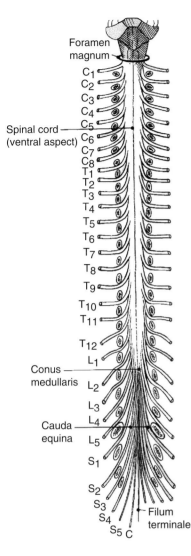

Foramen magnum

C1
C2
C3
C4
C5
Spinal cord (ventral aspect) — C6
C7
C8
T1
T2
T3
T4
T5
T6
T7
T8
T9
T10
T11
T12
L1
Conus medullaris — L2
L3
L4
Cauda equina — L5
S1
S2
S3
S4
S5 C
Filum terminale

Figure 11.1 The distribution of the nerve roots as they exit the spinal canal and their relation to the vertebrae. (From Melloni J, Dox I, Melloni H, Melloni B. *Attorney's Reference on Human Anatomy*. Cambridge: Cambridge University Press, 2008.)

Arterial

Both the anterior and posterior circulation systems of the cord receive contributions from the radicular and medullary arteries:

1. *Anterior arterial vessel*: The anterior spinal artery (from the union of the vertebral arteries), runs the entire length of the cord in the midline, supplies the anterior circumferential two thirds of cord and the central gray matter.

2. *Posterior arterial vessels* supply the remaining third circumferential of posterior cord.

The anastomotic flow between the anterior and posterior arterial systems is poor. Both arterial systems contribute to a net-like arterial plexus surrounding the thoracic, distal cervical, and proximal lumbar cord. While redundancy in the arterial supply of this area exists, this area is felt to be at greater risk of ischemia than the very upper and lower ends of the cord during episodes of hypotension (Figure 11.2).[16–18]

Venous

The venous system of the cord follows the arterial system, draining into the internal and external venous plexuses. The internal venous plexus passes superiorly and communicates with the dural sinuses and vertebral veins in the skull. The external venous plexus lies on the external surface of the vertebrae (Figure 11.3).[16]

The cord itself is made up of gray and white matter. White matter concentration is greatest in the cervical spinal segments (as a consequence of the large density of axonal fibers). The butterfly-shaped gray matter sits centrally and contains the nerve cell bodies and their processes, whereas the white matter is a collection of the myelinated ascending and descending axonal fibers known as tracts. Multiple tracts exist. Important spinal cord tracts are the posterior columns (medial and lateral), spinothalamic tract, and corticospinal tract. The tracts are named for their origins (i.e., corticospinal tract starts in the cortex, travels to the spine) (Table 11.1 and Figure 11.4).[17–19]

Classification of spinal cord injuries

The American Spinal Injury Association (ASIA) classification system is now used to describe the neurologic level of injury as well as the type of SCI (e.g., C8 ASIA A with zone of partial preservation of pinprick to T2). While not commonly used in actual emergency department (ED) practice, it may be used by consultants and in research (Figure 11.5). Copies may be found online and freely downloaded (http://www.asia-spinalinjury.org).[20]

Spinal cord injury terminology

Tetraplegia (formerly known as quadriplegia) is injury to the spinal cord in the cervical region with associated loss of muscle strength in all four extremities. It can be complete – lacking sensory and motor, or incomplete – having one or both of these neurologic functions partially or completely intact.[20]

Paraplegia is injury to the spinal cord in the thoracic, lumbar, or sacral regions, including the cauda equina and conus medullaris, sparing the upper extremities.[20]

169

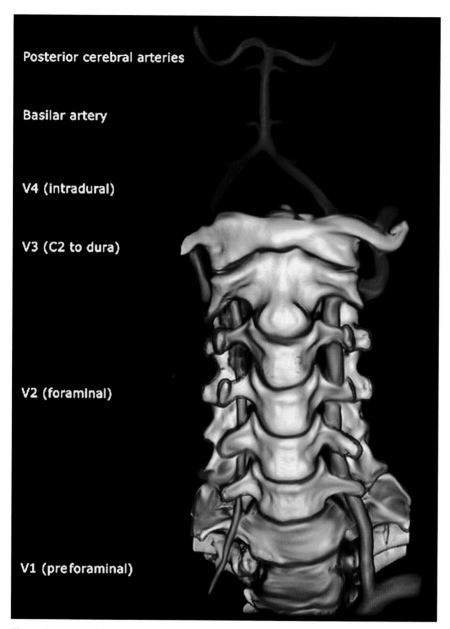

Posterior cerebral arteries

Basilar artery

V4 (intradural)

V3 (C2 to dura)

V2 (foraminal)

V1 (preforaminal)

Figure 11.2 Vertebral artery based on three-dimensional-surface rendered computed tomography angiogram (CTA). (Courtesy of Frank Gaillard.)

The extent of injury is defined by the ASIA Impairment Scale, using the categories listed in Table 11.2.

Digital rectal exam will help delineate between complete and incomplete SCIs. The presence of rectal tone or sacral sensation is considered sacral-sparing and this equates with an incomplete SCI. Accurate assessment of the type and level of SCI may be difficult in the acute period, especially if the patient is in spinal shock.

Pathology of spinal cord injury

Spinal cord injury can be sustained through multiple mechanisms. Research over the past 25 years has shown that the spinal cord suffers two distinct injuries: the initial or primary injury and a later secondary insult. The following list details common mechanisms (primary injuries) leading to tissue damage:

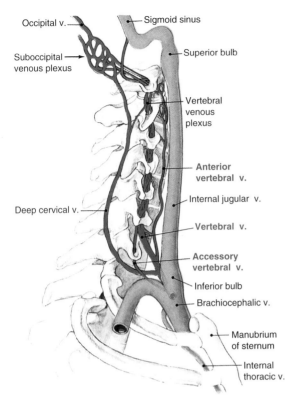

Figure 11.3 Venous drainage of the cervical spinal cord. (From Melloni J, Dox I, Melloni H, Melloni B. *Attorney's Reference on Human Anatomy*. Cambridge: Cambridge University Press, 2008.)

1. Destruction from direct trauma.
2. Compression by bone fragments, hematoma, or disk material.
3. Ischemia from damage or impingement on the spinal arteries.

Spinal cord edema could ensue secondary to any of the above.

The phenomenon of the secondary insult is still not entirely clear, but the various pathways are better understood now. Currently, secondary injury is believed to be a highly complex combination of cord hypoxia, calcium efflux, cell apoptosis, free radicals, and generalized inflammation.[21] Research will

Table 11.1 Major spinal cord nerve tracts

Tract	Function	Location of symptoms in acute cord injury
Corticospinal tract	Voluntary movement	Ipsilateral
Spinothalamic tract	Pain, temperature	Contralateral
Posterior columns	Proprioception, vibration	Ipsilateral

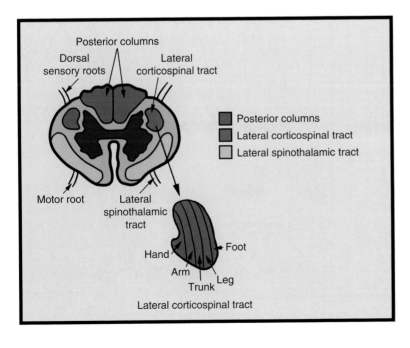

Figure 11.4 Illustration of the cross-section of cervical spinal cord showing ascending sensory and descending motor tracts and stereotopic organization of the lateral corticospinal tract. (From Mandavia D, Newton E, Demetriades D. *Colour Atlas of Emergency Trauma*. Cambridge: Cambridge University Press, 2003.)

171

Table 11.2 The American Spinal Injury Association (ASIA) Impairment Scale

ASIA classification	Injury	Sensation	Motor
A	Complete	Absent in S4–S5	Absent in S4–S5
B	Incomplete	Function preserved below neurologic level, extends through sacral segments S4–S5	Absent in S4–S5
C	Incomplete	Function preserved below neurologic level, extends through sacral segments S4–S5	Preserved below neurologic level, most key muscles below the neurologic level have muscle grade < 3
D	Incomplete	Function preserved below neurologic level, extends through sacral segments S4–S5	Preserved below neurologic level, most key muscles below neurologic level have muscle grade ≥ 3 but < 5
E	Normal	Function preserved below neurologic level, extends through sacral segments S4–S5	Motor preserved, muscle Grade 5 (*not used in acute injury*)

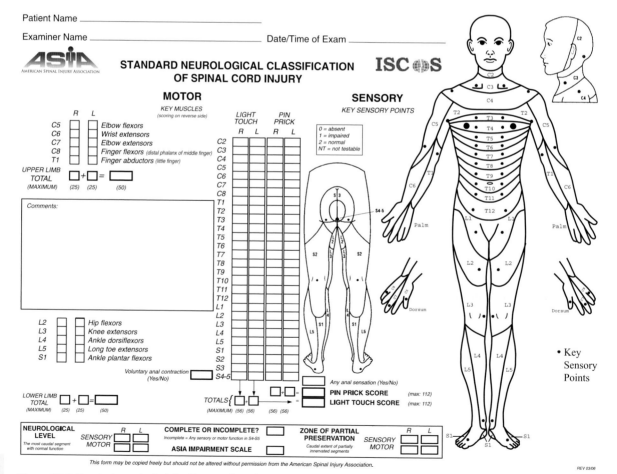

Figure 11.5 Standard neurological classification of spinal cord injury. (Courtesy of the American Spinal Injury Association.)

continue to search for new receptor targets, better pharmacologic therapies, and unravel the complicated pathway of neuronal death and regrowth.[22–24]

Prehospital interventions

Prehospital interventions are limited. Attention should be paid first to stabilization of the spine and the airway, breathing, and circulation (ABCs). In regards to the spine, emergency services personnel are tasked with stabilization and immobilization using a hard cervical collar, backboard, and other restraints to keep the patient as flat and still as possible. This can be difficult if the patient is intoxicated or combative.[25]

Emergency department evaluation and management

The emergency physician should be suspicious of a SCI if the patient:

1. States she or he cannot move a limb(s).
2. Has/had numbness/decreased sensation.
3. Complains of back or neck pain.
4. Has urinary or fecal incontinence.
5. Is intoxicated or has altered mental status and a traumatic mechanism.
6. Suffered a mechanism of injury which could lead to SCI. One should be alert for the presence of neurogenic shock. It is a diagnosis of exclusion, and typically presents with bradycardia and hypotension.

Initial evaluation

Assess the ABCs. If the patient is very combative and refuses to lie flat, they may require sedation and intubation to prohibit movement that may exacerbate a spinal cord injury. This should be balanced by the clinical suspicion for an injury and the risk/benefit of intubation or sedation. If the patient can be managed by sedation and observation in spinal precautions, this may be a more optimal approach, especially if suspicion is low by mechanism and exam findings. Some patients may require paralysis after intubation to facilitate acquisition of adequate imaging. When in doubt, treat the patient as if she or he has a spinal cord/column injury.

The initial goal is of patient stabilization, focusing on any life-threatening injuries. If the patient requires emergent surgery, that should take precedence over spinal cord imaging; however, the patient should remain in a cervical collar and be on spinal precautions until cleared.[25]

Secondary survey

During the secondary survey, be alert to the presence of other injuries as these are common in the SCI patient.[26] Injuries to the thoracic spine and cord require a very high amount of force and other severe injuries are not uncommon.[27] (The thoracic spine is the most stable section of the spine because of support from the rib cage.) Palpate the cervical spine for point tenderness and bony step-offs while a second person maintains in-line stabilization. Replace the cervical collar, log-roll the patient, repeat the same for the thoracic/lumbar/sacral bony spine. Look carefully for signs of penetrating and blunt trauma. At the end of the spinal examination is the best time to complete the rectal exam. Log-roll the patient to the supine position and complete the neurological evaluation. Ideally, the neurological exam is completed before sedation/paralysis occurs, however this may not be practical and a safe/secured airway takes precedence.

1. Assess **pupillary reflex** in both eyes (not crucial for evaluation of spinal cord injury).
2. Check for **gross movement** in all four extremities.
3. Assess **strength** by having the patient squeeze the examiner's fingers and plantar-flex both feet.

Muscle strengths are graded using a five-point scale. The patient should be supine. Muscle strength always should be graded according to maximum strength attained, regardless of the duration that level of strength was maintained during the examination. However, in the ED strength tends to be graded as normal, reduced, or absent. This may be a more appropriate initial description of a trauma patient's strength, with a more detailed exam being completed at a later time when the patient is stable enough to allow for a prolonged neurological exam:

5. Normal power
4. Moderate movement against resistance
3. Movement against gravity but not against resistance
2. Movement with gravity eliminated

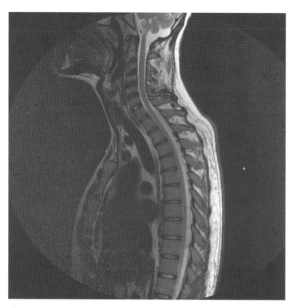

Figure 11.6 Magnetic resonance imaging (MRI) of the spine.

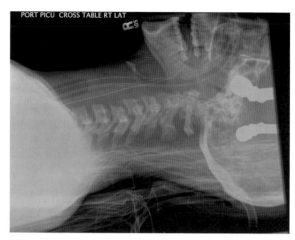

Figure 11.7 Cross-table lateral plain radiograph of the cervical spine.

1. Flicker of movement

0. No movement

4. While checking strength, quickly check **gross sensation** in hands and feet using light touch. If the patient is unable to feel anything distally, continue checking sensation while moving proximally towards the trunk. The goal is to identify the lowest level of sensation using the dermatomal scale (see ASIA Impairment Scale, Table 11.2.). Any toe movement defines the injury as incomplete.

5. Spinal *reflexes* should also be assessed. Again, quickly check the biceps/patellar reflexes bilaterally and assess for the presence of a Babinski sign bilaterally.

6. *Digital rectal exam* is performed to evaluate for rectal tone, perianal sensation, voluntary rectal contraction, and the bulbocavernosus reflex (BCR). The BCR can be done one of two ways – insert a finger into the anus and tug on the penis/foley or squeeze the glans. Anal sphincter contraction equals an intact BCR. The first three assess for sacral sparing, the BCR assesses for spinal shock.[28]

Trauma room studies based on severity

If the patient is stable enough, a spinal CT is the next appropriate study.[29] Although this is a general

Box 11.3 Summary of early ED evaluation and management for SCI

Acute interventions	1. Stabilize ABCs
	2. Find and treat life-threatening injuries
	3. Oxygen
	4. Avoid hypotension (intravenous fluid/blood/pressors)
	5. Stop hemorrhage
	6. Maintain spinal immobilization
Most important evaluation in the first 10 minutes	1. Assess and stabilize the ABCs
	2. Assess lowest level of sensation/movement

recommendation and clearly supported by the literature that spinal CT is much more sensitive, in reality, this is not always practical. In addition, there has been no definitive risk assessment of the increased sensitivity of CT compared with the increased radiation risks. Many institutions use some hybrid protocol where a lower risk patient will receive plain radiographs and a higher risk one will receive a CT. If the patient has spinal fractures or persistent neurological symptoms, an MRI of the spine is indicated. Magnetic resonance imaging provides the best visualization of the soft tissues, spinal cord, and

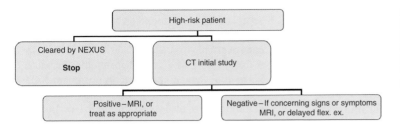

Figure 11.8 Radiologic evaluation of high-risk* patient. CT, computed tomography; flex. ex., flexion–extension; MRI, magnetic resonance imaging; NEXUS, National Emergency X-Radiography Utilization Study. *High risk: severe pain; elderly, significant mechanism; any signs or symptoms.

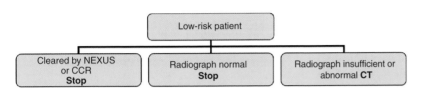

Figure 11.9 Radiologic evaluation of low-risk* patient. CCR, Canadian Cervical Spine Rule; CT, computed tomography; NEXUS, National Emergency X-Radiography Utilization Study. *Low risk: low mechanism; minimal findings; non-elderly.

spinous ligaments (Figure 11.6)[28,30,31]. At this time, MRI cannot predict neurological status at 6 weeks in cases of cord hemorrhage, edema, and contusion.[32] If a patient is very unstable, check a cross-table lateral cervical spine X-ray (Figure 11.7). It will provide basic information about the cervical spine. None of these diagnostic studies are therapeutic (Figures 11.8–11.10).

Treatment

The unfortunate reality is that there are few acute treatment options for SCI patients. Most SCI will be treated with supportive care and either surgery or watchful waiting, however it rarely changes the outcome. The following will discuss the management of the patient with acute SCI.

Medical

There are no pharmaceutical therapies at present that have been shown to convincingly improve the long-term outcome in SCI. Medical therapy's goal is to decrease/eliminate the secondary injury that affects the spinal cord. Although the biochemical pathways leading to the secondary injury (ischemia, free radical, calcium efflux, lipid peroxidation, apoptosis) are better understood, effective treatments are still lacking. Medications studied have included opiate receptor blockers, calcium channel blockers, GM1 ganglioside blockers, NMDA-

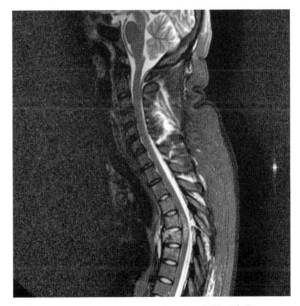

Figure 11.10 Magnetic resonance imaging (MRI) with T5 fracture.

receptor antagonists, growth factors, and glucocorticoids.[33–40]

Steroids

The treatment of spinal cord injury with corticosteroids remains controversial. To date, in the authors' opinion, there are no randomized, placebo-controlled trials that demonstrate significantly improved neurologic outcome in steroid-treated patients. Differing

175

interpretation of the current literature on steroids, as well as a lack of any other efficacious pharmacologic treatments, has fed the ongoing controversy.

The National Acute Spinal Cord Injury Studies (NASCIS I, II, and III)[41–43] were three large studies that looked at high-dose methylprednisolone in acute SCI. The original study showed no overall improvement in patient outcomes at 6 months or 1 year. However, looking deeper into the data of NASCIS II using post-hoc subgroup analysis, it appeared the group of patients treated within 8 hours of injury had a very small but statistically significant difference in motor function. These patients were only partially paralyzed and it is possible they would have improved without steroid therapy. The subsequent NASCIS III assumed the 8-hour subgroup was the important variable and subsequently tested different doses of methylprednisolone vs. other medications given within this 8-hour window. This conclusion from the post-hoc analysis has been questioned for its statistical validity.

A Cochrane review of corticosteroids for acute spinal cord injury in 2003 looked at eight trials (including NASCIS). None of these demonstrated any difference in motor scores at 6 weeks, 6 months, or 1 year.[44] Other authors note similar findings.[45,46] There are no studies subsequently that contradict these findings. At best, there is only weak support in the literature for the use of steroids. Furthermore, there appears to be a higher rate of severe pneumonia and sepsis in the steroid-treated groups, as well as higher frequency of arrhythmias, congestive heart failure, thromboembolism, and gastrointestinal bleeding.[47,48] Finally, the treatment has never been submitted for approval by the US Food and Drug Administration (FDA), and remains an off-label treatment. At this time, use remains variable and often institution-specific. The risk–benefit ratio should be weighed carefully when considering this treatment.

Box 11.4 Steriods in spinal trauma

- The treatment of spinal cord injury with corticosteroids remains controversial.
- No randomized, placebo-controlled trials demonstrate *significantly* improved neurologic outcome in steroid-treated patients.
- NASCIS i, ii, and iii were three large studies that looked at high-dose methylprednisolone in acute SCI.

- Some benefit was found in NASCIS II, but the findings remain questionable and highly controversial.
- A Cochrane review of corticosteroids for acute SCI in 2003 looked at eight trials (including NASCIS). None of these demonstrated any difference in motor scores at 6 weeks, 6 months, or 1 year.
- Severe pneumonia and sepsis in the steroid-treated groups appears greater, as well as higher frequency of arrhythmias, congestive heart failure, thromboembolism, and gastrointestinal bleeding.
- The risk–benefit ratio should be weighed carefully in considering this treatment.
- The authors of this chapter do not support its use.

Blood pressure control

Few major interventions are effective in the ED. One is blood pressure control. A mean arterial blood pressure of > 90 mmHg should be maintained to provide optimal circulation to the spinal cord.[17,49,50] Multiple animal studies have shown that hypotension worsens neurologic outcome and increases the secondary injury to the cord. Patients should be volume resuscitated first (with crystalloid and/or blood), then started on pressors (dopamine or phenylephrine) for fluid resistant hypotension and presumed neurogenic shock. Be cognizant of overaggressive fluid resuscitation.[51]

Oxygenation

Maintaining adequate oxygenation is also essential. Whereas adequate volume ensures perfusion of the spinal cord, sufficient oxygen levels are required for the spinal neurons' high metabolic needs. Maintain an oxygen saturation as close as possible to 100%.[50,51]

Surgical

Most patients with cord injuries will either undergo acute decompressive surgery or watchful waiting with repeated spinal imaging. There is no consensus in the literature regarding the optimal timing of surgical repair/decompression of spinal injuries. The general approach is to repair the bony lesion as soon as feasible. In studies where early decompression is considered < 3 days, late decompression > 5 days, generally no difference is found in the long-term neurological outcome, although there is some literature which supports early decompression (< 3 days).[52–54]

Concern exists regarding the "second hit" phenomenon: the theory postulates that the spinal cord suffers further ischemic damage when patients have early surgical repair, further worsening neurological outcome. In one study, a subset of five SCI patients with cervical lesions and early surgical repair, found that these patients had a worse neurological outcome than those who were repaired at a later time.[55]

Cervical traction in the ED is rarely done, but is an option for the patient with a cervical facet dislocation or fracture/dislocation causing severe cervical cord compression.[19,26,56] This is usually performed in conjunction with a spinal surgeon. The goal is the rapid reversal of the cord compression, which is done to restore anatomic alignment and ideally some neurologic function. Failure of closed reduction to restore alignment may be due to concurrent disc herniation.[57–60] Some studies recommend ventral decompression (surgery) before reduction if a significant disc herniation exists.[61]

If the patient has spinal column injury with worsening neurological deficits, the patient may require emergent operative decompression and stabilization. Urgent surgery should also be done for epidural lesions (hematoma) and cauda equina syndrome to decompress the spinal cord.[62,63]

Consultations

A patient with SCI will require consultations from a neurosurgeon, orthopedic surgeon, or both. Patients with SCI frequently require a trauma surgeon as most patients have other serious injuries in addition to SCI. The neurosurgeon/orthopedic surgeon will decide on the need for and timing of spinal surgery.

When to transfer for acute SCI

The indications for transfer are:

1. No trauma surgeon, orthopedic surgeon, or neurosurgeon available.
2. No CT or MRI scanner available.
3. A regional SCI center is within a reasonable transport time and the patient is stable for transfer (outcome has been found to be better for SCI patients at SCI centers).[64]

When to admit

Admit all patients with an acute SCI. The patient generally requires admission to an intensive care unit setting.

When to send home

If the patient has no documented spinal cord contusion, it is safe to discharge the patient to home. Symptoms such as subjective sensory complaints without objective sensory or motor signs on physical exam, are often temporary and resolve on their own over time. Although if there is doubt, the patient should be admitted for observation and further evaluation.

Prognosis

Providing an accurate prognosis for the patient with an acute SCI takes days and multiple imaging modalities. Rarely is this possible in the ED and should be avoided. Prognosis varies, depending on the exact injury to the spinal cord. Patients with a complete SCI currently have no chance of neurologic recovery. Spinal cord injured patients over the age of 50 have a dramatically higher mortality, especially if they are tetraplegic. In one paper, 90% of tetraplegic patients aged 1–24 years ($n = 1242$) lived for at least an additional 12 years, whereas only 27% of tetraplegic patients aged 50 years or older ($n = 187$) survived 12 years.[65] The prognosis is much better for the incomplete cord syndromes.

Complications

Patients with SCI are at risk for complications. Short-term complications include:[65–68]

1. Decubitus ulcers
2. Worsening of neurological symptoms
3. Aspiration/pneumonia/respiratory insufficiency
4. Other infections
5. Deep venous thrombosis/pulmonary embolism
6. Gastrointestinal hemorrhage
7. Depression.

Long-term complications include:[65,68]

1. Urinary tract infections
2. Pneumonia
3. Decubitus ulcers
4. Autonomic dysreflexia
5. Spasticity
6. Sepsis
7. Cardiac disease
8. Heterotopic ossification.

Medicolegal points

In one study of 20 cervical spine injury malpractice cases from 1987 to 2002, the types of errors were mixed and fairly evenly distributed. They were defined as Type I errors (inadequate or improper tests ordered), Type II errors (misreading or misinterpreting an appropriate test), and Type III (relying on a test insensitive to detect the injury). Those in which the jury found for the defendant were all Type I and III errors. Cases decided in favor of the plaintiff were a mix of Types I, II, and III errors.[69]

Basic areas to concentrate on from a risk management perspective are:

1. Diagnosis – perform a careful and well-documented neurological examination.
2. Proper spinal immobilization when SCI could be present – consider chemical and physical restraints as needed.
3. Consider neurogenic shock in the proper clinical picture.
4. Correct interpretation of imaging studies – this was the reason for the error in 10/12 malpractice cases found for the plaintiff.[69]

Documentation

Clearly document initial and serial neurological exams, noting the time of examination, lowest level of sensation, and movement. Medical decision making should also be documented.

Spinal shock and neurogenic shock

Confusion exists as to whether spinal shock and neurogenic shock are the same or different entities. Several papers define spinal shock as distinct from neurogenic shock. We suggest that they should remain separate for clarity's sake. Patients would be better served by defining the two terms separately, allowing for a more precise description of the degree of illness.[26] The term spinal shock refers solely to the loss of reflexes and muscle tone whereas neurogenic shock is defined as SCI with bradycardia and hypotension secondary to loss of sympathetic tone. It is useful to note that spinal shock does not denote any hemodynamic collapse.[26,55,70]

Spinal shock is only seen in complete cord injury and tends to occur more commonly in injuries above T6. Spinal shock is a state of transient physiological (rather than anatomical) reflex depression of cord function below the level of injury with associated loss of all sensorimotor functions. Flaccid paralysis, with bowel incontinence and urinary retention, is observed, and sometimes accompanied by sustained priapism. These symptoms tend to last several hours to days, rarely weeks, until the reflex arcs below the level of the injury begin to function again (e.g., BCR, muscle stretch reflex). Studies vary as to which physical finding is best to follow progress of spinal shock, but return of the BCR is considered a consistent exam finding signaling the resolution of spinal shock. Muscle tone and deep tendon reflexes (DTRs) will then follow.[70] Treatment is supportive.

Neurogenic shock implies a hemodynamically compromised patient.[26] Neurogenic shock is manifested by hypotension and bradycardia. Shock tends to occur more commonly in injuries above T6, secondary to the disruption of the sympathetic outflow and to unopposed parasympathetic tone. Loss of vascular tone leads to hypotension.[70] Rarely, atrioventricular block is present. Treatment of neurogenic shock is with fluid and vasopressors (e.g., norepinephrine or dopamine).[6,17]

Incomplete cord injuries

Many different types of incomplete cord syndromes exist. In incomplete injuries, the patient will have some preservation of sensory or motor function below the level of injury.

Central cord syndrome

This is the most common incomplete spinal cord syndrome, often seen in the elderly due to hyper-extension of the neck. One should suspect this in patients with spinal stenosis. As the vertebral column ages, degenerative changes occur (degenerative joint disease), leading to irregularities in the bony spine and hypertrophy of the ligamentum flavum. Hyperextension of the cervical spine pinches the cord between the hypertrophied arthritic surface of the anterior vertebral ridge and the thickened, bowing, posterior ligamentum flavum. Neurological symptoms (usually weakness) are most prominent in the upper extremities. Lower extremity symptoms tend to be more mild as compared to the upper extremities. The symptoms stem from damage within the central gray matter to the corticospinal and spinothalamic tracts. These range from weakness to paralysis. Sensory and bladder irregularities may be present. Sacral sparing will exist and the patient may have an associated spinal cord

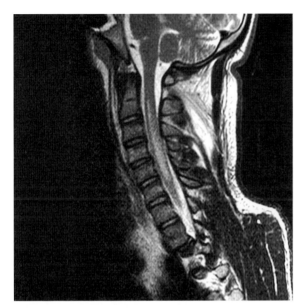

Figure 11.11 Central cord syndrome: cervical cord edema on magnetic resonance imaging (MRI). Sagittal, T2-weighted image. Spinal cord edema is present from C2–C7. This patient also has prevertebral hematoma (not well seen on this image) and C4 marrow edema secondary to vertebral fracture.

contusion.[17,18,71] See Figure 11.11 for MRI imaging of spinal cord edema. The prognosis depends in part on the patient's age at injury: if < 50 years, most retain bladder continence and the ability to walk; if > 50 years, a much smaller percentage regain bladder function and an ambulatory status.[72]

Brown-Séquard syndrome

In Brown-Séquard syndrome, hemisection of the cord occurs, from either penetrating trauma or lateral mass fractures of the cervical spine.[73] Blunt trauma is a very infrequent cause.[74] Neurological exam will reveal ipsilateral motor paralysis and proprioceptive loss with contralateral sensory deficit (pain and temperature). Bladder and bowel function remains intact, and the sacrum is spared.[17,18,71,75]

The prognosis of Brown-Séquard syndrome is the best of all incomplete cord syndromes. Most patients will have partial sensory and motor loss, but regain bowel and bladder continence, be able to walk, and to complete activities of daily living independently.[76]

Anterior cord syndrome

The mechanism of anterior cord syndrome is usually hyperflexion of the neck, commonly due to herniated discs or fragments of vertebral bone compressing the cord and/or anterior spinal artery. In addition, the spinal artery may be lacerated, or the aorta ruptured, leading to cord infarction from ischemia and subsequent anterior cord syndrome.[77] The intercostal arteries originate from the aorta, and terminate at the anterior spinal artery. Disruption of the aorta will halt or cause decreased blood flow to the anterior spinal artery. The gray matter has a higher metabolic rate and hence is more susceptible to ischemia.[78] Patients experience partial paralysis, decreased sensation (to light touch and pinprick), but maintain position, vibration, and touch sense.[17,18,71]

Most of the data regarding prognosis is from patients who suffered an ischemic insult to the cord. In a small study of five patients, three patients without lower extremity motor function at presentation all regained motor function at one year. Two with partial motor loss had improvement; one was able to walk independently at one year post-injury.[77] Another study showed motor improvement in two out of three patients with anterior spinal cord syndrome.[79] As these lesions may be operable, a neurosurgeon should be consulted as early as practical in the patient's course.

Posterior cord syndrome

Posterior cord syndrome is a very rare entity which involves the dorsal column. Patients will notice loss of proprioception and vibration. Strength is preserved. Many patients experience difficulty walking as a consequence of the loss of proprioception.[80]

Conus medullaris syndrome/cauda equina syndrome

Conus medullaris syndrome is associated with compression to the sacral cord (L1). Cauda equina syndrome is compression of the nerve roots at the terminus of the spinal cord.[17,18,71,80] Differentiating clinically between these two entities is not possible. The symptoms are the same: bladder and bowel overflow incontinence, lower limb weakness/paralysis, saddle anesthesia, and decreased or absent rectal tone. Sacral segments occasionally show preserved reflexes (e.g., BCR and ability to urinate voluntarily). Patients may also have unilateral or bilateral sciatica and back pain. Bilateral symptoms are more common with conus compression.[17,72,80] If the provider suspects cauda equina or conus syndrome, a lumbar MRI is indicated as it is the best way to see edema of the spinal cord.[81] A preliminary CT scan of the spine may be done, but the definitive study is MRI. If an MRI is not available at the treating facility, the patient should be transferred to a facility with an MRI.

The definitive treatment is surgical decompression of the cord/spinal nerves. While the standard teaching is to decompress the cord or nerve roots as soon as feasible, there is some research which shows that neither duration of symptoms nor early (within 6 hours) surgical intervention had any bearing on a patient's long-term bowel or bladder or sexual function.[82] The caregiver should consult a spine or neurosurgeon as soon as practical, as this is controversial, and the common practice is to perform early intervention.

Prognosis is generally good. Most patients do quite well after surgery, regaining most of their bladder or bowel function, sensation, and strength over weeks to months. However, in a small but significant percentage, urination, defecation, sexual function, motor, and sensation may still be altered enough to interfere with normal daily functions.[83,84]

Spinal cord injury without radiographic abnormality

Spinal cord injury without radiographic abnormality (SCIWORA) is defined as spinal cord deficit(s) in trauma patients with no observed bony abnormality on radiographs.[85] This entity has a higher incidence in children probably due to their anatomy and soft tissue pliability. In one study, up to 40% of children from birth to 17 years with varying ranges of traumatic myelopathy had SCIWORA.[86] The incidence of SCIWORA decreases with age as does the overall severity of the injury. Thoracic SCIWORA does not demonstrate a clearly age-related pattern, although it is usually related to a pedestrian being struck by a car.[86] Most recent research demonstrates that very few patients with neurological symptoms and negative cervical spine X-rays have negative spinal MRIs. In patients with spinal symptoms but normal radiographs, MRI of the spine often showed complete cord transection, cord contusion, hemorrhage, disc herniation, or cord edema.[87]

Although SCIWORA is felt to be more common in children, one large multicenter prospective observational study did not find any children with SCIWORA. Of the roughly 34 000 patients (from the National Emergency X-Radiography Utilization Study [NEXUS] trial data), 3000 patients were < 18 years old. Within the adult cohort, 27 (3%) of the 818 adults with cervical spine injury had SCIWORA, 0.08% overall.[88] The total pediatric population in this study may have been too small to derive any specific conclusions.

Causes of SCIWORA depend on a patient's age. In younger patients, pedestrian–motor vehicle collisions and falls predominate. Child abuse must also be considered. In older children, the injury is most often due to motor vehicle collisions or highly physical activities, such as gymnastics, diving, downhill skiing, and equestrianism.[86]

The mechanisms of injury include flexion, hyperextension, or longitudinal distraction with resultant spinal cord ischemia.[85] Children are felt to be at increased risk for this syndrome because of their inherent vertebral column elasticity and other age-related anatomical vertebral characteristics. One study of neonatal cadavers found that the spinal column stretched up to 2 inches without discernable damage whereas the spinal cord ruptured at a one quarter inch of elongation.[89] The juvenile vertebral column is extremely pliable, rendering it less prone to breakage but more likely to suffer ligamentous rupture. By 9 years of age, the spine is more like that of an adult: less deformable and at higher risk for bony fracture.

Children with upper cervical SCIWORA are more likely to have worse neurological injuries than children with lower cervical lesions. Neurological lesions in children under 9 years of age were generally more severe than those found in children of 9 years of age or older.[90]

Prehospital interventions include complete spinal immobilization, comforting the child, and rapid transport to the nearest appropriate treating facility. Spinal immobilization should include cervical collar and backboard, with care taken to minimize the movement of the child. In very young children the occiput is large enough to cause flexion of the neck when the child is supine on a backboard. Towels or blankets should be placed under the child's shoulders, torso, and hips to maintain the neck in a neutral position. Towels or blankets placed on either side of the head and secured with tape will maintain in-line cervical stabilization if the child is too small for a cervical collar.

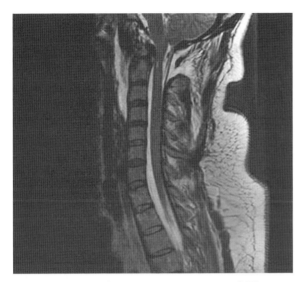

Figure 11.12 Cervical magnetic resonance imaging (MRI) showing prevertebral edema.

Presentations of SCIWORA can range from the very subtle to the overtly obvious. Symptoms may be transient, rendering the patient asymptomatic by the time they reach the ED. During the initial evaluation, the diagnosis may be missed, especially if more severe injuries exist.[86]

In children, there are several approaches to radiologic evaluation. While some physicians would recommend plain films initially, if the ultimate plan is to obtain a head CT, it makes sense to do a spinal CT at the same time. In order to decrease radiation, another option is to obtain plain films first and, if negative, follow with MRI in the symptomatic patient. If fractures are seen, CT is generally recommended. Data on adults supports omitting the full cervical spine X-ray series and going directly to cervical spine CT as the initial imaging modality.[91–95] Thin section axial scan with bone algorithms, including coronal and sagittal reconstructions should be done to identify occult fractures. The next step in patients with no radiologic findings but persistent spinal symptoms is to get the MRI of the spine as soon as possible. Transient symptoms with complete resolution in adults are unlikely to show clinically significant abnormalities (Figure 11.12).[86]

If the plain radiographs, CT, and MRI are all negative, it would be unlikely that an acute injury exists. The NEXUS subgroup analysis found that the flexion extension radiographs in the acute situations provided essentially no real change in management of patients with cervical spine injuries.[86] While a minimal percentage had new findings on this examination, they all had other significant injuries already known.[89] While new CT studies suggest that multidetector CT alone is good enough to clear the cervical spine, other studies found that there still is a small number of ligamentous injuries not diagnosed on CT.[96] These missed injuries are in unreliable patients (Glasgow Coma Scale score < 15).[96] If the CT is negative and MRI is not available in the patient with severe pain or minor neurologic finding, outpatient MRI is an option. The patient should be kept in a cervical collar such as a Philadelphia or Aspen collar until the studies can be completed. A neurology consult and possibly neurosurgical or orthopedics consult should be considered with objective findings or symptoms.

Finally, somatosensory evoked potentials (SSEPs) may be performed later in the course, but not as a part of the ED workup. These help separate SCI from head injury and brachial plexus injury, especially if the patient is unconscious.

Treatment of patients with SCIWORA may include spinal immobilization, neurosurgical intervention, steroids, supportive care, and treatment of concomitant injuries. Spinal immobilization should be maintained with a rigid collar, such as an Aspen or Philadelphia collar. The decision to implement steroid therapy should be made only after a complete discussion with the parent(s) or guardian(s) of the child, clearly explaining the risk–benefit profile and the lack of data in children. If used, current steroid therapy guidelines are intravenous methylprednisolone, 30 mg/kg over 15 minutes followed by 5.4 mg/kg per hour for the next 23 hours. Further, steroid treatment should be initiated within 8 hours of the injury.[86]

If one is unsure about an injury, it is prudent to admit the child for observation, repeated studies, and serial exams.

Cervical root syndrome

The deficit in cervical root syndrome results from an isolated nerve root impingement typically from acute disk herniation or a dislocated facet joint. Consequently, patients will have ipsilateral sensory and lower motor neuron deficits. Diagnosis is made with electromyography (EMG) and MRI. Treatment includes facet injection and surgery.[80]

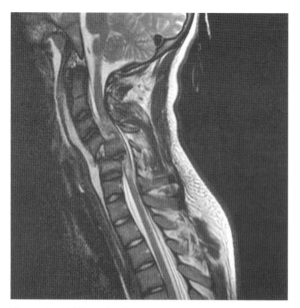

Figure 11.13 T2-weighted magnetic resonance imaging (MRI) image of C4–C5 complete cord transection. C3–C5 subluxation with anterolisthesis of C4 and C5 and concurrent retrolisthesis of C5 on C6. An epidural hematoma is visible, along with prevertebral and posterior paraspinous soft tissue hematoma/edema.

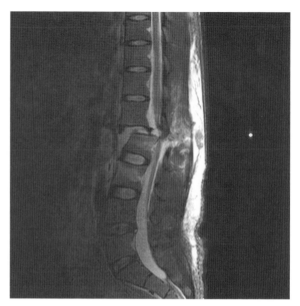

Figure 11.14 Magnetic resonance imaging (MRI) (stir image) of L1–L2 dislocation and cord compression with edema of hematoma within paraspinous tissues.

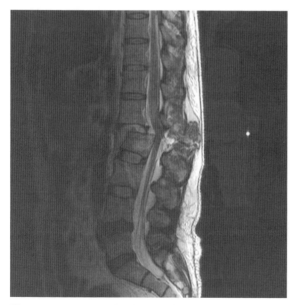

Figure 11.15 A T2-weighted image of the same patient in Figure 11.14.

Complete cord injury

Patients with complete cord injury experience a complete absence of sensory and motor functions from the level of injury caudad, from one of four causes:

1. Compression
2. Hemorrhage
3. Infarction
4. Transection.

Trauma is the most common reason for a person to incur a complete SCI.

The presentation of such an injury can vary. Reflexes may still be present as the DTR circuit is still intact, not requiring ascension in the spinal cord. Priapism and hypotension may exist. No sacral sparing will be present. Prognosis is very poor if symptoms of complete spinal cord syndrome persists past 24 hours; fewer than 5% of these patients will have a functional recovery. At 48 hours, virtually no chance of recovery exists (Figures 11.13–11.15 and Table 11.3).[17,80,97]

Penetrating injury to spine

Spinal stability is based upon the well-accepted three-column theory. The bony spine is separated into three columns: anterior, middle, and posterior columns (Table 11.4). Each is composed of bony and ligamentous structures. To create an unstable spine, one of two things must happen: either disruption of all columns or the anterior and middle columns.

Following this logic, a penetrating injury must traverse the spinal cord and break at least two columns to create an unstable spine fracture. A patient

Table 11.3 Spinal cord syndromes

Name	Usual cause	Neurologic deficit
Central cord syndrome	Hyperextension	Upper extremity weakness > lower extremity
		Distal > proximal
Brown-Séquard syndrome	Traumatic hemisection	Ipsilateral motor paralysis and proprioceptive loss.
		Contralateral pain and temperature decreased
Anterior cord syndrome	Hyperflexion	Partial paralysis
		Decreased pin and light touch sensation
Conus medullaris/cauda equina syndrome	Compression of distal spinal cord/cauda equina by masses/intervertebral disc	Saddle anesthesia
		Overflow incontinence of bladder and bowels
		Back pain
		Decreased or absent rectal tone
		Lower extremity weakness
Complete cord syndrome	Trauma	Complete loss of motor and sensation below level of lesion
		No rectal tone present.

Table 11.4 Three columns of the spine

Column	Contents
Anterior	Anterior longitudinal ligament and the anterior part of the vertebral body
Middle	Posterior part of the vertebral body and the posterior longitudinal ligament
Posterior	The bony and ligamentous structures posterior to the posterior longitudinal ligament

sustaining such a significant injury should have at minimum bony spine pain and tenderness, but more likely neurological signs and symptoms ranging from sensory changes to loss of motor function. Conversely, the lack of these symptoms should be able to rule out an unstable injury.[98–101] One study noted that three patients who sustained gunshot wounds to the face were found to have cervical spine fractures, despite presenting as alert and oriented without pain or neurological signs on physical exam.[101] However, none of these fractures required surgical repair. A single study noted patients presenting neurologically intact and asymptomatic after gunshot wounds to the spine, and were subsequently found to have bony spine injuries. Unfortunately, the study was a retrospective chart review, and one cannot ascertain what the true initial clinical presentation was for those patients.[102]

To date, there are no reports of unstable fractures occurring in the alert asymptomatic patients. An exceptionally cautious approach would be to CT all these patients, although this is not supported by any data. Negative plain films without bony injury are probably sufficient. Patients with neurological signs require CT of the spine in the region of concern, and may require MRI for assessment of ligamentous and spinal injury. Of note, while the data is limited, it appears that it is safe to perform MRI on patients with bullet fragments in the spine.[103]

Peripheral nerve injuries
Traumatic brachial plexus injury

The true incidence of traumatic brachial plexus injury (TBPI) is difficult to measure. However, it is likely increasing with the rising popularity of high velocity sports.[104] Traumatic brachial plexus injury occurs most commonly in males in their late teens to mid-twenties. Closed injury occurs more frequently than open. Motor vehicle crashes are the most common cause of TBPI; other causes include falls, bicycle/motorcycle crashes, gunshots/stabbings, or industrial accidents.[104–106]

The anatomy of the brachial plexus consists of combinations of nerves originating from C5–T1. Trauma can occur anywhere along the plexus and is divided into supraclavicular or infraclavicular injury.

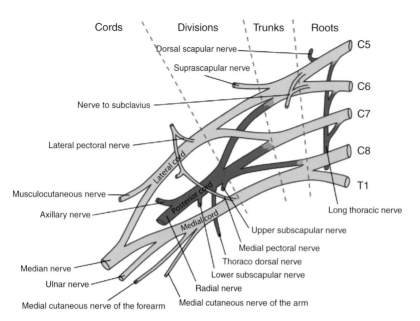

Figure 11.16 Anterior view of right brachial plexus.

The brachial plexus is organized into five zones/elements (Figure 11.16):[16]

1. Roots
2. Anterior branches of spinal nerves
3. Trunks
4. Cords
5. Terminal peripheral nerves.

Patients with brachial plexus injuries generally have other serious injuries and TBPI can easily be overlooked. Considerable traction on the upper extremity or neck is required to cause closed injury. Traumatic brachial plexus injury is associated with clavicular, shoulder, and first and second rib fractures.[107] Other physical findings which can signal TBPI include Horner syndrome, enophthalmos (if the avulsion is of ipsilateral preganglionic of T1), or winging of the scapula (injury to the long thoracic nerve or preganglionic C6 avulsion) (Table 11.5).[104,105]

Traumatic injury to the plexus may be induced by stretch/contusion, traction, compression (hematoma), or penetration. Supraclavicular injuries usually occur when a large amount of traction is applied to the head or ipsilateral shoulder, forcing them in opposite directions. Stretch/contusion injuries also tend to damage the plexus in the supraclavicular region, with the most rostral branches being affected first.[106] Infraclavicular injuries tend to result from extreme arm abduction (Figures 11.17 and 11.18).[104,108]

Patients can present with a wide range of symptoms, ranging from isolated neurological upper extremity complaints to "flail arm": complete paresis of the upper extremity.[107] Horner syndrome may be present as the sympathetic output to the head may be disrupted if the T1 root is avulsed. Diaphragmatic palsy, rhomboid, and serratus anterior weakness/palsy

Table 11.5 Physical exam findings in traumatic brachial plexus injury

Physical exam	Nerve
Elbow flexion/extension	Musculocutaneous N, Radial N
Shoulder abduction	Axillary N
Deltoid function	Posterior cord
Latissimus dorsi function	Thoracodorsal N
Pectoralis major and minor (have patient abduct against resistance)	Medial and lateral cords
Rotator cuff evaluation	Can mimic brachial plexus injury
Cranial nerve exam	CNIX – spinal accessory nerve, can be coinjured with brachial plexus
Sensory exam	Depends on location of findings
Tinel's sign/percussion of injured nerve	Acute pain with percussion of nerve suggests rupture

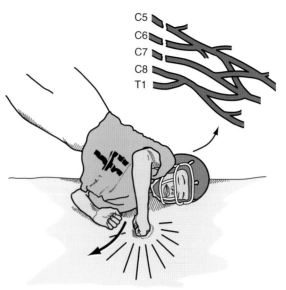

Figure 11.18 Stretch injury to superior elements of the brachial plexus (C5–C7).

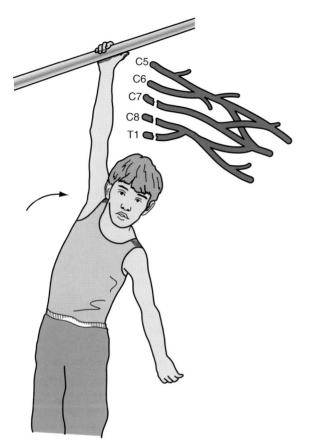

Figure 11.17 Traction injury to inferior elements of the brachial plexus (C7–T1).

suggest TBPI.[109] Be alert to other injuries, as these patients usually suffer polytrauma. Studies found the following major injuries associated with TBPI:[105,109]

1. Long bone fractures
2. Spinal fractures
3. Head injuries
4. Chest injuries
5. Axillary artery injury
6. Shoulder girdle injuries.

Imaging should be based on mechanism and other potential injuries. In regards to the brachial plexus injury, acute radiography is rarely helpful. The major concern is the presence of arterial injury. Arterial pressure indices should be completed first. In the arm, this is known as the Brachial–Brachial Index (BBI). In one study of 100 traumatized limbs (including upper and lower extremities), Arterial Pressure Index (API) had a sensitivity and specificity of 95% and 97%, respectively, for detecting significantly occult arterial damage. An abnormal API was a ratio of < 0.90. Of the 100 limbs, 17 had an API of < 0.90. Subsequently, 16 of those limbs had positive arteriograms.[110] There is limited research available, but what there is supports arterial angiography if there is a $> 10\%$ difference in forearm systolic blood pressure or in whom the ABI is < 0.90.[111]

Angiography of the axillary artery should also be considered as axillary arterial injury happens frequently with TBPI, roughly 20%. One study found 10 of 54 patients with TBPI had associated subclavian or axillary artery/vein injuries.[105] Another identified 13 of 58 patients with TBPI who had concurrent pseudoaneurysms or arteriovenous fistula.[112] A third study noted 17 of 100 patients with either a vascular tear or thrombosis, although the authors did not specify whether these were in patients with open, penetrating, or closed TBPI.[109] A CT angiogram or angiography should be performed. Eventually, the patient with TBPI will require CT myelography of the cervical spine to evaluate the extent of the injury, but again, this is not urgent and can wait weeks to months after the injury.[113,114] Magnetic resonance imaging of the brachial plexus shows promise as the technology evolves, but as yet does not have the sensitivity or specificity of CT myelography.[115,116]

Treatment is either urgent, if the injury is open or involves the artery, or delayed, with initial observation and physical therapy in all others.

185

Patients with open TBPI secondary to gunshot injuries appear to do well with conservative management as the nerves are rarely transected. Injury to the plexus is more often due to contusion or stretch injuries of the plexus.[117] In one study of 118 patients with TPBIs secondary to gunshot wounds, 40% resolved spontaneously and did not require surgery.[117] Surgery in most cases is delayed on the order of months. Patients with supraclavicular injuries tend to be better surgical candidates.[109,112,118]

Prognosis depends on what level of the plexus is injured (C5–T1), what type of injury occurred within the plexus (stretch vs. laceration), and where the injury occurred (supraclavicular vs. infraclavicular). Patients with injuries to more rostral elements of the plexus (especially C5–C6) have a better prognosis as the hand is neurologically intact and there appears to be a higher success rate with surgical repair of this zone.[106,109] Long-term neural prognosis of the arm/hand function is worse in patients with avulsion of the entire plexus. Open injuries have better outcomes than closed injuries.[109] Patients may also develop chronic pain syndromes.

Conclusion

Spinal cord injuries are common and devastating. While often the injuries do not benefit from acute management, correcting hypotension and hypoxia as well as managing the entire patient well may affect outcome.

References

1. Harvey C, Wilson SE, Greene CG, et al. New estimates of the direct costs of traumatic spinal cord injuries: results of a nationwide survey. *Paraplegia* 1992;**30**(12):834–50.

2. Sekhon LHS, Fehlings MG. Epidemiology, demographics, and pathophysiology of acute spinal cord injury. *Spine* 2001;**26**(suppl.):S2–12.

3. The National Spinal Cord Injury Statistical Center. Spinal cord injury. Facts and figures at a glance. *Spine* 2005;**28**(4):379–80. Also see: http://www.spinalcord.uab.edu, "Facts and Figures." June 4, 2008.

4. Berkowitz M, Harvey C, Greene CG, Wilson SE. *The Economic Consequences of Traumatic Spinal Cord Injury*. New York: Demos Publications, 1993.

5. Lowery DW, Wald MM, Browne BJ, et al. Epidemiology of cervical spine injury victims. *Ann Emerg Med* 2001;**38**(1):12–16.

6. Botterell EH, Jousse AT, Kraus AS, et al. A model for the future care of acute spinal cord injuires. *Can J Neurol Sci* 1975;**2**:361–80.

7. Kraus JF, Silberman TA, McArthur DL. Epidemiology of spinal cord injury. In Benzel ED, Cahill DW, McCormack P (eds.), *Principles of Spine Surgery*. New York: McGraw-Hill, 1996: pp. 41–58.

8. Tator CH, Ekong CEU, Rowed DW, et al. Changes in epidemiology of acute spinal cord injury from 1947 to 1981. *Surg Neurol* 1993;**40**:207–15.

9. Pickett GE, Campos-Benitez M, Keller JL, Duggal N. Epidemiology of traumatic spinal cord injury in Canada. *Spine* 2006;**31**(7):799–805.

10. Albin MS, White RJ. Epidemiology, physiopathology, and experimental therapeutics of acute spinal cord injury. *Crit Care Clin* 1987;**3**:441–52.

11. Carter RE, Jr. Etiology of traumatic spinal cord injury: statistics of more than 1100 cases. *Tex Med* 1977;**73**:61–5.

12. Kraus JF. Epidemiologic features of head and spinal cord injury. *Adv Neurol* 1978;**19**:261–79.

13. Holmes JF, Miller PQ, Panacek EA, et al. Epidemiology of thoracolumbar spine injury in blunt trauma. *Acad Emerg Med* 2001;**8**(9):866–72.

14. Fisher CG, Noonan VK, Dvorak MF. Changing face of spine trauma care in North America. *Spine* 2006;**31**(11 suppl.):S2–8.

15. Sansam KAJ. Controversies in the management of traumatic spinal cord injury. *Clin Med* 2006;**6**(2):202–4.

16. Moore KL, Dalley AF (eds.). Back. *Clinically Oriented Anatomy*, 4th edn. Baltimore: Lippincott, Williams, and Williams, 1999: pp. 431–502.

17. Wagner R, Jagoda A. Spinal cord syndromes. *Emerg Med Clin N Amer* 1997;**15**(3):699–711.

18. Maroon JC, Abla AA. Classification of acute spinal cord injury, neurological evaluation, and neurosurgical considerations. *Crit Care Clin* 1987;**3**(3):655–77.

19. Meyer PR, Cybulski GR, Rusin JJ, Haak MH. Spinal cord injury. *Neurol Clin* 1991;**9**(3):625–61.

20. American Spinal Injury Association. *Dermatome Map*. Available from http://www.asia-spinalinjury.org.

21. Luer MS, Rhoney DH, Hughes M, et al. New pharmacologic strategies for acute neuronal injury. *Pharmacotherapy* 1996;**16**(5):830–48.

22. Takeda H, Caiozzo VJ, Gardner VO. A functional *in vitro* model for studying the cellular and molecular basis of spinal cord injury. *Spine* 1993;**18**(9):1125–33.

23. Anderson DK, Hall ED. Pathophysiology of spinal cord trauma. *Ann Emerg Med* 1993;**22**:987–92.

24. Tator CH, Fehlings MG. Review of the secondary injury theory of acute spinal cord trauma with emphasis on vascular mechanisms. *J Neurosurg* 1991;**75**:15–26.

25. Green BA, Eismont FJ. Spinal cord injury – a systems approach: prevention, emergency medical services, and emergency room management. *Crit Care Clin* 1987;**3**(3):471–93.

26. Atkinson PP, Atkinson JL. Spinal shock. *Mayo Clin Proc* 1996;**71**:384–9.

27. Savitsky E, Votey S. Emergency department approach to acute thoracolumbar spine injury. *J Emerg Med* 1997;**15**(1):49–60.

28. Kirshblum SC, O'Connor KC. Predicting neurologic recovery in traumatic cervical spinal cord injury. *Arch Phys Med Rehabil* 1998;**79**:1456–66.

29. Brown CVR, Antevil JL, Sise MJ, et al. Spiral computed tomography for the diagnosis of cervical, thoracic, and lumbar spine fractures: its time has come. *J Trauma* 2005;**58**(5):890–6.

30. Slucky AV, Potter HG. Use of magnetic resonance imaging in spinal trauma: indications, techniques, and utility. *J Am Acad Orthop Surg* 1998;**6**(3):134–45.

31. Paleologos TS, Fratzoglou MM, Papadopoulos SS, et al. Posttraumatic spinal cord lesions without skeletal or discal and ligamentous abnormalities: the role of MR imaging. *J Spinal Disord* 1998;**11**(4):346–9.

32. Shepard MJ, Bracken MB. Magnetic resonance imaging and neurological recovery in acute spinal cord injury: observations from the National Acute Spinal Cord Injury Study 3. *Spinal Cord* 1999;**37**:833–7.

33. Takeda H, Caiozzo VJ, Gardner VO. A functional *in vitro* model for studying the cellular and molecular basis of spinal cord injury. *Spine* 1993;**18**(9):1125–33.

34. Anderson DK, Hall ED. Pathophysiology of spinal cord trauma. *Ann Emerg Med* 1993;**22**(6):987–92.

35. Tator CH, Fehlings MG. Review of the secondary injury theory of acute spinal cord trauma with emphasis on vascular mechanisms. *J Neurosurg* 1991;**75**:15–26.

36. Bracken MB, Shepard MJ, Collins WF, et al. A randomized, controlled trial of methylprednisolone or naloxone in the treatment of acute spinal-cord injury. *N Engl J Med* 1990;**322**(20):1405–11.

37. Liu D, Thnagnipon W, McAdoo DJ. Excitatory amino acids rise to toxic levels upon impact injury to the rat spinal cord. *Brain Res* 1991;**547**:344–8.

38. Haghighi SS, Chehrazi B. Effect of naloxone in experimental acute spinal cord injury. *Neurosurg* 1987;**20**:385–8.

39. Hall ED. The role of oxygen radicals in traumatic injury: clinical implications. *J Emerg Med* 1993;**11**:31–6.

40. Young W. Secondary injury mechanisms in acute spinal cord injury. *J Emerg Med* 1993;**11**:13–22.

41. Bracken MB, Collins WF, Freeman DF, et al. Efficacy of methylprednisolone in acute spinal cord injury. *JAMA* 1984; **251**:45–52.

42. Bracken MB, Shepard MJ, Collins WF, Jr., et al. Methylprednisolone or naloxone treatment after acute spinal cord injury: 1-year follow-up data. Results of the second National Acute Spinal Cord Injury Study. *J Neurosurg* 1992;**76**(1):23–31.

43. Bracken MB, Shepard MJ, Holford TR, et al. Administration of methylprednisolone for 24 or 48 hours or tirilazad mesylate for 48 hours in the treatment of acute spinal cord injury. Results of the Third National Acute Spinal Cord Injury Randomized Controlled Trial. National Acute Spinal Cord Injury Study. *JAMA* 1997;**277**(20):1597–604.

44. Spencer M. Are corticosteroids effective in traumatic spinal cord injury? *Annals of Emergency Medicine* 2003;**41**(3):410–13.

45. Hurlbert RJ. The role of steroids in acute spinal cord injury: an evidence-based analysis. *Spine* 2001;**26**(24 Suppl.):S39-46.

46. Coleman WP, Benzel D, Cahill DW, et al. A critical appraisal of the reporting of the National Acute Spinal Cord Injury Studies (II and III) of methylprednisolone in acute spinal cord injury. *J Spinal Disord* 2000;**13** (3):185–99.

47. Galandiuk S, Raque G, Appel S, et al. The two-edged sword of large-dose steroids for spinal cord trauma. *Ann Surg* 1993;**218**(4):419–25.

48. Short DJ, El Masry WS, Jones PW. High dose methylprednisolone in the management of acute spinal cord injury – a systematic review from a clinical perspective. *Spinal Cord* 2000;**38**(5):273–86.

49. Hadley MN. Blood pressure management after acute spinal cord injury. *Neurosurg* 2002;**50**(3 Suppl.):S58–62.

50. Hurlbert RJ. Strategies of medical intervention in the management of acute spinal cord injury. *Spine* 2006;**31** (11):S16–21.

51. Green BA, Eismont FJ. Spinal cord injury – a systems approach: prevention, emergency medical services, and emergency room management. *Crit Care Clin* 1987;**3** (3):471–93.

52. Fehlings MG, Perrin RG. The role and timing of early decompression for cervical spinal cord injury: update with a review of recent clinical evidence. *Injury* 2005;**36**:B13–26.

53. Mirza SK, Krengel WF, Chapman JR, et al. Early versus delayed surgery for acute cervical spinal cord injury. *Clin Ortho and Related Res* 1999;**359**:104–14.

54. Vaccaro AR, Daugherty RJ, Sheehan TP, et al. Neurologic outcome of early versus late surgery for cervical spinal cord injury. *Spine* 1997;**22**:2609–13.

55. Delamarter RB, Coyle J. Acute management of spinal cord injury. *J Amer Acad Ortho Surg* 1999;**7**(3):166–75.

56. Meyer PR, Cybulski GR, Rusin JJ, Haak MH. Spinal cord injury. *Neurol Clin* 1991;**9**(3):625–61.

57. Reindl R, Ouellet J, Harvey EJ, et al. Anterior reduction for cervical spine dislocation. *Spine* 2006;**31**(6):648–52.

58. Koivikko MP, Myllynen P, Santavirta S. Fracture dislocations of the cervical spine: a review of 106 conservatively and operatively treated patients. *Eur Spine J* 2004;**13**(7):610–16.

59. Cotler JM, Herbison GJ, Nasuti JF, et al. Closed reduction of traumatic cervical spine dislocation using traction weights up to 140 pounds. *Spine* 1993;**18**(3):386–90.

60. Star AM, Jones AA, Cotler JM, et al. Immediate closed reduction of cervical spine dislocations using traction. *Spine* 1990;**15**(10):1068–72.

61. American Association of Neurological Surgeons and the Congress of Neurological Surgeons. Initial closed reduction of cervical spine fracture–dislocation injuries. *Neurosurg* 2002;**50**(3 Suppl.):S44–50.

62. Ahn UM, Ahn NU, Buchowski JM, et al. Cauda equina syndrome secondary to lumbar disc herniation: a meta-analysis of surgical outcomes. *Spine* 2000;**25**(12):1515–22.

63. Liu WH, Hsieh CT, Chiang YH, Chen GJ. Spontaneous spinal epidural hematoma of thoracic spine: a rare case report and review of literature. *Am J Emerg Med* 2008;**26**(3):384.e1–2.

64. Heinemann AW, Yarkony GM, Roth EJ et al. Functional outcome following spinal cord injury. *Arch Neurol* 1989;**46**:1098–102.

65. DeVivo MJ, Stover SL, Black KJ. Prognostic factors for 12-year survival after spinal cord injury. *Arch Phys Med Rehabil* 1992;**73**:156–62.

66. VanBuren RL, Wagner FC. Respiratory complications after cervical spinal cord injury. *Spine* 1994;**19**(20):2315–20.

67. Matsumura JS, Prystowsky JB, Bresticker MA, et al. Gastrointestinal tract complications after acute spinal injury. *Arch Surg* 1995;**130**:751–3.

68. Ditunno JF, Formal CS. Chronic spinal cord injury. *N Engl J Med* 1994;**330**(8):550–6.

69. Lekovic GP, Harrington TR. Litigation of missed cervical spine injuries in patients presenting with blunt traumatic injury. *Neurosurg* 2007;**60**(3):516–23.

70. Ditunno JF, Little JW, Tessler A, Burns AS. Spinal shock revisited: a four-phase model. *Spinal Cord* 2004;**42**(7):383–95.

71. Harrop JS, Sharan A, Ratliff J. Central cord injury: pathophysiology, management, and outcomes. *Spine* 2006:**6**(6 Suppl.):198S–206S.

72. Dvorak MF, Fisher CG, Hoekema J, et al. Factors predicting motor recovery and functional outcome after traumatic central cord syndrome: a long-term follow-up. *Spine* 2005;**30**(20):2303–11.

73. Rumana CS, Baskin DS. Brown-Séquard syndrome produced by cervical disc herniation: case report and literature review. *Surg Neruol* 1996;**45**:359–61.

74. Henderson SO, Hoffner RJ. Brown-Séquard syndrome due to isolated blunt trauma. *J Emerg Med* 1998;**16**(6):847–50.

75. Koehler PJ, Lambertus JE. The Brown-Séquard syndrome. True or false? *Arch Neurol* 1986;**43**:921–4.

76. Roth EJ, Park T, Pang T, et al. Traumatic cervical Brown-Séquard and Brown-Séquard-plus syndromes: the spectrum of presentations and outcomes. *Paraplegia* 1991;**29**(9):582–9.

77. Waters RL, Sie I, Yakura J, et al. Recovery following ischemic myelopathy. *J Trauma* 1993;**35**:837–9.

78. Boggs JL, Waggener JD. The acute microvascular responses to spinal cord injury. *Adv Neurol* 1979;**22**:179.

79. Kim SW. The syndrome of acute anterior lumbar spinal cord injury. *Clin Neurol Neurosurg* 1990;**92**:249–53.

80. Lindsey RW, Gugala Z, Pneumaticos SG. Injury to the vertebrae and spinal cord. In Moore EE, Feliciano DV, Mattox KL (eds), *Trauma*, 5th edn. NewYork: McGraw-Hill, 2004: pp. 459–92.

81. Bell DA, Statham CD. Cauda equina syndrome – what is the correlation between clinical assessment and MRI scanning? *Br J Neurosurg* 2007;**21**(2):201–3.

82. McCarthy MJ, Aylott CE, Grevitt MP, Hegarty J. Cauda equina syndrome: factors affecting long-term functional and sphincteric outcome. *Spine* 2007;**32**(2):207–16.

83. Kostuik JP, Harrington I, Alexander D, et al. Cauda equina syndrome and lumbar disc herniation. *J Bone and Joint Surg* 1986;**68A**(3):386–91.

84. Delamarter RB, Sherman JE, Carr JB. Cauda equina syndrome: neurologic recovery following immediate, early, or late decompression. *Spine* 1991;**16**(9):1022–9.

85. Pang D, Wilberger JE, Jr. Spinal cord injury without radiographic abnormalities in children. *J Neurosurg* 1982;**57**(1):114–29.

86. Pang D. Spinal cord injury without radiographic abnormality in children, 2 decades later. *Neurosurgery* 2004;**55**(6):1325–42.

87. Nichols JS, Elger C, Hemminger L, et al. Magnetic resonance imaging: utilization in the management of central nervous system trauma. *J Trauma Inj Inf Crit Care* 1997;**42**(3):520–3.

88. Hendey GW, Wolfson AB, Mower WR. Spinal cord injury without radiographic abnormality: results of the

national emergency x-radiography utilization study in blunt cervical trauma. *J Trauma* 2002;**53**(1):1–4.

89. Leventhal HR. Birth injuries of the spinal cord. *J Pediatr* 1960;**56**:447–53.

90. Pang D, Pollack IF. Spinal cord injury without radiographic abnormality in children: the SCIWORA syndrome. *J Trauma* 1989;**29**:654–64.

91. Antevil JL, Sise MJ, Sack DI, et al. Spiral computed tomography for the initial evaluation of spine trauma: a new standard of care? *J Trauma* 2006;**61**(2):382–7.

92. Brown CV, Antevil JL, Sise MJ, Sack DI. Spiral computed tomography for the diagnosis of cervical, thoracic, and lumbar spine fractures: its time has come. *J Trauma* 2005;**58**(5):890–5.

93. Hauser CJ, Visvikis G, Hinrichs C, et al. Prospective validation of computed tomographic screening of the thoracolumbar spine in trauma. *J Trauma* 2003;**55**(2):228–34.

94. Gale SC, Gracias VH, Reilly PM, Schwab CW. The inefficiency of plain radiography to evaluate the cervical spine after blunt trauma. *J Trauma* 2005;**59**(5):1121–5.

95. McCulloch PT, France J, Jones DL, et al. Helical computed tomography alone compared with plain radiographs with adjunct computed tomography to evaluate the cervical spine after high-energy trauma. *J Bone Joint Surg Am* 2005;**87**(11):2388–94.

96. Menaker J, Philip A, Boswell S, Scalea TM. Computed tomography alone for cervical spine clearance in the unreliable patient – are we there yet? *J Trauma* 2008;**64**(4):898–904.

97. Savitsky E, Votey S. Emergency department approach to acute thoracolumbar spine injury. *J Emerg Med* 1997;**15**(1):49–60.

98. Connell RA, Graham CA, Munro PT. Is spinal immobilisation necessary for all patients sustaining isolated penetrating trauma? *Injury* 2003;**34**:912–14.

99. Cornwell EE, Chang DC, Bonar JP, et al. Thoracolumbar immobilization for trauma patients with torso gunshot wounds: is it necessary? *Arch Surg* 2001;**136**:324–7.

100. Rhee P, Kuncir EJ, Johnson L, et al. Cervical spine injury is highly dependent on the mechanism of injury following blunt and penetrating assault. *J Trauma* 2006;**61**(5):1166–70.

101. Medzon R., Rothenhaus T. Bono CM, Grindlinger G, Rathlev NK. Stability of cervical spine fractures after gunshot wounds to the head and neck. *Spine* 2005;**30**(20):2274–9.

102. Klein Y, Cohn SM, Soffer D, et al. Spine injuries are common among asymptomatic patients after gunshot wounds. *J Trauma* 2005;**58**:833–6.

103. Smugar SS, Schweitzer ME, Hume E. MRI in patients with intraspinal bullets. *J Magn Reson Imaging* 1999;**9**(1):151–3.

104. Moran SL, Steinmann SP, Shin AY. Adult brachial plexus injuries: mechanism, patterns of injury, and physical diagnosis. *Hand Clin* 2005;**21**:13–24.

105. Midha R. Epidemiology of brachial plexus injuries in a multitrauma population. *Neurosurg* 1997;**40**(6):1182–9.

106. Kim DH, Cho YJ, Tiel RL, et al. Outcomes of surgery in 1019 brachial plexus lesions treated at Louisiana State University Health Sciences Center. *J Neurosurg* 2003;**98**:1005–16.

107. Rankine JJ. Adult traumatic brachial plexus injury. *Clinical Rad* 2004;**59**:767–74.

108. Shin AY, Spinner RJ, Steinmann SP, Bishop AT. Adult traumatic brachial plexus injuries. *J Am Acad Orthop Surg* 2005;**13**:382–96.

109. Dubuisson AS, Kline DG. Brachial plexus injury: a survey of 100 consecutive cases from a single service. *Neurosurg* 2002;**51**(3):673–83.

110. Johansen K, Lynch K, Paun M, Copass M. Non-invasive vascular tests reliably exclude occult arterial trauma in injured extremities. *J Trauma* 1991;**31**(4):515–19.

111. Pillai L, Luchette FA. Upper-extremity arterial injury. *Am Surg* 1997;**63**(3):224–7.

112. Brophy RH, Wolfe SW. Planning brachial plexus surgery: treatment options and priorities. *Hand Clin* 2005;**21**:47–54.

113. Haninec P, Sámal F, Tomás R, et al. Direct repair (nerve grafting), neurontization, and end-to-side neurorrhaphy in the treatment of brachial plexus injury. *J Neurosurg* 2007;**106**:391–9.

114. Bertelli JA, Ghizoni MF. Use of clinical signs and computed tomography myelography findings in detecting and excluding nerve root avulsion in complete brachial plexus palsy. *J Neurosurg* 2006;**105**:835–42.

115. Amrami KK, Port JD. Imaging the brachial plexus. *Hand Clin* 2005;**21**:25–37.

116. Todd M, Shah GV, Mukherji SK. MR imaging of the brachial plexus. *Top Man Reson Imaging* 2004;**15**(2):113–25.

117. Kim DH, Murovic JA, Tiel RL, Kline DG. Penetrating injuies due to gunshot wounds involving the brachial plexus. *Neurosurg Focus* 2004;**16**(5):1–6.

118. Stewart MP, Birch R. Penetrating missile injuries of the brachial plexus. *J Bone Joint Surg Br* 2001;**83**B(4):517–24.

Chapter

12

Chest trauma

Alasdair Conn

Introduction

Many patients with severe chest trauma die before they reach the hospital; however, a large percentage will arrive alive and require emergency evaluation. Rapid evaluation and management is critical. The range of injuries varies from a mild thoracic contusion – which after evaluation can often be released from the emergency department (ED) – to a penetrating cardiac injury or a thoracic aortic injury in which the immediate assessment and management can make the difference between a successful outcome or a patient's demise. Fewer than 10% of blunt chest injuries and 30% of penetrating thoracic injuries will require operative intervention.

Motor vehicle crashes constitute the most common cause of major thoracic trauma. It is estimated that up to 20% of motor vehicle deaths may be attributed to blunt cardiac injury and a further 15% caused by thoracic aortic injury. Thoracic trauma accounts for about 16 000 deaths per year in the United States.[1] The most common severe thoracic injury is blunt aortic injury, typically the driver of a car involved in a motor vehicle crash. Blunt aortic injury is often associated with high speed crashes, lack of restraint use, and significant intrusion into the vehicle.

Major changes and developments

Over the last decade the evaluation of thoracic injury has dramatically improved with the advent of high-speed computed tomography (CT) scanning and, in conjunction with CT angiography, early diagnosis of thoracic vascular injury is now almost routine. A normal CT angiogram excludes a great vessel injury and in many centers the use of intra-arterial angiography to confirm the diagnosis has been abandoned.

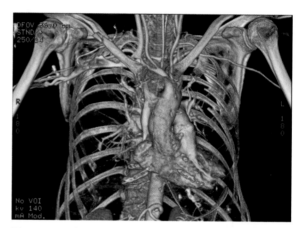

Figure 12.1 Three-dimensional multidetector computed tomography (MDCT). The use of CT is revolutionizing the diagnosis of thoracic injury. Multiple rib fractures and clavicular fracture can be easily seen.

This has allowed a more streamlined approach to the diagnosis. A thoracic CT with contrast may be ordered early in the course of a patient's evaluation, without the delays and costs associated with activating an angiographic team (Figure 12.1). Expanded use of multidetector CT scanning has also enabled identification of injuries such as pneumothoraces previously undetected by routine plain radiography. The treatment modality for injury to the thoracic aorta is also changing: thoracotomy and primary repair used to be the standard surgical approach but is being rapidly replaced by the endovascular placement of stents in selected patients. An additional major change has been the advent of portable ultrasonography; emergency physicians familiar with this technique can diagnose a cardiac effusion, cardiac tamponade, a hemothorax, and a pneumothorax within a few minutes of patient arrival. New research

Trauma: A Comprehensive Emergency Medicine Approach, eds. Eric Legome and Lee W. Shockley. Published by Cambridge University Press. © Cambridge University Press 2011.

on the evaluation of blunt cardiac injury has allowed risk stratification early in a patient's management and unnecessary intensive care monitoring can be avoided in these patients. Lastly the continued development and increasing sophistication of trauma systems have improved survival of the sickest patients.[2] Early identification and disposition to a designated trauma center is essential to this process.

Box 12.1   Essentials of chest trauma

- Fewer than 10% of blunt chest injuries and 30% of penetrating thoracic injuries will require operative intervention.
- Motor vehicle crashes constitute the most common cause of major thoracic trauma.
- The most common severe thoracic injury is blunt aortic injury.
- Blunt aortic injury is associated with high speed crashes, lack of restraint use, and significant intrusion into the vehicle.
- Over the last decade the rapid evaluation of thoracic injury has dramatically improved with the advent of high speed CT scanning.
- In conjunction with CT angiography, early diagnosis of thoracic vascular injury is now almost routine.
- A normal CT angiogram excludes a great vessel injury.

Clinical anatomy and pathophysiology

The thorax is the largest of the bony cavities of the body; it contains the heart, great vessels, and the lungs and is traversed by structures that pass from the neck to the abdomen. The following description is that of a normal anatomy, although there may be a variety of normal and abnormal variations.

Anatomy

The bony thorax comprises the 12 vertebrae, the 12th pairs of costae – the ribs and costal cartilages – and anteriorly, the sternum. Superiorly the entrance to the chest is bordered by the body of the first thoracic vertebra, the first rib and costal cartilages and the superior component of the manubrium. Inferiorly the thorax is limited by the two hemidiaphragms and is bordered by the lower costal cartilages and 12th rib on each side with the body of the 12th thoracic vertebra posteriorly. The hemidiaphragms have apertures which allow the aorta, esophagus, and vagal nerves to pass into the abdomen and the

inferior vena cava and thoracic duct to go from the abdomen into the chest. In expiration, the top of the diaphragm may reach up as high as the nipple so that penetrating injuries below this level may penetrate the diaphragm and damage the intra-abdominal contents.

Within the chest are the left and right lungs, the left lung has two lobes and the right has three; each lobe is further divided into segments. Superiorly the trachea enters the thorax and divides at the carina into the left and right mainstem bronchi; these mainstem bronchii then further divide to supply the lobes and then the segments of the lung. The heart is in the mediastinum and is enclosed by the fibrous pericardium.

The right atrium receives blood from the superior and inferior vena cavae; blood passes through the tricuspid valve into the right ventricle. The right ventricle is a lower pressure system than the left ventricle and hence the wall of the right ventricle is thinner than the left ventricle. Blood then emerges from the right ventricle through the pulmonary valve and into the main pulmonary artery; this divides into the left and right pulmonary arteries which subsequently branch to supply the lungs. After passing through the lungs, oxygenated blood returns to the left atrium through the pulmonary veins; blood then passes though the mitral valve into the left ventricle. During systole blood flows through the aortic valve into the proximal aorta. Initially the aorta passes superiorly and then, after giving off the innominate artery, left carotid and left subclavian arteries curves downward and lies anterior to the thoracic vertebral column. Superiorly the esophagus passes into the chest and lies posteriorly to the trachea as it enters the posterior mediastinum. It lies anteriorly to the vertebral column before entering the abdomen through the esophageal hiatus. The thoracic duct enters the chest through the diaphragm and courses superiorly in close proximity to the vertebral column before it ends by entering the left subclavian vein (Figure 12.2).

Physiology

Normal inspiration is effected by contraction of the diaphragm (innervated by the phrenic nerve which comes from the 3rd, 4th, and 5th cervical nerve roots) and the intercostal muscles; this creates a negative pressure within the pleural cavity and air at normal

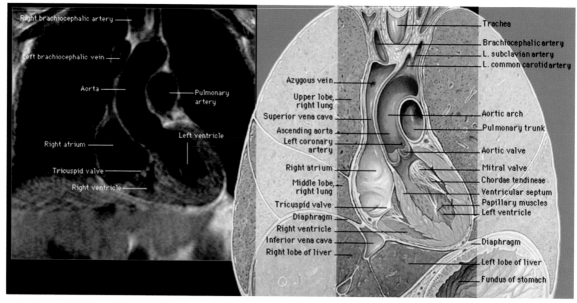

Figure 12.2 Overview of the anatomy of the thorax. Art., artery. (Courtesy of Patrick J. Lynch, in public domain.)

atmospheric pressure enters the lungs, provided the upper airway is not obstructed. Expiration is normally passive and caused by the relaxation of the musculature involved. If there is a large enough opening between the external environment and the pleural space, no such pressure gradient can be involved and the lung will not expand or be aerated. The reduced intrathoracic pressure during inspiration also assists with venous return, allowing a greater volume of blood to enter the chest during inspiration. If flow is obstructed by an increase in pressure within the chest (such as a tension pneumothorax) or constriction of the pericardium (such as cardiac tamponade) the patient may have clinically detectable distended neck veins.

Prehospital management

The prehospital management of the patient with thoracic injury is limited to two areas: the evaluation and triage component and acute intervention. Interventions permitted under the scope of practice for prehospital personnel will depend upon the local Emergency Medical Services (EMS) protocols but will usually include the administration of oxygen and the decompression of a tension pneumothorax using a large bore needle and inserted into the 2nd intercostal space midclavicular line or 5th intercostal space midaxillary line. For the patient that has

sustained a penetrating injury and the weapon is still impaled, prehospital providers will dress the wound to provide weapon immobilization until it can be removed in the ED or the operating room. For penetrating thoracic injuries without the object being impaled, the prehospital provider should provide an occlusive dressing whilst observing the patient for signs of a tension pneumothorax. These prehospital protocols are subject to the local medical direction and oversight, and hence may vary dependent upon locale. Appropriate prehospital evaluation and reporting of thoracic trauma should include the mechanism of injury together with the pertinent vital signs and physical exam of the chest. For the patient with blunt trauma the mechanism of injury may be important – the unrestrained driver who has compressed the steering wheel column is at risk for multiple rib fractures, pulmonary contusion, blunt aortic injury, and blunt cardiac injury. Likewise for penetrating injury, it is useful to obtain information of the nature of the weapon (gunshot wound or stabbing) and details of the exact weapon if this is available. Vital signs (including oxygenation), the adequacy of the upper airway, and the presence of bilateral breath sounds should all be reported. The prehospital providers should also be questioned as to the presence of stridor, subcutaneous emphysema, and the presence of any flail chest. Prehospital hypotension, especially if caused by a thoracic stab wound or gunshot

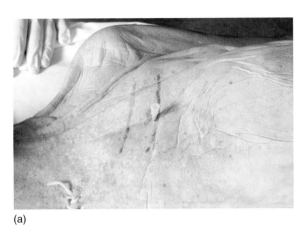 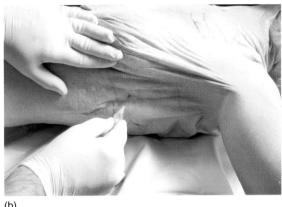

(a) (b)

Figure 12.3 Needle thoracostomy performed (on cadaver) with needle placed in the second intercostal space midclavicular line (a) and the fifth intercostal space midaxillary line (b).

wound, may require immediate operative intervention and under the appropriate circumstances the operating room should also be notified.

Needle thoracostomy

In most areas of the country advanced level prehospital providers can perform needle thoracostomy and insert a needle into the 2nd intercostal space midclavicular line or 5th intercostal space midaxillary line (Figure 12.3). A study suggests that untreated tension pneumothorax may have been the cause of death in 3.9% of casualties who died in the Vietnam conflict;[3] however, data from civilian experience is more difficult to obtain and some data suggests that this procedure is often overutilized.[4] It is also uncommon; in a retrospective review of the use of prehospital needle decompression of the chest by prehospital personnel brought to a Level I trauma center, of 20 330 advanced life support (ALS) calls only 39 patients (0.2%) had needle decompression for treatment of a tension pneumothorax.[5] Of these, 22 patients (56%) were in circulatory arrest. The conclusion of this article was that this appeared to be a safe procedure but an uncommon one – the authors did note that prehospital treatment resulted in four cases of unexpected survival over the one year of the study. In general it should be performed in the unstable patient (from respiratory or hemodynamic compromise) with clear signs or high suspicion for tension pneumothorax; e.g., unilateral breath sounds, subcutaneous emphysema, increasing difficulty in bagging the intubated patient.

Unless there is a contraindication to do so all thoracic trauma patients should be placed on supplemental oxygen. If it will not slow transport time, intravenous lines should also be initiated in the field as a component of prehospital trauma care.

Emergency department evaluation and management

The immediate life-threatening injuries associated with trauma to the chest include: ***upper airway obstruction***, ***tension pneumothorax*** (or a pneumothorax that is large enough to provide respiratory compromise but that is not under tension), ***large or tension hemothorax***, ***flail chest***, ***open chest wound***, and ***cardiac tamponade***. All of these injuries must be identified and managed by the emergency physician expeditiously; these conditions can frequently be identified and managed without the assistance of a chest radiograph.

Critical assessment

The initial assessment of the patient with chest trauma should concentrate on the airway, breathing, and circulation as it is related to traumatic chest injuries.

Upper airway assessment

The physician should examine the patient and determine if the upper airway is completely open, partially obstructed upper airway (indicated by stridorous breathing), or completely obstructed. Examine the

193

anterior neck for tracheal position and presence of hematomas; the removal of the anterior portion of the cervical collar may be necessary to facilitate this. Inspection of the neck veins should be performed; if they are prominent it indicates that a cardiac tamponade, pneumothorax, or venous obstruction might be present. Deviation of the trachea to one side is a late indication of a tension pneumothorax or a large hemothorax.

Breathing assessment

The presence or absence of cyanosis, the work of breathing and the symmetrical expansion of the chest can be confirmed rapidly. Auscultation should be quickly performed to confirm equal bilateral breath sounds. Decreased breath sounds on one side might indicate a pneumothorax or a hemothorax. The presence of paradoxical chest wall motion (on inspiration a portion of the rib cage moves in rather than out) confirms the clinical diagnosis of a flail chest. A low pulse oximetry measurement should alert the physician to look for an underlying cause. The physician should also palpate the chest for crepitus, deformity, or the presence of an open wound.

Circulation

Hypotension in the trauma patient should always be initially considered to be indicative of blood loss, however in chest trauma cardiac tamponade or tension pneumothorax can also cause hypotension. Hypotension is a late finding in both and is usually accompanied by distended neck veins.

In the elderly population a myocardial infarction may precipitate a motor vehicle crash; this will complicate both resuscitation and management. For the patient in extremis, emergency ultrasound should be used to visualize cardiac activity in the absence of a large cardiac tamponade. Portable ultrasonography may also be used for the detection of a hemothorax or a pneumothorax.

Box 12.2 Major life-threatening diagnoses in chest trauma

- Upper airway obstruction
- Tension pneumothorax
- Large or tension hemothorax
- Flail chest
- Open chest wound
- Cardiac tamponade

Severe injuries
Tension pneumothorax

A tension pneumothorax may arise from two mechanisms. In one, an injury to the lung allows air to pass into the pleural cavity on inspiration through a hole in the surface of the lung but on expiration the injury acts as a flap valve and so the air remains in the pleural space and cannot be expired. In the other, a patient with a simple pneumothorax or barotrauma to the lung is placed on positive pressure ventilation. In this instance, air is forced under pressure into the pleural space. In either mechanism, over the course of a few minutes the air in the pleural space pushes the heart and mediastinal structures to the opposite side, compressing the contralateral lung. Hypoxia results both from the collapsed lung on the affected side but also the compression of the contralateral lung; in addition, the decreased venous return from the dramatically increased intrathoracic pressure and the pressure on the thin walls of the atria cause a decrease in cardiac output eventually precipitating cardiac arrest and death. This is truly a dramatic event. The patient initially experiences increasing difficulty in breathing and chest pain, they will become confused and agitated as hypoxia progresses. The clinician will note tachycardia, tachypnea, and eventually hypotension. Cyanosis and a decrease in oxygen saturation are also common. Clinically the affected side of the chest is hyper-resonant and breath sounds are absent on the affected side, the trachea is deviated away from the side of the chest with tension although this is usually a late finding. The intercostal muscles on the affected side may also be "ballooned out" by the underlying dramatic increase in intrapleural pressure. A common misunderstanding amongst emergency providers is that a tension pneumothorax can arise in a few seconds or 1–2 minutes; this would be unusual. A recent comment states that the natural history of tension pneumothorax is that decompensation rarely takes < 20 minutes and most take about 30–60 minutes.[6] Hemodynamic and respiratory decompensation may take many hours to develop; the longest time on record is 4 days. However, this process can be rapidly accelerated in patients receiving positive pressure ventilation, especially in those with high airway pressures.

Treatment is by immediate decompression of the affected side; emergency practitioners should be familiar with the technique. A large bore needle (14–16 gauge will suffice) is inserted into the chest in the 2nd intercostal space anteriorly (or in the 5th intercostal space, anterior axillary line). A study in 2005 of 25 emergency physicians (21 of whom had completed ATLS® training) noted that only 60% were able to correctly identify the 2nd intercostal space.[7] The intercostal vessels and nerve lie just inferior to the rib and so needle decompression should be performed just over the top of the rib below to avoid damage to these structures. If the diagnosis is correct, a rush of high pressure air will be extruded through the needle: the symptoms related to the tension pneumothorax will resolve. Performance of needle decompression does not guarantee success even if tension is present; the catheter may not be long enough, or it may become kinked or obstructed. Success also depends upon the body habitus of the patient and the presence of subcutaneous emphysema. In a study of 111 patients the chest wall thickness was measured at the 2nd intercostal space, the mean chest wall thickness was 4.24 cm (95% confidence interval 3.97–4.52 cm) and almost 25% of patients had a chest wall thickness of > 5 cm. Further: the thickness was greater in women than men (4.90 cm for women; 4.16 cm for men; $P = 0.022$),[8] so that practitioners should ensure that the needles are long enough. Following this procedure in which the needle is placed into the pleural space, chest thoracostomy tube is generally necessary.

It is uncommon to see a patient with bilateral tension pneumothoraces, but in many patients with chest trauma the diagnosis may be of a tension pneumothorax on one side and a simple pneumothorax or a hemothorax on the other. In a small case series, three patients with bilateral tension pneumothoraces who presented in pulseless electrical activity (PEA) were reported; needle decompression failed to relieve the tension and cardiac output was only restored after chest tube insertion.[9] If there is doubt as to which side of the chest is affected, bilateral chest tubes may be inserted. Although not formally studied, it is likely that more patients succumb to the lack of a chest tube being inserted rather than the complications of chest tube insertion.

The insertion of a chest tube is not without complications: misplacement of the tube, infection, and further bleeding are the most common but rupture of the pulmonary vessels and of the heart have been reported.[10] The complication rate was studied by a Canadian group[11] and over a 12-month period a retrospective study of all chest tube insertions by residents at a regional trauma center demonstrated a complication rate of 30% – insertional, positional, and infective complications were identified. Computed tomography scanning was used to document the complications. The use of prophylactic antibiotics for tube thoracostomy is controversial: a prospective, multicentered, randomized trial of antibiotics in the prevention of empyema and pneumonia published in 2004 failed to show any benefit.[12] There were three arms, two antibiotic regimens, and a placebo group. Two hundred and twenty four patients were analyzed for a total of 229 thoracostomies; antibiotic use did not significantly affect the incidence of empyema or pneumonia.

Hemothorax

Hemothorax is blood in the pleural space and is common after thoracic trauma. A hemothorax is graded by the amount of blood in the pleural space; a massive hemothorax is a collection of 1500 cc or greater of blood. With rapid accumulations of this magnitude patients are usually hypotensive and tachycardic and often require volume resuscitation. Breath sounds are usually diminished on the side of the hemothorax and in the latter stages there may be deviation of the mediastinum and the trachea to the opposite side. Bleeding may be from lacerations of the lung parenchyma or from the intercostal vessels. Patients with complete transection of the aorta or other major vessels do not usually survive to reach the hospital. The treatment is twofold – to insert a chest tube relieving the hemothorax and to restore intravascular volume. In high volume trauma centers an autotransfuser may be available such that the blood can be collected, filtered, and then reinfused to the patient. Concerns as to bacterial contamination of autotransfused blood, in the case of a multiply injured patient, have not been realized in practice. There are not many reports in the literature of the use of autotransfusion in the management of a hemothorax but case reports do demonstrate that large volumes of up to 3000 ml may be autotransfused.[13,14] Often in these patients there is a large amount of blood that is lost as the tube is inserted. The chest tube should immediately be connected to an underwater seal so that the rate of bleeding from the chest tube can be monitored. The decision to proceed to thoracotomy for the management of a hemothorax depends upon the judgment of the individual thoracic or trauma surgeon. General guidelines for thoracotomy are as shown in Table 12.1. Some

Table 12.1 General guidelines for OR thoracotomy in patients with thoracic trauma

- If severe hemodynamic compromise, ED thoracotomy should be performed
- Hemodynamic instability in a patient with thoracic trauma despite aggressive resuscitation
- Immediate drainage of 20 ml/kg upon insertion of the first chest tube (approximately 1400 cc in a 70 kg patient)
- Continued drainage of > 3 ml/kg – or drainage increasing – over 4 hours. (200 ml/hour or above in a 70 kg patient)
- Cardiac tamponade or suspected cardiac injury, e.g., penetrating cardiac wound or rupture
- Severe tracheobronchial injury
- Impaled objects or intrathoracic retained bodies following trauma

surgeons will perform a thoracotomy based upon the absolute amount of drainage (about 1400 cc) on initial chest tube placement; others will examine the rate of blood loss and operate based upon the loss of 200–300 cc of blood per hour in an adult. If the blood loss is decreasing some surgeons may decide to monitor the patient and defer the decision to operate.

Flail chest

A flail chest is commonly noted clinically when three or more ribs are fractured in more than one location (Figure 12.4). On inspiration, when the chest normally expands, this segment will now be free floating and may cave into the chest. On expiration the positive pleural pressure will allow this free floating segment to bulge out – the so-called paradoxical respiration. Patients will experience pain when breathing because of the movement of the fractured ribs; clinically patients become tachypneic and will have rapid shallow breaths. Hypoxia is common but this is usually due to the underlying pulmonary contusion rather than the flail segment itself. Initial treatment includes supplemental oxygen and appropriate analgesics; regional (intercostals) nerve blocks or an epidural may be utilized in more severe cases. If the pulmonary contusion is severe and oxygenation compromised, intubation and ventilation may be required. Flail chest does seem to indicate a more severe pulmonary injury although the young are less likely to sustain rib fractures than the elder population whose ribs are more brittle. In an uncontrolled study, 22 patients with flail chest following trauma were compared with 90 patients with more than 2 fractured ribs.[15] Despite similar age and pulmonary contusion rates, patients with flail chest had higher needs for mechanical ventilation (86% vs. 42% $P < 0.01$), longer hospital length of stay (28 ± 21 days vs. 17 ± 19 days $P = 0.04$), and a higher incidence of

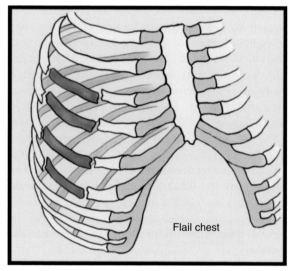

Figure 12.4 Illustration of flail chest. Double fractures of at least three adjacent ribs are required in order to produce a flail chest. (From Mandavia D, Newton E, Demetriades D. *Colour Atlas of Emergency Trauma*. Cambridge: Cambridge University Press, 2003.)

respiratory complications. (64% vs. 26%, $P < 0.01$). The authors concluded that flail chest was an independent marker of severe lung injury. For severe flail chest the use of internal fixation has been advocated.[16] This report documented operative fixation on seven patients with multiple rib fractures – five during the initial hospitalization and two delayed. They describe good results but the subset of patients who would benefit from such a procedure was not defined. In a further study in 2002, 37 consecutive flail chest patients were enrolled and identical respiratory management, analgesia, bronchial toilet were performed.[17] On day 5 of hospitalization the patients were randomly assigned to either conservative treatment or operative fixation. Analysis showed that the two groups appeared to be identical in terms of age, sex, and severity of lung injury; however, in the group that received fixation there was a shorter ventilatory period (10.8 ± 3.4 days vs. 18.3 ± 7.4 days) ($P < 0.05$), a shorter length of stay in the intensive care unit (fixation group 16.5 ± 7.4 days vs. 26.8 ± 13.2 days for the control group) ($P < 0.05$), and a decreased incidence of pneumonia (fixation group 24% and control 77%) ($P < 0.05$). They also noted that the fixation group returned faster to their job. The authors' conclusion was that operative fixation may be preferred in patients with severe flail chest but this technique has yet to receive wide acceptance; this second study also was not able to clearly define which subset of patients with rib fractures might best benefit from this technique.[17]

Open chest wound from penetrating injury

An open chest wound may not allow negative internal pleural pressure on inspiration. As a result, air passes in and out of the chest with each attempt at inspiration leading to hypoventilation of one lung, and resultant respiratory compromise. This type of injury is most common in penetrating trauma; however, blunt trauma can also cause open rib fractures with an open sucking chest wound. The patient will complain of pain around the chest wound site; tachycardia, tachypnea, and difficulty breathing will also be experienced. These injuries are commonly identified by the prehospital personnel. The treatment is to control the wound by applying an occlusive dressing (which can be performed in the prehospital phase) and then insert a chest tube. The chest tube should not be placed through the open wound, rather it should be placed in the intercostal space in the normal manner. Appropriate wound care with debridement and potentially closure of the primary wound can be performed in the ED.

Cardiac tamponade

Traumatic cardiac tamponade is caused by the accumulation of blood in the pericardial sac. As the blood accumulates it compromises the filling of the cardiac chambers, eventually leading to a restriction of cardiac output. Although most often seen in penetrating cardiac injury, it can also be seen in patients who have sustained blunt trauma where it is usually due to lacerations of the atrial appendage. Although the classic signs and symptoms are muffled heart sounds, systemic hypotension, and an elevated central venous pressure (noted clinically by distended neck veins) (Beck's triad), this may be a difficult clinical diagnosis. These signs and symptoms may be absent in the multiply injured patient or difficult to evaluate in a busy trauma resuscitation bay. The most reliable diagnostic modality is the portable ultrasound; a black stripe seen around the heart is indicative of fluid, however, acute clot in the pericardium may have a more echogenic appearance resembling liver parenchyma. Initially there may be no hemodynamic instability or compromise aside from tachycardia. As fluid accumulates, scalloping of the pericardium is seen, central venous pressure increases, and distended neck veins are noted. Initial therapy is to administer a bolus of intravenous fluid in an effort to increase central venous pressure and, hence, cardiac filling. If portable ultrasound detects a pericardial effusion following traumatic injury, early emergency surgical consultation is necessary. Case reports of incidental findings of pericardial fluid following abdominal trauma and subsequent emergency thoracotomy have been reported,[18] but, in general, patients with an ultrasound detected pericardial effusion should be further assessed in the operating room. A thoracotomy or a sternotomy is performed and the pericardial tamponade relieved; if there is doubt as to the diagnosis a small incision can be made in the upper abdomen with the removal of the xiphisternum and the pericardium opened. This is a so called "pericardial window" and if blood is found in the pericardial space further exposure is warranted. If the patient is experiencing severe hypotension in the ED then an emergency thoracotomy with relief of the tamponade should be considered.

Emergency department thoracotomy

A challenging situation for an emergency physician is the thoracic trauma patient who presents in the "pre-arrest" state or following cardiac arrest. The patient may have already been intubated and intravenous lines initiated and the emergency physician (perhaps with the assistance of a responding trauma team) will be faced with the question of whether to perform a resuscitative thoracotomy.

A thoracotomy in a patient in whom the efforts of resuscitation are futile will expose the trauma team to unnecessary exposure of potentially infected body fluids and may waste valuable resources.[19] However, in an appropriate patient this can be life saving (Table 12.2). The indications for ED thoracotomy are different for patients with blunt trauma and for patients with penetrating thoracic trauma. For patients that have sustained

Table 12.2 Potential benefits of ED thoracotomy

- Release of pericardial tamponade and tension pneumothorax
- Perform open chest CPR (with increased perfusion pressure than closed CPR)
- Control cardiac wounds
- Control wounds to great vessels
- Cross-clamp aorta to limit distal hemorrhage
- Cross-clamp hilum of lung to limit pulmonary hemorrhage
- Perform internal defibrillation and administer intracardiac resuscitation drugs

CPR, cardiopulmonary resuscitation; ED, emergency department.

blunt trauma and arrive to the ED in cardiac arrest the eventual successful outcome is poor. The vast majority of these patients have exsanguinated from severe injuries prior to hospital arrival and the heart is empty. Cardiopulmonary resuscitation (CPR) in these patients is not effective as the heart is empty (even though many of these patients will arrive with CPR in progress) and any attempt to open the chest, cross-clamp the aorta, and maintain some level of a cerebral perfusion is usually futile. The major injuries have not been controlled, cerebral perfusion has not been present for several minutes, and hypothermia and coagulopathy are usually present. Any resuscitative infusions of crystalloid and blood will continue to be lost through the injured organs. For this reason such heroic resuscitation efforts are usually not indicated; the risks and costs of performing this invasive procedure do not justify the means. The one exception is if the blunt trauma patient arriving in cardiac arrest has cardiac activity on ultrasound or has the presence of a cardiac tamponade. For patients who arrive with vital signs after blunt trauma but who have a cardiac arrest during resuscitation an ED thoracotomy is justified, these patients have only a short time when cerebral perfusion is compromised and with aggressive management may survive neurologically intact.

For patients who have sustained penetrating trauma to the chest and have vital signs upon arrival (and arrest either upon arrival or whilst they are being evaluated in the ED) or have had vital signs within 5 minutes of arrival, ED thoracotomy is justified. The survival for patients who have sustained this type of injury is between 20 and 60% depending upon the series.

For patients who have sustained prehospital cardiac arrest after trauma, data is available. In a study published in 2004, 26 years of ED thoracotomy were reviewed.[20] In total, 959 patients underwent ED thoracotomy and 62 patients survived to leave the hospital for a survival rate of 6.4%. Of the 62 who survived, 26 (42%) underwent prehospital CPR. The injury mechanism of these 26 was stab wound in 18, gunshot wound in 4, and blunt trauma in 4. Based upon analysis of the data it was proposed that resuscitative ED thoracotomy is futile in patients with blunt trauma requiring prehospital CPR for longer than 5 minutes and patients with penetrating trauma with more than 15 minutes of prehospital CPR.

The study was criticized because the authors did not comment on the use of portable ultrasound,[19] and the latest guidelines from the same authors indicate that they perform ED thoracotomy on patients who have sustained blunt trauma and arrive to the ED with CPR in process only if they can demonstrate electrical activity, or ultrasound detection of cardiac activity or tamponade.[21] Patients who have electrical activity or who have sustained penetrating trauma undergo thoracotomy; if, on direct visualization of the heart, there is no activity and no tamponade the patient is declared dead without further resuscitative efforts. There will be a few patients who have sustained blunt injury to the heart who will have a ruptured atrial appendage with subsequent tamponade; this should be obvious on ultrasound and with rapid identification and thoracotomy these patients can potentially be salvaged. It should also be noted that given the very small number of blunt trauma patients who survived ($n = 4$) it is hard to make a practice guideline using this number. Emergency department thoracotomy in penetrating trauma has much higher survival rate and the scientific and theoretical basis for it are much stronger.

For patients who arrive with vital signs and have sustained penetrating or blunt thoracic trauma but whose vital signs deteriorate in the ED, ED thoracotomy should be strongly considered (Table 12.3). Ultrasound may be used to identify the presence or absence of cardiac tamponade and hence to assist in appropriate decision making.

The exact surgical procedure will depend upon the mechanism and the suspected injuries. A general approach is as follows: The thoracotomy is performed by opening the left chest, a rib spreader is inserted and the contents of the chest quickly evaluated. If the

Table 12.3 Indications for emergency department thoracotomy (EDT)

Probably should perform an EDT

1. Patient with penetrating thoracic injury who has documented vital signs within 5 minutes of ED arrival

2. Patient with blunt or penetrating thoracic injury who has vital signs upon arrival but loses them in the ED

3. Patient with blunt or penetrating injury who has pericardial tamponade diagnosed on ultrasound and becomes unstable in the ED

Consider an EDT

1. Patient with abdominal, pelvic, or lower extremity trauma who becomes unstable in the ED and in whom proximal aortic control is considered justified

Probably should not perform an EDT

1. Patient with penetrating thoracic injury who has no vital signs for more than 5 minutes prior to hospital arrival

2. Patient with blunt thoracic trauma who has no vital signs within 5 minutes of ED arrival and has no cardiac activity or pericardial tamponade upon ED arrival

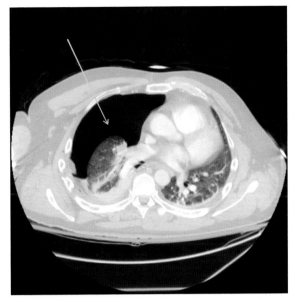

Figure 12.5 Computed tomography (CT) with tension pneumothorax. This should generally be diagnosed much earlier by physical examination or radiograph. The physician in this case reported that there were bilateral breath sounds and the oxygen saturation was above 90% on room air. The deviation of the mediastinum can be easily seen.

thoracotomy is being performed for a cardiac tamponade then the pericardium is open anterior to the phrenic nerve to relieve the tamponade and to identify the bleeding point in the myocardium. Penetrating myocardial injury can be initially controlled by pledgeted sutures, digital pressure, stapling, or Foley catheter tamponade.

The moderate injuries to be detected at this stage of the patient's evaluation include a simple pneumothorax, a hemothorax, blunt cardiac injury, pulmonary contusion, aortic or other great vessel injury, diaphragmatic rupture or penetration, and wounds that traverse the mediastinum in the patient with hemodynamic stability.

Pneumothorax

Pneumothorax is the presence of air in the pleural cavity, these may be small enough that they cannot be detected on a routine chest X-ray but only detected on subsequent CT scanning or so large that they encompass the collapse of the entire lung (Figure 12.5).

Normally the chest X-ray will show large pneumothoraces and these are then graded by the percentage of collapse. Many emergency chest radiographs initially ordered are performed on supine patients in the trauma bay and often do not demonstrate a large pneumothorax. In one study, only 52% of patients with a CT-proven pneumothorax had the pneumothorax detected on the initial supine chest radiograph.[22] An erect chest radiograph is more sensitive to detect a pneumothorax. This may not be practical in the unstable patient or in the patient with potential cervical, thoracic, or lumbar spine injuries. If hypoxia is present, then a pneumothorax decompression is indicated (Table 12.4). Ultrasound can also be used to diagnosis pneumothorax. An 18-month prospective study evaluated 109 conscious, spontaneously breathing patients who had been admitted to the ED with chest trauma and had a standard supine chest radiograph and a spiral thoracic CT scan within 1 hour of ED arrival.[22] All patients also had a lung ultrasound performed by an operator who was unaware of the other examination results. Twenty five traumatic pneumothoraces were detected in the 109 patients evaluated by CT scan (2 patients had bilateral pneumothoraces) and only 13 of 25 (52%) were detected by chest radiography. Twenty three of the 25 (92%) were detected by the lung ultrasound with one false positive (sensitivity 92%, specificity 99.4%).

Table 12.4 Indication for chest tube insertion without confirmatory radiograph

- Tension pneumothorax (hypotension, unilateral loss of breath sounds, increased airway pressures, tracheal deviation)

- Hemodynamically unstable patient with penetrating chest trauma

- Penetrating chest trauma and subcutaneous air

- Blunt chest trauma, subcutaneous air, and hypoxia or hypotension

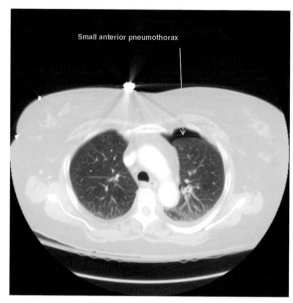

Small anterior pneumothorax

Figure 12.6 The initial chest X-ray and oxygenation is normal but the patient has a small pneumothorax detected by computed tomography (CT). The emergency physician should be cognizant of the management of these small pneumothoraces; this patient was managed conservatively.

Aspiration of spontaneous pneumothorax has been advocated.[23] In one series, aspiration was successful in 50% of cases in which it was attempted; many of these patients were sent home from the ED.[24] However, these series are for spontaneous pneumothoraces and not for traumatic pneumothoraces. Small trauma pneumothoraces may be observed, some may be aspirated, but at this time this observation should probably be in a hospital setting.

Not infrequently, small clinically inapparent or occult pneumothoraces are found only on CT scan (abdomen or thoracic) (Figure 12.6) or ultrasound. A common question is whether a chest tube should be inserted. Insertion of a chest tube may have significant complications and if not needed should be avoided. There have been only six published papers on this topic; three published since 1998. In one study the pneumothoraces were divided into miniscule, anterior, or anterolateral.[25] Of the 16 with miniscule pneumothoraces, 15 were observed without the need for a chest tube. Twelve of 20 with anterior were observed (1 developed a tension pneumothorax). The second paper was a prospective randomized clinical trial with 39 adult patients.[26] After randomization 18 patients received a chest tube and 21 were observed. Three patients who were observed developed respiratory distress with pneumothorax enlargement. The 3rd study was a prospective observational study involving 11 children who presented to a Level I trauma center; all were found to have an occult pneumothorax.[27] Only one patient had a chest tube placed: the rest were successfully observed.

Although all of these studies involve a small numbers of patients, it appears appropriate to manage small occult pneumothoraces with observation and monitoring. Overall, a small percentage (10–15%) will probably develop a significant pneumothorax.

Further research and definition is required as to what size and position of an occult pneumothorax required tube thoracostomy. Although there is some mixed evidence about how to proceed if positive pressure ventilation is being used, currently most physicians recommend prophylactic tube thoracostomy. Studies are being conducted to answer this question.

Hemothoraces may be seen in blunt or penetrating trauma (Figure 12.7). The exam may reveal decreased breath sounds or dullness to percussion, but they may be difficult to ascertain in the busy trauma bay. Large hemothoraces may present without initial instability, but can also present with hypotension due to hemorrhage or decreased cardiac return. In the stable patient a hemothorax may be detected by ultrasonography, chest radiograph, or CT scanning. For a supine film a hemothorax may appear as a diffuse opacity across all lung fields in the pleural space and breath sounds may be diminished on the appropriate side. Standard practice is to use chest radiograph and potentially CT scanning; however, evidence is showing a possible role for ultrasound. A report of 54 patients who underwent thoracic ultrasound following blunt trauma showed that 12 patients had a hemothorax detected by ultrasound and subsequently confirmed

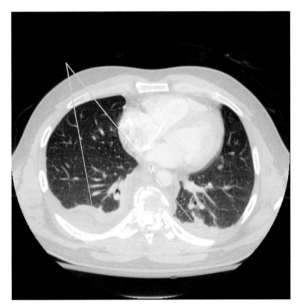

Figure 12.7 This radiograph shows a bilateral hemothoraces that was not immediately obvious on the supine admission chest X-ray. Sometimes one hemithorax is more opacified than the other on the initial X-ray, giving an indication that a hemothorax may be present. The blood appears to be draining posteriorly but this is because the patient is supine on the computed tomography (CT) table.

by CT or tube thoracostomy. Four of the hemothoraces were detected on ultrasound but were not apparent on the initial chest radiology. In this small series there were 12 true positives, 48 true negatives, no false positives, and 1 false negative. This led to a sensitivity of 92%, a specificity of 100% with a positive predictive value of 100%, and a negative predictive value of 98% for the detection for the hemothorax following blunt trauma. The conclusion of the authors was that ultrasound is a valuable tool and should be used to augment the immediate clinical assessment of trauma patients.[28] A review of the literature from 1996 to 2007 examining the use of ultrasonography to detect hemothorax following trauma came to the same conclusion, but also suggested that radiography should continue to be utilized in patient evaluation because it may provide additional information that ultrasonography cannot provide.[29] The treatment is to insert a chest tube in the appropriate side and record both the initial drainage and monitor the rate of bleeding. If the drainage is excessive a thoracic or trauma surgical consultation should be obtained. Unlike pneumothorax, aspiration is not indicated for hemothoraces.

Blunt cardiac injury

Blunt cardiac injury is a pathological diagnosis and is dependent upon the findings of acute inflammation and damage on autopsy, thoracotomy, or myocardial biopsy. The term "blunt cardiac injury" encompasses a range of pathology from clinically non-significant contusion through transient arrhythmias to fatal cardiac rupture. Previously used terms such as myocardial contusion or cardiac contusion have now been replaced by the broader term, blunt cardiac injury. The mechanism of injury is most commonly deceleration (e.g., a patient's chest impacting the steering wheel in a motor vehicle crash). The right ventricle is the most often injured chamber because of the relatively greater retrosternal area. Other rarer pathological findings may include valvular tears and ruptures, septal defects, and coronary artery thrombosis.[30] *Commotio cordis* is a rare cause of cardiac arrest, particularly noted in young athletes who sustain direct trauma to the anterior chest. A detailed review of this condition was conducted by the *Commotio Cordis* Registry.[31] Patients who have sustained blunt thoracic trauma should have a 12-lead electrocardiogram (ECG) performed as part of the initial evaluation; this may demonstrate sinus tachycardia, a new bundle branch block, ST depressions, or ST elevations. Patients with blunt cardiac injury have an increased risk of dysrhythmia compared with controls; the most common dysrhythmia outside of sinus tachycardia was atrial fibrillation.[32] In a patient with a new arrhythmia or with tachycardia out of proportion to the clinical status, echocardiography should be considered. Any complex dysrhythmias such as ventricular tachycardia or signs of instability should have an echocardiogram as soon as practical. Portable ultrasound may be used in the resuscitation bay to rule out pericardial tamponade; consultative echocardiography may demonstrate wall motion abnormalities, septal injuries, or valvular dysfunction.[33] The use of cardiac biomarkers in cardiac injury is controversial despite many studies. The lack of a gold standard for the diagnosis of blunt cardiac injury, the difficulty of interpretation of abnormal results, and the realization that biochemical measurements rarely effect clinical management decisions have led many centers to abandon the routine collection of cardiac biomarkers following acute injury. There are small subsets of patients who sustain a myocardial infarction related to their trauma; this should be detected by changes of acute myocardial infarction upon the initial ECG. Elevation of cardiac troponin I and T do not appear to be of prognostic value;[34] however, some experts have advocated that if the level is within normal range and the initial ECG is normal, significant cardiac injury can be safely excluded.[35] Patients who have valvular, septal, or ventricular injuries should receive a prompt consultation from a cardiologist or cardiac surgeon. Patients with complex cardiac dysrhythmias should be admitted to the intensive care unit for continuous cardiac monitoring for 24 hours. Those stable patients with persistent tachycardia alone may be managed on general telemetry. Intervention beyond the administration of antiarrythmic drugs for specific dysrhythmias is rarely required.

Pulmonary contusion

Blunt trauma to the lung parenchyma may result in hemorrhage into the lung and the inability of adequate gaseous exchange; this condition is termed pulmonary contusion. Although the initial chest radiograph may be non-diagnostic and initial measurements of gaseous exchange may be normal, pulmonary function may become compromised over the ensuing few hours. Subsequent radiographs taken over several hours may demonstrate the irregular opacification of the pulmonary parenchyma in a non-lobular pattern. Chest CT (often performed to rule out major vascular injuries) may demonstrate the contusion (Figure 12.8). Uncomplicated pulmonary contusions typically develop over the first 24 hours and resolve in approximately 1 week.[36] Patients with severe pulmonary contusions experience difficulty breathing and hypoxia. Repeat chest radiographs show an increasing opacity of the affected lung fields. The condition is exacerbated if extensive crystalloid fluid resuscitation has been performed. Blood gas evaluation reveals an increased a–A gradient. Treatment is initially supplemental oxygen administration to reverse hypoxia; however, subsequent intubation and ventilation with positive end-expiratory pressure may be required. Pulmonary toilet to prevent atelectasis and pneumonia, management of hypoxia, and analgesia are the mainstays of pulmonary contusion treatment.

Aortic and great vessel injury

Patients involved in severe decelaratative forces, such as high-speed motor vehicle crashes, may sustain aortic and great vessel injury. For blunt trauma the

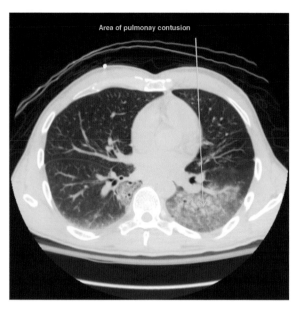

Figure 12.8 Computed tomography (CT) showing a pulmonary contusion. This is often better seen and delineated on the CT than it is on the plain X-ray.

most common site of aortic injury is just beyond the origin of the left subclavian artery near the ligamentum arteriosum. If the rupture involves all three layers of the aortic wall the patient will rapidly exsanguinate. Patients who survive to reach the hospital do so because the outer layer of the aorta (adventitia) remains intact; however, these patients are at great risk of subsequent rupture if the injury remains untreated. It is estimated that if undiagnosed and untreated, 50% of these patients will succumb in the first 24 hours. Plain chest radiography may demonstrate an abnormality consistent with a hematoma around the aorta or great vessels; these patients should undergo further diagnostic investigation. Up to 7% of patients who had a rupture of the aorta will have no mediastinal abnormality detected on the initial chest X-ray. For this reason CT scanning with intravenous contrast is often used to evaluate the patient who has sustained severe thoracic injury (Figures 12.9–12.12). A normal CT examination of the chest excludes major thoracic vessel injury.[37] For patients in which an aortic rupture is suspected, the heart rate should be maintained below 100 and the systolic blood pressure kept around 90–100 mmHg. Intra-arterial pressure monitoring and intravenous beta-blockade should be used to prevent systolic hypertension with subsequent rupture of the periaortic hematoma and immediate

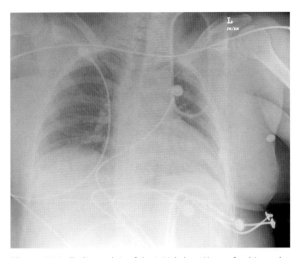

Figure 12.9 Radiograph is of the initial chest X-ray of a driver who was unrestrained and involved in a high-speed motor vehicle crash. Even on the supine X-ray there is the suggestion of a widening of the mediastinum. Figure 12.10 shows the computed tomography (CT) images.

exsanguination. If beta-blockade is contraindicated, calcium channel blockers may be used. The physician should first lower the heart with beta-blockade to prevent reflex tachychardia, and then the blood pressure with nitroprusside if the beta-blockade alone does not do so. Appropriate consultation should be made as soon as the diagnosis is seriously considered; in smaller facilities this will include consideration for transfer to a trauma center that has the capability and experience of managing this type of injury. Over the last 10 years CT angiography has overtaken the need for intravascular angiography to confirm the diagnosis;[38] 70% of trauma centers will now use the CT arteriography findings as confirming the diagnosis. The management of this injury has also changed as more centers become experienced in endovascular repair;[39–42] while the long-term outcomes are not yet known, more recent experience seems to indicate a decreased immediate mortality and morbidity. With appropriate beta-blockade and control of the systolic blood pressure, operation can be delayed and emergency transfer effected.

Diaphragmatic rupture

Diaphragmatic injury following blunt trauma is a diagnosis that is often missed in the multiply injured patient and occurs in approximately 1% of thoracic trauma patients. The diagnosis can be missed especially if the patient has not sustained a significant intra-abdominal or thoracic injury requiring surgery. The diagnosis appears to be increasing as the diagnostic accuracy of multidetector CT scanners becomes more widely available.[43] The mechanism of injury is most commonly that of a high-speed motor vehicle crash. Increased intra-abdominal pressure from the forceful impact causes a pressure pulse leading to acute rupture of the diaphragm: this is most commonly on the left side because the right side hemidiaphragm is protected by the liver. In a series of 65 patients, the rupture was on the left in 66%, on the right in 32%, and bilateral in 1.5%.[44] The diaphragm does not usually bleed sufficiently to cause a large hemothorax or hemoperitoneum. The classic findings of the gastric bubble being in the chest or the nasogastric tube being above the diaphragm are only seen in 44% of patients. Other findings are of an elevated hemidiaphragm and a hemothorax. The initial chest radiograph of patients proven to have a traumatic diaphragmatic rupture have a normal or non-diagnostic chest radiograph up to 50% of the time. Because of the difficulty of diagnosis different modalities have been examined in an effort to improve diagnostic accuracy. Diagnostic peritoneal lavage is helpful, but highly non-specific and relying on this may lead to non-therapeutic laparotomies. However, DPL fluid that comes out a chest tube is diagnostic. Helical CT scanning has improved the accuracy of the diagnosis (Figure 12.13).

Once a traumatic rupture of the diaphragm is diagnosed following blunt trauma, expeditious repair is warranted. The late complications include herniation through the diaphragmatic defect leading to bowel obstruction and gangrene of the bowel.

For penetrating injury the average length of laceration is only approximately 1 cm compared to 5 or 6 cm in blunt trauma. Detection of these injuries it is usually by inference, a penetrating wound to the lower chest on the left side has a significant likelihood of penetrating the diaphragm and producing an intra-abdominal injury. The detection in these cases of intra-abdominal injury by CT scanning or other modality from a penetrating chest wound infers penetration of the diaphragm. Many of these patients may be observed if the intra-abdominal injury does not require surgery. The long-term risk of complications such as adhesions or diaphragmatic herniation of such a traumatic laceration of approximately 1–2 cm is not known.

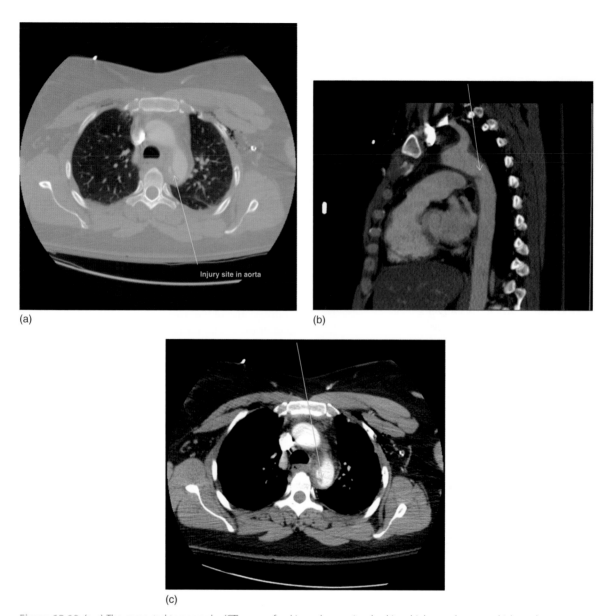

(a)

(b)

Injury site in aorta

(c)

Figure 12.10 (a–c) The computed tomography (CT) scans of a driver who was involved in a high-speed motor vehicle crash. The arrows show the area of aortic injury.

Transmediastinal wounds

For patients who have sustained gunshot wounds that have traversed the mediastinum and who are unstable, immediate operative repair is necessary. For those patients who are hemodynamically stable the question is somewhat controversial, some surgeons would advocate immediate exploration whilst other would advocate a more conservative approach with CT scanning.[45] Advocates of the conservative approach indicate that 68% of patients who were stable following a transmediastinal gunshot wound had no injuries on CT scanning and were safely observed, no late complications were reported.[45]

Minor injuries

Patients may complain of chest pain from trauma but have a normal chest radiograph and normal vital signs – including oximetry. Minor injuries include fractured ribs and small pulmonary contusions.

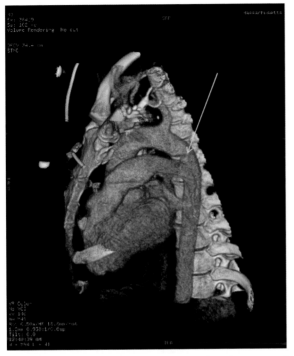

Figure 12.11 This image is the reconstruction from the computed tomography (CT) scan of the same driver.

Fractured ribs

Rib fractures are common injuries resulting from blunt thoracic trauma. Fractures often occur at the site of impact; however, the posterolateral bend of the rib, the weakest point, is also vulnerable. Fractured ribs which are out of alignment (displaced) are more readily seen on plain radiographs than non-displaced fractures. Displaced rib fractures have a higher risk of injury to the underlying lung and intercostal vessels.[46] Patients will often have localized tenderness over the site of the fracture. An isolated single rib fracture does not usually require hospitalization; however, a patient who has sustained two or more rib fractures (especially in the elderly) is at risk for complications including respiratory compromise, atelectasis, pneumonia, and moderate to severe pain. In such a case, consider hospitalization. If palpation demonstrates tenderness of multiple adjacent ribs a thoracic CT is justified to define the diagnosis, identify associated injuries, and determine if hospitalization is required. Patients with fractures of the lower ribs should be evaluated for potential intra-abdominal injuries. In general, fractures of the superior ribs are associated with greater forces and have a higher potential for underlying pulmonary contusion than other ribs. Fractured ribs are common in the elderly

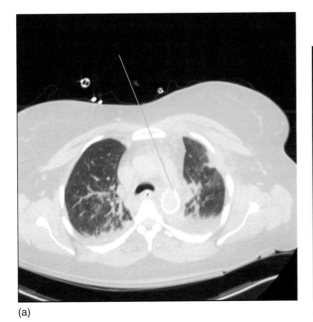

(a)

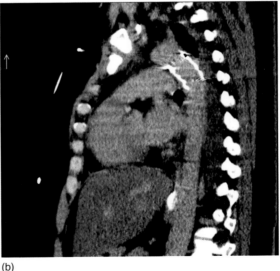

(b)

Figure 12.12 (a and b) The same patient after endovascular stent placement in the aorta. The patient was doing well in follow up 2 years after the injury.

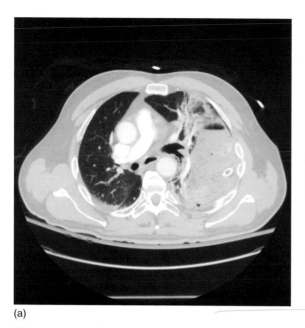

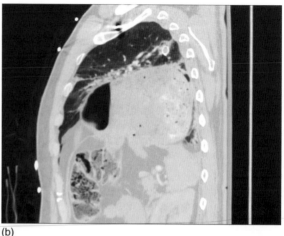

(a) (b)

Figure 12.13 Diaphragmatic rupture of the left hemidiaphragm. (a and b) These computed tomography (CT) slices demonstrate traumatic rupture of the left hemidiaphragm. Here the stomach is clearly seen in the left hemithorax on both coronal (a) and sagittal (b) views of the CT.

due to the high incidence of osteoporosis in this age group; conversely, children have more pliable ribs and fractures are less common with similar forces.

The diagnosis of rib fracture is often made on a chest radiograph; detailed rib views may increase the yield but are often not indicated unless detection of additional fractures would alter the patient's management.

If other injuries can be excluded the treatment of a non-displaced rib fracture is symptomatic. Pain control may be achieved with non-steroidal anti-inflammatory drugs (NSAIDs) but often opiates are required; local nerve blocks may also assist in management. Generally, patients should be admitted if they have three or more rib fractures because these are associated with a higher morbidity.[47]

Sternal fracture

Fractures to the sternum are usually associated with blunt force trauma to the chest. A typical patient is a driver who was not wearing a safety belt and the airbag either was not present or it did not deploy. Patients will complain of localized pain in the anterior chest and often a step-off or crepitus is felt at the site. Usually

fractures are not grossly displaced, management will be symptomatic although recognition should be made of the severity of traumatic injury and appropriate evaluation should be performed looking for pulmonary contusion, aortic rupture, or blunt cardiac injury. A fractured sternum is more common in the elderly because the sternum is more brittle and requires less force to fracture (Figure 12.14).

Occult injuries

Even after an appropriate initial evaluation in the ED some injuries may be difficult to diagnose. Physicians should be aware of the following five particular conditions whose diagnosis may be delayed: (1) aortic rupture; (2) pulmonary contusion; (3) rib fractures; (4) diaphragmatic injury; and (5) pneumothorax (Figure 12.15).

Radiography

Most patients who have sustained thoracic trauma will require a chest radiograph to determine if the patient has sustained a pneumothorax, hemothorax, pulmonary contusion, or injury to the mediastinum or great vessels. However, chest radiography alone is not highly sensitive for the detection of small

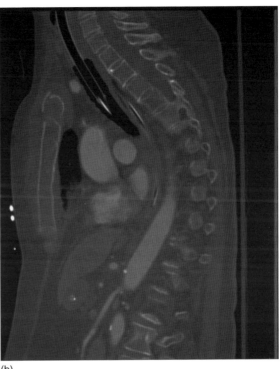

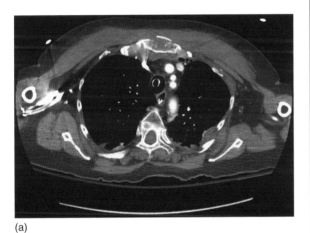

(a)

(b)

Figure 12.14 Computed tomography (CT) images (a) and (b) show a fractured sternum. Fractured sternums are often not obvious on an anteroposterior (AP) chest X-ray and may be seen best on lateral chest X-ray. However, a CT will give a better definition and delineation of a sternal injury.

pneumothoraces, small hemothoraces, early pulmonary contusions, non-displaced fractured ribs, and subtle aortic injuries. In high-risk patients CT scanning may be necessary to define these injuries.

Ultrasound

Ultrasonography for the evaluation of thoracic trauma is divided into the use of portable ultrasound at the bedside and consultative ultrasonography to assess cardiac function to visualize aortic injuries. Portable ultrasonography may be used for the rapid detection of cardiac tamponade, pneumothorax, and hemothorax.

CT scanning in blunt trauma: The majority of patients who have sustained severe blunt thoracic trauma undergo CT scanning expeditiously. Often this is in conjunction with the CT scan of the head, neck, abdomen, and pelvis. Prior to the administration of intravenous contrast media, it is prudent to consider a patient's renal function and potential for pregnancy. However, in the patient in which a rapid means of diagnosis is critical and the information

obtainable by CT scanning is necessary and not easily obtainable by other means with less risk, the physician should not delay the study for considerations of renal function or pregnancy.

For the chest CT, intravenous contrast is usually administered in a timed fashion such that the CT scan can be performed when the contrast bolus has entered the great vessels. This will allow detection of aortic or great vessel injuries. A normal thoracic CT angiogram will exclude great vessel injury, injuries to the thoracic wall, pneumo and hemothoraces, the presence of cardiac tamponade, and most intrathoracic injuries. If the CT of the aorta is indeterminate in the high-risk patient, it should be followed by angiogram.

CT scanning in penetrating trauma: The majority of stab wounds to the chest, particularly to the right chest, do not require CT scanning. However, CT scanning does have the ability to visualize small pneumothoraces and hemothoraces. Stab wounds below the nipple line on either side of the chest may penetrate through the diaphragm and into the abdominal cavity. A CT scan will be able to detect significant

207

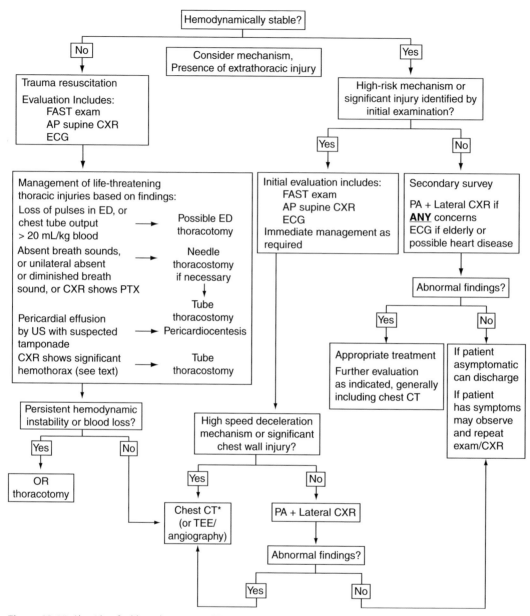

Figure 12.15 Algorithm for blunt chest trauma ED management. AP, anteroposterior; CT, computed tomography; CXR, chest X-ray; ECG, electrocardiogram; ED, emergency department; FAST, focused assessment with sonography in trauma; OR, operating room; PA, posteroanterior; PTX, pneumothorax; TEE, transesophageal echocardiography; US, ultrasound. *This algorithm is a general guide; sophisticated imaging may not be necessary in all circumstances (From Legome L. General approach to blunt thoracic trauma in adults. Available from http://www.uptodate.com, with permission.)

intra-abdominal injury. For stable patients with gunshot wounds, CT scanning of the chest is being increasingly used to follow the track of the projectile. This may be particularly important in cases in which bullets enter the thoracic cavity and strike bone; the wound track may not be clinically obvious in such a case. An unsuspected thoracic injury, vascular injury, or an intra-abdominal injury can be detected using this technique. A CT scan evaluation of transmediastinal gunshot wounds may help alleviate the need for surgery in approximately 70% of stable patients (Table 12.5).[48,49]

Table 12.5 Phases of thoracic evaluation

First phase: during the primary survey

Identification of:

- Upper airway obstruction
- Tension pneumothorax
- Large hemothorax
- Flail chest
- Open chest wound from penetrating injury
- Cardiac tamponade
- Decision if an emergency department thoracotomy is justified

Second phase – after initial stabilization

Identification of:

- Simple pneumothorax
- Hemothorax
- Blunt cardiac injury
- Pulmonary contusion
- Aortic or great vessel injury
- Diaphragmatic injury or penetration
- Wounds traversing the mediastinum

Third phase (may be in the hospital phase of care and evaluation)

Identification of:

- Fractured ribs
- Sternal fractures
- Other less common intrathoracic injuries such as esophageal injury

Laboratory evaluation

A suitable evaluation for the patient with thoracic trauma will include consideration of the following laboratory analyses.

Complete blood count: The hematocrit or hemoglobin determination is often normal initially in major trauma patients because significant hemodilution takes time. However, a baseline measurement may be helpful in interpreting future measurements. The white count may be elevated, but is rarely helpful for clinical decision making.

Coagulation measurements: Twenty-five to fifty percent of severely injured patients have coagulation abnormalities evident upon their arrival at the hospital.[50,51] For this reason, many trauma centers make these tests a portion of their initial laboratory studies. On the other, healthy patients not significantly injured probably have little or no benefit from these studies.

Electrolytes (Chem 7): Routine measurement of electrolytes and renal function is warranted in all moderate or severe thoracic trauma patients. Electrolyte abnormalities, metabolic acidosis, metabolic alkalosis, and renal function can be rapidly assessed.

Beta human chorionic gonadotrophin (hCG) (or a urine hCG) in all women of childbearing years unless there is unquestionable evidence of pregnancy, such as seeing the fetus on abdominal ultrasonography or no possibility of pregnancy such as a previous hysterectomy.

Blood typing is indicated in all cases of severe and moderate chest injury. Clinical guidelines stratify the use of type O-negative blood, type-specific blood, and cross-matched blood.

Toxicology (serum or the urine) in appropriate patients.

Serum troponin and myocardial creatinine kinase: The use of cardiac markers has not shown clear utility in the absence of an abnormal ECG or hemodynamic cardiac instability. They are not generally recommended.

Blood gases are indicated for patients that are intubated or are hypoxic on pulse oximetry.

Serum lactate levels: Many trauma centers advocate a baseline serum lactate level for moderate or severe thoracic injury. The initial serum lactate level in the resuscitation bay is an indication of the amount of tissue hypoperfusion. The rate of clearance of lactate gives an indication of prognosis.

Documentation

The presenting history, symptoms, evaluation and assessment, response to therapy, and medications administered should be carefully documented. If possible the previous medical history, previous surgical history, medications, and allergies should also be recorded. These details are often not available during the initial assessment. If the patient is to be transferred, copies of records (including the laboratory and radiological findings) and consents should accompany the patient.

Table 12.6 Indications for ED surgical consultation

Depending on the capabilities of the ED and the hospital the following should be considered for surgical consultation:

1. **All indications for transfer** as noted in Table 12.7

2. Detection of a **traumatic hemothorax or pneumothorax**

3. **Multiple fractured ribs** – especially in the extremes of age

4. **New cardiac arrhythmia** following trauma

5. **Pulmonary contusion** as detected by X ray, CT scan, oximetry, or by mechanism of injury

6. **Sternal fracture**

7. **Hypotension** at any stage in the patient management

8. **Stab wounds to the chest** (isolated non-life-threatening stab wound can often be managed at the local level)

Management can be completely performed in the ED but if a chest tube is inserted or if the patient is admitted to the hospital for observation then the appropriate service (trauma service; acute care surgery service; general surgery service, or thoracic service) should be notified and physician transfer of patient responsibility performed

CT, computed tomography; ED, emergency department.

Table 12.7 Indications for transfer

Although the exact indications for an interfacility transfer will depend upon the capabilities of the sending and receiving institution, the following may be used as guidelines for transfer to a higher level of care (Level I or a Level II trauma center)

1. **Thoracic injury associated with other multiple severe injuries** (severe head injury, intra-abdominal injury, or multiple long bone or severe pelvic fractures). These would normally be patients with an Injury Severity Score of > 15

2. **Aortic or intrathoracic great vessel injury**

3. **Gunshot wounds to the chest**

4. **Severe pulmonary contusion requiring** continued pulmonary support

5. **Flail chest**

6. **Thoracic injury at the extremes of age** (geriatric and pediatric)

7. **Multiple rib fractures with pulmonary contusion**

8. **Thoracic trauma with severe underlying medical condition** (severe hepatic, renal, or cardiac disease, chronic obstructive pulmonary disease [COPD], advanced pregnancy)

Disposition

Many patients with uncomplicated stab wounds that produce small pneumothoraces or hemothoraces can usually be managed at a non-trauma center, community hospital. More severe injuries (particularly great vessel and cardiac injuries) should be considered for transfer to a major trauma center. Transfer criteria and referral patterns should be developed at the local and regional level; the exact criteria will depend upon the capabilities of the initial hospital receiving the patient. A guideline of which thoracic trauma injuries should be considered for transfer is shown in Tables 12.6 and 12.7.

References

1. LoCicero J, Mattox KL. Epidemiology of chest trauma. *Surg Clin North Am* 1989;**69**:15.

2. MacKenzie EJ, Rivara FP, Jurkovich GJ, et al. A national evaluation of the effect of trauma-center care on mortality. *N Engl J Med* 2006;**354**(4):366–78.

3. McPherson J, Feigin D, Bellamy R. Prevalence of tension pneumothorax in fatally wounded combat casualties. *J Trauma* 2006;**60**:573–8.

4. Cullinane DC, Morris JA, Jr., Bass JG, et al. Needle thoracostomy may not be indicated in the trauma patient. *Injury* 2001;**32**:749–52.

5. Warner KJ, Copass MK, Bulger EM. Paramedic use of needle thoracostomy in the prehospital environment. *Prehosp Emerg Care* 2008;**12**(2):162–8.

6. Leigh-Smith S, Davies, G. Indications for thoracic needle decompression. *J Trauma* 2007;**63**(6):1403–4.

7. Ferrie EP, Collum N, McGobern S. The right place in the right space? Awareness of site for needle thoracocentesis. *Emerg Med J* 2005;**22**(11):788–9.

8. Givens ML, Ayotte K, Manifold C. Needle thoracostomy: implications of computed chest wall thickness. *Acad Emerg Med* 2004;**11**:211–13.

9. Givens N, Tagg A, Owen R. Bilateral tension pneumothorax. *Resuscitation* 2005;**65**:103–5.

10. Kao C l, Lu MS, Chang JP. Successful management of pulmonary artery perforation after chest tube insertion. *J Trauma* 2007;**62**(6):1533.

11. Ball CG, Lord J, Laupland KB, et al. Chest tube complications: how well are we training our residents? *Can J Surg* 2007;**50**(6):450–8.

12. Maxwell RA, Cambell DJ, Fabian TC, et al. Use of presumptive antibiotics following tube thoracostomy for traumatic hemopneumothorax in the prevention of empyema and pneumonia – a multi-center trial. *J Trauma* 2004;**57**(4):742–8.

13. Singh K, Kaur A, Singh A, et al. Intraoperative autotransfusion – a simple and cost effective method. *J Indian Med Assoc* 2007;**105**(12):668–90.

14. Kamiyoshihara M, Ibe T, Takeyoshi I. The utility of an autologous blood salvage system in emergency thoracotomy for a hemothorax after chest trauma. *Gen Thorac Cardiovasc Surg* 2008;**56**(5):222–5.

15. Velamhos GC, Vassiliu P, Chan LS, et al. Influence of flail chest on outcome among patients with severe thoracic cage trauma. *Int Surg* 2002;**87**(4):240–4.

16. Richardson JD, Franklin GA, Heffley S, et al. Operative fixation of chest wall fractures: an underused procedure? *Am Surg* 2007;**73**(6):591–6.

17. Tanaka H, Yukioka T, Yamaguti Y, et al. Surgical stabilization or internal pneumatic stabilization? A prospective randomized study of management of severe flail chest patients. *J Trauma* 2002;**52**(4):727–32.

18. Menaker J, Cushman J, Vermillion JM, Rosenthal RE, Scalea TM. Ultrasound-diagnosed cardiac tamponade after blunt abdominal trauma-treated with emergent thoracotomy. *J Emerg Med* 2007;**32**(1):99–103.

19. Sikka R, Millham FH, Feldman JA. Analysis of occupational exposures associated with emergency department thoracotomy. *J Trauma* 2004; **56**(4):867–72.

20. Powell DW, Moore EE, Cothren CC, et al. Is emergency department resuscitative thoracotomy futile care for the critically injured patient requiring prehospital cardiopulmonary resuscitation? *J Am Coll Surg* 2004;**199**(2):211–15.

21. Buchman TG. Letter: emergency department resuscitative thoracotomy. *J Am Coll Surg* 2005; **200**(1):148.

22. Soldati G, Testa A, Sher S, et al. Diagnostic accuracy of lung ultrasonography in the emergency department. *Chest* 2008;**133**(1):204–11.

23. Chan SS. The role of simple aspiration in the management of primary spontaneous pneumothorax. *J Emerg Med* 2008;**34**(2):131–8.

24. Kelly AM, Kerr D, Clooney M. Outcomes of emergency department patients treated for primary spontaneous pneumothorax. *Chest* 2008; **134**(5):1033–6.

25. Wolfman NT, Myers WS, Glauser SJ, Meredith JW, Chen MY. Validity of CT classification on management of occult pneumothorax. *Am J Roentgenol* 1998;**171**(5):1317–20.

26. Brasel KJ, Stafford RE, Weigelt JA, Tenquist JE, Borgstrom DC. Treatment of occult pneumothoraces from blunt trauma. *J Trauma* 1999;**46**(6):987–90.

27. Holmes JF, Brant WE, Bogren HG, London KL, Kuppermann N. Prevalence and importance of pneumothoraces visualised on abdominal CT scan in children with blunt trauma. *J Trauma* 2000; **50**(3):516–20.

28. Brooks A, Davies B, Smethhurst M, Connolly J. Emergency ultrasound in the acute assessment of haemothorax. *Emerg Med J* 2004;**21**:44–6.

29. McEwan K, Thompson P. Ultrasound to detect haemothorax after chest injury. *Emerg Med J* 2007;**24**:581–2.

30. Schultz TM, Trunkey DD. Blunt cardiac injury. *Crit Care Clin* 2004;**20**:57–70.

31. Barry J, Maron MD, Thomas E, et al. Clinical profile and spectrum of *commotio cordis*. *JAMA* 2002;**287**:1142–6.

32. Ismailov RM, Ness RB, Redmond CK, et al. Trauma associated with cardiac dysrhythmias: results from a large matched case-control study. *J Trauma* 2007;**62**:1186–91.

33. Elie MC. Blunt cardiac injury. *Mt Sinai J Med* 2006;**73**:542–52.

34. Bertinchant JP, Polge A, Mohty D, et al. Evaluation of incidence, clinical significance, and prognostic value of circulating cardiac troponin I and T elevation in hemodynamically stable patients with suspected myocardial contusion after blunt chest trauma. *J Trauma* 2000;**48**:924–31.

35. Velmahos GC, Karaiskakis M, Salim A, et al. Normal electrocardiography and serum troponin I levels preclude the presence of clinically significant blunt cardiac injury. *J Trauma* 2003;**54**:45–51.

36. Wanek S, Mayberry JC. Blunt thoracic trauma: flail chest, pulmonary contusion, and blast injury. *Crit Care Clin* 2004;**20**:71–81.

37. Mirvis SE, Shanmuganathan K, Buell J, et al. Use of spiral computed tomography for the assessment of blunt trauma patients with potential aortic injury. *J Trauma* 1998;**45**:922–30.

38. Demetriades D, Velmahos GC, Scalea TM, et al. Diagnosis and treatment of blunt thoracic aortic injuries: changing perspectives. *J Trauma* 2008; **64**(6):1415–18; discussion 18–19.

39. Karmy-Jones R, Nicholls S, Gleason TG. The endovascular approach to acute aortic trauma. *Thorac Surg Clin* 2007;**17**(1):109–28.

40. Kasirajan K, Marek J, Langsfeld M. Endovascular management of acute traumatic thoracic aneurysm. *J Trauma* 2002;**52**(2):387–90.

41. Demetriades D, Velmahos GC, Scalea TM, et al. (American Association for the Surgery of Trauma Thoracic Aortic Injury Study Group.) Operative repair or endovascular stent graft in blunt traumatic thoracic aortic injuries: results of an American Association for the Surgery of Trauma Multicenter Study. *J Trauma* 2008;**64**(3):561–70; discussion 70–1.

42. Bent CL, Matson MB, Sobeh M, et al. Endovascular management of acute blunt traumatic thoracic aortic injury: a single center experience. *J Vasc Surg* 2007; **46**(5):920–7.

43. Killeen KL, Mirvis SE, Shanmuganathan K. Helical CT of diaphragmatic rupture caused by blunt trauma. *AJR Am J Roentgenol* 1999;**173**:1611–16.

44. Mihos P, Potaris K, Gakidis J, et al. Traumatic rupture of the diaphragm: experience with 65 patients. *Injury* 2003;**34**(3):169–72.

45. Stassen NA, Lukan JK, Spain DA, et al. Reevaluation of diagnostic procedures for transmediastinal gunshot wounds. *J Trauma* 2002;**53**(4):635–8; discussion 8.

46. Ashrafian H, Kumar P, Sarkar PK, et al. Delayed penetrating intrathoracic injury from multiple rib fractures. *J Trauma* 2005;**58**:858–9.

47. Sirmali M, Turut H, Topcu S, et al. A comprehensive analysis of traumatic rib fractures: morbidity, mortality and management. *Eur J Cardio Thorac Surg* 2003;**24**(1):133–8.

48. Magnotti LJ, Weinberg JA, Schroeppel TJ, et al. Initial chest CT obviates the need for repeat chest radiograph after penetrating thoracic trauma. *Am Surg* 2007;**73** (6):569–72.

49. Mirvis SE. Imaging of acute thoracic injury: the advent of MDCT screening. *Semin Ultrasound CT MR* 2005;**26**(5):305–31.

50. Brohi K, Singh J, Heron M, Coats T. Acute traumatic coagulopathy. *J Trauma* 2003;**54**(6):1127–30.

51. MacLeod JB, Lynn M, McKenney MG, Cohn SM, Murtha M. Early coagulopathy predicts mortality in trauma. *J Trauma* 2003;**55**(1):39–44.

Chapter 13

Abdominal trauma

Jennifer Isenhour and John Marx

Introduction

Abdominal trauma is frequently encountered in the emergency department (ED) and emergency physicians (EP) must be prepared to identify and expeditiously manage these patients, avoiding the most serious pitfall of missed or delayed diagnosis. Newer high resolution computed tomography (CT), bedside ultrasound (US), diagnostic laparoscopy (DL) and the ability to serially evaluate patients augments the armamentarium of the EP and trauma surgeon in identifying injury associated with blunt and penetrating abdominal trauma.

Blunt abdominal trauma (BAT) while frequent in the ED, is often difficult to diagnose with accuracy; it is commonly associated with extra-abdominal injuries. Most commonly blunt injuries occur after a motor vehicle collision (MVC), followed in decreasing frequency by a pedestrian being struck, a direct abdominal blow, or a fall.[1,2] In addition, intimate partner violence, elder abuse, and child abuse may all result in BAT. All intra-abdominal solid organs are at risk, but the spleen is most often injured and may be an isolated finding in nearly two thirds of abdominal trauma patients. The liver is the next most common, and hollow viscera, usually the intestine, are less frequently involved.[3]

The number of homicides committed with a firearm exceeds the number of homicides from all other forms of violence. This is due to their greater velocity and potential for widespread damage. Firearm deaths are greatest among African-Americans aged 15–34 years, closely followed by Hispanics in the same age range.

Box 13.1   Essentials of abdominal trauma

- Most commonly blunt injuries occur after a MVC, followed in decreasing frequency by a pedestrian being struck, a direct abdominal blow, or a fall.

- In blunt trauma the spleen is most often injured and may be an isolated finding in nearly two thirds of abdominal trauma patients. The liver is the next most common, and hollow viscera, usually the intestine, are less frequently involved.
- Penetrating abdominal trauma (PAT) is less commonly observed in the ED when compared to BAT, but it still carries a high morbidity and mortality.
- Stabbings are encountered three times more often than firearm injuries, but the latter have greater associated morbidity and account for up to 90% of mortality for PAT.

Clinical anatomy and pathophysiology

Blunt abdominal trauma

There are three main physiologic entities which lead to injury after BAT.

First, outward forces from a seat belt may create a sudden or pronounced increase in intra-abdominal pressure resulting in rupture or burst of a hollow viscus. Second, abdominal organs may be compressed between the abdominal wall and the spinal column. This crushing effect usually injures solid viscera such as the spleen and liver. Those with lax abdominal wall musculature, for instance the elderly, children, or alcoholics, are at increased risk for this type of injury. Finally, both hollow and solid organs, and their vascular pedicles, are at risk of injury from shearing forces that may cause laceration. Areas of fixed organ attachment are especially vulnerable to this type of injury, particularly following sudden acceleration–deceleration as occurs in head-on MVCs.

Seat belt injuries deserve special mention, as their use, while shown to decrease morbidity after MVC, is associated with some specific injury patterns. For example, three-point restraint systems when positioned incorrectly (for example, placing the shoulder restraint under the arm) may cause intrathoracic and intra-abdominal organs to be compressed and injured. Lap-belt only restraint systems create a fulcrum for compression of bowel against the vertebral column or bowel upon bowel creating a closed loop, which may in turn rupture due to an increase in intraluminal pressure.[4] During the second and third trimesters of pregnancy, improperly worn lap belts (those placed over the uterus rather than under it) place the fetus and mother at risk.

Ecchymosis of the abdominal wall in the distribution of the lap belt (a seat belt sign) is found in relatively few patients with BAT, but its presence correlates with a significantly increased risk of underlying intra-abdominal injury, compared to similar patients without the finding.[5,6]

Penetrating abdominal trauma

Knives, hand guns, shotguns, and rifles are the traditional implements of penetrating trauma. However, flying glass, arrows, fence posts, horned animals, scissors, arrows, grenades, and bombs may all create nonconventional PAT. Gunshot wounds (GSWs) have the highest mortality due to their increased kinetic energy, but SWs are encountered more frequently. In either case, the bowel, and then the liver, are most commonly injured.[7]

Stab wounds

Stab wounds are most commonly located in the left upper quadrant followed by the right upper quadrant then the lower quadrants. Ten percent will involve the chest and up to 20% of patients will have more than one SW. Most SWs don't cause serious intra-abdominal injury even with penetration through the peritoneum. Anterior abdominal SWs enter the peritoneum in up to 70% of cases, but only half of these will inflict serious injury.[8] Flank and back wounds penetrate 44% and 15% of the time, respectively. Low chest wounds have increased rates of diaphragmatic injury, pneumothorax, and pericardial tamponade and nearly a 15% rate of coincident intra-abdominal injury.[9,10]

Gunshot wounds

The wounding potential is most closely correlated with the amount of kinetic energy (KE = 1/2 MV

Table 13.1 Muzzle velocity

Type	Approximate velocity	Weapon
Low velocity	< 1100 fps	Pistol
Medium velocity	1100–2000 fps	Lever action rifle
High velocity	> 2000 fps	Assault rifle

fps, feet per second.

where M = mass and V = velocity) imparted by the bullet to the patient.[2] The greater the mass of the bullet and the faster it travels, the more energy present and thus increased potential for tissue destruction. Additionally the viscoelastic properties of the tissue transversed and the stability of the missile also contribute to the amount of destruction.

Impact velocity, which is the main contributor to the kinetic energy of the bullet in the patient, is based on the distance of the firearm from the patient, the muzzle velocity of the firearm and characteristics of the bullet itself, and is the most important factor in determining the potential for injury (Table 13.1).

High and medium velocity ballistics have an "explosive" effect on tissues. This can create cavities for temporary passage which may in turn indirectly injure nearby organs. There are case reports of intra-abdominal injury even with extra-abdominal missile passage.[11]

Missiles may also contaminate wounds by "dragging in" foreign material such as shotgun wadding and clothing. The wound tract or permanent cavity may be much smaller than the temporary cavity the bullet passed through. This may lead to underestimation of injury. Finally, the bullet may fragment once inside the abdominal cavity causing increased destruction.

Shotgun wounds

Shotguns are designed to shoot small rapidly moving targets. The shape of the pellets (round) experience a large amount of drag through the air and thus decelerate rapidly after leaving the barrel. The kinetic energy imparted to the patient is based on the pellet size (mass) used, the number of pellets, the type and amount of powder and the barrel choke (constriction); but the most important variable is the distance of the victim from the weapon to the victim. The closer the range the more tightly clustered the pellets and the more lethal the shot (Table 13.2).

Tissue damage is proportional to the specific gravity and inversely proportional to the elastic properties of the affected organ (as such, the liver is more vulnerable to injury than the lungs). The brain is the most vulnerable organ for several reasons: its specific gravity 1.01–1.02 is the same as the liver, the brain tissue is irreplaceable, and the brain is encased in the skull, which must be shattered with resultant secondary missiles (bone fragments) when penetrated. Wadding and other contaminants may be driven into Type II or III shotgun wounds (Figure 13.1).

Prehospital

The basics of prehospital medicine applies to both BAT and PAT. Patients must be expeditiously evacuated to the closest appropriate facility. Death from uncontrolled hemorrhage and ensuing shock is the major threat.

Traditionally early and aggressive initiation of intravenous (IV) fluid resuscitation was standard in these patients. However there is concern that this may lead to increased bleeding secondary to dilution of clotting factors as well as loss of soft clot with increased blood pressure. Currently there are no authoritative studies to support or refute use of early crystalloid resuscitation in patients with hemorrhagic shock. Only a few studies have addressed the question in human trauma patients, and the data, while suggesting that the less aggressive approach may be better, is not definitive. Further research may define the best approach.[12]

Covering open wounds and eviscerations, and securing implements in situ, help prevent further contamination and injury.

Emergency Medical Service personnel are important in providing historical factors surrounding the mechanism of injury. For BAT due to vehicular collision, the number of fatalities at the scene, type of vehicles involved, velocity of the vehicles, amount of intrusion, rollover, steering wheel deformity, use of seat belts and airbags, and patient location within the vehicle may assist the EP needs in assessing the patient.[13,14] In PAT, the weapon involved, the size and length of a blade, the number of gunshots heard, the distance of the patient from the gun, and the position of the patient are all important facts prehospital care providers can supply.

Table 13.2 Shotgun wounds

Type	Distance	Pellet spread	Injuries
Type I	> 7 yards	> 25 cm	Subcutaneous and fascia penetration
Type II	3–7 yards	10–25 cm	Large number of perforated structures
Type III	< 3 yards	< 10 cm "point blank" range	Mass destruction/ highest mortality

Box 13.2 Essentials of prehospital care in abdominal trauma

- The basics of prehospital medicine applies to both BAT and PAT.
- Expeditiously evacuate to the closest appropriate facility; death from uncontrolled hemorrhage and ensuing shock is the major threat.

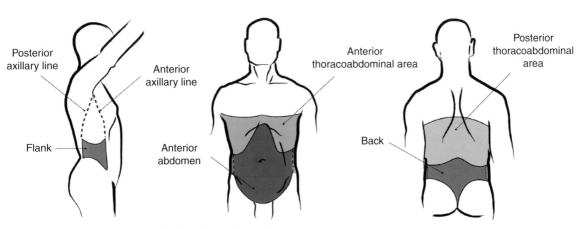

Figure 13.1 Anatomic drawings of the boundaries of the abdomen.

Box 13.2 (cont.)

- There are no definite answers whether more or less aggressive fluid resuscitation is best in the field in the patient with ongoing hemorrhage, although some data (especially in penetrating trauma) suggests less aggressive may be better.
- Covering open wounds and eviscerations, and securing implements in situ, help prevent further contamination and injury.

Emergency department evaluation and management

Blunt abdominal trauma

Common presentations

Depending on the severity of injury, patients sustaining BAT present with a variety of findings ranging from inconsequential up to shock and coma. Patients with abdominal tenderness or peritonitis, evidence of gastrointestinal bleeding, and hypotension without signs of extra-abdominal hemorrhage suggest presence of intraperitoneal injury. However, sometimes these signs are not evident early in the resuscitation. Some patients, seemingly uninjured, have occult intra-abdominal trauma, and can only be discovered through additional testing or serial evaluation.

Initial evaluation

Physical examination

Patients should be fully undressed and exposed for a complete evaluation. Unstable patients may require resuscitation concurrent with physical examination.

Even though the physical examination in stable alert patients has a reported sensitivity $< 65\%$ for detecting intra-abdominal injury, it remains the first line of evaluation. In the proper patient population, e.g., otherwise healthy and no other injuries, it is probably an excellent definitive test.[15] In patients with altered mental status, intoxication, closed head injury, or a distracting injury, physical examination is even less reliable and close, frequent re-evaluation as well as diagnostic testing based on clinical suspicion warranted.

Hypotension in the absence of extra-abdominal causes of blood loss usually results from splenic or liver injury. However, even if an extra-abdominal cause of hemorrhage is present, evaluation for concomitant intra-abdominal injury is warranted if the

mechanism fits. Up to 10% of those with closed head injury and 7% of those with extra-abdominal injuries will have an intra-abdominal injury.[16]

Certain physical exam findings portend intra-abdominal injuries. Patients with left lower rib fractures may have associated splenic injury and those with right lower rib fractures may have associated liver injury.[17] Patients with abdominal wall ecchymosis from a lap belt have injury, typically hollow viscus, up to one third of the time.[6]

While the presence of concerning physical exam findings is helpful, their absence does not rule out intraperitoneal injury. Adjuvant laboratory and radiology testing, as well as serial evaluation, helps to avoid missed intra-abdominal injuries.

A nasogastric tube placed in those without concern for facial trauma, decompresses the stomach and identifies upper gastrointestinal hemorrhage. Similarly a Foley catheter detects gross hematuria and provides a means to follow urine output. The information gleaned from these studies should be balanced with the invasiveness, discomfort, and risk. These should be reserved for patients with a real concern for occult injury or known significant traumatic injury.

Trauma room studies

Radiology: A chest radiograph is a useful adjuvant test. It may demonstrate the presence of rib fractures, mediastinal air, hemothorax, and pneumothorax, allowing for directed interventions and raising suspicion for coincident intra-abdominal injury. In those patients able to sit upright, free air under the diaphragm strongly suggests hollow viscous perforation.

Pelvis X-rays are helpful in identifying those patients with open book or shear fractures in which severe hemorrhage occurs. Emergent interventions such as pelvic wrapping may limit blood loss in these patients. Furthermore, the knowledge that a pelvic fracture exists helps direct resuscitation and evaluation for concomitant intra-abdominal injury. On the other hand, stable patients with no pelvic pain or patients with a stable pelvis and normal blood pressure who are getting a rapid CT scan may forego the trauma room pelvic film.

Laboratory: Patients with signs of more than minimal injury should have a baseline hematocrit or hemoglobin, and those with hypotension or indications for emergent laparotomy should have their blood typed and screened and often cross-matched. Other testing such as base deficit is frequently utilized, but these values may lag behind physical examination findings.[18] White blood cell count, pancreatic enzymes, liver function testing, and amylase have historically been part of the panel of laboratory tests ordered for those with BAT, but these are unreliable indicators of intraperitoneal injury.[19,20] These should be ordered based on clinician judgment rather than empirically on every patient. All women of childbearing age with unknown pregnancy status should have a urine pregnancy test. Gross hematuria in patients with shock indicates abdominal injury in 65% of patients, while microscopic hematuria in unstable patients portend intra-abdominal injury 29% of the time.[21] Microscopic hematuria alone, however, does not necessarily indicate a higher risk of important intra-abdominal injury. Toxicologic screening adds little to the initial clinical assessment of abdominal trauma patients, except in those patients with altered mental status in whom closed head injury is a possibility.[22]

Ultrasound: The advent of bedside US has changed the emergent management of BAT. It rapidly detects the presence of hemoperitoneum and has a reported sensitivity of up to 95% for distinguishing as little as 100 cc of fluid.[23] Serial bedside US increases its sensitivity in patients with BAT.[24,25] Recent small studies adding sonographic contrast demonstrate accuracy for identifying solid viscus injury with active bleeding, although this is not actively performed in most centers at this point.[26–28] It is non-invasive, portable, and imparts no radiation to the patient. Visualization of the mediastinum and pericardium may be concurrently performed.

Disadvantages of US include the inability to differentiate ascites from hemoperitoneum. Therefore, its value in patients with liver disease and known ascites is limited. It cannot provide any information about the retroperitoneum, and diaphragmatic, hollow viscus, and subcapsular solid viscus injuries are not well visualized due to their minimal bleeding.[29] Uncooperative, agitated, and obese patients are not ideal candidates and results may not be accurate in these patients. If an US is indeterminate, then further diagnostic studies are warranted.[25]

Ultrasound is particularly helpful in the rapid triage of hypotensive patients with BAT who have no other signs of extra-abdominal injury or cause of hypotension.[30] It is replacing diagnostic peritoneal aspirate in the initial evaluation of these patients and typically those with a positive US in this setting

proceed to exploratory laparotomy. However, US is not as sensitive as DPL and its availability should not preclude the use of DPL.

Box 13.3 Advantages and disadvantages of bedside US

Advantages	Disadvantages
• It rapidly detects the presence of hemoperitoneum.	• Inability to differentiate ascites from hemoperitoneum.
• It is non-invasive, portable, and imparts no radiation to the patient.	• It cannot provide any information about the retroperitoneum, and diaphragmatic, hollow viscus, and subcapsular solid viscus injuries are not well visualized due to their minimal bleeding.
• Ultrasound is particularly helpful in the rapid triage of hypotensive patients with BAT and has largely supplanted DPL.	• Uncooperative, agitated, and obese patients are not ideal candidates and results may not be accurate in these patients.

Diagnostic peritoneal tap: For hemodynamically unstable patients with multiple injuries and a negative or indeterminate US, a diagnostic peritoneal tap (DPT) rapidly determines the presence of hemoperitoneum. When 10 ml or greater of gross blood is aspirated in these patients, emergent operative intervention to control hemorrhage from solid viscus or vascular injury is indicated (Figure 13.2).

Acute interventions

Initial management is focused on stabilization and identification of those patients with hemoperitoneum requiring emergent intervention.

Intubation: Unstable patients with evidence of airway compromise or severely compromised hemodynamics or anticipated ED course requiring them to leave the department (losing the ability to closely monitor their airway status) need emergent intubation. This is a clinical decision based on suspicion of underlying pathology, patient conditions, skills, and available resources.

Intravenous access: Obtain IV access for fluid and blood administration. In patients with hemodynamic

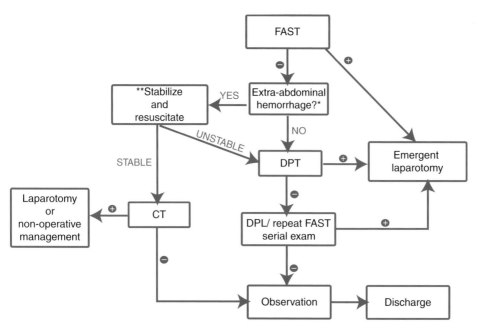

Figure 13.2 Algorithm for unstable blunt abdominal trauma. CT, computed tomography; DPL, diagnostic peritoneal lavage; DPT, diagnostic peritoneal tap; DPT+, > 10 ml blood aspirated; FAST, focused abdominal sonography in trauma. *Long bone fracture, hemothorax, scalp laceration, pelvic fracture. **Pelvic wrapping, splinting, whipstitch, tube thoracostomy.

instability or potential for this, obtain a minimum of two IV lines, although they may need addition when critically ill.

Tube thoracostomy: Patients with BAT in the thoracoabdominal region are at increased risk for concomitant chest trauma including pneumothorax or hemothorax. In unstable patients and those undergoing positive pressure ventilation, these injuries require emergent tube thoracostomy to prevent further hemodynamic compromise and, in the case of hemothorax, to monitor blood loss.

Thoracotomy: While a rare procedure in the ED for those with BAT, in patients with traumatic arrest or "pre-arrest" in the ED, thoracotomy with cross-clamping of the aorta may help control bleeding and shunt blood to the heart and brain while resuscitative measures ensue.

Emergent laparotomy: Using trauma room studies such as chest and pelvic radiographs, US, and DPL/DPT, coupled with physical examination identifies those patients requiring emergent laparotomy. The five parameters in Table 13.3 guide operative intervention.

Uncontrolled intraperitoneal hemorrhage is an immediate life threat and should be a priority among diagnostic and therapeutic interventions. For example, the altered patient with hypotension and

Table 13.3 Indicators for emergent laparotomy in blunt abdominal trauma (BAT)

1. Continued profound hypotension despite resuscitation in a patient strongly suspected to have intra-abdominal injury

2. Presence of unequivocal peritonitis on physical examination

3. Pneumoperitoneum suggesting viscous rupture as visualized on radiographs

4. Diaphragmatic rupture visualized on radiographs

5. Persistent gastrointestinal bleeding as evidenced by nasogastric tube output or hemetemesis not felt to be due to swallowed blood

hemoperitoneum should have laparotomy prior to CT scan of the head. Likewise radiographs of extremities can also wait, and if needed emergent fasciotomy can be done empirically in the operating room if a serious concern. However, in patients who are stable, who may have intra-abdominal injury that does not require immediate operative intervention (e.g., bladder rupture, hollow viscus injury, diaphragmatic injury), other life-threatening extra-abdominal injuries such as severe closed head trauma and pelvic fractures may assume precedence (Table 13.3).

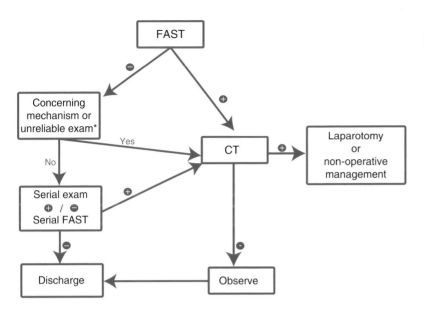

Figure 13.3 **Algorithm for stable blunt abdominal trauma.** CT, computed tomography; FAST, focused abdominal sonography in trauma. *Concerning mechanism: fatality at scene, rollover, intrusion, prolonged extrication, ejection. Unreliable exam: altered mental status, intoxication, distracting injury.

Secondary evaluation

Stable patients require continued evaluation once an immediate need for operative intervention has been removed. Computed tomography is the preferred diagnostic test for these patients as it allows for detection of specific organ injury, active intraperitoneal hemorrhage and evaluation of extra-abdominal structures. Ultrasound and DPL may also be utilized. Diagnostic laparoscopy is rarely utilized in evaluation of BAT unless there is suspicion for diaphragmatic injury or HVI (Figure 13.3).

Computed tomography: Multislice scanners with high resolution and the ability to rapidly perform studies make them the most often used test for the evaluation of BAT.[31] While it doesn't have 100% sensitivity for detecting all intra-abdominal injuries (especially hollow viscus and pancreatic injury), it does provide invaluable data for solid organ injury while additionally providing information about the retroperitoneal space, diaphragm, vascular structures, and vertebrae.[32,33] Some centers advocate CT for all patients with BAT regardless of physical examination findings, citing a change in management in up to 19% of patients when CT was utilized, although this study is not consistent with usual findings and does not reflect current standard of care.[34] As non-operative management for many splenic and hepatic injuries has become the most common approach, CT is important in delineating

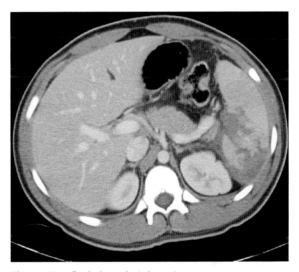

Figure 13.4 Grade 3–4 splenic laceration.

those injuries amenable to this treatment algorithm (Table 13.4[35] and Figure 13.4).[36–39] It decreases the number of non-therapeutic laparotomies and therefore morbidity and mortality associated with liver and spleen injuries.[40] Detection of hollow viscus injuries is improving, even when no oral contrast is given and only IV contrast is utilized.[41,42]

Disadvantages include significant radiation exposure and cost associated with the increased use of CT. Additionally, patients must leave the trauma bay and

219

Table 13.4 Splenic and hepatic injury grades by computed tomography (CT) findings[35]

	CT finding
Splenic injury grade	
1	Capsular tear; laceration < 1 cm; subcapsular hematoma < 10%
2	Laceration 1–3 cm not involving trabecular vessel; subcapsular hematoma 10–50%; intraparenchymal hematoma < 5 cm
3	Laceration > 3 cm or involving trabecular vessels; subcapsular hematoma > 50% or expanding; ruptured subcapsular or parenchymal hematoma
4	Laceration involving segmental or hilar vessels producing major devascularization (> 25% of spleen);
5	Completely shattered spleen; hilar vascular injury which devascularizes spleen
Hepatic injury grade	
1	Subcapsular hematoma < 10%; laceration < 1 cm in depth
2	Subcapsular hematoma 10–50%; laceration 1–3 cm in depth; parenchymal hematoma ≤ 10 cm in length
3	Subcapsular hematoma > 50%; laceration > 3 cm in depth; parenchymal hematoma > 10 cm in length
4	Laceration 25–75% of lobe or 1–3 Couinaud segments
5	Laceration > 75% of lobe or > 3 Couinaud segments; retrohepatic inferior vena cava or major hepatic vein injury

travel to the CT scanner, making it less ideal in those who may be uncooperative, have tenuous hemodynamic status, or other extra-abdominal injuries requiring emergent interventions.[43] Finally, coincidental hollow viscus and mesentery injury in patients with BAT and splenic or liver injuries is still possible. While CT is improving, it still has decreased sensitivity for these injuries as well as those to the diaphragm and pancreas.[41,42]

Ultrasound: Stable patients with a positive US, require further delineation of their injuries usually via CT, as many solid viscus injuries are managed non-operatively. Ultrasound is not well suited for identifying subcapsular solid viscus injuries, bowel, retroperitoneal, and diaphragmatic injuries.[44–46] But for many patients, US can decrease the need for CT or DPL.[47,48] A negative focused abdominal sonography in trauma (FAST) coupled with negative serial physical examinations during an observation period of up to 24 hours typically excludes injury.[49]

Diagnostic peritoneal lavage: As mentioned above, DPT is best utilized in unstable patients to help triage them to laparotomy. If a DPT does not show > 10 ml of blood or EI contents then further evaluation for intra-abdominal injury is needed. Diagnostic peritoneal lavage is a bedside test which detects the presence of hollow viscus and diaphragmatic injury in addition to solid organ injury.[50,51] It is especially useful in those patients in whom CT is not amenable due to other injuries or instability and whose physical examination is not reliable (those with severe closed head injury or intubated sedated patients). It also can be useful with an equivocal or unclear ultrasound and a suspicion of serious intra-abdominal injury.

A positive test is one with > 100 000 red blood cells per high powered field (RBC/hpf) present in the lavage effluent. Gross bowel or bladder contents is also considered a positive lavage. If there are concerns for diaphragmatic injury, the threshold for positivity is dropped to 5000 RBC/hpf, which increases the sensitivity of the test at the expense of specificity. False negatives occur when the lavage catheter is placed into the preperitoneal space, or omentum obstructs egress of fluid, or there are large diaphragmatic tears allowing fluid to enter the thoracic cavity instead of returning, or adhesions compartmentalize the lavage fluid. Inadequate control of hemostasis when introducing the catheter into the peritoneal cavity, or passage of the catheter into a hematoma create false positive studies.

The DPT portion of DPL may be revealing in patients with multisystem injury and hypotension. Otherwise DPL has had decreasing value in the BAT patient as many of the injuries it previously found are non-operative. However, in addition to serving as a rapid triage instrument in patients with hypotension and blunt multisystem injury, it can also be used to detect hollow viscus rupture in the severely obtunded patient in whom the CT either shows solid organ injury and there is ongoing concern for hollow viscus or it shows only isolated free fluid.

Special cases

Pelvic fracture: Patients with pelvic fractures are at greater risk for concomitant and potentially life-threatening intra-abdominal hemorrhage. In a patient found to have active intraperitoneal hemorrhage and hypotension, laparotomy should ensue. If the search for intraperitoneal hemorrhage is negative in the unstable patient, the presumption should be that the source of hypotension is retroperitoneal hemorrhage secondary to the pelvic fracture, in which case interventional angiography and embolization or "damage control" exploration and packing is undertaken. External fixators and various methods of attempting to stabilize and compress the pelvis, particularly with open book fractures, are adjuncts that may be undertaken in the patient with unstable pelvic fractures.

Closed head injury: Patients with concomitant closed head injury and hemorrhagic shock ascribed to intraperitoneal hemorrhage can pose a conundrum. In patients without lateralizing findings, the need for emergent craniotomy is extremely low. If there are lateralizing findings and the patient can be stabilized, CT is indicated to determine whether active intracranial hemorrhage amenable to intervention is present. If the patient with intra-abdominal injury cannot be stabilized hemodynamically and has lateralizing neurologic signs, exploratory laparotomy prior to CT is indicated. While under anesthesia, if intracranial hemorrhage with herniation is strongly suspected clinically, concomitant intracranial monitoring device or craniotomy may be performed by neurosurgeons without prior neuroimaging. In some centers, mobile CT scan may be available.

Treatment

Solid organ injury

Most injuries to the spleen and liver are amenable to non-operative management.[52] A CT scan of the abdomen allows accurate grading of the severity of injury. Knowing the extent of injury allows the clinician to rely upon serial physical examination and monitoring of hemodynamic status and hematocrit to make further operative decisions in these patients.[53]

Most Grade 1 and 2 injuries are managed non-operatively. Some centers advocate this approach for Grade 3 and higher injuries as well.[54] Therapeutic angiography and embolization of vessels may augment

this approach. Centers advocating non-operative management of high-grade injuries should anticipate the need for possible operative intervention and have the personnel available to quickly convert to this treatment plan. Patients with distracting extra-abdominal injuries or altered mental status rendering their exams unreliable are less optimal candidates for this less conservative approach.

Pitfalls include increased use of blood products, underestimation of severity of injury, missed concurrent HVI, and unsuccessful attempts at embolization of hemorrhage which therefore must be operatively repaired. Those patients with rare blood types, those who refuse blood products, or those with underlying coagulopathy should undergo operation sooner rather than later when non-operative management fails. Non-operative management is more likely to fail when the patient has a non-hepatic injury (i.e., a spleen or renal injury), a positive FAST at presentation, > 300 ml of intra-abdominal free fluid on CT and requires a blood transfusion.[38]

Hollow viscus injuries

All of these injuries with perforation or devascularization must be managed operatively. Some minor contusion or bowel wall hemorrhage may be observed. As previously mentioned, diagnosis of hollow viscus injuries is difficult and thus the physician must be vigilant, especially in the multi-injured patient.[55] Patients with persistent significant abdominal tenderness, peritoneal signs, and CT presence of free fluid without evidence of solid organ injury should raise the suspicion for the presence of a HVI.[45] However, even those patients with negative CTs may have undetected HVI in up to 13% of cases, and as time to diagnosis increases, so do complications. Those patients with concerns cited above and a negative CT should generally remain for a period of observation.[45,56]

Penetrating abdominal trauma

Initial evaluation

Physical examination

As with all trauma patients, those with PAT must be fully undressed and exposed to ensure complete evaluation. Wounds may be obscured by clothing, body habitus or blood, or "hidden" in the axilla, groin, buttocks, skin folds, or scalp. In those sustaining GSWs, finding the number and area of wounds may help elucidate whether there is a retained missile as well as the potential of underlying abdominal injury. However, bullets do not always maintain a straight path and it is difficult, if not sometimes impossible, to ascertain whether a wound is an entrance or exit in the ED.[57] Both a nasogastric tube and foley catheter should be placed if no contraindications exist. If the patient will clearly require the operating room, this may be done there.

Hemodynamic instability: Shock usually results from massive hemorrhage due to solid viscus or vascular injury. These patients should proceed from the ED directly to the operating room if there is PAT and no other signs of extra-abdominal causes of hypotension and shock such as tension pneumothorax, hemothorax, pericardial tamponade, or significant blood loss from lacerations involving the scalp or other extra-abdominal areas.[58]

Peritoneal signs: While several studies have noted that physical examination can be inprecise, most centers agree that if unequivocal peritonitis is present (i.e., involuntary guarding/abdominal rigidity), particularly in those with delayed presentation in whom hollow viscus perforation may be present, these patients should undergo exploratory laparotomy.[59]

Evisceration: This used to be an unequivocal criterion for mandatory laparotomy, however, newer studies show this practice may be unnecessary.[60] Up to one third of patients with evisceration after PAT may have a non-therapeutic laparotomy. Therefore some advocate serial examinations instead of mandatory laparotomy, especially in those stable patients with only omental evisceration.[58] Others cite an incidence of up to 80% of patients having major intraperitoneal injury requiring operative repair when omentum or viscus herniation is found. They advocate exploratory laparotomy as the next step in these patients.[61] Evisceration after GSWs generally require exploratory laparotomy. The GSW mechanism typically imparts greater energy and greater risk for substantial injury than stab wounds.

Gastrointestinal hemorrhage: Hollow viscus perforation results in bleeding which may be detected in nasogastric tube effluent, hematemesis or rectal bleeding. These injuries require operative repair.[58,59]

Implement in situ: These are typically removed in the operating room because if the implement is in a vascular structure, removal may cause sudden and substantial hemorrhage. If, however, the implement is interfering with necessary resuscitative measures, it may have to be removed in the ED.[43]

Box 13.4 Indications for immediate laparotomy in PAT

Indication	Likely findings or concerns
Hemodynamic instability	Solid organ or vascular injury
Unequivocal peritoneal signs	Solid organ or HVI
Evisceration*	Bowel injury
Evidence of gastrointestinal hemorrhage	Hollow viscus perforation
Implement in situ	Possible hemorrhage when removed

*Some centers will replace eviscerated omentum and then serially examine the patient rather than proceed to emergent laparotomy.

Trauma room studies

Initial trauma room studies augment the above criteria to determine the need for emergent laparotomy and include radiographs, laboratory tests, and ultrasound.

Radiology: A chest radiograph (CXR) may rapidly detect the presence of significant pneumothoraces and hemothoraces. If these are present, interventions such as tube thoracostomy may stabilize a hemodynamically compromised patient and avoid the perceived need for mandatory laparotomy. A CXR illustrating free air under the diaphragm indicates peritoneal penetration. However, these patients do not necessarily have peritoneal organ injury and as such do not need mandatory exploration (unless the criteria above are present). This is especially true for anterior SWs as implements may draw in air as they penetrate the peritoneal cavity.[60] However, for GSWs, free air connotes peritoneal transgression. This, in turn, usually prompts laparotomy although some centers, in patients without other indications for operation, will undertake additional testing, serial observation, or both. Other radiographs, when obtained in two planes, can help locate retained missiles, estimate missile path and potential organ injury. One rare occurrence to keep in mind is the potential for embolization of a ballistic missile, particularly shotgun pellets. In addition, tracking of multiple missiles and ones that have ricocheted can create considerable confusion and misinterpretation. Estimation of bullet caliber based on film appearance is often wrong and unhelpful.

Laboratory: Initial testing is helpful to establish baseline values. These may include a hemoglobin/hematocrit, lactate, and base excess. All women of child-bearing age with the possibility of unknown pregnancy should have a urine pregnancy test. In patients with torso injuries, a urinalysis indicating the presence of microscopic hematuria suggests urologic injury. Urine drug screens and blood alcohol levels typically do not add to the initial evaluation of these patients. However, if positive, these may allow an opportunity for substance abuse intervention in follow up. Finally, in unstable patients and those requiring mandatory exploratory laparotomy, type and crossed matched blood is usual practice.

Ultrasound: Bedside US is now a mainstay in the evaluation of trauma patients. In patients with PAT, its utility is in quickly assessing for evidence of hemoperitoneum, pneumothorax, and pericardial tamponade.[62,63] The presence of hemoperitoneum has a high (> 90%) positive predictive value for a therapeutic laparatomy.[64] However an US which is negative for hemoperitoneum is insensitive for peritoneal penetration and potential injury, especially to the diaphragm and hollow viscus; Further studies will be necessary.[65,66]

Acute interventions

Initial management is focused on stabilization and identification of those patients with hemoperitoneum requiring emergent intervention.

Intubation: Unstable patients with evidence of airway compromise or severely compromised hemodynamics or anticipated ED course requiring them to leave the department (losing the ability to closely monitor their airway status) need emergent intubation. This is a clinical decision based on suspicion of underlying pathology, patient conditions, skills, and available resources.

Intravenous access: Obtain IV access for fluid and blood administration. In patients with hemodynamic instability or potential for this, obtain a minimum of two IV lines, although they may need additional lines when critically ill.

Tube thoracostomy: Radiographic confirmation is not necessary prior to tube placement in the unstable patient with clinical signs of pneumothorax or hemothorax. These may include subcutaneous emphysema or loss of unilateral breath sounds.

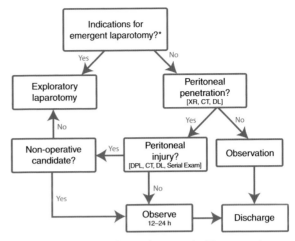

Figure 13.5 Algorithm for gunshot wounds. CT, computed tomography; DL, diagnostic laparoscopy; DPL, diagnostic peritoneal lavage; Serial exam, frequent abdominal examination; XR, plain radiographs in two planes. *Indications for emergent laparotomy.

Thoracotomy: For those with penetrating injury to the thoracoabdominal area and cardiac arrest, thoracotomy allows the emergent identification and mitigation of intrathoracic injury, the ability to perform open chest cardiopulmonary resuscitation, as well as the ability to cross-clamp the aorta and limit hemorrhage below the diaphragm.

Secondary evaluation

Once those patients not meeting criteria for mandatory laparotomy (Figure 13.5) are stabilized, the secondary evaluation should answer the following questions. First, is there peritoneal penetration? Second, if there is peritoneal penetration, is there intraperitoneal organ injury requiring operative intervention?

Stab wounds (Figure 13.6)

Is there peritoneal penetration? –– If the wound tract is definitively found to be superficial to the entire abdominal cavity, including the retroperitoneum, pleura, and pericardium, then these patients may be discharged after appropriate wound care.[67–70]

Plain radiographs: An upright CXR, especially for those with thoracoabdominal wounds, or a lateral decubitus abdominal film showing free air indicates peritoneal violation. The converse of this, lack of free air, does not guarantee no penetration (Figure 13.7).

Local wound exploration (LWE): This is best utilized in those patients with anterior abdominal wall SWs. However it has been utilized in those with back

223

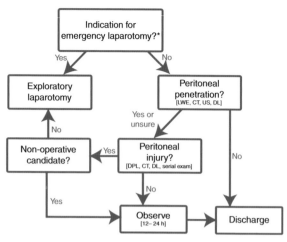

Figure 13.6 Algorithm for stab wounds. CT, computed tomography; DL, diagnostic laparoscopy; DPL, diagnostic peritoneal lavage; LWE, local wound exploration; Serial exam, frequent abdominal examination; US, ultrasound. *Indications for emergent laparotomy.

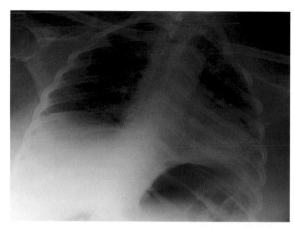

Figure 13.7 Chest radiograph shows free air under the diaphragm.

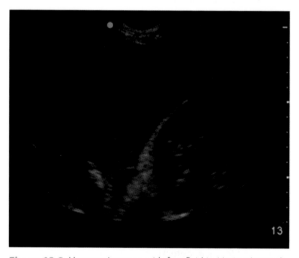

Figure 13.8 Hemoperitoneum with free fluid in Morison's pouch.

and flank wounds with some success.[9,10] Those with heavy musculature or obesity may be poor candidates for local wound exploration as localizing the abdominal fascia is challenging in these patients. In addition, if there are multiple wound tracts present, LWE may not be an efficient means of determining peritoneal penetration. Slash wounds to the chest may be carefully inspected to determine if the thoracic cavity is penetrated; however, deeper wounds on the chest wall should not be explored due to the presence of neurovascular structures and pleura. Blind probing with cotton swabs, fingers, or instruments is dangerous and may lead to inaccurate results.[71]

Ultrasound: Hemoperitoneum indicates peritoneal penetration; however, a negative US does not rule out penetration (Figure 13.8). There is recent limited use of US in conjunction with LWE to evaluate intactness of abdominal fascia.[72] If fascial violation is not found using US, other methods must be pursued, as US is specific in determining fascial violation, but not very sensitive.

Direct laparoscopy: This is a reliable means of diagnosing peritoneal penetration; however, it is mainly performed in the operating room by the surgeon. It is best utilized in those patients with wounds to the left thoracoabdominal area to inspect and repair diaphragm injuries. Those with right-sided wounds have fewer incidences of diaphragmatic injury and evisceration due to protection of that area by the liver. But, if peritoneal injury is concurrently found, repair may quickly ensue.[73–75]

Is there peritoneal injury requiring operative intervention? -- Some patients have known or equivocal peritoneal penetration and require further diagnostic studies to determine if operative injury exists. Even if these studies show no evidence of injury, an observation period of at least 12–24 hours should follow as hollow viscus and pancreatic injuries which may not be detected on initial evaluation typically demonstrate peritonitis within this time frame.[67,68]

Diagnostic peritoneal lavage: This is an invasive but rapid procedure that can be easily performed at the bedside.[71] It allows for immediate detection of hemoperitoneum. However, because it is a highly sensitive test, it has only fair specificity for injuries requiring operative intervention, as it will also identify organ injury that is amenable to non-operative management.

For anterior SWs, the initial return of 10 ml or more of gross blood or lavage effluent of > 100 000 RBC/hpf indicates visceral injury in > 90% of patients.[76,77] Most agree that when 20–100 000 RBC/hpf are found there is need for continued evaluation and observation for injury.[77,78] Injuries to hollow viscera typically produce such results and usually declare themselves clinically within a 12–24 hour observation period. Others suggest decreasing the threshold to 5000–10 000 RBC/hpf to better detect hollow viscus injury (HVI) or diaphragmatic injuries, which bleed minimally, but this would conversely increase the negative laparotomy rate.[79] Another approach is to couple the presence of > 100 000 RBC/hpf with the presence of > 500 WBC/hpf or bile or amylase in the effluent to better detect HVI.[80]

For thoracoabdominal SWs with a specific concern for diaphragmatic injuries, the threshold is lowered to 5–10 000 RBC/hpf to better detect these injuries which are more common in these patients.[71,80]

As other diagnostic modalities have evolved and become more accurate, the routine use of DPL has diminished. It is best employed in those patients with unreliable examinations or thoracoabdominal wounds.

Computed tomagraphy: Multislice scanners are gaining favor as the test of choice in stable patients. It not only detects peritoneal injury, but provides the extent of the injury allowing some patients non-operative management.[31,81] Studies cite a sensitivity of up to 97% for detecting peritoneal violation and specificity of 95% for predicting the need for operation.[81–83] Newer studies suggest oral contrast is not necessary to detect HVI as free intraperitoneal air, free intraperitoneal fluid in the absence of solid organ injury, localized bowel wall thickening, and wound tracts close to the hollow viscus suggest injury; operative repair is indicated (Figure 13.9).[84,85]

Diagnostic laparoscopy: This remains most useful for patients with thoracoabdominal wounds, as it allows inspection and repair of the diaphragm.[75,86,87] In those patients with equivocal peritoneal penetration, it can identify violation of the peritoneum and visceral injury. However DL has poor sensitivity for detecting HVI and retroperitoneal injuries.[74,88] Some injuries to the diaphragm, solid viscera, stomach and small bowel may be concurrently repaired, leading to decreased length of stay, cost, and morbidity when DL

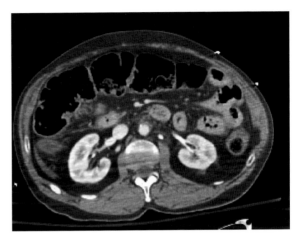
Figure 13.9 Hollow viscus injury.

is employed.[74,75] But most centers are not adept at its routine use for PAT.[73–75]

Gunshot wounds

Is there peritoneal penetration? –– Abdominal GSWs enter the peritoneal cavity in approximately 80% of cases, and in more than 90% of those involving penetration there is intraperitoneal damage.[89] Given the increased velocity and chance for ricochet, even those whose missile path appears to have traveled extra-abdominally warrant close inspection and suspicion for peritoneal injury.

Plain radiographs: While two views of the abdomen in perpendicular planes showing presence of an intra-abdominal missile are helpful, when there are multiple GSWs or through-and-through wounds, this modality is less useful. Additionally missiles may travel outside the peritoneal cavity and make tracking and anticipation of injury difficult.

Local wound exploration: If a wound is deemed to be low velocity and suspected to be tangential, then LWE may be carefully employed, otherwise this approach is not recommended.[90]

Ultrasound: This modality is best utilized to identify hemoperitoneum and hemopericardium rather than the path of wound tracts.[91] A negative ultrasound cannot rule out intra-abdominal injury.

Direct laparoscopy: This approach to assess peritoneal penetration is more costly and invasive than imaging. Also, if penetration is found, most surgeons will proceed to open laparotomy.[75,90]

Computed tomography: CT scanning is becoming the modality of choice for evaluation of peritoneal

225

penetration especially in those stable patients with seemingly tangential GSWs. Several studies demonstrate its ability to exclude transperitoneal and transpelvic trajectories thus preventing negative laparotomies.[82,92] One small study suggests injecting water-soluble contrast into the wound tract to better delineate its path on CT.[93]

Is there peritoneal injury requiring operative intervention? -- Most patients sustaining an abdominal GSW will be assumed to have intraperitoneal injury requiring operative intervention. However, more recent studies indicate that there may only be injury requiring operative repair in 70–80% of the time. Therefore, certain centers will continue their evaluation utilizing DPL, CT, and DL to search for those injuries requiring operative repair.[85,90,94]

Diagnostic peritoneal lavage: This is a rapid, reliable means of determining peritoneal injury with a sensitivity of 96%.[95,96] All positive criteria remain the same, as in stab wounds, except that the presence of RBCs is lowered to 5–10 000/hpf in order to increase the sensitivity of the procedure due to the greater incidence of hollow viscus and diaphragmatic injuries.[71,77,95]

Computed tomography: High resolution CT scanners are sensitive for identifying hollow viscus and diaphragmatic injuries, as well as delineating the extent of solid viscus injury and the missile pathway. Several studies now show that in penetrating injury CT with IV contrast alone has a sensitivity approaching that of CT with triple contrast (IV, PO, and rectal).[85,95] Thus, triple contrast is reserved for those patients with suspected colorectal injury. The use of CT also allows for better selection of those patients with GSWs who may be amenable to non-operative management.[81,90,94,97–99]

Diagnostic laparoscopy: As with patients sustaining SWs, DL for GSWs is not routinely utilized due to its invasive nature, need to convert to open laparotomy, and difficulty visualizing some injuries. However, for those with GSWs to the left thoracoabdominal area or tangential GSWs, without the need for other operative intervention, it is useful in inspecting the diaphragm and may avoid laparotomy.[75,88,90,100]

Patients who sustain a high velocity (i.e., bullets at > 2000 fps [feet per second] such as a .308, 30–06) GSW are at risk for intraperitoneal injury despite the path of the missile being near the abdominal cavity but entirely extraperitoneal. This is attributed to the shock wave created by the high forces caused by the sudden opening and closing of the cavity created

by the missile. As such, these patients should be managed as if the peritoneal space had been transgressed.[11]

Special cases

Thoracoabdominal -- Penetrating trauma to the thoracoabdominal area potentially violates not only the peritoneal cavity, but also the mediastinum, thoracic, and retroperitoneal cavities. Risk of occult diaphragmatic injury is 7%,[87] but patients with GSWs to this area have intraperitoneal injury 45% of the time, and 17% of those with SWs to the left thoracoabdominal area will have concurrent diaphragmatic injury.[73] The most conservative approaches still recommend exploratory laparotomy in all patients with left lower chest SWs and all thoracoabdominal GSWs. While this ensures a lower missed injury rate, it leads to increased negative and non-therapeutic laparotomy rates.

For those patients not undergoing emergent laparotomy, US is a useful modality to quickly rule in the presence of hemopericardium or hemoperitoneum.[91] Diagnostic peritoneal lavage, utilizing a lowered RBC criterion to 5–10 000 RBC/hpf, may be helpful in evaluating patients at risk for diaphragmatic and intraperitoneal injury. A negative DPL markedly lowers risk, although a positive one by lower end RBC criterion simply rules in the possibility of having this injury.[77] As mentioned previously, DL can visualize and repair the diaphragm and some other organs, but is invasive, time consuming, and best utilized in those centers adept at its use in trauma.[86,87]

Computed tomography is becoming the diagnostic test of choice for stable patients. In some centers is has test characteristics markedly improved from previous with sensitivities of 94% and specificity approaching 96% for diaphragmatic injury.[83] As this is not consistent everywhere, those with negative CTs should be closely monitored for potentially undetected hollow viscus and diaphragmatic injury, and those with equivocal scans require further diagnostic testing.

Flank and back: Evaluation of these wounds is particularly difficult as retroperitoneal structures are at greatest risk; however, isolated or concomitant intraperitoneal injuries are seen in up to 40% of cases.[9] Local wound exploration should be the first step for SWs, however, it is often difficult due to paraspinous musculature and should not be used for GSWs in this area. Physical examination may be unreliable and DPL less likely to detect retroperitoneal injuries.[10] Computed tomography is gaining favor in stable patients as it allows evaluation of both the peritoneal and

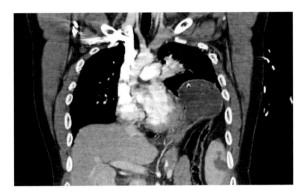

Figure 13.10 Computed tomography (CT) shows diaphragmatic injury with stomach herniation into the thoracic cavity.

Table 13.5 Evaluation of shotgun wounds

Type	Injuries	Diagnostic modality
I	Dermal wounds	Serial examination
II	Small HV perforations No peritoneal fluid	Usually exploratory laparotomy Some utilize serial examination
III	Multiple organ injury Severe tissue destruction Shock	Emergent exploratory laparotomy

HV, hollow viscus.

retroperitoneal structures. Multislice scanners have the ability to detect most but not all bowel and diaphragmatic injury (Figure 13.10).[59,75,92,97]

Once again, conservative centers mandate operative evaluation for these wounds, however, others advocate for initial non-operative management with serial examinations and CT.[85]

Shotgun wounds -- Type I injuries are low velocity and have greatest pellet spread, therefore injury is less likely. Serial examination and operation on only those with peritoneal signs or increasing pain is standard. Type II wounds may injure intraperitoneal structures, however often these are small hollow viscus puncture wounds that have no intraperitoneal spillage and may heal without surgical repair. Thus some centers utilize non-operative management in these patients, but most proceed to exploratory laparotomy. Significant tissue destruction, multiorgan injury, and shock are common with type III wounds leading to emergent laparotomy for all cases (Table 13.5).[96]

Treatment

Selective non-operative management-stab wounds

Traditional treatment for PAT advocated mandatory exploratory laparotomy; however, this led to a high negative laparotomy rate. In the 1960s Shaftan published a small study evaluating non-operative management of SWs.[101] Stable patients were serially examined and only proceeded to laparotomy if peritonitis or instability developed.[101] This influential study changed the usual practice of mandatory exploratory laparotomy operative management and most trauma centers have adopted this approach coupled with the diagnostic tests described previously (see Figure 13.6).[58,59,67,94,97]

Therefore it should only be used at those centers able to provide the intense monitoring needed. Numerous studies demonstrate this.[58,59,67,94,97]

Box 13.5 Essentials of non-operative management of stab wounds

- Most anterior stab wounds do not require intervention.
- Non-operative management requires the ability to serially examine the patient and expeditiously move to operative intervention if peritoneal signs or hemodynamic compromise develops; therefore, it requires significant resources.
- Non-operative management in appropriate patients leads to decreased non-therapeutic and negative laparotomy rates, reduction in overall length of hospital stay, and costs.

Selective non-operative management GSWs

If there is no need for emergent laparotomy some centers are pursuing non-operative management of GSWs. Serial examination in awake, stable patients coupled with judicious use of diagnostic testing such as CT, DPL, and DL, allows for patient stratification to operative or non-operative treatment.[82,85] Again, this requires a setting where frequent examination and expeditious transition to operation when needed is available.[90,92]

Documentation

Penetrating abdominal trauma

Careful documentation of the location and size of each wound is optimal. Do not attempt to determine entry vs. exit wounds.

Blunt abdominal trauma

All patients selected for non-operative management must have their repeat evaluations documented. Changes in hemodynamic status, increasing abdominal tenderness, and decreases in hematocrit are all indications that operative intervention may be required.

Disposition

Patients with serious abdominal trauma, especially those requiring operative repair do better at regional trauma centers.[102,103] Consult and transfer early. A small subset with hemodynamic instability and known hemoperitomenum may do better with damage control laparotomy and control of hemorrhage at the presenting hospital and then transfer to a trauma center.[104]

References

1. Demetriades D, Murray JA, Brown C, et al. High-level falls: type and severity of injuries and survival outcome according to age. *J Trauma* 2005;**58**:342–5.

2. Demetriades D, Murray JA, Martin M, et al. Pedestrians injured by automobiles: relationship of age to injury type and severity. *J Amer Coll Surg* 2004;**199**:382–7.

3. Davis JJ, Cohn I, Jr., Nance FC, et al. Diagnosis and management of blunt abdominal trauma. *Ann Surg* 1976;**183**:672–8.

4. Rivara FP, Koepsell TD, Grossman DC, Mock C. Effectiveness of automatic shoulder belt systems in motor vehicle crashes. *JAMA* 2000;**283**:2826–8.

5. Sokolove PE, Kuppermann N, Holmes JF. Association between the seat belt sign and intraabdominal injury in children with blunt torso trauma. *Acad Emerg Med* 2005;**12**:808–13.

6. Velmahos GC, Tatevossian R, Demetriades D, et al. The "seat belt mark" sign: a call for increased vigilance among physicians treating victims of motor vehicle accidents. *Am Surg* 1999;**65**:181–5.

7. Nicholas JM, Rix EP, Easley KA, et al. Changing patterns in the management of penetrating abdominal trauma: the more things change, the more they stay the same. *J Trauma* 2003;**55**:1095–110.

8. Demetriades D, Rabinowitz B, Demetriades D, Rabinowitz B. Indications for operation in abdominal stab wounds. A prospective study of 651 patients. *Ann Surg* 1987;**205**:129–32.

9. McCarthy M, Lowdermilk GA, Canal D, et al. Prediction of injury caused by penetrating wounds to the abdomen, flank and back. *Arch Surg* 1991;**128**:926.

10. Boyle EM, Jr., Maier RV, Salazar JD, et al. Diagnosis of injuries after stab wounds to the back and flank. *J Trauma* 1997;**42**:260–5.

11. Velitchkov NGM. Delayed small bowel injury as a result of penetrating extraperitoneal high-velocity ballistic trauma to the abdomen. *J Trauma* 2000;**48**:169–70.

12. Kwan I, Bunn F, Roberts I. Timing and volume of fluid administration for patients with bleeding. *Cochrane Database Syst Rev* 2003;**3**:CD002245.

13. Brasel KJ, Nirula R. What mechanism justifies abdominal evaluation in motor vehicle crashes. *J Trauma* 2005;**59**:1057–61.

14. Newgard CD, Lewis RJ, Kraus JF. Steering wheel deformity and serious thoracic or abdominal injury among drivers and passengers involved in motor vehicle crashes. *Ann Emerg Med* 2005;**45**:43–50.

15. Brown CK, Dunn KA, Wilson K, et al. Diagnostic evaluation of patients with blunt abdominal trauma: a decision analysis. *Acad Emerg Med* 2000;**7**:385–96.

16. Ferrera PC, Verdile VP, Bartfield JM, Snyder HS, Salluzzo RF. Injuries distracting from intraabdominal injuries after blunt trauma. *Am J Emerg Med* 1998;**16**:145–9.

17. Holmes JF, Ngyuen H, Jacoby RC, et al. Do all patients with left costal margin injuries require radiographic evaluation for intraabdominal injury. *Ann Emerg Med* 2005;**46**:232–6.

18. Davis JW, Kaups KL, Parks SN, et al. Base deficit is superior to pH in evaluating clearance of acidosis after traumatic shock. *J Trauma* 1998;**44**:114–18.

19. Asimos AW, Gibbs MA, Marx JA, et al. Value of point-of-care blood testing in emergent trauma management. *J Trauma* 2000;**48**:1101–8.

20. Takishima T, Sugimoto K, Hirata M, et al. Serum amylase level on admission in the diagnosis of blunt injury to the pancreas. Its significance and limitations. *Ann Emerg Med* 1997;**226**:70–6.

21. Knudson MM, McAninch JW, Gomez R, et al. Hematuria as a predictor of abdominal injury after blunt trauma. *Am J Surg* 1992;**164**:482–5.

22. Sloan EP, Zalenski RJ, Smith RF, et al. Toxicology screening in urban trauma patients: drug prevalence and its relationship to trauma severity and management. *J Trauma* 1989;**29**:1647–53.

23. Dolich MO, Mckenney MG, Varela JE, et al. 2576 ultrasounds for blunt abdominal trauma. *J Trauma* 2001;**50**:108–12.

24. Blackbourne LH, Soffer D, Mckenney MG, et al. Secondary ultrasound examination increases the sensitivity of the FAST exam in blunt trauma. *J Trauma* 2004;**57**:934–8.

25. Henderson SO, Sung J, Mandavia D, et al. Serial abdominal ultrasound in the setting of trauma. *J Emerg Med* 2000;**18**:79–81.

26. Poletti PA, Mirvis SE, Shanmuganathan K, et al. Blunt abdominal trauma patients: can organ injury be excluded without performing computed tomography? *J Trauma* 2004;**57**:1072–81.

27. Catalano O, Sandomenico F, Raso MM, et al. Real-time, contrast-enhanced sonography: a new tool for detecting active bleeding. *J Trauma* 2005;**59**:933–9.

28. Valentino M, Serra C, Zironi G, et al. Blunt abdominal trauma: emergency contrast-enhanced sonography for detection of solid organ injuries. *AJR Am J Roentgenol* 2006;**186**:1361–7.

29. Miller MT, Pasquale MD, Bromberg WJ, Wasser TE, Cox J. Not so fast. *J Trauma* 2003;**54**:52–60.

30. Melniker LA, Leibner E, McKenney MG, et al. Randomized controlled clinical trial of point-of-care, limited ultrasonography for trauma in the emergency department: the first sonography outcomes assessment program trial. *Ann Emerg Med* 2006;**48**:227–35.

31. Miller LA, Shanmuganathan K, Miller LA, Shanmuganathan K. Multidetector CT evaluation of abdominal trauma. *Radiol Clin North Am* 2005;**43**:1079–95.

32. Haan JM, Biffl W, Knudson MM, et al. Splenic embolization revisited: a multicenter review. *J Trauma* 2004;**56**:542–7.

33. Hauser CJM. Prospective validation of computed tomographic screening of the thoracolumbar spine in trauma. *J Trauma* 2003;**55**:228–35.

34. Salim A, Sangthong B, Martin M, et al. Whole body imaging in blunt multisystem trauma patients without obvious signs of injury: results of a prospective study. *Arch Surg* 2006;**141**:468–73.

35. Moore EE, Shackford SR, Pachter HL, et al. Organ injury scaling: spleen, liver, and kidney. *J Trauma.* 1989;**29**:1664–6.

36. Lee SK, Carrillo EH, Lee SK, Carrillo EH. Advances and changes in the management of liver injuries. *Am Surg* 2007;**73**:201–6.

37. Harbrecht BG. Is anything new in adult blunt splenic trauma? *Am J Surg* 2005;**190**:273–8.

38. Velmahos GC, Toutouzas KG, Radin R, et al. Nonoperative treatment of blunt injury to solid abdominal organs: a prospective study. *Arch Surg* 2003;**138**:844–51.

39. Mele TS, Stewart K, Marokus B, O'Keefe GE. Evaluation of a diagnostic protocol using screening of diagnostic peritoneal lavage with selective use of abdominal computed tomography in blunt abdominal trauma. *J Trauma* 1999;**46**:847–52.

40. Weninger P, Mauritz W, Fridrich P, et al. Emergency room management of patients with blunt major trauma: evaluation of the multislice computed tomography protocol exemplified by an urban trauma center. *J Trauma* 2007;**62**:584–91.

41. Elton C, Riaz AA, Young N, et al. Accuracy of computed tomography in the detection of blunt bowel and mesenteric injuries. *Br J Surg* 2005;**92**:1024–8.

42. Stuhlfaut JW, Soto JA, Lucey BC, et al. Blunt abdominal trauma: performance of CT without oral contrast material. *Radiology* 2004;**233**:689–94.

43. Marx JA, Isenhour JL. Abdominal Trauma. In Marx JA (ed.), *Rosen's Emergency Medicine: Concepts and Clinical Practice*. 6th edn. Philadelphia, PA: Mosby, 2006: pp. 414–34.

44. Holmes JF, Harris D, Battistella FD. Performance of abdominal ultrasonography in blunt trauma patients with out of hospital or emergency department hypotension. *Ann Emerg Med* 2004;**43**:354–61.

45. Fakhry SM, Watts DD, Luchette FA, et al. Current diagnostic approaches lack sensitivity in the diagnosis of perforated blunt small bowel injury: analysis from 275 557 trauma admissions from the EAST multi-institutional HVI trial. *J Trauma* 2003;**54**:295–306.

46. Lorente-Ramos RM, Santiago-Hernando A, Del Valle-Sanz Y, et al. Sonographic diagnosis of intramural duodenal hematomas. *J Clin Ultrasound* 1999;**27**:213–16.

47. Branney SW, Moore EE, Cantrill SV, et al. Ultrasound based key clinical pathway reduces the use of hospital resources for the evaluation of blunt abdominal trauma. *J Trauma* 1997;**42**:1086–90.

48. Ollerton JE, Sugrue M, Balogh Z, et al. Prospective study to evaluate the influence of FAST on trauma patient management. *J Trauma* 2006;**60**:785–91.

49. Sirlin CB, Brown MA, Andrade-Barreto OA, et al. Blunt abdominal trauma: clinical value of negative screening US scans. *Radiology* 2004;**230**:661–8.

50. Williams MD, Watts D, Fakhry S. Colon injury after blunt abdominal trauma: results of the EAST multi-institutional hollow viscus injury study. *J Trauma* 2003;**55**:906–12.

51. Mendez C, Gubler KD, Maier RV, et al. Diagnostic accuracy of peritoneal lavage in patients with pelvic fractures. *Arch Surg* 1994;**129**:477–81.

52. Clancy TV, Ramshaw DG, Maxwell JG, et al. Management outcomes in splenic injury: a statewide trauma center review. *Ann Surg* 1997;**226**:17–24.

53. Malhotra AK, Fabian TC, Croce MA, et al. Blunt hepatic injury: a paradigm shift from operative to nonoperative management in the 1990s. *Ann Emerg Med* 2000;**231**:804–13.

54. Kozar RA, Moore JB, Niles SE, et al. Complications of nonoperative management of high-grade blunt hepatic injuries. *J Trauma* 2005;**59**:1066–71.

55. Kaban G, Somani RA, Carter J, et al. Delayed presentation of small bowel injury after blunt abdominal trauma: case report. *J Trauma* 2004;**56**:1144–5.

56. Fakhry SM, Brownstein M, Watts DD, et al. Relatively short diagnostic delays (< 8 hours) produce morbidity and mortality in blunt small bowel injury: an analysis of time to operative intervention in 198 patients from a multicenter experience. *J Trauma* 2000;**48**:408–14.

57. Apfelbaum JD, Shockley LW, Wahe JW, et al. Entrance and exit gunshot wounds: incorrect terms for the emergency department? *J Emerg Med* 1998;**16**:741–5.

58. Arikan S, Kocakusak A, Yucel AF, et al. A prospective comparison of the selective observation and routine exploration methods for penetrating abdominal stab wounds with organ or omentum evisceration. *J Trauma* 2005;**58**:526–32.

59. Ertekin C, Yanar H, Taviloglu K, et al. Unnecessary laparotomy by using physical examination and different diagnostic modalities for penetrating abdominal stab wounds. *Emerg Med J* 2005;**22**:790–4.

60. Leppaniemi AK, Voutilainen PE, Haapiainen RK et al. Indications for early mandatory laparotomy in abdominal stab wounds. *Br J Surg* 1999;**86**:76–80.

61. Nagy KK, Roberts RR, Joseph KT, Gary A, Barrett J. Evisceration after abdominal stab wounds: is laparotomy required. *J Trauma* 1999;**47**:1–9.

62. Boulanger BRM. The routine use of sonography in penetrating torso injury is beneficial. *J Trauma* 2001;**51**:320–5.

63. Tayal VS, Beatty MA, Marx JA, et al. FAST (focused assessment with sonography in trauma) accurate for cardiac and intraperitoneal injury in penetrating anterior chest trauma. *J Ultrasound Med* 2004;**23**:467–72.

64. Boulanger BR, Kearney PA, Tsuei B, et al. The routine use of sonography in penetrating torso injury is beneficial. *J Trauma* 2001;**51**:320–5.

65. Udobi KF, Rodriguez A, Chiu WC, et al. Role of ultrasonography in penetrating abdominal trauma: a prospective clinical study. *J Trauma* 2001;**50**:475–9.

66. Soto JA, Morales C, Munera F, et al. Penetrating stab wounds to the abdomen: use of serial US and contrast-enhanced CT in stable patients. *Radiology* 2001;**220**:365–71.

67. Tsikitis V, Biffl WL, Majercik S, et al. Selective clinical management of anterior abdominal stab wounds. *Am J Surg* 2004;**188**:807–12.

68. Alzamel HA, Cohn SM, Alzamel HA, Cohn SM. When is it safe to discharge asymptomatic patients with abdominal stab wounds? *J Trauma* 2005;**58**:523–5.

69. Sugrue M, Balogh Z, Lynch J, et al. Guidelines for the management of haemodynamically stable patients with stab wounds to the anterior abdomen. *ANZ J Surg* 2007;**77**:614–20.

70. Mitra B, Gocentas R, O'Reilly G, et al. Management of haemodynamically stable patients with abdominal stab wounds. *Emerg Med Australas* 2007;**19**:269–75.

71. Marx JA. Peritoneal Procedures. Roberts JR, Hedges JR (eds), *Clinical Procedures in Emergency Medicine*, 4th edn. Philadelphia, PA: Elsevier, 2004: pp. 851–6.

72. Murphy JT, Hall J, Provost D. Fascial ultrasound for evaluation of anterior abdominal stab wound injury. *J Trauma* 2005;**59**:843–6.

73. Leppäniemi A, Haapiainen R. Diagnostic laparoscopy in abdominal stab wounds: a prospective, randomized study. *J Trauma* 2003;**55**:636–45.

74. Simon RJ, Rabin J, Kuhls D. Impact of increased use of laparoscopy on negative laparotomy rates after penetrating trauma. *J Trauma* 2002;**53**:297–302.

75. Ahmed N, Whelan J, Brownlee J, et al. The contribution of laparoscopy in evaluation of penetrating abdominal wounds. *J Am Coll Surg* 2005;**201**:213–16.

76. Gonzalez RP, Ickler J, Gachassin P. Complementary roles of diagnostic peritoneal lavage and computed tomography in the evaluation of blunt abdominal trauma. *J Trauma* 2001;**51**:1128–36.

77. Nagy KK, Roberts RR, Joseph KT, et al. Experience with over 2500 diagnostic peritoneal lavages. *Injury* 2000;**31**:479–82.

78. Otomo Y, Henmi H, Mashiko K, et al. New diagnostic peritoneal lavage criteria for diagnosis of intestinal injury. *J Trauma* 1998;**44**:991–7.

79. Sriussadaporn S, Pak-Art R, Pattaratiwanon M, et al. Clinical uses of diagnostic peritoneal lavage in stab wounds of the anterior abdomen: a prospective study. *Eur J Surg.* 2002;**168**:490–3.

80. Thacker LK, Parks J, Thal ER. Diagnostic peritoneal lavage: is 100 000 RBCs a valid figure for penetrating abdominal trauma? *J Trauma* 2007;**62**:853–7.

81. Shanmuganathan K, Mirvis SE, Chiu WC, et al. Penetrating torso trauma: triple-contrast helical CT in peritoneal violation and organ injury–a prospective study in 200 patients. *Radiology* 2004;**231**:775–84.

82. Chiu WC, Shanmuganathan K, Mirvis SE, Scalea TM. Determining the need for laparotomy in penetrating torso trauma: a prospective study using triple contrast enhanced abdominopelvic computed tomography. *J Trauma* 2001;**51**:860–9.

83. Stein DMM. Accuracy of computed tomography (CT) scan in the detection of penetrating diaphragm injury. *J Trauma* 2007;**63**:538–43.

84. Demetriades D, Hadjizacharia P, Constantinou C, et al. Selective nonoperative management of penetrating abdominal solid organ injuries. *Ann Surg* 2006;**244**:620–8.

85. Velmahos GC, Constantinou C, Tillou A, et al. Abdominal computed tomographic scan for patients with gunshot wounds to the abdomen selected for nonoperative management. *J Trauma* 2005;**59**:1155–61.

86. Friese RS, Coln CE, Gentilello LM, et al. Laparoscopy is sufficient to exclude occult diaphragm injury after penetrating abdominal trauma. *J Trauma* 2005;**58**:789–92.

87. Leppäniemi A, Haapiainen R. Occult diaphragmatic injuries caused by stab wounds. *J Trauma* 2003;**55**:646–50.

88. Poole GV, Thomae KR, Hauser CJ, et al. Laparoscopy in trauma. *Surg Clin North Am* 1996;**76**:547–56.

89. Moore EE, Marx JA, Moore EE, Marx JA. Penetrating abdominal wounds. Rationale for exploratory laparotomy. *JAMA* 1985;**253**:2705–8.

90. Pryor JP, Reilly PM, Dabrowski GP, Grossman MD, Schwab CW. Nonoperative management of abdominal gunshot wounds. *Ann Emerg Med* 2004;**43**:344–53.

91. Tayal VS. FAST accurate for cardiac and intraperitoneal injury in penetrating chest trauma. *Acad Emerg Med.* 2000;**7**:493.

92. Ginzburg E, Carrillo EH, Kopelman T, et al. The role of computed tomography in selective management of gunshot wounds to the abdomen and flank. *J Trauma* 1998;**45**:1005–9.

93. Bruckner BA, Norman M, Scott BG, et al. CT Tractogram: technique for demonstrating tangential bullet trajectories. *J Trauma* 2006;**60**:1362–3.

94. Velmahos GC, Demetriades D, Toutouzas KG, et al. Selective nonoperative management in 1856 patients with abdominal gunshot wounds: should routine laparotomy still be the standard of care? *Ann Emerg Med* 2001;**234**:395–403.

95. Nagy KK, Krosner SM, Joseph KT, et al. A method of determining peritoneal penetration in gunshot wounds to the abdomen. *J Trauma* 1997;**43**:242–6.

96. Brakenridge SC, Nagy KK, Joseph KT, et al. Detection of intra-abdominal injury using diagnostic peritoneal lavage after shotgun wound to abdomen. *J Trauma* 2003;**54**:329–31.

97. Conrad MF, Patton JH, Jr., Parikshak M, et al. Selective management of penetrating truncal injuries: is emergency department discharge a reasonable goal? *Am Surg* 2003;**69**:266–72.

98. Demetriades D, Hadjizacharia P, Constantinou C, et al. Selective nonoperative management of penetrating abdominal solid organ injuries. *Ann Surg* 2006;**244**:620–8.

99. Demetriades D, Hadjizacharia P, Constantinou C, et al. Selective nonoperative management of penetrating abdominal solid organ injuries. *Ann Surg* 2006;**244**:620–8.

100. Friese RS, Coln E, Gentilello LM. Laparoscopy is sufficient to exclude occult diaphragm injury after penetrating abdominal wounds. *J Trauma* 2005;**58**:789–92.

101. Shaftan GW. Indications for operation in abdominal trauma. *Am J Surg* 1960;**99**:657–64.

102. Mullins RJ, Veum-Stone J, Helfand M, et al. Outcome of hospitalized injured patients after institution of a trauma system in an urban area. *JAMA* 1994;**271**:1919–24.

103. Shackford SR, Hollingworth-Fridlund P, Cooper GF, et al. The effect of regionalization upon the quality of trauma care as assessed by concurrent audit before and after institution of a trauma system: a preliminary report. *J Trauma* 1986;**26**:812–20.

104. Weinberg JA, McKinley K, Petersen SR, et al. Trauma laparotomy in a rural setting before transfer to a regional center: does it save lives? *J Trauma* 2003;**54**:823–8.

Chapter

14

Genitourinary trauma

James F. Holmes

Epidemiology

Following splenic and hepatic injuries, renal injuries are the third most commonly injured abdominal structure, affecting 10% of patients with major traumatic injuries.[1,2] As with most injuries, genitourinary (GU) trauma is most common in those 20–35 years of age and in the male sex.[1] Most GU injuries (90%) result from blunt mechanisms of injury with penetrating accounting for the remainder. The most frequent blunt mechanisms resulting in GU injury include motor vehicle collisions, automobile vs. pedestrians or bicycles, and falls; less commonly occurring after assaults and sports-related injuries. Genital specific injuries have a high prevalence of self-infliction.

Box 14.1 Essentials of GU trauma

- The kidneys are the third most injured abdominal organ.
- Renal injuries are most common after blunt mechanisms (especially deceleration injuries and direct blows).
- Ureteral, bladder, urethral, and genital injuries are significantly less common than renal injuries.

Clinical anatomy and pathophysiology

The urinary system can be divided into an upper and lower portion, which is not only anatomic but is also appropriate as the evaluation varies by location. The upper urinary tract consists of the kidney and ureter (both evaluated with contrast-enhanced computed tomography [CT] scan). The kidney is located in the upper portion of the retroperitoneum. It consists of an outer core of renal parenchyma that feeds into a central collecting system at the renal hilum. The kidneys are

positioned from the 11th thoracic to the 3rd lumbar vertebrae and are partially protected by the posterior aspect of the lower costal margin. Further protection is provided by the posterior musculature. The left kidney is adjacent to the spleen and the right kidney is adjacent to the liver (and is displaced more inferiorly by the right lobe of the liver). Due to the proximity of the kidneys to the liver and spleen, injuries to these organs are often associated with hematuria and renal injuries. The adrenal glands are positioned immediately superior to the kidneys. The renal artery and vein enter the kidney at the hilum with the renal artery rapidly separating to supply the five different segments of the kidney, although significant anatomic variation in the renal vasculature does occur. The ureter travels from the renal pelvis to the bladder in the retroperitoneal space. Its location, mobility, and small size limit the chances of injury.

The lower urinary tract consists of the urinary bladder and urethra (both structures evaluated with focused radiographic testing). The bladder resides in the anterior portion of the pelvis and is protected from injury by the pubic bones (except during the second and third trimester of pregnancy when the gravid uterus displaces the bladder outside of the pelvis). The dome of the bladder is covered with peritoneum and injury to the dome results in intraperitoneal spillage of urine. The bladder neck is secured to the pelvic floor by pelvic fascia.

The urethra is divided by the urogenital diaphragm into anterior and posterior portions. Male and female urethral anatomies are significantly different. The male urethra is significantly longer than the female urethra (which is not firmly attached to the pelvic floor), and thus more susceptible to injury. The anterior portion of the male urethra (distal to the diaphragm and located external to the pelvis) is additionally divided into penile and bulbous

Trauma: A Comprehensive Emergency Medicine Approach, eds. Eric Legome and Lee W. Shockley. Published by Cambridge University Press. © Cambridge University Press 2011.

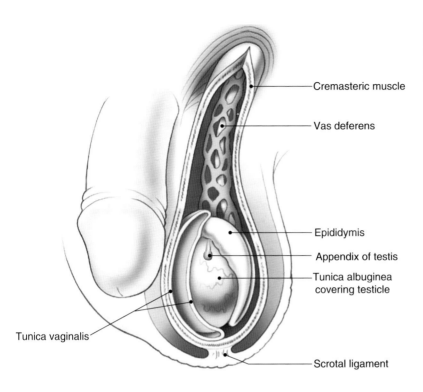

Figure 14.1 Anatomy of the scrotum. (From Mahadevan S, Garmel G. *An Introduction to Clinical Emergency Medicine.* Cambridge: Cambridge University Press, 2005.)

Cremasteric muscle

Vas deferens

Epididymis

Appendix of testis

Tunica albuginea covering testicle

Tunica vaginalis

Scrotal ligament

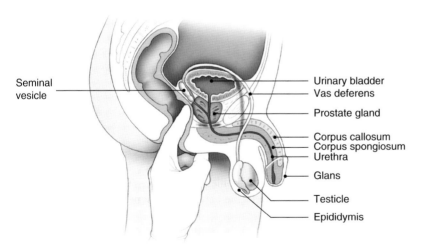

Figure 14.2 Lateral view of digital rectal examination with male genitalia anatomy. (Adapted from National Institutes of Digestive and Kidney Diseases, National Institutes of Health.)

Seminal vesicle

Urinary bladder
Vas deferens

Prostate gland

Corpus callosum
Corpus spongiosum
Urethra

Glans

Testicle

Epididymis

segments. The posterior portion (proximal to the diaphragm and located within the pelvis) is divided into the prostatic and membranous segments.

The male external genitalia consists of the penis and scrotum. The scrotum is composed of multiple layers of protective tissue (Figure 14.1).

These layers (from external to internal) include the scrotal skin, dartos fascia, spermatic fascia (including the cremasteric muscle), tunical vaginalis (two layers – parietal and visceral), and the tunica albuginea. The tunica albuginea is a thick, white fibrous layer that encapsulates the seminiferous tubules of the testes and is important as injury through the tunica albuginea results in testicular rupture. The penis consists of the penile urethra which is surrounded by the corpus spongiosum and Buck's fascia (Figure 14.2).

Table 14.1 Grading scales for renal injuries[4]

Grade	Findings
I	**Contusion:** Normal urologic imaging with hematuria (microscopic or gross) **Hematoma:** Subcapsular hematoma without parenchymal laceration
II	**Hematoma:** Perirenal hematoma, non-expanding and confined to retroperitoneum **Laceration:** Renal cortex parenchymal laceration < 1 cm, without urinary extravasation
III	**Laceration:** Renal cortex parenchymal laceration > 1 cm, without urinary extravasation or collecting system rupture
IV	**Laceration:** Parenchymal laceration through renal cortex, medulla, and collecting system **Vascular:** Renal artery or vein injury with contained hemorrhage
V	**Laceration:** Completely shattered kidney **Vascular:** Avulsion of renal hilum with devascularized kidney

The female urethra, due to its internal and shortened anatomy compared to the male, is rarely injured outside of significant pelvic trauma, usually with an associated pelvic fracture.

Renal trauma results from a variety of mechanisms but is most common after direct blows or sudden decelerations (especially motor vehicle collisions). Renal injuries associated with penetrating trauma (particularly gunshot wounds) often have additional injuries present. Blunt renal injuries are frequently isolated. Certain injury patterns occur within the GU tract. Renal injuries are associated with lumbar spine fractures, most commonly lumbar spine transverse process fractures.[3] Bladder and urethral injuries occur in conjunction with pelvic fractures, especially those with pubic symphysis and sacroiliac joint diastasis. Urethral injuries most often occur from straddle injuries as the urethra is compressed against the symphysis pubis. Male genital injuries are frequently from self-inflicted mechanisms.

Over half of all GU injuries involve the kidney. Renal injuries are graded based on the American Association for the Surgery of Trauma Grading Scale (Table 14.1 and Figure 14.3).[4]

The majority of renal injuries are Grade 1. Ureter, bladder, and urethra injuries also have established grading scales (Table 14.2),[5] as does the penis, scrotum, and testicles (Table 14.3).[6] All injury-grading scales were developed to standardize treatment, injury reporting, and to assist in research and comparing outcomes between trauma centers. Although the Renal Grading Scale is generally well accepted and widely used, the grading scales for the ureter, bladder, urethra, penis, scrotum, and testicles are less applicable.

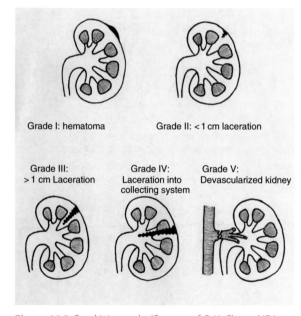

Grade I: hematoma   Grade II: < 1 cm laceration

Grade III:
> 1 cm Laceration

Grade IV:
Laceration into
collecting system

Grade V:
Devascularized kidney

Figure 14.3 Renal injury scale. (Courtesy of C. H. Chang, MD.)

Prehospital care

Standard prehospital care of the trauma patient is appropriate for those patients with GU injuries. No specific intervention by prehospital providers is generally necessary. For the rare instances of penile amputation, direct pressure (no tourniquet) is applied to stop active bleeding. The amputated penis is transported with the patient to the treating facility. Placement of the amputated penis in a sterile dressing, then in a container with ice but not in direct contact with the ice, enhances the chance of successful reimplantation.

Table 14.2 Grading scales for ureter, bladder, and urethral injuries[5]

Ureter Injury Scale	
I	**Hematoma:** Contusion or hematoma without devascularization
II	**Laceration:** Transection < 50%
III	**Laceration:** Transection > 50%
IV	**Laceration:** Complete transaction with < 2 cm devascularization
V	**Laceration:** Avulsion with > 2 cm devascularization

Bladder Injury Scale	
I	**Hematoma:** Contusion, intramural hematoma **Laceration:** Partial thickness laceration
II	**Laceration:** Extraperitoneal bladder wall, < 2 cm
III	**Laceration:** Extraperitoneal bladder wall, > 2 cm; intraperitoneal bladder wall, < 2 cm
IV	**Laceration:** Intraperitoneal bladder wall, > 2 cm
V	**Laceration:** Laceration extending into the bladder neck or ureteral orifice

Urethral Injury Scale	
I	**Contusion:** Blood at urethral orifice, normal radiographs
II	**Stretch injury:** Urethral elongation, no extravasation on urethrography
III	**Partial disruption:** Contrast extravasation on urethrography with contrast in bladder
IV	**Complete disruption:** Contrast extravasation on urethrography, no contrast in bladder; separation < 2 cm
V	**Completed disruption:** Complete transaction with > 2 cm of separation, extension into prostate/vagina

Table 14.3 Grading Scales for penile and testicular injuries[6]

Penile Injury Scale	
I	Cutaneous laceration or contusion
II	Laceration through Buck's fascia without tissue loss
III	Cutaneous avulsion, laceration through glans/meatus, cavernosal or urethral defect < 2 cm
IV	Partial penectomy, cavernosal or urethral defect > 2 cm
V	Total penectomy

Testicular Injury Scale	
I	Contusion or hematoma
II	Subclinical laceration of tunica albuguinea
III	Laceration of tunica albuguinea with < 50% parenchymal loss
IV	Laceration of tunica albuguinea with ≥ 50% parenchymal loss
V	Testicular avulsion or destruction

Emergency department evaluation and management

History and physical examination

The GU tract is unlikely to provide an immediate life-threatening injury, although active bleeding from a renal artery injury can produce hemodynamic instability. Thus, the primary survey does not routinely involve specific evaluation of the GU tract.

Once the primary survey is completed, the GU tract is assessed during the secondary survey; at this time appropriate historical information is obtained. As with all trauma patients, the history includes specific information on the mechanism of injury and the patient's medical history. In regards to GU trauma, the history should also focus on any problems with the patient's renal function or patients with higher risk for renal insufficiency, e.g., diabetes, hypertension, heart failure; most trauma patients now undergo one or more contrast-enhanced CT scans. Although the instance is rare, it may be imperative to identify those patients with a known solitary kidney if going immediately to the operating suite, as this may prevent removal of the kidney. If the emergency department (ED) presentation is delayed from the time of injury, the patient is queried for gross hematuria or difficulty voiding since the time of injury.

The physical examinations of the flank provide important clinical information regarding the risk of direct trauma to the kidneys. Lower costal margin injury predicts injury to the kidney, in addition to the liver and spleen. The thoracolumbar spine is carefully palpated to identify patients with potential thoracic or lumbar spine fractures. Those diagnosed with transverse process fractures are at increased risk of renal injury. Although the bladder can not be palpated on examination, determining pelvic stability provides information as to the risk of bladder injury as pelvic instability increases the risk of bladder injury.

Increasing evidence suggests that the rectal examination is not useful in all trauma patients, but only in those with pelvic fractures, penetrating injuries to the lower abdomen and to confirm rectal tone in suspected spinal cord injuries.[7,8] When performed in cases of actual or suspected pelvic fracture, the rectal examination provides information on the prostate. Although a rare finding a high riding or boggy prostate suggests urethral injury. Examination of the perineum for a perineal hematoma and edema also suggests urethral injury. A detailed examination of the external genitalia is standard to evaluate for both penile and urethral injury, looking for edema, laceration, deformity, or blood at the urethral meatus, respectively. Palpation of both the testicles is performed to evaluate for direct testicular injury.

Following penetrating trauma, determining the trajectory of the penetrating object guides appropriate evaluation and management. If the trajectory is in close proximity to the GU system, then definitive evaluation is indicated regardless of the presence or absence of hematuria. Penetrating flank injuries posterior to the anterior axillary line of the abdomen and lower chest place the kidneys at risk.

Foley catheter placement

Critically injured trauma patients generally require Foley catheter placement. Placement of a Foley catheter allows immediate urine testing for blood and close monitoring of urine output in patients with circulatory compromise. In addition, patients requiring supine positioning for prolonged time periods benefit from Foley catheter for ease of urination. Stable patients less seriously injured but supine for a prolonged time may use a Condom catheter. Care must be taken with placement of a Foley catheter in patients with potential urethral injuries. Initial placement of a Foley catheter via the penile urethra is contraindicated in patients with blood at the urethral meatus, boggy or "high-riding" prostate, or a perineal hematoma due to the risk of worsening a possible urethral injury. In such patients, a retrograde urethrogram is indicated to rule out urethral injury prior to Foley catheter placement. Urologic consultation is also advised if practical. Difficulty in passing a Foley catheter raises the suspicion of urethral injury but also occurs in patients with urethral strictures or prostatic hypertrophy or cancer. If significant resistance is met on Foley catheter placement, consideration is given to a retrograde urethrogram to evaluate for possible urethral injury before additional attempts are made. Traumatic Foley catheter placement will result in hematuria; however, hematuria > 4 red blood cells per high powered field (RBC/hpf) should not be attributed to Foley catheter placement.[9]

The secondary survey includes:

- Questioning the patient on renal function and risk factors.
- Identifying specific trauma to the flank or GU structures.
- Determining pelvic bone instability, increasing suspicion of bladder injury.
- Foley catheter placement once determined safe (assessment of blood at the urethral meatus, prostate integrity, and perineal hematoma).

Urinalysis and hematuria

The primary initial screening test for evaluating GU trauma is assessing the patient's urine for hematuria. In addition, the female patient's urine may be quickly tested for beta human chorionic gonadotrophin (hCG) to determine pregnancy status. Urine is initially inspected for gross blood and then assessed via dipstick for potential microscopic hematuria, to be confirmed in the laboratory. As both hemoglobin and myoglobin result in a urine dipstick positive for blood, all urine testing positive for blood by dipstick is sent to the laboratory to determine the presence and amount of microscopic red blood cells.

Nearly 50% of patients with gross hematuria are identified with renal injuries and another 15% are identified with other intra-abdominal injuries. Gross hematuria should prompt the evaluation of both the urinary tract (kidneys and bladder) and the remaining organs of the abdominal cavity. Fortunately, abdominal CT scanning with delayed images of the kidney adequately evaluates most of these structures. A cystogram is then indicated to evaluate bladder injury. Despite the importance of hematuria, approximately 5% of renal injuries lack hematuria and significant GU injury occurs without hematuria. Renal artery injury and disruption of the ureteropelvic junction may occur without hematuria, however these injuries are unlikely to be overlooked due to the patient's clinical status.[10,11]

Controversy exists over the importance of microscopic hematuria in the blunt trauma patient. In the pediatric trauma population, several studies identify microscopic hematuria as an important screen for intra-abdominal injury.[12–14] Pediatric emergency physicians routinely utilize the urinalysis to risk stratify injured children for both GU tract injuries and other intra-abdominal injuries. However, the degree of microscopic hematuria warranting further abdominal diagnostic testing (abdominal CT scan) in children remains debatable. Studies suggest hematuria levels as low as 5 RBC/hpf warrant abdominal imaging.[13] Clinicians have advocated hematuria cut-off levels for abdominal imaging from 5 to 50 RBC/hpf, but no consensus currently exists. With regards solely to the urinary system in children, the vast majority of significant urinary tract injuries have more than 50 RBC/hpf.[15–18] It is prudent for the clinician to recognize that with increasing levels of hematuria the risk of intra-abdominal injury increases. The level of hematuria must be considered with the mechanism of injury, the physical examination findings, and the possibility of non-GU intra-abdominal injuries to determine the appropriate ED evaluation.

The evaluation of microscopic hematuria in adults is more controversial. It is a long-held belief that adult blunt trauma patients require upper urinary tract (kidney and ureter) imaging solely for gross hematuria or microscopic hematuria in the presence of shock. This practice is generated from older studies focusing solely on identifying renal injuries requiring intervention.[19–25] These prior studies, however, accept missing renal injuries (mainly Grade I and Grade II injuries) not requiring therapeutic intervention, ignore the ability of microscopic hematuria to predict non-GU intra-abdominal injuries, and fail to consider the importance of hematuria to predict lower urinary tract injuries (bladder and urethra). Recent evidence indicates that, like the pediatric population, microscopic hematuria predicts the presence of non-urinary tract intra-abdominal injuries.[26–28] Again, the degree of hematuria warranting abdominal imaging is controversial as investigators suggest patients are at increased risk for renal and non-urinary tract intra-abdominal injuries with urinalysis results of > 10 RBC/hpf[27] or > 25 RBC/hpf.[26,28] Certainly, as the degree of hematuria increases, the risk of both urinary tract and intra-abdominal injuries increases. In addition, the clinician must realize that perhaps the most serious renal injury (renal vascular injury) may present without any hematuria. Thus, like the pediatric population, the presence of microscopic hematuria must alert the physician to the possibility of non-urinary tract injuries, in addition to urinary tract injuries. It is, however, one piece of information among many that will help the clinician decide further evaluation. For example, 10 RBC/hpf in the healthy male who fell from standing and has no physical complaints or findings can probably be safely followed up. The same amount in the patient who fell from height and has flank pain should probably prompt further imaging. The clinician must evaluate the degree of hematuria, mechanism of injury and additional physical findings to determine the need for further diagnostic evaluation (e.g., abdominal CT scanning).

Additional laboratory testing

A complete blood count and type and screen are indicated in all trauma patients with suspicion of injury that may result in significant blood loss. Serum creatinine is important to screen for pre-existing renal disease. Delaying contrast CT scanning to screen patients for renal insufficiency is a low-yield practice in patients with no risk factors (elderly, chronic hypertension, long-term diabetes, or known renal disease). Contrast CT scanning is performed as soon as possible in the critically injured. In the less critically injured, those at high risk of renal disease should probably wait for the results if it may change the plan of diagnosis. Increasing BUN and creatinine in the hospitalized trauma patient suggests renal insult or urea reabsorption, from unidentified bladder or ureteral injury.

Box 14.3 Essentials of laboratory testings

- Gross hematuria often indicates significant GU trauma and mandates evaluation of the upper and lower GU tract.
- Controversy exists as to the degree of microscopic hematuria (or any) that warrants abdominal imaging. More than 25 RBC/hpf increases the risk of injury to the spleen, liver, and kidney, but should be used in conjunction with history and physical in planning the potential need for further evaluation.
- Rising BUN and creatinine levels indicates loss of renal function or spillage (and subsequent reabsorption) of urine into the peritoneal cavity from bladder injury.

Specific injuries of the GU tract and treatment

Upper urinary tract

Renal injuries

Injury grade and type of renal trauma is the most predictive of need for surgical therapy. A decision guideline further predicts the need for surgical

therapy of renal injuries based on the following factors: devitalized tissue, active hemorrhage, and significant injury to the collecting system/ureteral disruption.[29] Low grade renal injuries (Grades I, II, and III) are almost always managed non-operatively in both adults and children.[30] Nearly half of Grade IV injuries require surgery and Grade V injuries always require surgery.[29]

Routine follow-up imaging is not necessary for the majority of renal injuries, however, evidence of urine extravasation on the initial radiographic study is an indication for repeat imaging to document resolution of the urinoma.[31] Patients with Grade I or II renal injuries heal without subsequent radiographic evidence of prior injury; however, Grade III and higher injuries leave evidence of renal scarring on subsequent imaging studies.[32] Acute complications of renal injury include hemorrhage, urinoma, hydronephrosis, arterial pseudoaneurysm, and infection. Long-term complications in those with high-grade injuries include loss of kidney function and hypertension.

Renovascular injuries are classified as either Grade IV or Grade V depending on the extent of injury. These are potentially the most debilitating of all renal injuries, but fortunately they are rare, composing only 2% of renal injuries.[33] The most common renovascular injury is renal artery thrombosis from a minor intimal tear of the renal artery. These injuries occur in the most severely injured patients. Again, hematuria is present in most cases but it may be absent in up to 20% of renovascular injuries.[33] However, these patients have apparent clinical findings, e.g., significant pain, bruising, hemodynamic instability. Abdominal CT scanning is the initial screening test. Findings suggesting renovascular injury include extravasation of contrast from the renal pedicle, a non-enhancing kidney, focal nonenhancement of the kidney, and hematoma at the renal hilum (Figure 14.4).

Renal vein injuries are suggested by a hematoma at the renal hilum with a normal enhancing kidney (indicating contrast successfully delivered to the kidney).

Treatment of renovascular injury is aimed at salvaging renal function and has traditionally involved surgical repair. Emergent intervention is often attempted if complete devascularization of the kidney has occurred. However, results are not promising as most require nephrectomy.[34] Angiographic embolization is now an acceptable, alternative treatment for

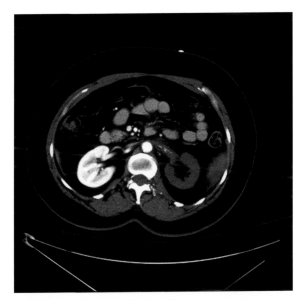

Figure 14.4 Devascularized kidney. The right kidney demonstrates contrast enhancement whereas the left kidney is devascularized and demonstrates no evidence of contrast enhancement. Renal vein injuries are suggested by a hematoma at the renal hilum with a normal enhancing kidney (indicating contrast successfully delivered to the kidney).

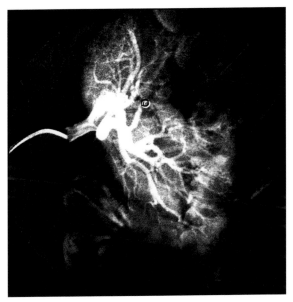

Figure 14.5 Angiographic embolization of a segmental renal arterial injury coil is easily visualized with no flow distal to the coil.

vascular injuries to abdominal solid organs. Angiographic embolization is a viable treatment option for active extravasation of contrast from a renal artery injury or in cases of traumatic pseudoaneurysm (Figure 14.5).[35] Furthermore, endovascular stent placement has been successfully employed in patients with renal artery dissections.[36] Hypertension develops in nearly 50% of patients with renovascular injuries, thus close follow up is indicated in these patients.

Ureteral injury

Traumatic ureteral injuries are exceedingly rare making up only 1% of GU injuries. Most non-iatrogenic ureteral injuries occur from gunshot wounds (94%), followed by stab wounds (5%), and blunt mechanisms (1%).[37] Blunt injuries to the ureter usually result from a sudden deceleration that disrupts the ureter, especially at the ureterovesical and ureteropelvic junctions. No specific physical examination findings can be expected with this injury. Hematuria is insensitive, present in only 75% of patients with ureteral injuries.[37] Computed tomography scanning is the diagnostic screening test of choice and delayed imaging is critical to demonstrate urine extravasation in cases of ureteral tears.[38] However, retrograde pyelography is the most sensitive diagnostic test and is indicated if there is high suspicion on CT scanning. Due to the difficulty in diagnosis, delayed diagnosis is common. The grading scale for ureteral injuries has not been well accepted. This is likely due to the rarity of the injury and the difficulty in grading the injury by radiographic techniques (ureteral injury is best graded at laparotomy).

Ureteral injuries with active extravasation of urine require stenting, primary closure, or ureteroneocystostomy. Ureteroureterostomy (connecting the injured ureter to the uninjured ureter) is now performed with much less frequency due to risks of damage to the uninjured ureter. Complications from ureteral injury occur in 15–25% of cases and include urinoma, abscess, stricture, hydronephroma, fistula, and ileus.[37] Small urinomas may be observed for resolution but large urinomas are treated with percutaneous drainage until definitive repair can be safely performed.

Box 14.4 Essentials of upper urinary tract injuries

- Most renal injuries are minor, simply observed, and result in no long-term complications.
- Renovasclar injuries require prompt diagnosis and urologic consultation.
- Ureteral injuries are rare and most often the result of penetrating trauma.

239

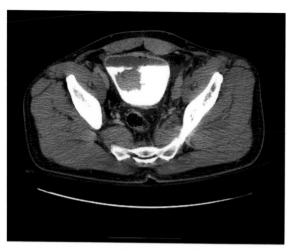

Figure 14.6 Bladder hematoma on computed tomography (CT) scan. Contrast is present in the inferior aspect of the bladder with urine layering in the superior aspect. The hematoma is present in the mid-right portion of the bladder.

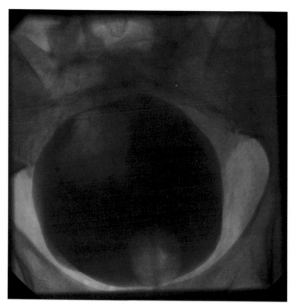

Figure 14.7 Intraperitoneal bladder rupture and bladder hematoma on plain radiograph The radiograph demonstrates a large bladder clot (right side of bladder) and contrast filling the intraperitoneal cavity from the dome of the bladder.

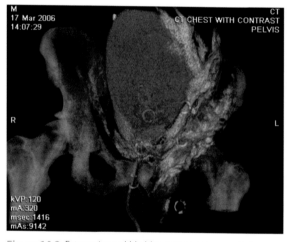

Figure 14.8 Extraperitoneal bladder rupture on computed tomography (CT) scan. Contrast extravasation is identified anterior to the bladder demonstrating the flame-like appearance characteristic of extraperitoneal bladder rupture.

Lower urinary tract

Bladder injuries

Bladder injuries are much less common than renal injuries. The classic triad is gross hematuria, suprapubic pain, and inability to void. Pelvic fractures (especially pubic symphysis diastasis, sacroiliac diastasis, and, to a lesser extent, pubic rami fractures) increase risk of bladder injuries and 85% of bladder injuries occur in conjunction with pelvic fractures. In addition, pregnant women beyond their first trimester (due to uteral displacement of the bladder outside of the protection of the pelvic bones) and intoxicated patients (due to a distended bladder at their time of injury) are at increased risk. Gross hematuria is present in two thirds of patients with bladder injuries. Bladder injury is rare if there is < 25 RBC/hpf.[39] Standard abdominal CT scanning for trauma may identify only 50–67% of patients with bladder injuries.[40] Dedicated bladder CT scanning or plain film cystogram is required for definitive diagnosis.[41,42]

Although a scale with five grades of bladder injury exists,[5] these injuries are best divided into three types: (1) contusion/hematoma (Figure 14.6); (2) intraperitoneal rupture (Figure 14.7); and (3) extraperitoneal rupture (Figure 14.8).

This definition is not only anatomically appropriate, but it is also treatment appropriate. Extraperitoneal bladder ruptures account for 70% of bladder injuries while 10% have both intraperitoneal and extraperitoneal rupture (especially in cases of penetrating trauma). Lacerations superior to the peritoneal reflection (along the dome of the bladder) cause intraperitoneal urine extravasation whereas lacerations inferior to the peritoneal reflection result in extraperitoneal extravasation. In blunt trauma, extraperitoneal injuries are directly related to bony fragment tearing the bladder wall or from the shearing force of the injury. Intraperitoneal bladder ruptures occur at the dome of the bladder because this is the weakest portion of the bladder and the only portion covered by the peritoneum. Injuries to this location occur with a sudden increase in intra-bladder pressure (especially in a bladder distended with urine). When diagnosis is delayed, increased BUN and creatinine levels are noted as urine (urinary ascites) is reabsorbed from the peritoneal cavity.

Patients with gross hematuria or with high-risk pelvic fractures and microscopic hematuria > 25 RBC/hpf require evaluation for bladder injury. Those patients with microscopic hematuria without other evidence of lower abdominal and pelvic trauma are unlikely to have a bladder injury.[43]

Bladder contusions and hematomas are simply observed for resolution of the hematuria. Bladder laceration management is dependent on the location of rupture. Extraperitoneal rupture is managed conservatively with observation for approximately 7 days with urinary catheter drainage. After 7 days and resolution of the hematuria, a repeat cystogram is obtained to document healing of the bladder tear. Intraperitoneal bladder rupture requires operative repair with catheter drainage for 14 days. Two weeks post-operatively, the patient undergoes a repeat cystogram to document the presence or absence of urine leakage. The Foley catheter is then removed if the injury has healed. Broad spectrum antibiotics are administered during this time to prevent infection. Extended bladder drainage is necessary for cases with continued extravasation on repeat cystograms. Controversy exists over the need for a suprapubic bladder catheterization in patients with bladder rupture, but a large sample suggests simple urethral catheterization is effective.[44] Patients with bladder injuries treated and discharged from the hospital who subsequently present to the ED with urinary retention after bladder catheter removal, a Foley catheter is placed (consultation with the urologist is advised) and urine is tested for infection. Complications of bladder injury include infections, urinomas, inability or difficulty voiding, and development of fistulous tracts.

Urethral injuries

Urethral injuries are rare but may contribute to significant patient morbidity from complications including urethral stricture, impotence, and incontinence.[45]

Patients with high-risk pelvic fractures, straddle injuries, penetrating trauma in proximity to the urethra, and penile fractures are at risk and warrant evaluation. Due to anatomic length (males 4–5 times that of females), males account for over 95% of urethral injuries.[45] Pediatric patients with pelvic fractures are at higher risk for urethral injuries than adult patients due to different pelvic fracture patterns.[46] Pubic symphysis diastasis, sacroiliac diastasis, straddle fracture, and Malgaigne's fracture all increase risk of urethral injury.[46] Certain physical examination findings heighten the clinician's suspicion of a urethral injury. Blood at the urethral meatus, perineal hematoma or edema, a "high-riding" or boggy prostate on rectal examination all warrant urethral evaluation for injury prior to Foley catheter placement. All these physical examination findings are rare, however, and the most common finding is gross hematuria.[47] Any difficulty placing a Foley catheter in the patient with gross hematuria alone should still prompt a urethral evaluation before proceeding further. Anterior urethral injuries most often occur after penetrating trauma or with direct blunt trauma to the penis or perineum (straddle injuries). Anterior urethral injuries with an intact Buck's fascia result in penile shaft edema and ecchymosis as the bleeding and edema is contained within the fascia. Disruption of Buck's fascia allows urine and blood to leak into the perineum, scrotum and lower abdominal wall (ultimately limited by Colles' fascia). As with the ureter and bladder, the grading system by Moore is not well accepted. Again, this is partially due to the rarity of the injury but also the existence of a competing scale.[48] The key factors in determining the severity of injury are the location of the injury and whether the injury is a complete or incomplete transection of the urethra.

Urethral injuries are evaluated with a retrograde urethrogram prior to placement of a Foley catheter. Placement of the Foley catheter potentially worsens a pre-existing urethral injury causing extension of the urethral laceration, increase bleeding, and contamination of the hematoma. Once urethral injury is identified, urologic consultation is mandatory and the decision of Foley catheter placement via the urethral approach or a suprapubic approach is determined in consultation. Because there is limited evidence that Foley catheterization via the penile urethra worsens urethral injuries, some advocate catheterization via the penile urethra.[47]

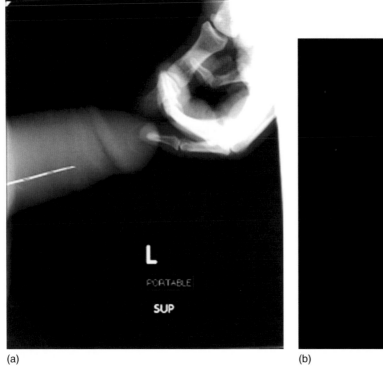

(a)

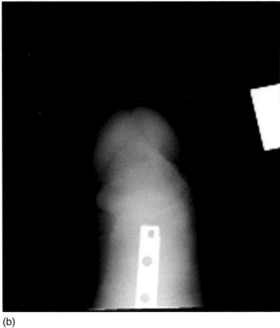

(b)

Figure 14.9 Foreign body in the penis: (a) lateral; (b) anteroposterior (AP) demonstrating razor blade.

Box 14.5   Essentials of lower GU tract injuries
- Suspect bladder injuries in patients with pelvic fractures and > 25 RBC/hpf on urinalysis.
- Intraperitoneal bladder rupture is treated surgically whereas extraperitoneal bladder rupture is treated conservatively with Foley catheter drainage.
- Foley catheter placement is ideally performed by a urologist in patients with urethral injuries as it may worsen the degree of injury.

External genitalia injuries

The combination of both penile and scrotal injuries occur in 20% of patients with external genitalia injuries.[49] Additional unique traumatic injuries occurring to the penis include penile fracture and self-inflicted penile injuries. Penile injuries occur following both blunt and penetrating mechanisms. Self-inflicted penile injuries are most often in patients with psychiatric disorders and include penile amputation or placement of foreign bodies into the urethral tract (Figure 14.9).

Simple superficial penile lacerations may be repaired in the ED. Complex or extensive lacerations require urologic consultation and operative repair with debridement and possible skin grafting. Violation of Buck's fascia requires urologic consultation.

Penile fractures occur in the erect penis (during coitus or masturbation) and present with penile pain, loss of erection, deformity, swelling, and difficulty with voiding. The injuries are commonly limited to the corpus cavernosum and Buck's fascia,[50] but may involve the urethra (5–20%). A small fraction of penile fractures are managed non-operatively (those superficial to Buck's or dartos fascia) but most benefit from early surgical treatment.[49,51]

Penile amputation is best treated with reimplantation if warm ischemic time is < 6 hours. On arrival to the ED, the amputated penis is kept cold (in dry gauze on ice) and immediate urologic consultation is indicated. Complications of penile injuries include urethral stricture, painful erection, and impotence.

Penile foreign bodies require urologic consultation and emergent removal. Blunt foreign bodies in the distal urethra are often removed blindly in the ED, but sharp or those not easily visualized in the more proximal urethra are taken to the operative suite for removal by the urologist.

Testicular injuries, like penile injuries, are uncommon; they occur most commonly in men 15–30 years of age. Blunt mechanisms are most common (80–90%) and usually involve a single testicle, whereas penetrating injuries often involve both testicles. Testicular rupture (laceration to the tunica albuginea with extrusion of the inner contents of the testicle – seminiferous tubules) is the most severe injury. Hemorrhage into the tunica vaginalis is known as a hematocele. Testicular dislocation (or luxation), where the testicle is forced from the scrotum, is rare, and occurs most often with motorcycle collisions, and is frequently missed during ED evaluation.[52] Manual reduction of testicular dislocation in the ED is recommended with surgery in cases unable to be reduced. Ultrasound is the diagnostic test of choice for most testicular injuries.[53] Abdominal CT scan will also demonstrates testicular dislocation in nearly all cases.[52]

Treatment of minor testicular injuries is supportive and includes scrotal elevation, ice, non-steroidal anti-inflammatory drugs (NSAIDs), and limited activity until resolution of symptoms. Operative therapy is indicated for patients with testicular rupture, expanding hematocele, inability to reduce testicular dislocation, and scrotal degloving. Prompt diagnosis is imperative although only testicular salvage may occur in 40% of cases.[54] Complications include bleeding, abscess, skin necrosis, infertility, testicular atrophy, or necrosis.

Box 14.6 Essentials of penile and testicular injuries

- Simple superficial penile and scrotal skin lacerations may be repaired in the ED. More complex injuries should prompt urologic consultation.
- Penile fractures require emergent urologic consultation.
- Minor testicular injuries (contusions) are treated conservatively with rest, ice, NSAIDS, and elevation.

Radiographic imaging of GU injuries

Intravenous pyelography (IVP) was once the standard method for diagnostic evaluation of the upper urinary system,[55,56] although its sensitivity for identifying significant injury is only 90%. With the introduction and expansion of abdominal CT scanning, IVP is essentially a historical test. However, a few indications for IVP remain, including: (1) lack of available CT scanner in a patient with concern for upper urinary tract injury; (2) identification or follow up of a ureteral injury; or (3) to confirm renal anatomy in an unstable patient taken directly to the operating suite and not undergoing abdominal CT scanning. This "one-shot" IVP provides the surgeon with immediate knowledge of the patient's renal anatomy (presence of two functioning kidneys) and evidence of major renal vascular injury or urinary extravasation. The actual utility in clinical practice of the "one-shot" IVP is unclear. Given the rarity of a unilateral kidney or bilateral injuries, the likehood of finding pathology that changes practice is low. In some centers, the "one-shot" IVP is often withheld, especially in the ED setting. Some surgeons may opt for one in the operating suite, whereas others will manually explore the renal bed during laparotomy. The delay in the hypotensive trauma patient to perform a "one-shot" IVP is not likely justified due to the low likelihood of finding a solitary kidney. One benefit of this test, however, is allowing the surgeon to withhold exploring a perinephric hematoma if the kidney is otherwise well perfused.[57–59] Findings on IVP predictive of renal injury include loss of the psoas margin, displaced kidney, loss of renal cortical outline, failure of a kidney to enhance, and contrast extravasation.

Ultrasonography: The role of abdominal ultrasonography in patients with GU trauma has not been definitively clarified. The focused assessment with sonography for trauma (FAST) examination identifies intraperitoneal fluid in patients but does not image organs well, and thus does not generally identify the organ injured. Injury on ultrasound scanning is suggested by changes in echogenicity of the renal parenchyma or decreased echogenicity surrounding the kidney (indicating perinephric hematoma). The largest renal ultrasound study (99 patients with renal injuries) indicated ultrasonography identified only 67% of renal injuries; it failed to identify 20% of patients undergoing surgical repair for their renal injury.[60] Areas of future research includes contrast-enhanced ultrasound and Doppler ultrasonography of the renal vasculature.

Testicular ultrasonography is the diagnostic test of choice in patients with testicular trauma.[53,61] Doppler flow evaluates vascular flow to both testicles. Heterogeneous echogenicity to the testicular parenchyma (Figure 14.10a) and absence of Doppler flow (Figure 14.10b) both indicate significant testicular injury.

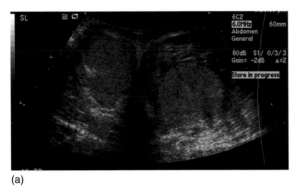

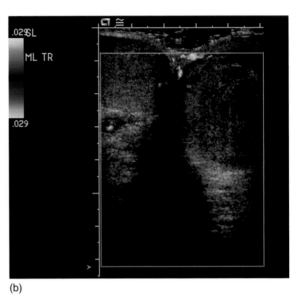

(a)   (b)

Figure 14.10 Testicular ultrasound with Doppler: (a) hematocele in right testes with (b) no flow on Doppler ultrasound.

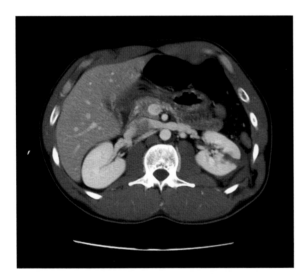

Figure 14.11 Penetrating flank trauma. The patient sustained a stab wound to the left flank. The computed tomography (CT) demonstrates extension of the stab wound through the flank musculature through the renal parenchyma and to the renal hilum.

Abdominal CT is now the principle method for imaging the kidneys and ureters after blunt trauma[62] and is used with increasing frequency in patients with penetrating injuries that may involve the kidneys (Figure 14.11).

In addition to providing information regarding the abdominal organs, the spine, and the pelvis, abdominal CT provides detailed visualization of the renal anatomy and ureter and appropriately grades the renal injury. Administration of intravenous contrast is important to appropriately visualize renal and ureteral injuries. Although not included in some trauma abdominal CT protocols, delayed renal CT images allow concentration of the intravenous contrast in the kidney and excretion into the ureter. These delayed images identify subtle renal and ureteral injuries. Not obtaining delayed renal images may result in failure to correctly diagnose the severity of injury (Figure 14.12).

A viable alternative to delayed renal images is reviewing the renal images in real time and obtaining delayed renal images if abnormalities are identified while the patient remains on the CT table. The CT findings suggesting ureteral injury include extravasation of intravenous contrast, peri-ureteral stranding, and failure of the distal ureter to opacify. Unfortunately, CT scanning does not adequately grade the severity of ureteral injury. Furthermore, a standard trauma abdominal/pelvic CT scan does not identify all bladder injuries, since the bladder is not intentionally distended during the CT.

Magnetic resonance imaging (MRI) does not offer significant benefit over CT scanning.[63,64] It may be a viable option in those with severe contrast allergies who are stable and can not undergo contrast-enhanced CT scanning. In these instances, gadolinium-enhanced MRI is indicated.

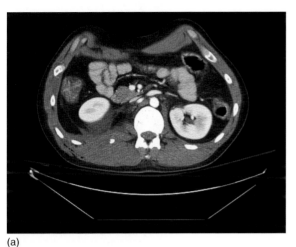 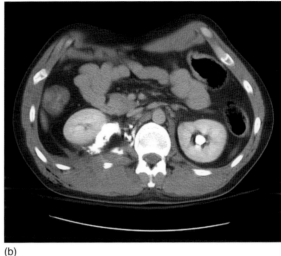

(a)   (b)

Figure 14.12 Urinoma on computed tomography (CT) scan. (a) CT image obtained at the time of intravenous contrast demonstrates a traumatic abnormality posterior to the right kidney. (b) Delayed image demonstrates contrast extravasation of urine collection posterior to the right kidney consistent with urinoma.

Cystogram: A cystogram is the primary diagnostic test for bladder injury. Although routine trauma abdominal/pelvic CT is the initial screening test, CT only identifies up to 67% of bladder injuries.[65] In patients at very high risk for bladder injury, a cystogram may be planned at the time of initial CT scanning. In these instances, a Foley catheter is inserted and the bladder distended with contrast prior to the CT scan. Another technique that may be used is to clamp the Foley catheter and allow the bladder to fill with excreted contrast. Then, a CT cystogram is obtained with the standard abdominal CT images.

Significant hematuria (> 25 RBC/hpf) with pelvic fractures is an indication for bladder imaging.[43] Cystograms may be obtained either as plain radiographs (see Figure 14.6) or using CT technology (Figure 14.13).

Both radiographs generally involve the same technique whereby the bladder is fully distended with contrast (from 300 to 400 cc instilled under gravity).[66] Radiographic images are obtained with a contrast-enhanced distended bladder. A CT cystogram provides better images and more fully evaluates the injury, but results in more radiation exposure to the pelvic region than plain radiographs. With plain film cystograms, both bladder distention radiographs and drainage radiographs (radiographs taken after the bladder is drained) maximize sensitivity.[66] Drainage radiographs identify contrast extravasation into the

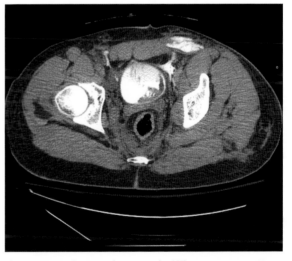

Figure 14.13 Computed tomography (CT) cystogram contrast leaking into the extraperitoneal space.

cul-de-sac which is otherwise missed on the distended bladder film (Figure 14.15).

Complete distention of the bladder is necessary for both CT and plain film studies because small tears are not noted if the bladder detrusor muscle has temporarily "sealed" the laceration.

Intraperitoneal bladder rupture is diagnosed by identification of contrast within the abdomen. Signs of this include contrast from dome of bladder, surrounding the intestines and within the paracolic gutters and the cul-de-sac (Figure 14.14).

245

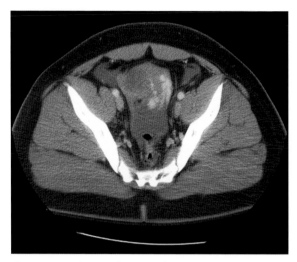

Figure 14.14 Computed tomography (CT) cystogram contrast leaking from the dome of the bladder. Intraperitoneal fluid (urine) is additionally visualized.

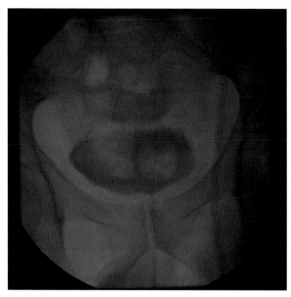

Figure 14.15 Plain cystogram post-voiding image. Image confirms the intraperitoneal leak as contrast remains in the rectal vesicular fossa.

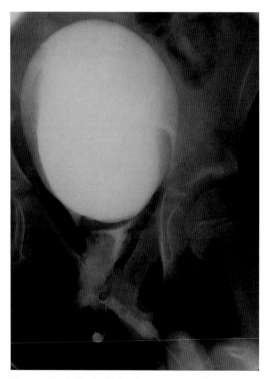

Figure 14.16 Urethral injury. Large amount of contrast extravasation occurring at the proximal urethra (bladder opacified from prior contrast computed tomography [CT]).

Extraperitoneal rupture is noted by flame-like contrast material lateral or superior to the bladder, as it transverses along the fascia (see Figure 14.8). Either plain radiography or CT, when technically adequate, is acceptable for identifying important bladder injuries.[41,42]

Retrograde urethrogram is a plain radiographic test identifying injuries to the urethra. Technique is as follows: After sterile preparation, a Foley catheter is placed at the urethra tip with the balloon partially inflated in the fossa navicularis. The penis is subsequently stretched and held at a 45° angle over the proximal thigh. Approximately 30 ml of contrast material is injected and an anteroposterior radiograph is obtained. A normal urethrogram demonstrates consistent flow of contrast into the bladder. At the time of normal urethrogram, the Foley catheter is directly placed through the urethra and into the bladder. An abnormal retrograde urethrogram is identified by the extravasation of contrast from the urethra during the examination (Figure 14.16). Once contrast extravasation is identified, the Foley catheter is not advanced. In those instances where a Foley catheter has been previously placed and urethral injury is subsequently suspected, a peri-catheter urethrogram is performed.

Arteriography: With the increased use of abdominal CT scanning and the speed of the new generation CT scanners, the need for arteriography as a diagnostic test has significantly decreased. Currently, arteriography is a therapeutic option (embolization) in patients with active bleeding identified from the renal

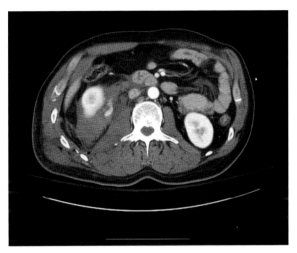

Figure 14.17 Active contrast extravasation. Contrast extravasation from the right renal artery into the large hematoma.

vasculature on CT scan or with renal pseudoaneurysms (Figure 14.17).

Box 14.7 Essentials of imaging the GU tract
- The upper GU tract is initially imaged with abdominal CT scanning.
- Obtaining delayed renal CT images (at the time of contrast concentration within the kidney) maximizes sensitivity of CT for renal injury.
- Ultrasound only identifies two thirds of renal parenchymal injuries.
- Ultrasound is the standard for diagnosing testicular injuries.
- Dedicated bladder images (cystogram) are required to definitively evaluate the bladder.
- Retrograde urethrogram is the diagnostic test for urethral injury.

Documentation

Documenting a complete (as possible) trauma history and physical examination covers most of the appropriate issues for the GU tract. However, certain unique issues to the GU tract also require documentation. Examination of the penis and testicles, especially in the high-risk patient (e.g., victims of motorcycle collisions) should be documented. Urine is obtained and identified for the presence and degree of hematuria. Results of diagnostic testing and decisions based on those tests are included in the medical record. As with all consultations, the discussion with the urologist and their comments are reflected in the medical record.

Disposition

The ED physician's primary goal in patients with GU injuries is to ensure prompt diagnosis through knowledge of the anatomy, injury patterns, and appropriate diagnostic testing. The ED physician then initiates timely treatment, including urologic consultation and appropriate antibiotics when indicated. It is not uncommon for patients with GU injuries to return to the ED after initial hospitalization and treatment. Delayed complications (especially infection and rebleeding) are aggressively evaluated and urologic consultation is indicated.

Box 14.8 Admission criteria

Consider admission/consultation	Admission/consultation mandatory
Grade I renal injury	Renal injury ≥ Grade II
Gross hematuria without other injury	Ureteral injury/urinoma on CT scan
Bladder hematoma/contusion	Any bladder laceration
Urethral contusion/stretch injury (normal RUG)	Urethral extravasation of contrast
	Significant penile injury

Transfer criteria*

Gross hematuria and inability to image kidneys and bladder

Suspected significant testicular injury and unable to image testicle with ultrasound Gross hematuria and inability to image kidneys and bladder

Meets admission criteria (as above) and no urologic consultation available

Suspected significant testicular injury and unable to image testicle with ultrasound

	Significant testicular injury

*Standard transfer protocols must be followed. Meets admission criteria (as above) and no urologic consultation available

References

1. Dreitlein DA, Suner S, Basler J. Genitourinary trauma. *Emerg Med Clin North Am* 2001;**19**:569–90.

2. McAninch JW, Federle MP. Evaluation of renal injuries with computerized tomography. *J Urol* 1982;**128**:456–60.

3. Patten RM, Gunberg SR, Brandenburger DK. Frequency and importance of transverse process fractures in the lumbar vertebrae at helical abdominal CT in patients with trauma. *Radiology* 2000; **215**:831–4.

4. Moore EE, Shackford SR, Pachter HL, et al. Organ injury scaling: spleen, liver, and kidney. *J Trauma* 1989;**29**:1664–6.

5. Moore EE, Cogbill TH, Jurkovich GJ, et al. Organ injury scaling. III: Chest wall, abdominal vascular, ureter, bladder, and urethra. *J Trauma* 1992;**33**:337–9.

6. Moore EE, Malangoni MA, Cogbill TH, et al. Organ injury scaling VII: cervical vascular, peripheral vascular, adrenal, penis, testis, and scrotum. *J Trauma* 1996;**41**:523–4.

7. Esposito TJ, Ingraham A, Luchette FA, et al. Reasons to omit digital rectal exam in trauma patients: no fingers, no rectum, no useful additional information. *J Trauma* 2005;**59**:1314–19.

8. Porter JM, Ursic CM. Digital rectal examination for trauma: does every patient need one? *Am Surg* 2001;**67**:438–41.

9. Sklar DP, Diven B, Jones J. Incidence and magnitude of catheter-induced hematuria. *Am J Emerg Med* 1986;**4**:14–16.

10. Boone TB, Gilling PJ, Husmann DA. Ureteropelvic junction disruption following blunt abdominal trauma. *J Urol* 1993;**150**:33–6.

11. Stables DP, Fouche RF, de Villiers van Niekerk JP, et al. Traumatic renal artery occlusion: 21 cases. *J Urol* 1976;**115**:229–33.

12. Holmes JF, Sokolove PE, Brant WE, et al. Identification of children with intra-abdominal injuries after blunt trauma. *Ann Emerg Med* 2002;**39**:500–9.

13. Isaacman DJ, Scarfone RJ, Kost SI, et al. Utility of routine laboratory testing for detecting intra-abdominal injury in the pediatric trauma patient. *Pediatrics* 1993;**92**:691–4.

14. Stalker HP, Kaufman RA, Stedje K. The significance of hematuria in children after blunt abdominal trauma. *AJR Am J Roentgenol* 1990;**154**:569–71.

15. Fleisher G. Prospective evaluation of selective criteria for imaging among children with suspected blunt renal trauma. *Pediatr Emerg Care* 1989;**5**:8–11.

16. Lieu TA, Fleisher GR, Mahboubi S, Schwartz JS. Hematuria and clinical findings as indications for intravenous pyelography in pediatric blunt renal trauma. *Pediatrics* 1988;**82**:216–22.

17. Perez-Brayfield MR, Gatti JM, Smith EA, et al. Blunt traumatic hematuria in children. Is a simplified algorithm justified? *J Urol* 2002;**167**:2543–6; discussion 6–7.

18. Santucci RA, Langenburg SE, Zachareas MJ. Traumatic hematuria in children can be evaluated as in adults. *J Urol* 2004;**171**:822–5.

19. Cass AS, Luxenberg M, Gleich P, Smith CS. Clinical indications for radiographic evaluation of blunt renal trauma. *J Urol* 1986;**136**:370–1.

20. Eastham JA, Wilson TG, Ahlering TE. Radiographic evaluation of adult patients with blunt renal trauma. *J Urol* 1992;**148**:266–7.

21. Guice K, Oldham K, Eide B, Johansen K. Hematuria after blunt trauma: when is pyelography useful? *J Trauma* 1983;**23**:305–11.

22. Kisa E, Schenk WG, 3rd. Indications for emergency intravenous pyelography (IVP) in blunt abdominal trauma: a reappraisal. *J Trauma* 1986;**26**:1086–9.

23. McAndrew JD, Corriere JN, Jr. Radiographic evaluation of renal trauma: evaluation of 1103 consecutive patients. *Br J Urol* 1994;**73**:352–4.

24. Mee SL, McAninch JW, Robinson AL, Auerbach PS, Carroll PR. Radiographic assessment of renal trauma: a 10-year prospective study of patient selection. *J Urol* 1989;**141**:1095–8.

25. Nicolaisen GS, McAninch JW, Marshall GA, Bluth RF, Jr., Carroll PR. Renal trauma: re-evaluation of the indications for radiographic assessment. *J Urol* 1985;**133**:183–7.

26. Holmes JF, Wisner DH, McGahan PJ, Mower WR, Kuppermann N. Clinical prediction rules for identifying adults at very low and high risk for intraabdominal injuries after blunt trauma. *Ann Emerg Med* 2009;**54**:575–89.

27. Richards JR, Derlet RW. Computed tomography and blunt abdominal injury: patient selection based on examination, haematocrit and haematuria. *Injury* 1997;**28**:181–5.

28. Sirlin CB, Brown MA, Andrade-Barreto OA, et al. Blunt abdominal trauma: clinical value of negative screening US scans. *Radiology* 2004;**230**:661–8.

29. Shariat SF, Trinh QD, Morey AF, et al. Development of a highly accurate nomogram for prediction of the need for exploration in patients with renal trauma. *J Trauma* 2008;**64**:1451–8.

30. Henderson CG, Sedberry-Ross S, Pickard R, et al. Management of high grade renal trauma: 20-year experience at a pediatric Level I trauma center. *J Urol* 2007;**178**:246–50; discussion 250.

31. Malcolm JB, Derweesh IH, Mehrazin R, et al. Nonoperative management of blunt renal trauma: is routine early follow-up imaging necessary? *BMC Urol* 2008;**8**:11.

32. Dunfee BL, Lucey BC, Soto JA. Development of renal scars on CT after abdominal trauma: does grade of injury matter? *AJR Am J Roentgenol* 2008; **190**:1174–9.

33. Knudson MM, Harrison PB, Hoyt DB, et al. Outcome after major renovascular injuries: a Western trauma association multicenter report. *J Trauma* 2000;**49**:1116–22.

34. Haas CA, Dinchman KH, Nasrallah PF, Spirnak JP. Traumatic renal artery occlusion: a 15-year review. *J Trauma* 1998;**45**:557–61.

35. Dinkel HP, Danuser H, Triller J. Blunt renal trauma: minimally invasive management with microcatheter embolization experience in nine patients. *Radiology* 2002;**223**:723–30.

36. Schwartz JH, Malhotra A, Lang E, Sclafani SJ. One-year followup of renal artery stent graft for blunt trauma. *J Urol* 2008;**180**:1507.

37. Elliott SP, McAninch JW. Ureteral injuries from external violence: the 25-year experience at San Francisco General Hospital. *J Urol* 2003;**170**:1213–16.

38. Mulligan JM, Cagiannos I, Collins JP, Millward SF. Ureteropelvic junction disruption secondary to blunt trauma: excretory phase imaging (delayed films) should help prevent a missed diagnosis. *J Urol* 1998;**159**:67–70.

39. Morgan DE, Nallamala LK, Kenney PJ, Mayo MS, Rue LW, 3rd. CT cystography: radiographic and clinical predictors of bladder rupture. *AJR Am J Roentgenol* 2000;**174**:89–95.

40. Udekwu PO, Gurkin B, Oller DW. The use of computed tomography in blunt abdominal injuries. *Am Surg* 1996;**62**:56–9.

41. Peng MY, Parisky YR, Cornwell EE, 3rd, Radin R, Bragin S. CT cystography versus conventional cystography in evaluation of bladder injury. *AJR Am J Roentgenol* 1999;**173**:1269–72.

42. Quagliano PV, Delair SM, Malhotra AK. Diagnosis of blunt bladder injury: a prospective comparative study of computed tomography cystography and conventional retrograde cystography. *J Trauma* 2006;**61**:410–21; discussion 21–2.

43. Morey AF, Iverson AJ, Swan A, et al. Bladder rupture after blunt trauma: guidelines for diagnostic imaging. *J Trauma* 2001;**51**:683–6.

44. Parry NG, Rozycki GS, Feliciano DV, et al. Traumatic rupture of the urinary bladder: is the suprapubic tube necessary? *J Trauma* 2003;**54**:431–6.

45. McAninch JW. Traumatic injuries to the urethra. *J Trauma* 1981;**21**:291–7.

46. Koraitim MM, Marzouk ME, Atta MA, Orabi SS. Risk factors and mechanism of urethral injury in pelvic fractures. *Br J Urol* 1996;**77**:876–80.

47. Shlamovitz GZ, McCullough L. Blind urethral catheterization in trauma patients suffering from lower urinary tract injuries. *J Trauma* 2007;**62**:330–5; discussion 4–5.

48. Colapinto V, McCallum RW. Injury to the male posterior urethra in fractured pelvis: a new classification. *J Urol* 1977;**118**:575–80.

49. Phonsombat S, Master VA, McAninch JW. Penetrating external genital trauma: a 30-year single institution experience. *J Urol* 2008;**180**:192–5; discussion 5–6.

50. El-Taher AM, Aboul-Ella HA, Sayed MA, Gaafar AA. Management of penile fracture. *J Trauma* 2004;**56**:1138–40; discussion 40.

51. Eke N. Fracture of the penis. *Br J Surg* 2002; **89**:555–65.

52. Ko SF, Ng SH, Wan YL, et al. Testicular dislocation: an uncommon and easily overlooked complication of blunt abdominal trauma. *Ann Emerg Med* 2004;**43**:371–5.

53. Buckley JC, McAninch JW. Use of ultrasonography for the diagnosis of testicular injuries in blunt scrotal trauma. *J Urol* 2006;**175**:175–8.

54. Mohr AM, Pham AM, Lavery RF, et al. Management of trauma to the male external genitalia: the usefulness of American Association for the Surgery of Trauma organ injury scales. *J Urol* 2003;**170**:2311–15.

55. Monstrey SJ, Vander Werken C, Debruyne FM, Goris RJ. Rational guidelines in renal trauma assessment. *Urology* 1988;**31**:469–73.

56. Uehara DT, Eisner RF. Indications for intravenous pyelography in trauma. *Ann Emerg Med* 1986; **15**:266–9.

57. Nagy KK, Brenneman FD, Krosner SM, et al. Routine preoperative "one-shot" intravenous pyelography is not indicated in all patients with penetrating abdominal trauma. *J Am Coll Surg* 1997;**185**:530–3.

58. Patel VG, Walker ML. The role of "one-shot" intravenous pyelogram in evaluation of penetrating abdominal trauma. *Am Surg* 1997;**63**:350–3.

59. Stevenson J, Battistella FD. The 'one-shot' intravenous pyelogram: is it indicated in unstable trauma patients before celiotomy? *J Trauma* 1994;**36**:828–33; discussion 33–4.

60. McGahan PJ, Richards JR, Bair AE, Rose JS. Ultrasound detection of blunt urological trauma: a 6-year study. *Injury* 2005;**36**:762–70.

61. Guichard G, El Ammari J, Del Coro C, et al. Accuracy of ultrasonography in diagnosis of testicular rupture after blunt scrotal trauma. *Urology* 2008;**71**:52–6.

62. Park SJ, Kim JK, Kim KW, Cho KS. MDCT Findings of renal trauma. *AJR Am J Roentgenol* 2006;**187**:541–7.

63. Leppaniemi AK, Kivisaari AO, Haapiainen RK, Lehtonen TA. Role of magnetic resonance imaging in blunt renal parenchymal trauma. *Br J Urol* 1991;**68**:355–60.

64. Marcos HB, Noone TC, Semelka RC. MRI evaluation of acute renal trauma. *J Magn Reson Imaging* 1998;**8**:989–90.

65. Rehm CG, Mure AJ, O'Malley KF, Ross SE. Blunt traumatic bladder rupture: the role of retrograde cystogram. *Ann Emerg Med* 1991;**20**:845–7.

66. Carroll PR, McAninch JW. Major bladder trauma: the accuracy of cystography. *J Urol* 1983;**130**:887–8.

Pelvic fracture

Jean Hammel

Introduction

Fractures of the pelvis are a major cause of morbidity and mortality in trauma patients. Significant disruptions of the pelvic ring generally result from high-energy blunt trauma, such as motor vehicle collisions (MVCs), and are frequently associated with injuries to other major organs. Comparatively minor pelvic injuries include pubic ramus fractures, acetabular fractures, and pelvic avulsion fractures. These tend to be isolated and due to simple falls or athletic activities.

Significant advances in the diagnosis and management of pelvic fractures have been made over the past decade. Innovations include more selective use of plain radiography, earlier and more aggressive angiography with embolization, and newer modalities for mechanical stabilization of the pelvis. In addition, the widespread use of bedside ultrasound has enabled emergency physicians to more accurately rule out significant hemoperitoneum and focus resuscitative efforts on the pelvic injury. Thus, the rapid identification, stabilization, and treatment of pelvic fractures in the context of a multiply injured patient are critical skills for the emergency physician.

Epidemiology

The most common mechanisms that lead to major pelvic ring fractures are motor vehicle and motorcycle collisions, falls from height, and pedestrians struck by motor vehicles.[1,2] Among MVCs, certain risk factors have been associated with an increased incidence of pelvic fractures, including side-impact collisions and vehicle size discrepancy.[3,4] Motor vehicle collisions involving a sport utility vehicle vs. a car carry a four-times greater mortality than a car vs. car in head-on collisions, and 27-times greater mortality in side-impact collisions.[5] Furthermore, the use of seat

belts appears to be protective against pelvic fracture only in front-end, but not in side-impact, MVCs.[6] Open pelvic fractures, which account for roughly 5% of all pelvic fractures, are most common after motorcycle and MVCs.[7,8]

In addition, pelvic fractures are frequently associated with injuries to other organs – most frequently the bladder and urethra (5–20%), spleen and liver (12%), and bowel (4%).[1,9,10] Urethral injuries tend to occur with disruptions of the anterior pelvic ring; they are far more common in men due to the longer course of the male urethra and its attachment to the prostate.[11] Intracranial and intrathoracic injuries are also common.

Mortality in patients with major pelvic fractures ranges from 10% to 30%.[12–20] Deaths within the first 24 hours after injury tend to be due to exsanguination from the pelvic vessels, whereas later deaths are caused by associated injuries and sepsis.[21] Open pelvic fractures are particularly prone to infectious complications and higher mortality, up to 45% in some series.[22] Open pelvic fractures that communicate with either the rectum or vagina are correlated with a significantly increased incidence of sepsis.[8]

Long-term morbidity is a similarly significant consequence of pelvic fractures, particularly those associated with a high degree of ligamentous disruption.[1] Overall, fewer than half of patients who recover from a pelvic fracture will regain their prior level of function.[2,23] In women, pelvic fractures are associated with impaired reproductive function and an increased rate of subsequent cesarean deliveries.[23]

In addition to the major pelvic ring disruptions, there are also several classes of comparatively minor pelvic fractures which are seen far more commonly in the emergency department (ED). These include isolated pubic ramus fractures, pelvic avulsion fractures,

---

Trauma: A Comprehensive Emergency Medicine Approach, eds. Eric Legome and Lee W. Shockley. Published by Cambridge University Press. © Cambridge University Press 2011.

and acetabular fractures. The epidemiology of these fractures is quite varied. Pubic ramus fractures are the most common type of pelvic fracture overall, the vast majority of which occur in elderly women after a minor fall.[24,25] These fractures are usually unilateral, and the incidence is approximately evenly divided between inferior, superior, and both ipsilateral rami.[24]

Pelvic avulsion fractures are injuries that occur primarily in adolescents and young adults, as a result of their immature apophyseal ossification centers. Most such fractures are sports-related and occur in patients between 14 and 25 years of age.[26] The most common sites for pelvic avulsions are the anterior superior iliac spine, followed by the ischial tuberosity, the anterior inferior iliac spine, and the iliac crest.[25]

Lastly, acetabular fractures are caused by either direct lateral trauma to the greater tuberosity of the femur, or indirect longitudinal trauma to the distal femur that is transmitted proximally to the acetabulum via a flexed hip (i.e., the so-called "dashboard injuries"). These fractures can be associated with a significant degree of morbidity. Such fractures generally occur in the setting of MVC or falls. Associated injuries are common, particularly hip dislocations and ipsilateral knee injuries.

Box 15.1 Essential Information/highlights

- Pelvic ring fractures result from massive blunt trauma and are commonly associated with other organ injuries.
- Early mortality from pelvic fractures is due to exsanguination from pelvic vessels.
- As computed tomography (CT) becomes more commonly used for multisystem trauma, plain radiography has taken on a limited role in the diagnosis of pelvic fractures.
- The role of the emergency physician is to rapidly identify the most immediately life-threatening injuries, mechanically stabilize the pelvis, and resuscitate the patient while determining the need for definitive therapy.
- Persistent hemodynamic instability due to pelvic fractures requires either immediate angiography with embolization or laparotomy for other injuries with packing of the retroperitoneum.
- Minor pelvic fractures, such as pubic ramus fractures in the elderly after a fall or a pelvic avulsion fracture in a young athlete, are generally treated conservatively.
- Acetabular fractures are stable injuries that require surgical repair in most cases.

Clinical anatomy and pathophysiology
Anatomy

The pelvis is an extremely strong structure which contributes to the load-bearing ability of the body. It consists not only of bony elements, but also an intricate network of ligaments, soft tissues, and an abundance of blood vessels.

The three main bones of the pelvis are the ischium, the ilium, and the pubis (Figure 15.1). These bones are fused via the triradiate cartilage at the acetabulum; together they make up the innominate bone (Figure 15.2). The sacrum is bound to the pelvis via the posterior ligaments, and this ligamentous complex contributes significantly to the overall stability and weightbearing capacity of the pelvis.

The acetabulum is a concave bony structure lined with articular cartilage to accommodate the femoral head. The dome of the acetabulum, particularly the superior portion, contributes significantly to weightbearing and mobility. Anatomically, the acetabulum is divided into the anterior and posterior columns, which provide its structural support; this can be conceptualized as an inverted "Y" encasing the dome. The anterior column is comprised of the iliac crest, symphysis pubis, and the anterior wall of the acetabular dome. The posterior column includes the ischial tuberosity, the inferior pubic ramus, and the posterior wall of the acetabular dome.

Ligaments bind the bones of the pelvis together into the pelvic ring (Figure 15.3). The posterior ligamentous complex confers the greatest strength and stability to the pelvis.[9] This complex is composed of the sacro-iliac (SI) joints, as well as the sacrotuberous

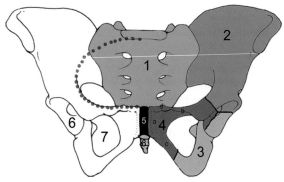

Figure 15.1 The bony pelvis: (1) sacrum; (2) ilium; (3) ischium; (4) pubis; (5) pubic symphysis; (6) acetabulum; (7) obturator foramen; (8) coccyx; (red dotted line) linea terminalis.

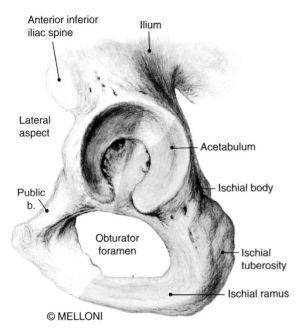

Anterior inferior iliac spine

Ilium

Lateral aspect

Acetabulum

Public b.

Ischial body

Obturator foramen

Ischial tuberosity

Ischial ramus

© MELLONI

Figure 15.2 Innominate bone. (From Melloni J, Dox I, Melloni H, Melloni B. *Attorney's Reference on Human Anatomy*. Cambridge: Cambridge University Press, 2008.)

and sacrospinous ligaments. As the name implies, the SI joints hold the posterior iliac wings to the sacrum and are the strongest joints in the body. Within the SI joints are both anterior and posterior elements, the latter being particularly important to pelvic ring stability. The sacrotuberous ligament runs from the inferomedial aspect of the sacrum to the ischial tuberosity, and the sacrospinous ligament binds the inferior sacrum and coccyx to the ischial spine. Anteriorly, the pubic symphysis holds the two pubic bones together in the midline and is the weakest part of the pelvic ring, conferring only 15% of its total strength.[9] The lumbosacral and iliolumbar ligaments provide additional stability by affixing the lumbar spine to the pelvis.

In addition, extremely strong tendons bind the pelvic bones to associated musculature, which can lead to avulsion fractures when forcefully contracted or stretched (Figure 15.4). The sartorius muscle runs from the anterior superior iliac spine to the medial aspect of the proximal tibia; it causes hip flexion, hip external rotation, and knee flexion. The hamstrings attach to the ischial tuberosity and insert along the posterior femur, and result in hip extension with contraction. The rectus femoris muscle inserts at the anterior inferior iliac spine and contributes to hip flexion.

The pelvis also houses a massive amount of vasculature, providing blood supply to its own structures as well as the lower extremities (Figures 15.5 and 15.6).

The pelvic bones are primary cancellous, with a large network of veins within the bones themselves. The iliac veins and arteries branch numerous times within the pelvis to supply the genitourinary system, anus, rectum, and lower extremities. Many smaller, thin-walled veins form a venous plexus that directly overlies the pelvic girdle. Exsanguination from these many sources is one of the most acutely life-threatening sequelae of pelvic fracture.

The soft tissues of the pelvis include the pelvic diaphragm as well as several major organ systems. The diaphragm composes the floor of the pelvis via a complex network of muscles. The rectum, bladder, urethra, uterus, and vagina in women, or prostate in men are also within the pelvis. Injury to these structures is important to diagnose, as violation of the rectum or vagina constitutes an open pelvic fracture.

Lastly, many major nerves course through the pelvis and sacrum. The cauda equina terminates in the sacrum, with nerve roots exiting through their respective foramina. In addition, the femoral and obturator nerves pass through the pelvic ring itself and are often damaged by displaced fractures. Similarly, autonomic innervation to the bowel, bladder, and reproductive organs is contained within the pelvic girdle and can be affected by pelvic injuries.

Pathophysiology: pelvic fracture classification

Fractures of the pelvis can be divided into significant disruptions of the pelvic ring vs. more minor, isolated pelvic bone fractures. The latter category includes acetabular fractures, avulsion fractures, and isolated pubic ramus fractures. These are both mechanically and hemodynamically stable injuries and generally result from athletic activities in young people or minor falls in the elderly. No classification systems exist for pubic ramus and avulsion fractures; simply describing the fracture is sufficient.

Acetabular fractures can be the result of low- or high-energy trauma, and are classified according to the Letournel and Judet system. In simple terms, this system divides acetabular fractures into simple and "associated," or more complex, types (Table 15.1). The five simple fractures are seen in Figure 15.7.

253

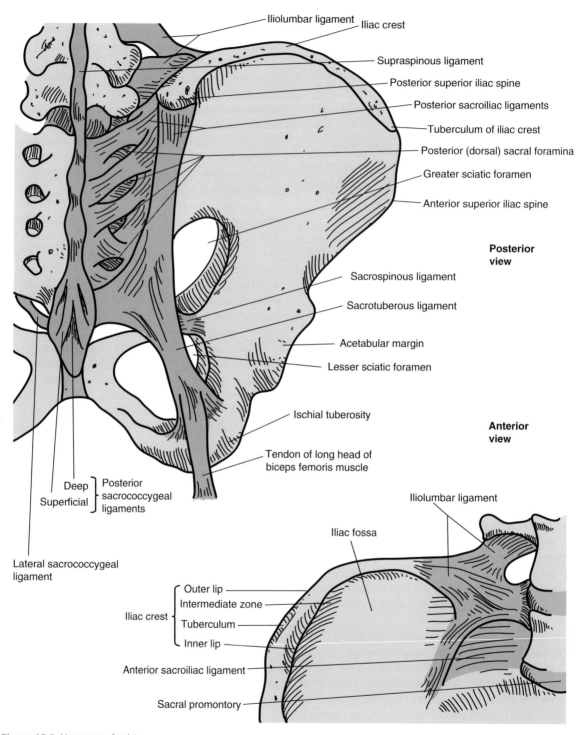

Iliolumbar ligament
Iliac crest
Supraspinous ligament
Posterior superior iliac spine
Posterior sacroiliac ligaments
Tuberculum of iliac crest
Posterior (dorsal) sacral foramina
Greater sciatic foramen
Anterior superior iliac spine

Posterior view

Sacrospinous ligament
Sacrotuberous ligament
Acetabular margin
Lesser sciatic foramen

Ischial tuberosity

Anterior view

Tendon of long head of biceps femoris muscle

Deep
Superficial
Posterior sacrococcygeal ligaments

Lateral sacrococcygeal ligament

Iliolumbar ligament
Iliac fossa

Iliac crest
Outer lip
Intermediate zone
Tuberculum
Inner lip

Anterior sacroiliac ligament
Sacral promontory

Figure 15.3 Ligaments of pelvis.

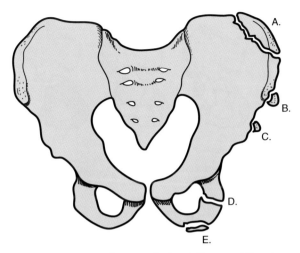

Figure 15.4 Avulsion fractures of pelvis. A: Fracture of iliac wing. B: Avulsion of anterosuperior iliac spine. C: Avulsion of anteroinferior iliac spine. D: Fracture of ischial ramus. E: Avulsion of ischial tuberosity.

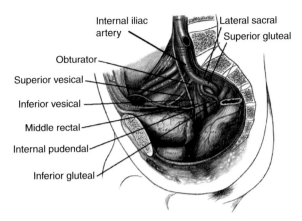

Figure 15.5 The arteries of the pelvis. Right side (distal from spectator).

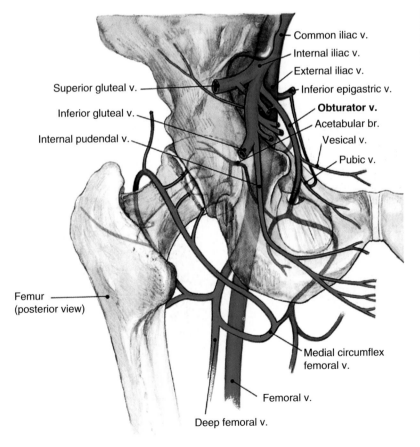

Figure 15.6 Venous supply to the pelvis. (From Melloni J, Dox I, Melloni H, Melloni B. *Attorney's Reference on Human Anatomy.* Cambridge: Cambridge University Press, 2008.)

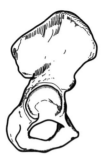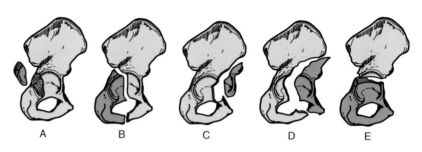

Figure 15.7 Simple acetabular fractures classification. A: Posterior wall fracture. B: Posterior column fracture. C: Anterior wall fracture. D: Anterior column fracture. E: Transverse fracture.

Table 15.1 Acetabular Fracture Classification – Letournel and Judet System

Simple fractures	Associated fractures
Posterior wall	T-shaped
Posterior column	Posterior column and posterior wall
Anterior wall	Transverse and posterior wall
Anterior column	Anterior column and posterior hemitransverse
Transverse	Both column

The both column fracture is the most complex associated fracture, resulting in the so-called "floating acetabulum" (Figure 15.8).

The type of acetabular fracture correlates with the mechanism of injury. Transverse fractures, for instance, tend to result from force directed at the greater trochanter of the femur; an abducted femur leads to a low transverse acetabular fracture, whereas an adducted femur leads to a high transverse fracture. The degree of internal or external rotation of the femur at the time of impact determines whether the fracture involves the posterior or anterior columns, respectively. In the same vein, "dashboard" injuries that transmit force from the distal femur to the acetabulum via a flexed hip cause fractures of the posterior wall. The posterior wall can be disrupted either superiorly or inferiorly, depending on the degree of hip flexion at the time of impact.

Pelvic ring disruptions, in contrast to the aforementioned isolated injuries, run the spectrum from stable to life-threatening. Several classification systems have been devised for these fractures in the

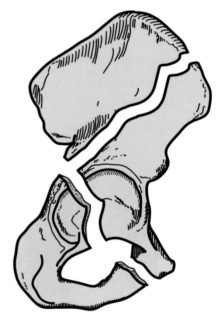

Figure 15.8 Both column complex acetabular fracture.

orthopedic and trauma literature. In general, pelvic fracture subtype does not impact ED management of these patients – the clinical picture is far more important. However, for emergency physicians, understanding the general approach to pelvic fracture classification will facilitate collaboration with our surgical colleagues and enable us to anticipate common injury patterns.

First, the Tile classification system was developed based on the concept of mechanical stability, regardless of vector of force. Tile type A fractures are completely mechanically stable and involve no disruption of the pelvic ring. These include the minor avulsion fractures and isolated pubic ramus fractures. Tile type B fractures encompass a wide array of pelvic fractures that are mechanically unstable to

Table 15.2 Young and Burgess classification of pelvic ring fractures

Anterior–posterior compression	APC I	Pubic symphysis diastasis < 2.5 cm	Mechanically stable
	APC II	Pubic symphysis diastasis > 2.5 cm, anterior SI disruptio.	Rotationally unstable Vertically stable
	APC III	Pubic symphysis diastasis > 2.5 cm: SI joints completely disrupted	Completely unstable
Lateral compression	LC I	Transverse pubic rami fractures, impaction of the sacrum	Mechanically stable
	LC II	LC I + posterior SI disruption	Rotationally unstable Vertically stable
	LC III	LC II + external rotation of contralateral hemipelvis	Completely unstable
Vertical shear	VS	Vertical disruption of bony and ligamentous supports	Completely unstable
Combined mechanism	CM	Massive pelvic fractures which do not fit any other category	Completely unstable

APC, anterior–posterior compression; CM, combined mechanism; LC, lateral compression; SI, sacro-iliac; VS, vertical shear.

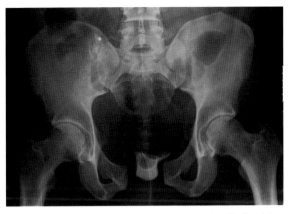

Figure 15.9 Type II anterior–posterior compression (APC) pelvic fracture plain radiograph. (Courtesy of Mark Bernstein, MD.)

The Young and Burgess classification system was devised based on mechanism of injury and secondarily mechanical stability. This system is most relevant to clinical practice and is now more widely used than the Tile classification. The four main categories are: anterior–posterior compression (APC), lateral compression (LC), vertical shear (VS), and combined mechanism (CM). Each mechanism of injury causes a predictable spectrum of pelvic fracture patterns and associated injuries. The APC and LC fractures are further subdivided into Types I, II, and III by mechanical stability; VS and CM are all unstable (Table 15.2).

APC injuries are the so-called "open-book" pelvic fractures, generally caused by front-end collisions resulting in some degree of external rotation of the pelvic ring. Type I APC fractures involve diastasis of the pubic symphysis of < 2.5 cm. Examples of common APC I injuries are ipsilateral vertical superior and inferior pubic ramus fractures with minimal displacement and isolated pubic symphyseal diastasis. By definition, there is no disruption of the posterior pelvic ring, and therefore these are both mechanically and hemodynamically stable. Type II APC fractures are defined by diastasis of the pubic symphysis of > 2.5 cm as well as disruption of the anterior SI joint. These fractures are rotationally unstable to lateral force, but vertically stable. Type III APC injuries involve total disruption of the posterior ligamentous complex, and are completely unstable (Figures 15.9–15.11).

The second category in the Young and Burgess classification system is lateral compression (LC) (Figure 15.12). These fractures are usually associated with side-impact collisions and cause internal rotation of the pelvic ring. Type I LC injuries are mechanically

rotational force, but stable to vertical force. Finally, Tile type C includes those fractures which are both rotationally and vertically unstable.

stable and involve transverse fractures of one or two pubic rami with impaction of the sacrum on the side of injury. Type II LC injuries result from forces directly both medially and anteriorly. In LC II injuries, in addition to the injuries found in LC I fractures, the posterior aspect of the SI joint is disrupted and the iliac wing is often fractured. These are rotationally unstable to medial stress but are vertically stable. Finally, LC III fractures result from such high-energy force that the contralateral side of the pelvis suffers an external rotation injury in addition to the ipsilateral LC II fractures. These injuries tend to result from crush or rollover mechanisms and are completely mechanically unstable.

Vertical shear (VS) fractures are caused by falls from height or head-on MVCs with force directed onto an extended lower extremity. Virtually all ligamentous supports are disrupted with multiple associated fractures. Therefore, these are both rotationally and vertically unstable fracture patterns. Lastly, combined mechanism injuries (CM) are not easily categorized in any of the previously discussed Young and Burgess classifications. These injuries are also completely

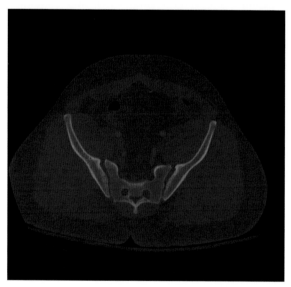

Figure 15.10 Same fracture as Figure 15.9 with computed tomography (CT) reconstructions. (Courtesy of Mark Bernstein, MD.)

mechanically unstable with multiple fractures and widespread ligamentous damage (Figure 15.13).

Considerable research has focused on whether fracture pattern is predictive of hemorrhage, associated injuries, or overall outcome. Initially, the Young and Burgess classification scheme was embraced as a way to predict such clinical variables. In the landmark 1990 study by Burgess et al, of the 210 patients studied, those with APC fractures had greater transfusion requirements and associated mortality than patients with other fracture patterns.[15] Other small retrospective studies followed, which attempted to correlate fracture pattern with injury severity and had varying results.[14,27,28]

More recent literature, however, has shown that fracture pattern does not accurately predict the presence of arterial hemorrhage or mortality.[29–34] While mechanically unstable fractures of all types more commonly cause life-threatening bleeding,[35] up to 10% of so-called "stable" Young and Burgess APC and LC class I fractures can cause significant arterial hemorrhage.[30] Thus, the entire clinical picture rather than just the pelvic radiograph must be taken into account when determining the next step in the patient's management.

Pelvic fracture type may, however, predict where arterial hemorrhage is likely to occur. That is, APC fractures generally cause posterior bleeding, particularly from the superior gluteal and internal iliac arteries, whereas LC fractures more commonly caused anterior bleeding from the pudendal and obturator arteries.[36]

Prehospital

Patients with pelvic fractures have often suffered multisystem trauma. In all patients with high-energy pelvic fractures, two large-bore intravenous lines should be obtained and frequent vital sign monitoring performed en route to the ED. All such patients should be placed in full spinal immobilization with a rigid back-board and cervical collar in place. Transport should be as expeditious as possible.

In patients with obviously unstable pelvic fractures, mechanical pelvic stabilization can be applied

Figure 15.11 Young–Burgess anterior–posterior compression (APC) pelvic fracture classifications.

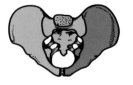

I.

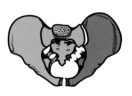

II.

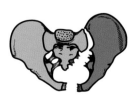

III.

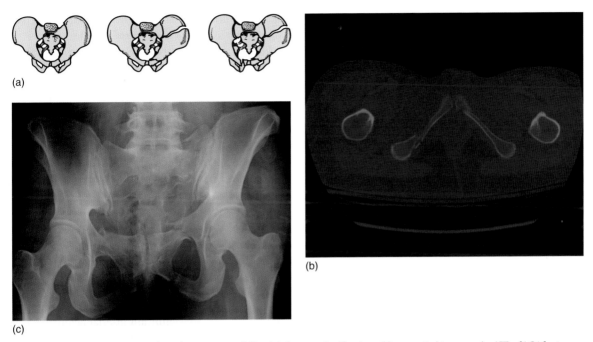

(a)

(b)

(c)

Figure 15.12 (a) Young–Burgess lateral compression (LC) pelvic fracture classifications; (b) computed tomography (CT) of LC I fracture pattern; (c) X-ray of LC I fracture pattern.

by prehospital personnel. The two main modalities available in the prehospital setting are the pneumatic anti-shock garment (PASG) and the pelvic binder, e.g., a simple sheet wrapped around the pelvis.

Much controversy has surrounded the use of the PASG, sometimes called the military anti-shock trouser (MAST) from its widespread use in the Vietnam war. The PASG is a set of inflatable trousers that compresses the lower extremities, pelvis, and most of the abdomen. The goal of this intervention is to tamponade hemorrhage, improve venous return, and to stabilize pelvic and lower extremity fractures. However, the risks of the PASG are significant, and studies have repeatedly shown that this intervention does not improve outcomes.[37,38] Adverse effects of the PASG include compartment syndromes, respiratory compromise due to increased intra-abdominal pressure, limited vascular and operative access, increased bleeding from thoracic injuries, metabolic acidosis, and profound hypotension after removal. There are a few instances in the prehospital setting where a PASG may be appropriate; these are limited to patients with obvious pelvic fractures, hypotension, poor intravenous access *and* prolonged transport times. If it is used for pelvic fractures, only the pelvic compartment should be inflated, leaving the

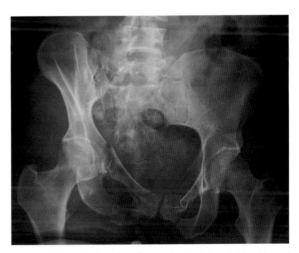

Figure 15.13 Combined mechanism (vertical shear [VS] and lateral compression [LC]) fractures.

leg compartments deflated. In the vast majority of cases, however, the PASG no longer plays a role; this is reflected in the fact that most prehospital systems do not carry the device.

Conversely, wrapping the pelvis with a sheet is a reasonable and easily performed intervention for prehospital providers. While the evidence supporting this technique will be discussed below, our recommendation is in favor of pelvic binding in patients with unstable pelvic fractures and hypotension in the prehospital setting. Performing this intervention should in no way delay transport to the ED for definitive care.

Emergency department evaluation and management

Common presentations

Severe and moderate

Disruptions to the pelvic ring are generally the result of major blunt trauma and will usually present to the ED by ambulance. Most awake patients will be able to communicate that they have pain at the fracture site, though this is dependent on mental status and the degree of distracting injuries. Patients may perceive the pain from a pelvic fracture as lower abdominal pain, hip pain, or lumbosacral pain; such complaints should alert the emergency physician to a potential injury to the pelvic ring.

More severely injured patients, however, often cannot communicate effectively or may not perceive the pain of their pelvic injury. They are frequently hypotensive and intubated early. Therefore, it is important to keep pelvic fracture high in the differential diagnosis when evaluating any multiply injured patient.

Minor

Low-energy pelvic fractures generally occur in the young and active, or the elderly and osteoporotic. Avulsion injuries occur suddenly during athletic activity in young adults and adolescents. The acute onset of hip pain with forceful muscle contraction, such as taking off for a sprint, jumping, or kicking is a common historical finding. Patients also often report a "pop" at the time of injury. Physical examination findings include localized tenderness, decreased range of motion, and worsened pain with stretching of the affected muscle.

Pubic ramus fractures are seen often in elderly patients after a minor fall from standing. Patients may complain of hip or pelvic pain, although they do not have any shortening or rotation of the affected lower extremity. In the absence of other major injuries, patients are generally hemodynamically stable. Examination reveals localized tenderness over the anterior pubic bone and occasionally limitation of hip motion due to pain. Up to a quarter of patients will have a second fracture, most commonly the distal radius, lumbar spine, and proximal humerus[24] – consistent with the mechanism of a fall from standing.

Acetabular fractures may result from a variety of mechanisms ranging from low energy such as a simple fall to high energy such as a MVC. Patients generally complain of hip, rather than pelvic, pain. In the setting of an isolated acetabular fracture, the affected lower extremity is generally not shortened or rotated. The sciatic nerve can be injured in posterior acetabular fractures. Concomitant injuries of the ipsilateral lower extremity are common, especially when increased force is involved. Posterior acetabular fractures are associated with patellar fractures, posterior knee ligamentous injuries, and hip dislocations – which correlate with the common "dashboard" mechanism of injury.

Occult

A common problem for the emergency physician is the patient who presents with hip or pelvic pain after minor trauma, negative radiographs, and persistent difficulty ambulating. While avulsion injuries are easily seen radiographically, both pubic ramus fractures and acetabular fractures can be missed with plain radiography. One series showed that up to 17% of isolated pubic ramus fractures were not seen on the initial X-ray.[24] Clinically, it may be difficult to differentiate between occult femoral neck, acetabular, and pubic ramus fractures. For patients with inability to ambulate despite normal plain films, definitive imaging studies such as CT or magnetic resonance imaging (MRI) are warranted.

Initial evaluation

Physical examination

The examination of the traumatized pelvis is a focused process. Detecting an injury to the pelvic structures on physical examination entails more than simply "rocking the pelvis." The fully-undressed patient should be examined for ecchymoses, bony deformities, leg-length discrepancies, and abdominal distention. The perineum should be inspected for blood at the urethral meatus, the vaginal introitus, or any lacerations that could indicate an open pelvic fracture. Vaginal and rectal examinations should be performed when a major pelvic fracture is confirmed to look for internal lacerations, gross blood or abnormal tone.

The pelvis should be evaluated for tenderness not only at the iliac spines, but also over the pubic symphysis, the posterior and lateral iliac crests, and the posterior SI joints. The spine should be palpated for tenderness, extending inferiorly to include the sacrum and coccyx. Gross mechanical stability of the pelvis is assessed by applying a gentle external and internal rotational force to the anterior superior iliac spines. Any motion is abnormal and denotes an unstable fracture. Of note, this part of the examination should be performed once and without great force; repeatedly moving an unstable pelvic fracture risks further exacerbating the injury, increasing blood loss as well as causing severe pain for the conscious patient. Motor strength, deep tendon reflexes, pulses, and sensation in the lower extremities should be tested. Perineal sensation as well as rectal tone should similarly be noted.

Trauma room studies

Severe

Pelvic fractures can be a cause of hemodynamic instability in trauma patients. While the pelvic radiograph directly assesses only bony injury, severe disruptions of the pelvic ring are an indirect indication of hemorrhage into the pelvis and retroperitoneum. A completely normal AP pelvic radiograph, though not sufficiently sensitive for all pelvic fractures, remains a reasonable first test to rule out unstable pelvic ring fracture as a cause of hypotension.[39]

The focused abdominal sonography in trauma (FAST) exam, similar to the pelvic X-ray, is not a highly sensitive test for subtle injuries such as occult hemoperitoneum or abdominal injuries not associated with intraperitoneal bleeding. However, the FAST exam has been shown to be extremely accurate at detecting clinically significant hemoperitoneum.[40] Emergency physicians are now routinely trained in this procedure and have been shown to be accurate in performing and interpreting the results.[38] In the setting of pelvic ring fracture, FAST may be slightly less specific due to bladder injuries and pelvic hematomas, but it is still a highly accurate tool.[41]

In those few trauma centers that do not regularly use the FAST exam or in patients with an equivocal FAST and hypotension, diagnostic peritoneal lavage (DPL) can be performed to detect hemoperitoneum. The supraumbilical approach is recommended in order to avoid false positives due to retroperitoneal hemorrhage tracking into the fascia below the umbilicus. The FAST exam is preferable to DPL because it is non-invasive, quicker, and more accurate for hemodynamically significant intra-abdominal bleeding.[42]

Moderate and minor

In contrast, hemodynamically stable patients do not routinely require immediate trauma bay pelvic radiography. While the chest X-ray (CXR) and FAST examination should be performed on most victims of significant blunt trauma even if stable, the pelvic radiograph can often be deferred. Several studies have shown that a normal physical exam is sufficient, and perhaps better than an X-ray, to exclude pelvic fracture in awake and alert trauma patients.[3,39,43] In a large prospective study of blunt trauma patients with a Glasgow Coma Score of 14 or 15, the physical examination had a sensitivity of 93% for pelvic fracture.[39] None of the injuries missed by physical exam required surgery or other change in management. Another recent prospective study found a thorough physical exam to have a sensitivity of 100% for pelvic fractures.[43]

The reliability of the physical exam appears to be maintained in mildly intoxicated patients, i.e., those with a normal neurologic examination and mental status. In several studies of patients who were deemed "clinically sober" but with ethanol levels over 100 mg/dl, the history and physical examination detected 91–95% of pelvic fractures.[3,39] This was comparable to control patients with lower ethanol levels. Pelvic fractures missed on clinical grounds alone were either clinically insignificant or in the context of painful distracting injuries.

In contrast, data on the reliability of the physical examination in children are mixed. Studies cite the sensitivity for pelvic fracture between 69 and 92%.[44,45] Thus, in this younger population, pelvic X-ray is still recommended as part of the routine workup of major blunt trauma patients, even if hemodynamically stable.

In addition to demonstrating the accuracy of the physical examination, these studies have also demonstrated the comparatively poor performance of the plain radiograph in detecting more subtle pelvic ring disruptions. Using CT as the gold standard, pelvic X-ray is only 54–87% sensitive for pelvic fracture in both adults and children.[39,46–48] Therefore, in any stable patient for which CT of the abdomen and pelvis is planned, a pelvic radiograph is not necessary.

For those patients *not* undergoing pelvic CT scan for other reasons, evidence supports obtaining a pelvic radiograph in patients with any of the following: history or physical exam findings suggestive of pelvic injury, altered mental status, distracting injury, or in children. This radiograph may be performed in the trauma room or the radiology suite. Stable patients with no pelvic pain, a normal physical examination, and normal mental status need no pelvic imaging.

Acute interventions

For the patient with a high-energy pelvic fracture, the initial resuscitation should proceed as it would for any other multiply injured patient. In cases of obvious pelvic fracture or trauma to the lower extremities, venous access should be obtained above the diaphragm. Unless signs of urethral transection such as blood at the urethral meatus are found on physical examination, a urethral catheter should be placed to obtain urine and monitor urine output.

Early mechanical pelvic stabilization may decrease the hemorrhage from torn pelvic veins and the fractured cancellous pelvic bones, though some debate surrounds this issue in the literature. Mechanical stabilization theoretically decreases venous hemorrhage through two mechanisms: (1) by reapproximating the bones; and (2) by reducing the pelvic volume to create tamponade. In a cadaveric model, however, mechanical stabilization was shown to only minimally increase the pressure within the pelvis, potentially enough to control venous but not arterial hemorrhage.[49] In addition, in the case of the conscious patient, early stabilization will also decrease discomfort.

There are several means of achieving rapid mechanical stabilization of pelvic fractures in the ED. Most common is the "pelvic binder," or a sheet tied around the pelvis circumferentially from the femoral greater tuberosities to the anterior superior iliac spines (Figure 15.14). Surgical hemostats can be used to secure the sheet to prevent slippage that can occur from a knot alone. In addition, several studies have looked at various commercial pelvic stabilizers, including a C-clamp or other devices such as the SAM® sling (Figure 15.15a), the T-Pod® (Figure 15.15b), or a neoprene belt. Proposed advantages to these are the ability to stabilize the posterior pelvic ring and to allow access to the groin and abdomen for angiography and laparotomy. The PASG has no role in the ED care of these patients. Lastly, a few trauma centers are capable of rapid and sterile application of an external fixator in the trauma room.

The evidence supporting one means of stabilization over another is scarce. Few trauma centers have access to specialized devices, thus no clinical trials have compared different means of stabilization. In theory, the posterior pelvic ring disruptions of LC and VS fracture patterns might be further displaced with a sheet alone, though there is no evidence to support that contention. Some centers will withhold this treatment in these types of disruptions. No clear guidance based on the literature is available. In a cadaveric model analyzing the effect of a C-clamp, circumferential sheet, and external fixation on different pelvic fracture patterns, all significantly increased the mechanical stability of the pelvic ring, but external fixation was by far the most effective.[50] Interestingly, no significant differences were found in the stabilization achieved by the C-clamp vs. the wrapped sheet, even in lateral compression injuries.

In summary, in cases of significant pelvic fractures (i.e., all but Young and Burgess APC and LC Class 1), we recommend early mechanical stabilization in the ED. A wrapped sheet appears to be equally as efficacious as other compression devices. Early external fixation may be optimal in those few centers capable of rapidly applying the device in the ED, although this has never been proven *in vivo*.

> **Box 15.3 Acute emergency department interventions**
>
> - Fluid and blood resuscitation for signs of hypovolemia.
> - Intravenous access above the diaphragm.
> - Mechanical stabilization of the pelvis via pelvic binder.
> - Chest radiograph, pelvis radiograph, and FAST exam in the trauma room for all unstable patients to rapidly determine the source of most life-threatening hemorrhage.

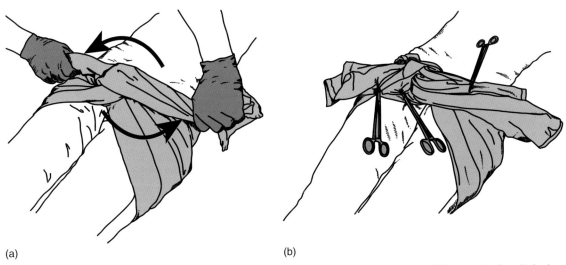

(a)　　　　　　　　　　　　　　　　　　(b)

Figure 15.14 (a) Patient wrapped circumferentially around pelvis with sheet tightened clockwise, and (b) secured with multiple clamps.

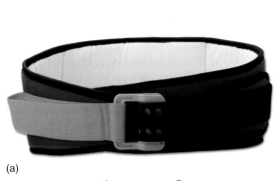

(a)

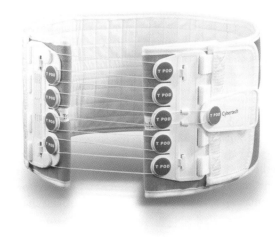

(b)

Figure 15.15 (a) SAM® sling; (b) T-Pod®.

Secondary evaluation

Severe

Radiologic

In hemodynamically unstable patients with pelvic fractures, initial pelvic imaging should be accomplished with portable AP radiograph. Likewise, portable chest radiography and FAST are complementary studies in determining the extent of injuries and are usually sufficient to plan ongoing treatment. Transportation to the radiology suite and prolonged CT scanning is contraindicated. In the unstable patient, further imaging is rarely necessary before life-saving interventions are performed, e.g., embolization or laparotomy with pelvic packing.

Laboratory

For these unstable trauma patients, although rarely impacting immediate management, common laboratory tests include those listed in Box 15.4.

The blood bank should be alerted to make several units of packed red blood cells and fresh frozen plasma available as soon as possible. Again, none of these will affect the ED management of the patient.

Box 15.4   Recommended testing
- Definite tests
  - Complete blood count
  - Full electrolyte panel
  - Coagulation panel
  - Type and cross-match (4–8 units)
  - Urinalysis
  - Beta human chorionic gonadotrophin (beta-hCG) for women of childbearing age
- Optional tests
  - Urine toxicology screen
  - Serum ethanol level
  - Serum lactate
  - Arterial blood gas

Moderate

Radiologic

In stable patients for whom intra-abdominal injury is not a concern but pelvic fracture is suspected, a plain pelvic X-ray is indicated. If positive, this may be followed by CT to better define the fractures and any associated injuries. In well-appearing, ambulatory patients with a low initial suspicion for fracture, a negative X-ray is sufficient to rule out clinically significant fracture.

For stable blunt trauma patients with high clinical suspicion of abdominal and pelvic injuries, CT of the abdomen and pelvis should be done, which can obviate the need for a pelvic radiograph. Reconstructions of the lumbar spine and pelvis can also be done from this imaging study. These patients will usually have undergone a chest radiograph and FAST exam in the trauma room. The results of these studies and the physical exam will determine which additional CTs are indicated.

Patients with pelvic fractures have a high incidence of concomitant genitourinary injuries.[1,9,11] If gross hematuria is present, the CT should be modified to include thin cuts through the kidneys and CT cystograms to assess the integrity of the upper and lower urinary tracts.

Abdominal-pelvic CT provides a tremendous amount of information. For the bony pelvis, CT will detect many more fractures than plain radiography alone.[39,47] In addition, CT will show associated visceral and soft tissue injuries, pelvic and retroperitonal hematomas, as well as contrast "blush" consistent with active arterial hemorrhage. Even in the hemodynamically stable patient, such hematomas and extravasation of contrast correlate with significant hemorrhage from the pelvic vessels.[34,51–53] Thus, CT can better define not only the bony injuries to the pelvis but also help determine further management strategies to control internal hemorrhage.

Laboratory

Laboratory tests should be the same as those for severely injured patients, although type-and-cross may be replaced by type-and-screen in some cases. This depends on the patients underlying medical problems, concomitant injuries, and whether ongoing hemorrhage is suspected.

Minor

Radiologic

Plain radiographs are the initial study of choice to detect pelvic avulsion fractures, pubic ramus fractures, and acetabular fractures. For the latter two, hip radiographs should also be performed, as it is often difficult to distinguish clinically between occult femoral neck fractures and minor pelvic injuries.

Standard pelvic X-ray views include the anterior-posterior, inlet, outlet, and oblique or "Judet" views. The inlet view is taken with the X-ray beam at a 45° angle directed caudal to the patient, visualizing the widest opening of the pelvic ring superiorly. Conversely, the outlet view aims 45° cephalad, providing more detail of the obturator ring and SI joints. For pelvic avulsion injuries and pubic ramus fractures, the AP view is usually adequate, though inlet and outlet views may slightly increase the sensitivity for ramus and ischial tuberosity fractures. To detect acetabular fractures, AP and oblique views are generally recommended. Oblique views image the pelvis at 45° angles from each side, thus visualizing the acetabulum straight-on. However, positioning for these views can be very uncomfortable for injured patients.

In recent years, CT scan has largely replaced complicated plain film views for all types of pelvic fractures. In a patient for whom there remains a high suspicion for acetabular fracture after negative plain radiographs, a non-contrast pelvic CT with detailed reconstructions should be performed.

For patients in whom pubic ramus fracture is suspected despite negative plain films, the next step is generally an MRI or bone scan looking for occult femoral neck or pubic ramus fracture. Depending on institutional capabilities, these patients are often admitted to the hospital for these time-consuming studies.

Laboratory

In stable patients with clinical presentations concerning for minor pelvic fracture, laboratory tests are of little clinical utility in the ED. All women of childbearing age should have a bedside qualitative beta-hCG performed prior to radiography. Only in patients being admitted or surgically repaired should basic preoperative blood tests be done.

Box 15.5 Key emergency department evaluation

Pelvic ring fractures

Pelvis X-ray indicated:
- Hemodynamic instability
- Altered mental status
- Distracting injuries
- Children
- CT not being done for another reason

Skip the pelvis X-ray:
- Pelvic CT being done for any other reason

No pelvic imaging:
- Normal exam
- Normal mental status *AND* ambulatory

Pubic ramus fractures
- Pelvis and hip radiographs
- MRI or bone scan for "occult" injuries (pain and inability to bear weight)
- Clinically may be difficult to distinguish from occult femoral neck fractures

Acetabular fractures
- Pelvic radiographs, AP, and oblique
- CT if radiographs negative and high clinical suspicion

Pelvic avulsion fractures
- Pelvic radiograph only

Treatment

Essential emergency department treatment

Severe

The most important treatment for significant pelvic fractures in the ED is rapid stabilization, both hemodynamic and mechanical. Fluid and blood product administration should be initiated promptly. Mechanical stabilization of the pelvis via a pelvic binder or C-clamp should also be achieved.

Moderate

Patients with pelvic ring disruptions have a potential for rapid hemodynamic deterioration. Therefore, large-bore intravenous access and blood product preparation (type and screen) should be routine. Mechanical stabilization is unnecessary, unless obvious pelvic instability is noted on physical examination. Adequate analgesia is important in these patients.

Minor

No major ED interventions are necessary in patients with minor pelvic fractures other than ensuring non-weightbearing status until the fracture is defined and providing pain control.

Post-emergency department treatment

Severe

After the initial ED resuscitation, optimal management strategies for significant pelvic fractures have been the subject of considerable debate. Accepted practices vary widely both within the United States and in Europe for the treatment of unstable pelvic fractures.

The common goal in severely injured pelvic fracture patients is to control hemorrhage from pelvic vessels and to prioritize the definitive treatment of their injuries. Severely injured, hemodynamically unstable patients are not appropriate for extensive CT scanning. If intrathoracic or intra-abdominal injuries appear to be the most immediate life threat, the patient is best treated by operating room thoracotomy or laparotomy, respectively. However, if pelvic or retroperitoneal hemorrhage is the most pressing concern, then further management must focus on the pelvic injuries. In practice, the choice may not always be so clear, and this difficult decision should be made collaboratively amongst the emergency physicians, trauma surgeons, and orthopedic surgeons.

There are three generally accepted strategies for controlling pelvic bleeding: angiography with selective arterial embolization, mechanical stabilization via external fixation, and laparotomy with surgical packing of the retroperitoneum. The latter two treatment modalities are thought to control venous hemorrhage, whereas the former targets arterial bleeding.

Hemorrhage from pelvic vessels can be both arterial and venous in origin. In all patients presenting with pelvic fractures, the majority of bleeding is from the pelvic veins, presacral plexus, and the large, cancellous pelvic bones.[21,33] However, hypotensive pelvic fracture patients who do not respond to initial resuscitation are more often suffering from an arterial hemorrhage.[33-35,54]

Historically, external fixation has been the primary modality of stabilizing pelvic fractures. Unlike the pelvic binder and C-clamp, external fixation must be applied under sterile conditions using fluoroscopic guidance. The external fixator reapproximates the bony fragments and reduces the pelvic volume.[50] Typically, this device is applied in the angiography suite or in the operating room during thoracotomy or laparotomy. Few trauma centers have the capability of applying external pelvic fixation in the ED.

Direct packing of the retroperitoneum during laparotomy is an alternative means to control venous bleeding. This approach is very popular in Europe and is gaining acceptance in the United States.[55] Protocols in many European trauma centers incorporate routine external fixation followed by surgical packing for unstable pelvic fractures, using angiography only after these two modalities have failed to stabilize the patient.[20,55] Obvious arterial hemorrhage can be controlled through direct visualization and ligation during this same procedure. The abdomen is left open, and the patient returns to the operating room in 48 hours for either removal or replacement of the packing. A disadvantage to this approach is that it exposes patients to the physiological stress of a major surgical procedure. Moreover, laparotomy runs the risk of dislodging any clot that may have formed and releasing tamponade within the pelvis. However, in those patients requiring exploratory laparotomy for intra-abdominal injuries, this procedure can be done concomitantly.

Lastly, angiography with selective arterial embolization has become routine for hemodynamically unstable patients with pelvic fractures in the United States. The angiographer catheterizes the femoral artery to gain access to the abdominal aorta. From there, radio-opaque contrast is injected to detect extravasation from the pelvic arteries. Depending on how cephalad in the aorta the catheter is inserted, the hepatic and renal arteries may be visualized as well. Transcatheter arterial embolization can then be performed for each site of extravasation.

Arterial embolization for pelvic fractures has been shown to be very successful, though not without complications. Most authors cite a 90–100% success

rate, and < 6–7% complication rate.[51,56] Such complications include hepatic necrosis, femoral artery occlusion, unilateral gluteal infarction, contrast-induced nephropathy, and injury to smaller arteries during embolization.[56,57] The procedure can be quite time-consuming, and mortality in these critically ill patients while on the angiography table has been reported up to 15%.[57] Despite a high initial success rate, several studies have also shown that some patients require repeat angiography for recurrent or new bleeding.[58,59]

Thus, physicians must decide between the operating room and the angiography suite for persistently hypotensive patients with severe pelvic fractures. Even though evidence is limited, venous hemorrhage appears to be more common in pelvic fracture patients overall, but arterial hemorrhage predominates in those who are persistently hypotensive.[33,34] Therefore, in the absence of other life-threatening injuries, angiography with embolization may be the best initial intervention after ED resuscitation in unstable patients. However, in the setting of intra-abdominal injuries requiring immediate laparotomy, retroperitoneal packing may be performed as a first-line therapy. If the patient remains hypotensive after these interventions, angiography should follow laparotomy. In either case, the orthopedic team should be consulted early for consideration of applying an external fixation device.

Definitive care of pelvic fractures often requires open reduction and internal fixation. This is rarely indicated in the acute setting. "Damage-control" orthopedics aims at rapid stabilization with lengthy surgical procedures being deferred until after clinical stabilization is achieved. This approach has been shown to decrease pulmonary complications, late-onset organ failure, and mortality.[60]

Moderate

A pelvic CT scan is useful in making management decisions in hemodynamically stable patients with pelvic ring disruptions. Computed tomography provides information about bony displacement, soft tissue injuries, hematomas, and active bleeding. The majority of these patients undergo urgent external fixation; if no signs of bleeding or other injuries exist, definitive open reduction and internal fixation may be delayed at the discretion of the orthopedic surgeon.

However, controversy exists regarding the best treatment of stable patients with large pelvic hematomas or active extravasation seen on CT. These patients may benefit from early angiography with embolization to prevent further blood loss and clinical deterioration. Blackmore et al. developed a receiver-operating-characteristic curve correlating volume of pelvic hematoma with likelihood of positive angiography: 99% of patients with hematomas > 600 ml had arterial bleeding on angiography, whereas fewer than 5% of patients with hematomas < 200 ml had arterial bleeding.[12] Other studies have shown that active arterial extravasation seen on CT is highly specific for positive angiography.[34,52,53,61] The sooner the CT is done after the injury, the more predictive these markers are.

Thus, based on this data, some trauma centers in the United States have taken a more aggressive approach to early angiography with promising preliminary results. Kimbrell et al. describe their experience with early angiography for "soft" signs of ongoing hemorrhage, including pelvic hematoma on CT, decreasing serial hematocrits, tachycardia, or certain fracture patterns.[51] Whereas their rate of successful hemorrhage control was 95%, their rate of negative angiography was over 35%.[56] Opponents argue that the natural course of pelvic hemorrhage in most patients would be resolution with supportive care alone; thus, angiography for "soft signs" exposed patients to the risks of the procedures without real benefits. To date, no trials have compared these two approaches.

Minor

The treatment of pubic ramus fractures is supportive; patients may ambulate with assistance as they can tolerate. However, because many of these injuries occur in the frail and elderly, most will not be able to ambulate safely and may require inpatient rehabilitation.

Similarly, avulsion fractures are almost always treated non-operatively. Patients should be advised to rest, apply ice, and gradually ambulate with assistance. Surgical fixation is only considered in serious athletes with significantly displaced ischial tuberosity fractures. Even in those cases, no clear benefit has been shown over conservative management.[26]

Lastly, management of acetabular fractures is more complex. They are repaired surgically unless very minimally displaced and not involving the weightbearing acetabular dome. This surgery is non-emergent and can be done within the following few days after the injury. Those few acetabular fractures for which surgery is not necessary require 4–8 weeks of skeletal traction and non-weightbearing status.

Box 15.6 Common post-emergency department interventions

- Expeditious external fixation for all significant pelvic ring fractures.
- Unstable pelvic ring fractures → angiography vs. laparotomy with retroperitoneal packing based on the results of the pelvic radiograph and FAST.
- Hemodynamically stable pelvic ring fractures → consider selective angiography for clinical or radiographic signs of arterial hemorrhage.
- Pubic ramus and avulsion fractures → supportive care.
- Acetabular fractures → non-weightbearing, non-emergent surgical repair.

Special populations

Like many traumatic injuries, pelvic fractures in children, pregnant women, and the elderly merit special attention. Children tend to sustain pelvic fractures far less often than adults with similar mechanisms of injury.[1,62] This is presumably due to their strong cartilage, elastic joints, and somewhat flexible bones.[62,63] Pelvic fractures most commonly occur in children as a result of pedestrian vs. MVCs; lateral compression is the most common fracture type.[44,4] The rate of severe hemorrhage and mortality from pelvic fracture in children is very low.[4,44,45,63,64] Associated injuries are common, presumably because the small flexible pelvis confers little protection to pelvic and abdominal viscera.[4,63] Surgical repair is rarely needed in children, as the thick periosteum tends to stabilize the fractures.[4,64]

Pregnant women are of particular concern in the setting of pelvic fracture. Both direct uterine trauma as well as maternal hemorrhage can compromise the fetus; however, neither fracture type nor gestational age appears to affect fetal outcome.[65] Whereas maternal mortality is comparable to non-pregnant controls, overall fetal mortality is as high as 37% in the setting of pelvic fracture.[65]

Elderly patients fare worse than their younger counterparts with similar pelvic injuries. Pelvic ring fractures can result from extremely minor mechanisms in this population, and mortality is much higher.[66,67] Furthermore, elderly patients suffer a disproportionate amount of late mortality due to comorbid diseases.[67]

For unclear reasons, elderly patients sustain more lateral compression fractures than other patients.[66,67] Moreover, advanced age is a risk factor for arterial bleeding requiring angiography, perhaps due to brittle and atherosclerotic vessels incapable of adequate vasoconstriction.[51,56] Thus, the emergency physician must be especially vigilant for occult injuries and pelvic bleeding in elderly patients.

Documentation

Thorough documentation is extremely important for both patient care and medicolegal reasons in pelvic trauma. First, the mechanism of injury should be described, including the patient's position in the vehicle, protective equipment (e.g., helmet, airbags, seat belt), speed of the collision, or height of the fall. If brought in by ambulance, the patient's condition in the field and any interventions performed en route should also be documented. Next, a full but concise description of the primary and secondary surveys, with particular attention to the pelvic injuries should be noted. Neurovascular status of the lower extremities and groin is very important and should be reassessed after any intervention such as pelvic binding. All ancillary studies and their interpretations should be recorded in the ED chart.

The patient should be reassessed frequently, particularly if unstable or in the ED for a prolonged period of time. The medical record should accurately reflect the patient's course in the ED. Reassessments as well as the final condition of the patient upon leaving the ED should be documented in the chart.

Last and perhaps most important, is documentation of the decision-making process. Management of pelvic fractures is complex; thus, explaining the rationale behind these often difficult management decisions in the ED chart is critical. In addition, it is important to note whether our trauma or orthopedic colleagues were present during the ED resuscitation, and what role they had in any collaborative decision-making processes.

Disposition

All significant pelvic ring disruptions should be admitted to a trauma service. This may require the transfer of the patient to another facility for intensive care unit care after initial stabilization. Orthopedic and trauma surgery consultation should be obtained early in the ED course of these patients.

Pelvic fractures which are both hemodynamically and mechanically stable, with no signs of hemorrhage on CT or clinically, may be admitted to the floor or step-down unit based on the patient's clinical picture. These patients may be best served at a hospital with extensive experience in pelvic injuries. Similarly, orthopedic and trauma surgery should be consulted from the ED for these patients.

Isolated pubic ramus fractures are extremely common and do not require specialized trauma center care. These patients may be allowed to bear weight with assistance as they tolerate it. However, patients with pubic ramus fractures who are elderly or who have significant comorbidities are generally admitted to the hospital for rehabilitation and physical therapy. Depending on institutional practices, these patients can either be admitted to the orthopedic surgery service or the internal medicine service with orthopedic consultation. Patients with pubic ramus fractures who are relatively young and otherwise healthy, have safe home environments, ample assistance, and close follow up may be discharged.

Pelvic avulsion fractures, similarly, require supportive care only. As these patients tend to be young and athletic, discharge with crutches and close follow up is appropriate. However, patients who have difficulty ambulating or need significant analgesia may be admitted to the hospital for those reasons. Orthopedic consultation is not always required, provided that close follow up can be arranged.

Acetabular fractures generally require surgical fixation and should be admitted. Unless other injuries exist, patients with isolated acetabular or pubic ramus fractures may be admitted to the floor on the orthopedic surgery service.

Box 15.7   Disposition and transfer criteria

Admission criteria

Discharge with follow up*	Consider admission	Admission necessary
Pelvic avulsion fractures	Pubic ramus fractures in the elderly	Acetabular fractures
Selected pubic ramus fractures		Pelvic ring fractures

Transfer criteria

- All hemodynamically unstable pelvic fractures should be transferred to a trauma center as early as possible.
- Significant disruptions of the pelvic ring, even if hemodynamically stable, should generally be transferred to a trauma center or hospital with extensive experience in such injuries.

*All patients being discharged must be ambulatory, have adequate pain control with oral analgesics, and close follow up arranged.

Summary

Pelvic fractures encompass a wide spectrum of injuries from stable to life-threatening and are commonly encountered in emergency medicine practice. In major pelvic trauma, it is important to understand common injury patterns, the techniques for stabilization in the ED, and the options for definitive care after the ED resuscitation. More minor pelvic injuries such as pubic ramus, avulsion, and acetabular fractures present to the ED far more commonly and often much more subtly. Emergency physicians should be readily familiar with the clinical presentations as well as the appropriate diagnostic workup of these occasionally occult injuries.

References

1. Demetriades D, Karaiskakis, M, Toutouzas, K, et al. Pelvic fractures:epidemiology and predictors of associated abdominal injuries and outcomes. *J Am Coll Surg* 2002;**195**(1):1–10.

2. Oliver CW, Twaddle B, Agel J, et al. Outcome after pelvic ring fractures: evaluation using the medical outcomes short form SF-36. *Injury* 1996;**27**(9):635–41.

3. Tien IY, Dufel SE. Does ethanol affect the reliability of pelvic bone examination in blunt trauma? *Ann Emerg Med* 2000;**36**(5):451–5.

4. Silber JS, Flynn JM, Koffler KM, et al. Analysis of the cause, classification, and associated injuries of 166 consecutive pediatric pelvic fractures. *J Ped Orthop* 2001;**21**:446–50.

5. Rowe SA, Sochor MS, Staples KS, et al. Pelvic ring fractures: implications of vehicle design, crash type, and occupant characteristics. *Surgery* 2004;**136**(4):842–7.

6. Stein D, O'Connor J, Kufera J, et al. Risk factors associated with pelvic fractures sustained in motor vehicle collisions involving new vehicles. *J Trauma* 2006;**61**(1):21–30.

7. Brenneman FD, Katyal D, Boulanger BR, et al. Long-term outcomes in open pelvic fractures. *J Trauma* 1997;**42**(5):773–7.

8. Jones AL, Powell JN, Kellam JF, et al. Open pelvic fractures. *Orthop Clin North Am* 1997;**28**(3):345–50.

9. Durkin A, Sagi HC, Durham R, et al. Contemporary management of pelvic fractures. *Am J Surg* 2006;**192**(2):211–23.

10. Routt ML, Jr., Kregor PJ, Simonian PT, et al. High-energy pelvic ring disruptions. *Orthop Clin North Am* 2002;**33**(1):59–72.

11. Basta AM, Blackmore CC, Wessells H. Predicting urethral injury from pelvic fracture patterns in male patients with blunt trauma. *J Urol* 2007;**177**(2):571–5.

12. Blackmore CC, Jurkovich GJ, Linnau KF, et al. Assessment of volume of hemorrhage and outcome from pelvic fracture. *Arch Surg* 2003;**138**(5):504–8.

13. Poole GV, Ward EF. Causes of mortality in patients with pelvic fractures. *Orthopedics* 1994;**17**(8):691–6.

14. Cryer HM, Miller FB, Evers BM, et al. Pelvic fracture classification: correlation with hemorrhage. *J Trauma* 1988;**28**(7):973–80.

15. Burgess AR, Eastridge BJ, Young JW, et al. Pelvic ring disruptions: effective classification system and treatment protocols. *J Trauma* 1990;**30**(7):848–56.

16. O'Sullivan RE, White TO, Keating JF. Major pelvic fractures: identification of patients at high risk. *J Bone Joint Surg Br* 2005;**87**(4):530–3.

17. Poole GV, Ward EF, Muakkassa FF. Pelvic fracture from major blunt trauma. *Ann Surg* 1991;**213**(6):532–9.

18. Biffl WL, Smith WR, Moore EE, et al. Evolution of a multidisciplinary clinical pathway for the management of unstable patients with pelvic fractures. *Ann Surg* 2001;**233**(6):843–50.

19. Gilliland MD, Ward RE, Barton RM, et al. Factors affecting mortality in pelvic fractures. *J Trauma* 1982;**22**(8):691–3.

20. Cothren CC, Osborn PM, Moore EE, et al. Preperitoneal pelvic packing for hemodynamically unstable pelvic fractures: a paradigm shift. *J Trauma* 2007;**62**(4):834–42.

21. Gylling SF, Ward RE, Holcroft JW, et al. Immediate external fixation of unstable pelvic fractures. *Am J Surg* 1985;**150**:721–4.

22. Dente CJ, Feliciano DV, Rozycki GS, et al. The outcome of open pelvic fractures in the modern era. *Am J Surg* 2005;**190**(6):830–5.

23. Copeland CE, Bosse MJ, McCarthy ML, et al. Effect of trauma and pelvic fracture on female genitourinary, sexual, and reproductive function. *J Orthop Trauma* 1997;**11**(2):73–81.

269

24. Hill RM, Robinson CM, Keating JF. Fractures of the pubic rami: epidemiology and 5-year survival. *J Bone Joint Surg Br* 2001;**83**(8):1141–4.

25. Koval KJ, Aharonoff GB, Schwartz MC, et al. Pubic rami fracture: a benign pelvic injury? *J Orthop Trauma* 1997;**11**(1):7–9.

26. LaBella CR. Common acute sports-related lower extremity injuries in children and adolescents. *Clin Pediatr Emerg Med* 2007;**8**(1):31–42.

27. Siegel JH, SA Dalal, AR Burgess, et al. Pattern of organ injuries in pelvic fracture: impact force implications for survival and death in motor vehicles. *Accid Anal Prev* 1990;**22**(5):457–66.

28. Metz CM, Hak DJ, Goulet JA, et al. Pelvic fracture patterns and their corresponding angiographic sources of hemorrhage. *Orthop Clin North Am* 2004;**35**(4):431–7.

29. O'Sullivan E, White TO, Keating JF, et al. Major pelvic fractures: identification of patients at high risk. *J Bone Joint Surg Br* 2005;**87**(4):530–3.

30. Eastridge BJ, Starr A, Minei JP, et al. The importance of fracture pattern in guiding therapeutic decision-making in patients with hemorrhagic shock and pelvic ring disruptions. *J Trauma* 2002;**53**(3):446–50.

31. Sarin EL, Moore JB, Moore EE, et al. Pelvic fracture pattern does not always predict the need for urgent embolization. *J Trauma* 2005;**58**(5):973–7.

32. Lunsjo K, Tadros A, Hauggaard A, et al. Associated injuries and not fracture instability predict mortality in pelvic fractures: a prospective study of 100 patients. *J Trauma* 2007;**62**(3):687–91.

33. Cook RE, Keating JF, Gillespie I. The role of angiography in the management of hemorrhage from major fractures of the pelvis. *J Bone Joint Surg Br.* 2002;**84**(2):178–82.

34. Miller PR, Moore PS, Mansell E, et al. External fixation or arteriogram in bleeding pelvic fracture: initial therapy guided by markers of arterial hemorrhage. *J Trauma* 2003;**54**(3):437–43.

35. Blackmore CC, Cummings P, Jurkovich GJ, et al. Predicting major hemorrhage in patients with pelvic fracture. *J Trauma* 2006;**61**(2):346–52.

36. O'Neill PA, Riina J, Sclafani S, et al. Angiographic findings in pelvic fractures. *Clin Orthop and Rel Res* 1996;**329**:60–6.

37. Chang FC, Harrison PB, Beech RR, et al. PASG: Does it help in the management of traumatic shock? *J Trauma* 1995;**39**(3):453–6.

38. Brooks A, Davies B, Smethhurst M, et al. Prospective evaluation of non-radiologist performed emergency abdominal ultrasound for haemoperitoneum. *Emerg Med J* 2003;**21**:e5.

39. Gonzalez RP, Fried PQ, Bukhalo M. The utility of clinical examination in screening for pelvic fractures in blunt trauma. *J Am Coll Surg* 2002;**194**(2):121–5.

40. Dolich MO, McKenney MG, Varela JE, et al. 2576 ultrasound for blunt abdominal trauma. *J Trauma* 2001;**50**(1):108–12.

41. Tayal VS, Neilsen, A, Jones AE, et al. Accuracy of trauma ultrasound in major pelvic injury. *J Trauma* 2006;**61**(6):1453–7.

42. Boulanger BR, McLellan BA, Brenneman FD, et al. Prospective evidence of the superiority of a sonography-based algorithm in the assessment of blunt abdominal injury. *J Trauma* 1999;**47**(4):632–7.

43. Duane TM, Tan BB, Golay D, et al. Blunt trauma and the role of routine pelvic radiographs: a prospective analysis. *J Trauma* 2002;**53**(3):463–8.

44. Junkins EP, Furnival RA, Bolte RG. The clinical presentation of pediatric pelvic fractures. *Ped Emerg Care* 2001;**17**(1):15–18.

45. Junkins EP, Jr., Nelson DS, Carroll KL, et al. A prospective evaluation of the clinical presentation of pediatric pelvic fractures. *J Trauma* 2001;**51**:64–8.

46. Guillamondegui OD, Mahboubi S, Stafford PW, et al. The utility of pelvic radiograph in the assessment of pediatric pelvic fractures. *J Trauma* 2003;**55**(2):236–9.

47. Guillamondegui OD, Pryor JP, Gracias VH, et al. Pelvic radiography in blunt trauma resuscitation: a diminishing role. *J Trauma* 2002;**53**(6):1043–7.

48. Berg EE, Chebuhar C, Bell RM. Pelvic trauma imaging: a blinded comparison of computed tomography and roentgenograms. *J Trauma* 1995;**41**(6):994–8.

49. Grimm MR, Vrahas MS, Thomas KA. Pressure–volume characteristics of the intact and disrupted pelvic retroperitoneum. *J Trauma* 1998;**44**(3):454–9.

50. Bottlang M, Krieg JC, Mohr M, et al. Emergent management of pelvic ring fractures with the use of circumferential compression. *J Bone Joint Surg Am* 2002;**84A**(Suppl. 2):43–7.

51. Kimbrell BJ, Velmahos GC, Chan LS, et al. Angiographic embolization for pelvic fractures in older patients. *Arch Surg* 2004;**139**(7):728–32.

52. Stephen DJ, Kreder HJ, Day AC, et al. Early detection of arterial bleeding in acute pelvic trauma. *J Trauma* 1999;**47**(4):638–42.

53. Shanmuganathan K, Mirvis SE, Sover ER. Value of contrast-enhanced CT in detecting active hemorrhage in patients with blunt abdominal or pelvic trauma. *AJR Am J Roentgenol* 1993;**161**:65–9.

54. Wong YC, Wang LJ, Ng CJ, et al. Mortality after successful transcatheter arterial embolization in patients with unstable pelvic fractures. *J Trauma* 2000;**49**(1):71–4.

55. Smith WR, Moore EE, Osborn P, et al. Retroperitoneal packing as a resuscitation technique for hemodynamically unstable patients with pelvic fractures: report of two representative cases and a description of technique. *J Trauma* 2005; **59**(6):1510–14.

56. Velmahos GC, Toutouzas KG, Vassiliu P, et al. A prospective study on the safety and efficacy of angiographic embolization for pelvic and visceral injuries. *J Trauma* 2002;**53**(2):303–8.

57. Hak DJ. The role of pelvic angiography in evaluation and management of pelvic trauma. *Orthop Clin North Am* 2004;**35**(4):439–43.

58. Shapiro M, McDonald AA, Knight D. The role of repeat angiography in the management of pelvic fractures. *J Trauma* 2005;**58**(2):227–31.

59. Gourlay D, Hoffer E, Routt M, et al. Pelvic angiography for recurrent traumatic pelvic arterial hemorrhage. *J Trauma* 2005;**59**(5):1168–73.

60. Taeger G, Ruchholtz S, Waydhas C, et al. Damage control orthopedics in patients with multiple injuries is effective, time-saving, and safe. *J Trauma* 2005; **59**(2):409–16.

61. Cerva DS, Mirvis SE, Shanmuganathan K, et al. Detection of bleeding in patients with major pelvic fractures: value of contrast-enhanced CT. *AJR Am J Roentgenol* 1996;**166**:131–5.

62. Heeg M, de Ridder VA, Tornetta P, et al. Acetabular fractures in children and adolescents. *Clin Orthop Relat Res* 2000;**376**:80–6.

63. Chia JP, Holland AJ, Little, D, et al. Pelvic fractures and associated injuries in children. *J Trauma* 2004; **56**(1):83–8.

64. Blasier RD, McAtee J, White R, et al. Disruption of the pelvic ring in pediatric patients. *Clin Orthop Relat Res* 2000;**376**: 87–95.

65. Leggon RE, Wood G, Indeck M. Pelvic fractures in pregnancy: factors influencing maternal and fetal outcomes. *J Trauma* 2002;**53**(4):796–804.

66. Henry SM, Pollak AN, Jones AL, et al. Pelvic fracture in geriatric patients: a distinct clinical entity. *J Trauma* 2002;**53**(1):15–20.

67. O'Brien DP, Luchette FA, Pereira SJ, et al. Pelvic fracture in the elderly associated with increased mortality. *Surgery* 2002;**132**(4):710–14.

16

Upper extremity orthopedic trauma

Moira Davenport and Tamara A. Scerpella

Introduction

Fractures and dislocations of the upper extremity are commonly seen in the emergency department (ED). Although the mechanisms vary, a fall on the outstretched hand (FOOSH) is responsible for many of these injuries, as forces are transmitted proximally from the point of impact along the entire length of the extremity. Early diagnosis and proper management may help prevent long-term adverse sequelae. To achieve optimal outcomes, emergency physicians should be familiar with current management concepts for upper extremity bony trauma.

Prehospital

Prehospital care of the extremity injured patient includes basic trauma resuscitation followed by stabilization of the injury site. Although a variety of splinting devices are available to Emergency Medical Services (EMS) providers, improvisation is common. Pillows and tape are often used to stabilize extremities as an acceptable alternative to pre-made devices. In general, prehospital providers should not attempt reduction of the injury, other than to grossly align the extremity, whenever possible. An open fracture wound should be covered with gauze soaked in sterile saline. Undiluted Povidone–Iodine should not be placed in the wound. As these are painful injuries, many prehospital systems have protocols in place to allow for early analgesia.

Emergency department evaluation

Emergency department evaluation begins with the standard primary survey (airway, breathing, circulation, and disability) followed by a rapid neurovascular examination of the injured extremity. A fractured or dislocated extremity that has compromised circulation requires rapid reduction in an attempt to improve perfusion. In circumstances of cold, pulseless extremities or significant tenting of skin, reduction should be carried out without the delay of pre-reduction imaging. Post-reduction reassessment of perfusion status and expedited surgical consultation is required if the vascular status does not normalize following reduction.

Analgesics are administered as soon as practical to maximize patient comfort and to allow for an adequate physical examination. Field immobilization should be temporarily taken down during the examination and reapplied to prevent fracture movement during the evaluation and resuscitation phase. Injuries which have not been splinted by the prehospital providers should optimally be splinted in the trauma resuscitation room prior to transporting the patient; however, the treatment of life-threatening injuries must take priority. Physical examination of the injured extremity should include the injury site as well as the joints above and below that site, as forces are frequently transmitted along the length of the extremity. It is imperative that radiographs are obtained in at least two planes, in order to avoid missing subtle injuries. Furthermore, the joints proximal and distal to a fracture should be considered for radiographic evaluation in order to rule out associated injury. This practice is particularly important when the mechanism of injury is suspicious for significant transmission of forces and for patients with multiple injuries and are unable to actively participate in the examination. Wounds associated with open fractures should be covered with gauze soaked in sterile saline. Avoid placing undiluted iodine, alcohol, or hydrogen peroxide-based solutions, into open wounds as these solutions cause tissue toxicity and may affect wound healing. Furthermore, such solutions may also increase the difficulty of surgical intervention, particularly in large wounds that may communicate with surrounding joint spaces. Intravenous antibiotics should be administered to patients with open fractures;[1] a first-generation cephalosporin is sufficient in most cases, and supplemented with an aminoglycoside in the case of Grade II or III open fractures (wound of comminution > 1 cm).[1] Gross contamination of the wound dictates the addition of an anti-anerobic antibiotic such as penicillin to prophylax against *Clostridium*.[1] The patient's tetanus status should be ascertained and updated if deficient or indeterminate.

Box 16.1 Essentials of upper extremity injury

- FOOSH is responsible for a great many of upper extremity injuries, as forces are transmitted proximally from the point of impact along the entire length of the extremity.
- In general, prehospital providers should not attempt reduction of the injury, other than to grossly align the extremity when possible.
- An open fracture wound should initially be covered with gauze soaked in sterile saline.
- A fractured or dislocated extremity that has compromised circulation requires rapid reduction in an attempt to improve perfusion.
- In circumstances of cold, pulseless extremities or significant tenting of skin, reduction should be carried out without the delay of pre-reduction imaging.

Specific injuries

Shoulder

The shoulder is a diarthrodial joint formed by the articulation of the humeral head and the glenoid fossa of the scapula. The glenoid fossa is relatively shallow; its depth is increased by the circumferential labrum, and shoulder stability is greatly dependent upon soft tissue constraints. The supero-lateral aspect of the scapula is the acromion; it articulates with the distal clavicle via the acromioclavicular joint (ACJ) which is stabilized by the acromioclavicular ligaments. Together, the ACJ and acromion form the "roof" of the shoulder joint. The coronoid process projects anteriorly from the scapula and serves as the origin of the coracoclavicular (CC) ligaments and the coracoacromial (CA) ligament; the former provides vertical stability to the distal clavicle. The shoulder has

greater range of motion than any joint in the body, and is the most frequently dislocated (Figure 16.1).[2]

Shoulder dislocations may occur as the result of direct trauma or due to indirect forces applied more distally to the upper extremity. Injuries are most

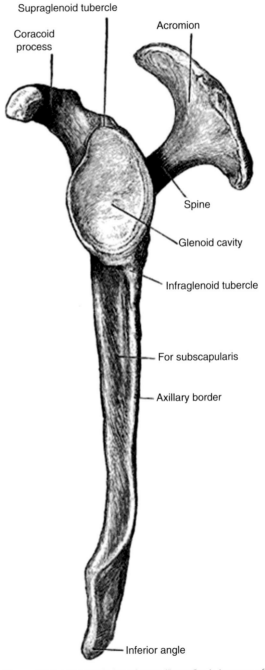

Figure 16.1 Left scapula lateral view. (From *Gray's Anatomy of the Human Body*, 20th edn, in Public Domain.)

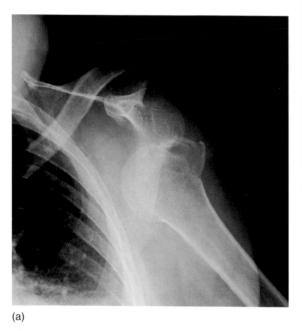

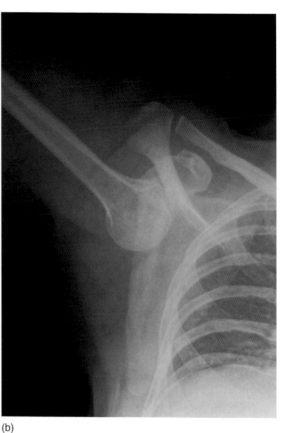

(a)   (b)

Figure 16.2 (a) Anterior shoulder dislocation with Hill–Sachs deformity. (b) Inferior shoulder dislocation (luxatio erecta). (Courtesy of Mark Bernstein, MD.)

common in young males who tend to participate in more aggressive, high velocity activities than those in other demographic groups.[2] Younger patients are more likely to sustain recurrent dislocations; recurrence rates approach 100% in patients who sustain their first injury before age 18.[3] With increasing age, recurrence rates decrease, but the likelihood of associated rotator cuff injury increases.[4] Associated bony injuries are common in young patients (Hill–Sachs and glenoid rim fractures), but can occur in any age group (Figure 16.2).

Dislocations are defined based on the position of the humeral head relative to the glenoid. Anterior dislocations account for 97% of all dislocations,[5] and can be further defined as subacromial, subcoracoid, subglenoid, or subclavicular. They typically occur when force is applied to the arm while it is abducted and externally rotated. Posterior dislocations are rare; they are more commonly associated with seizure activity, electrical injury or psychotic behavior, but may

also result from a fall or a motor vehicle collision. Also uncommon (~1–2%) are inferior shoulder dislocations, also known as luxio erecta. These occur with severe hyperabduction of the arm or axial loading when the arm is fully abducted. Patients with an anterior shoulder dislocation often present with the affected extremity slightly abducted and externally rotated. A posteriorly dislocated shoulder, though typically adducted and internally rotated, often seems to be normally positioned. However, both groups of patients have significantly decreased ranges of motion and usually resist attempts to move the extremity. Physical exam findings may include an obvious alteration in bony landmarks. Sensory deficits are common; however, the axillary nerve, which provides sensation over the lateral deltoid, is particularly at risk. If they occur, these injuries are typically neuropraxic in nature and are an indication for immediate reduction.[6] If the neurovascular status is intact, pre-reduction radiographs should be obtained in order to identify the location of the humeral head and any associated fractures. One reasonable exception to this rule is the chronic dislocator who redislocates with minimal trauma. However, no specific, validated guidelines exist to assist the physician in deciding which patients to radiograph.[7] Radiographs should be obtained in anteroposterior (AP) and lateral planes. The axillary view is the preferred lateral view and provides particularly important information regarding the location of the humeral head in relation to the glenoid. *Failure to obtain an axillary view can result in a missed posterior dislocation, as the AP view presents only subtle abnormalities with this injury.* The technique required to obtain an axillary view is often painful when the shoulder is dislocated. Thus, Geusens et al. proposed a modified axillary view which is performed with the patient standing but forward flexed 45° at the hips.[8] The radiograph beam is directed in a 30–45° craniocaudal direction. Additional views, particularly the scapular Y view, may be helpful if the AP and axillary are inadequate or unobtainable or fail to show expected pathology.

Several options exist for reduction of a shoulder dislocation. Choice of a technique depends upon patient safety, pain control, and sedation requirements, as well as physician skill and current staffing needs.

The ***traction–countertraction method*** is performed with the patient in a supine position. A sheet is wrapped around the patient's torso, with the free ends directed away from the affected extremity. After procedural sedation is initiated, one provider applies countertraction on the sheet while the physician distracts the affected arm in line with the humerus, attempting to disengage the humeral head from its position. Constant traction should be applied to prevent muscle spasm, which further complicates the reduction (Figure 16.3).

The ***Kocher method*** can often be completed without sedation. The physician flexes the elbow of the affected extremity and then gently adducts the arm. Upon reaching full adduction, the extremity is externally rotated as far as the patient can tolerate, and then elevated in the forward plane. This sequence of movements usually achieves reduction in a quick, less painful manner; however, care should be taken to avoid undue force which can result in glenoid rim fracture (Figure 16.4). Kocher's original paper was mistranslated; there was no mention of the downward traction on the humerus typically described with this technique (and associated with a high rate of humeral

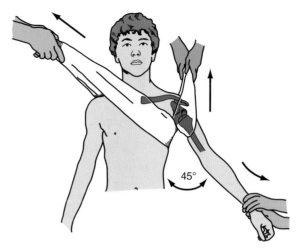

Figure 16.3 Traction–countertraction method.

head fractures). The modified Hennepin technique is a variation of the correctly translated Kocher method. The modified Hennepin technique is started like the Kocher method. However, instead of performing forward elevation, the modified Hennepin technique relocates the humeral head by abducting the extremity (Figure 16.5).

The ***Milch method*** is performed by abducting and externally rotating the extremity; reduction is often achieved by 90–105° of abduction. This technique is often performed quickly and without sedation. O'Connor et al. published a case series of 76 consecutive patients with anterior shoulder dislocations that were treated with the Milch method.[9] Reduction was successful on the first attempt in all cases and no sedation was required. ***Scapular manipulation*** can be attempted with the patient prone or sitting with the hips flexed. The physician gently pushes the inferior border of the scapula medially, thereby rotating the glenoid and allowing the humeral head to relocate (Figure 16.6).

The ***Stimson method*** uses gravity to achieve reduction. The patient is placed prone with the affected extremity hanging off the stretcher. In some cases, muscle relaxation in this position will allow reduction to occur. Typically, weights are required; these are attached to the dangling extremity tied via a loop of cast stockinette about the wrist. This technique can be quite time consuming and is not appropriate for many trauma patients or for those with the potential for respiratory compromise.

Orthopedic consultation should be sought when reduction is not obtained after several attempts under

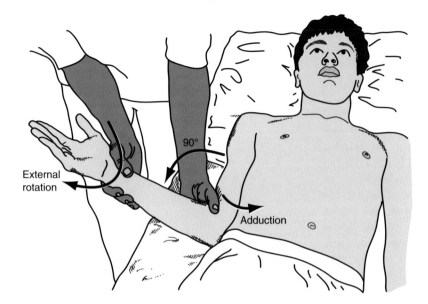

Figure 16.4 Kocher method.

External rotation

90°

Adduction

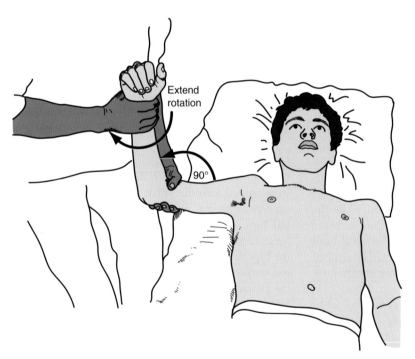

Figure 16.5 Modified Hennepin technique.

Extend rotation

90°

appropriate conditions; all discharged patients should have orthopedic follow-up care arranged in 7–10 days. Orthopedic surgeons should also be involved in the care of patients with a fracture–dislocation of the shoulder; reduction in this patient population should be performed by these specialists. The exception to this standard is the Hill–Sachs fracture. The emergency physician may appropriately attempt to reduce dislocations associated with this injury. The patient should be informed that the presence of the defect increases the likelihood of the shoulder dislocating again.

Posterior dislocations are usually associated with considerably more muscle spasm than anterior injuries.[10] Thus, these are rarely reduced without procedural sedation. The patient is positioned in a fashion

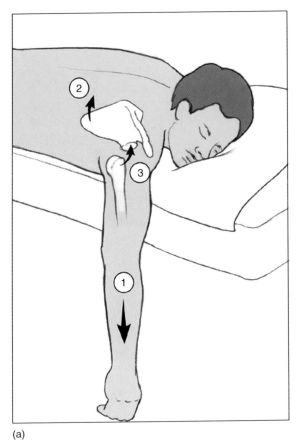

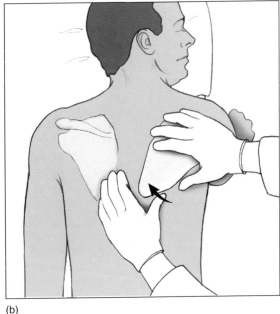

(a)　　　　　　　　　　　　　　　　　　　(b)

Figure 16.6 Scapular manipulation.

similar to that described above for the traction–countertraction method. An assistant applies countertraction while one physician applies longitudinal traction (in the axis of the humerus) and a second provider applies a constant, anteriorly directed force on the humeral head in an attempt to dislodge it from behind the glenoid.[11]

Post-reduction care of all shoulder dislocations begins with a thorough neurovascular examination. Axillary nerve injuries may occur with shoulder dislocation and are typically detected post-reduction. Repeat radiographs in both AP and lateral planes (axillary view) should be completed to ensure reduction of the joint and to evaluate for associated fractures (fractures may be associated with a dislocation, or may be incurred during reduction). Several fractures can occur in conjunction with a shoulder dislocation; these are usually visible on both pre- and post-reduction radiographs. A Hill–Sachs fracture results from impaction of the posterolateral humeral

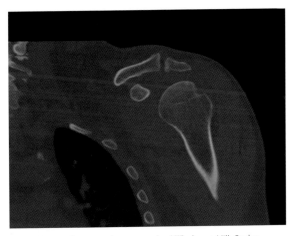

Figure 16.7 Computed tomography (CT) shows Hill–Sachs fracture after a reduction. (Courtesy of Mark Bernstein, MD.)

head against the rim of the glenoid during the course of anterior dislocation (Figure 16.7). A *reverse* Hill–Sachs fracture occurs when the anteromedial aspect of

277

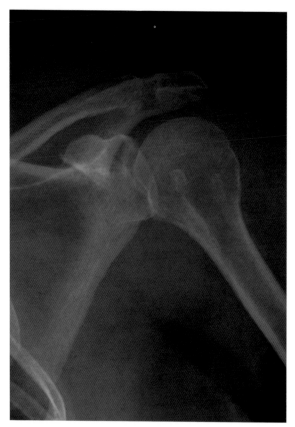

Figure 16.8 Reverse Hill–Sachs deformity is seen on anteromedial aspect of humeral head. (Courtesy of Mark Bernstein, MD.)

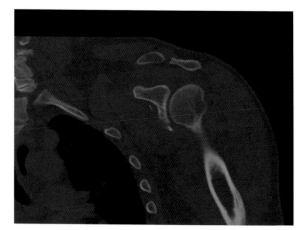

Figure 16.9 Hill–Sachs and Bankhart lesions are seen on this scan.

the humeral head impacts against the posterior rim of the glenoid during a posterior dislocation (Figure 16.8). A bony Bankart lesion, an avulsion of the glenoid rim, may occur with either anterior or posterior dislocations. Although usually visible on post-reduction films, special views (e.g., West Point or Stryker notch) may be necessary to delineate these sometimes subtle fractures.[12] Computed tomography (CT) scanning may be a useful diagnostic adjunct, particularly when concurrent injuries are present and necessitate such studies. Magnetic resonance imaging (MRI) scanning remains the definitive diagnostic study and is often performed on an outpatient basis (Figure 16.9).

Post-reduction positioning for anterior dislocations is controversial. Traditionally, the affected extremity was placed in an adducted, internally rotated position and the patient discharged with either a shoulder immobilizer or a sling for comfort. In contrast, Itoi proposed immobilization of the arm in 45° of external rotation.[13] This position maximizes

contact between the anterior glenoid and the avulsed capsulolabral tissues, theoretically enhancing non-operative healing of the pathologic Bankart lesion. These authors demonstrated decreased recurrence rates with this protocol, but their results have not been duplicated. Until these findings have been replicated, it is appropriate that patients should still be discharged in internal rotation. All patients who have sustained more than one dislocation (and first-time dislocators with physically demanding lifestyles) should be seen in follow up by an orthopedic surgeon. There is a trend toward earlier surgical intervention to restore stability through capsulolabral reconstruction, thereby reducing the morbidity associated with repeat dislocations.[5]

Acromioclavicular (AC) joint injuries are common athletic injuries. They typically result from direct trauma, usually a fall on the adducted shoulder. Patients present with tenderness over the AC joint, with or without deformity, depending upon the extent of the injury. Range of motion (particularly abduction) may be limited by pain. Neurovascular deficits are rare with this injury but a thorough examination should be performed to rule out concomitant injuries. Both AP and axillary shoulder radiographs are obtained to assess the extent of ACJ injury. Additional views such as clavicle or specific AC joint may be helpful as well; however, stress views are not recommended as they do not add useful information and can cause significant pain. Comparison of the injured and uninjured AC joints on the chest radiograph or bilateral films can be helpful in determining the patient's normal anatomy, if necessary. Injuries were previously classified into a

Table 16.1 AC joint injuries

Type i	Partial tear of the AC ligaments, no disruption of CC ligaments
Type ii	Complete disruption of the AC ligaments, partial or no disruption of CC ligaments
Type iii	Complete disruption of AC and CC ligaments resulting in superior displacement of the distal clavicle
Type iv	Complete disruption of the AC and CC ligaments with posterior displacement of the distal clavicle into or through the trapezius fascia
Type v	Marked superior displacement (subcutaneous) of the distal clavicle due to complete disruption of the AC and CC ligaments and deltoid/trapezius muscle/fascial injury
Type vi	Complete disruption of the AC and CC ligaments with subcoracoid displacement of the distal clavicle (exceedingly rare)

AC, acromioclavicular; CC, coracoclavicular.

Table 16.2 Distal clavicle fracture classifications

Classification	Fracture pattern
Type i	Fracture occurs between CC ligaments and ACJ; because at least one of the CC ligaments remains attached to the clavicle, displacement is minimal
Type ii	Fracture occurs medial to CC ligaments resulting in superior displacement of the clavicle
Type iii	Intra-articular fracture

ACJ, acromioclavicular joint; CC, coracoclavicular.

three part grading scale (Type I: minimal, Type II: partial, and Type III: unstable). However, injuries are now classified into six types (Table 16.1).

With the exception of the rare Type VI injury, all patients with isolated AC separations may safely be discharged from the ED with analgesics, a sling for comfort, and orthopedic follow up. Type I and II injuries are managed non-operatively and have an excellent prognosis for full recovery. These patients do benefit from follow up as physical therapy is often needed to restore pre-injury range of motion and strength. The treatment of Type III injuries is controversial, with proponents of both operative and non-operative management.[14] Subacute operative management typically occurs within the first 7–10 days following injury; chronic reconstruction may also be performed for patients that fail non-operative care.[15] Type IV–VI injuries generally require operative repair.[15]

Clavicle fractures are common sequelae of falls and motor vehicle crashes. Patients present with tenderness over the fracture site and crepitus and deformity if the fracture is displaced. Shoulder range of motion is decreased due to pain. In polytrauma cases, the diagnosis is often made on the routine chest radiograph series; the posteroanterior (PA) view, in particular, allows good visualization of both clavicles. Care should be taken to rule out associated intrathoracic injuries

depending on the direction of dislocation. Chest CT scan with intravenous contrast under a vascular protocol should be obtained if there is concern for damage to the subclavian vasculature or lung.[16] Patients with isolated midshaft clavicle fractures may be safely discharged in a sling with analgesics and instructions for orthopedic follow up in 1–2 weeks. Physical therapy is often needed to restore pre-injury range of motion and strength. Use of the figure of eight harness is no longer recommended, as multiple studies have shown the device to cause increased pain while failing to accelerate healing.[17] Although bony union typically occurs over 6–8 weeks with conservative therapy, markedly displaced fractures (> 5 mm)[15] may result in non-union. Therefore, marked displacement is considered an indication for surgical repair;[15] additionally, surgical repair may be considered to minimize cosmetic deformity in the case of moderately displaced fractures.

Distal clavicle fractures may mimic AC separation in both the mechanism of injury and in their presentation. Radiographs in the AP and axillary plane are diagnostic. Fractures are subdivided into three types (Table 16.2).

Patients with these fractures may be discharged from the ED with a sling and analgesics for comfort and instructions for orthopedic follow up. Type I and III fractures are typically treated conservatively, while Type II fractures require surgical repair to avoid non-union and chronic pain due to significant displacement.[18]

Medial clavicle fractures are much less common, representing < 5% of all clavicle fractures.[19] They are usually the result of motor vehicle trauma and are found in patients with multisystem injury; they are typically treated non-operatively.[19]

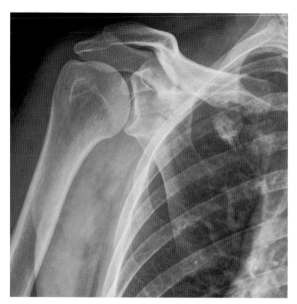

Figure 16.10 Scapular glenoid fracture. (Courtesy of Mark Bernstein, MD.)

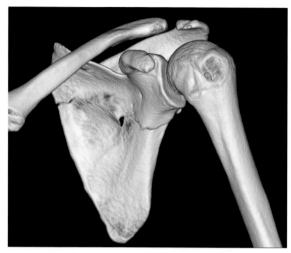

Figure 16.11 Three-dimensional computed tomography (CT) reconstruction of scapula fracture. (Courtesy of Mark Bernstein, MD.)

The "floating shoulder" describes a relatively rare injury that includes ipsilateral glenoid neck and clavicle fractures. This definition has been expanded to include ipsilateral glenoid neck fracture and either sternoclavicular or acromioclavicular dissociation.[20] The combination of these injuries can produce instability of the entire shoulder suspensory complex, leading to malunion, non-union, and other long-term adverse sequelae.

Scapular fractures are incurred under considerable amounts of trauma, and concurrent injuries to the chest and abdomen are frequent. Both scapular and clavicular fractures are usually detected initially on the portable (AP) chest radiograph which should be followed by either a complete shoulder series or CT scan after potentially life-threatening injuries have been stabilized. Floating shoulders with minimal displacement may be treated non-operatively in a shoulder immobilizer.[21] Pain control is essential in the initial phase of recovery, allowing initiation of a gradual stretching and strengthening program at 3 weeks after injury. Unstable fractures with anteromedial glenoid displacement should be treated surgically.[21] The amount of glenoid displacement considered significant is controversial in the orthopedic literature. A recent summary of management protocols suggests that patients with < 5 mm scapular neck displacement are appropriate candidates for non-operative

management while patients with > 30 mm medial glenoid displacement should undergo operative fixation.[21] No long-term studies have been published to document the ultimate functional, cosmetic, or pain outcomes of patients with a floating shoulder. The functional needs of the patient should be considered concomitantly with radiographic appearance when planning definitive management (Figures 16.10 and 16.11).

Humerus fractures

Proximal humerus fractures have a bi-modal age distribution, occurring in adolescents and the elderly, often the result of a fall.[22] These injuries are the third most common fracture in the elderly (after hip and distal radius fractures).[23] Fractures in the adolescent population occur at the growth plate (Salter–Harris fractures) prior to physeal closure. In addition, adolescents taken into police custody appear to be at increased risk for proximal humeral fractures during handcuff placement.[24]

Patients with proximal humerus fractures present with pain at the shoulder and demonstrate tenderness, sometimes with crepitus (just distal to the shoulder). Decreased range of motion in all planes is common. Up to 50% of proximal humerus fractures are associated with neurologic injury; the highest incidence occurs in anterior fracture–dislocation.[25] As with shoulder dislocations, the axillary nerve is the most frequently affected nerve.[26] Fractures are classified based upon the integrity of the greater and lesser

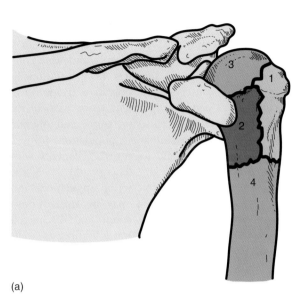

	Two-part	Three-part	Four-part

(a)

(b)

Figure 16.12 (a) Humeral parts in Neer classification. (b) Examples of displaced fractures using the Neer classification.

tuberosities and the head-shaft relationship; degree of displacement is also considered. The common Neer classification system uses four parts, the greater tuberosity, lesser tuberosity, the surgical neck and the anatomic neck. Fractures are classified based on displacement of fracture part(s) from the rest, with displacement charactized by > 1 cm of separation or > 45° of angulation (Figure 16.12). Fracture displacement is primarily due to the force exerted through muscular and tendinous insertions on the bony fragments. Because vascularity to the humeral head is supplied through these muscular attachments, tuberosity displacement predicts risk of avascular necrosis. Routine shoulder radiographs (the AP, axillary, and scapular Y view) are adequate to diagnose most proximal humerus fractures. The relationship between the humeral head and glenoid should be carefully evaluated; a CT scan may be necessary if an adequate axillary or modified axillary view cannot be obtained (Figure 16.13). Most patients with isolated proximal humerus fractures can be safely discharged from the ED with a sling and analgesics. Follow up should be arranged with an orthopedic surgeon for final disposition. Physical therapy is often needed to restore pre-injury range of motion and strength. Although minimally displaced fractures are treated non-operatively, displaced one-, two-, and three-part fractures are surgically repaired;[27] bone quality should be considered in

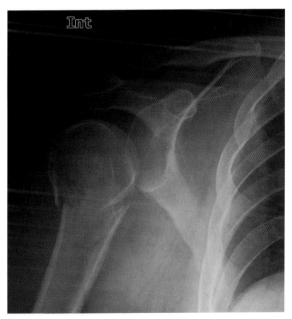

Figure 16.13 Two-part humeral head fracture. (Courtesy of Mark Bernstein, MD.)

surgical decision making for elderly patients. Four-part fractures are typically treated with surgical repair where bone quality is good or with hemi-arthroplasty in the elderly or in patients with poor bone quality.[28] Fracture dislocations require orthopedic consultation

281

in the ED and are usually treated with expeditious surgical repair.[27]

Isolated greater tuberosity fractures are common. The mechanism for this injury is abduction and external rotation of the upper extremity, the same force that often results in rotator cuff disruption and shoulder dislocation.[29] These fractures are commonly seen in conjunction with anterior shoulder dislocation. Reduction of the glenohumeral joint usually improves the position of a displaced tuberosity fragment. However, to avoid a mechanical block to range of motion or subacromial impingement, only minimal displacement is acceptable; thus surgical repair may be necessary.[30] Concomitant rotator cuff tears are also common with this injury and should be considered at follow up; MRI scan may be necessary for the diagnosis.[31] Emergency department management of isolated greater tuberosity fractures is the same as for proximal humerus fractures.

Diaphyseal humerus fractures account for 1–3% of all fractures and only 20% of humerus fractures.[32] Falls provide the most common mechanism for diaphyseal humerus fractures and the incidence increases with increasing age. Both AP and lateral radiographs of the humerus are obtained as part of the secondary survey. Patients typically present with pain at the fracture site. Range of motion at both the shoulder and elbow are usually limited by pain; movement below the fracture may also be decreased by associated neurologic deficits. The neurovascular examination is of particular importance in this group as damage to the radial nerve occurs in 2–18% of these injuries.[33] The course of the nerve and its lack of anatomic protection predisposes it to injury in the distal third of the humerus; in this region, it is tethered by the intermuscular septum and closely follows the contour of the bone. Regional variation in fracture pattern further explains the incidence of nerve injury. Midshaft fractures tend to be transverse, thereby limiting the likelihood of contact with the radial nerve. Fractures through the distal diaphysis tend to be spiral or oblique fractures, increasing the potential for contact between the fracture and the nerve. Proximal and middle third radial nerve injuries are likely to be neuropraxic in nature and carry a significantly better prognosis for full recovery of nerve function than do distal injuries where permanent neurologic deficits are more common.[34]

Patients presenting to the ED with a diaphyseal humerus fracture and a radial nerve deficit should be evaluated expeditiously by an orthopedic surgeon as these injuries require urgent operative exploration and fracture fixation.[35] Treatment of patients with a normal neurovascular examination is somewhat controversial. While these fractures have traditionally been treated conservatively, operative fixation has become more common in recent years, particularly with specific fracture patterns (spiral and oblique fractures) and in certain patient populations (cancer patients with pathologic fractures).[36] Patients with no appreciable neurologic deficits and < 3 cm of shortening, 20° anteroposterior angulation, and 30° varus/valgus angulation may be treated non-operatively in a coaptation splint and discharged with orthopedic follow up.[37] During healing as swelling decreases with increasing fracture stability, the coaptation splint is replaced by a functional brace. In some cases, adequate reduction cannot be maintained, and delayed operative fixation is necessary. Jawa et al. performed a retrospective comparison of functional bracing and plate fixation for treatment of extra-articular distal third humeral diaphyseal fractures.[33] Patients who underwent operative fixation had more predictable alignment and slightly quicker return to function but had higher the risk of infection and iatrogenic nerve injury. Those who were treated with functional bracing were more likely to have skin breakdown and angular deformity; however, this angulation did not effect function or range of motion. Neither group sustained significant loss of motion at the shoulder or the elbow.

Non-diaphyseal distal humerus fractures are relatively rare in adults. Unlike pediatric supracondylar fractures, there is no consensus regarding a classification scheme. The most current scheme classifies injuries as extra-articular, metaphyseal extending to the articular surface and primarily intra-articular.[38] Injury is typically due to a fall; fractures may occur with minimal trauma in those with osteopenia, while a greater force is required to produce this injury in healthy bone. Patients present with a flexed, adducted elbow with painful, limited motion. Range of motion in the shoulder is usually limited by pain; however, this motion may be normal if the extremity is supported from the elbow to the hand. Tenderness is expected at the elbow but it may be difficult to localize. Antecubital ecchymosis may be indicative of associated brachial artery injury and should prompt consideration of angiographic evaluation of the affected extremity, especially in the case of decreased pulses.[39] Thorough neurovascular examination should be performed at the time of presentation and at regular intervals (30–45 minutes), as neurologic injuries are not uncommon with these fractures.[35] If a neurovascular deficit is detected on the initial exam, expeditious orthopedic consultation should be obtained. A markedly displaced fracture with a neurovascular deficit should undergo an immediate attempt at reduction. Reduction is achieved by flexing the elbow and digitally reducing the distal fragment with the thumbs while distracting the forearm inferiorly. The extremity is splinted with the elbow in 90° of flexion. Patients without neurovascular injury but suspicion of this fracture and significant pain can be splinted while awaiting radiograph. (Further attempts at reduction may be performed using radiographic results to facilitate efforts.) Displaced fractures typically require operative reduction and fixation; those with intra-articular involvement frequently require olecranon osteotomy.[40] Total elbow arthroplasty is an alternative for patients with intra-articular involvement and poor bone quality.

Elbow dislocation

The elbow joint is formed by the articulation of the humerus with the radial head and the ulna. Flexion and extension occur at the ulnohumeral articulation, while pronation and supination occur at the radioulnar and radiohumeral articulations (normal range of pronation/supination is 75–85°/80–90°)[41]. The interosseous membrane connects the shafts of the radius and ulna, allowing forces to be transmitted the length of the forearm. While this improves the efficiency of motion, it also predisposes to distinct injury patterns. The trochlea and capitellum increase the articular surface of the humerus, while the coronoid and olecranon processes increase the ulnar articular surface. The coronoid and the anterior capsule serve as the main anterior stabilizers of the joint while the olecranon plays a role in both varus and valgus stability. The ulnar collateral ligament (UCL) is the primary medial stabilizer of the joint. Injuries to the UCL significantly increase the structural demands placed on the radial head and apply a tensile stress to the ulnar nerve which crosses the joint adjacent to the UCL. The lateral collateral ligament complex is composed of the annular ligament, the radial collateral ligament and the lateral ulnar collateral ligament. The annular ligament tethers the radial head to the ulna, which is critical for maintaining joint stability during pronation and supination. Injury to the radial collateral ligament often accelerates annular ligament degeneration, further destabilizing the joint; although this is often a chronic process, it can be seen in the acute phase as well. The numerous muscle groups that cross the elbow serve as dynamic stabilizers for the joint. Dislocation of the elbow is a very common injury; it is the most common dislocation in children and is second only to shoulder dislocations in adults.[42] The most common mechanism of injury is FOOSH, followed closely by direct trauma, which is usually related to sports participation. Injury patterns are described based upon the location of the forearm relative to the humerus: anterior, posterior, medial, lateral, and divergent (includes separation of the proximal radius and ulna). Posterior injuries are much more common. Although further subdivided as straight posterior, posterolateral, and posteromedial injuries, this distinction can be difficult to make and seldom influences treatment. Presentation to the ED varies based upon the type of dislocation sustained. An obvious deformity is usually noted but may be obscured by soft tissue swelling. Associated rupture of the joint capsule may lead to marked swelling in the forearm; thus, the physician should be alert to the possibility of compartment syndrome. Open injuries are rare but should be considered if lacerations are present, especially when displacement is large. The presence of skin tenting suggests the possibility of an impending open injury necessitating prompt reduction to avoid an open dislocation. The neurovascular examination is important, and should be carefully assessed prior to manipulation and again after manipulation; injury to the median or ulnar nerve may occur by entrapment in the joint during reduction. If nerve entrapment is suspected, rapid orthopedic consultation should be obtained. The ulnar nerve is particularly vulnerable in the case of medial dislocation, whereas median nerve injuries are more likely to occur in elbow dislocations that are complicated by compartment syndrome.[41] Careful examination of the entire upper extremity is important, particularly in those who have sustained a FOOSH mechanism, as other injuries may be present. Initial radiographic evaluation includes AP and lateral views of the elbow. Computed tomography scanning should be performed in the ED if no fracture is detected on plain radiograph and reduction cannot be performed as small intra-articular fragments may be blocking the joint. Outpatient CT scanning may be

283

necessary to facilitate operative planning if large fracture fragments are seen on plain radiographs. If fractures are detected, CT scanning will help to delineate the extent of injury and identify small intra-articular fragments that may impede closed reduction.[43]

Box 16.2 Overview of CT requirements in elbow dislocations

No CT necessary	Outpatient CT	CT in ED
• Easily reduced	• Easily reduced	• Difficult reduction
• No fragments	• Neurologically intact	• Neurovascular compromise
• Neurologically intact	• Fracture fragments identified	

Simple (isolated) dislocations can be reduced by the emergency physician, but complex dislocations, with associated bone, open, or extensive soft tissue, or neurovascular injury, may be best managed by orthopedic consultation. This may not be practical at all hospitals. Inability to reduce or post-reduction findings above should be considered for transfer. Due to the significant forces required to cause an anterior dislocation, and the associated damage from concomitant injuries, orthopedic consultation and reduction in the operating room is recommended.[44]

Several methods are available to reduce the posterior injury; all include distraction followed by anterior translation of the proximal forearm. Muscle relaxation and pain control are essential; procedural sedation may be required. Intra-articular injection of anesthetic agents may be attempted but the procedure is not as well tolerated due to the smaller joint space involved. Multidirectional dislocations should first be reduced in the varus/valgus plane through application of a force on the forearm in the direction opposite of the dislocation, while stabilizing the distal humerus; the posterior dislocation is then reduced using one of the following methods. A simple, less painful method of reduction includes exertion of an anterior force on the dislocated fragment with one hand, while the other hand is used to apply traction along the longitudinal axis of the forearm by gripping the patient's supinated hand. Reduction is usually achieved as the elbow is slowly flexed while maintaining traction. If this method fails to achieve reduction, traction/countertraction may be performed. An assistant applies countertraction to the humerus while the physician applies longitudinal traction to the forearm, reducing the dislocation. Reduction may be facilitated by flexing the elbow as traction is applied. In addition, the assistant may exert an anteriorly directed force on the olecranon while holding countertraction, further assisting the reduction. As with shoulder dislocations, patients with elbow dislocations may also be placed prone with the affected extremity hanging off the stretcher. Gravity alone may be enough to reduce the dislocation or the process may be performed with weights hanging from the wrist. Anterior pressure on the olecranon and/or slight elbow flexion will typically achieve reduction after 15–20 minutes.[45] This procedure may not be appropriate for patients with concurrent injuries or underlying respiratory difficulties. Once reduction is achieved, the arm is placed in either a sugar-tong or posterior splint with the elbow at 90° flexion. Documentation of an adequate reduction should be confirmed via repeat radiographs. Range of motion should be assessed in all planes to detect an intra-articular block that may not be visible on plain films. Orthopedic consultation is necessary in the ED if a confirmed radiographic reduction is not obtained or if a block in motion is present on physical examination; these cases may require urgent surgical exploration and reduction.[41] Ligamentous stability is assessed through the application of varus and valgus forces to the elbow in full extension and in 15° of flexion. Although most dislocations are relatively stable following reduction, elbows with significant ligamentous disruption may be so unstable that a reduction cannot be maintained.[46] Such cases also require orthopedic consultation; surgical treatment to restore stability is usually carried out on an urgent basis. Patients with stable, reductions may be discharged from the ED in the splint and sling with instructions for orthopedic follow up.

Because loss of motion is the most common sequelae of this injury, it is important that discharge instructions include splint removal for the performance of basic elbow range of motion exercises beginning 2–3 days after injury. Repeat radiographs are recommended at 3–5 days from the time of injury; assuming maintenance of the reduction, a hinged brace is typically applied and physical therapy is instituted. Chronic instability (leading to subluxation or

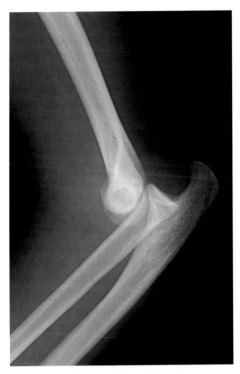

Figure 16.14 Posterior elbow dislocation.

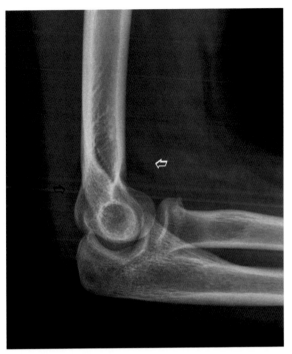

Figure 16.15 Elbow injury with effusion caption posterior fat pad (black arrow) and anterior sail sign (white arrow) suggest radial head fracture. (Courtesy of Mark Bernstein, MD.)

recurrent dislocation) and heterotopic ossification are less frequent long-term complications of this injury. Either may necessitate operative management (Figure 16.14).

Elbow and forearm fractures

Fractures about the elbow are quite common and usually result from indirect trauma, typically the FOOSH. Radial head fractures may occur as an isolated injury, or in conjunction with elbow dislocations. Patients present with a flexed elbow and pain with range of motion, particularly pronation and supination. Subtle elbow effusions are common. Tenderness, and sometimes crepitus, is elicited if the examiner palpates the radial head while pronating and supinating the forearm. In some cases, full range of motion in these planes is blocked by a displaced radial head fragment. Diagnosis is confirmed with AP and lateral radiographs of the elbow. In order to be sufficient, the lateral radiograph of the elbow optimally will be in the true lateral plane with the elbow at 90° flexion. The presence of either a posterior fat pad or an enlarged anterior fat pad (the sail sign) on the lateral radiograph should produce strong suspicion

for a radial head fracture, even if a discrete fracture line is not visible (Figure 16.15).

As opposed to adult, however, this finding in children is more likely to be a supracondylar fracture. It is important to perform a thorough examination to identify associated injuries. If a moderate or large effusion is present, therapeutic arthrocentesis and intra-articular injection of lidocaine, bupivicaine, or morphine sulfate should be considered to allow adequate examination. Elbow stability should be assessed, particularly to valgus stress, as ulnar collateral ligament injury is frequently associated with radial head fracture. The forearm and wrist should also be examined; tenderness and swelling suggest injury to the interosseous membrane and/or distal radioulnar joint (Essex–Lopresti injury).

Patients with occult or non-displaced radial head fractures may be placed in a sling and discharged from the ED with orthopedic follow up. Patients with exquisite pain are occasionally discharged from the ED is sugar-tong splints for additional support; however there is no literature to support this practice. Patients should be encouraged to perform gentle range of motion exercises of the shoulder and elbow to avoid stiffness. The can be started almost immediately. Minimally displaced radial head fractures may be treated similarly, although persistent loss of pronation/supination may require surgical treatment. Fractures typically requiring operative fixation include: (1) mechanical block to range of motion; (2) greater than one-third involvement of the articular surface; (3) significant (> 2–3 mm) displacement or articular depression; (4) extension to the radial neck; and (5) comminution.[47] Although simple excision is historically the surgical procedure of choice, many surgeons are advocating various fixation techniques.[48]

The Essex–Lopresti injury is the combination of a radial head fracture with disruption of the interosseous membrane and dislocation of the distal radio-ulnar joint (DRUJ).[49] This constellation of injury is frequently overlooked in the ED, and should be considered in any patient who sustains a radial head fracture. A missed diagnosis, leading to delayed treatment, produces inferior results, including decreased range of motion and decreased strength, particularly grip strength.[49] Physical exam findings include wrist tenderness, instability of the DRUJ, and ulnar prominence. These findings should prompt the EP to obtain radiographs at the wrist. Management is significantly different than that of the isolated radial head fracture, requiring operative fixation of the DRUJ and radial head fracture fixation or replacement.[49]

Forearm fractures may be associated with ipsilateral ligamentous injuries, resulting from transmission of force along the interosseous membrane. The Galeazzi eponym classically described the combination of DRUJ disruption and distal radial shaft fracture, but has been expanded to include fractures anywhere along the radial shaft or fractures of both radial and ulnar shafts in combination with DRUJ injury (Figure 16.16). Patients present with pain at the fracture site and wrist, but DRUJ instability may be difficult to distinguish on exam, particularly when the fracture is distal. Thus, a high index of suspicion is necessary when pain and tenderness are identified at the wrist. Both AP and lateral radiographs of the entire forearm, elbow, and wrist should be obtained. Signs of injury to the DRUJ include ulnar styloid fracture, widening of the DRUJ joint space on the AP film, dislocation of the DRUJ on the lateral film, and radial shortening of > 5 mm.[50] Orthopedic consultation should be obtained in the ED, as operative fixation is the definitive treatment. When badly displaced, attempted reduction of the radial fracture may

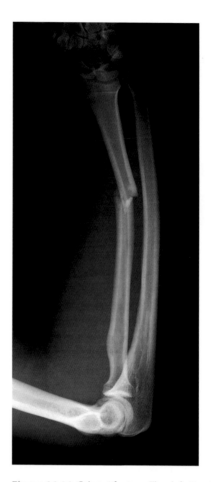

Figure 16.16 Galeazzi fracture. The definition has expanded to include fractures anywhere along the radial shaft or fractures of both radial and ulnar shafts in combination with distal radioulnar joint (DRUJ) injury. (Courtesy of Mark Bernstein, MD.)

be performed for patient comfort while awaiting consult. This is accomplished by applying traction through the distal fragment to correct shortening, then in the direction opposite of the displacement of the distal fragment (radial or ulnar) to correct angulation, while stabilizing the proximal forearm. A sugar-tong splint is applied to maintain position while awaiting definitive management.

The Monteggia fracture–dislocation similarly occurs through transmission of forces along the interosseous membrane, resulting in the combination of radial head dislocation and a fracture of the proximal ulna or ulnar diaphysis (or proximal diaphysis of both bone radius and ulna) (Figure 16.17). This relatively rare injury accounts for 1–2% of all forearm fractures and typically results from the FOOSH mechanism.[51]

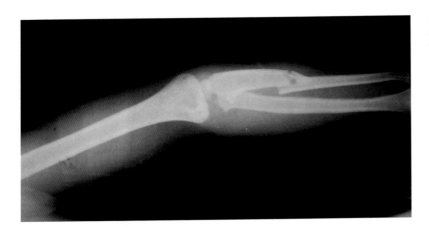

Figure 16.17 Montaggia fracture. The radiograph reveals radial head dislocation and a fracture of the ulnar diaphysis.

Patients present with the elbow flexed and the forearm pronated. Obvious deformity may be visible at the ulnar fracture site. Although deformity may also be present at the elbow, the more important physical examination finding is pain and reduction in motion associated with pronation and supination of the forearm. These physical findings should prompt AP and lateral radiographs of both forearm and elbow. Dislocation of the radial head is confirmed radiographically if a line drawn through the center of the radial shaft and head fails to align with the capitellum in all projections. Posterior interosseous nerve injury is not uncommon with this fracture–dislocation, and presents with loss or weakness of wrist extension. The prognosis for nerve recovery is good. Because surgical treatment is necessary in most cases, orthopedic consultation is recommended at the time of presentation; the arm may be splinted for comfort while awaiting further management.

The floating elbow describes a combination of humeral shaft fracture and both-bone forearm fracture; elbow dislocation (usually posterior) may also be involved. These injuries are the result of high-energy direct trauma. Significant deformity is evident on physical examination, and neurovascular deficits are common (25–45%).[52] Reduce deformities to relieve neurovascular deficits. Arteriography is indicated to evaluate for vascular injury if pulses are not restored upon limb realignment. Orthopedic consultation should be obtained as these injuries require urgent operative exploration and repair.

Isolated radial neck fractures are relatively uncommon in adults, most occur in conjunction with radial head fractures, frequently as a result of elbow dislocation. Isolated radial neck fractures displaced < 4 mm have excellent outcome when treated nonoperatively.[53] Larger displacement should be operatively reduced, as should those with concomitant radial head fractures.[54]

Fracture of the coronoid process of the ulna is rarely an isolated injury. These fractures typically occur as part of the "terrible triad," which includes posterior elbow dislocation and radial head fracture.[55] The coronoid presents a bony block to posterior translocation of the ulna, and provides the origin for the anterior bundle of the medial collateral ligament, and the middle portion of the anterior capsule, further contributing to joint stability. Thus, fracture of the coracoid process in association with elbow dislocation can result in an unstable reduction. Coronoid fractures have been described by two classification schemes (Table 16.3).[56]

Fractures may be missed on plain AP and lateral radiographs, as the radial head overlaps the coronoid process on the lateral view; oblique views are useful. In cases where coronoid process fractures are suspected (such as unstable elbow dislocations), a CT scan with

Table 16.3 Different descriptions of coronoid fractures[56]

Type 1 being an avulsion fracture of the tip	Type I fractures are transverse at the tip type
Type II fractures involving < 50% of the body	Type II fractures are through the anteromedial facet
Type III involving > 50% of the coronoid process	Type III fractures involving the base

287

three-dimensional reconstruction is the preferred diagnostic modality.[57,58] Current recommendations include operative fixation of any coronoid fracture that is associated with an unstable elbow reduction, regardless of the size of the fracture fragment.[59] Thus, unstable elbow reductions require orthopedic consultation in the ED. All other patients with coronoid fractures may be safely discharged in a sling with early orthopedic follow up for operative consideration.

Olecranon fractures may occur from a direct blow, FOOSH, or as high-energy injuries in combination with other fractures or dislocations. Several classification systems describe fracture patterns, and are useful for consideration of the mechanical requirements of internal fixation. Orthopedic consultation is required for all displaced (> 2 mm) fractures, as surgical treatment is indicated.[60] Surgical repair may involve fracture fixation or excision of the fracture fragment and triceps reattachment. Displaced fractures in patients with severe comorbid medical conditions, dementia, or severe osteopenia may be treated non-operatively with the expectation of marked loss of elbow extension power. For such patients, treatment is focused on protecting contused skin with padding and an Ace wrap.[61] Non-displaced fractures are rare; these can be managed non-operatively with splinting in midflexion (45–90°).[62] Orthopedic follow up should be planned at 7–10 days for repeat radiographs to evaluate the possibility of fracture displacement.

Both bone forearm fractures typically occur as a result of high energy trauma, following a direct blow or a fall from a height. Associated injuries are common. Patients may have abrasions or lacerations overlying the fracture. A careful evaluation of the soft tissues is indicated in order to identify an open fracture, if present. Neurovascular deficits are rare with closed forearm fractures, but common in open injuries. The forearm may be splinted for comfort in the ED, using either posterior or sugar-tong splinting. Orthopedic consultation should be obtained expeditiously, as definitive management of these fractures is nearly always surgical. Significant loss of forearm rotation and grip strength has been reported in patients with as little as 5° of malalignment.[63]

Wrist fractures

Distal radius fractures

Distal radius fractures account for more than 15% of all adult fractures.[64] The age distribution is bimodal, peaking in early adolescence and again in the elderly; these injuries typically occur from the FOOSH mechanism. In addition, high-energy injuries following a fall or motor vehicle accident occur in older adolescents and adults of all ages. Women sustain seven times as many distal radius fractures as men (7 : 1).[65] Patients present with pain and, often deformity at the wrist. Range of motion is typically limited. A thorough neurovascular exam should be documented. Vascular injuries and injury to the radial and ulnar nerves are rare, but acute injury to the median nerve may be associated with significant fracture displacement.[66] Carpal tunnel syndrome has been reported to occur in up to 20% of patients with distal radial fractures, although it may be a delayed.[67] The presence of an acute nerve injury is an indication for orthopedic consultation in the ED as immediate operative reduction, fixation, and nerve decompression has been advocated.[67] Evaluation of distal tendon function is important, as tendon laceration or entrapment can occur with these injuries.

Several schemes exist for fracture classification of the distal radius and ulna; these are based on mechanism of injury or anatomy of the fracture. However, the historical use of eponyms to describe these fractures remains a common practice: Colles fractures result from a FOOSH and the distal fragment displaces dorsally; Smith fractures ("Reverse Colles") displace volarly and result from a fall on the supinated hand (Figure 16.18).

True PA and lateral radiographs are important in distinguishing fracture pattern and determining treatment (Figure 16.19). It is important to distinguish extra-articular from intra-articular fractures, as the latter may require operative treatment if more than minimally displaced. Metaphyseal comminution, particularly on the dorsal aspect, and increased ulnar variance, have been found to predict fracture instability when identified on initial films.[68] Furthermore, fracture stability decreases with increasing age, due to poor bone quality. Unstable fractures are more likely to require operative management.

The emergency physician may attempt reduction of displaced fractures. A hematoma block provides excellent pain control by the injection of lidocaine directly into the fracture hematoma. The skin over the fracture site is sterilely prepped and draped; injection is typically made from the dorsum of the forearm in order to avoid neurovascular structures. A 22-gauge needle attached to a syringe containing

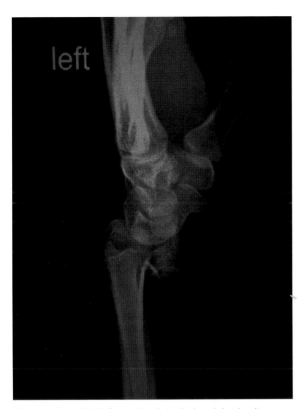

Figure 16.18 "Smith fracture": volarly displaced distal radius fracture.

8–10 cc of 1% lidocaine is directed perpendicularly into the center of the hematoma. Blood is aspirated from the hematoma confirming needle placement; lidocaine is then injected. While allowing the hematoma block to take effect (10–15 minutes), material for a sugar-tong splint may be prepared based on measurements of the uninjured extremity. Alternatively, the Bier block, regional nerve block, and procedural sedation may also be used to achieve anesthesia for the reduction. However, the hematoma block is the easiest to perform and requires fewer additional physicians/extenders to perform. Reduction is achieved by distracting the distal fragment while applying a force in the direction opposite fragment displacement. If this method fails to achieve adequate reduction, traction may be applied via the use of finger traps, suspending the arm in a vertical fashion, and allowing the physician to focus on correction of angulation. When reduction is complete, the splint is applied and molded to maintain a slight palmar flexion, ulnar deviation, and neutral rotation. Post-reduction radiographs should be obtained to demonstrate the reduction and

to serve as a point of comparison for follow-up radiographs. Patients may be discharged from the ED with instructions for elevation of the extremity, finger movement exercises, and orthopedic follow up in 3–5 days. There is considerable debate in the orthopedic literature regarding the long-term disability resulting from subtle alteration in radial geometry.[69,70] Thus, treatment decisions for extra-articular fractures will vary based upon patient age and bone quality, comorbidities that may affect outcome (such as rheumatoid arthritis), recreational and vocational activities of the patient, and hand dominance.[71]

Carpal fractures: The bones of the wrist are arranged in two carpal rows. The proximal row contains the scaphoid, lunate, triquetrum, and the pisiform (from radial to ulnar aspect) while the distal row contains the trapezium, trapezoid, capitate, and hamate.

The interosseous membrane partially overlaps the proximal row, contributing to wrist stability. A key anatomic structure is the triangular-fibrocartilage complex (TFCC) which originates at the ulnar aspect of the radius and extends to the ulnar styloid. This complex further anchors the DRUJ and ulnar aspect of the carpus. The carpal ligaments are both extrinsic (radius to carpus) and intrinsic (between carpal bones); they maintain overall carpal alignment and support the relationship between carpal bones, particularly, the position of the lunate. This is important as a negative radiograph cannot fully exclude a significant injury to the ligamentous structures.

A scaphoid fracture should be considered in any patient who presents with dorsal-radial wrist pain following a FOOSH. Significant deformity is rare, as is any associated acute neurovascular injury. Range of motion is often limited by pain. Tenderness in the anatomic snuff box should heighten the physician's suspicion for scaphoid fracture, as should recreation of symptoms with axial loading of the thumb. Initial radiographs should include PA, lateral, and oblique views of the wrist (Figure 16.20). In addition to obvious fracture lines and bony displacement, an abnormal scaphoid fat pad may be seen. However, the significance of this finding has been debated. A dedicated scaphoid view can also be added to provide further detail. This view is obtained by directing the beam perpendicular to the scaphoid while the wrist is held in an ulnarly deviated position. Barring significant displacement of fracture fragments, scaphoid fractures are notoriously difficult to diagnose acutely.

289

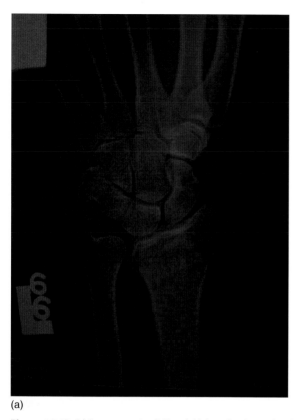

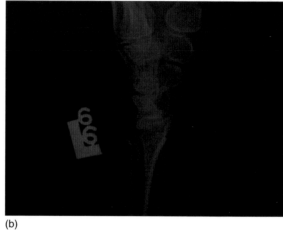

(a)   (b)

Figure 16.19 (a) Posteroanterior (PA) and (b) lateral radiographs of distal radius fracture.

In those patients with radiographs without acute fracture, there are several options. One option is to place the patient in a non-removable thumb spica short arm splint with re-evaluation in 1–2 weeks. This immobilization is critical in the maintenance of adequate vascularity to the proximal scaphoid, as blood supply enters distally (in a retrograde fashion) and most fractures occur at the scaphoid waist. Failure to adequately immobilize fractures on an acute basis is associated with increased non-union rates and increased need for surgical treatment. Thus, temporary immobilization of an injury that is **not** a fracture is much preferred over failure to treat an actual fracture. Orthopedic follow up should be arranged in about 2 weeks. At that point, if there is still pain or tenderness, repeat radiographs are obtained. Another acceptable approach would be to obtain additional imaging including an MRI or CT scan acutely or a bone scan in several days. However, CT or bone scanning limit evaluation of potential ligamentous injury.[72]

When a scaphoid fracture is evident in the ED, it can be managed with application of a thumb spica

splint or short arm cast (based upon the amount of swelling present). There is some debate in the literature regarding the benefits of long vs. short arm thumb spica splints. Although long arm spicas tend to reduce the time to healing and the rate of non-union, the differences were not found to be significant. Orthopedic follow up should be arranged within 3–5 days for definitive care. Displaced fractures, many proximal pole fractures (which are predisposed to avascular necrosis), and fractures in patients who cannot afford a long period of immobilization are treated surgically. Fractures that are treated non-operatively require up to 3 months of immobilization.

Carpal dislocations are also common sequelae of a FOOSH injury and should be considered in the differential of wrist pain. The scapholunate dislocation presents similarly to the scaphoid fracture, with tenderness in the anatomic snuff box and decreased wrist motion. Unlike scaphoid fractures, however, a subtle deformity may be detected over the dorsum of the proximal carpal row, and tenderness is typically greatest in this location. Neurovascular deficits are

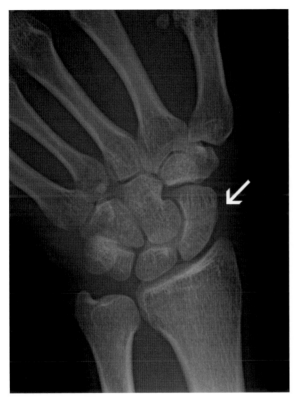

Figure 16.20 Scaphoid wrist fracture. (Courtesy of Mark Bernstein, MD.)

rare. A standard wrist radiograph series should be obtained, but the diagnosis is made primarily on the PA view. Key findings include a short, dense scaphoid and > 3 mm space between the scaphoid and the lunate.[73] This gap between bony structures is referred to as the Terry Thomas sign (a.k.a. the David Letterman sign). Attempts at non-operative reduction are rarely successful. Orthopedic consultation should be obtained in the ED, but patients may be discharged in a thumb spica splint while awaiting definitive management.

The FOOSH mechanism may also result in injury *about* the lunate. A sequence of injury follows forceful hyperextension and ulnar deviation of the hand. First, scapholunate dissociation occurs; continued force produces damage to intrinsic and extrinsic ligaments, culminating in perilunate dislocation or, ultimately, lunate dislocation. Although these dislocations are most commonly dorsal in nature (distal carpus displacement relative to the radius), dislocations can occur in the opposite direction. Perilunate and lunate dislocations can include fractures to the radial styloid,

scaphoid, capitates, and/or triquetrum; scaphoid fractures are most common of these fractures. These injuries present with pain and tenderness at the dorsum of the wrist, particularly at the proximal carpal row. Deformity may be obvious; alternatively clinical presentation may be innocuous. The latter presentation is responsible for the delay in diagnosis that has been reported to occur in up to 25% of cases.[74] Median nerve compromise is the most commonly associated neurovascular injury; delayed reduction may result in permanent neurologic sequelae. Standard wrist radiographs, particularly the lateral view, provide the key to diagnosis. A break in the colinear alignment of the radius, lunate, capitate and metacarpals on the lateral radiograph is diagnostic. In the case of perilunate dislocation, the lunate maintains its position atop the radius while the capitate and remaining carpal bones are displaced (Figure 16.21a and b). With lunate dislocation, the lunate has the appearance of a "spilled teacup," lying volar to the radius while the remaining carpal bones maintain normal alignment (Figure 16.21c).

In addition, on the PA radiograph, the normally "square" appearance of the lunate becomes "triangular" in the case of lunate dislocation. Orthopedic consultation should be obtained promptly, as both lunate and perilunate dislocations require urgent reduction. Attempts at reduction should be made by the emergency physician in cases of neurovascular compromise when orthopedic consultation will be delayed. Reduction should be performed by maintaining longitudinal traction on the flexed fingers while gently reversing the direction (either volar or dorsal) of the dislocation. However, given the rotational component of the lunate displacement in anterior lunate dislocations, closed reduction is usually not possible. Surgical stabilization is typically required following closed reduction; this may be performed acutely, or may be delayed if the neurovascular status is normal. Some dislocations are not reducible by closed methods and should be taken urgently to the operating room.

Patients who have sustained FOOSH injuries may present with pain along the ulnar aspect of the wrist. Tenderness in this anatomic distribution with normal wrist radiographs should prompt the physician to consider TFCC injuries. Patients may note a clicking with wrist motion, particularly ulnar deviation. Pain may be produced with pronation and supination of the forearm. Further diagnostic evidence is provided

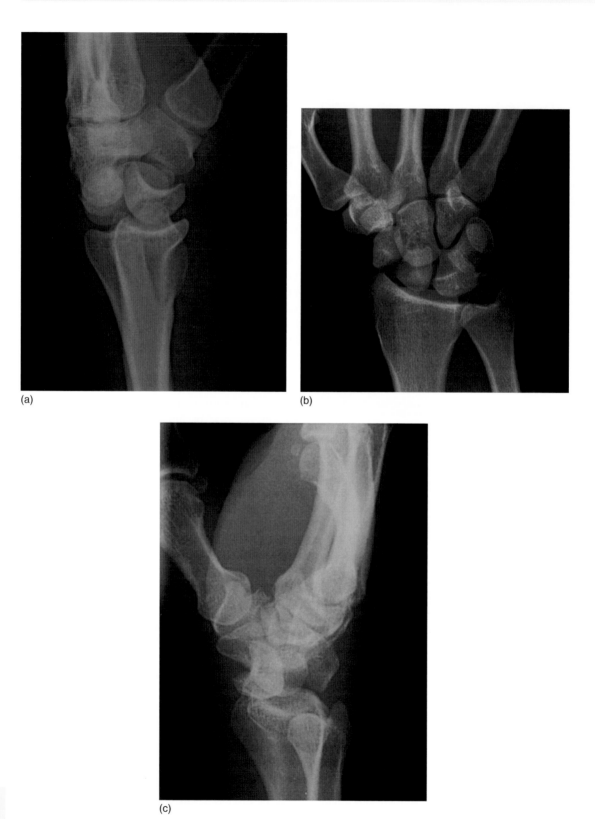

(a)

(b)

(c)

Figure 16.21 Perilunate dislocations: (a) lateral; (b) posteroanterior (PA) radiographs; (c) lunate dislocation lateral view with spilled teacup sign.

via the ulnar abutment test which is sensitive for TFCC tears. This test is performed with the forearm pronated. The examiner stabilizes the distal forearm while placing the hand in maximal ulnar deviation. Production of pain or the appreciation of a click is diagnostic of a TFCC injury. A volar splint should be applied to patients with persistent pain and edema and a negative radiograph, particularly when the physical examination is concerning for potential TFCC injuries. This will comfort and protect while awaiting orthopedic follow up, preferably within a week of the injury.

Hand injuries

Hand fractures may result from axial load or direct trauma. An adequate history should be performed to elicit the mechanism of injury; open fractures via any mechanism and fractures resulting from human bites are at high risk. Neurovascular status should be carefully evaluated. In cases where inadequate perfusion is a concern, capillary refill should be assessed and generally be expected to return in < 2 seconds in all digits. Sensation via light touch and two-point discrimination should be assessed; normal for the latter is < 6 mm. Abnormal findings should be compared to the uninjured hand, as a perceived abnormality may be the patient's baseline. This is particularly true for manual laborers, who may exhibit decreased sensation due to repetitive trauma. Rotational deformity should be assessed by examination of the palmar aspect of the patient's hand during active flexion of the MCP and PIP joints of all fingers. The distal aspect of each finger should point toward the scaphoid; deviation is an indication of rotational displacement of the fracture. It should be noted that rotational deformities are usually not evident with the fingers in extension. Flexor and extensor function at the MCP, PIP, and DIP joints should be assessed for all fingers of the affected hand, as displaced fracture fragments may disrupt tendon mechanisms. Deficits are defined based on the extensor and flexor zones. Orthopedic consultation should be obtained for all injuries involving the flexor tendons as these usually require operative repair. Injuries to the extensor mechanism without associated laceration (i.e., central slip injuries) can usually be splinted with the affected digit in extension, and orthopedic follow up arranged in 3–5 days. The longer the delay from time of injury to time of definitive repair, the more

likely the tendon fragments are to retract, complicating repair and lowering chances of a successful repair and return to normal function. Local custom may dicatate whether the lacerated extensor tendon is repaired by the emergency physician or by a hand surgeon. If the tendon is to be repaired in the ED, non-absorbable, low-reactive material such as ethibond or nylon or longer acting absorbable sutures should be used. Figure of eight, modified Kessler or horizontal mattress stitches may all be performed to reapproximate the tendon ends. While evidence is extrapolated from flexor tendon injuries, general custom dictates that a laceration > 50% of the width is repaired. Less can probably be splinted without repair. At least PA and lateral radiographs of the involved part should be obtained if there is any concern for possibility of fracture or foreign body; 10° pronated or supinated views may be helpful in visualizing the 2nd and 5th metacarpal fractures.

Patients with displaced metacarpal fractures usually present with pain at the fracture site, obvious deformity, edema, and ecchymosis. Metacarpal fractures may involve the neck, shaft, or base of the metacarpal. The former typically occurs as a result of an axial load against a clenched fist; these fractures exhibit apex dorsal angulation. Up to 35° and 45° of angulation can be accepted in the ring and little fingers, respectively, but < 15° is acceptable for index and long fingers, due to more rigid carpometacarpal joints.[75] There is evidence to support immediate mobilization (i.e., discharge with buddy taping or without any taping/splinting) of 5th metacarpal fractures, without reduction, even with high degrees of apex dorsal angulation.[76,77] At this time, no definitive treatment for 5th metacarpal fractures is proven superior. Options include splinting or buddy taping. Choice is often determined by local practice patterns. Rotational and lateral deformity should be corrected, when present. Metacarpal shaft fractures also typically present with apex dorsal angulation; considerable shortening may occur in the index and 5th metacarpals because they lack the suspensory effect of the intermetacarpal ligaments. Guidelines for acceptable dorsal angulation and shortening with shaft fractures are as follows:[75] Up to 0.5 cm of shortening is acceptable, but rotational malalignment is not.[75] Fractures at the base of the metacarpal may be missed because of inadequate radiographs. Tenderness in this location should prompt additional oblique views if not seen on initial films. Although these fractures are

Table 16.4 Acceptable angulation for metacarpal shaft fractures

Finger	Acceptable angulation of shaft
Little (small)	< 30°
Ring	< 20°
Long	0°
Index	0°

typically stable, rotational alignment must be corrected. Reduction of displaced fractures is best carried out after adequate analgesia is achieved. A hematoma block (or other forms of anesthesia as described in the section for distal radius fractures) usually provides excellent analgesia; 3–5 cc of lidocaine 1% is required. Reduction is performed by applying gentle traction to the distal fragment while directing the same fragment in the direction opposite to the displacement (Table 16.4). Digital pressure over the dorsal apex is helpful in reducing deformity in that plane. Gentle rotation while performing the traction/manipulation maneuver may correct rotational deformity. Once fracture reduction is obtained the affected extremity is immobilized. An ulnar gutter splint is used for 4th and 5th metacarpal fractures. A custom splint is prepared with volar and dorsal slabs for index and middle metacarpal fractures. Both the volar and dorsal components are needed for index and middle metacarpal fractures given the relative difficulty associated with limiting the range of motion of the centrally located bones. In all cases, the MCP joints should be immobilized in full flexion and the IP joints in extension. Patients can be discharged with orthopedic follow up arranged in 5–7 days. Displaced intra-articular fractures, unstable fractures, and multiple metacarpal fractures typically require surgical treatment. However, this may be set up as an outpatient, and patients may be safely discharged with a splint orthopedic follow up in 3–5 days. Open fractures or those with considerable associated soft tissue injury require immediate consultation with a hand specialist in the ED.

Non-displaced phalangeal fractures may present with only swelling and tenderness over the fracture site while comminuted, displaced fractures may feature swelling, ecchymosis, and significant deformity. The latter may be associated with digital nerve or tendon injuries or skin lacerations. If an isolated distal injury is suspected, radiographs may be limited to a finger series (AP, lateral, and oblique views). However, if multiple injuries are suspected, obtain a complete hand series, Although complex intra-articular fractures should be reduced by hand specialists, the emergency physician may safely reduce extra-articular fractures or attempt reduction of simple minor intra-articular ones using the same methods as for metacarpal fractures. A digital block provides excellent anesthesia in most cases. With multiple finger fractures, regional anesthesia may be more appropriate than multiple digital blocks. Angulation > 10° is unacceptable in any plane.[78] Fractures with ulnar or radial deviation may be buddy taped, after reduction, to the adjacent digit in the direction opposite the original displacement; this minimizes risk of recurrence. Stable fractures can be immobilized in malleable finger splints; buddy taping may also be performed for additional comfort and improved functionality. However buddy taping alone does not provide substantial protection during everyday activity. Unstable fractures should be splinted similarly to metacarpal fractures. Patients may be discharged from the ED with hand specialty follow up in 3–5 days to assess for maintenance of reduction.

Dislocations of the MCP and IP joints are extremely common. Dorsal PIP dislocations represent the most frequent articular injury in the hand.[79] These involve injury to the collateral ligaments and volar plate, but are typically stable after reduction, allowing immediate mobilization via buddy taping to the adjacent digit. Volar dislocations are less common, but more severe, and may include disruption of the central slip of the extensor tendon.[80] Pre- and post-reduction radiographs (AP, lateral, and oblique views) should be obtained to evaluate for associated fractures. It is particularly important to identify intra-articular fractures as these may require operative fixation regardless of the success of reduction attempts.[79] Pre-reduction radiography is also helpful to identify small intra-articular foreign bodies, the presence of which may make adequate closed reduction difficult. Reduction may be blocked due to interposition of the central slip or the collateral ligaments. Reduction attempts should be made with the MCP and PIP joints in a flexed position to allow relaxation of the lateral bands. The extensor mechanism should be assessed post-reduction; if full active extension of the PIP joint is not possible, the joint should be immobilized in full extension to treat a presumptive central slip injury. If closed reduction is unsuccessful, open reduction is required. The PIP dislocations may be associated with volar avulsion fractures or dorsal avulsion fractures at the central slip insertion; these injuries should be evaluated by a hand specialist, as special splinting techniques or surgical treatment may be required. All other patients may be discharged from the ED following reduction and splinting, with appropriate follow up arranged in 7–10 days.

Injuries to MCP and DIP joints are less common than PIP injuries. The MCP dislocations are treated with closed reduction. Care should be taken in assessing these injuries radiographically, adding oblique views to evaluate for intra-articular fractures that require specialty consultation and likely surgical treatment. DIP joint injuries frequently involve disruption of the tendon bone unit. *Mallet finger* injury occurs when the extensor tendon is avulsed from the base of the distal phalanx when the DIP joint is forcibly flexed against a taut tendon (e.g., catching a ball). Diagnosis is based upon the inability to fully extend the DIP joint in an active manner. Patients may be treated with a dorsal, volar, or stack splint holding the DIP joint in full extension, and appropriate follow up in 1–2 weeks. *It is imperative that the patient does not remove the splint for any reason. If the splint is removed and the finger flexed, any previous time spent in the splint is negated and the treatment time starts over.* When associated with a fracture, specialty consultation is required, as open treatment may be necessary. *Jersey finger* is the name applied to avulsion of the flexor digitorum profundus tendon from the volar base of the distal phalanx. It is most commonly an athletic injury, occurring during the course of a missed tackle, when a flexed finger is forcibly extended.[81] Patients usually present with the DIP extended and are not able to actively flex the DIP. Careful evaluation of active joint motion should be carried out to avoid missing this injury. A potential pitfall is ascribing loss of flexion to pain and swelling. Early referral is necessary. If the tendon retracts, it must be repaired early to obtain a good result and this cannot often be diagnosed clinically.

The thumb is also vulnerable to injury via the FOOSH mechanism, particularly when the thumb is abducted. Patients with thumb trauma often present with tenderness at the MCP joint, edema, and ecchymosis. Fractures typically occur at the base of

the 1st metacarpal, and are often intra-articular. Shaft fractures are uncommon due to the lack of rigid fixation at the 1st CMC joint. A Bennett's fracture is an intra-articular metacarpal fracture with a small volar metacarpal fragment. A Rolando fracture is a comminuted metacarpal intra-articular fracture, resulting from a greater force application. These fractures are typically highly unstable and the majority require operative fixation. Patients may be safely discharged from the ED in a thumb spica splint while awaiting definitive management; operative repair usually takes place within a week of injury. The physician should also consider trapezium dislocation when evaluating patients with acute thumb pain. Although reduction may be achieved in the ED, this rare injury often requires K wire fixation for definitive treatment.[82]

Pure dislocations of the 1st MP joint are usually dorsal, resulting from forcible hyperextension. A simple dislocation is reducible by closed means, while a complex dislocation requires open reduction. This distinction can be made by careful inspection: with a simple dislocation the phalanx rests atop the metacarpal head in ~90° of hyperextension; a complex dislocation is associated with a skin dimple on the volar aspect of the thenar eminence and the proximal phalanx lies in only slight hyperextension[83]. Specialist consultation in the ED is required for treatment of complex dislocations. *It is important to note that a simple dislocation can be converted into a complex dislocation with an improper reduction maneuver.* The application of traction may cause entrapment of the volar plate, rendering the dislocation irreducible. Reduction is properly performed by hyperextending the proximal phalanx on the metacarpal, flexing the IP joint and pushing the dorsal base of the proximal phalanx back into place. Wrist flexion during this maneuver relaxes the flexor tendons, facilitating reduction. Following successful reduction, the collateral ligaments should be assessed for stability; evidence of complete rupture should prompt consultation for definitive treatment. If stable, thumb spica immobilization is applied and the patient is discharged with orthopedic follow up.

Ulnar collateral ligament injuries (gamekeeper's or skier's thumb) should be suspected when patients present with pain at the thumb MCP joint but negative radiographs. This ligament is injured when a valgus-extension force is applied to the thumb resulting in partial or complete rupture of the UCL. Integrity of the ligament is assessed through the

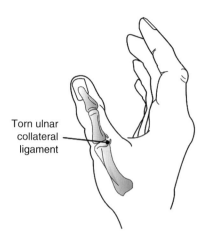

Figure 16.22 Ulnar collateral injury (Courtesy of National Institutes of Health National Institute of Arthritis and Musculoskeletal and Skin Diseases [NIH-NIAMS]).

Torn ulnar collateral ligament

application of valgus stress (radial deviation) to the MP joint at neutral and at 30° of flexion, using the other thumb for comparison.[84] There are several options to evaluate. Local anesthesia may be required to allow for full examination. Another possibility is that because laxity may be difficult to detect, if injury is suspected, forego ED stress of joint and immobilization in a thumb spica splint is appropriate. Repeat evaluation can be done as an outpatient. Patients may be discharged with appropriate follow up for definitive treatment, which may be surgical in cases of complete rupture (Figure 16.22).

Finger amputations are commonly seen in the ED. Patients often present accompanied by the amputated part. It is imperative that prehospital providers attempt to gently decontaminate the fragment and then place it in a sealed plastic bag. The bag may then be floated on ice; however, the amputated part should not come into direct contact with ice. A thorough neurovascular examination should be performed. Radiographs of the hand and the amputated part should be performed to evaluate the viability of the fragment. Intravenous antibiotics, typically a first generation cephalosporin,[1] and analgesics should be administered and tetanus updated as needed while radiographic studies are obtained. The critical question to be addressed early in the management of this injury is whether or not reimplantation will be attempted, thus early involvement of the hand specialists is neccesary. The decision to attempt reattachment is multifactorial. Injuries to the thumb almost always lead to reattachment attempts, as does involvement of the index finger (from the PIP distally) of the dominant hand. While more proximal injuries are arguably more important to reimplant, distal injuries have better outcomes. Multiple amputations also increase the likelihood of operative attempts, as does amputations in children. The patient's career also impacts the decision to reattach. This decision may be swayed by patients who have professions that rely upon fine motor skills. Reattachment is most successful when the repair is performed < 6 hours from the time of injury; however, there are isolated reports of success up to 24 hours after the amputation.[85] Simple, clean-cut amputations are more likely to be successfully reimplanted than those associated with crush injuries. *It is imperative that the decision to attempt reimplantation be made as quickly as possible to maximize tissue viability.*[85] As rapidity of reimplantation correlates with success, transfer to a reimplation center as soon as possible is the best option. Once there is a judgment that the patient is a possible candidate, efforts should be made to rapidly transport. All non-essential treatment, such as radiographs for simple amputations or tetanus can be performed at the receiving center if they will delay transport.

Pediatric considerations

The evaluation and treatment of pediatric fractures are influenced by the presence of open physes. This is particularly true in the case of periarticular fractures that can result in growth arrest or articular incongruity. Fracture lines are easily obscured in epiphyseal cartilage, and fracture diagnosis may rely upon indirect evidence of altered anatomy. When evaluating an injured pediatric extremity, comparison radiographs of the unaffected extremity are extremely useful, particularly in the case of periarticular fractures. In addition, a radiographic reference detailing the age of epiphyseal ossification for major joints is helpful. Although many periarticular pediatric fractures require anatomic reduction, diaphyseal fractures may tolerate greater angulation than would be tolerated in adults, due to the ability of pediatric bone to remodel with growth.[86,87] This is particularly true for fractures that are close to the physis.

The Salter–Harris classification describes physeal fractures (Figure 16.23). It discriminates between fracture patterns that require surgical treatment and carry a high risk of poor outcome vs. those that may be treated non-operatively with little risk of adverse sequelae. Type I and II fractures can often be managed non-operatively; splinting is typically

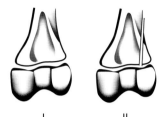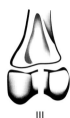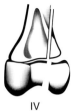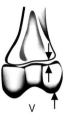

I II III IV V

Figure 16.23 The Salter–Harris classification of growth plate injury. See text for more details. (Courtesy of National Institutes of Health National Institute of Arthritis and Musculoskeletal and Skin Diseases [NIH-NIAMS])

sufficient for upper extremity fractures. These injuries do not usually result in growth disturbance. Type III injuries require operative fixation when displaced; accurate determination of displacement may require CT evaluation. Type IV fractures almost universally require operative fixation; even so, limb length discrepancies are common. Type V fractures are relatively rare but carry a high likelihood of growth disturbance. Treatment decisions regarding physeal fractures are best made in consultation with orthopedic surgeons and are based primarily on the size of the fragment and the amount of displacement.

The pediatric population is particularly susceptible to supracondylar humerus fractures. This injury accounts for up to 80% of pediatric elbow fractures and approximately 5% of all fractures in children.[88] As with most upper extremity fractures, the common mechanism of injury is the FOOSH, accounting for 98% of all supracondylar humeral fractures.[89] Children often present with the elbow flexed and the extremity adducted. The injured child is unlikely to use the affected extremity for any purpose, and resists attempts to manipulate the elbow through a range of motion. It is often difficult to locate a point of maximum tenderness. As with adults, antecubital ecchymosis is indicative of associated brachial artery injury and should prompt the physician to consider angiographic evaluation of the affected extremity even in the presence of normal pulses. The neurovascular examination is of paramount importance, as nerve injuries are commonly associated with this fracture. The radial nerve is most commonly injured, followed closely by the anterior interosseous branch of the median nerve.[90] Patients with the former will present with wrist drop and inability to abduct the thumb (the "hitchhiker's sign"). Patients with the latter injury are unable to oppose the thumb and index finger (the "ok sign"). Orthopedic consultation should be obtained immediately for any child with a supracondylar humerus fracture and a vascular deficit.

Children with significant pain or with a presumed unstable injury should be splinted with the elbow in 45–90° flexion prior to obtaining radiographs. Frequent (every 30–45 minutes) neurovascular checks should be performed in order to identify an evolving neurovascular injury due to progressive swelling; compartment syndrome with permanent neurovascular deficit is a disastrous sequelae of this fracture. Radiographic evaluation for this injury consists of AP and lateral views of the elbow and forearm. Due to the variable ossification of the elbow, contralateral extremity films may be helpful for comparison in unclear cases. The anterior humeral line is key in diagnosing the supracondylar humeral fracture. On the lateral radiograph, a line drawn down the anterior cortex of the humerus should transect the midpoint of the capitellum. Any variation in this relationship should heighten suspicion for a supracondylar fracture (Figure 16.24).

Supracondylar fractures that occur with an extension mechanism are classified according to the Gartland scheme.[91] Type I injuries are non-displaced while Type III fractures are completely displaced. Type II injuries feature either posterior angulation with the posterior cortex intact or malrotation of the distal fragment. Flexion injuries are relatively rare (~2% of all supracondylar fractures) and are classified with a modification of Gartland's scheme[92]: Type I are non-displaced; Type II are in contact but angulated or rotated; Type III are completely displaced. These fractures are notoriously unstable and require surgical treatment when displaced.

Treatment of supracondylar humerus fractures is based upon fracture type and the presence of neurovascular deficits. Non-displaced (Type I) fractures are treated in a posterior splint with the elbow flexed to 90° and arrangements made for orthopedic follow up in 5–7 days. All other fractures require orthopedic consultation in the ED; those with neurovascular compromise require urgent consultation.

297

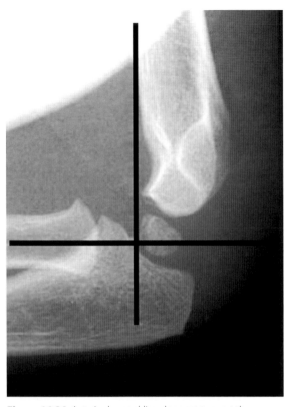

Figure 16.24 Anterior humeral line does not transect the midpoint of the capitellum, raising the suspicion for a Type I supracondylar fracture.

An attempt at closed reduction of a displaced fracture with neurovascular compromise can be carried out by the emergency physician if orthopedic consultation is delayed > 1 hour.[90] Reduction for extension fractures is as detailed in the adult section. Type II fractures may be reduced in the ED under appropriate sedation; stabilization of the reduction requires splinting in 120° of elbow flexion. Failure to flex the elbow to 120° is associated with a high likelihood of loss of reduction; however, this position increases the risk of Volkmann's ischemia.[93] Therefore, Type II fractures are typically treated under general anesthesia with closed reduction and percutaneous pinning to stabilize the fracture and allow splinting in less elbow flexion. Type III fractures are treated in the operating room with closed reduction and percutaneous pinning; rarely, open reduction is required for an irreducible fracture. All patients with displaced fractures should be admitted for 24 hour observation of the neurovascular status, with frequent neurovascular checks during the admission (Figure 16.25).

Isolated fractures of the lateral humeral condyle are the second most common fracture in the pediatric elbow and typically occur between 5 and 10 years of age.[94] In comparison to the supracondylar fracture, this injury typically results from a fall on a supinated, extended elbow. Presentation is similar to that for supracondylar fractures, although swelling and tenderness may be relatively concentrated at the lateral

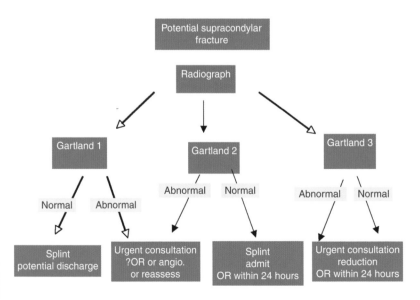

Figure 16.25 Algorithm for treatment of supracondylar fracture. angio., angiography; OR, operating room.

Table 16.5 Milch Classification by displacement lateral condyle fracture

Stage	Displacement	Treatment
Stage I	< 2 mm displacement and an intact articular surface	Splinted with the elbow flexed to 90° and the forearm supinated. Close follow up by an orthopedic surgeon is mandatory because the incidence of late displacement is high
Stage II	Disruption of the articular surface and rotation of the condylar fragment	Closed reduction and percutaneous pinning to avoid late loss of reduction
Stage III	Complete displacement and rotation, and associated with elbow instability	Closed reduction and percutaneous pinning to avoid late loss of reduction

Table 16.6 Medial condyle fracture classification

Type	Description	Treatment
Type I	Impacted	Elbow splinted in 90° of flexion with neutral rotation and early orthopedic follow up (3–5 days)
Type II	Non-displaced with intra-articular extension	Elbow splinted in 90° of flexion with neutral rotation and early orthopedic follow up (3–5 days)
Type III	Displaced and rotated	Orthopedic consultation in the ED for definitive management involving closed vs. open reduction and percutaneous pinning

aspect of the elbow. Initial evaluation is the same as for supracondylar fractures, and includes imaging with standard AP and lateral radiographs. Internal and external oblique views may enhance evaluation of fracture displacement. Addition of the internal oblique view, in particular, has been shown to alter management of these fractures, prompting operative treatment in a larger percentage of patients.[95] Fractures are classified historically according to Milch (Table 16.5).[96] Type I fractures extend through the ossification center of the lateral condyle and exit the joint at the radiocapitellar groove. Type II fractures track through the physis, exiting the joint at the trochlear notch, making the joint unstable; these fractures may be associated with an elbow dislocation (primarily posterior). Because of the high incidence of complications, all patients with lateral condylar fractures require orthopedic consultation.

Medial condyle fractures are rare, accounting for < 2% of all pediatric elbow fractures.[97] These injuries occur from a direct blow on the apex of the elbow, or with valgus stress to the elbow. Children present with swelling and tenderness localized to the medial aspect of the elbow and decreased range of motion because of

pain. This fracture should be distinguished from a medial epicondyle fracture, described below. Standard AP and lateral radiographs of the elbow should be sufficient to make the diagnosis: a Thurston–Holland metaphyseal fragment (i.e. a small separated bone fragment from the growth plate) suggests a medial condylar fracture rather than a medial epicondylar fracture (Table 16.6).[97]

Medial epicondyle fractures typically occur during early adolescence; they represent about 10% of pediatric elbow fractures.[98] This injury results when a valgus force is applied to an extended elbow; the medial epicondyle is avulsed from the distal humerus by the wrist flexors. Alternatively, forced flexion of the forearm against an extended elbow can result in medial epicondylar fracture. This injury may occur along with posterolateral elbow dislocation; the medial epicondylar fragment can become entrapped within the joint following reduction of the dislocation, and should be extracted surgically.[98] Incidence of this injury has increased significantly due to increasing participation in youth baseball; the forces associated with pitching are sufficient to produce this apophyseal avulsion fracture. Neurovascular examination is particularly important with this fracture due to a relatively high incidence of associated ulnar nerve injury. The fracture is usually clearly delineated on the AP radiograph; the lateral radiograph is useful in determining whether the dislocated fragment is intra-articular, as occurs following reduction of a concomitant elbow dislocation. Non-displaced fractures may be treated by placement of the elbow in a posterior splint with the joint flexed to 90°. Motion is initiated early to avoid stiffness; therefore orthopedic follow up should be arranged in 5–7 days. Intra-articular displaced fractures or those displaced > 5 mm should be operatively reduced.[98]

The nursemaid's elbow is commonly seen in the pediatric population between the ages of 1–4 years; however, it has been reported in both infants and early adolescents. This injury involves a subluxation of the radial head over the annular ligament. It typically occurs with traction on an extended elbow, often in an attempt to pull a child from a situation of potential danger. The injured child often presents with the forearm pronated and the extremity hanging at the side. The child is reluctant to use the extremity for any purpose. There may be tenderness around the elbow but this is usually difficult to localize, particularly in younger children. Neurovascular deficits are not expected. Radiographs are not necessary (they typically show no evidence of displacement) unless immediate reduction can not be obtained or the history is unclear or suggestive of other injuries. Reduction is usually easily achieved by supinating and flexing the affected elbow, which is cupped in the physician's hand with the physician's thumb over the patient's radial head. An alternate method uses hyperpronation and extension. In most cases a snapping sensation is palpable and audible with reduction. Pain is typically completely relieved over the ensuing 5–10 minutes and full motion and use of the extremity return. Children may be discharged without immobilization after instructing the parents regarding the mechanism of injury and the possibility of home treatment if the subluxation recurs. There should be no long-term effects on the patients; however, they are more likely to have a recurrent nursemaid's elbow.

The radial head ossifies late in adolescence. For this reason, radial head fractures are rare in children. However, the radial neck is susceptible to fractures from indirect trauma, particularly the FOOSH mechanism; these injuries can also occur concomitant with elbow dislocations. Radial neck fractures occur at an average age of 10 years and typically result from a fall on an outstretched, supinated hand.[99] The majority of these fractures are through the relatively weak region of metaphyseal bone; Salter–Harris fractures

are less common. Angulation of < 30° with minimal translocation can be treated in a posterior splint, followed by early motion as pain decreases.[99] Displaced fractures are reduced under general anesthesia, with open reduction usually required in fractures with > 60° of angulation or significant translocation.[100] Attempts at closed reduction are usually not attempted due to the presence of open physes and the high likelihood of fracture to these structures during reduction attempts.

Forearm fractures account for approximately 5% of all pediatric fractures,[101] most in the distal third. As in adults, the majority of forearm fractures result from FOOSH. Patients often present with pain at the fracture site; crepitus and obvious deformity are variable findings. Range of motion should be assessed in all joints of the affected extremity. The neurovascular examination is important. Abrasions or lacerations may be indicative of an open fracture, necessitating further treatment. Standard AP and lateral radiographs should include the surrounding joints as dissipation of forces may result in injuries in these areas as well. Reduction is performed based upon the displacement visible on plain radiographs. In general, the extremity is either pronated or supinated to correlate with the direction of angulation (i.e., extremities with apex volar fragments should be supinated for reduction and those with apex dorsal fractures should be pronated for reduction). Following adequate analgesia and sedation, gentle longitudinal traction is applied to correct shortening and a simultaneous force is applied to the distal fragment in a direction opposite to the displacement. Once reduction is achieved, the extremity is placed in a long arm splint with the elbow flexed to 90° and in neutral rotation. Post-reduction radiographs in the AP and lateral projection should be obtained to ensure adequate reduction in all planes. Surgical reduction is typically reserved for open fractures, those associated with compartment syndrome or other significant soft tissue injuries and those with multiple fractures.

Distal radius fractures are common in the pediatric population; the distal radial metaphysis is the most commonly fractured pediatric bone.[102] Metaphyseal fractures may be incomplete and non-displaced, termed "buckle," or "torus" fracture. The hallmark of the buckle fracture is disruption of one cortex while the opposite side remains intact. Treatment paradigms for this injury have recently changed. Although these fractures have traditionally been immobilized for 3 weeks in a short arm cast, multiple prospective studies have shown quicker return to normal activity and normal range of motion after treatment in a removable short arm splint, with no difference in pain levels or radiographic healing. Based on several studies, discharge in a removable splint is appropriate. "Greenstick" fractures occur when one cortex fails under tension, as compared to compression with a torus fracture. Any volar angulation and dorsal angulation > 10° should be corrected.[103] Reduction is typically carried out under sedation as hematoma blocks are difficult to perform due to the presence of an intact dorsal cortex. Immobilization in a sugar-tong or long arm splint to prevent rotation, with orthopedic follow up in 3–5 days is appropriate. Completely displaced fractures typically overlap in "bayonet apposition" due to muscle pull. These fractures require a hematoma block and sedation or general anesthesia [104] for muscle relaxation to allow hyperextension at the fracture site, allowing for apposition of fracture ends, followed by correction of angulation, and application of a sugar-tong or long arm cast or splint.

The distal radial physis is the most commonly injured physis in the body.[103] Most are Salter–Harris II fractures, and most occur from a fall on a dorsiflexed wrist. These fractures are usually associated with a fracture of the distal ulnar metaphysis or an avulsion of the ulnar styloid. Median nerve injury may occur with significantly displaced physeal fractures.[105] Non-displaced fractures are immobilized in a short arm splint. Displaced fractures are reduced with longitudinal traction and gentle reversal of the angulation, under adequate sedation in order to minimize injury to the physis. The fracture is immobilized in a long-arm or sugar-tong splint; a cast is placed in 2–3 weeks. Recent evidence suggests that a sugar-tong splint provides adequate immobilization in pediatric distal radius fractures, with excellent maintenance of reduction, obviating the need for long arm splinting in these patients.[106]

In summary, any pediatric patient who sustains an injury to the area of the physis and has persistent tenderness and/or swelling but negative radiographs should be presumed to have a Salter–Harris I fracture and placed in a splint. Children with injuries to the lower extremity should be made non-weightbearing as practical. Orthopedic follow up is essential to arrange the subsequent imaging required to make a definitive diagnosis.

Emergency physicians can treat the vast majority of upper extremity trauma in adults and children. However, this should be carefully orchestrated with the orthopedists for optimal results. It is important to adequately and fully examine the extremity, be familiar with common radiographic presentations, and demand expeditious consultation in the ED for those injuries that require operative management or immediate orthopedic specialists.

References

1. Jaeger M, Maier D, Kern W, Sudkamp N. Antibiotics in trauma and orthopedic surgery–a primer of evidence-based recommendations. *Injury* 2006;**37** (Suppl. 2):S74–80.

2. Hovelius L. The natural history of primary anterior dislocation of the shoulder in the young. *J Orthop Sci* 1994;**4**:307–17.

3. Kovacic J, Bergfeld J. Return to play issues in upper extremity injuries. *Clin J Sports Med* 2005;**15** (6):448–52.

4. Simank H, Dauer G, Schneider S, Loew M. Incidence of rotator cuff tears in shoulder dislocations and results of therapy in older patients. *Arch Orthop Trauma Surg* 2006;**126**(4):235–40.

5. Good C, MacGillivary J. Traumatic shoulder dislocation in the adolescent athlete: advances in surgical treatment. *Current Opin Peds* 2005;**17**(1):25–9.

6. Kuhn J. Treating the initial anterior shoulder dislocation–an evidence based-medicine approach. *Sports Med Arthroscopy Rev* 2006;**14**(4):192–8.

7. Emond M, LeSage N, Lavoie A, Rochette L. Clinical factors predicting fractures associated with an anterior shoulder dislocation. *Acad Emerg Med* 2004;**11**(8):853–8.

8. Geusens E, Pans S, Verhulst D, Brys P. The modified axillary view of the shoulder, a painless alternative. *Emerg Radiol* 2006;**12**:227–30.

9. O'Connor DR, Schwarze D, Fragomen AT, et al. Painless reduction of acute anterior shoulder dislocations without anesthesia. *Orthopaedics* 2006;**29** (6):528–32.

10. Perron A, Jones R. Posterior shoulder dislocation; avoiding a missed diagnosis. *Am J Emerg Med* 2000;**18** (2):189–91.

11. McCarty E, Ritchie P, Gill H, McFarland E. Shoulder instability: return to play. *Clin Sports Med* 2004;**23** (3):335–51.

12. Pavlov H, Warren R, Jr. The roetgenographic evaluation of anterior shoulder instability. *Clin Orthop* 1995;**194**:153–8.

13. Itoi E. A new method of immobilization after traumatic anterior dislocation of the shoulder: a cadaveric study. *J Shoulder Elbow Surg* 2003;**12**:413–15.

14. Spencer JE. Treatment of Grade III AC joint injuries: a systemic review. *Clin Ortho and Rel Res* 2007;**455**:38–44.

15. Chernchujit B, Tischer T, Imhoff A. Arthroscopic reconstruction of the AC joint disruption: surgical technique and preliminary results. *Arch Orthop Trauma Surg* 2006;**126**(9):575–81.

16. Stokkeland P, Soreide K, Fjetland L. Acute endovascular repair of right subclavian artery perforation from clavicular fracture after blunt trauma. *J Vasc Intervent Radiology* 2007;**18**(5):689–90.

17. Anderson K, Jensen P, Lauritzen J. Treatment of clavicle fractures. Figure of eight bandages versus a simple sling. *Acta Orthop Scand* 1987;**58**:71–4.

18. Potter J, Jones C, Wild L, Schemitsch E, McKee M. Does delay matter? The restoration of objectively measured shoulder strength and patient oriented outcome after immediate fixation versus delayed reconstruction of displaced midshaft clavicle fractures. *J Shoulder Elbow Surg* 2007;**16**(5):514–18.

19. Throckmorton T, Kuhn J. Fracture of the medial end of the clavicle. *J Shoulder Elbow Surg* 2007;**16**(1):49–54.

20. Owens B, Goss T. The floating shoulder. *J Bone Joint Surg-Br* 2006;**88**-B(11):1419–24.

21. DeFranco M, Patterson B. The Floating Shoulder. *J American Acad Ortho Surg* 2006;**14**(8):499–509.

22. Bengner U, Johnell O, Redlund-Johnell I. Changes in the incidence of fracture of the upper end of the humerus during a 30-year period a study of 2125 fractures. *Clin Orthop and Relat Res.* 1988;**231**:179–82.

23. Palvanen M, Kannus P, Niemi S, et al. Update in the epidemiology of proximal humeral fractures. *Clin Ortho and Rel Res* 2006;**442**:87–92.

24. Hilton M, Yngve DA, Carmichael KD. Proximal humerus fractures sustained during the use of restraints in adolescents. *J Pediatr Orthop* 2006;**26**:50–2.

25. Sperling J, Cuomo F, Hill J, et al. The difficult proximal humerus fracture: tips and techniques to avoid complications and improve results. *Instr Course Lect* 2007;**56**:45–57.

26. Steinmann S, Moran E. Axillary nerve injury: diagnosis and treatment. *J American Acad Ortho Surg* 2001;**9**(5):328–35.

27. Braunstein V, Wiedemann E, Piltz W, et al. The difficult proximal humerus fracture: tips and techniques to avoid complications and improve results. *Instr Course Lect* 2007;**56**:45–57.

28. DeFranco MJ, Brems JJ, Williams GR, Jr., et al. Evaluation and management of valgus impacted four-part proximal humerus fractures. *Clin Ortho and Rel Res* 2006;**442**:109–14.

29. Bahrs C, Lingenfelter E, Fischer F, et al. Mechanism of injury and morphology of the greater tuberosity. *J Shoulder Elbow Surg* 2006;**15**(2):140–7.

30. Fuchtmeier B, May R, Hente R, et al. Operative treatment of greater tuberosity fractures of the humerus-a biomechanical analysis. *Clin Biomech* 2007;**22**(6):652–7.

31. Hewins E, Gofton W, Dubberly J, et al. Innovations in the management of displaced proximal humerus fractures. *J American Acad Ortho Surg* 2007;**15**(1):12–26.

32. Ekholm R, Adami J, Tidermark J, et al. Fractures of the shaft of the humerus: an epidemiological study of 401 fractures. *J Bone Joint Surg-Br* 2006;**88**-B(11):1469–71.

33. Jawa A, McCarty P, Doornberg J, et al. Extra-articular distal-third diaphyseal fractures of the humerus. *J Bone Joint Surg-A* 2006;**88**-A(11):2343–7.

34. DeFranco M, Lawton J. Radial nerve injuries associated with humeral fractures. *J Hand Surg-A* 2006;**31**(4):655–63.

35. Livani B, Belangero WD, Castro de Medeiros R. Fractures of the distal third of the humerus with palsy of the radial nerve. *J Bone Joint Surg-Br* 2006;**88**-B(12):1625–8.

36. Frassica F, Frassica D. Metastatic bone disease of the humerus. *J American Acad Ortho Surg* 2003;**11**(4):282–8.

37. Zehms CT Balsamo L, Dunbar R. Coaptation splinting for humeral shaft fractures in adults and children: a modified method. *Am J Orthopaedics* 2006;**35**(10):452–4.

38. Davies M, Stanley D. A clinically applicable fracture classification for distal humeral fractures. *J Shoulder Elbow Surg* 2006;**15**(5):602–8.

39. Novak V, Baratz M. Anteromedial ecchymosis about the elbow in an adult with a distal humerus fracture. *J Hand Surg-A* 2006;**31**A(5):860–3.

40. Lewicky Y, Sheppard J, Ruth J. The combined olecranon osteotomy, lateral paratricepital sparing, deltoid insertion splitting approach for concomitant distal intra articular and humeral shaft fractures. *J Orthop Trauma* 2007;**21**(2):133–9.

41. Maripuri SN, Debnath UK, Rao P, et al. Simple elbow dislocation among adults: a comparative study of 2 different methods of treatment. *Injury* 2007;**35**(10):452–4.

42. Hickey D, Loebennerg M. Elbow instability. *Bull NYU Hospital Jt Dis* 2006;**64**(3–4):166–71.

43. Buckwalter K, Farber J. Application of multidetector CT in skeletal trauma. *Semin Musculoskelet Radiol* 2004;**8**(2):147–56.

44. Venkatram N, Wurum V, Houshian S. Anterior dislocation of the ulnar-humeral joint in a so-called 'pulled elbow'. *Emerg Med J* 2006;**23**(6):e37.

45. Scheps DM, Hildebrand KA, Boorman RS. Simple dislocations of the elbow: evaluation and treatment. *Hand Clinics* 2004;**20**:389–404.

46. Tashjian R, Katarincic J. Complex elbow instability. *J Am Acad Ortho Surg* 2006;**14**:278–86.

47. Tejwani N, Metha H. Fractures of the radial head and neck: current concepts in management. *J Am Acad Ortho Surg* 2007;**15**(7):380–7.

48. Roidis NT, Papadakis SA, Rigopoulos N, et al. Current concepts and controversies in the management of radial head fractures. *Orthopaedics* 2006;**29** (10):904–16.

49. Jungbluth P, Frangen TM, Arens S, et al. The undiagnosed Essex-Lopresti injury. *J Bone Joint Surg-Br* 2006;**88**-B(12):1629–33.

50. Giannoulis F, Sotereanos D. Galeazzi fractures and dislocations. *Hand Clinics* 2007;**23**(2):153–63.

51. Eathiirajn S, Mugdal C, Jupiter J. Monteggia hand fractures. *Hand Clinics* 2007;**23**(2):165–77.

52. DeCarli P, Boretto JG, Bourgeois WO, et al. Floating dislocated elbow: a variant with articular fracture of the humerus. *J Trauma* 2006;**60**(2):421–2.

53. Akesson T, Herbertsson P, Josefsson PO, et al. Displaced fractures of the neck of the radius in adults. *J Bone Joint Surg-Br* 2006;**88**B(5):642–4.

54. Navali A, Sadigi A. Displaced fracture of the neck of the radius with complete 180 rotation of the radial head during closed reduction. *J Hand Surg-Br* 2006;**31**B(6):689–91.

55. Doornberg JN, van Duijn J, Ring D. Coronoid fracture height in terrible-triad injuries. *J Hand Surg-A* 2006;**31** (5):794–7.

56. Regan W, Morrey B. Fractures of the coronoid process of the ulna. *J Bone Joint Surg-A* 1989;**71**(9):1348–54.

57. Doornberg J, Ring D. Coronoid fracture patterns. *J Hand Surg-A* 2006;**31**A(1):45–52.

58. Ring D. Fractures of the coronoid process of the ulna. *J Hand Surg-A* 2006;**31**(10):1679–89.

59. Sanchez-Sotelo J, O'Driscoll SW, Morrey BF. Medial oblique compression fracture of the coronoid process of the ulna. *J Shoulder Elbow Surg* 2005;**14** (1):60–4.

60. Nork S, Jones C, Henley M. Surgical treatment of olecranon fractures. *Am J Orthopaedics* 2001;**30** (7):577–86.

61. Ikeda M, Fukushima Y, Kobayashi Y, Oka Y. Comminuted fractures of the olecranon. Management by bone graft from the iliac crest and multiple tension-band wiring. *J Bone Joint Surg-Br* 2001;**83**(6):805–8.

62. Monte LV, Vercher MS. Conservative treatment of displaced fractures of the olecranon in the elderly. *Injury* 1999;**30**(2):105–10.

63. LaStayo P, Lee M. The forearm complex: anatomy, biomechanics and clinical considerations. *J Hand Ther* 2006;**19**:137–45.

64. Nijs S, Broos P. Fractures of the distal radius: a contemporary approach. *Acta Chir Belg* 2004; **104**(4):401–12.

65. Newport M. Upper extremity disorders in women. *Clin Ortho and Rel Res* 2000;**372**:85–94.

66. Turner R, Farber K, Athwal G. Complications of distal radius fractures. *Orthop Clin North Am* 2007;**38** (2):217–28.

67. Bienek T, Kusz D, Cleinski L. Peripheral nerve compression neuropathy after fractures of the distal radius. *J Hand Surg-Br* 2006;**31**B:256–60.

68. Mackenney PJ, McQueen MM, Elton R. Prediction of instability in distal radial fractures. *J Bone Joint Surg-A* 2006;**88**A(9):1944–51.

69. Anzarut A, Johnson JA, Rowe BH, et al. Radiologic and patient-reported functional outcomes in an elderly cohort with conservatively treated distal radius fractures. *J Hand Surg-A* 2004;**29**(6):1121–7.

70. Kreder HJ, Agel J, McKee MD, et al. A Randomized, controlled trial of distal radius fractures with metaphyseal displacement but without joint incongruity: closed reduction and casting versus closed reduction, spanning external fixation, and optional percutaneous K-wires. *J Orthop Trauma* 2006;**20** (2):115–21.

71. Hardy P, Gomes N, Chebil M, et al. Wrist arthroscopy and intra-articular fractures of the distal radius in young adults. *Knee Surg Sports Traumatol Arthrosc* 2006;**14**:1225–30.

72. Cunningham P. MR imaging of trauma: elbow and wrist. *Semin Musculoskelet Radiol* 2006;**10**(4):284–92.

73. Vitello W, Gordon D. Obvious radiographic scapholunate dissociation: Xray the other wrist. *Am J Orthopaedics* 2005;**34**(7):347–51.

74. Goldfarb C. Traumatic wrist instability: what's in and what's out? *Instruct Course Lect* 2007;**56**:65–8.

75. Birndorf M, Daley R, Greenwald D. Metacarpal fracture angulation decreases flexor mechanical efficiency in human hands. *Plast Reconst Surg* 1997;**99** (4):1079–83.

76. Bansal R, Craigen M. Fifth metacarpal neck fractures: is followup required? *J Hand Surg-Br* 2007;**32**(1):69–73.

303

77. Statius-Muller M, Poolman R, van Hoogstraten MJ, Steller E. Immediate mobilization gives good results in boxer's fractures with volar angulation up to 70°: a prospective randomized trial comparing immediate mobilization with cast immobilization. *Arch Orthop Trauma Surg* 2003;**123**(10):534–7.

78. Agee J. Treatment principles for proximal and middle phalangeal fractures. *Orthop Clin North Am* 1992;**23**(1):35–40.

79. Freiberg A, Pollard B, MacDonald M, Duncan M. Management of PIP joint injuries. *Hand Clinics* 1995;**22**(3):235–42.

80. Lo I, Richards R. Combined central slip and volar plate injury at the PIP joint. *J Hand Surg-Br* 1995;**20**(3):390–1.

81. Peterson J, Bancroft L. Injuries of the fingers and thumb in the athlete. *Clin Sports Med* 2006;**25**(3):527–42.

82. Wintman B, Fowler J, Baratz M. Traumatic dislocation of the trapezium: case report and review of the literature. *Am J Orthopaedics* 2000;**3**:229–32.

83. Hirata H, Tsujii M, Nakao E. Locking of the MCP joint of the thumb caused by a fracture fragment of the radial condyle of the metacarpal head after dorsal dislocation. *J Hand Surg-Br* 2006;**31**(6):635–6.

84. Heim D. The skier's thumb. *Acta Orthop Belg* 1999;**65**(4):440–6.

85. Morrison W, McCombe D. Digital replantation. *Hand Clinics* 2007;**23**(1):1–12.

86. Rodriguez-Merchan E. Pediatric fractures of the forearm. *Clin Ortho and Rel Res* 2005;**432**:65–72.

87. Mashru R, Herman M, Pizzutillo P. Tibial shaft fractures in children and adolescents. *J Am Acad Ortho Surg* 2005;**13**(5):345–52.

88. Mahan S, May C, Kocher M. Operative management of displaced flexion supracondylar humerus fractures in children. *J Pediatr Orthop* 2007;**27**(5):551–6.

89. Bhatnagar R, Nzegwu NI, Miller NH. Diagnosis and treatment of common fractures in children: femoral shaft fractures and supracondylar humeral fractures. *J Surg Ortho Advances* 2006;**15**(1):1–15.

90. Heras JDL, Duran D. Supracondylar fractures of the humerus in children. *Clin Ortho and Rel Res* 2005;**432**:57–64.

91. Heal J, Bould M, Livingstone J, Blewitt N, Blom A. Reproducibility of the Gartland classification for supracondylar humeral fractures in children. *J Orthop Surg* 2007;**15**(1):12–14.

92. Barton KL, Kaminsky CK, Green DW, et al. Reliability of a modified Gartland classification of supracondylar humerus fractures. *J Pediatr Orthop*. 2001;**21**(1):27–30.

93. Storm S, Williams D. Elbow deformities after fracture. *Hand Clinics* 2006;**22**(1):121–9.

94. Sullivan J. Fractures of the lateral condyle of the humerus. *J Am Acad Ortho Surg* 2006;**14**(1):58–62.

95. Song KS, Kang CH, Min BW, et al. Internal oblique radiographs for diagnosis of nondisplaced or minimally displaced lateral condylar fractures of the humerus in children. *J Bone Joint Surg-A* 2007;**89**:58–63.

96. Mirsky E, Karas E. Lateral condyle fractures in children: evaluation of classification and treatment. *J Orthop Trauma* 1997;**11**(2):117–20.

97. Leet A, Yound C. Medial condyle fractures of the humerus in children. *J Pediatr Orthop* 2002;**22**(1):2–7.

98. Haxhija E, Mayr J. Treatment of medial epicondylar apophyseal avulsion in children. *Oper Orthop Traumatol* 2006;**18**(2):120–34.

99. Waseem M, Devas G. Fell on outstretched hand. *Pediatr Emerg Care* 2006;**22**(9):647–9.

100. Ursei M, Sales de Gauzy J. Surgical treatment of radial neck fractures in children by intramedullary pinning. *Acta Orthop Belg* 2006;**72**(2):131–7.

101. Carmichael K, English C. Outcomes assessment of pediatric both bone forearm fractures treated operatively. *Orthopedics* 2007;**30**(5):379–83.

102. Al-Ansari K, Howard A. Minimally angulated pediatric wrist fractures: is immobilization without manipulation enough? *Can J Emerg Med* 2007;**9**(1):9–15.

103. Rodriguez-Merchan E. Pediatric skeletal trauma: a review and historical perspective. *Clin Ortho and Rel Res* 2005;**432**:8–13.

104. Luhmann JD, Schootman M, Luhmann SJ, et al. A randomized comparison of nitrous oxide plus hematoma block versus ketamine plus midazolam for emergency department forearm fracture reduction in children. *Pediatrics* 2006;**118**:e1078–86.

105. Binfield P, Sott-Minkas A. Median nerve compression associated with displaced Salter–Harris type II distal radius epiphyseal fracture. *Injury* 1998;**29**(2):93–4.

106. Denes A, Goding R, Tamborlane J, Schwartz E. Maintenance of reduction of pediatric distal radius fractures with a sugar-tong splint. *Am J Orthopaedics* 2007;**36**(2):68–70.

Chapter

17

Lower extremity orthopedic trauma

Moira Davenport and Tamara A. Scerpella

Introduction

Due to the length of the lower extremity and the significant forces to which the limb is subjected during weight bearing, fractures and dislocations are relatively common. Care of the lower extremity fracture in the emergency department (ED) is directed at diagnosis, hemorrhage, and pain control, splinting when appropriate, and decision making regarding inpatient treatment (usually operative) or outpatient referral.

Prehospital care

Prehospital care of the extremity injured patient requires basic trauma resuscitation followed by stabilization of the injured extremity. A variety of splinting devices are available to Emergency Medical Services (EMS) providers. However, depending on the circumstances surrounding the injury, the use of formal equipment is not always practical; improvisation is common. Patients often arrive in the ED with extremity injuries stabilized with pillows and tape in addition to prefabricated splints. It is not generally recommended that prehospital providers attempt reduction. Indications for prehospital reduction of fractures include vascular compromise (i.e., cold pulseless extremity distal to fracture site) or potential for or actual hemodynamic compromise such as would be seen with a mid-shaft femur fracture. If an open fracture is identified in the field, the wound should be covered with gauze soaked in sterile saline.

Initial evaluation in the emergency department

Upon arrival in the ED a rapid neurovascular examination is performed. Analgesics are administered as soon as practical in order to maximize patient comfort and allow for an adequate physical examination. Field immobilization may be temporarily taken down for the examination and reapplied during the radiograph process. Radiographs are best taken with the splint off; however, this is not always practical. The presence of a neurovascular deficit requires an expeditious attempt at reduction even prior to radiographs. In the case of an open fracture, the wound should be covered with gauze soaked in sterile saline. While dilute povidone iodine (0.1%–1.0%) is sometimes used and has proponents, generally undiluted povidone iodine (10%) should not be used because of its propensity to cause tissue toxicity. Antibiotics should be administered, preferably a first-generation cephalosporin with an aminoglycoside added for wounds that are > 1–2 cm in size. Penicillin should be added as prophylaxis against *Clostridium* in the case of barnyard injuries or gross contamination.[1–3] The patient's tetanus status should be updated as needed.

Box 17.1   Essentials of the initial evaluation

- Full evaluation of the patient is performed to avoid missing important injuries.
- Analgesics are provided early to allow for patient comfort and full evaluation.
- Radiographs should be performed with splinting taken down (if practical and safe).
- Reductions of obvious dislocations may be performed prior to radiographs with neurovascular deficits or potential for conversion to open fracture.

Hip fractures

Although the hip joint is the articulation formed by the acetabulum and the femoral head, the term "hip fracture" typically refers only to fractures involving the

---

Trauma: A Comprehensive Emergency Medicine Approach, eds. Eric Legome and Lee W. Shockley. Published by Cambridge University Press. © Cambridge University Press 2011.

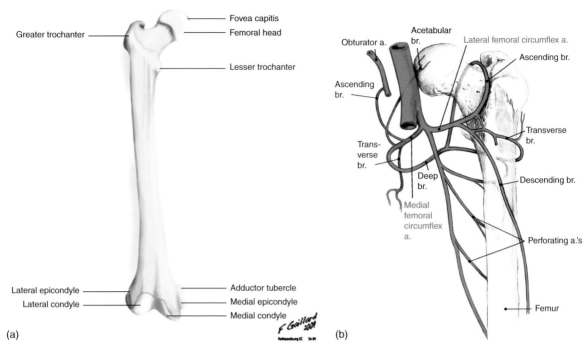

Figure 17.1 (a) Anterior view of the femur. (Courtesy of F. Gaillard, MD.) (b) Arterial supply to the proximal femur. (From Melloni J, Dox I, Melloni H, Melloni B. *Attorney's Reference on Human Anatomy*. Cambridge: Cambridge University Press, 2008.)

proximal femur. The proximal femur is comprised of the femoral head, the femoral neck, the intertrochanteric region (including greater and lesser trochanters), and the subtrochanteric region (Figure 17.1a).

Blood supply to the proximal femur is from the deep femoral artery (profunda branch) that arises from the femoral artery and subsequently divides to form the medial and lateral circumflex arteries. These circumflex branches wrap around the neck of the femur and are the primary arterial supply for the femoral head and neck. The integrity of these arteries figures prominently in the treatment algorithm for hip fractures. Smaller perforating arteries (arising from the profunda branch) provide the vascular supply to the subtrochanteric region of the femur and the femoral shaft (Figure 17.1b).

Innervation to the femur is provided via branches of the lumbar plexus.

Hip fractures are increasingly common in the United States. Current estimates put the annual incidence at 330 000 fractures per year with a marked increase anticipated as the baby boomer generation ages.[4] Although women now sustain fractures at a rate of 3 : 1 relative to men, this ratio is expected to equalize by the year 2025.[5] Several risk factors are associated with hip fracture. Increasing age produces increased risk, largely due to decreasing bone density. Corticosteroid use decreases bone density, thus increasing fracture risk. Intermittent doses of > 30 mg of prednisone, with a cumulative dose > 5 g, increases the risk of hip fracture 3.13-fold. Married individuals are less likely to sustain hip fractures than those who are unmarried. Data regarding the financial status of the patient and the neighborhood in which the patient lives have not been conclusive.[6]

The vast majority of hip fractures occur in the elderly; in the younger population these injuries are the result of high-energy trauma such as a fall from a height or a motor vehicle crash. Elderly patients present to the ED noting hip pain after a fall; between 90 and 95% of hip fractures are due to this mechanism.[4] The intermittent use of corticosteroids also increase a patient's risk of fracture following a relatively minor fall.[7] The emergency physician should attempt to determine if the fall was strictly mechanical or if it was the result of a cardiac or neurologic event. It is particularly important to identify these potential comorbidities, as hip fracture alone increases mortality by 20% in women and 40% in men in the 2 years following fracture.[6,8,9]

Imaging of a suspected hip fracture includes an anteroposterior (AP) pelvis radiograph, allowing assessment of the general condition of the hip joints and providing a standard against which to compare the injured side. Improper technique for this film may result in missed fractures. Ideal positioning requires 5–10° of internal rotation of the legs; prominence of the lesser trochanter indicates slight external rotation. Inadequate films must be repeated. A dedicated AP view of the injured hip may provide additional detail, and should be obtained. A cross-table lateral radiograph completes the evaluation, providing imaging in a second plane. This image is preferred to a frog leg lateral view, which requires difficult, painful positioning and risks fracture displacement. Patients with the presumptive clinical diagnosis of hip fracture, but negative radiographs, should undergo further diagnostic imaging. Magnetic resonance imaging (MRI) is the preferred modality, particularly in those older than 70 years.[10] A computed tomography (CT) scan with narrow cuts may be performed if MRI is not available; however, the small amount of evidence to date suggests that if negative, it is not fully possible to exclude hip fracture.[10–12] When concomitant fractures are present, particularly those that require external fixation in order to achieve hemodynamic stability, a CT scan is the preferred modality if circumstances allow. Orthopedic surgery consultation should be obtained when the fracture is confirmed on radiograph, or earlier in the examination process if neurovascular deficits are identified.

Patients with displaced *femoral neck fractures* typically present with the extremity shortened and externally rotated. Depending upon the age of the injury, ecchymoses may be present at the anatomic area that contacted the ground; this is more likely if the patient is on warfarin or another blood-thinning medication. If neurovascular deficits are detected on initial examination, immediate reduction should be performed through the application of gentle downward traction in line with the long axis of the leg. The leg must be internally rotated to recreate the normal lie of the lower extremity, using the unaffected extremity as a measure of reduction. A pillow is placed between the legs and taped in place to function as a splint and maintain reduction while awaiting radiograph confirmation. If the neurologic exam is unremarkable, the leg should be splinted where it lies with pillows placed beside the leg to minimize further movement. *Avoid range of motion or manipulation of*

Table 17.1 Garden Classification for hip fractures

Type	Description
I	Incomplete or impacted
II	Complete but without displacement
II	Partially displaced
IV	Completely displaced

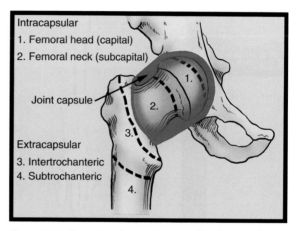

Figure 17.2 Illustration of anatomic types of hip fractures. (From Mandavia D, Newton E, Demetriades D. *Colour Atlas of Emergency Trauma.* Cambridge: Cambridge University Press, 2003.)

the hip that may further injure the vascular supply to the femoral head. Radiographs are obtained for confirmation of the injury.

Fractures of the femoral neck may be described based on anatomic location of the injury. Subcapital fractures occur adjacent to the femoral head, transcervical fractures are through the midportion of the femoral neck and basilar neck fractures are adjacent to the intertrochanteric region (Figure 17.2).

Fractures may also be described according to the Garden Classification (Table 17.1).

All femoral neck fractures require orthopedic consultation; the vast majority undergo operative treatment.[13] Avascular necrosis (AVN) is a complication of these intracapsular fractures; the incidence is related to age, degree of displacement, level of the fracture (subcapital > basilar neck), interval from injury to surgery, and other factors.[14] Non-displaced fractures are typically treated with internal fixation, as are displaced fractures in most patients < 70 years of age; fixation is performed on an urgent basis to lessen the likelihood of AVN.[15] Displaced fractures,

307

Table 17.2 Intertrochanteric fracture description

Part	Description
1 part	Avulsion of the greater or lesser trochanter
2 part	Fracture line through the intertrochanteric region separating the head–neck fragment from the shaft fragment
3 part	Intertrochanteric fracture line and fracture of either greater or lesser trochanter
4 part	Intertrochanteric fracture line and fracture of both greater and lesser trochanters

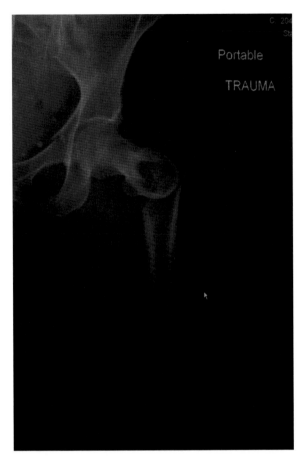

Figure 17.4 Left subtrochanteric hip fracture.

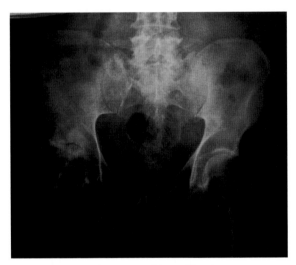

Figure 17.3 Avascular necrosis of femoral head.

particularly Garden IV fractures in the elderly or the infirm, may be treated with hemi-arthroplasty (i.e., replacement of the femoral head with an artificial prothesis). Patients with significant pre-existing degenerative joint disease may, alternatively, be treated with primary total hip arthroplasty (THA) (replacement of the femoral head and the acetabulum.). Basilar neck fractures are physiologically akin to intertrochanteric fractures, and are treated as such (Figure 17.3).

Patients who sustain *intertrochanteric fractures* are typically a decade older than those who sustain femoral neck fractures; they are common in elderly women, probably because of a higher incidence of osteoporosis. The limb presents in a position of extreme shortening and external rotation (greater than that seen with femoral neck fractures). Fractures are typically classified as listed in Table 17.2.

When the main fracture line is at or below the level of the lesser trochanter, the fracture is classified as *subtrochanteric*. Except in the case of non- or minimally displaced one-part fractures, these fractures require reduction and fixation (Figure 17.4).

Box 17.2 Essentials of hip fractures

- Risk factors associated with hip fracture include elderly age, corticosteroid use, and unmarried individuals.
- The vast majority of hip fractures in the elderly are due to a fall.
- Basic imaging of a suspected hip fracture includes an AP pelvis radiograph, a dedicated AP view of the injured, and a cross-table lateral radiograph of the hip.
- A negative radiograph series in a patient with a high clinical suspicion (e.g., severe pain, inability to ambulate) should prompt further imaging.

- MRI is the preferred modality for occult fractures, particularly in those > 70 years.
- Hip fractures may be femoral head fractures, femoral neck fractures, the trochanteric fractures, or subtrochanteric fractures, with multiple subclassifications.
- The majority require an operative procedure.

Hip dislocation

Hip dislocations occur as the result of high-velocity trauma (motor vehicle accidents or falls from a height) or lower-velocity trauma associated with sporting injuries. Dislocations are classified based on the final position of the femoral head relative to the acetabulum: anterior, posterior, or central. Each has a characteristic presentation (Table 17.3). Native (non-prosthetic) hip dislocations are true orthopedic emergencies due to the tenuous nature of the blood supply to the femoral head. Prosthetic hip dislocations are common. They are typically the result of improper positioning of the leg, and may involve little actual force or trauma.

Patients with hip dislocations usually present with severe pain. Range of motion is markedly limited by anatomic distortion and pain; an alert patient resists any attempts at leg movement. A thorough neurovascular examination should be performed, and rapid reduction attempted in the face of any deficit. Sciatic nerve injury is most common, occurring in 10–15% of posterior dislocations. Anterior dislocations place the femoral artery or vein at risk. An AP pelvis and a cross-table lateral radiograph of the hip should be obtained as soon as possible. Comparison of the involved hip to the normal hip allows detection of subtle dislocations. In cases of multiple trauma, particularly when an ipsilateral femur fracture is present, hip dislocation may **not** be obvious on clinical examination. A high index of suspicion, and examination of the joint above and below the site of injury, will help identify a hip dislocation in these cases. Reduction is performed as soon as possible after the completion of radiographs. Prolonged dislocation increases the risk of avascular necrosis that occurs from disruption of the blood supply to the femoral head. In addition, prolonged dislocation significantly increases the extent of muscle spasm, further complicating reduction.

Closed reduction is usually possible in the ED using procedural sedation. Once reduction is achieved, the leg is splinted with the hip in neutral

Table 17.3 Types of hip dislocation

Dislocation	Mechanism	Presentation
Anterior	Occur when the hip is flexed and externally rotated	The degree of external rotation dictates the ultimate lie of the femoral head: antero-inferiorly in the obturator foramen or antero-superiorly over the pubic ramus. An antero-inferior dislocation results in a limb position of flexion, abduction, and external rotation. Patients with an antero-superior dislocation present with shortening and severe external rotation of the limb, similar to the presentation of a femoral neck fracture
Posterior	A posteriorly directed force applied to a flexed knee ("dashboard injury") associated with vehicular trauma. Lower energy injury commonly occurs when forces are transmitted across an extended knee along the femoral shaft with the hip in a position of flexion, adduction, and internal rotation	Present with the affected extremity shortened and internally rotated
Central	Occur in conjunction with acetabular fracture, and result in	The significant forces required to produce this injury may result

Table 17.3 *(cont.)*

Dislocation	Mechanism	Presentation
	intrapelvic dislocation of the femoral head	in concomitant life-threatening intra-abdominal injuries. Leg is shortened. Other findings depend on penetration into pelvis

position; this can be done with a formal splint or with a pillow taped between the legs (with the hips extended). A post-reduction neurovascular examination is performed, and radiographs are obtained to confirm reduction. Anteroposterior pelvis, cross-table lateral, and Judet views (45° internal/external rotation) are obtained to confirm reduction and evaluate for associated fracture. If fracture is suspected, or a reduction cannot be obtained, a CT scan provides further diagnostic assistance. Patients with uncomplicated dislocations can be discharged with instructions for non-weightbearing ambulation and orthopedic follow up. Orthopedic consultation in the ED is required for cases with neurovascular involvement, where closed reduction is not successful, or in the event of associated fracture. In such cases, open reduction may be necessary to remove interposed soft tissue or bony fragments and/or to perform internal fixation.

Posterior dislocations account for 90% of all hip dislocations. Closed reduction is facilitated by placement of the stretcher mattress on the floor, maximizing physician positioning and safety. An assistant stabilizes the patient's pelvis while the physician performing the reduction provides gentle traction in line with the long axis of the femur. Steady traction may be required to overcome muscle spasm. After the femoral head has been disengaged from behind the acetabulum, gentle flexion of the hip, with continued traction, allows relocation of the femoral head. Slight internal and external rotation may also assist with femoral head relocation (Figure 17.5).

Anterior hip dislocations: An anterior dislocation is reduced in a similar fashion to that described above for posterior dislocation. Longitudinal traction to overcome muscle spasm, accentuation of the deformity to disengage the femoral head and repositioning of the limb usually result in a successful reduction.

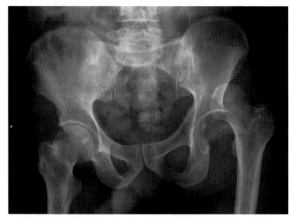

Figure 17.5 Posterior hip dislocation.

Central dislocations: Closed reduction of a central dislocation is not recommended in the ED, as significant vascular injury is usually present, necessitating angiographic or operative intervention. Orthopedic and general or trauma surgery consultation must be obtained immediately to manage the dislocation and any concomitant pelvic ring injuries.

Dislocation of a prosthetic hip may occur from a low-energy fall or with simple position change, such as flexion and adduction associated with crossing of the legs in a seated position. Anterior dislocations are much less common than posterior. Both types of dislocation are usually reducible with procedural sedation; although general anesthesia may be necessary if the dislocation time is prolonged. Reduction maneuvers are similar as for native dislocations. Irreducible dislocations are typically due to displacement of the plastic acetabular liner; these require open reduction. Most patients can be discharged from the ED following reduction of the prosthetic hip, with instructions for positioning precautions and orthopaedic follow up. A markedly unstable prosthetic hip requires admission of the patient for surgical revision.

Subtrochanteric and midshaft femur fractures typically result from significant blunt force injury, and are most commonly the result of vehicular trauma or a fall from a height. Femur fractures have also been reported following prolonged athletic activity, particularly marathon running.[16] Patients with femur fractures present with significant pain at the site of the fracture and variable amounts of edema, ecchymosis, crepitance, spasm, and deformity. Displaced or comminuted fractures can result in significant blood loss into the thigh. Patients with a neurovascular deficit or with signs of hypovolemic

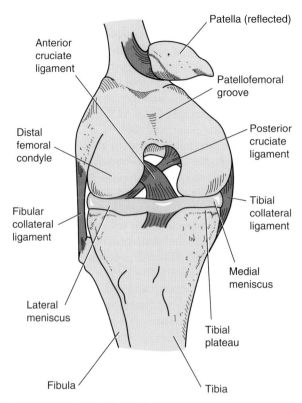

Anterior cruciate ligament

Patella (reflected)

Patellofemoral groove

Distal femoral condyle

Posterior cruciate ligament

Fibular collateral ligament

Tibial collateral ligament

Medial meniscus

Lateral meniscus

Tibial plateau

Fibula

Tibia

Figure 17.6 Anterior view of knee.

shock are treated with immediate reduction of the fracture, utilizing manual traction, a Hare® traction splint, or external fixation. Initial radiographic evaluation includes AP and lateral views of the femur. Given the significant trauma required to produce a femur fracture, both pelvic and knee series should be obtained to rule out injury to these joints. Orthopedic consultation is obtained in the ED, as definitive fixation is performed on a semi-urgent basis for isolated fractures in stable patients, and on an urgent basis in the multiply injured or hemodynamically unstable patient.

Knee injuries

The distal femur, proximal tibia, and patella comprise the knee joint; it is subdivided into three compartments: the medial (medial femoral condyle-medial tibial plateau articulation); lateral (lateral femoral condyle-lateral tibial plateau articulation), and patellofemoral compartments. Four ligaments stabilize the tibio-femoral articulation. The anterior and posterior cruciate ligaments (ACL and PCL) prevent anterior and posterior displacement of the tibia on the femur,

respectively, while the medial and lateral collateral ligaments (MCL and LCL) prevent valgus and varus angulation, respectively. The posterolateral corner of the knee contributes to varus and rotatory stability of the knee; it is commonly injured in conjunction with ACL and/or PCL tears. This complex region is comprised of three distinct tissue layers; the important deep layer includes the popliteus, the popliteofibular ligament, the LCL, the arcuate ligament and the posterolateral capsule. The patellofemoral joint is stabilized by the medial and lateral retinaculum and by the medial patellofemoral ligament. The medial and lateral menisci are "C"-shaped cartilaginous structures that lie within the tibio-femoral articulation and provide stability, and shock absorption. The popliteal artery and tibial nerve are tethered to the distal femur by the adductor magnus muscle, predisposing them to injury (Figure 17.6).

Patients who have sustained trauma to the knee may present with joint pain, effusion or hemarthrosis, and decreased range of motion. A careful history, elucidating the mechanism, may help predict type and extent of injury. Key historical points include the position of the knee at the time of injury and the direction of force(s) applied (i.e., varus force or force to the medial side of the knee or valgus force, or force to the lateral aspect of the knee). Further considerations include the ability to bear weight, the presence of locking or giving way, and the history of prior knee injury.

Knee injuries are frequently associated with effusions, which may limit range of motion; small effusions limit flexion, while larger effusions limit both flexion and extension. Arthrocentesis may be considered in cases of large effusions that produce significant pain and limit the examination. Because effusions may result from the accumulation of synovial fluid, inflammatory cells, or blood (hemarthrosis), aspiration is both diagnostic and therapeutic. Hemarthroses occur most commonly with ACL tears, patellar dislocations, extensor mechanism (quadriceps/patellar tendon) ruptures, and intra-articular fractures. Visible deformity in the absence of crepitance is typically due to dislocation of the patella or the knee (tibiofemoral joint). Where crepitance is noted on examination, fracture must be suspected, and further physical examination avoided until radiographs are obtained. Initial radiographs include AP and lateral views (Figure 17.7). Specialized views of the patella (sunrise or Merchant's view) may be helpful in cases of patellofemoral injury.

311

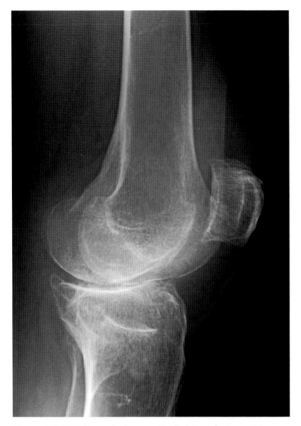

Figure 17.7 Radiograph shows a tibial plateau fracture with associated layered lipohemarthrosis.

Knee stability is assessed in all four planes; the uninjured knee is used as a baseline, as there is considerable variability in joint laxity between patients. The Lachman test assesses anterior displacement of the tibia in relation to the femur at 15–20° of knee flexion; it is the most sensitive test for diagnosing ACL injury (Figure 17.8). An ACL injury will lack a definite stopping point, and seem "soft" compared to the opposite extremity. Injury to the PCL is most effectively detected using the posterior drawer test, whereby a posterior force is applied to the proximal tibia with the knee flexed to 90°, assessing posterior translation of the tibia in relation to the femur (Figure 17.9). The external recurvatum test is used to identify potential injury to the posterolateral corner of the knee (Figure 17.10). This test is performed by lifting the supine patient's leg at the foot or ankle, allowing the knee to fully extend and maintaining neutral rotation at the hip.[17] A varus deformity (bowleg appearance) is indicative of posterolateral injury. Because these injuries are commonly associated with cruciate ligament injury; AP stability must be carefully evaluated. When concomitant cruciate and posterolateral injury are identified, suspicion for a spontaneously reduced knee dislocation must be high. A careful neurovascular exam, to detect subtle injury, is paramount. Evaluation should proceed as described for knee dislocations.

Figure 17.8 Lachman test.

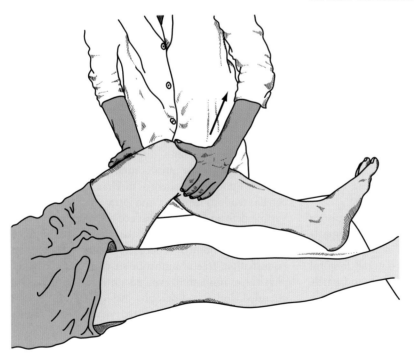

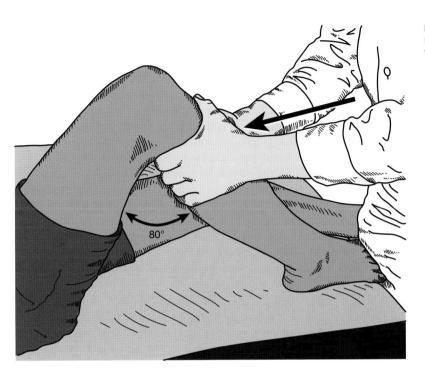

Figure 17.9 Posterior drawer test. Posterior force is applied to the proximal tibia with the knee flexed to 90°.

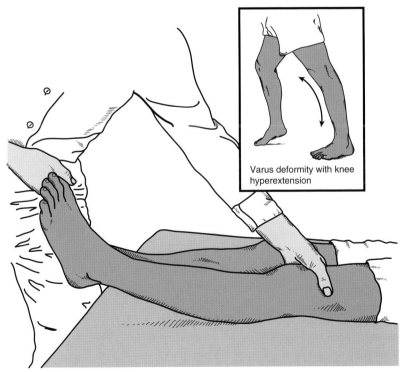

Figure 17.10 External recurvatum test.

Varus deformity with knee hyperextension

If meniscal injury is suspected, a McMurray test is performed. With the patient supine, the examiner lifts the affected extremity off the stretcher, flexing the knee to 90°. The examiner supports the flexed knee with one hand, placing his or her thumb on the medial or lateral joint line and the fingers on the other joint line. The examiner's other hand grasps the patient's foot or ankle and applies a rotational force across the knee. Simultaneous application of a varus or valgus force compresses the medial or lateral joint line, respectively, catching a torn meniscal fragment between the tibia and femur. This test is positive if a palpable or audible pop occurs when the meniscus disengages from the joint space as the knee is extended from the flexed position. In many cases, recreation of the patient's symptoms occurs without a pop; although this is not considered a true positive, it is a noteworthy finding that is frequently indicative of a meniscus tear. This maneuver may be difficult to tolerate in the acute

Box 17.4 Common knee tests for stability

Test	Use
Lachman test	Assesses anterior displacement of the tibia in relation to the femur at 15–20° of knee flexion; it is the most sensitive test for diagnosing ACL injury.
McMurray test	A rotational force is placed across the flexed knee with concomitant varus or valgus force. Assesses for meniscal tear.
Varus and valgus stress test	These maneuvers are performed with the knee unflexed and at 30° of flexion. They assess the medial and lateral collateral ligaments. Instability at extension also suggests cruciate instability.
Posterior Drawer Test	A posterior force is applied to the proximal tibia with the knee flexed to 90°, assessing posterior translation of the tibia in relation to the femur to evaluate PCL injury.
External recurvatum test	The extended leg is lifted observed for varus or valgus deformity. A varus deformity is used to identify potential injury to the posterolateral corner of the knee.

setting and is not helpful in the presence of concomitant patellofemoral or multiple ligament injuries.

Patellar dislocation occurs following a direct blow to the medial aspect of the patella or as the result of a valgus or external rotation force applied to a semi-flexed knee while the foot is fixed. Patients with patellar dislocations present with the knee flexed and the patella dislocated laterally. Some experts recommend pre-reduction radiographs (AP, lateral, and sunrise views) for medicolegal reasons to document the absence of fracture prior to the reduction attempt. There is no clear evidence that this is medicolegally necessary. Reduction is obtained by slowly extending the knee while exerting a medially directed force on the lateral aspect of the patella. Analgesia and sedation may be required. Injection for local analgesia is reasonable, however, it may interfere with the interpretation of an MRI which is performed in the following 1–2 weeks due to difficulty discerning between physiologic and non-physiologic effusion. A knee immobilizer is applied following reduction, and post-reduction AP and lateral films are obtained to ensure anatomic reduction and rule out fractures associated with the reduction. The extensor mechanism must be examined to determine its integrity; the quadriceps and patellar tendons should be palpably intact and the patient should be capable of full active knee extension. Orthopedic consultation must be obtained in the rare case where reduction is unsuccessful or in the case of fracture–dislocation. Patients with uncomplicated dislocations may be discharged from the ED with analgesics, instructions for full-time use of the knee immobilizer, and orthopedic follow up within 1–2 weeks.

Patellar fracture usually results from a fall onto a flexed knee, or from vehicular trauma (dashboard injury). Patients present with a knee effusion and ecchymosis. A palpable defect may be appreciated when fragments are displaced. The neurovascular examination is usually unremarkable. The examiner must be cautioned not to interpret inability to perform a straight leg raise as a neurovascular deficit as it is due to loss of continuity of the extensor mechanism. Anteroposterior, lateral, and patellar radiographs identify the fracture (Figure 17.11). Orthopedic consultation should be obtained for patients with displaced fractures or for those who are unable to perform a straight leg raise; operative fixation may be required, and is typically performed within 24–48 hours. All other patients can be discharged from the ED with a

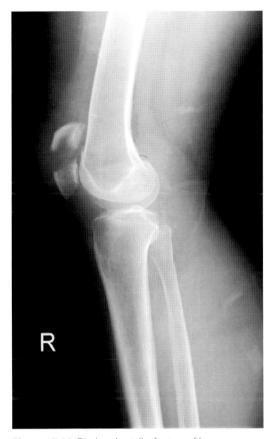

Figure 17.11 Displaced patellar fracture of knee.

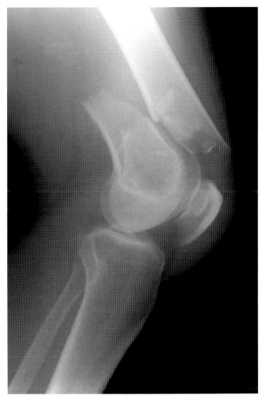

Figure 17.12 Displaced supracondylar fracture of the femur. (Courtesy of Mark Bernstein, MD.)

knee immobilizer, crutches, and orthopedic follow up within 7–10 days of the injury.

Supracondylar and intercondylar fractures of the distal femur generally are seen with two common mechanisms: direct trauma to a flexed knee, often seen in young adults (high energy) and from axial loading in combination with rotational or varus/valgus force, more common in the elderly (low energy). Fractures are classified as extra-articular, unicondylar or bicondylar with further subdivisions based upon degree of comminution and plane of the fracture. Evaluation of the extremity includes neurovascular examination. Due to tethering of the popliteal artery ~10 cm proximal to the joint at Hunter's canal, vascular injury must be suspected in association with a supracondylar fracture. Examination of the soft tissues follows, with particular attention paid to differentiating abrasions and puncture wounds from open fractures. Initial radiographs include AP and lateral views of the distal femur, as well as the hip and knee (Figure 17.12). Orthopedic consultation is optimal in the ED for

evaluation and formulation of a treatment plan; displaced fractures require surgical stabilization. Non-displaced or impacted fractures, fractures in severely osteopenic bone (precluding stable fixation) and fractures in patients with significant underlying comorbidities, may be treated non-operatively in a knee immobilizer with conversion to a fracture brace when swelling has decreased.

Tibial plateau fractures may occur when varus (medial) or valgus (lateral) forces are applied to the knee. Low-energy injuries result from a minor fall, while high energy injuries are the result of a major fall or vehicular trauma. Patients with these injuries typically present with hemarthrosis and tenderness to palpation over the affected joint line, as well as ecchymosis and crepitance. Lateral plateau fractures occur most frequently, however medial plateau and bicondylar fractures are not uncommon. If the initial AP and lateral radiographs are non-diagnostic but suspicion is high for a plateau fracture, additional imaging should be obtained. Internal and external oblique films may identify the fracture. A cross-table

315

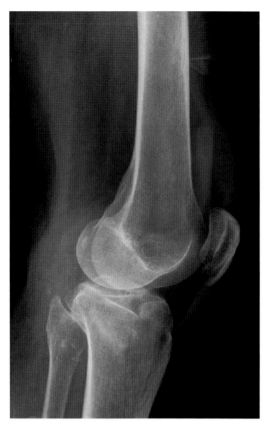

Figure 17.13 Depressed tibial plateau fracture that will require operative treatment. (Courtesy of Mark Bernstein, MD.)

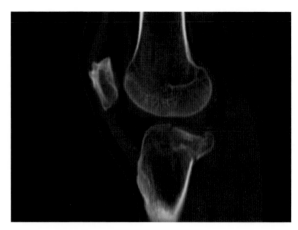

Figure 17.14 Computed tomography (CT) of tibial plateau fracture. (Courtesy of Mark Bernstein, MD.)

lateral view, performed with the knee fully extended (as compared to the traditional lateral in which the knee is flexed 15°), may demonstrate a lipohemarthrosis, (distinct layering of fat, blood, and synovial fluid) pathognomonic of a tibial plateau fracture. It is not uncommon to perform arthrocentesis on a traumatic knee effusion to relieve pressure and pain. Occasionally the aspirate will contain blood and fat globules. This should be considered diagnostic of a periarticular fracture, most likely a tibial plateau. Where possible, CT scanning with 1–2 mm windows is the imaging modality of choice. The CT scan is also crucial in formation of a treatment plan, as tibial plateau fractures with > 2–3 mm of displacement require operative treatment (Figures 17.13 and 17.14). Tibial plateau fractures may be associated with collateral ligament injury on the side opposite the fracture. Plateau fractures may also occur in conjunction with combined ligament injuries to the knee or with knee dislocation, and care must be taken to rule out these more serious injury combinations by gentle examination of the collateral ligaments. Orthopedic consultation should be obtained in the ED for determination of the treatment plan. Grossly unstable, or open fractures may be stabilized with a spanning external fixator, or treated with immediate internal fixation. Most fractures are treated semi-electively, with internal fixation several days post-injury, when soft tissue swelling has decreased. Thus, patients with relatively stable fracture patterns are often discharged from the ED with a knee immobilizer or hinged knee brace, crutches for non-weightbearing ambulation, and orthopedic follow up in 5–7 days.

Tibial spine fractures are avulsion fractures that occur when an axial load is applied to a slightly flexed knee, the same mechanism that usually produces an ACL tear. Radiographic findings may be subtle; signs of ACL laxity and large hemarthrosis on physical examination should heighten physician suspicion for this injury. Truly non-displaced fractures (Type I) may be treated with a knee immobilizer and orthopedic follow up in 3–5 days. Hinged (Type II) or displaced (Type III) fractures require orthopedic consultation in the ED. The former may be reducible by closed methods; if this fails, surgical reduction and fixation are required. All Type III fractures require surgical treatment (Figure 17.15).

Knee dislocation involves disruption of at least three of the four major ligaments of the knee (ACL, PCL, LCL, and MCL) and subsequent joint dislocation, thus constituting a true orthopedic emergency.[18] These injuries may occur following high velocity trauma (vehicular trauma or fall from a height) or sporting injury. Less commonly, knee dislocation occurs in

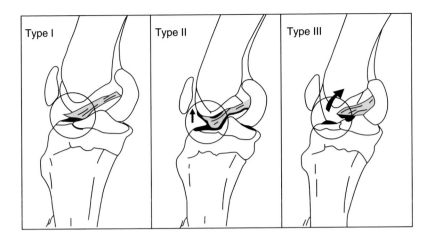

Figure 17.15 Classification of tibial spine avulsion. (Courtesy of Mark Bernstein, MD.)

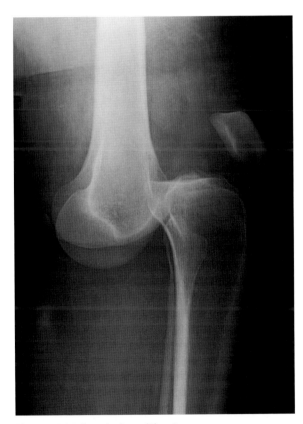

Figure 17.16 Posterior knee dislocation.

an obese individual following minor trauma, such as stepping off a curb.[19] Knee dislocations are described by the position of the tibia relative to the femur: anterior, posterior, medial, lateral, and rotary. Posterior dislocation is most common (Figure 17.16). A newer classification system is based upon the associated ligament injuries and fractures. This method is now preferred, as spontaneously reduced knees are difficult to classify with the former system.

Presentation includes severe pain, deformity (in cases where the joint is still dislocated), marked laxity (post-reduction), swelling, and ecchymosis. Although a hemarthrosis is common with this injury, disruption of the joint capsule may allow dissipation of fluid into the leg, preventing formation of a detectable effusion. Similarly, capsular disruption often allows spontaneous reduction of the dislocated knee, initially masking the severity and extent of the patient's injury. Thus, in cases of marked laxity, the ED physician must have a high index of suspicion that a dislocation has occurred. Ligamentous examination may confirm this suspicion. Failure to diagnose a knee dislocation may be devastating, as vascular injury is seen in approximately 20% of these injuries and may lead to a compartment syndrome. Orthopedic consultation should be obtained expeditiously as operative fixation may be emergently indicated. While there is not absolute standard, prudence would strongly suggest that even low-energy trauma injuries should be admitted for at least overnight observation.

Initial evaluation must include neurovascular examination; deficits require immediate reduction of a dislocated knee. In the absence of neurovascular injury, AP and lateral radiographs are rapidly obtained to assess for associated fractures. If unable to obtain radiograph in a reasonable time frame, e.g., under 15 minutes, attempted reduction is reasonable. The Segond fracture is a capsular avulsion of the lateral tibial plateau; it is pathognomonic for ACL disruption, and is frequently present with a knee dislocation. Due to the associated capsular disruption, most dislocations are easily reduced without procedural sedation; analgesia or local anesthesia, i.e., joint injection, may be warranted. This procedure should be performed as quickly as feasible; dislocation time > 6 hours significantly increases the likelihood of neurovascular compromise. Reduction is accomplished through the application of gentle longitudinal traction to the lower leg. Force is then applied at the proximal tibia in the direction opposite of the dislocation, while an assistant stabilizes the femur. Angular, translational, and rotational displacements must all be corrected for proper reduction. The reduced knee is immobilized in a hinged knee brace locked at 15–20° of flexion. If no hinged brace is available, a posterior leg splint should be applied with the knee in 20 degrees of flexion. Care should be taken to adequately pad the bony prominences (especially at the proximal fibula). On occasion, a button-hole deformity occurs, with the medial femoral condyle protruding through the capsule, locking the dislocation and necessitating open reduction. This deformity is most commonly seen with posterolateral dislocations.

Appropriate post-reduction evaluation of the dislocated knee is crucial. The detection of vascular injury is of paramount importance in preventing morbidity from this injury. Popliteal artery injury is identified in 9–40% of knee dislocations, and requires immediate consultation with a vascular surgeon.[20] Although in prior years angiography was performed routinely following knee dislocation, this test is now reserved for patients with absent pulses or an abnormal ankle–brachial index (ABI).[21] Multiple studies have shown that patients with a normal neurovascular examination immediately pre- and post-reduction and an ABI > 0.9 do not require emergent angiography.[22] In fact, a pre-reduction ABI < 0.9 has been shown to have a positive predictive value of 100% for vascular injuries requiring surgical exploration and repair. While no absolute consensus exists, the authors recommend that patients with normal vascular examinations should be admitted for at least 24 hours of observation with frequent (every 2–3 hours) neurovascular checks. Any change in the vascular exam is an indication for immediate angiography.

Peroneal nerve injury is also associated with approximately 25% of knee dislocations.[20] This injury produces sensory deficits over the lateral aspect of the leg, dorsum of the foot, or first web space. Motor deficits may include weakness of the extensor hallucis

longus, anterior tibialis, and peroneal tendons, producing loss of great toe extension, foot drop, and weakness of ankle eversion, respectively. Patients with a suspected peroneal nerve injury should have the foot splinted in 90° flexion at the ankle to reduce stretch to the nerve and avoid contracture. Compartment syndrome must also be considered in the ED and throughout the period of observation. It is more likely to occur in cases where dislocation time is prolonged, or where there is complete capsular rupture, resulting in extravasation of blood and synovial fluid into the lower leg. If undetected, elevation of compartment pressure will result in nerve and muscle death.

Most orthopedic surgeons recommend a staged repair and reconstruction of the ligamentous and capsular injuries. Posterolateral ligament injuries are usually repaired within 10–14 days of the injury, typically in conjunction with PCL reconstruction. Any ACL reconstruction can be delayed until the effusion resolves and range of motion approaches normal. In cases requiring vascular repair or those with marked instability of the knee, an external fixator may be applied to provide immediate, temporary stabilization.

Box 17.5 Essentials of knee dislocations

- Knee dislocation involves disruption of at least three of the four major ligaments of the knee (ACL, PCL, LCL, and MCL) and subsequent joint dislocation.

- Hemarthrosis is common but disruption of the joint capsule may allow dissipation of fluid into the leg, preventing a detectable effusion. Capsular disruption often allows spontaneous reduction of the dislocated knee, masking the severity of the patient's injury.

- In cases of marked laxity, the ED physician must have a high index of suspicion that a dislocation has occurred. Ligamentous examination may confirm this suspicion. Failure to diagnose a knee dislocation may be devastating, as vascular injury is seen in approximately 9%–40% of these.

- Popliteal artery injury is identified in 9%–40% of knee dislocations, and requires immediate vascular surgical consultation.

- Angiography had been performed routinely following knee dislocation in prior years, this test is now reserved for patients with absent/abnormal pulses or an abnormal ankle–brachial index (ABI).

Isolated ligament injuries: The MCL is the most commonly injured knee ligament. Disruption typically occurs when a valgus force is applied to the knee, either by direct blow, or by indirect force such as valgus stress on a planted foot. Greater force produces greater injury, ranging from Grade I (stretch), to Grade II (partial rupture), to Grade III (complete rupture). Although Grade III injury typically includes a small effusion, Grade I and II injuries may present without effusion. Ecchymosis may be present over the disrupted ligament as well as over the location where the force was applied (coup–contracoup injuries). Range of motion is minimally affected. Tenderness is present at the site of ligament disruption, which may be within the ligament or at the femoral or tibial insertions. Assuming a normal neurovascular examination and normal radiographs, patients may be safely discharged in a hinged knee brace or knee immobilizer with instructions for orthopedic follow up in 7–10 days.

Isolated *LCL injuries* are uncommon. The most common mechanism for such an injury involves manual application of a varus force to the knee as may occur in a wrestling match. Usually, an LCL tear is found in association with either ACL or PCL tear, representing a multi-ligament injury. Posterolateral soft tissue injury may occur in association with an LCL tear.[23] Care should be taken to examine for the presence of these other ligamentous injuries, as the combination is more serious and requires orthopedic evaluation for consideration of surgical reconstruction. The patient can be safely discharged in a knee immobilizer or hinged knee brace with crutches for non-weight bearing ambulation and orthopedic follow up in 7–10 days.

Anterior cruciate ligament tears occur most commonly during athletic participation, but may also result from a misstep or jump. Patients frequently report hearing or feeling a "pop" at the time of injury. A mild to moderate effusion typically develops over the first few hours post-injury; ecchymosis is rare. Weightbearing is often possible immediately after the injury, but becomes more difficult as the effusion accumulates. Patients with ACL tears may be safely discharged in a hinged knee brace or knee immobilizer. If full range of motion (ROM) (particularly extension) is blocked, a displaced meniscal tear may be present and weight-bearing must be avoided. It is particularly important that patients with ACL tears receive orthopedic follow up; early referral to physical therapy is required to maximize range of motion, particularly extension,

Table 17.4 Immobilization vs. hinged knee brace

Immobilization	Hinged knee brace
Non-displaced patellar fracture	ACL/PCL injury
Patellar dislocation	LCL/MCL injury
Non-displaced tibial plateau fracture	Meniscal tear

before reconstruction is carried out. These patients should be discharged with instructions to perform heel props (i.e., place heel on rolled towel, when thigh is elevated off surface, allow leg to relax) and basic quadriceps contraction exercises to initiate this process.

Isolated PCL injuries are relatively rare. These occur with hyperextension of the knee or following a fall on the flexed knee. Because the PCL is extracapsular, these injuries typically present without a knee effusion. A careful examination must be made in order to rule out other ligamentous injury, particularly posterolateral corner injuries.[24] Patients with PCL tears are usually discharged from the ED in a hinged knee brace or knee immobolizer, with orthopedic follow up in 7–10 days.

Patients with suspected posterolateral corner disruptions merit early orthopedic consultation. Recent studies have demonstrated significantly reduced morbidity and higher functioning when repair and reconstruction of the posterolateral corner is performed within 10 days. Thus, a heightened suspicion for this injury will allow the diagnosis to be made and orthopedic consultation to be sought in the ED. The external recurvatum test can easily detect posterolateral corner injuries. The patient should be supine on the stretcher with both knees extended. The examiner lifts both legs off the stretcher, holding the patient's extremities by the toes. If the affected extremity has a varus deformity while it is being lifted, the examiner should suspect posterolateral corner injury.

Table 17.4 summarizes the indications for knee immobilization and hinged knee braces. These are optimal uses. If a knee brace is unavailable, immobilization may be used temporarily for all.

Lower leg fractures

The lower leg is composed of two bones, the tibia and the fibula. The tibia articulates proximally with the femoral condyles and distally with the talus, at the tibial plafond, to form the ankle joint. The fibula

Table 17.5 Compartments of the lower extremity

Compartment	Components	Function
Anterior	Tibialis anterior muscle	Foot dorsiflexion
	Extensor hallicus longus	Toe dorsiflexion
	Anterior tibial artery	Sensation to the first web space
	Deep peroneal nerve	
Lateral	Peroneus longus	Foot eversion
	Peroneus brevis	Sensation to the dorsum of the foot (lateral aspect)
	Superficial peroneal nerve	
Superficial posterior	Gastrocnemius	Foot plantar flexion
	Plantaris	Sensation to the lateral heel
	Soleus	
	Sural nerve	
Deep posterior	Tibialis posterior	Toe plantar flexion
	Flexor hallicus longus	Sensation to plantar surface of foot
	Tibial nerve	

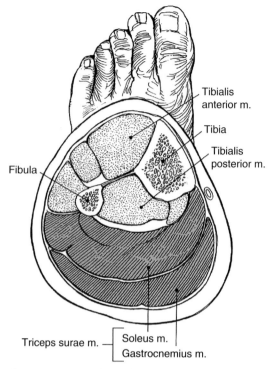

Figure 17.17 Musculature of lower extremity. (From Melloni J, Dox I, Melloni H, Melloni B. *Attorney's Reference on Human Anatomy.* Cambridge: Cambridge University Press, 2008.)

articulates proximally with the tibia at the proximal tibio-fibular joint. Distally, the fibula forms the lateral portion of the ankle joint, and articulates with the distal tibia via the syndesmosis. The tibia and fibula are connected along the length of their shafts via the interosseous membrane and distally via the syndesmotic ligaments. The tibia is the larger of the two bones and is responsible for the majority of weightbearing (80%). The fibula lies posterolateral to the tibia and is much narrower than the tibia (Figure 17.17). Muscle and neurovascular structures in the lower leg travel in four fascial compartments; these compartments and their key components are listed in Table 17.5.

The presentation of patients with lower leg fractures is predicated on the mechanism of injury. Low-energy twisting injuries typically result in spiral fractures; such fractures may have little associated displacement, but result in edema and ecchymosis at the fracture site. Direct trauma results in discrete fracture lines; higher velocity injuries may present with skin tenting and open fracture. The physical exam must include an assessment of soft tissue damage concentrating on open vs. closed, and a careful neurovascular examination. This assessment should be performed early in the evaluation, as significant neurovascular disruption or extensive crush injury may alter the treatment algorithm, necessitating amputation rather than limb salvage. If no neurovascular deficits are detected, the affected leg may be splinted for comfort while awaiting radiographs (AP and lateral views). The presence of any neurovascular insult or tenting of the skin should prompt expeditious attempts at reduction prior to radiographs. With an assistant stabilizing the leg proximal to the fracture, either at the tibia or the knee, the physician applies longitudinal traction to the distal extremity, correcting angular and rotational deformities.

Orthopedic consultation should be obtained for all tibial fracture patients; the consult should be prompt when an open fracture or neurovascular injury is present. Open fractures have high infection rates and require operative debridement and washout before definitive fixation is performed.[25,26] These fractures may be stabilized intra-operatively by internal or external fixation, depending upon fracture pattern and degree of contamination. Early stabilization is paramount in the management of neurovascular injuries; operative treatment may include exploration of the neurovascular bundle. Vascular injuries producing ischemia require revascularization within 6 hours, necessitating rapid evaluation and progression through the ED. Closed fractures with significant displacement are also typically managed with operative fixation. Non-displaced fractures are treated with cast immobilization, while minimally displaced fractures may be managed via open or closed means.

Increasing compartment pressures may occur in association with tibia fracture, particularly those with significant fracture displacement or associated crush injury. This entity presents a true emergency. Fascial compartments in the lower leg cannot accommodate expanding volume due to bleeding or swelling. Increased pressure within the fascial compartment results; neurologic and muscular damage occurs rapidly. A high index of suspicion is key to the prevention of this potentially devastating sequelae of tibia fracture. Increasing pain, or pain greater than expected for the injury, is the first sign of compartment syndrome in an alert patient. Pain with passive movement of the toes should prompt further testing for elevated compartment pressures. Other signs of compartment syndrome include tense compartments, pallor, paresthesias, and pulselessness. By the time these findings develop, pressures are significantly elevated, and, when untreated, permanent neurologic and muscular damage occur. An even higher index of suspicion must be maintained when a trauma patient is not alert; tense compartments must be measured, and pre-emptive fasciotomies are often performed at the time of operative fracture fixation. Measurement of compartment pressure is performed with a manometer, and, when elevated, fasciotomy is performed rapidly. A two-incision technique is typically employed in order to adequately decompress all four compartments of the leg. The anterior and lateral compartments are typically released through a longitudinally oriented incision starting at the midpoint of the lower leg and located

2–3 cm anterior to the body of the fibula while the two posterior compartments (deep and superficial) should be decompressed using a longitudinal incision in the midportion of the lower leg starting 2–3 cm posteromedial to the medial aspect of the tibia. Fracture stabilization, typically with an external fixator, is performed simultaneous with compartment release.

Pilon fractures are intra-articular distal tibia fractures that occur as a result of axial loading and high velocity trauma. Fractures occur when the talus abuts the tibia; The fracture pattern depends on foot position at the time of axial loading. A plantar flexed foot results in a posterior shear fragment while a dorsiflexed foot results in an anterior shear fragment. An axial load to a neutral foot typically results in multiple fragments, usually in a T or Y formation. Approximately 80% of pilon fractures have associated fibular fracture.[27] Systemic injury occurs in 30% of cases.[27] A neurovascular and soft tissue examination should be performed and immediate reduction carried out in the case of neurovascular compromise or tenting of the skin. A splint should be applied prior to radiographic evaluation. Radiographs of the tibia/fibula and ankle should be obtained. CT scanning with three-dimensional reconstruction is frequently used to delineate fracture lines, displacement, impaction, and to assist in operative planning. Multiple classifications schemes are used by orthopedic surgeons to define these fractures; the AO system is most widely used. Orthopedic consultation should be obtained expeditiously in cases of suspected pilon fracture. Definitive operative management may be delayed based upon the extent of soft tissue damage; external fixation may be required for temporary stabilization.

The fibula is fractured more easily and frequently than the tibia. *Isolated proximal fibular fractures* may be treated with a simple elastic bandage or, with a knee immobilizer if associated with significant pain and swelling. These patients may weightbear as tolerated, and should follow up with an orthopedic surgeon 2–3 weeks later.

Midshaft fibular fractures occur less frequently than those at extremes of the bone but are treated similarly to the proximal injury. Distal fibular fractures are discussed with ankle injuries.

Ankle injuries

The bony composition of the ankle joint includes the talus and distal portions of both tibia and fibula. The ankle joint moves only in plantar flexion and dorsiflexion; the subtalar joint (the articulation of the talus with the calcaneus) is responsible for inversion and eversion of the heel. The geometry of the talus makes the ankle particularly unstable as plantar flexion increases; the majority of injuries to the joint occur in this position. Joint stability is enhanced by soft tissue structures:

- Lateral ligamentous complex
  - (anterior talofibular (ATFL)
  - calcaneofibular (CFL)
  - posterior talofibular (PTFL) ligaments)
- Medial ligamentous complex
  - deltoid ligament (superficial and deep portions),
- Syndesmotic complex
  - anterior and posterior inferior tibiofibular ligaments
  - distal interosseous membrane.

Ankle sprains are among the most common injuries seen in the ED. The degree of injury depends on the position of the foot at the time of injury and both the extent and direction of rotation applied. With normal ambulation, the foot is slightly supinated or inverted (lateral malleolus towards the ground, medial aspect elevated) at heel strike, and progresses towards pronation or eversion (medial malleolus towards the ground, lateral malleolus elevated) as the foot approaches push off. Forces applied to the supinated foot typically result in injuries to the lateral ligamentous complex while forces on the pronated foot result in disruption of the deltoid ligament. Patients who have sustained an ankle sprain present with varying degrees of edema and ecchymosis. This is most common over the lateral malleolus. Range of motion is usually limited by pain. Neurovascular injuries are rare but a thorough examination should be performed. Tenderness is present directly over the injured structure; therefore, tenderness in atypical locations should raise suspicion for other injury. Fifth metatarsal fractures, talus fractures, and fractures of the anterior process of the calcaneus can all masquerade as ankle sprains.

Radiographs are obtained in many cases. However, the Ottawa Foot and Ankle Rules were designed to decrease the number of radiographs taken in the ED without missing any clinically significant fractures. Radiographs of the acutely injured ankle and foot are not needed if the patient could walk 4 steps at the scene of injury and again in the ED **and** if the distal 6 cm of both medial and lateral malleolus, the base of the 5th metatarsal, and the navicular are nontender. If radiographs are indicated, a standard series should include AP, lateral, and mortise views. Ultrasound (using a high-frequency transducer) can also be used to detect periarticular fractures and to evaluate the lateral ankle ligaments, particularly the ATFL and the CFL.[28] The ATFL stability is clinically assessed via the anterior drawer: the examiner stabilizes the tibia with one hand while applying an anteriorly directed force to the calcaneus with the foot in a neutral position. The CFL stability is assessed with the talar tilt test: the examiner stabilizes the tibia with one hand while attempting to supinate the neutrally positioned foot. The lack of a definitive end-point on either maneuver, or increased excursion in comparison to the contralateral side, should heighten physician suspicion for ligamentous disruption and prompt orthopedic follow up within a week in order to expedite referral to physical therapy and limit long-term instability. The routine use of stress X-rays is no longer recommended as advanced imaging techniques, MRI in particular, provides better detail of soft tissue anatomy.[29,30]

Patients with ankle sprains should be discharged from the ED with a commercially available splinting device (if available) rather than with an elastic bandage. The preformed splints provide better resolution of edema while decreasing stress to the injured ligaments through control of subtalar motion.[31] A three-way plaster splint should be applied if there is suspicion for complete ligamentous disruption. For the preformed splints, crutches are not required but may be dispensed as needed based on the patient's ability to ambulate. Range of motion exercises should be started as soon as tolerated; alphabet and marble exercises have been shown to accelerate the return of normal proprioception. Alphabet exercises are performed by placing the toes on the floor and then tracing the letters of the alphabet without removing the toes from the floor. Marble exercises are performed by placing marbles on the floor and then having the patient pick them up with his or her toes and place the marbles in a container located medially and then laterally to the foot.[32] Orthopedic or primary care follow up should be arranged for all patients, as formal physical therapy is often required for rapid and full return to activity.[33]

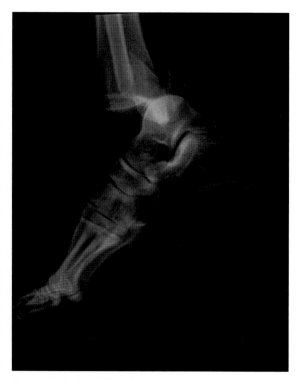

Figure 17.18 Talar dislocation.

Subtalar dislocation The subtalar joint allows inversion and eversion of the foot, and is most stable in slight eversion. Subtalar dislocations typically result from high-speed mechanisms, usually athletic activity or motor vehicle collisions. Fractures of the talus, calcaneus, or navicular may be associated with subtalar dislocation. The direction of the dislocation is described as the position of the calcaneus relative to the talus; it may be medial, lateral, or anterior, depending upon the injury-inducing force. Medial dislocations are most common; they typically follow an extreme inversion injury. Lateral dislocations are most likely to be associated with significant morbidity.

Patients present with significant pain and an obvious deformity of the foot. The presence of any neurovascular deficit necessitates immediate reduction. If no deficits are present, plain X-rays should be obtained to evaluate for associated fractures (Figure 17.18). Reduction is performed under conscious sedation. The knee is flexed and longitudinal traction is applied through the hindfoot. Once the calcaneus is distracted, a gentle force opposite to the direction of the dislocation is applied to reduce the joint. Some dislocations are irreducible due to soft tissue interposition, requiring

operative intervention for open reduction. Post-reduction X-rays and CT scan should be performed to confirm full reduction and to identify any fractures. A short leg splint is applied (with conversion to short leg cast once edema decreases) and the patient is instructed to remain non-weightbearing for 3–4 weeks. Some orthopedic surgeons favor initiation of range of motion therapy and protected weightbearing at 4 weeks while others prefer a full 8 weeks of immobilization. Current literature does not definitively support either treatment protocol.

Peroneal tendon subluxation must be considered in a patient who has sustained an inversion injury to the foot. Patients with these injuries present with tenderness along the course of the tendons and may have weak eversion, depending on the extent of the injury. To assess for subluxation, the physician places a hand over the lateral malleolus and asks the patient to evert the foot; the tendons can be appreciated sliding anteriorly over the lateral malleolus if the peroneal retinaculum is ruptured. Standard ankle radiographs should be performed to evaluate for avulsion fractures. Ultrasound may also be used in the diagnostic process. This modality allows dynamic assessment of the soft tissue structures and may capture the actual tendon subluxation. Patients with peroneal tendon subluxation should be placed in a posterior splint or boot. Operative repair may be necessary in some cases, based upon the size of the retinacular defect; this determination is usually made after failure of conservative treatment. *Peroneal tendon rupture* may also occur with inversion injury. Extreme pain with active eversion should arouse suspicion for this injury. However, this entity is often diagnosed secondarily, via MRI scanning, when recovery fails to progress as expected following inversion injury.

Syndesmotic injuries occur with forced plantar flexion of the foot; these injuries are also termed "high ankle sprains." Patients present with pain in the anterior aspect of the ankle, tenderness over the syndesmosis, and pain at the anterior ankle with either the squeeze test (compression of the tibia and fibula at mid-calf) or with external rotation of the foot. Radiographs (AP, lateral, and mortise) are taken to rule out fracture and to evaluate for widening of the syndesmosis or medial clear space. Widening of the medial clear space or loss of the distal tib-fib overlap indicates significant disruption of the syndesmosis requiring operative fixation. Emergency care for

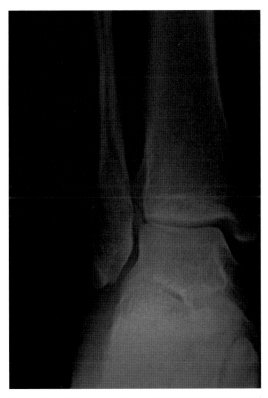

Figure 17.19 Syndesmotic and deltoid ligament injury with associated fibula fracture.

Table 17.6 The Danis–Weber classification system

Type	Location
A	Distal to the syndesmosis
B	At the level of the syndesmosis
C	Proximal to the syndesmosis

Table 17.7 The Lauge–Hansen classification system. The Lauge–Hansen classification describes fractures based upon the mechanism of injury[34]

Mechanism	Injury
Supination-adduction (SAD)	Distal fibular fractures and medial malleolar fractures
Supination-eversion (SEM)	Fractures at the level of the syndesmosis
Pronation-eversion (PER)	Fractures proximal to the ankle joint

syndesmotic sprains without widening is similar to that for traditional lateral ankle sprains, but "high ankle sprains" typically require 6–8 weeks longer to heal compared to the 4–6 week healing time usually required for lateral ankle sprains.

When syndesmotic and deltoid ligament tenderness is combined, a *Maisonneuve fracture* must be suspected. This constellation of injuries results when a foot is subjected to excess pronation; forces are transmitted along the intraosseous membrane from the ankle to the proximal fibula. The presence of deltoid and syndesmotic tenderness should prompt assessment for proximal fibular tenderness and performance of the squeeze test, providing presumptive evidence of a Maisonneuve fracture. In the event of positive examination findings, standard tibia/fibula radiographs should be obtained to visualize the length of the fibula. The mortise view of the ankle radiograph series may demonstrate widening of the medial clear space, a classic sign of syndesmotic disruption. A stress view of the ankle taken with the joint in dorsiflexion–external rotation, or more commonly, an MRI, assesses deltoid ligament integrity; a medial clear space of > 4 mm is indicative of deltoid injury. All patients with syndesmotic disruption, with or without associated fibular fracture, should be seen by an orthopedist within 2–3 days, as operative fixation is necessary to restore normal joint anatomy (Figure 17.19).

Ankle fractures result from the same basic mechanisms responsible for ligamentous injury. Fractures have previously been termed "bimalleolar" and "trimalleolar." Two other classification systems are considered more precise. The Danis–Weber system describes all fractures about the ankle based on the location of the fibular fracture (Table 17.6).[34] The Lauge–Hansen classification system describes injuries based on mechanism (Table 17.7).[34]

Gradations of each pattern further describe the associated injuries. Patients with ankle fractures should undergo evaluation for associated neurovascular deficits and soft tissue injury. Immediate reduction should be performed in the face of neurovascular injury or skin tenting. The latter signals impending open injury or soft tissue compromise that can greatly complicate post-operative management. After reduction is obtained, the extremity should be splinted while awaiting post-reduction films. A posterior splint is preferred in order to avoid translation of the talus in the sagittal plane; combined use of a sugar-tong splint will improve control in the coronal plane, especially in a large patient. External fixation may be required in some unstable injury patterns. Orthopedic

consultation must be obtained for all patients, as operative fixation provides definitive management, particularly where fracture displacement is present.[35,36] The one exception to this maxim is the minimally displaced Danis–Weber A injury, which can be managed in the fashion of a lateral ankle sprain.

Foot injuries

The bony anatomy of the foot is complex, with over 20 bones contributing to its structure. The subtalar joint, which provides heel inversion and eversion, is formed by the articulation of the inferior surface of the talus with the superior surface of the calcaneus. The head of the talus articulates distally with the navicular bone on the medial column of the foot, and the calcaneus articulates distally with the cuboid bone within the lateral column. The distal navicular bone articulates with the medial, middle, and lateral cuneiforms; the lateral cuneiform bone also articulates with the cuboid bone. The tarso-metatarsal joints are formed by the articulation of the proximal metatarsals with the three cuneiforms and the cuboid bones. In order to accommodate the range of motion the foot experiences during the normal gait cycle, these joints are particularly mobile. The most stable of these interfaces is the Lisfranc joint, formed by the articulation of the middle cuneiform bone with the second metatarsal bone and reinforced by the plantar ligament.

Calcaneal fractures result from axial loading, usually after a fall from a height with the patient landing on the feet. Edema, ecchymosis, and tenderness are common; crepitance may be present depending on the number of fracture fragments and the extent of displacement. Routine foot radiographs (AP, lateral, and oblique views) should be obtained after physical examination. If a fracture is suspected by mechanism and examination but radiographs reveal no obvious fracture, calculation of Bohler's angle may be productive. This angle is assessed using the lateral radiograph; it measures the height of the posterior facet of the calcaneus. The angle formed by the intersection of a line drawn from the highest point on the anterior tuberosity to the highest point on the posterior facet, with a line drawn from the latter to the highest point on the posterior tuberosity should measure 20–40°. Smaller angles are indicative of a compression fracture and should prompt further imaging; comparison views are useful in determining "normal" for each individual (Figure 17.20). The Harris axial view is useful for

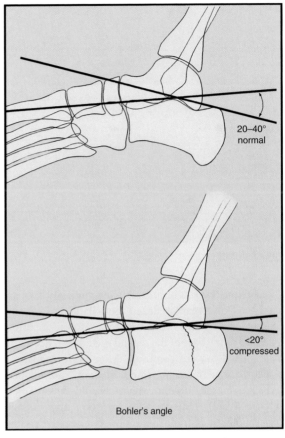

Figure 17.20 Illustration of Bohler's angle. This angle is seen on the lateral view and is the angle between lines connecting the three highest points of the calcaneus. (From Mandavia D, Newton E, Demetriades D. *Colour Atlas of Emergency Trauma.* Cambridge: Cambridge University Press, 2003.)

visualization of fractures in the sagittal plane. This view is obtained by placing the plantar aspect of the foot (and heel) on the radiograph cassette with the ankle dorsiflexed approximately 10°; the radiograph beam is angled ~45° to the cassette (Figure 17.21). In cases of displaced fracture, CT scanning provides further delineation of bony injury, assisting in decision making for definitive management. The fractured calcaneus should be immobilized in a posterior AO splint with extra padding and layers around the calcaneus. Orthopedic consultation is warranted for all patients with calcaneal fractures. The emergency physician must perform a careful evaluation of the lumbosacral spine, because concomitant lumbosacral spine fractures are identified in 15% of patients with calcaneal fractures.[37] Evaluation should include AP, lateral, and oblique films if lumbosacral pain or tenderness are present or unable to be evaluated.

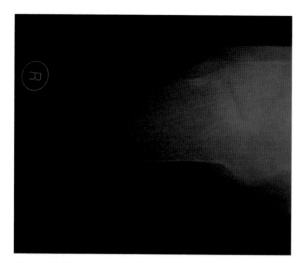

Figure 17.21 Harris axial radiograph.

Lisfranc injuries occur following application of an axial load to a plantar flexed foot. Patients typically present with pain across the entire forefoot, often localized to the base of the second metatarsal. Ecchymosis and edema are common. After performance of a neurovascular exam, standard foot radiographs (AP, lateral, and oblique views) should be obtained (Figure 17.22). Patients with an exam and history concerning for Lisfranc disruption, but negative radiographs, should undergo further imaging. A relatively high index of suspicion must be present in order to avoid missing this injury, as findings can be subtle and poor results follow missed or delayed diagnosis. Stress radiographs are obtained by anchoring the hindfoot and applying pronation and supination forces to the forefoot. This manipulation is particularly painful; procedural sedation may be required. These views are rarely performed as CT has obviated the need for these studies. A CT scan with narrow cuts will delineate the extent of injury, particularly when fracture–dislocation is suspected. Lastly, MRI can be used to define partial vs. complete ligamentous disruption. Patients with known Lisfranc injuries should be immobilized in a posterior AO splint while awaiting evaluation by an orthopedic surgeon; it is recommended that the patient be evaluated by an orthopedist at the time of injury based on the instability associated with this injury pattern. Patients must remain non-weightbearing because even partial weightbearing can cause further displacement of fracture fragments. Due to the significant instability associated with these injuries, the majority of cases require operative fixation.

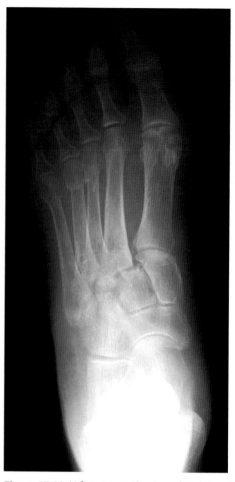

Figure 17.22 Lisfranc injury. (Courtesy of Mark Bernstein, MD.)

Fractures of the 5th metatarsal are particularly common. The typical mechanism of injury is inversion; three types of injury may result, each affecting different portions of the metatarsal. All three injuries present with pain at the base of the 5th metatarsal, edema, and ecchymosis. Thus, radiograph examination (AP, lateral, and oblique views of the foot) is necessary for definitive diagnosis (Figure 17.23). Ottawa Ankle Rules, described above, apply to the clinical examination of this region. A pseudo-Jones fracture is a vertical fracture at the base of the 5th metatarsal (Figure 17.23b). Previously termed "peroneal avulsion fracture," controversy regarding the true anatomic insertion of the peroneus brevis tendon has caused this term to fall out of favor. A Jones fracture is a horizontally oriented fracture at the metaphyseal-diaphyseal junction (Figure 17.23a). A diaphyseal stress fracture is a horizontally oriented

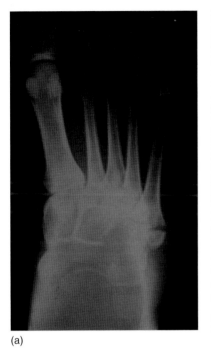 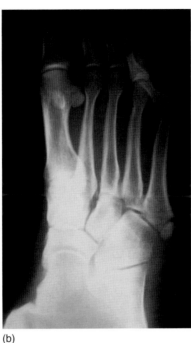

Figure 17.23 (a) Jones and (b) pseudo-Jones 5th metatarsal fractures.

(a) (b)

midshaft fracture that results from repetitive micro-trauma. It is critical for the emergency physician to identify the type of fracture as treatment varies. Patients with pseudo-Jones fractures may be placed in a hard-soled shoe and allowed to fully weight bear in the protective device. In contrast, Jones fractures have a high rate of non-union, often requiring internal fixation. Many orthopedists advocate early surgical treatment in active patients, as this decreases the complication rate and speeds the return to normal activity. Jones fractures can occur as acute injuries, or as completion of a stress fracture (pre-existing symptoms are present in the latter cases). The presence of pre-existing symptoms increases the indication for surgical treatment, as closed treatment is less likely to be successful. Patients with Jones fractures and diaphyseal stress fractures may be placed in a posterior splint or short leg cast and discharged from the ED. They should be instructed to remain non-weightbearing and orthopedic follow up should be arranged within 5–7 days for determination of definitive treatment.

References

1. Kondo F, Kuroki H. The effects of subminimal inhibitory concentrations of beta-lactam antibiotics against *Clostridium perfringens*. *Microbios* 2001;**105** (412):163–74.

2. Drake A, King A, Slack W. Gas gangrene and related infections: classification, clinical features and etiology, management and mortality. *Br J Surg* 1977;**64**:104–12.

3. Hitchcock C. Gas gangrene in the injured extremity. In Gustilo R (ed.), *Management of Open Fractures and Their Complications*. Philadelphia, PA: WB Saunders, 1982: p. 183.

4. Cummings S, Rubin S, Black D. The future of hip fractures. *J Gerontol* 1989;**44**:M107–11.

5. Reimers A, Laflamme L. Hip fractures among the elderly: personal and contextual social factors that matter. *J Trauma* 2007;**62**(2):365–9.

6. Mortimore E, Haselow D, Dolan M, Hawkes W. Amount of social contact and hip fracture mortality. *J Am Geriatr Soc* 2008;**56**(6):1069–74.

7. deVries F, Bracke M, Leufkens H, et al. Fracture risk with intermittent high-dose oral glucocorticoid therapy. *Arthritis Rheum* 2007;**56** (1):208–14.

8. Cummings S, Cawthon P, Ensrud K, et al. BMD and risk of hip and nonvertebral fractures in older men: a prospective study and comparison with older women. *J Bone Min Res* 2006;**21** (10):1550–6.

9. Orwig D, Chan J, Magaziner J. Hip fracture and its consequences: differences between men and women. *Orthop Clin N Am* 2006;**37**:611–22.

327

10. Chana R, Noorani A, Ashwood N, et al. The role of MRI in the diagnosis of proximal femoral fractures in the elderly. *Injury* 2006;**37**:185–9.

11. Lubovsky O, Liebergall M, Mattan Y, Weil Y, Mosheiff R. Early diagnosis of occult hip fractures MRI versus CT scan. *Injury* 2005;**36**(6):788–92.

12. Evans P, Wilson C, Lyons K. Comparison of MRI with bone scanning for suspected hip fracture in elderly patients. *J Bone Joint Surg* 1994;**76**:158–9.

13. Probe R, Ward R. Internal fixation of femoral neck fractures. *J Am Acad Orthop Surg* 2006;**14**(9):565–71.

14. Tornetta P, Kain M, Creevy W. Diagnosis of femoral neck Fractures in patients with a femoral shaft fracture. *J Bone Joint Surg* 2007;**89**-A(1):39–43.

15. Iorio R, Schwartz B, Macaulay W, et al. Surgical treatment of displaced femoral neck fractures in the elderly. *J Arthroplasty* 2006;**21**(8):1124–33.

16. Farkas T, Zane R. Comminuted femur fracture secondary to stress during the Boston Marathon. *J Emerg Med* 2006;**31**(1):79–82.

17. Davies H. The posterolateral corner of the knee anatomy, biomechanics and management of injuries. *Injury* 2004;**35**:68–75.

18. Reckling F, Peliter L. Acute knee dislocations and their complications. *Clin Orthop and Rel Res* 2004;**422**:135–41.

19. Robertson A, Nutton R, Keating J. Dislocation of the knee. *J Bone Joint Surg* 2006;**88**-B(6):706–11.

20. Stannard J. Vascular injuries in knee dislocations: the role of physical examination in determining the need for arteriography. *J Bone Joint Surg* 2004;**86**-A (5):910–15.

21. Mills W. The value of the ankle–brachial index for diagnosing arterial injury after knee dislocation: a prospective study. *J Trauma* 2004;**56**(6):1261–5.

22. Klineberg E. The role of arteriography in assessing popliteal artery injury in knee dislocation. *J Trauma* 2004;**56**(4):786–90.

23. Bahk M, Cosgarea A. Physical examination and imaging of the lateral collateral ligament and posterolateral corner of the knee. *Sports Med Arthrosc Rev* 2006;**14**(1):12–19.

24. Freeman R. Combined chronic posterior cruciate and posterolateral corner ligamentous injuries: a comparison of posterior cruciate ligament reconstruction with and without reconstruction of the posterolateral corner. *Knee* 2002;**9**:309–12.

25. Cole P. Open tibia fracture: amputation versus limb salvage; opinion limb salvage. *J Orthop Trauma* 2006;**21**(1):68–9.

26. Dougherty P. Open tibia fracture: amputation versus limb salvage; opinion: below-the-knee amputation. *J Orthop Trauma* 2006;**21**(1):67–8.

27. Dickson K. Tibial plafond fracture. In Wheeless CR III, (ed.), *Wheeless' Textbook of Orthopaedic Surgery*. Available from http://www.wheelessonline.com/ortho/tibial_plafond_fracture.

28. Hsu C, Tsai W, Chen C, et al. Ultrasonic examination for inversion ankle sprains associated with osseous injuries. *Am J Phys Med Rehabil* 2006;**85**(10):785–92.

29. Kragh J, Ward J. Radiographic indicators of ankle instability: changes with plantarflexion. *Foot Ankle Int* 2006;**27**(1):23–8.

30. McConnell T, Creevy W, 3rd. Stress examination of supination external rotation-type fibular fractures. *J Bone Joint Surg* 2004;**86**-A(10):2171–8.

31. Kerkhoffs GMMJ, Rowe BH, Assendelft WJJ, et al. Immobilisation and functional treatment for acute lateral ankle ligament injuries in adults. *Cochrane Database Syst Rev* 2002;**3**:CD003762.

32. Chorley J. Ankle sprain discharge instructions from the emergency department. *Ped Emerg Care* 2005;**21**:498–501.

33. Anandacoomarasamy A. Long term outcomes of inversion ankle injuries. *Br J Sports Med* 2005;**39**:14–18.

34. Gardner M, Demetrakapoulos D, Briggs S, Helfet D, Lorich D. The ability of the Lauge–Hansen Classification to predict ligament injury and mechanism in ankle fractures: an MRI study. *J Orthop Trauma* 2006;**20**(4):267–72.

35. Egol K, Amirtharage M, Tejwani N, Capla E, Koval K. Ankle stress test for predicting the need for surgical fixation of isolated fibular fractures. *J Bone Joint Surg* 2004;**86**A(11):2393–8.

36. Park S, Kubiak E, Egol K, Kummer F, Koval K. Stress radiographs after ankle fracture. *J Orthop Trauma* 2006;**20**(1):11–18.

37. Teh J, Firth M, Sharma A. Jumpers and fallers: a comparison of the distribution of skeletal injury. *Clin Radiol* 2003;**58**(6):482–6.

18

Cutaneous injuries

E. Parker Hays, Jr. and D. Matthew Sullivan

Introduction

Lacerations, avulsions, bites, burns, and puncture wounds are among the most common complaints in US emergency departments (EDs). Approximately 12 million lacerations are treated in US EDs annually.[1] Countless more wounds present in multiply injured patients and are part of the overall management of trauma. Practitioners can improve outcomes by seeing each wound as an opportunity to alter the course of wound healing toward the ideal and away from complications. A wound's end result is affected by the mechanism of wounding, various host factors, prehospital care and timing, management techniques, and aftercare. The goal for the clinician is to create optimal conditions in which the wound does its healing.

Clinical anatomy and pathophysiology

The largest organ in the body, skin multitasks in protection and structural integrity, heat exchange, prevention of infection, and tactile interface with the person's environment.

While all layers of skin – epidermis, dermis, and connective tissue – contribute to functional wound healing, the relative contribution of any layer changes over the course of healing. The dermis is the thickest layer and provides structural integument, carries vascular structures and the cutaneous nerves (Figure 18.1). Its apposition in wound repair may strongly influence the quality of the repair the most.

A predictable sequence of coagulation, hemostasis, inflammation, tissue formation, and tissue remodeling follows skin injury; the patient or clinician may modify each of these steps.

The thickness, color, and height or degrees of depression all influence the aesthetic outcome of a

scar. The thickness depends on the width of the initial wound and the necessity of additional granulation tissue to fill gaps (secondary intention). Vascularity and pigmentation of the scar, compared to surrounding tissue, determine color. The alignment and apposition of healing skin edges, the tensile and shear forces across the wound, and the amount of inflammation preceding the formation of scar tissue may alter the scar's height. Depressed scars create shadowing that makes them appear darker than the neighboring reflective surfaces, as commonly demonstrated by normal age-associated wrinkles (Figure 18.2).

Awareness of the factors in scar formation helps in repair decisions and counseling patients in aftercare, particularly in patients prone to keloid formation. However, many steps of general wound management remain the same.

Prehospital

Cutaneous injuries are subject to the environmental conditions present at the time of the trauma, and thus may be grossly contaminated, bleeding, or have ongoing wounding in the case of some chemical burns. Prehospital care should be directed toward hemostasis, typically with direct pressure, and coverage with clean dressings to prevent further contamination.

Emergency department evaluation and management

Careful evaluation of the patient as a whole is critical since a wound represents only the entry point of injurious force. Certain questions should be addressed: What is the mechanism of cutaneous injury (shear, compression, abrasion, burn)? Can

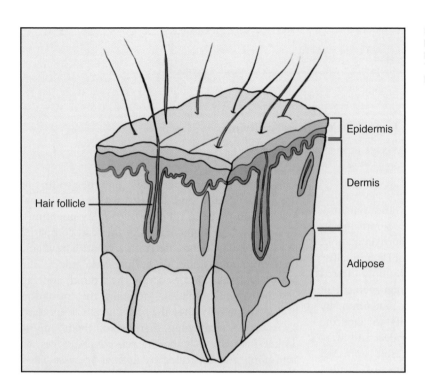

Figure 18.1 Illustration of normal skin layers. (From Mandavia D, Newton E, Demetriades D. *Colour Atlas of Emergency Trauma.* Cambridge: Cambridge University Press, 2003.)

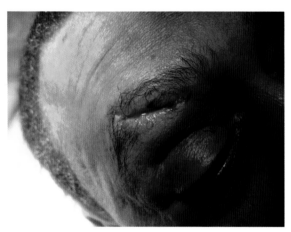

Figure 18.2 Skin tension lines or wound contraction make wounds prone to depression of the edges. In this repair, meticulous suture placement was needed to elevate the edges to better apposition.

you document the functional status of the patient before and after injury? What general characteristics of the patient (host), or the wound, suggest higher or lower risk of infection or poor healing? Concentration on a wound to the exclusion of the full patient can be a major misstep in managing a traumatized patient with a cutaneous injury.

A consideration of host and wound factors helps predict the overall risk of infection and the likelihood of complications. An identically sized linear wound on the scalp of a normal child carries much lower risks for complications than on the shin of an elderly person with diabetes and peripheral vascular disease.[2]

Host factors

Each patient is a unique environment for wound healing due to age, various medical conditions, and overall health. The skin changes with time, largely related to thinning of the dermis. Hosts also have varying degrees of vascular function, bony strength, and immune disorders or medication effects.

Wound factors

Major wound factors are location including association with other structures, contamination, and timing to presentation. Further, patients have often altered wound factors by attending to the injury themselves. Placing a cut finger in the mouth, pressure dressings, or hopeful neglect can theoretically affect a wound's prognosis (Table 18.1).

Foreign bodies

Any break in the skin's barrier means a foreign body could be introduced.

Table 18.1 Factors affecting wound healing

Host factors	Wound factors
Age	Location
Diabetes	Mechanism of injury
Peripheral vascular disease	Age of wound
Other immunocompromise	Degree and type of contaminants
Tetanus status	Involvement of underlying structures
Latex allergy	Foreign body risk

Common presentations include shattered glass in a motor vehicle crash, organic material in wounds during outdoor activities, and "puncture particles" introduced through footwear. Foreign bodies increase infection risk and may prevent healing.

Underlying structure injury

Skin can fail in its protective role if sufficiently breached allowing underlying tendon, nerves, muscle, bone, or other structures to be injured. Perform a diligent assessment of the function of the structures near a wound site.

Assess tendon function throughout a range of motion. Ask the patient to estimate the position of a body part at the time of injury, especially in hand injuries. Range of motion may remain intact in partial tendon injuries, potentially misleading the practitioner. Pain or decreased range of motion with movement of a tendon may be the best clues to raise suspicion for a partial injury (Figure 18.3). Nerves can be injured by the wounding mechanism itself or by indiscriminate iatrogenic maneuvers. Avoid clamping, blind probing, and unnecessary debridement as all can worsen the trauma to adjacent nerves. Nerves run in close proximity to vasculature, especially in the hands and face, and zealous attempts to control a bleeding vessel can result in damage to the neighboring nerve. Injected anesthetics also may injure nerves through pressure necrosis in finite spaces, including a large nerve's own sheath. Injections into the olecranon groove or foramina of the hard palate of the mouth are good examples. Patients may report excessive pain with

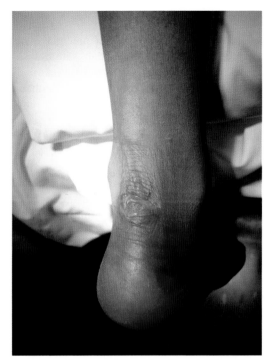

Figure 18.3 Although the visible laceration appears innocuous, the underlying Achilles tendon proved transected by the Thompson test and required operative repair. More subtle examples in the hand, forearm, knee, and foot could be missed without an adequate evaluation.

intraneural needle placement. In general, good measures to avoid nerve injury include following aseptic technique to avoid infection, injecting near nerves with some surrounding soft tissue rather than a bony foramen, and using the lowest effective anesthetic volume.

Muscles are highly vascular tissue and may be involved in deep cutaneous wounds. A muscle is a dynamic unit, and subsequent hematomas, scars, or infection can result in dysfunction. Control bleeding with direct pressure and avoid unnecessary debridement. Muscle can usually be repaired by securing the surrounding supportive structures (fascia, skin) which place the cut surfaces of muscle in direct contact. Muscle tissue should only be sutured directly when this is insufficient.

Cutaneous injuries may be the only sign of an underlying fracture, either because the skin was injured and the force carried through to the bone, or because the broken bone edges tore the skin from within. Perform an evaluation of the bones in areas with skin injury in the trauma patient.

331

Immunization status

With all cutaneous injuries where the potential exists for contamination, ask about the patient's immunization status. Patients who have sustained dirty wounds and who may have never received standard childhood immunizations, should be given tetanus immunoglobulin and tetanus vaccination. If the patient has previously received a full series of immunizations then tetanus toxoid booster is warranted based on the time interval since last vaccination. For dirty wounds (e.g., those that have a high suspicion for soil contamination), use 5 years as the appropriate time frame for updating their tetanus immunization. For simple cutaneous injuries that are clean (e.g., bread knife to the hand), then this to 10 years between each tetanus toxoid boosters.

Treatment

Preparing the wound can be tantamount to or surpass closure in importance in order to meet the goals of reducing infection risk, minimizing underlying structure damage, and forming a functional and cosmetically acceptable scar. The properly prepared wound has been anesthetized, decontaminated of large particles or foreign bodies, minimized bacterial counts through irrigation, and has edges amenable to optimal repair if indicated.

Sterile gloves

Studies have shown that the use of sterile vs. non-sterile boxed gloves in the routine wound may not have a significant effect on infection rate.[3] However, infection is not the only factor to consider in choosing gloves. For example, the quality of gloves packaged in sterile format may be of a higher quality and sizable fit compared to boxed non-sterile models. Avoid powdered gloves due to their association with granuloma formation and be aware of possible latex allergy. While fastidious attention to sterile technique may still be indicated in managing some complex or high-risk wounds, its universal use with routine wounds may not be necessary.

Anesthesia

In general, anesthesia should precede significant efforts at cleansing, irrigation, exploration, and closure. In spite of long held dogma, lidocaine with epinephrine can be safely used in most areas of the body, including most hand wounds and digital blocks.[4]

Wound cleansing and irrigation

The goals of wound cleansing and irrigation are to: (1) remove gross contaminants and particulate matter; (2) reduce bacterial counts in the wound; and (3) avoid impeding the host's responses and natural defenses.

Ideal wound irrigation requires sufficient pressure and volume while providing drainage and not exposing the clinician to body fluids. If large particles are present, perform gross decontamination prior to pressure irrigation. Leaves, dirt, and other large contaminants may be removed with a water spray in the sink or simply poking holes in the plastic top of a saline bottle. Even in the context of the multiply injured trauma patient, initial gross decontamination and dressing application is indicated and may facilitate later management. Regardless of the method used, at some point the pressure of the irrigating stream should be sufficient to overcome the adhesive forces of bacteria (around 5–12 psi) for most wounds.[5]

This pressure can be produced with a 35 cc syringe and a 19 g catheter or a commercial device with an integrated splash cup. The volume of irrigant sufficient to decontaminate wounds is unknown. However, since bacteria may be present in all sections of a wound, expose all surfaces of a wound to the irrigating stream. In general, the composition of the fluid is much less important than its mechanical action in decontaminating a wound of bacteria.[6]

Wound edge preparation

Hair does not generally need removal and shaving has been shown to increase infection rate. If directly and substantially interfering with proper suture placement, hair can be clipped near the wound edge with scissors. A common scenario in trauma is a bleeding scalp wound on a multiply injured patient who requires further testing or intervention. These wounds can be rapidly closed with a running suture, achieving hemostasis.

In general, do not debride any more than is absolutely necessary to remove clearly devitalized tissue. The irregular, undulating wound may actually be superior to the straight linear excised wound because the wound's natural skin marks, corners, and contours demonstrate exactly how the wound should be repaired. Further, longer surface area results in better tensile strength across the healing wound. If debridement is necessary, use quality forceps and a number 15 blade scalpel or a small iris scissors.

Aftercare

Compared to the emphasis placed on actively managing the wound, aftercare sometimes receives little attention and instruction. The aims of aftercare are to optimize the chances of a wound healing without infection and with a functional, aesthetically acceptable scar. Generally established principles that promote wound healing include maintaining an uncontaminated milieu, immobilization, and elevation to reduce edema.

Application of an antibiotic ointment is commonly recommended. At least one emergency medicine study supports using an ointment, although it is unclear whether the benefit is derived from the antibiotic itself or the petrolatum vehicle that promotes a moist environment for epithelialization.[7]

Immobilize injured parts, at least until epithelialization occurs (usually about 24–36 hours), or longer in wounds (i.e., until sutures are removed) subjected to high tension (e.g., a laceration over the kneecap or the wrist).

Patients often ask, "Will there be a scar?" Various factors influence scar formation. Histologically, reorganization of the reticular layers of the dermis and epithelialization can result in different types of scars. A "normal" scar is at first immature with some itch, redness, and width, but matures to a light colored, pliable, narrow scar. A *hypertrophic* scar has raised, heaped-up cells, but remains within the borders of the original wound. A *keloid* extends its scar tissue beyond the margins of the initial wound, and can become quite large. Any depression from the surrounding plane of skin causes shadowing and makes a scar more noticeable (Figure 18.4). Examine the patient for prior scars, giving clues to how they might heal their acute wound. Patients who have a tendency to form hypertrophic or keloid scars should be identified by the emergency practitioner and informed of treatment options available to decrease scarring. Pressure with paper taping and massage over developing scars is simple and may be begun soon after initial wound healing. Many other methods have been studied, but the only treatments with sufficient prospective data to support their use are silicone gel sheets and intralesional corticosteroid injections, although these are generally performed in

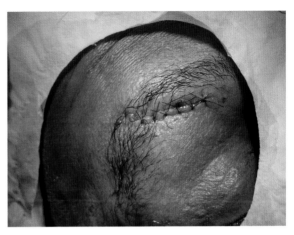

Figure 18.4 Eyebrow laceration.

the outpatient setting.[8] Other topical preparations have been promoted to aesthetically improve scars. Vitamin E cream is popular and is available over-the-counter, yet no good study exists to show its effectiveness in acute lacerations and at least one study showed a detrimental effect.[9]

Documentation

"If you saw it, did it, or said it – write it" guides documentation. A description of the mechanism, history, prehospital care, surrounding functions prior to and after any medical maneuvers, steps taken to reduce infection, evaluation for foreign bodies, and closure of the wound are all important elements of record keeping. Proper instructions given the patient should include precautions for return, infection signs, and explicit instructions for the short- and long-term aftercare of the wound. Common significant pitfalls in documentation are inadequately addressing the search for a foreign body, omitting irrigation or assessment of surrounding function, or failure to describe the wound's length and complexity of repair.[10]

Since patients largely direct and conduct the aftercare of wounds themselves, they need a thorough list of "if-thens." The signs of infection (including increased redness, pus from the wound, more swelling than they think is appropriate, excessive pain), persistent foreign body sensation, or any significant concern about the wound should be reason to return to the ED. While some EDs use a routine wound check at 48 hours, for uncomplicated wounds in the informed patient this is not necessary. Suture removal times are also important as are avoiding direct sunlight on the wound (usually by using sun block) for about 6 months.

Preprinted sheets detailing expected occurrences and instruction are useful, especially if they allow custom information to be added about specific wounds.

Specific wound types

Lacerations

Lacerations are the sharp division of tissue with no or minimal tissue loss. They may be linear, irregular, jagged, stellate, oblique, or adjacent to an area of abrasion. They may be so superficial as to only involve some of the skin layers or deep enough to have lacerated the underlying connective tissue, fascia, muscle, or other structures.

In the setting of trauma, achieve hemostasis by direct pressure. Ongoing blood loss must on occasion be staunched by rapid closure, either with sutures or staples. If possible, avoid staple closures adjacent to areas that may require computed tomography (CT) scanning (e.g., scalp wounds in the potentially brain-injured patient) as they may cause scatter artifact and make the scan difficult to interpret.

Some wounds may not warrant immediate closure. A study of uncomplicated hand lacerations, < 2 cm in length, showed that functional and cosmetic outcomes were similar at 3 months whether the wound was sutured on not.[11] However, factors such as returning to specific work tasks and functional facility during the healing period were not measured. Therefore, a cook with a lacerated hand might prefer suture closure even if long-term outcome of the wound is similar if not repaired.

Primary vs. delayed primary vs. secondary intention

Primary closure is the repair of wounds within the initial day or two after injury. Most uncomplicated or clean lacerations, including almost all on the head and neck, can be closed primarily. Because of the myriad of host and wound factors that portend risk, no definite rules for parts of the body exist. A simple rationale recommendation from one wound care text is that any wound that, ". . . regardless of time from injury, can be converted to a fresh-appearing, slightly bleeding, non-devitalized wound, with no visible contamination or debris after aggressive cleansing, irrigation, and debridement, can be considered for primary closure."[12]

Delayed primary closure may be appropriate for contaminated wounds or compromised hosts when repair is functionally or cosmetically desired (e.g., a contaminated forearm wound on a person with diabetes). After good wound preparation and irrigation, apply a sterile gauze packing dressing, recheck as necessary in 1–2 days, and evaluate for suture repair 4–5 days after injury There are no definitive studies addressing whether antibiotics are beneficial for delayed closure. However, many of the same factors that prompt delayed closure (bite wounds, immunocompromised host, gross contamination, evidence of infection) may be indications for antibiotics at the initial evaluation and should guide the clinical decision.

Secondary intention is the filling of gaps in skin and tissue by coagulation, granulation, contraction, and scar formation. The practitioner may rely on secondary intention to heal wounds that do not have sufficient skin remaining to repair or are deemed too risky for primary or delayed primary repair.

Box 18.1 Lacerations: essential points

- Different mechanisms on different hosts create differing degrees of risk for complications.
- The goals of management are initial hemostasis and decontamination, thorough assessment of surrounding neurovascular and musculoskeletal structures and their functioning, and repair of tissue in a manner that minimizes complications and maximizes cosmetic and functional outcome.
- Lacerations are the relatively sharp division of skin tissue. They can be repaired using mechanical closure methods (sutures, staples, adhesive) by acute or delayed primary closure, or allowed to heal by secondary intention depending on underlying host and wound factors that modify risks for infection.

Avulsions

Introduction

The loss of tissue in conjunction with the division of skin is an avulsion. Avulsions present a variety of challenges in their evaluation, preparation, and particularly their management to achieve adequate tissue coverage or promotion of secondary intention healing.

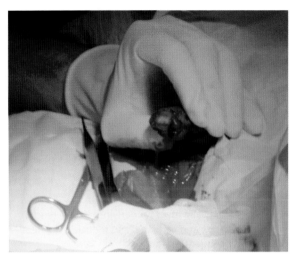

Figure 18.5 Exposed bone in the fingertip can be judiciously trimmed to allow soft tissue coverage.

Clinical anatomy and pathophysiology

Avulsions often have greater degrees of devitalized tissue, contamination, and underlying structural injury than cutaneous lacerations. Relatively fastidious decontamination, evaluation of the surrounding function, and wound repair techniques (if performed) are indicated. Any area of the body may suffer avulsion injury, but common presentations involve facial structures, including lip, ear, and nose, and fingertips, toes, or extremity soft tissue.

Prehospital

If practical, avulsed tissue should be preserved and brought to the hospital wrapped in saline-moistened gauze in a plastic bag. Similar to amputations, the tissue may be of use in the repair or coverage of the wound even if it is not "reattached" per se.

Emergency department evaluation and management

Basic management must include achieving hemostasis, removing contaminants and grossly devitalized tissue, and stabilization of viable but loosely attached parts.

What can be saved? Should you debride? What structures must be covered up? -- The decision to undermine and close, rotate a flap, autologously graft, or let heal by secondary intention is variable based on the involved structures. In general, after the above basic management, neurovascular structures, bone, and cartilage need to be covered by soft tissue. If avulsed tissue is not obviously devitalized or grossly

contaminated, and has been well preserved, it may be used in the initial management. In some cases the avulsed tissue, once replaced may remain viable, but in others it serves as a "bandage" that maintains anatomy and coverage until subsequent surgical management is performed. Most examples of this will be when the avulsed tissue remains connected by a stalk or thin section. If it can stay in place and allow some wound granulation and contraction, it is reasonable to leave attached in the repair.

Some areas simply cannot be closed adequately with the available skin, even with undermining and plastic advancement techniques, and are candidates for subsequent skin grafting. Plastic surgery referral is often warranted. Some body areas that are particularly difficult to undermine and close include the shin, scalp, knee, palm of the hand, and sole of the foot.

Common presentations

In the case of fingertip avulsions, using a *rongeur* instrument to remove protuberant distal phalanx bone and allow soft tissue coverage of the remaining bone is necessary (Figure 18.5). Tendon insertion is on the proximal surface of the distal phalanx and should be avoided. Distal fingertip avulsion may also be treated by skin grafting or by rotational flaps. This is dependent on both the injury and the patient's desires and occupation. A flap may preserve length, however, will prolong the healing process. If this is desired, a hand surgeon is generally consulted. Rongeuring the bone back with primary coverage may be done by a hand surgeon or by an emergency physician (Figure 18.6).

With ear avulsions, cartilage should not be removed unless obviously devitalized. However, skin coverage of cartilage is ideal. Subsequent reconstruction by plastic surgery may utilize any saved cartilage (Figure 18.7).

Gaping extremity injuries, although daunting at first, often merit an attempt at closure by undermining, tension-reducing suture techniques, and frequent wound checks (Figure 18.8).

Documentation

Documentation of avulsions is similar to other wounds with the exception that more of these patients will require documentation of the need for frequent rechecks or a referral plan with plastic surgery for ongoing reconstruction. Digital photography is increasingly being utilized to document before and after repairs, however, if used in the ED, it should be in conjunction with a departmental policy.

335

Disposition and transfer

Avulsions that are stabilized and do not require emergent consultation may be candidates for discharge if appropriate in the context of the trauma patient. Some avulsion wounds are managed as inpatients surgically largely because other orthopedic or traumatic operative procedures are necessary and can be

done simultaneously. Wounds that have hemostasis, have been appropriately decontaminated, and do not have exposed bone or cartilage may be followed up in 24–36 hours.

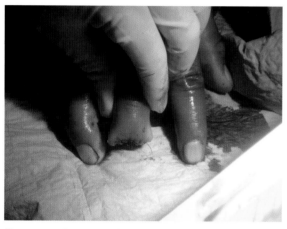

Figure 18.6 Fingertip avulsion treated by roungeuring the bone with primary coverage.

> **Box 18.2 Avulsions: essential points**
>
> - Avulsions result from the division of skin with a loss of tissue and may pose higher risk of associated structure injury, dysfunction, infection, and cosmetic deformity.
> - Beyond the usual management goals, avulsion repair involves achieving adequate tissue coverage, especially over underlying bone, tendon, vasculature, and cartilage, and reducing the need for subsequent grafting.
> - They have a higher incidence of requiring specialized care.

Puncture wounds

Introduction

By their nature, puncture wounds are different than lacerations in mechanism, risk, and prognosis. Although extremely common, the available data on

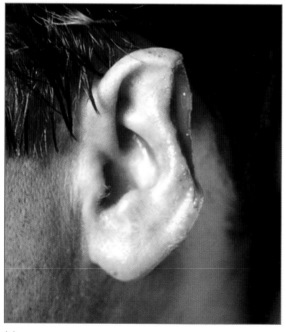

(a)

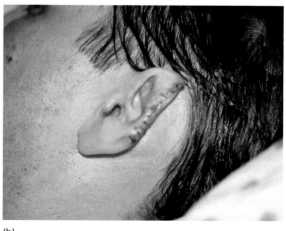

(b)

Figure 18.7 (a) Ear avulsion laceration with loss of cartilage. (b) Ear avulsion after primary closure may require revision in the future for improved cosmesis.

practitioner will encounter this entity and should be well versed in the basics of management.

Clinical anatomy and pathophysiology

The pathophysiology relating to puncture wounds is often substantially different than that of any other types of cutaneous injury. In some cases, the disruption of the tissues and destruction of the underlying structure is actually far less in puncture wounds than it is in other wounds. Conversely, puncture wounds seen in the hands and feet, where the bones, tendon sheaths, and vessels are in close proximity to the skin, may be more at risk by the mechanism of injury. In addition, it has been assumed that puncture wounds have a higher rate of infection than other wounds, but the true incidence is not known. Mechanisms associated with puncture wounds often include the penetration of a sock and shoe by a nail or other object of varying degree of contamination, and may include the weight of the body coming down on the penetrating object with significant force. All of these factors in combination require a detailed examination and specialized approach to the puncture wound.

Prehospital

The prehospital management of puncture wounds is similar to other cutaneous injury in that hemorrhage control is of primary importance. The protection of underlying neurovascular structures through the use of splinting may be of benefit if a foreign body is in place. If a foreign body is present, it should not be extracted in the field.

Emergency department evaluation and management

Puncture wounds can be categorized as minor to severe, but typically that categorization relates to the amount of ongoing hemorrhage and blood loss sustained at the time of injury. More commonly, non-life-threatening puncture wounds should be categorized as *early presenters* vs. *late presenters*.

As is the case with all wounds, early wound cleansing should begin at the earliest possible time – even as the encounter begins. Early dogma which preached that high-pressure irrigation may "drive particles deeper" is unsubstantiated. As has been discussed earlier, the evidence clearly points to better outcomes with wound irrigation at the correct pressure and this should not be ignored in the case of a puncture wound even if the opening for irrigation is very small. Anesthesia can be achieved locally, as in other types of cutaneous

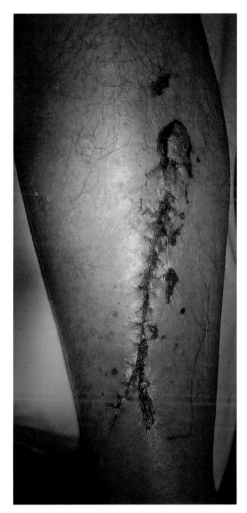

Figure 18.8 Skin laceration of the shin. Even in this difficult area, careful undermining and the use of tension-reducing suture techniques allowed skin coverage without grafting.

treatment and prognosis is retrospective and observational. One survey indicated that 44% of persons had experienced a plantar puncture wound at some time during their life but only half of these present for care.[13] The early condition of the injury may dictate whether patients will present to the ED for evaluation: some will present nearly 100% of the time (infected puncture wounds) and others rarely present at all (routine nail puncture of the foot). Unfortunately, unlike other cutaneous injuries, there is a paucity of literature to help guide emergency practitioners in their evaluation, acute management, or risk stratification of these wounds. Despite the lack of evidence-based guidelines and the varying practice patterns that exist for puncture wounds, almost every emergency

Table 18.2 Concerns with early and late presentations with puncture wounds

Early presenters	Late presenters
Uncontrolled hemorrhage or retained foreign body	Infectious symptoms
Concerns over tetanus status or exposure to blood-borne pathogens	Persistent foreign body symptoms or concerns
Pain control	Neurovascular abnormality (e.g., persistent numbness)
Stab wounds or assault	
Work mandated evaluation	

wounds, but may also be achieved with the use of peripheral nerve blocks to ensure adequate analgesia throughout the evaluation and wound irrigation.

Soaking the puncture wound has been a past treatment in many EDs. Similar to irrigation in these wounds, the benefits of soaking remain unproven. In addition, if performed, there is controversy over whether dilute povidone iodine should be used or if saline is the best solution. There remains a trade off between the anti-bacterial properties of povidone iodine and the cytotoxic properties of the solution. The one small ED study that compared soaking plantar puncture wounds in 1% povidone iodine vs. no soaking or saline soaking found that after 10 minutes, saline-soaked wounds had a slight increase in bacterial number, and the povidone-soaked wound had slightly less bacteria than the untreated. The clinical significance is unclear, but it is concerning that the saline soaked wounds actually increased bacterial count. Furthermore, many practitioners may not dilute the povidone appropriately. The beneficial effects proven with irrigation suggest this may be a better method for the decontamination of puncture wounds.

Assessing a puncture wound includes a detailed understanding of the historical presentation. In addition to significant host factors (Table 18.2), care should be taken to fully understand the specific circumstances of the puncture: what location in the body, was there overlying clothing, what protective gear may have been in place, what implement caused the puncture wound, the timing of the injury, and any type of delay to presentation are all helpful components of the history.

As with all wounds, evaluation of the underlying structures and their function should be undertaken. The vascular function should be evaluated and any deficits in motor or sensory function should be documented. With damage to underlying arterial structures, bleeding may be fairly profuse and require immediate intervention. In actuality, simple puncture wounds bleed far less than other, larger cutaneous injuries due to the limited opening of the injury itself. The small aperture makes evaluation for foreign body or underlying structure injury more difficult as well. Ultimately, the practitioner must establish a pretest probability for retained foreign body or "puncture particles" that have been forced into the wound with the injury. In an *early presentation* of a knife stab wound to the bare arm, the pretest probability of a retained foreign body may be extremely low, while *late presentation* of an infected foot after a puncture wound through a shoe should raise a very high suspicion of a potentially retained foreign body.

Due to a higher than normal likelihood for foreign material in these types of cutaneous injuries, diligently search for foreign bodies at the onset of wound evaluation. Any obvious foreign body should be removed immediately unless a case can be made that the puncture is near critical structures and the offending foreign body might best be removed in the operating room. If for any reason, there is concern for an unrecognized retained foreign body then radiographic exploration should be used. There is growing literature to support the use of bedside ultrasonography for the identification of embedded foreign bodies and as this modality becomes more commonplace, this entity will become an increasingly valuable tool.[14] For those without bedside ultrasonography, plain radiographs will reveal most foreign bodies including wood, metal, plastics, glass, and some vegetative matter. Radiographic testing should be guided by the practitioner's pretesting probability of a retained foreign body as well as the location of the wound and how much of the wound can be visually inspected at the time of examination. For *late presenters* with evidence of cellulitis or infection, radiographic imaging should be undertaken in almost all cases. In some cases, extension of the wound by incision to allow for removal of the foreign body may be required. However, removing large areas of tissue to ensure that material is not embedded in the wound is no longer common practice and may lead to further destruction and disability; it should be discouraged.

Controversy remains regarding the value and timing of antibiotic use with puncture wounds. There have been no randomized trials using antibiotics for puncture wounds.[15] Trying to discern which wounds are contaminated typically results in a high level of intraobserver disagreement. Despite that it is only one minor component of the spectrum of the disease, classic teaching has been that puncture wounds occurring through the sole of a tennis shoe carry a high risk of *Pseudomonas*. This literature is unfortunately anecdotal case-reporting paired with studies aimed at identifying which bacteria grow in a tennis shoe. While these studies may make intuitive sense, their correlation to clinical practice is unknown. A more practical approach utilizes the same categorization of wounds as described above. *Early presenters* with puncture wounds should have standard wound care, immobilization of the injured structures, and a re-evaluation at 36–48 hours. *Late presenters*, who already have an infection, should be thoroughly re-examined for a nidus of infection and treated with antibiotics. If antibiotics are required, it is then appropriate to consider an antibiotic that covers *Pseudomonas* in cases where the puncture wound occurred through an athletic shoe.

Disposition and transfer

It is important to clearly explain the significant risks of puncture wounds, provide accessible aftercare and follow up, and make sure the patient understands fully the importance. Nearly all routine puncture wounds are typically discharged home with follow up. For those patients where foreign body material is identified, and despite best efforts, can't be fully removed, prompt surgical referral should be made within 24–48 hours. Antibiotic use in these rare instances should be considered in consultation with your surgical referral. All patients should be informed about the possibility for infection and retained foreign body and that the wound may heal with scar and some persistent discomfort.

Box 18.3   Puncture wounds: essential points

- Only a fraction of puncture wounds present to the emergency practitioner.
- The management of these injuries is limited and variable secondary to the relatively small size of the cutaneous opening and the paucity of literature to guide the management.
- Early presentations of *simple* punctures require standard wound care and early follow up.

- The late presentation of infected wounds should raise suspicion for retained foreign body and may require radiographic and wound exploration in addition to antibiotic coverage.

Bites

Introduction

Almost half of all people will receive a mammalian bite within their lifetime, although like puncture wounds, the true incidence is unobtainable due to a substantial number of pet owners managing their bite injuries at home. Despite that, almost 5 million present for emergency care each year; the spectrum of wounds seen range from minor abrasions to fatal injuries. Children are more commonly bitten than adults and the younger the child, the more likely the injury will occur in the head and neck region.[16] Of wounds which present for care, dog bites are most common and typically result from a male dog who has been provoked.[17]

Clinical anatomy and pathophysiology

Bite wounds differ from more commonplace cutaneous injuries in that often these injuries are a mixed presentation of laceration, puncture, and avulsion type wounds. Regardless of the external appearance, almost all of these wounds are crush injuries. A large dog is able to exert a bite force of about 450 pounds per square inch while animals with smaller teeth injure with a pattern more consistent with puncture wounds. Due to the flora of the mammalian mouth, infection is a serious consideration in all bite wounds.

Prehospital

Depending on the circumstances of the bite, the prehospital care may require resuscitative efforts in the manner of multisystem trauma. However, the majority of bite wounds in patients over 5 years of age are located on the extremities and should be managed with prehospital analgesia, control of bleeding, immobility, and, if circumstances permit, early wound cleansing.

Emergency department evaluation and management
Common presentations

Minor bite wounds are seen in every emergency setting and are most often from domesticated animals, frequently living in the same home as the patient, and

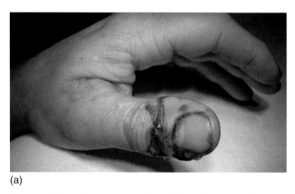

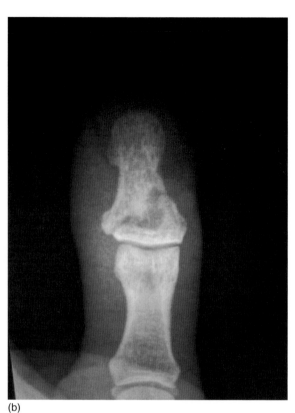

(a)   (b)

Figure 18.9 (a) Dog bite wound and (b) dog bite wound radiograph. Dogs can produce tremendous compressive force with their jaws. This injury should be treated as an open fracture with thorough wound care, pressure irrigation, splinting, and antibiotic treatment.

require similar management as any routine laceration. In addition to the standard historical wound factors ask about the risk factors for infection and rabies, type and breed of animal, who owns the animal, what caused the bite (provoked vs. unprovoked), where the bite geographically occurred, the vaccination and health record for both the patient and the animal involved, and if law enforcement has already been contacted. Some of these historical elements are required by state law to be reported by the provider to animal control authorities, even in what may be a common low-risk injury.

Initial evaluation

The initial evaluation of the bite injury is similar to that of other wounds, but place emphasis on the evaluation of the underlying structures and their function due to the crush and tear mechanism inherent in these wounds. Because of these forces, bite wounds tend to be very painful and thus prompt analgesia via local or peripheral nerve

blocks is in order. As with all other wounds, prompt attention to irrigation is the best practice (Figure 18.9).

Acute interventions

One major pitfall of focusing on the obvious external wounds is not recognizing shock from ongoing hemorrhage or other life or limb threat. The principles of trauma resuscitation should be followed and, if need be, involve your surgical consultants earlier if the need for operative intervention is likely. Control of hemorrhage can be difficult if there are multiple, deep, scattered wounds.

Secondary evaluation

Host factors and wound factors should continue to guide the evaluation and risk stratification of each bite wound as they do for the other types of cutaneous wounds. Due to the crushing force that may have been present, clinicians should have concerns that underlying bones may have been injured.

Table 18.3 Bite wound antimicrobials – options for therapy

Recommended therapy options

Amoxicillin–clavulanate

Second-generation cephalosporin

Penicillin plus first-generation cephalosporin

Penicillin plus dicloxacillin

Penicillin plus trimethoprim–sulfamethoxazole

Penicillin or cephalosporin-allergic patients

Clindamycin plus ciprofloxacin

Additionally, smaller animals (gerbils, cats, etc.) may have had teeth avulsed off into the wound. There should be a clear reason when you do not perform a radiograph. In general these wounds should be X-rayed. Any suspicion for foreign body mandates meticulous inspection of the wound. Crush injury may manifest in neurovascular dysfunction and a full neurovascular exam should be performed. Bites that have occurred over joints may require intra-operative inspection and irrigation if there is evidence that the joint capsule has been violated with a substantial contamination. Special consideration should be given to anyone with a laceration just proximal to the metacarpal phalangeal joint of the hand as this is the characteristic "fight bite" injury of the street pugilist and this wound carries a higher than average likelihood of joint capsule inoculation, extensor tendon injury, and often has a concomitant underlying fracture.

Treatment

Rigorously apply the basic tenets of wound care to bite wounds. Beyond this, bite wounds that present in delayed fashion with evidence of cellulitis or underlying infection are typically infected with *Staphylococcus*, *Streptococcus*, and *Pasteurella* and therefore require antibiotic coverage for polymicrobial bacteria (Table 18.3).[18]

However, there are additional considerations for antibiotics for each presenting case. The literature supports a clear delineation of those bites that present to the ED between cat and dog bites, with a much higher likelihood of cat bites resulting in infection compared to dog bites. Within the subset of dog bites, multiple studies have not shown evidence that antibiotic administration at the time of initial

presentation is beneficial in preventing the development of infection. However, a meta-analysis of 8 prospective trials demonstrated a benefit (relative risk [RR] 0.56) in the pooled data for dog bites in antibiotics preventing infection.[19] Additionally, subset analysis in various trials have shown a trend where bites to the hand ultimately developed less infections if given antibiotics.[20] The overall data suggests that cat bites benefit from antibiotics and dog bites may not as a whole, although some subsets may. Bites from other animals are poorly studied. This includes data relating to human bites where a referral bias exists in that complicated human bites more likely present for care (assaults) than the non-complicated bite (child daycare).[21] In the final recommendation, it is prudent to cover all but the most superficial non-canine bites with antibiotics. Uncomplicated dog bites may be managed based on the location of the wound. Hand bites are appropriate to cover while other locations on the body likely do not benefit from empiric antibiotic therapy.[22] Early treatment (within 3 hours from the time of the bite) lowers the risk, and the ability to ensure close follow up for serial re-examinations (24–36 hours) may prompt a more conservative approach to giving antibiotics. For patients who present in delayed fashion after a bite wound with signs of sepsis, *Capnocytophaga canimorsus* is a cited cause of hemodynamic collapse.[23] Antibiotic administration should aim to cover the various aerobic and anaerobic pathogens. Most commonly, this can be achieved with amoxicillin–clavulanate (Augmentin®). The combination of cephalexin (Keflex®) and dicloxacillin is an effective, low-cost alternative.

Closure of these wounds is often debated. If appropriate wound care is instituted early, and the risk–benefit related to infection and scar formation is clearly outlined to the patient, then the primary closure of non-puncture wounds is warranted – particularly in cosmetically sensitive areas. Deep wounds through multiple tissue planes or into deep compartments may benefit from delayed primary closure. Any additional steps that can be taken to further risk for infection (reduce expedient irrigation, avoiding unnecessary deep sutures) will help mitigate the overall risk.

Finally, considering the high rate of extremity bites, immobilization of the injury part assists in both comfort and healing and should be considered in every injury.

Documentation

The documentation of bite wounds often crosses into the medicolegal realm and therefore, should be descriptive and complete. Depending on state regulations, documentation may be needed to be duplicated for law enforcement (animal control), and sent to enforcement agencies at the time of patient care.

Disposition and transfer

The majority of bite wounds encountered in the ED are able to be managed as outpatients with close follow up. Bite injuries should be re-evaluated in 24–36 hours to ensure that any infectious complications are noted and quickly managed. Bite injuries that occur in patients with significant **host factors** (e.g., immunocompromise, diabetes mellitus, asplenia) and signs of local infection, those patients with signs of systemic infection, and those patients who fail outpatient antibiotic therapy should be admitted. Patients who have life-threatening or cosmetic injuries beyond the capabilities of the initial hospital of presentation should be transferred to a tertiary facility with the appropriate resources.

Box 18.4 Bite wounds: essential points

- Bite wounds have a wide spectrum of injury pattern and a higher than normal risk for infection.
- Despite that, standard wound management practices still provide for the best outcomes and an understanding of the risks relating to infection is necessary to care for and counsel patients.
- Early wound irrigation, the judicious use of antibiotics in select cases, attention to rabies risk and tetanus immunization, and close follow up will result in the best patient outcomes.
- Bites outside the common spectrum of human, dog, cat, and suburban or park denizens may have unique microbial spectrum and standard emergency or infectious disease references should be checked for specific requirements.

Superficial burns

Introduction

Burns represent a large spectrum of disease and at times require specialized care and critical resuscitation. Superficial cutaneous thermal and chemical burns account for almost half-a-million burns seen in EDs annually.[24] Although less common,

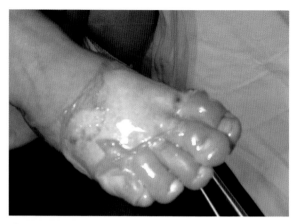

Figure 18.10 Second-degree burn with blistering. In partial thickness burns, the dermis is involved to varying degrees. Superficial involvement of the dermis results in characteristic blistering, often seen at the time of presentation to the emergency department.

chemical burns may present for emergent care. Understanding the presentation, treatment, and disposition of burns is part of trauma management and emergency care.

Clinical anatomy and pathophysiology

Knowledge of the underlying structure of the skin is the foundation for understanding the classifications of burns (Figure 18.1). The most common superficial burns are **first-degree burns** that are limited to the most external portion of the skin – the epidermis. Unless the injury is work related or associated with another emergency presentation, these injuries rarely present for emergency care and are self-limited and can be managed at home (e.g., sunburn). However, the **second-degree burns** that involve the dermal layer are common presentations for emergency care. These injuries are both work and home injuries and are often subcategorized as superficial second-degree burns (e.g., steam burns, scald burns) and deep second-degree burns (e.g., grease burns, ember burns) and involve the superficial layer and the deep layer of the dermis, respectively. The characteristic blisters of the second-degree burn help the clinician rapidly recognize this entity (Figure 18.10). Deeper burns that extend through both the epidermal and dermal layers are categorized as **third-degree burns** and, if underlying structures of muscle, tendon, or bone are involved, these most serious injuries are referred to as **fourth-degree burns**. A further distinction can be made based on the patient's perception of the locally painful first- and second-degree burns and the insensate third and fourth-degree burns. For thermal burns, the hotter the offending agent and the longer the duration of exposure dictate the depth and, therefore, the degree of burn. Chemical burn severity is also related to the potency of the offending agent and duration of exposure. Categorizing the burn is helpful to address specific aspects of management and help with communicating the correct clinical picture for consultants.

Prehospital

For cutaneous burns of significance, burn management begins by addressing the ABCs. Standard, non-life-threatening burn care begins in the prehospital setting with prompt removal of the offending agent. In the case of chemical burns, an identification of the offending agent and, if possible, obtaining the hazardous Material Safety Data Sheet (MSDS) aids the prompt care of the burn. Prompt irrigation of the burned area may also begin in the prehospital setting in all cases except chemical burns caused by elemental material where the addition of water to the chemical reaction might worsen the burn via exothermic reaction (i.e., elemental sodium, potassium, lithium, magnesium, aluminium, and calcium). Finally, the patient's pain should be addressed; prehospital protocols should ensure that this step is not overlooked.

Emergency department evaluation and management

Common presentations

Most commonly, the emergency practitioner will encounter a patient with a household burn that results in a significant superficial second-degree burn. Pain and blistering usually influences patients to seek care. Third- and fourth-degree burns are handled primarily at trauma and burn centers but will occasionally require initial stabilization in the community ED. Chemical burns from industrial work or household hobbies may present at any time, often hours after occurring.

Initial evaluation

The recognition of airway involvement is of primary importance. Due to the nature of the burn and a paucity of symptoms immediately following the incident this may be overlooked. Smoke inhalation, carbon monoxide poisoning, and even cyanide toxicity may be part of the larger clinical picture in the patient with a third-degree burn. Once attention to the ABCs and secondary injury is complete, then address the burn itself.

Acute interventions

As with prehospital intervention, ensuring that the offending agents are correctly identified and have been removed is necessary to halt the burn process. In the case of chemical burns, standard hospital gowns and gloves may not provide a sufficient barrier to many harsh chemicals. Refer to the MSDS when practical for the offending agent before placing yourself or emergency staff at risk for burns. After removal and identification of the source of the burn, irrigation of the affected area and pain management should follow quickly. While irrigating the burn, debris should be removed from the injured skin judiciously. Once primary assessment has completed, the focus of attention should be turned to fluid management to maintain adequate urine output. Cooling the area of the burn with cool water-soaked pads along with elevation of the injured area will help to slow edema formation and inflammation. Exercise caution to avoid hypothermia. Ice may actually worsen the injury if placed directly on the burn or left on for too long even if wrapped. While once advocated, the use of high-dose non-steroidal medications is now not routinely promoted but their value in standard doses for acute pain relief persists.[25]

Secondary evaluation

The secondary evaluation of cutaneous wounds is primarily focused on the search for injured underlying structures and effects on the body relative to the environment in which the burn was sustained (inhalational injury, hypocalcemia, etc.). Typically, most burn care does not require diagnostic testing beyond the occasional need to manage electrolyte balance in the face of fluid resuscitation.

Treatment

Do not underestimate the total body fluid loss with larger areas of tissue destruction from a burn. Formulas and tables exist (Parkland, Galveston, Lund and Browder) to help the clinician quickly assess how much of the total body surface area (TBSA) has been burned and help guide fluid resuscitation. The BSA burned is based on the area of second- and third-degree burns. Both formulas guide fluid replacement for a 24 hour period, where half of the recommended amount is given in the first 8 hours and the remainder given over the later 16 hours to achieve a urine output of 0.5 ml/kg per hour in adults and twice that urine output for children.

Table 18.4 Chemical burns and specific therapies

Formic acid	Bicarbonate administration to counteract acidosis
	Consider hemodialysis
Hydrofluoric acid	Calcium gluconate gel 2.5% superficially
	Calcium gluconate 10% intravenous infiltration
	Calcium gluconate 5% intra-arterial infiltration
Nitrates	Methylene blue for methemoglobinemia
Nitrogen mustards	Prolonged irrigation
	Steroid and antibiotic dressings
Phosphorous	Prolonged irrigation
	5% Sodium bicarbonate and 3% copper sulfate, in 1% hydroxyethyl cellulose

Chemical burns from certain offending agents have specific treatments that merit brief discussion as the toxicity that these chemical convey can be mitigated in certain circumstances (Table 18.4).

After the initial stabilization and acute interventions are underway, apply dressings, both for comfort and to help prevent ongoing external fluid loss. For simple first-degree burns, there is likely no significant advantage to a topical dressing unless patients perceive it as analgesic. Off-the-shelf topical lotions are adequate. For second-degree burns the use of silver sulfadiazine has been advocated, but the literature suggests that it is no more effective than other topical antimicrobials and silver sulfadiazine also carries a risk of skin discoloration.[26] As such, simple moist dressings with topical antimicrobial ointment and a gauze dressing change three to four times a day is preferable and cost-effective.[27] (Prepackaged commercially available dressings are available and may have some benefit for a subset of more serious burns; however, data is limited and the cost of care should be evaluated in select cases of superficially burned patients.)[28] Bedside teaching for blister debridement at home should reinforce that moist gauze and gentle traction is all that is required to remove sloughed skin. Unless burn center referral is arranged, many patients will mange superficial burns locally with their primary physician. Thus, the burden of education may fall on the emergency practitioner and emphasis on pain control, frequent rechecks, signs of infection, and early range of motion are essential. Patients with hand burns may benefit by using nylon gloves as a protective barrier and dressing to allow an early to return to work.

Documentation

Documentation of these wounds is critical for ongoing follow up and referral. With burn care, illustrations and pictures provide the best descriptors of the initial findings.

Disposition and transfer

Burn transfer is highly recommended for centers that are not equipped for the specialized care required for the management of third- and fourth-degree burns. The American Burn Association recommends that certain burns be referred to a burn center (Table 18.5).[29]

These guidelines should be interpreted on an institution specific basis. For emergency practitioners who have limited access to plastic surgery or burn surgery consultants, particularly far from regional centers, management of intermediate type burns can be a challenge. Conservative management via burn center transfer may be warranted unless local physicians are comfortable in following these burns. As an example, near circumferential hand burns in a young patient without significant host factors may not require emergent transfer to a burn center if there are systems in place to ensure that adequate follow up and urgent referral on an as-needed basis is available.

Box 18.5 Burns: essential points

- Cutaneous thermal burns should be managed aggressively with specific attention to pain management, irrigation and cooling, wound dressings, referral to a burn center if the burn is outside the scope of the stabilizing center, and fluid management to ensure against ongoing loss.
- Proper identification of the offending agent with a focus on potentially reversible toxicity is important in the management of chemical burns.
- Regardless of the type of burn, patient education and serial follow up is an important part of ensuring a good outcome.

Table 18.5 American Burn Association Recommendations – Burn Center Referral Guidelines[29]

- Partial thickness burns > 10% total body surface area (TBSA)

- Burns that involve the face, hands, feet, genitalia, perineum, or major joints

- Third-degree burns in any age group

- Electrical burns, including lightning injury

- Chemical burns

- Inhalational injury

- Burn injury in patients with pre-existing medical disorders that could complicate management, prolong recovery, or affect mortality

- Any patient with burns and concomitant trauma (such as fractures) in which the burn injury poses the greatest risk of morbidity or mortality. In such cases, if the trauma poses the greater immediate risk, the patient's condition may be stabilized at the trauma center before the transfer to a burn center

- Burned children in hospitals without qualified personnel or equipment for the care of children

- Burn injury in patients who will require special social, emotional, or rehabilitation intervention

Cutaneous injuries: summary

Restoring the major functions of the body's largest organ (protection and structural integrity, heat exchange, prevention of infection, and tactile interface with the environment) is the overarching tenet of cutaneous injury management. Creating optimal conditions for this to occur is the challenge posed by traumatized patients and regularly met by emergency caregivers.

- See the patient's presentation in its entirety before focusing specifically on wounds.
- Most mistakes are in the evaluation and preparation, not the actual repair.
- Beware of underlying structural injury and retained foreign body.
- Some wounds are better off not being repaired immediately.
- Avulsions, punctures, bites, and burns have mechanism-specific tenets of management.
- Create optimal conditions for wound healing to progress.

References

1. Singer AJ, Hollander JE, Quinn JV. Evaluation and management of traumatic lacerations. *N Engl J Med* 1997;**337**(16):1142–8.

2. Hollander JE, Singer AJ, Valentine SM, et al. Risk factors for infection in patients with traumatic lacerations. *Acad Emerg Med* 2001;**8**(7):716–20.

3. Perelman VS, Francis GJ, Rutledge T, et al. Sterile versus nonsterile gloves for repair of uncomplicated lacerations in the emergency department: a randomized controlled trial. *Ann Emerg Med* 2004;**43**(3):362–70.

4. Denkler K. A comprehensive review of epinephrine in the finger: to do or not to do. *Plast Reconstr Surg* 2001;**108**(1):114–24.

5. Stevenson TR, Thacker JG, Rodeheaver GT, et al. Cleansing the traumatic wound by high pressure syringe irrigation. *JACEP* 1976;**5**(1):17–21.

6. Fernandez R, Griffiths R. Water for wound cleansing. *Cochrane Database Syst Rev* 2008;**1**:CD003861.

7. Dire DJ, Coppola M, Dwyer DA, et al. Prospective evaluation of topical antibiotics for preventing infections in uncomplicated soft-tissue wounds repaired in the ED. *Acad Emerg Med* 1995;**2**(1):4–10.

8. Mustoe TA, Cooter RD, Gold MH, et al. International clinical recommendations on scar management. *Plast Reconstr Surg* 2002;**110**(2):560–71.

9. Baumann LS, Spencer J. The effects of topical vitamin E on the cosmetic appearance of scars. *Dermatol Surg* 1999;**25**(4):311–15.

10. Sullivan D. Wound care: retained foreign bodies and missed tendon injuries. *ED Legal Letter*. 1998; **9**(5):45–6.

11. Quinn J, Cummings S, Callaham M, et al. Suturing versus conservative management of lacerations of the hand: randomised controlled trial. *BMJ* 2002;**325** (7359):299.

12. Trott A. Decisions before closure: timing, débridement, and consultation. In Trott AT (ed.), *Wounds and Lacerations:Emergency Care and Closure*, 3rd edn. Philadelphia, PA: Mosby, 2005: p. 108.

13. Weber EJ, Plantar puncture wounds: a survey to determine the incidence of infection. *J Accid Emerg Med* 1996;**13**(4):274–7.

14. Orlinsky M, Knittle P, Chan L, et al. The comparative accuracy of radiolucent foreign body detection using ultrasonography. *Am J Emerg Med* 2000;**18**(4):401–3.

15. Harrison M, Thomas M. Towards evidence based emergency medicine: best BETs from the Manchester Royal Infirmary. Antibiotics after puncture wounds to the foot. *Emerg Med J* 2002;**19**(1):49.

16. Weiss HB, Friedman DI, Coben JH. Incidence of dog bite injuries treated in emergency departments. *JAMA* 1998;**279**(1): 51–3.

17. Schalamon J, Ainoedhofer H, Singer G, et al. Analysis of dog bites in children who are younger than 17 years. *Pediatrics* 2006;**117**(3):e374–9.

18. Talan DA, Citron DM, Abrahamian FM, et al. Bacteriologic analysis of infected dog and cat bites. Emergency Medicine Animal Bite Infection Study Group. *N Engl J Med* 1999;**340**(2):85–92.

19. Cummings, P. Antibiotics to prevent infection in patients with dog bite wounds: a meta-analysis of randomized trials. *Ann Emerg Med* 1994;**23**(3):535–40.

20. Zubowicz VN, Gravier M. Management of early human bites of the hand: a prospective randomized study. *Plast Reconstr Surg* 1991;**88**(1):111–14.

21. Rittner AV, Fitzpatrick K, Corfield A. Best evidence topic report. Are antibiotics indicated following human bites? *Emerg Med J* 2005; **22**(9):654.

22. Medeiros I, Saconato H. Antibiotic prophylaxis for mammalian bites. *Cochrane Database Syst Rev* 2001; **2**:CD001738.

23. Van der Klooster JM, Grootendorst AF. *Capnocytophaga canimorsus* sepsis in an immune-competent patient: tiny dog, major sepsis. *Neth J Med* 2002;**60**(4):186–7; author reply 8.

24. National Burn Association. *Repository 2007 Report*. Available from http://www.ameriburn.org/ 2007NBRAnnualReport.pdf.

25. Stubhaug A, Romundstad L, Kaasa T, et al. Methylprednisolone and ketorolac rapidly reduce hyperalgesia around a skin burn injury and increase pressure pain thresholds. *Acta Anaesthesiol Scand* 2007;**51**(9):1138–46.

26. Fisher NM, Marsh E, Lazova R. Scar-localized argyria secondary to silver sulfadiazine cream. *J Am Acad Dermatol* 2003;**49**(4):730–2.

27. Ang ES, Lee ST, Gan CS, et al. Evaluating the role of alternative therapy in burn wound management: randomized trial comparing moist exposed burn ointment with conventional methods in the management of patients with second-degree burns. *Med Gen Med* 2001;**3**(2):3.

28. Caruso DM, Foster KN, Blome-Eberwein SA, et al. Randomized clinical study of Hydrofiber dressing with silver or silver sulfadiazine in the management of partial-thickness burns. *J Burn Care Res* 2006; **27**(3):298–309.

29. American College of Surgeons Committee on Trauma. Guidelines for the operation of burn centers. In *Resources for Optimal Care of the Injured Patient 2006*. Chicago, IL: American College of Surgeons, 2006, pp. 79–86.

Soft tissue trauma

Kaushal Shah and Omar Bholat

Introduction

Soft tissue injuries are a very common presentation to the emergency department (ED) and encompass a wide array of traumatic injuries that need to be considered in the acute evaluation. They range from minor contusions and ligamentous injuries to an initially subtle compartment syndrome or dramatic open fractures and vascular injuries that immediately threaten the viability of the limb. The diagnosis can be particularly difficult when the trauma patient presents altered.

Clinical anatomy and pathophysiology

Injury to soft tissue can occur at many levels from superficial lacerations or hematomas to cellular ischemia from arterial injury or compartment syndrome. It is important to understand the underlying pathophysiology of the common injury patterns in order to reverse or mitigate the process.

Compartment syndrome is a rare but serious complication of trauma, surgery, or repetitive muscle overuse that leads to muscle swelling and results in increased pressure within a fascial compartment. As compartment pressure increases, loss of viability of nerve and muscle tissue results. With the death of muscle cells, and the liberation of myoglobin, renal failure can occur. The increased pressure can occur from three mechanisms: increase in content of the compartment, decrease in the volume of the compartment, or external pressure on the compartment. It should be considered in a situation where pain is out of proportion to the exam or paresthesias are present. Although it is more common in the setting of fractures, compartment syndrome can occur with isolated soft tissue trauma; in a study of 164 patients in the United Kingdom, 69% involved a fracture

(half involving the tibial shaft) but 31% had soft tissue injury without a fracture.[1]

> **Box 19.1   Essentials of compartment syndrome[2]**
>
> Causes of compartment syndrome
> - Increased content
> - Trauma – fracture, bleeding, soft tissue swelling
> - Bleeding – vascular injury, coagulation disorder
> - Intensive muscle use – exercise, seizures
> - Burns
> - Snake bites
> - Decreased volume
> - Excessive traction of fractured limbs
> - Closure of facial defects
> - External pressure
> - Restrictive casts, splints, or braces
> - Lying on limb

The most common scenario is traumatic injury causing soft tissue to become more edematous and swollen thereby increasing the content of the compartment and decreasing blood flow. The normal physiologic response to rising intra-compartmental pressure is elevation of the perfusion pressure. However, autoregulatory mechanisms become overwhelmed. Instead, blood flow becomes restricted through several mechanisms: loss of vasomotor tone of arterioles, collapse of thinner-walled veins, and the overall loss of the pressure gradient between the arterial and venous system. In addition, as the tissues become more ischemic, histamine-like substances are released locally that dilate the capillary beds and improve blood flow. Histamine also increases capillary permeability thereby resulting in leakage of fluid and proteins into the soft tissue.[2] The subsequent transudative process leads to an increased concentration of erythrocytes within the capillary bed, increased vascular viscosity, and serves

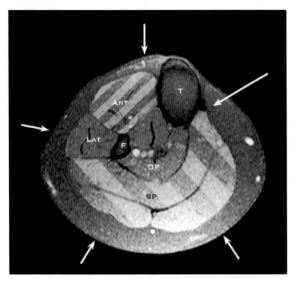

Figure 19.1 Compartments of the lower leg. ANT, anterior compartment; DP, deep posterior compartment; F, fibula bone; LAT, lateral compartment; SP, superficial posterior compartment; T, tibial bone. (From Shah K, Mason C. *Essential Emergency Procedures*. Philadelphia, PA: Lippincott, Williams and Wilkins, 2008: p. 200, with permission.)

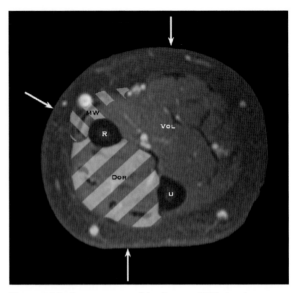

Figure 19.2 Compartments of the forearm. DOR, dorsal compartment; MW, mobile wad; R, radial bone; U, ulna bone; VOL, volar compartment. (From Shah K, Mason C. *Essential Emergency Procedures*. Philadelphia, PA: Lippincott, Williams and Wilkins, 2008: p. 200, with permission.)

to even further decrease microvascular blood flow.[3] The swelling leads to even higher pressures within the fascial compartment. Eventually, blood flow at the level of the arteriole is compromised to the point of ischemia and necrosis of the muscles and nerves in the compartment.[4]

The normal compartment pressure is theoretically zero but the range of normal measurements during the relaxed state is 0–8 mmHg. Capillary perfusion pressure (CPP) is a determinant of tissue perfusion and is measured by subtracting compartment pressure from mean arterial pressure (MAP). The metabolic requirements of myocytes necessitate an oxygen tension of 5–7 mmHg. This requisite is accomplished by maintaining a CPP of 25 mmHg. When the compartment pressure exceeds the diastolic blood pressure, perfusion is certainly compromised and compartment syndrome is inevitable. Although there is individual variability, as a general rule of thumb, when pressures exceed 30 mmHg or when within 30 mmHg of the diastolic pressure, there is a high concern for compartment syndrome. On the other hand, this must also be evaluated in the overall clinical picture, as at least one study has shown that patients clearly without compartment syndrome did not develop it despite these abnormal pressures.[5] It is estimated that muscles and nerves can tolerate ischemia for 4–6 hours without significant

sequelae; after 8 hours, necrosis of tissue is certain and a non-functional limb is likely.[6]

In trauma, the anterior compartment of the leg is the most common location of compartment syndrome; however, it is possible for it to occur in any extremity compartment, including the buttocks.[2] There are four compartments in the lower leg and three compartments in the forearm as depicted by Figure 19.1 and Figure 19.2.

The pathophysiology of *crush injuries* is similar to compartment syndrome. While motor vehicle collisions, pedestrians struck by motor vehicles, and industrial accidents are the most common causes of a crush injury, a large number of life-threatening crush injuries occur as a result of natural disasters. *Crush injury* occurs when a limb is compressed resulting in direct tissue injury and disruption of vascular supply that may lead to tissue necrosis. The cause of the damage is from an external force but the ischemic injury to the limb is due to disruption of blood vessels nourishing the limb. The severity of injury is directly related to the force applied to an extremity and to the degree and duration of the compression. When the external force is removed from the extremity, a cascade of events called "crush syndrome" occurs. The internal components of cells (potassium, calcium, and myoglobin) are liberated into the circulation, fluid is sequestered into the third space, and acidosis occurs from release of lactate and other organic acids.

At the cellular level, mechanical stresses result in disruption of the Na/K pump and an influx of calcium eventually leading to cellular edema and death. The microtrauma results in a decrease in serum calcium and an elevation in all of the following: myoglobin, creatinine kinase, uric acid, potassium, lactic acid, phosphorus, and blood urea nitrogen (BUN). On the clinical level, the patient can develop hypovolemia, shock, compartment syndrome, lactic acidosis, or renal failure from traumatic rhabdomyolysis. While creatine kinase (CK) is used as a marker for the presence of rhabdomyolysis, renal failure occurs when precipitation of the myoglobin molecules occurs within the renal tubules and prevents glomerular filtration.[6]

Open fractures are complex injuries of not only bone but the surrounding neurovascular structures. These fractures require a great deal of force and usually significantly disrupt the original anatomy. The communication with the outside world results in contamination and the gross deformity may result in compromised vascular supply. This combination places the wound at very high risk of infection and wound healing complications. Open fractures almost always occur with high-energy trauma, e.g., motorcycle and motor vehicle accidents or auto vs. pedestrian injuries. Associated injuries to the skull, chest, abdomen, or pelvis are present in 50% of open fracture cases and almost 10% are complicated by compartment syndrome when involving the lower extremity.[2,7,8] The main concerns due to the fracture itself are arterial injury compromising the viability of the extremity and deep tissue and joint space contamination that can lead to long-term complications, such as osteomyelitis. The risk of infection is stratified by the severity of injury. Although the severity of injury is a continuum, Gustilo et al. has established a helpful classification system (Table 19.1).[8,9]

Degloving injuries of the extremities can occur from a variety of traumatic mechanisms. Exposure of the underlying tendons, nerves, and bones can lead to infection, necrosis, and malfunction. The ultimate goal of treatment is coverage of the exposed area with viable skin; however, often initial management is important for long-term return of function and cosmetics.

Ligamentous sprains are extremely common in the emergency setting and can occur at various joints

Table 19.1 Open fracture classification system

	Injury	Risk of infection
I	Puncture wound < 1 cm with minimal contamination or crushing	0–2%
II	Laceration > 1 cm with moderate soft tissue injury	2–10%
IIIA	Extensive soft tissue damage, severe crush component, massive contamination. Bone coverage adequate	10–50%
IIIB	Extensive soft tissue damage with periosteal stripping and exposure. Severe contamination and bone comminution. Flap coverage required	10–50%
IIIC	Arterial injury requiring repair	10–50%

with the ankle, wrist, and knee being the most common. The degree of injury can vary greatly from mild swelling and pain to severe ecchymosis, inability to bear weight, and unstable joints.

Prehospital

Soft tissue injuries are common and occur from a variety of different causes. After scene safety assessment, prehospital providers should always follow the ABC (airway, breathing, circulation) principles without being distracted by significant soft tissue injuries. As part of the circulatory assessment, however, life-threatening exsanguinating external hemorrhage must be managed before the head-to-toe secondary survey. Treatment of active significant bleeding can be achieved with a step-wise approach outlined by Lee and Porter: direct pressure, elevation, wound packing, windlass technique, indirect pressure, and finally a tourniquet, if necessary (see Box 19.2).[10]

Direct pressure and elevation of the limb will usually control most external bleeding. If the wound is large, packing the wound with gauze and applying pressure may be necessary. If blood continues to soak through, a windlass technique can be utilized: tie a large, broad bandage (e.g., crepe bandage) over the packing and insert a pen under the knot; rotate the pen and tighten the bandage until hemorrhage is controlled. If the windlass diminishes distal pulses, it can be loosened until pulses return but the risk is rebleeding. Alternatively, the windlass can simply act as a tourniquet in which case the time of placement should be noted. There are no clear guidelines on how long a tourniquet can be placed on an extremity; the general recommendation is to take them off as soon as possible and should generally not be left in place > 1 hour.

In cases of gross deformity (including open fractures) of an extremity, there are two critical issues for the prehospital provider: hemorrhage control and neurovascular status. The simplest method to reduce hemorrhage from a long bone deformity is to apply traction to gently reduce the deformity and splint the extremity. If there is loss of perfusion to the distal end, manipulation of the deformity can be limb saving. In most instances, simple realignment to neutral position is all that is necessary and can be achieved with axial traction. Frequent neurovascular checks should be performed en route to the hospital.

Degloving injuries or amputations should be handled carefully. Wrapping the exposed extremities in wet gauze (preferably cold saline soaked) and immobilization as necessary (for protection or comfort) is ideal. An amputated finger should be wrapped in wet gauze and placed in a dry plastic bag. The bag should then be placed on ice because 1 hour of warm ischemia is equivalent to 6 hours of cold ischemia.[11]

Analgesia for patient comfort should be considered in all cases. In one study of children with extremity injuries, only 37% received pain medications prior to arrival in the ED; there was no difference in the group that had a fracture or soft tissue injury only.[12] Pain from minor soft tissue injuries may only require oral acetaminophen or ibuprofen to achieve comfort but more serious injuries should receive intravenous (IV) narcotics assuming there are no allergies and the patient is not hemodynamically unstable.

There is controversy whether trauma patients should receive aggressive fluid resuscitation or whether permissive hypotension should be allowed; however, crush soft tissue injuries lead to significant muscle damage with the possibility of subsequent rhabdomyolysis and hyperkalemia. These patients benefit from aggressive fluid resuscitation. Without penetrating trauma or concern for "popping the clot," prehospital providers should administer copious fluids.

Box 19.2 Essential prehospital interventions

Prehospital approach to exsanguination

- Direct pressure
- Elevation
- Wound packing
- Windlass technique
- Indirect pressure
- Tourniquet

Emergency department evaluation and management

Initial presentation

Initial evaluation and management of soft tissue injuries requires the same systematic approach implemented for all trauma patients regardless of whether the patient has a major crush injury or a dramatic degloving injury. Evaluation of ABCs, fluid resuscitation, hemorrhage control, and treatment of life threats should take priority. Address the hypotension with appropriate IV fluids before focusing on the crushed extremity. The leading cause of death after crush injury is hypovolemic shock.[13]

If a trauma patient requires airway management, rapid sequence intubation is the treatment of choice but the commonly used paralytic, succinylcholine, should be avoided in cases of major crush injury because of the possibility of hyperkalemia. The crush injury can cause an up-regulation of the acetylcholine receptor, with increased number, sensitivity, and distribution of receptors, leading to an increase in potassium with succinylcholine administration. While the exact timing is unclear, it seems that it may happen quite early in the patient's course. Hyperkalemia is a contraindication for use of succinycholine. A non-depolarizing neuromuscular blocker should be used instead with a large crush injury.

Hemorrhage control should be via direct pressure. If a bleeding vessel can be identified, it should be isolated and a non-crushing vascular clamp should be utilized to control the bleeding. Blind clamping of bleeding vessels should never be attempted because the likelihood of injuring associated nerves and tendons is high. Angulated or dislocated fractures should be reduced and splinted as soon as possible to decrease hemorrhage and correct any pulse deficits.

In *compartment syndrome*, the initial presentation is also the hallmark presentation: pain in an injured limb that is out of proportion to injury or findings. Patients often describe the pain as "deep," "burning," and "unrelenting" with difficulty in localization. Pain with passive stretching of the muscle groups or tightness of the compartment is also common; the compartment may feel "woody." Fracture blisters are very suggestive of increased compartment pressure but are not consistently present.[6] Paresthesia or decreased sensation in the distribution of the nerves in the compartment is also highly suggestive of increased pressures within the compartment. Symptoms commonly arise within 2 hours of injury but can also present up to 6 days later.[14]

The clinical presence of the five "Ps" (pain, pallor, pulselessness, paresthesias, and paralysis) early in the course should be attributed to **arterial injury** and not compartment syndrome. Compartment syndrome presents with pain first and foremost. The other findings of pallor, paresthesias, paralysis, and pulselessness are late findings.

In limb trauma, it is important to evaluate capillary refill time, temperature and color of skin, and presence or absence of distal pulses, as they may indicate reduced arterial flow and possible vascular trauma. An arterial injury should be suspected when there are weak or no palpable pulses in the traumatized extremity or significant asymmetry with the contralateral side. If there is any ambiguity, a Doppler pulse exam is more reliable. If there is gross deformity of the limb, manipulation to reduce the limb to anatomic position should be performed immediately. This may relieve the compression on the artery with return of circulation.

Rarely, in cases of major **crush injury**, patients can present with cardiac arrhythmias or even cardiac arrest due to elevated potassium levels. Assessing the heart rhythm with an electrocardiogram (ECG) and obtaining a stat potassium level with arterial blood should be considered. Alternatively, administering calcium empirically in treating the arrest is appropriate.

Secondary evaluation

A thorough evaluation of the neurovascular status of the injured or crushed limb is important and serial exams are often warranted. A delay in the diagnosis of vessel and nerve injury or compartment syndrome may lead to poor outcomes for the limb and the patient. If the pulses are not immediately palpable, use a Doppler and compare to the opposite limb.

Compartment syndrome is a complication of trauma with serious consequences; a delay in diagnosis

Table 19.2 Findings in lower leg compartment syndrome

General findings

Pain out of proportion to injury

Analgesia use out of proportion to injury

Anterior compartment

Weakness of toe extension

Pain on passive toe flexion

Diminished sensation in the first web space

Deep posterior compartment

Weakness of ankle inversion and toe flexion

Pain on passive toe extension referred to the posterior leg

Diminished sensation over medial sole of foot

correlates directly with worse outcomes. For this reason, compartment pressures should be measured in all cases where history and physical exam are suggestive of compartment syndrome. Pain out of proportion to expectation and increasing use of analgesia out of proportion to expectation for the injury should immediately raise the suspicion of compartment syndrome. It is important to note that compartment syndrome can occur when the compartment is open, such as open fractures and stab wounds.[15] Table 19.2 describes the physical findings consistent with the most common site of compartment syndrome, the lower leg.

Commercially available devices exist (e.g., Stryker) that accurately measure pressures. If the index of suspicion is high but the number is less than expected, consider serial measurements. Doppler ultrasound of the extremity is not indicated because arterial blood flow can appear normal in cases of clear compartment syndrome. Orthopedic consultation is also recommended in cases of elevated compartment pressures or cases that are concerning.

There is no blood or radiologic test to diagnose compartment syndrome. Necrotic muscle tissue will produce lactic acid and creatinine phosphokinase but these are not specific and they are late findings. The physician must rely on clinical judgment.

The treatment goal of compartment syndrome is the immediate relief of the pressure. This starts with removing any constricting devices, bandages, or casts followed by definitive treatment with fasciotomy of all

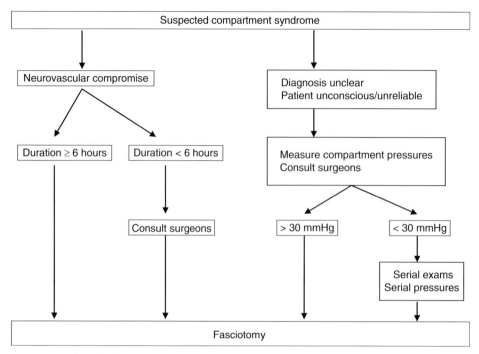

Figure 19.3 Algorithm for suspected compartment syndrome.

involved compartments if necessary. This is generally done in the operating room (OR).

When there are clear clinical findings (i.e., neurovascular compromise) in suspected compartment syndrome, and the duration of compartment syndrome with deficit is > 6 hours and rapid subspecialty consultation is not available or requires transfer, the emergency physician should optimally perform the limb-saving procedure in the ED. If the compartment syndrome is < 6 hours, it is reasonable to consult the orthopedic and trauma surgeons or perform a transfer to facilitate a controlled fasciotomy in the OR. When the diagnosis is unclear or the patient is unconscious or unreliable, it is advisable to measure compartment pressures and consult the appropriate surgeons. An algorithm for treatment of suspected compartment syndrome is shown in Figure 19.3.

Although the initial instinct is to elevate the limb to reduce swelling prior to surgery, it is not advisable. Raising the limb above the heart decreases perfusion without decreasing compartment pressures; one study found that, for each centimeter of leg elevation, there is a 0.8 mmHg drop in arterial pressure.[16] Neutral elevation, i.e., at the level of the heart., is the preferred position.

In addition to a rapid diagnosis and facilitating OR fasciotomy within 6 hours, ideally, or performing emergent fasciotomy, the emergency physician should administer timely prophylactic antibiotics and analgesia. Prophylactic antibiotics have been promoted as appropriate, however, the necessity of antibiotics is based predominantly on expert opinion, and has not been rigorously studied. Inpatient post-fasciotomy management includes continued debridement of necrotic tissue, monitoring renal function, continuing antibiotics and analgesia, and considering skin flaps or grafts. Delay in treatment can lead to permanent nerve damage, myonecrosis, and muscle contractures.

Box 19.3 Essential ED interventions for compartment syndrome

- Rapid diagnosis of compartment syndrome
- Remove casts and occlusive dressings
- Place extremity in neutral position
- Prophylactic antibiotics
- Analgesia
- Emergent fasciotomy or facilitating OR fasciotomy
- Inpatient post-fasciotomy care
- Debridement
- Monitoring renal function
- Continued antibiotics and analgesia
- Considering skin flaps or grafts

Crush injuries can result in "crush syndrome" or damage to bones, muscle, nerves, and vascular structures. These should all be assessed carefully, especially when the patient is unconscious or has altered mental status.

The "crush syndrome" comprises all the problems that arise as a result of a crush injury. These are typically categorized into electrolyte abnormalities, metabolic acidosis, and rhabdomyolysis. The serum potassium, calcium, phosphate, and uric acid should be tested for possible hyperkalemia, hypocalcemia, hyperphosphatemia, and hyperuricemia that results from massive cellular damage. Hypoperfusion and cellular starvation result in a metabolic acidosis and elevation in lactic acid. An initial and serial lactate levels have been demonstrated to be diagnostic and prognostic in traumatic injuries.[17,18] Massive muscle damage results in release of myoglobin into the circulation; the surrogate marker tested to assess the extent of muscle damage is the creatinine phosphokinase (CPK). The biggest concern of the circulating large myoglogin molecules is disruption of the renal filtration system. Rhabdomyolysis can cause acute renal failure in up to 40% of patients with crush injuries.[19] Although a CPK level is not routinely obtained in victims of trauma, it is very helpful to stratify injury severity in crush injuries.[13] Serial CPK measurements can be monitored to determine improvement or worsening of rhabdomyolysis. The primary reason for the use of CPK as a surrogate for the presence of crush syndrome is that a serum myoglobin cannot be obtained rapidly in the clinical arena. Clinically, its presence can be determined indirectly. Myoglobin in the urine will be detected as "blood" on the urine dipstick but there will be no red blood cells noted on the urine analysis; this should also suggest the diagnosis of possible rhabdomyolysis if not initially considered.

Box 19.4 Crush injury evaluation

- "Crush syndrome" evaluation
- Electrolyte abnormalities
- Metabolic acidosis
- Rhabdomyolysis and acute renal failure
- Orthopedic
- Plain radiographs
- Muscular
- Compartment syndrome evaluation
- Peripheral nerve injury
- Arterial injury

- Hard and soft signs
- Ankle–brachial index (ABI)
- Duplex ultrasound
- Computed tomography angiography (CTA)
- Arteriography

Crush injury treatment is multifaceted. It entails addressing metabolic, orthopaedic, and neurovascular issues while simultaneously trying to prevent the sequelae of rhabdomyolysis and compartment syndrome. The majority of the metabolic derangements can be addressed with IV fluid hydration; it will address the hypoperfusion, reduce the lactic acidosis, and flush out the myoglobin and CPK. Consider placement of a Foley catheter to monitor urine output carefully. Low urine output suggests ongoing hypovolemia or acute renal failure.

If rhabdomyolysis develops, early hydration is the key to prevent or lessen the severity of acute renal failure;[20] the earlier the IV fluid resuscitation, the better the outcome.[21,22] In severe cases of rhabdomyolysis with crush injury it may be necessary to administer both blood products and IV fluids to affectively address a patient's hypovolemia.[23,24] Sodium bicarbonate is often used to alkalinize the urine to prevent the breakdown of myoglobin into its nephrotoxic metabolites (i.e., ferrihemate).[20,25] Sodium bicarbonate can be administered by adding one ampule to 1 L ½ NS or 2–3 ampules in 1 L D5W and infuse at a rate of 100 ml/h. The urine pH should be maintained at a level > 6.5 while the plasma pH should be kept between 7.4 and 7.45 to help prevent acute renal failure.[25,26] Alkaline urine with a pH of 7.0 or higher also reduces the crystallization of uric acid, decreasing damage to renal tubules.[27] This therapy is still controversial as there are those who argue against the alkalinization of urine.[28,29] Knochel argues that the large volume of infused crystalloid alkalinizes the urine sufficiently, and that the amount of added sodium bicarbonate needed to reach the suggested urine pH of 6.5 or greater is so large that it will increase hypocalcemia, and can cause more harm than benefit to the patient.[30]

There are no large, randomized trials to demonstrate that alkalinization of urine is better than early, aggressive hydration for the treatment of rhabdomyolysis.

The increase in serum potassium is most severe in the first 12–36 hours after muscle injury. Life-threatening hyperkalemia must be addressed quickly and effectively. Hyperkalemic cardiac arrest contributes to a large percentage of early deaths in crush injury patients.[31] The ECG should guide the clinician's decision to begin emergent administration of serum potassium lowering agents. Classic signs of hyperkalemia on ECG are peaked T waves, widened QRS complexes and flattened p waves; with rising potassium levels, these changes continue until the ECG looks like a sinusoidal wave followed by cardiac arrest. Calcium administration to stabilize the cardiac membranes is first-line treatment for severe hyperkalemia with ECG changes. However, in the setting of hyperphosphatemia that may be present in rhabdomyolysis, IV calcium may be less effective as it may bind to extracellular phosphate leading to metastatic calcification.[32] Temporary reduction in the potassium can be achieved with IV insulin with glucose, IV sodium bicarbonate, and inhaled beta-2 agonists, all of which act to drive extracellular potassium into the intracellular compartment. Kayexalate given by mouth or per rectum will remove the potassium from circulation but will take many hours. If hyperkalemia persists despite these treatments, emergent dialysis will be necessary.

Plain radiographs are essential for diagnosis of underlying fractures. The degree of damage to bone will also provide a qualitative assessment of the magnitude of the forces that caused the injury. Comminuted, displaced, and *open fractures* usually require a significant mechanism of injury. Wounds in the vicinity of a fracture should be considered an "open fracture" until proven otherwise. In cases of a clear open fracture (e.g., bone visibly protruding through soft tissue), arterial flow to the distal extremity should be checked and dislocations should be reduced as soon as possible. Wound cultures prior to debridement are not necessary as they have been found to have low predictive value.[33] Compartment syndrome can occur with open fractures as well; in one series, compartment syndrome was more common with open than closed fractures.[34] This reflects the fact that a great amount of energy/force is necessary to cause an open fracture leading to significant soft tissue trauma in addition to a fracture.

A thorough sensory and motor exam is all that is necessary to identify a peripheral nerve injury. Further evaluation depends on the suspected cause. Closed crushed nerve injuries without suspicion of compartment syndrome do not require immediate evaluation by the specialist. Serial exams should be performed and documented. The majority of these cases have recovery of nerve function within 3 months. If the nerve injury is complete and associated with a laceration or open wound, surgical consultation in the ED or within 12–24 hours for exploration is recommended. If partial or a minor sensory issue, early follow up within the week would be appropriate.

Management of the orthopedic issues is based on the plain radiographs. If the fracture is dislocated or significantly displaced, it should be reduced. Reduction of a dislocated joint or an angulated fracture will likely reduce the bleeding and eliminate the secondary insult to the crushed limb. Open fractures involve significant displacement of bone and injury to the soft tissue that is very painful; IV analgesia is often necessary and should be given early. In hypotensive patients, fentanyl may be the most appropriate choice. The fracture/dislocation should be reduced and placed in a splint as soon as possible to reduce the amount of bleeding and pain. If there is any hypoperfusion of the extremity or concern for arterial injury, the fracture/dislocation should be reduced emergently. Open dislocations with gross contamination and intact pulses should have thorough irrigation and reduction of the joint in the OR. If a significant delay to the OR is anticipated (e.g., transfer to specialty care is required), risk–benefit analysis of early reduction of the joint should be discussed with the orthopedic consultant. Broad spectrum IV antibiotics should be started in the ED; early administration (within 3 hours) of cephalosporins has been demonstrated to reduce the infection rate significantly.[35] Betadine at full strength should not be instilled into the wound. Gentle cleansing with saline may be appropriate in the ED. Tetanus toxoid is the standard treatment for patients who have completed the primary tetanus immunization series. Those who have not received the series should receive the tetanus immune globulin in addition to the toxoid.

Box 19.5 Essential treatment of open fractures in the ED

- Analgesia
- Reduction of the fracture/dislocation
- Antibiotics intravenously
- Tetanus prophylaxis
- Orthopedic consultation
- Surgical open fracture treatment

- Irrigation and debridement
- Wound closure
- Soft tissue reconstruction
- Fracture stabilization
- Secondary procedures: bone grafting to stimulate healing

Open fractures do not require immediate attention unless there is an associated pulse deficit. In this scenario the deformity is likely compressing arterial flow. Immediate reduction to the anatomical position in an attempt to improve perfusion to the limb is necessary. If the pulse does not return to normal, an arterial injury should be suspected.

If an *arterial injury* is suspected, the initial goals of the emergency physician are to diagnose the injury by considering the "hard" and "soft" signs (see Box 19.6) and consult the appropriate surgeons to perform the arterial repair. Given that pulses can be maintained in 42% of arterial injuries and no arterial injury is found in up to 27% of cases with no palpable pulse, the consulting surgeon may prefer to have an arteriogram to locate and define the injury before operating.[36] "Proximity wounds" defined as wounds within 1 cm or 1 inch of a major vessel was once thought to require further investigation; however, without soft or hard findings of arterial injury, arteriography is likely negative when the sole indication is "proximity wound."

Patients with hard findings almost always require surgical exploration; if the ischemic time is minimal, preoperative arteriography is reasonable. There are many more options for evaluation of limbs with soft findings: ABI, duplex ultrasound, or CTA. The ABI index is determined by checking the pulse pressure of the injured lower extremity with that of the upper extremity. First, record the highest Doppler sound of the brachial pulse present in the arms or comparing it to the highest Doppler sound of the posterior tibial or dorsalis pedis artery. The ankle Doppler pressure is then divided by the brachial Doppler pressure to calculate the index. An ABI of < 0.9 or a difference between two sides is considered abnormal.[37] A normal ABI, on the other hand, is good for ruling out a lesion. Duplex ultrasound detects both venous and arterial blood flow and can be performed at the bedside. This has clear advantages in significant trauma situations where the patient may be unstable or is actively being resuscitated. Transport outside of the emergency room or intensive care unit is fraught with risk. The overall use of multislice CTA has increased tremendously over the last decade and is now showing promise for detection of arterial injury. Busquets et al. found no missed injuries in their study of 97 CTAs,[38] and Inaba et al. reported 100% sensitivity and specificity in their retrospective review of CTAs for penetrating arterial injury.[39]

Contrast arteriography is the gold standard imaging evaluation of potential arterial injury. It can detect the exact location and type of injury. However, it is not without risk. The procedure is invasive, requires contrast dye, and cannot be done at the bedside. It is also more costly than the alternative modalities.

Two special circumstances in potential arterial injuries are shotgun wounds and knee dislocations. Given the nature of shotgun wounds (multiple missiles in various trajectories), there should be a low threshold for arteriography to rule out arterial injury. The same was once true for knee dislocations. Given the likelihood of popliteal injury and the associated morbidity (i.e., amputation) of a missed popliteal injury in the setting of a knee dislocation, routine arteriography was once advocated; however, a selective approach is now considered reasonable. Physical exam with ABI and Doppler ultrasound are sensitive tests to determine which patients need immediate angiography.[40] Computed tomography angiography is also being utilized more frequently in place of contrast angiography.

> **Box 19.6 Findings in arterial injury**
>
> **Hard findings of arterial injury**
> - Pulsatile or rapidly expanding hematoma
> - Obvious pulsatile arterial bleeding
> - Bruit or thrill with arterial palpation
> - 5 "Ps" of arterial insufficiency: pulseless, pallor, pain, paresthesia, paralysis
>
> **Soft findings of arterial injury**
> - Diminished pulse compared to opposite limb
> - Delayed capillary refill
> - Isolated peripheral nerve injury
> - Non-pulsatile, stable hematoma

Management of potential *arterial injuries* is stratified into two pathways based on the physical exam. If there are "hard signs" of arterial injury, an

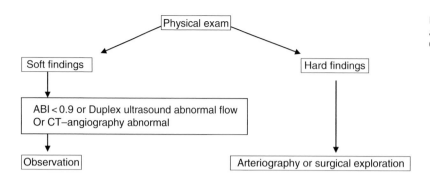

Figure 19.4 Extremity arterial injury algorithm. ABI, Ankle–Brachial Index; CT, computed tomography.

emergent vascular surgery consultation is necessary for exploration and repair. The surgeons may opt for a preoperative arteriogram but surgical exploration is virtually inevitable. If there are "soft signs" of arterial injury, further imaging is usually necessary to determine the need for arteriography or surgical exploration. The four main options are: determination of an ABI, color-flow Doppler ultrasound, or CTA or conventional angiography. The choice is dependent on where the injury lies, the availability of tests, stability of the patient, and surgeon preference

In one study of 100 consecutive injured limbs in 93 trauma victims, ABI was calculated but only contrast arteriography was used in clinical decision making.[41] An ABI < 0.90 had a sensitivity of 87% and a specificity of 97% compared to arteriography; when compared with clinical outcome, sensitivity and specificity rose to 95% and 97%.[41]

Based on these numbers, it is reasonable to rely on ABI in the absence of obvious signs of arterial injury when assessing a traumatized extremity. Duplex ultrasound, if available, can be used reliably to rule in and rule out arterial injury when soft findings are present (Figure 19.4).

Degloving injuries of the extremities require a thorough evaluation of the underlying structures. If possible, evaluate the degree of perfusion and distal sensation. Plain films to assess for fractures and foreign bodies should be obtained as soon as possible. Immediate consultation with an orthopedist or hand surgeon is of utmost importance because mobilization of the appropriate resources is critical for potential limb salvage.[42] Degloving injuries should be treated as a surgical emergency. After radiographs are obtained, cover the limb with saline-soaked gauze and splint for comfort. The patient should receive IV antibiotics depending on the nature, severity, and timing of the injury. If there is any likelihood of bacterial contamination (i.e., dirty wound or delay in presentation to the ED > 6 hours), antibiotics should be given prophylactically. Administer tetanus toxoid as appropriate.

In the setting of significant soft tissue injuries, the diagnosis of **ligamentous sprain** or soft tissue strain is one of exclusion. If there is edema and/or ecchymosis without an underlying fracture or signs of compartment syndrome or crush injury, a ligamentous injury should be suspected and treated appropriately. The severity of ligamentous injuries are graded by the degree (e.g., mild, moderate, or severe) of edema/ecchymosis and laxity of the joint on exam. Table 19.3 is provided as an example of sprain severity classification with regard specifically to the ankle joint.

Ligamentous sprains and muscle strains should be treated with analgesia (oral ibuprofen, acetaminophen, or IV or IM ketorolac are appropriate in the ED). Opioids may be necessary. It was shown in one study that patients with non-fracture soft tissue injuries are less likely to receive appropriate analgesia in the ED, although the pain scores were similar to those with fractures.[43] The general management is often remembered by the "*RICE*" mnemonic: *r*est and avoid re-injury which may entail use of crutches or splints; *i*ce the injury for 20 minutes 3–4 times per day for the first day to reduce swelling; *c*ompress with an elastic ACE wrap or brace to reduce swelling and pain; *e*levate the extremity as often as possible to reduce swelling. As an example, Table 19.3 describes the management of ankle sprains based on the grade of the injury. If serious ligamentous injury is suspected, resulting in joint laxity (i.e., Grade II and higher sprains), more rigid splinting methods should be considered.

Table 19.3 Classification of ankle sprains

Severity	Symptoms	Signs	Examination	Treatment
Grade I	Mild pain and swelling, able to bear weight	Slight edema	Negative anterior drawer and talar tilt	RICE* and referral to primary care physician in 1 week
Grade II	Moderate pain and swelling, difficulty bearing weight	Moderate edema and ecchymosis	Positive anterior drawer (4–14 mm) and talar tilt test (5–15°)	Rigid splint and referral to orthopedist in a week
Grade III	Severe pain and swelling, inability to bear weight	Severe edema and ecchymosis	Positive anterior (> 15 mm) and tilt test (> 15°)	Rigid splint and referral to orthopedist within a week

*Rest, ice, compressive dressing, and elevation.

Documentation

Documentation is always important. The most import-ant piece of information to document in cases of soft tissue injury is the neurovascular exam. Whether the patient had perfusion, sensation, or function when you evaluated the patient is an important piece of data. Documentation of serial exams is likewise important.

Even if you do everything a reasonable clinician would do, there will be a certain small number of patients that will develop cellulitis, compartment syn-drome, increased pain, deep venous thrombosis, or ischemia after you have discharged the patient or transferred care to a primary care or specialist phys-ician. Proper documentation is the best way to prove that the standard of care was met.

Disposition

The disposition of most of the serious soft tissue injuries (compartment syndrome, crush injury, open fractures, arterial injury, and degloving injury) is admission to the hospital for continued care or obser-vation. In fact, many of these injuries often cross multiple medical disciplines. It is advisable for the emergency physician to enlist the help of the any necessary consultants: orthopedic surgeons, trauma surgeons, vascular surgeons, burn care specialists, and intensivists.

Injuries resulting in a significantly swollen limb without a fracture may be considered for discharge home, but with several caveats: clear instructions should be provided and understood and the patient must be able to follow up appropriately. Acute compartment syndrome as well as muscle necrosis can occur, and there is usually a greater delay to definitive treatment (i.e., fasciotomy).[44] These patients should have close follow up assured.

Patients with suspected crush injury and rhabdo-myolysis should be admitted for continued IV hydra-tion, management of complications, and any necessary treatment of the underlying etiology. If there are significant complications or metabolic derangements, admission to an intensive care bed is advisable. A nephrology consult is indicated if there are signs of acute renal failure or a need for dialysis.

Patients with open fractures need admission to the hospital for IV antibiotics and possible irrigation and debridement in the OR.

Suspected arterial injury evaluation is not an out-patient process. These patients should be evaluated in the hospital. If the complete evaluation cannot be done from the ED, the patient should be admitted to the hospital. Patients found to have no injuries may be discharged home safely but should be given instructions for follow-up care and clear instructions on when to return to the ED.

Patients with ligamentous sprains can be dis-charged home but should have appropriate follow up in about a week. Although pain, swelling, and the ability to ambulate should improve with time, occult fractures and high-grade sprains may require further orthopedic, rehabilitation, or sports medicine care including surgical treatment. Other indications for orthopedic referral include: (1) a "pop" that is heard or felt; (2) a history of several previous injuries; (3) persistent focal tenderness; (4) a positive stress test of the joint; and (5) Grade II and higher sprains

357

in children with open growth plates.[11] In children, less force is required to sustain a Salter–Harris I fracture than is required to tear a ligament. Thus, any child who is suspected of having a significant ankle sprain and no clear fracture on X-ray should be splinted and referred to an orthopedic surgeon for follow up.

References

1. McQueen MM, Gaston P, Court-Brown CM. Acute compartment syndrome. Who is at risk? *J Bone Joint Surg Br* 2000;**82**(2):200–3.

2. Geiderman JM. General principles of orthopedic injuries. In Marx JA (ed.), *Rosen's Emergency Medicine*, 6th edn.St. Louis: Mosby, 2006: pp. 549–76.

3. Haller P. Compartment syndromes. In Tintinalli J, Kelan G, Stapczynski J (eds), *Emergency Medicine, A Comprehensive Study Guide*, 4th edn. New York: McGraw Hill, 2004: pp. 1746–9.

4. Slater MS, Mullins RJ. Rhabdomyolysis and myoglobinuric renal failure in trauma and surgical patients: a review. *J Am Coll Surg* 1998;**186**(6):693–716.

5. Prayson MJ, Chen JL, Hampers D, et al. Baseline compartment pressure measurements in isolated lower extremity fractures without clinical compartment syndrome. *J Trauma* 2006;**60**(5):1037–40.

6. Newton EJ, Love J. Acute complications of extremity trauma. *Emerg Med Clin North Am* 2007; **25**(3):751–61, iv.

7. Blick SS, Brumback RJ, Poka A, Burgess AR, Ebraheim NA. Compartment syndrome in open tibial fractures. *J Bone Joint Surg Am.* 1986;**68**(9):1348–53.

8. Zalavras CG, Patzakis MJ, Holtom PD, Sherman R. Management of open fractures. *Infect Dis Clin North Am* 2005;**19**(4):915–29.

9. Gustilo RB, Anderson JT. Prevention of infection in the treatment of 1025 open fractures of long bones: retrospective and prospective analyses. *J Bone Joint Surg Am* 1976;**58**(4):453–8.

10. Lee C, Porter KM. Prehospital management of lower limb fractures. *Emerg Med J* 2005;**22**(9):660–3.

11. Kazzi Z, Langdorf MI. *Replantation*. Available from http://www.emedicine.com/emerg/topic502.htm.

12. Rogovik AL, Goldman RD. Prehospital use of analgesics at home or en route to the hospital in children with extremity injuries. *Am J Emerg Med* 2007;**25**(4):400–5.

13. Malinoski DJ, Slater MS, Mullins RJ. Crush injury and rhabdomyolysis. *Crit Care Clin* 2004;**20**(1):171–92.

14. Siefert JA. Acute compartment syndrome. In Wolfson AB (ed.), *Clinical Practice of Emergency Medicine*.

15. Philadelphia, PA: Lippincott, Williams and Wilkins; 2005: pp. 1109–12.

15. Gillooly JJ, Hacker A, Patel V. Compartment syndrome as a complication of a stab wound to the thigh: a case report and review of the literature. *Emerg Med J* 2007;**24**(11):780–1.

16. Matsen FA, 3rd, Wyss CR, Krugmire RB, Jr., Simmons CW, King RV. The effects of limb elevation and dependency on local arteriovenous gradients in normal human limbs with particular reference to limbs with increased tissue pressure. *Clin Orthop Relat Res* 1980;**150**:187–95.

17. Baron BJ, Sinert RH, Sinha AK, et al. Effects of traditional versus delayed resuscitation on serum lactate and base deficit. *Resuscitation* 1999; **43**(1):39–46.

18. Abramson D, Scalea TM, Hitchcock R, et al. Lactate clearance and survival following injury. *J Trauma* 1993;**35**(4):584–8; discussion 8–9.

19. Gonzalez D. Crush syndrome. *Crit Care Med* 2005; **33**(1 Suppl.):S34–41.

20. Bonventre J, Shah S, Walker P, Humphreys M. Rhabdomyolysis-induced acute renal failure. In Jacobson HR, Striker GE, Klahr S (eds), *The Principles and Practice of Nephrology*, 2nd edn. St Louis: Mosby, 1995: pp. 569–73.

21. Abassi ZA, Hoffman A, Better OS. Acute renal failure complicating muscle crush injury. *Semin Nephrol* 1998;**18**(5):558–65.

22. Shimazu T, Yoshioka T, Nakata Y, et al. Fluid resuscitation and systemic complications in crush syndrome: 14 Hanshin-Awaji earthquake patients. *J Trauma* 1997;**42**(4):641–6.

23. Knochel JP. Pigment nephropathy. In Greenberg A (ed.), *Primer on Kidney Diseases*, 2nd edn. Boston: Academic Press, 1998: pp. 273–6.

24. Russell TA. Acute renal failure related to rhabdomyolysis: pathophysiology, diagnosis, and collaborative management. *Nephrol Nurs J.* 2000; **27**(6):567–75; quiz 76–7.

25. Ron D, Taitelman U, Michaelson M, et al. Prevention of acute renal failure in traumatic rhabdomyolysis. *Arch Intern Med* 1984;**144**(2):277–80.

26. Richards JR. Rhabdomyolysis and drugs of abuse. *J Emerg Med* 2000;**19**(1):51–6.

27. Mallinson RH, Goldsmith DJ, Higgins RM, Venning MC, Ackrill P. Acute swollen legs due to rhabdomyolysis: initial management as deep vein thrombosis may lead to acute renal failure. *BMJ* 1994;**309**(6965):1361–2.

28. Knochel JP. Rhabdomyolysis and myoglobinuria. *Annu Rev Med* 1982;**33**:435–43.

29. Knottenbelt JD. Traumatic rhabdomyolysis from severe beating–experience of volume diuresis in 200 patients. *J Trauma* 1994;**37**(2):214–19.

30. Knochel JP. Neuromuscular manifestations of electrolyte disorders. *Am J Med* 1982;**72**(3):521–35.

31. Better OS, Stein JH. Early management of shock and prophylaxis of acute renal failure in traumatic rhabdomyolysis. *N Engl J Med* 1990;**322**(12):825–9.

32. Visweswaran P, Guntupalli J. Rhabdomyolysis. *Crit Care Clin* 1999;**15**(2):415–28, ix-x.

33. Zalavras CG, Patzakis MJ. Open fractures: evaluation and management. *J Am Acad Orthop Surg* 2003;**11**(3):212–19.

34. DeLee JC, Stiehl JB. Open tibia fracture with compartment syndrome. *Clin Orthop Relat Res* 1981;**160**:175–84.

35. Patzakis MJ, Harvey JP, Jr., Ivler D. The role of antibiotics in the management of open fractures. *J Bone Joint Surg Am* 1974;**56**(3):532–41.

36. Fields CE, Latifi R, Ivatury RR. Brachial and forearm vessel injuries. *Surg Clin North Am* 2002;**82**(1):105–14.

37. Hood DB, Weaver FA, Yellin AE. Changing perspectives in the diagnosis of peripheral vascular trauma. *Semin Vasc Surg* 1998;**11**(4):255–60.

38. Busquets AR, Acosta JA, Colon E, Alejandro KV, Rodriguez P. Helical computed tomographic angiography for the diagnosis of traumatic arterial injuries of the extremities. *J Trauma* 2004;**56**(3):625–8.

39. Inaba K, Potzman J, Munera F, et al. Multi-slice CT angiography for arterial evaluation in the injured lower extremity. *J Trauma* 2006;**60**(3):502–6; discussion 6–7.

40. Treiman GS, Yellin AE, Weaver FA, et al. Examination of the patient with a knee dislocation. The case for selective arteriography. *Arch Surg* 1992;**127**(9):1056–62; discussion 62–3.

41. Lynch K, Johansen K. Can Doppler pressure measurement replace "exclusion" arteriography in the diagnosis of occult extremity arterial trauma? *Ann Surg* 1991;**214**(6):737–41.

42. Adani R, Castagnetti C, Landi A. Degloving injuries of the hand and fingers. *Clin Orthop Relat Res* 1995;**314**:19–25.

43. Pines JM, Perron AD. Oligoanalgesia in ED patients with isolated extremity injury without documented fracture. *Am J Emerg Med* 2005;**23**(4):580.

44. Hope MJ, McQueen MM. Acute compartment syndrome in the absence of fracture. *J Orthop Trauma* 2004;**18**(4):220–4.

Phillip L. Rice, Jr. and Jonathan S. Gates

Introduction

Penetrating extremity vascular trauma comprise a minority of traumatic injuries in the civilian population; however, the morbidity can be serious. A higher proportion of these injuries in an urban environment are due to penetrating trauma than is seen in the rural setting. In military trauma, 54% of penetrating injuries are extremity wounds, mainly caused by explosive devices. The higher percentage in extremities are presumably due to the protective effects of body armor which leave exposed the face, neck, and extremities.[1] Deaths due to extremity vascular trauma still do occur, either directly from the injury or indirectly (renal failure from rhabdomyolysis and sepsis). Deaths due directly from the vascular injury are usually from exanguination and coagulopathy secondary to blood loss. Morbidity due to vascular injuries can result from delayed identification and diagnosis, resulting in thrombosis and ischemia of the extremity.

Death from vascular extremity trauma catches the attention of many due to the conception that it should always be preventable. Death from exanguination of an extremity seems very treatable, either from refined surgical technique or by cruder methods such as tourniquets. Once the bleeding has been controlled, resuscitation measures should keep the patient alive with definitive management to follow. Although this theoretically makes sense, there continue to be deaths from either exsanguination when the bleeding is not controlled rapidly enough or sepsis, often after multisystem dysfunction from prolonged hypoperfusion due to these injuries.

The evolution in the evaluation of vascular trauma over the last 10 years has centered on imaging. Initially angiography was the cornerstone of the evaluation; however, this was time and resource intensive and required coordination between the vascular surgeon and interventionalist.[2] Newer modalities, which are non-invasive and faster, are replacing angiography in certain cases.

Anatomy and pathophysiology

Peripheral vascular injuries refer to injuries in the extremities where proximal control can be obtained without an intra-abdominal or thoracic operation. These injuries include: the axillary, brachial, radial, ulnar, femoral, popliteal, posterior tibial, and anterior tibial arteries and their branches. In particular there are two transition points where proximal control of the peripheral vascular injury becomes difficult: the femoral artery just distal to the inguinal ligament and the axillary artery just distal to the clavicle.

The type of vascular injury varies: complete transection, partial transection, laceration (axially as well as longitudinally), contusion with thrombosis, crush injury, arteriovenous fistula, or pseudoaneurysm of the artery (Figure 20.1).

The major implements causing penetrating injuries include bullets (high and low velocity gunshots), stabbings (knives, glass, machetes, ice picks), shotgun pellets, explosion (secondary blast injuries), and animal bites (snakes and cats). Blunt injury causes include crush injuries from industrial machine accidents, animal bites (dog and marine animals), motorcycle and car crashes, pedestrian vs. auto injuries, and falls from heights as well as joint dislocations.

Prehospital treatment will vary depending on the nature of the injury encountered. Most commonly a compressive dressing is employed, but in some localities tourniquets can be used to control severe hemorrhage. Use of tourniquets to control hemorrhage has

Trauma: A Comprehensive Emergency Medicine Approach, eds. Eric Legome and Lee W. Shockley. Published by Cambridge University Press. © Cambridge University Press 2011.

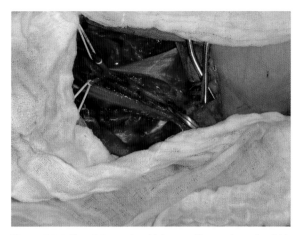

Figure 20.1 Blunt injury to brachial artery. Picture shows brachial artery at operative exploration with contusion and thrombosis.

also been validated in combat related injuries.[3] Quick and expeditious transport to an emergency department (ED) from the field is the goal for prehospital personnel. A thorough description of the scene environment should be told to the emergency physician including the mechanism of injury and estimated blood loss. Hemorrhage control is an early priority in trauma treatment; it is preceded only by airway control and management of breathing. Knowledge of the mechanism may assist the physician attempting hemorrhage control (e.g., glass vs. gunshot).

Box 20.1 Essentials of vascular trauma

- Peripheral vascular injuries refer to injuries in the extremities where proximal control can be obtained without an intra-abdominal or thoracic operation.
- The types of vascular injury include: complete transection, partial transection, laceration (axially as well as longitudinally), contusion with thrombosis, crush injury, arteriovenous fistula, or pseudoaneurysm of the artery.

Emergency department management

The history taken from prehospital personnel, the patient, and family should focus on the mechanism and time of the incident. This can clue the clinician into potential critical injuries. Hand dominance should be ascertained along with time of last meal and allergies. In shotgun blasts, knowledge of the distance from the shooter to the patient may help in determining likelihood of serious injury.[4]

While much of the evaluation in many patients ultimately involves diagnostic imaging, the history in conjunction with the physical examination still plays a role. That is, a normal physical examination, including that of the vascular system, can rule out a clinically significant injury in the low velocity penetrating injury trauma patient.[5]

In the patient with persistent bleeding, there are several variations of pressure application for hemorrhage control. These include: digital pressure, instrument pressure, and tourniquet application. Blind application of hemostats into a wound is discouraged as the vascular and nerve bundles often lie next to each other, and there is a high potential for injury of these nerves.

Tourniquets applied by prehospital personnel can vary from commercial tourniquets, to blood pressure cuffs or improvised windlass dressings, e.g., circumferential dressings with a stick used to tighten the dressings. Tourniquet application is a very effective management tool limited by time constraints before ischemia of the limb sets in.[3,6] The other limitation is in very proximal injuries, where the application of a tourniquet is not technically feasible (axilla or proximal thigh) or effective. If a prehospital applied tourniquet is present, query Emergency Medical Services (EMS) on length of time applied. The decision on whether to remove in the ED depends on the amount and force of bleeding and difficulty with control. There are no absolutes. If you are going to take the tourniquet down preparations should be made to control the bleeding.

The most common approach to hemorrhage control is digital pressure. Digital pressure should be applied with caution due to the potential for sharp objects to be in the wound. Digital pressure with use of an interposed gauze is preferable to gloved fingers. An advantage of direct digital pressure is the ability to feel the pulsatile origin of the blood loss and thus achieve effective pressure application.

If the decision is made in the ED to apply a tourniquet, use a manual blood pressure cuff, and place it proximal to the injury. Inflate the cuff above the systolic pressure and use a hemostat to clamp the air tubing to the cuff to minimize air leak. Another option is to use a pneumatic cuff set to a certain pressure (e.g., > 200 mmHg for the upper extremity). Note the time of tourniquet application. Once the tourniquet is applied, the neurological exam should commence since the ischemia from the tourniquet

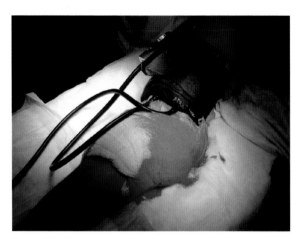

Figure 20.2 Pneumatic cuff used as a tourniquet.

will alter the exam findings. The tourniquet should remain in place < 120 minutes (Figure 20.2).

A hemostat with a gauze-in-teeth applied to the spurting wound with sufficient pressure should be able to temporize the bleeding in most cases. Sometimes several of these are needed in the wound to achieve hemostasis. Once hemostasis is achieved, then one by one each gauzed hemostat may be removed in a four quadrant fashion. One mentally divides the wound into four quadrants if it is not clear as to the exact origin of the bleeder within the wound. Then after releasing pressure in one quadrant of the wound, one inspects for bleeding while keeping pressure on the other three quadrant areas. If none is present, then the same is done for each successive quadrant until the bleeder is localized within the wound. This may be a very painful procedure so local anesthetics should be used as soon as is practical. Once the bleeding is controlled a rapid evaluation of the limb should proceed. If the extremity is deformed, fractured, or dislocated, these should be reduced and splinted. Often this reduction will reduce ischemia to the distal limb if present. In addition to local anesthesia, intravenous opioids, moderate sedation, or endotracheal intubation may often be required for further management.

Further assessment of the limb should include the determination of distal pulses and perfusion. The examiner should evaluate for a thrill or bruit, expanding hematoma, or motor or sensory deficits in the affected limb. Motor deficits not explained by tendon injuries should be suspected of being of ischemic origin or due to direct nerve injury. The quality of peripheral perfusion may help distinguish. The presence of these examination findings or arterial

bleeding is generally an indication for operative management of the wound. These are often described as "hard signs."

> **Box 20.2 Hard signs of arterial injury**
> - Diminished or absent pulses
> - Bruit or thrill
> - Active or pulsatile hemorrhage
> - Signs of limb ischemia/compartment syndrome (paresthesias, paralysis, pain, pulselessness, pallor [seen mainly in light-complexioned individuals], and pain on passive extension)
> - Pulsatile or expanding hematoma

The use of Doppler ultrasound is common when pulses are palpably diminished or absent. Comparison with the contralateral limb will help in the assessment to make sure that a congenitally anomalous arterial formation is not present

If there are no hard signs, the examiner should proceed to evaluate for the presence of external signs of injury (bruises, lacerations, or abrasions) and "soft" signs of vascular injury.[7,8]

> **Box 20.3 Soft signs of vascular injury**
> - Proximity of injury tract to the vascular bundle
> - Major single nerve deficit (sciatic, femoral, median, ulnar, and radial)
> - Non-expanding hematoma
> - Diminished pulses
> - Posterior knee or anterior elbow dislocation
> - Hypotension or history of moderate blood loss at the scene

In general, proximity alone is not an indication for vascular imaging. Vascular imaging for proximity injuries (i.e., wound tract within a cm of a major vessel) is warranted for a mechanism of blast force, high velocity missile injury, or in a shotgun wound.[9] Otherwise, there should be clinical signs of injury or an ankle–brachial index (ABI) of < 0.9.

Frykberg et al. published a prospective study of penetrating extremity injuries ($N = 366$) over the course of a year. All hard signs of vascular injury (6%) were taken to the operating room, all proximity injuries (78%) were observed clinically. The remaining 16% were extremity wounds without hard signs and without proximity and were discharged. The proximity wound category ($N = 286$) had 2 patients who slowly went on to develop evidence for vascular injury requiring repair for a missed injury rate of 0.7% (2/286); the diagnostic accuracy of physical exam in this subset of patients was 99.45% (364/366).[5] This experience has been corroborated with additional studies and now serves as the basis for our continued observation of penetrating wounds of the extremities in the absence of clinically apparent vascular injuries. Given the generous collateral circulation and the presence of major vascular structures around the groin and thoracic outlet, this approach is not applicable to these areas. It is possible to have injury to the profunda femoris or profunda brachii or other major vascular structure in these proximal locations with the preservation of adequate peripheral perfusion. Hence, the wait and see approach without radiologic evaluation for proximity wounds to the extremity is best suited for injuries distal to the mid-thigh or mid-brachium.

Neurological status should include a full evaluation of all motor and sensory function distal to the injury. A tourniquet that has been placed on the limb will produce numbness and paresthesias distal to the tourniquet after a period of 15 minutes. If the prehospital personnel have applied a tourniquet, note the time of application and interpret the neurological examination in this light. The neurologic changes due to ischemia from a tourniquet do not reverse quickly after releasing the tourniquet, often taking 20–30 minutes or longer to fully resolve; longer times of tourniquet application correlating with more widespread and prolonged ischemic effects.

Presentation

The presentations of extremity injuries with vascular trauma can be dramatic and varied. Industrial accidents, railroad accidents, and blast injuries commonly produce proximal amputations: exposed bone, muscle, vessels, and nerves. Often bleeding is not severe as the proximal vessel may have retracted and closed off due to spasm. Bleeding may have also been controlled prior to arrival by a tourniquet placed by prehospital personnel. If bleeding has been controlled, place saline gauzes over the exposed soft tissue. Large injured/severed nerves are exposed and exquisitely sensitive.

Near amputations can present with a large bone fracture deformity accompanied by large soft tissue injury. Partial transections of a large artery can occur causing heavy bleeding. The inability of the artery to retract and close off by spasm allows it to profusely bleed. Direct pressure should be applied; if insufficient, a tourniquet may be necessary.

Penetrating injuries to the wrist may involve the radial artery, ulnar artery, or palmar arch. These have a propensity to bleed heavily since they bleed from both directions.

Both gunshot and stab wounds may present with a small external wound with an underlying hematoma.

Stab wound hematomas are often larger than gunshot wound hematomas as the stab wound can retract around the exiting sharp (knife or glass) whereas the gunshot wound may leave a tract that cannot close, allowing for active external bleeding rather than contained hematoma. Care must be taken with injuries from glass, because of the risk of injury to the treating staff.

Crush injuries may be deceptive. The crushed segment may extend for significant length. The thin and loose skin of an elderly patient is at particular risk for degloving injuries. A force producing this injury can easily cause a crushing vascular injury that extends over a long segment of the extremity.

Animal bites can cause arterial injury from crush injuries (e.g., dog bite) or puncture injuries (e.g., cat bite or a snake).[10] Certain snake bites can additionally be complicated by thrombosis or coagulopathy caused by venom in the bite.[11]

Several blunt trauma mechanisms are also associated with vascular extremity injury. Highly suspicious are the extremity dislocations that involve "swelling" of the joint or hematoma formation. Traumatic shoulder, knee, and elbow dislocations can develop vascular injuries during dislocation or reduction.[12,13] Knee dislocations produce a potential for both popliteal arterial and venous injury with thromboembolic sequelae such as compartment syndrome and eventual need for amputation.[14] The previously routine practice of angiography for all knee dislocations revealed that the incidence of popliteal artery injury was between 16 and 30%. Treiman et al. examined 22 patients with knee dislocation and normal peripheral vascular exams by angiography.[15] They found that 3/22 (13.6%) of those patients had angiographic evidence for minor arterial injury.[15] Continued observation revealed that the natural history of these clinically occult lesions was benign hence did not warrant detection through angiography. Others verified similar results using duplex ultrasound. General current practice is to observe those patients with

Table 20.1 How to perform ankle–brachial index (ABI)

- The patient is placed supine with the cuff placed on the injured arm (or lower extremity)

- The ipsilateral brachial artery is insonated with the Doppler device until the brachial artery is clearly heard

- The cuff is pumped up 20 mmHg past the point where the Doppler sound disappears. The cuff is slowly released until the Doppler device picks up the arterial sound again (the systolic pressure)

- The pressure at which this sound occurs is recorded and the procedure is repeated for the opposite uninjured upper extremity

- A similar procedure is then done with both lower extremities, comparing the systolic pressure at the ankle (insonating the dorsalis pedis or posterior tibial artery with the Doppler device; the cuff is placed just above the ankle) in the injured lower extremity with the systolic pressure in the uninjured lower extremity

- The ABI = the systolic pressure of the injured extremity (ankle or forearm) divided by the brachial systolic pressure in the uninjured extremity

- ABI > 0.9 is highly unlikely to have a vascular injury and may be observed

- ABI < 0.9 indicates possible vascular injury: requires further evaluation, preferably by computed tomography angiogram (CTA)

knee dislocation and a normal peripheral vascular exam, i.e., normal perfusion, pulses, and ABIs. There is no standard for how long, but at maximum, 24 hours seems sufficient.

Secondary evaluation

Plain film radiography

The purpose of plain films is to identify fractures, dislocations, and foreign bodies in the wound. The plain films assist with the expeditious reduction of fractured long bones and dislocations. The location of the dislocation or fracture may prompt a greater concern for certain neurovascular injuries. Isolated injuries to the extremity may generally undergo radiography in the radiology suite. Patients with multiple trauma or concerning dislocations may require bedside radiography.

Ankle–Brachial Index or Arterial Pressure Index

Patients with soft signs may be evaluated using the ABI or the Arterial Pressure Index (API). The APIs use has been validated by numerous studies as a screening tool for vascular trauma that offers improved sensitivity over the pulse exam alone. An API < 0.9 indicates possible vascular injury warranting further evaluation such as an angiogram or computed tomography angiogram (CTA).

The API probably will not detect all injuries, such as those to the peroneal and profunda arteries, or

those that do not obstruct flow. Those patients with significant peripheral vascular disease and those in shock may also have abnormal APIs without an acute injury.[16]

Some centers have incorporated the API into their extremity injury protocol (Table 20.1).[16–18] Lynch and Johansen studied ABI use in penetrating and blunt trauma in 100 patients and found, using an ABI of 0.9 or lower for ruling in a lesion, a sensitivity of 87% and specificity of 97%.[19] An ABI of 0.9 or higher had a negative predictive value of 96%. Mills et al. evaluated 38 patients and found 100% sensitivity, specificity, and positive predictive value for arterial injury in patients with knee dislocations.[20] However, none of those with ABI above 0.9 had arteriography (duplex ultrasound or clinical follow up were the standards used in those patients) so the study was limited by its methodology.[20] Its comparison with duplex ultrasonography revealed that it is less sensitive in one well-controlled trial.[21]

Conventional angiography

Historically, angiography was the preferred imaging study in most centers for the evaluation of vascular trauma. However, many of these studies do not demonstrate pathology that requires intervention. In 1989, Frykberg studied 152 patients by angiography whom had a normal vascular exam; he found 27 injuries (18%) to the vascular structures.[5] These injuries included spasm, minor intimal flaps (image), and pseudoaneurysms (image) of named arteries. He followed those patients with clinically unapparent but angiographically demonstrated vascular injuries. Subsequent angiography showed that all but one lesion resolved completely. One small pseudoaneurysm continued to enlarge and was electively repaired. Therefore, 96% of the injuries in his series resolved without operative intervention.[5]

The complication rate of angiography is 1–2%.[22] The advantages of angiography are the ability to intervene endovascularly to control hemorrhage by embolization or stenting and the high sensitivity achieved by dynamic imaging from multiple angles. Consequently, conventional angiography has been the gold standard by which other modalities are measured.[23–25] However, angiography has a false negative rate and a false positive rate as high as 2% with some shotgun injuries becoming apparent years after the event.[26,27] In particular, arteriography, the gold standard, has been found to miss shotgun injuries that show up years later.[27]

Magnetic resonance imaging

The investigation of vascular trauma with magnetic resonance angiography (MRA) is currently being evaluated.[28] Compared with conventional or CTA, MRA is non-invasive, does not use ionizing radiation, and has less risk of renal injury due to contrast injection. An MRA typically involves the use of paramagnetic contrast materials such as a gadolinium chelate. Gadolinium has minimal nephrotoxicity and anaphylaxis risk compared to iodinated X-ray contrast.[29] In patients with renal insufficiency, however, there is a risk of developing nephrogenic systemic fibrosis (NSF) after exposure to the extracellular, non-ionic, low-osmolar, gadolinium-based contrast agent, gadodiamide. The typical patient who develops NSF is middle-aged with end-stage renal disease on chronic dialysis. The highest glomerular filtration rate (GFR) in which NSF has been reported was 20 ml/min (normal ~100 ml/min).[30] A study of high-dose gadolinium in a population with a high prevalence of baseline renal insufficiency showed no renal failure associated with its administration.[29] The most common adverse reaction in a study of 9528 patients was nausea and vomiting (40% of adverse reactions) and rash (33%). One patient (0.01%) had an anaphylactoid reaction.[29] It is unclear whether premedication has any role in attenuating an adverse reaction. Patients pretreated with prednisone and diphenhydramine still developed the same adverse reaction with gadolinium.

The acquisition time for MRA images is greater than that for CTA.

Duplex ultrasonography

Duplex ultrasonography is an imaging modality that uses both Doppler and B mode. It is non-invasive and it visualizes arterial as well as venous injuries. The ultrasonographer is able to distinguish the vessel anatomy as well as flow velocities and direction. Duplex ultrasonography provides information about pseudoaneurysms, flow velocities, intraluminal clot formation, and arteriovenous malformations. Duplex ultrasonography provides dynamic imaging; it compares well with angiography. However, the accuracy of duplex ultrasonography is operator-dependent and the studies may be time consuming.[31,32] Some injuries may be missed if the entire arterial tree is not imaged.[33] Large wound defects, casted extremities, external hardware, subcutaneous air, and injuries near the clavicle or inguinal ligament can limit the ability of the study to detect vascular injuries.[34] Further, detecting vascular injuries distal to an existing high-grade lesion is difficult.[35]

Duplex ultrasonography is not as sensitive as angiography in identifying intimal defects and small vessel occlusions. In a prospective randomized blinded trial, Bergstein et al. showed that duplex ultrasound was 99% specific and 50% sensitive, compared with digital subtraction angiography; the positive predictive value was 66% and the negative predictive value was 97%.[33] Two pseudoaneurysms were missed in this study because they were more proximal in the vessel than the area studied. Bergstein's recommendation was to scan the entire arterial tree in the injured extremity; however, this adds to the time required to perform the study. Duplex ultrasonography is particularly time consuming in evaluations of the legs below the level of the trifurcation of the popliteal artery.[33] It's ability to evaluate venous injury is excellent.[14]

CT angiography

Computed tomography angiography has multiple advantages to all other modalities: rapidity, three dimensionality, sensitivity, and specificity.[36,37] The major downside to CTA is that it is a diagnostic modality alone that does not allow for treatment such as stenting or embolizations. Compared with digital subtraction angiography, CTA is faster, exposes the

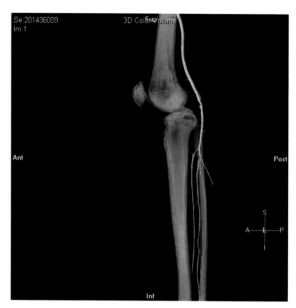

Figure 20.3 Computed tomography angiography (CTA) of popliteal vessel injury.

patient to only about 25% of the radiation, is less costly, allows a greater ability to change the volumetric raw data, and has fewer complications.[38] In addition, CTA can assess luminal plaques, thrombus, inflammation, and perivascular disease.[39] Multidetector row CT (MDCT) can capture arterial and venous phases within a few minutes.[40] The 64- and 128-row detector CTA produce images that are of similar quality to conventional angiography. Soto et al. compared conventional angiography with CTA; the sensitivity was 90–100% and the specificity was 100% with an inter-observer agreement of 0.9 (Figure 20.3).[36]

Trauma from penetrating injuries with retained foreign bodies can cause imaging artifacts. Similarly, implanted medical devices and artificial joints can also produce imaging artifacts. Such artifacts may create difficulty in visualizing segments of the vascular structures.[40] Other pitfalls to CTA include the difficulty in differentiating spasm in a normal vessel from occlusion and mistaken appearance of a thrombus if the venous phase is imaged too early.[40]

Compared with duplex ultrasound, CTA is less operator-dependent, can evaluate the presence of collateral vessels and evaluate the distal vascular bed. Compared with magnetic resonance imaging (MRI), CTA is faster and the image signal is less influenced by vessel tortuosity and slow flow, and has higher spatial resolution.[39]

Box 20.4 Summary of radiologic modalities

Modality	Use and characteristics
Plain films	Identify fractures, dislocations, and foreign bodies in the wound
	Insensitive for arterial injury, but location of injury may prompt further evaluation
Angiography	Gold standard allowing interventional procedures: stenting and embolization
	Allows for a dynamic evaluation of the arterial tree
Ultrasound	Duplex ultrasonography may be useful in detecting lower extremity venous injuries and delayed aneurysms
	If contrast allergy present, may be used in place of CTA or angiography
	Limited sensitivity in some small injuries and intimal defects
	Non-therapeutic
MRI	Non-invasive, does not use ionizing radiation, and has less risk of renal injury due to contrast injection
	High accuracy but expensive and not practical for unstable patients
	Not therapeutic
CT angiography	64 slice and above are as comparable to digital subtraction angiography with lower complications, faster, and less expensive
	Major limitation is that it is diagnostic only, not therapeutic

Treatment of vascular injuries of the extremities

Initial therapy

Initial ED treatment for active bleeding consists of direct pressure, hemostatic bandages or application of a tourniquet. The first step in control of active arterial or venous bleeding in the ED is with direct pressure. Blind application of surgical clamps is contraindicated if the operative field is obscured by blood. Direct local pressure may allow temporary control of the bleeding to allow time to transport the patient to the operating room. At times, the bleeding may be so brisk that the direct pressure cannot be removed; in these cases the skin should be prepped with iodine around the compressing hand until definitive control can be done in a more sterile and controlled setting to achieve proximal and distal control.

Recently, three variations of hemostatic bandages have become available for both military and civilian use. The most prevalent is the HemCon® bandage, made from the complex carbohydrate chitin. This bandage has been distributed to over 600 000 troops, with uncontrolled retrospective data reporting 97% effectiveness. ChitoFlex® is a softer, more compliant variation of HemCon® designed to be stuffed into smaller wounds, such as those from small caliber low velocity injuries. QuickClot® is an inert porous zeolite powder that absorbs water, concentrating clotting factors through dehydration. The initial reports suggested that due to an exothermic reaction when used, a large amount of heat was generated, which limited its effectiveness. Some of that heat generation has now been tempered through the use of pre-hydration of the crystals.

The tourniquet has not been positively received throughout the years. During World War I, the use of the tourniquet was discouraged because of misuse, the potential for prolonged application, possible contribution to limb loss and the possible relationship with infection. In retrospect, this was probably more a function of the minimal prehospital care, prolonged evacuation, primitive understanding of resuscitation, and lack of antibiotics rather than the device itself. Today, support for its use is widespread, yet remains mostly anecdotal and poorly studied. It is readily available and easily applied by the injured victim. It may be highly valuable in the event of mass casualties to allow the delivery of care to multiple victims by a limited number of caregivers.

Systemic therapy

The control and therapy for active arterial bleeding is both local and systemic. Once local control is achieved, systemic therapy may involve either volume resuscitation or volume restriction, depending on the specific circumstances. The commonly cited approach is the administration of 2 L of crystalloid with the expectation that normotension will be restored. In the event of severe bleeding and moderate hypotension, however, it may be more prudent to maintain

minimal volume expansion with crystalloid and move the patient directly to the operating room for definitive care. Continued aggressive crystalloid resuscitation in the absence of control of bleeding will lead to the dilution of coagulation factors, hypothermia, and acidosis as well as restoration of circulatory volume with fluid that is unable to transport oxygen. In the event that the patient had been able to clot off the injured vessel, aggressive fluid resuscitation may raise the blood pressure, and increase the risk of "popping off" the previously protective clot. In the injured actively bleeding patient, it may be best to wait until control of hemorrhage has occurred to provide aggressive replacement with warmed packed red cells, fresh frozen plasma, and platelets with minimal use of crystalloid. There is ample animal laboratory evidence and some clearly suggestive human data that this modern day damage-control resuscitation is far more physiologic and results in less hypothermia, coagulopathy, and acidosis.[41,42]

Patients with hard signs require surgical consultation and operative management. These patients do not need vascular imaging unless the point of injury is unclear. After an initial decision is made that operative treatment is not immediately necessary, further evaluation and management can proceed. If the patient has soft signs, a decision is required about the need for vascular imaging. If the injury is distal, the use of a normal exam and normal ABIs can rule out the need for imaging. The patient with an ABI of < 0.9 should be studied by conventional or CT angiogram to evaluate the injured extremity. Evidence of arterial injury by imaging in conjunction with soft signs usually result in operative management, although some have been conservatively managed.[33] The patient who is asymptomatic and has an ABI > 0.9 can be safely observed or discharged depending on the injuries (Figure 20.4).

Local wound exploration, cleansing the wounds, identification of other injured structures (tendons), and local hemorrhage control are the next steps. If a partially transected or lacerated artery is encountered during closure, pass thick silk suture under the vessel proximally and distally and then gently tent up. This will usually achieve enough hemostasis for either repair or ligation. If there is good distal and proximal flow in the injured radial or ulnar artery, it may be ligated, although if practical a vascular or hand surgeon should be consulted. Wounds should be closed early unless the patient is going to the operating

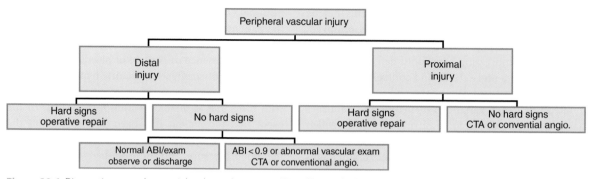

Figure 20.4 Diagnostic approach to peripheral vascular trauma. ABI, Ankle–Brachial Index; angio., angiography; CTA, computed tomography angiography.

room; they can be closed there. Deep stab wounds or wounds into multiple muscle compartments, especially if dirty, should be closed by delayed primary closure or secondary intention. The clean wound should not be left open for hours (increasing the likelihood of infection). The transition to the operating room should not be delayed to close minor wounds.

Tetanus toxoid should be administered as well as tetanus immune globulin if there is a lack of previous immunization.

Although not well studied, antibiotics are usually given with a typical agent being cefazolin 1 g intravenously. Those allergic to cephalosporins can be given a macrolide and vancomycin.

Operative management

Operatively, the surgeon has several choices: Direct repair, interposition graft, or ligation.[43]

Preoperative preparation includes the treatment or prevention of hypothermia, adequate vascular access and blood typing. The injury may be tamponaded by local clot and tissues. Disruption of this protective environment should not occur until adequate control of the vessels leading into and out of the hematoma has been achieved. Proximal and distal control of the artery prior to exposing the actual injury avoids sudden uncontrolled blood loss. Proximal control of the brachial vessels may include supraclavicular subclavian artery exposure or infraclavicular axillary artery exposure. Proximal control of the common femoral artery may require the extraperitoneal exposure of the external iliac artery.

Small, distal, and redundant injured arteries may be ligated; however, the majority of larger arterial injuries should be repaired. During the American Civil War, extremity amputation was the most common operation and the named vessels were routinely ligated. Prior to the turn of the twentieth century, injured arteries were routinely ligated necessitating amputations. It was not until DeBakey began repairing arteries toward the end of World War II that there was proof that it was feasible and beneficial to do so. DeBakey et al. demonstrated that with repair, the amputation rate dropped from 50% to 35%.[44,45]

In patients with the hemodynamic instability damage control surgery may be more appropriate than a prolonged reconstruction. In these situations, liberal uses of intravascular shunts allow immediate restoration of prograde blood flow into the injured extremity limiting the total duration of limb ischemia. A recent report from Iraq found that the use of shunts in 23 patients with arterial injuries allowed 100% limb salvage at short-term follow up (2–30 days). In addition, the avoidance of aggressive resuscitation to normotension prior to operative repair may avoid disruption clot and dilution of clotting factors.[46,47]

Repairs to arterial defects are performed with sutures, patch angioplasty, interposition grafting, or vein patches depending on the type, location, and size of injury.

Documentation

Patients with extremity trauma should have the physical examination documented including the neurovascular evaluation. This aspect should be repeated and documented after splinting, reduction of dislocations, and release of tourniquets. Tourniquet time should be estimated and documented also. Hand dominance should be documented as it may assist with rehabilitation planning.

Box 20.5   Essentials of documentation

- Neurovascular examination including pulses, sensation, perfusion, and motor (comparison to contralateral side if applicable)
- Repeat evaluation after splinting, dislocation reduction, tourniquet release, etc.
- Estimated tourniquet time (if used)
- Hand dominance (if upper extremity injury)

Disposition

Any patients with hard signs of injury need emergent operative intervention; if this cannot be provided at the initial hospital then the patient should be transferred to a trauma center. If there are soft signs of arterial injury, surgical consultation and ED evaluation are the appropriate next steps. If the trauma evaluation yields no injuries other than the extremity injury with soft signs but the ABI/exam or imaging is negative the patient may be discharged or observed. If there are proximal soft signs requiring imaging or abnormal ABIs and no imaging modality is available at the base hospital, then the patient should be transferred to a facility that can perform these studies. Patients with amputations should be sent to a replantation center with efforts to preserve the amputated limb.

References

1. Owens BD, Kragh JF, Wenke JC, et al. Combat wounds in operation Iraqi freedom and operation enduring freedom. *J Trauma* 2008;**64**(2):295–303.

2. Sirinek KR, Gaskill HV, 3rd, Dittman WI, et al. Exclusion angiography for patients with possible vascular injuries of the extremities–a better use of trauma center resources. *Surgery* 1983;**94**:598–603.

3. Beekley AC, Sebesta JA, Blackbourne LH, et al. Prehospital tourniquet use in Operation Iraqi Freedom: effect on hemorrhage control and outcomes. *J Trauma* 2008;**64**(2):s28–37.

4. Bender J, Hoekstra S, Levison M. Improving outcome from extremity shotgun injury. *Am Surg* 1993;**59**: 359–64.

5. Frykberg ER, Dennis JW, Bishop K, Laneve L, et al. The reliability of physical examination in the evaluation of penetrating extremity trauma for vascular injury: results at one year. *J Trauma* 1991; **31**(4):502–11.

6. Gazmuri RR, Munoz JA, Ilic JP, et al. Vasospasm after use of a tourniquet: another cause of postoperative limb ischemia? *Anesth Analg* 2002;**94**:1152–4.

7. Gomez GA, Kreis DJ, Jr., Ratner L, et al. Suspected vascular trauma of the extremities: the role of arteriography in proximity injuries. *J Trauma* 1986; **26**:1005–8.

8. Frykberg ER, Crump JM, Vines FS, et al. Reassessment of the role of arteriography in penetrating proximity extremity trauma: a prospective study. *J Trauma* 1989;**29**(8):1041–52.

9. Wolf YG, Rivkind A. Vascular trauma in high-velocity gunshot wounds and shrapnel-blast injuries in Israel. *Surg Clin N Am* 2002;**82**(1):237–44.

10. Levis JT, Garmel GM. Radial artery pseudoaneurysm formation after cat bite to the wrist. *Ann Emerg Med* 2008;**51**(5): 668–70.

11. Thomas L, Chausson N, Uzan J, et al. Thrombotic stroke following snake bites by the "Fer-de-Lance" Bothrops lanceolatus in Martinique despite antivenom treatment: a report of three recent cases. *Toxicon* 2006;**48**(1):23–8.

12. Bravman JT, Ipaktchi K, Biffl WL, et al. Vascular injuries after blunt upper extremity trauma: pitfalls in the recognition and diagnosis of potential "near miss" injuries. *Scand J Trauma Resusc Emerg Med* 2008;**16**:16–24.

13. Kuhn MA, Ross G. Acute elbow dislocations. *Orthop Clin N Am* 2008;**39**:155–61.

14. Gagne PJ, Cone JB, McFarland D, et al. Proximity penetrating extremity trauma: the role of duplex ultrasound in the detection of occult venous injuries. *J Trauma* 1995;**39**(6):1157–63.

15. Treiman GS, Yelliin AE, Weaver FA, et al. Examination of the patient with a knee dislocation. The case for selective arteriography. *Arch Surg* 1992;**127**(1):1056–62; discussion 62–3.

16. Redmond JM, Levy BA, Dajani KA, et al. Detecting vascular injury in lower-extremity orthopedic trauma: the role of CT angiography. *Orthopedics* 2008;**31**:761–9.

17. Peng PD, Spain DA, Tataria M, et al. CT angiography effectively evaluates extremity vascular trauma. *Am Surg* 2008;**74**:103–7.

18. Conrad MF, Patton JH, Parikshak M, et al. Evaluation of vascular injury in penetrating extremity trauma: angiographers stay home. *Am Surg* 2002;**68**:269–74.

19. Lynch K, Johansen K. Can Doppler pressure measurement replace arteriography in the diagnosis of occult extremity arterial trauma? *Ann Surg* 1991;**214**:737–41.

20. Mills WJ, Barei DP, McNair P. The value of the ankle–brachial index for diagnosing arterial injury after knee dislocation: a prospective study. *J Trauma* 2004; **56**(6):1261–5.

21. Heijboer H, Butler HR, Lensing A, et al. A comparison of real-time compression ultrasonography with impedance plethysmography for the diagnosis of deep-vein thrombosis in symptomatic outpatients. *N Engl J Med* 1993;**329**:1365–9.

22. Hessel SJ, Adams DF, Abrams HL. Complications of angiography. *Radiology* 1981;**138**:273–81.

23. Sclafani SJA, Cooper R, Shaftan GW, et al. Arterial trauma: diaagnostic and therapeutic angiography. *Radiology* 1986;**161**:165–72.

24. Rose SC, Moore EE. Angiography in patients with arterial trauma: correlation between angiographic abnormalities, operative findings, and clinical outcome. *Am J Roentgenol* 1987;**149**:613–19.

25. Rose SC, Moore EE. Emergency trauma angiography: accuracy, safety, and pitfalls. *Am J Roentgenol* 1987;**148**:1243–6.

26. Busquets AR, Acosta JA, Colon E, et al. Helical computed tomographic angiography for the diagnosis of traumatic arterial injuries of the extremities. *J Trauma* 2004;**56**(3):625–8.

27. Lipchik EO, Kaebnick HW, Beres JJ, et al. The role of anteriography in acute penetrating trauma to the extremities. *Cardiovasc Intervent Radiol* 1987;**10**:202–4.

28. Yaquinto JJ, Harms SE, Siemers PT, et al. Arterial injury from penetrating trauma: evaluation with single-acquisition fat-suppressed MR imaging. *AJR Am J Roentgenol* 1992;**158**:631–3.

29. Li A, Wong CS, Wong MK, et al. Acute adverse reactions to magnetic resonance media-gadolinium chelates. *Br J Radiol* 2006;**79**:368–71.

30. Thomsen HS. Nephrogenic systemic fibrosis: a serious late adverse reaction to gadodiamide. *Eur Radiol* 2006;**16**(12):2619–21.

31. Knudson MM, Lewis FR, Atkinson K, et al. The role of duplex ultrasound arterial imaging in patients with penetrating extremity trauma. *Arch Surg* 1993;**128**:1033–8.

32. Schwartz M, Weaver F, Yellin A, et al. The utility of color flow Doppler examination in penetrating extremity arterial trauma. *Am Surg* 1993;**59**:375–8.

33. Bergstein JM, Blair J, Edwards J, et al. Pitfalls in the use of color-flow duplex ultrasound for screening of suspected arterial injuries in penetrating extremities. *J Trauma* 1992;**33**(3):395–402.

34. Gaitini D, Razi NB, Ghersin E, et al. Sonographic evaluation of vascular injuries. *J Ultrasound Med* 2008;**27**:95–107.

35. Zierler RE, Zierler BK. Duplex sonography of lower extremity arteries. *Sem Ultrasound CT MRI* 1997;**18**(1):39–56.

36. Soto JA, Munera F, Morales C, et al. Focal arterial injuries of the proximal extremities: helical CT arteriography as the initial method of diagnosis. *Radiology* 2001;**218**:188–94.

37. Soto JA, Munera F, Cardoso N, et al. Diagnostic performance of helical CT angiography in trauma to large arteries of the extremities. *J of Comput Assist Tomogr* 1999;**23**(2):188–96.

38. Katz DS, Hon M. CT angiography of the lower extremities and aortoiliac system with a multi-detector row helical CT scanner: promise of new opportunities fulfilled. *Radiology* 2001;**221**:7–15.

39. Kalva SP, Mueller PR. Vascular imaging in the elderly. *Radio Clin N Am* 2008;**46**:663–83.

40. Fishman EK, Horton KM, Johnson PT. Multidetector CT and three-dimensional CT angiography for suspected vascular trauma of the extremities. *Radiographics* 2008;**28**:653–67.

41. Fabian T. Damage control in trauma: laparotomy wound management acute to chronic. *Surg Clin N Am* 2007;**87**:73–93.

42. Blackbourne L. Combat damage control surgery. *Crit Care Med* 2008;**36**(7 Suppl.):s304–10.

43. Arthurs ZM, Sohn VY, Starnes BW. Vascular trauma: endovascular management and techniques. *Surg Clin N Am* 2007;**87**:1179–92.

44. Debakey ME, Simeone FA. Battle injuries of the arteries in World War II: an analysis of 2471 cases. *Ann Surg* 1946;**123**(4): 534–79.

45. DeBakey ME, Carter NB. Current considerations of war surgery. *Ann Surg* 1945;**121**(5): 545–63.

46. Dutton RP, Mackenzie CF, Scalea TM. Hypotensive resuscitation during active hemorrhage: impact on in-hospital mortality. *J Trauma* 2002;**52**(6):1141–6.

47. Stern SA. Low-volume fluid resuscitation for presumed hemorrhagic shock: helpful or harmful? *Curr Opin Crit Care* 2001;**7**(6):422–30.

Chapter

21

Trauma in pregnancy

Diana Felton and Carrie D. Tibbles

Introduction

Trauma complicates approximately 5% of pregnancies.[1] Many factors, including physiologic changes in pregnancy, concerns over radiation and medication effects on the fetus, the necessity of fetal monitoring, and the need to recognize and treat specific pregnancy-related complications, can make these cases very challenging to manage. Motor vehicle collisions, followed by falls and assaults, are the most common cause of maternal trauma.[2] As expected, more severe injuries are associated with poor outcomes for both the mother and developing fetus.[3] While many pregnant women suffer minor injuries, that do not require hospitalization, even apparently minor injuries like extremity fractures, are linked to poor perinatal outcomes.[4–6] Therefore, all pregnant trauma patients require careful evaluation.

A few general principles are helpful in the management of the pregnant trauma patient. First, a developing fetus is very susceptible to maternal hypoxia and hypovolemia, and the initial resuscitation should focus on stabilizing the mother. The majority of the time, the evaluation of the mother follows general trauma protocols, similar to non-pregnant patients. The physiologic changes in pregnancy can make the identification of shock more difficult and the clinician must be aware of subtle signs of hemodynamic instability. Finally, placental abruption is the most common cause of fetal loss following trauma, and is best evaluated by initiating cardiotocographic monitoring early in the emergency department (ED) course.

> **Box 21.1 Essential principles in caring for the pregnant patient with traumatic injury**
> - Adequate resuscitation of the mother is essential, as fetal well-being is largely dependent on the stability of the mother.

- In the second half of pregnancy, patients should be placed in the left lateral decubitus position to avoid supine hypotension from compression of the inferior vena cava by the uterus.
- Placental abruption can occur even after minor trauma. If the fetus is viable, continuous fetal monitoring should be initiated as soon as possible, and continued for a minimum of 4–6 hours.
- In general, necessary radiologic studies should not be withheld from the mother because of concerns of radiation exposure to the fetus.
- All Rh-negative mothers should receive RhoGAM following trauma to prevent maternal isoimmunization.

Clinical anatomy and physiology

The enlarging uterus remains inside the confines of the pelvis until week 12, reaching the umbilicus at week 20, and the costal margins between weeks 34 and 36 (Figure 21.1). This expanding uterus pushes the bowel into the upper abdomen, and also displaces the bladder anteriorly, increasing its susceptibility to injury. In the later stages of pregnancy, the uterus may compress the vena cava when the patient is lying on her back. This phenomena, known as supine hypotension, has a significant impact on the blood return to the heart, subsequently reducing cardiac output.

The perfusion requirements of the uterus and placenta result in a number of significant alterations in maternal physiology beginning in the middle of the first trimester and continuing throughout the pregnancy. Resting heart rate is typically elevated 10–15 beats/min. Because of decreased vascular resistance, both systolic and diastolic blood pressure typically

Trauma: A Comprehensive Emergency Medicine Approach, eds. Eric Legome and Lee W. Shockley. Published by Cambridge University Press. © Cambridge University Press 2011.

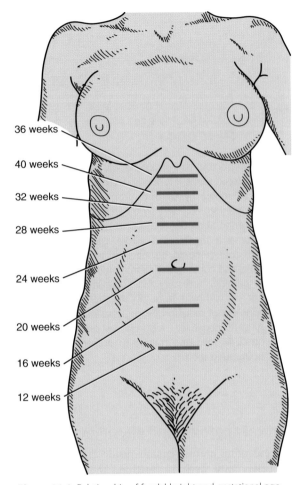

36 weeks
40 weeks
32 weeks
28 weeks
24 weeks
20 weeks
16 weeks
12 weeks

Figure 21.1 Relationship of fundal height and gestational age.

at 30 mmHg. Oxygen consumption is increased. All this translates to lower pulmonary reserves in situations of respiratory distress.

Pregnancy increases progesterone levels which relaxes smooth muscle throughout the body. In addition to decreased vascular resistance, important effects include relaxation of the lower esophageal sphincter and decreased gastric motility, with subsequent increased aspiration risk.[7] Progesterone also increases ligament laxity, which may leave a pregnant patient more prone to orthopedic injuries.

Recognition of these alterations in anatomy and physiology are important for accurate assessment of the pregnant trauma patient and are summarized in Box 21.2.

Box 21.2 Important physiologic changes in pregnancy			
System	Change	Approx. change	Onset change
Cardiovascular	Increased cardiac output	40%	First to second trimester
	Increased blood volume	40%	First to second trimester
	Elevated resting heart rate	15%	First trimester
	Systemic vascular resistance (SVR)	−20%	
	Decreased blood pressure	−30%	Second trimester
Pulmonary	Increased respiratory rate	15%	First to second trimester
	Decreased functional residual capacity	−20%	Third trimester
	Increased tidal volume	40%	First to second trimester

falls 5–15 mmHg in the second trimester. Cardiac output is increased by 1.0–1.5 L/min, with the enlarging uterus receiving 20% of the total cardiac output. Maternal blood volume increases in pregnancy, without a proportional increase in red blood cell production, resulting in a dilutional anemia. Because of this increased volume, a pregnant trauma patient may lose up to 1500 ml of blood before exhibiting signs of hypovolemia such as tachycardia and hypotension. However, this amount of hemorrhage is sufficient to cause fetal distress.

Respiratory dynamics change significantly in pregnancy starting as early as 6–8 weeks of gestation. The pregnant woman effectively exchanges more gas per breath. Her tidal volume will increase by 40% in conjunction with a 25% drop in functional residual volume beginning midway through the second trimester. Consequently, baseline PCO_2 will run lower

	Increased minute ventilation	50%	First to second trimester
	Respiratory alkalosis (decreases PCO_2)	$Paco_2$ average of 32 mmHg	Throughout
Gastrointestinal	Decreased gastric motility		First trimester
	Decreased esophageal sphincter tone		
Musculoskeletal	Increased ligament laxity		First trimester

Prehospital

Overall, standard protocols for prehospital care of trauma patients apply to pregnant patients, with a few specific considerations. In a patient > 20 weeks pregnant requiring spine immobilization, the backboard should be tilted 15° to the left to prevent hypotension from the compression of the vena cava by the uterus. Positioning towels or blankets under the backboard is easy and effective.[8] Supplemental oxygen should be provided and intravenous access placed. Any pregnant patient at risk for complications of traumatic or obstetrical complications should be transferred to a trauma center with obstetric capabilities whenever possible. Patients with a viable pregnancy (> 24 weeks) plus abnormal vital signs, chest pain, loss of consciousness, or a significant mechanism, should be transported to a trauma center if practical.[9] Blunt abdominal trauma, uterine tenderness, vaginal bleeding, or leakage of amniotic fluid is predictive of obstetric complications.[10] Hemodynamically stable patients with pre-viable pregnancies and no apparent serious injury, can be safely managed at the nearest facility based on local Emergency Medical Services (EMS) protocols.

Box 21.3   Essential prehospital interventions
- If spine precautions are required, the backboard should be tilted 15° to avoid supine hypotension

- Supplemental oxygen
- Intravenous fluids, especially if signs of hemodynamic compromise or serious injury
- Transport (when practical) to a Level I trauma center with obstetric capabilities if serious injuries, major mechanism, or signs of obstetrical complications including uterine contractions, uterine tenderness, vaginal bleeding, leakage of amniotic fluid.
- Greater than 20 weeks pregnancy should be determined by history or by fundal height at or above umbilicus.

Emergency department evaluation and management

Common presentations

Pregnant patients present with a full range of potential injuries, and are generally evaluated in the same manner as non-pregnant patients, with consideration of a few specific pregnancy-related conditions, the most common of which is abruption of the placenta. Early in pregnancy, the uterus and fetus are entirely within the pelvis, affording direct protection from all but the most severe blunt trauma. As the pregnancy progresses, the fetus itself remains fairly well protected from blunt trauma forces, bathed in amniotic fluid. However, the placenta, being a more fixed structure, can be negatively affected by traumatic forces. Placental abruption can be subtle and difficult to diagnose. Abdominal pain is present in almost all cases. Vaginal bleeding is uncommon. Ultrasound is insensitive for the diagnosis of placental abruption as the bleeding is often indistinguishable from the placenta itself. Signs of fetal distress on fetal heart rate monitoring, including late decelerations, loss of variability and persistent tachycardia or bradycardia, are the best indication of placental abruption, although they may be somewhat non-specific. A normal monitor strip, however, provides a considerably increased probability that there is no significant fetal distress (Figure 21.2). If abruption is expected, and there are signs of fetal distress, an emergency cesarean may be indicated.

Preterm labor, defined as, uterine contractions with progressive cervical dilation, is another potential complication following trauma. Similar to placental abruption, even minor injuries can precipitate

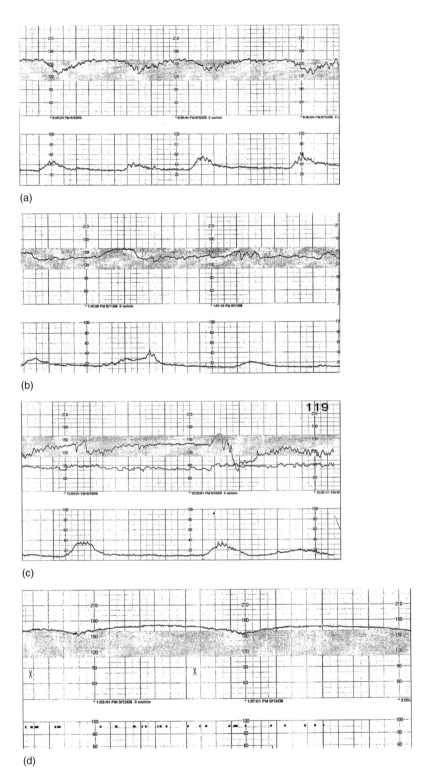

(a)

(b)

(c)

(d)

Figure 21.2 Fetal monitor tracings: (a) early decelerations; (b) normal decelerations; (c) normal with increased variability; (d) late decelerations (X marks area of contractions). (Courtesy of George Musalli, MD.)

preterm labor. Uterine rupture is a devastating complication of severe trauma and is almost always uniformly fatal for the fetus. Uterine rupture presents in a similar manner as placental abruption. Physical exam is notable for uterine tenderness and may reveal palpable fetal parts.

Penetrating injuries to the abdomen during pregnancy are associated with a high rate of complications for both the mother and the developing fetus. As the uterus enlarges, the bowel is displaced superiorly, changing the pattern of injury following penetrating trauma. The large, muscular uterus also offers some protection to the mother. For example, a gunshot wound to the abdomen has a 19% incidence of visceral injury in pregnant patients, compared to an 82% incidence in non-pregnant patients.[11] A large proportion of fetal deaths from trauma are the result of penetrating injuries, primarily gunshot wounds.[12]

Initial evaluation

The primary survey is performed according to Advanced Life Support protocols, with careful consideration of the cardiopulmonary alterations described earlier. Pregnancy increases the risk of aspiration because of decreased esophageal sphincter tone and elevation of the diaphragm. Pregnant patients also have decreased oxygen reserves, and given the susceptibility of the fetus to hypoxia, early intubation should be considered. Additionally, the fluid retention typically associated with pregnancy can cause swelling of the soft tissues of the airway. Given all these factors, the emergency physician must be prepared for a potential difficult airway when intubating a pregnant patient in the third trimester. Rapid sequence induction agents may be used in pregnancy; however, if delivery is imminent, a flaccid, apneic, infant may result, as paralytics do cross the placenta.[13] Careful attention to oxygenation and subtle signs of respiratory compromise is essential. If tube thoracostomy is required, the chest tube should be placed two intercostal spaces higher to avoid entering the abdominal cavity.[8] When evaluating hemodynamics, the physiologic changes of pregnancy must be kept in mind. The changes in vital signs that accompany the different phases of pregnancy should not mislead the physician into a false sense of security. Because of increased maternal blood volume, a pregnant patient may lose a large amount of blood before demonstrating signs of hemodynamic instability. The patient should be placed in the lateral decubitus position or have the gravid uterus manually displaced to avoid supine hypotension. Fluid resuscitation and transfusion of O-negative blood should be initiated early.

After evaluation of potential immediate life threats, a secondary survey is performed, and should include a complete evaluation of any potential maternal injuries and fetal monitoring should be initiated. The bedside focused abdominal sonography in trauma (FAST) exam is highly sensitive for intraperitoneal blood, as in non-pregnant patients, and should be performed early in the resuscitation.[14,15] A FAST exam in the pregnant patient is performed with the same technique as the non-pregnant patient. It may be useful to add additional views of the uterus to assess fetal location, presence of amniotic fluid, and fetal heart tones. A pelvic exam should be performed on all patients with major blunt trauma to the abdomen, pelvic fracture, signs of fetal distress, uterine contractions, vaginal bleeding, or leakage of clear fluid. This should be done to evaluate for presenting parts, intravaginal trauma, cervical dilation, or rupture of membranes. In the second and third trimester, a sterile speculum examination as the initial evaluation is appropriate. If there is a known or suspected concomitant placenta previa, do not perform the examination until an obstetrician is present. A positive nitrazine paper test or ferning of the vaginal fluid on a slide is suggestive of amniotic fluid. Consider the possibility of eclamptic seizures in the patient with altered mental status, particularly if the mechanism of the trauma is unclear.[8]

Acute interventions

In addition to the initial resuscitation of the mother, fetal heart tones and uterine activity should be monitored for a minimum of 4–6 hours, if the gestational age is > 20 weeks.[16,17] As mentioned above, signs of fetal distress include persistent tachycardia or bradycardia, decelerations, and loss of beat-to-beat variability (see Figures 21.2b and c above).

Secondary evaluation
Radiology studies

One of the most challenging aspects of managing a pregnant trauma patient is balancing the need to diagnose injuries in the mother, while avoiding unnecessary radiation exposure to the fetus. The

Diagnostic study	Fetal dose of radiation
Chest radiograph	0.02–0.07 mrad
Pelvis radiograph	100 mrad
Head CT	< 1 rad
Chest CT	< 1 rad
Abdominal/lumbar spine CT	3.5 rads
Cervical spine CT	< 1 rad
Pelvis CT	250 mrads

CT, computed tomography.

American College of Obstetrics and Gynecology has issued a consensus bulletin summarizing guidelines regarding diagnostic imaging during pregnancy that are very applicable to the pregnant trauma patient. In summary, the guidelines conclude that a pregnant woman should be counseled that X-ray exposure from a single diagnostic study does not result in harmful effects to a fetus. Specifically, exposure to < 5 rads has not been associated with an increase in fetal anomalies or pregnancy loss.[18] In a similar statement, the American College of Radiology concluded that:

> The risk of abnormality is considered to be negligible at 5 rads or less when compared to other risks of pregnancy, and the risk of malformations is substantially increased above control levels only at doses above 15 rads. Therefore, radiation exposure to the fetus arising from diagnostic procedures would very rarely, by itself, be a cause for terminating the pregnancy.[19]

Table 21.1 lists the approximate dose of fetal radiation, without lead shielding, from standard imaging studies obtained in trauma patients. A pregnant trauma patient can receive multiple studies and still be well below the 5 rads threshold. The American College of Obstetrics and Gynecology guidelines also recommend that alternative forms of imaging be considered when feasible, and that a radiologist (or radiation safety officer) may be of assistance in calculating the radiation dose of multiple studies.[18]

As discussed above, the FAST exam has the same sensitivity as in non-pregnant patients, and should be used routinely in the assessment of pregnant trauma patients. Ultrasonography can also be used for a quick assessment of the fetus, noting the fetal heart rate and the presence of amniotic fluid.[20] Ultrasound may demonstrate a placental abruption, but has a reported sensitivity of 50% and should not be used to routinely rule out an abruption. Computed tomography should be used in the pregnant trauma patient in the same manner as the non-pregnant trauma patient. If spleen or liver injury is the most likely diagnosis, a radiologist ultrasound looking for intraparenchymal injury as well as free fluid may be substituted as a screening examination; however, it is much less useful if hollow viscus or retroperitoneal injury is in the differential. While it is important to limit unnecessary computed tomography (CT) scans, especially in early pregnancy, the benefit of timely identification of maternal injuries far outweighs the risks of radiation to the fetus. In stable patients, magnetic resonance imaging (MRI) may be considered for the evaluation of the abdominal injuries, although this is not routinely performed in most centers because of lack of availability and the time required to obtain the images.

Laboratory tests

Hematocrit and coagulation studies including prothrombin time (PT), partial thrombin time (PTT), and fibrinogen, should be initially drawn, as disseminated intravascular coagulation (DIC) can be a devastating complication of placental abruption. Pregnancy alters several laboratory values starting as early as week 6 of gestation. White blood cell count is increased, as are fibrinogen and D-dimer levels. Hematocrit, blood urea nitrogen (BUN), and platelets are decreased. All pregnant trauma patients should have their blood type determined. Even minor trauma can result in mixing of maternal and fetal blood, therefore possibly exposing the Rh-negative mother to Rh-positive blood.[21] A Kleihauer–Betke (KB) test can be useful to estimate the amount of transplacental hemorrhage and therefore the amount of Rho (D) immunoglobulin needed to protect the Rh-negative mother. Additionally, in a recent study, significant amounts of transplacental hemorrhage and a positive KB test have been accurately used as a risk factor of preterm labor after trauma, helping to identify patients that need prolonged monitoring.[22] The KB test is performed by adding an acidic solution to a maternal blood smear. The red cells containing fetal hemoglobin are resistant to the acid and remain pink, while red cells containing adult hemoglobin are clear on the smear. A ratio of fetal : adult red cells is then used to estimate the amount of transplacental hemorrhage. The test is somewhat operator dependent, and its ability to predict complications from trauma is debated in the literature.[23]

Increased	Decreased
• White blood cell count	• Hematocrit
• Clotting factors	• BUN
• D-dimer, fibrinogen	• Platelets

Procedures

If intra-abdominal hemorrhage is strongly suspected and the FAST exam is indeterminate or negative, diagnostic peritoneal lavage (DPL) can be performed in the pregnant patient. During pregnancy, this should be done utilizing an open, supra-umbilical technique. This modification helps to avoid injury to the uterus.[24]

Treatment

In general, treatment of traumatic injuries during pregnancy is similar to the standard trauma patient. Box 21.5 outlines the ED management priorities.

Box 21.5 Emergency department essential interventions

- Identify and treat any injuries in the mother, in most cases, in the same manner as non-pregnant patients.
- Initiate fetal monitoring as soon as possible.
- Adequate fluid resuscitation and stabilization of the mother
- Consult obstetrics early if the patient is in the second or third trimester, or if there is evidence of fetal distress.
- Consider a perimortem cesarean section in cases of maternal cardiac arrest and a potentially viable fetus.

Most medications routinely given to trauma patients, including tetanus, are safe to give in pregnancy and should be administered as indicated (Table 21.2).

Rh immunoglobulin should be given to all Rh-negative pregnant women experiencing trauma, even without clear evidence of fetal hemorrhage. The standard dosage of Rho (D) immune globulin (RhoGAM) is 300 mcg (1 vial) intramuscularly. This covers roughly 15 ml of Rh-positive blood transferred from the fetus to maternal circulation. In an Rh-negative mother with extensive injuries, a Kleihauer–Betke test can help estimate the amount

Table 21.2 Safety in pregnancy of common medications used in trauma patients

Medications	Considerations in pregnancy
Tetanus	Safe to give in pregnancy
Antibiotics	Fluoroquinolones and gentamycin should not be given in pregnancy, most others are safe
RSIs	RSI medications may be used in pregnancy
Analgesia	Unless delivery is imminent, narcotic medications may be used. NSAIDS should be avoided because of potential compromise of the uterine blood supply
Sedation	Propofol may be given in pregnancy, benzodiazepines are contraindicated
Seizure medications	Dilantin and benzodiazepines should not be given in pregnancy. Remember to consider eclampsia as a potential etiology in the seizing patient
DVT prophylaxis	Pregnant patients are at increased risk for DVT. Lovenox and SQ heparin can be used in pregnancy

DVT, deep vein thrombosis; NSAIDS, non-steroidal anti-inflammatory drug; RSI, rapid sequence medication.

of fetal hemorrhage, and the need for additional doses of Rho (D) immunoglobulin.[22]

Emergent cesarean section may be performed with evidence of fetal distress. This also depends on the particular constellation of injuries to the mother, and the age of the fetus. Signs of fetal distress include late decelerations, persistent tachycardia or bradycardia, and loss of variability noted on fetal heart rate monitoring.

In the event of maternal cardiac arrest or a prearrest state, a perimortem cesarean section should be considered. Although even in the best cases outcome is generally poor, delivery of the fetus within 5 minutes of arrest is associated with better fetal outcomes and improved chances of an intact neurological status. Additionally, removing the fetus may actually improve maternal circulation and hemodynamics because of the improved blood return to the heart achieved when the weight of the fetus is removed from the vena cava.[25,26] Because of the extreme time sensitivity, emergency physicians should be familiar with the indications and technique of this procedure. To perform a perimortem cesarean, a No. 10 scalpel is used to make a midline, vertical incision from the symphysis pubis to the umbilicus. This incision should proceed into the peritoneal cavity, exposing the uterus. Exposure can be improved using retractors, and with Foley catheter decompression of the bladder if time allows. At this point, a small vertical incision should be made in the lower uterine segment, allowing fingers and scissors to enter the uterine cavity and extend the incision to the fundus. The fetus should then be delivered, nose and mouth suctioned, and the umbilical cord clamped and cut. It should be emphasized that this procedure is done as a last resort, with variable survival rates and resultant neurologic function of the newborn.[27,28]

Documentation

The medical record should reflect the full evaluation of maternal injuries and assessment of the fetus, including cardiotocomonitoring. Consultations with obstetrics should also be included on all patients with viable pregnancies. Trauma surgery consultation should be performed based on injuries.

Disposition

As described above, cardiotocomonitoring should continue for 4–6 hours in any pregnant patient > 20 weeks gestation (generally considered the lower limit of viability although not standardized), following multisystem or even minor abdominal trauma. Patients with evidence of uterine contractions, vaginal bleeding, non-reassuring fetal monitor strip, or uterine tenderness should be admitted for further monitoring.[1,16] Some investigators have attempted to determine specific risk factors for adverse fetal outcomes that warrant longer periods of monitoring. However, at this time, no independent predictive factors have emerged clinically useful.[29] As a general rule, clinicians should maintain a low threshold for admitting pregnant trauma patients, especially in the third trimester and following a significant mechanism of injury. Patients with minor injuries may be discharged after appropriate fetal monitoring, in consultation with obstetrics and gynecology. Close outpatient follow up should be arranged.

Finally, injury prevention and patient education are an important element of discharge instructions. All pregnant patients should be informed of the importance of seat belt use. Proper seat belt use has been shown to greatly impact outcomes for both the mother and fetus.[30–32] In pregnancy, the lap belt should be worn low across the pelvic rim and the shoulder restraint

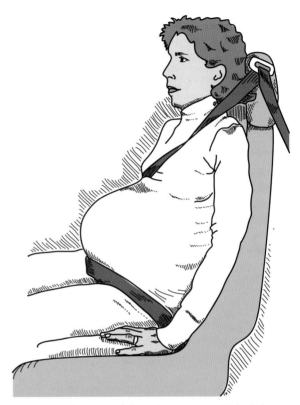

Figure 21.3 Proper seat belt use in pregnancy with lap belt worn low across the pelvic rim and the shoulder restraint placed between the breasts, above the uterus.

should be placed between the breasts, above the uterus (Figure 21.3). The safety of airbags in pregnancy is less clear. Known to improve outcomes in non-pregnant adults, there is concern that airbags may cause blunt abdominal trauma to the gravid uterus and fetus as they are often within 10 inches of the origination of the airbag. A recent study of 30 pregnant patients reported no increase in placental abruption or fetal mortality with airbag use.[33] The National Highway Safety Administration currently recommends the use of airbags in pregnancy, stating that the origin of the airbag should be > 10 cm from the abdomen.[33]

Box 21.6 Consultation/disposition/transfer criteria

- Obstetrics should be consulted for the large majority of pregnant trauma patients, including anyone at risk for traumatic or obstetrical complications. This is a must for any patient with a viable pregnancy and blunt abdominal trauma.
- Most pregnant trauma patients with viable pregnancies should be admitted to the hospital for treatment of their injuries and monitoring of the fetus.

- Patients with isolated minor injuries and viable pregnancies may be discharged after appropriate monitoring, usually 4–6 hours of cardiotocomonitoring. Close follow up with an obstetrician as an outpatient is important.
- A pregnant trauma patient should be transferred to a trauma center if practical following a high energy mechanism or with significant injuries, especially if they have a viable pregnancy.

In conclusion, management of trauma in pregnancy is challenging. Care of these patients is optimized by careful attention to the unique physiology and potential injuries associated with pregnancy, and careful monitoring of both the mother and developing baby.

References

1. Mattox KL, Goetzl L. Trauma in pregnancy. *Crit Care Med* 2005;**33**(10 Suppl.):S385–9.

2. Van Hook JW. Trauma in pregnancy. *Clin Obstet Gynecol* 2002;**45**(2):414–24.

3. Schiff MA, Holt VL, Daling JR. Maternal and infant outcomes after injury during pregnancy in Washington state from 1989 to 1997. *J Trauma* 2002;**53**(5):939–45.

4. Cahill AG, Bastek JA, Stamilio DM, et al. Minor trauma in pregnancy- is the evaluation warranted? *Am J Obstet Gynecol* 2008;**198**:208.e1–5.

5. Greenblatt JF, Dannenberg AL, Johnson CJ. Incidence of hospitalized injuries among pregnant women in Maryland, 1979–1990. *Am J Prev Med* 1997;**13**(5): 374–9.

6. El Kady D, Gilbert WM, Xing G, Smith LH. Association of maternal fractures with adverse perinatal outcomes. *Am J Obstet Gynecol* 2006;**195**(3): 711–16.

7. Hawkins JL. Anesthesia-related maternal mortality. *Clin Obset Gnecol* 2003;**46**(3):679–87.

8. Shah AJ, Kilcline BA. Trauma in pregnancy. *Emerg Med Clin North Am* 2003;**21**(3):615–29.

9. Rogers FB, Rozycki GS, Osler TM, et al. A multi-institutional study of factors associated with fetal death in injured pregnant patients. *Arch Surg* 1999;**134**(11): 1274–7.

10. Goodwin TM, Breen MT. Pregnancy outcome and fetomaternal hemorrhage after noncatastrophic trauma. *Am J Obstet Gynecol* 1990;**162**:665–71.

11. Lavery JP, Staten-McCormick M. Management of moderate to severe trauma in pregnancy. *Obstet Gynecol Clin North Am* 1995;**22**(1):69–90.

12. Chames MC, Pearlman MD. Trauma during pregnancy. *Clin Obset Gynecol* 2008;**51**(2):398–408.

13. Abouleish EI, Abboud TK, Bikhazi G, et al. Rapacuronium for modified rapid sequence induction in elective caesarean section: neuromuscular blocking effects and safety compared with succinylcholine, and placental transfer. *Br J Anaesth* 1999;**83**:862–7.

14. Ma OJ, Mateer JR, DeBehnke DJ. Use of ultrasonography for the evaluation of pregnant trauma patients. *J Trauma* 1996;**40**(4):665–8.

15. Goodwin H, Holmes JF, Wisner DH. Abdominal ultrasound examination in pregnant blunt trauma patients. *J Trauma* 2001;**50**(4):689–93; discussion 94.

16. Curet MJ, Schermer CR, Demarest GB, Bieneik EJ, 3rd, Curet LB. Predictors of outcome in trauma during pregnancy: identification of patients who can be monitored for less than 6 hours. *J Trauma* 2000; **49**(1):18–24; discussion 24–5.

17. Dahmus MA, Sibai BM. Blunt abdominal trauma: are there any predictive factors for abruptio placentae or maternal-fetal distress? *Am J Obstet Gynecol* 1993; **169**(4):1054–9.

18. ACOG Committee Opinion. Guidelines for diagnostic imaging during pregnancy. Number 299, September 2004 (replaces No. 158, September 1995). *Obstet Gynecol* 2004;**104**(3):647–51.

19. Gray JE. Safety (risk) of diagnostic radiology exposures. In *American College of Radiology. Radiation Risk: A Primer*. Reston, VA: American College of Radiology, 1996: pp. 15–17.

20. Brown MA, Sirlin CB, Farahmand N, Hoyt DB, Casola G. Screening sonography in pregnant patients with blunt abdominal trauma. *J Ultrasound Med* 2005; **24**(2):175–81; quiz 83–84.

21. Fisher M. Acute Rh isoimmunization following abdominal trauma associated with late abruption placenta. *Acta Obstet Gynecol Scand* 1989;**68**(7):657–9.

22. Muench MV, Baschat AA, Reddy UM, et al. Kleihauer-Betke testing is important in all cases of maternal trauma. *J Trauma* 2004;**57**(5):1094–8.

23. Dhanraj D, Lambers D. The incidences of positive Kleihauer-Betke test in low-risk pregnancies and maternal trauma patients. *Am J Obstet Gynecol* 2004;**190**(5):1461–3.

24. Rothenberger DA, Quattlebaum FW, Zabel J, Fischer RP. Diagnostic peritoneal lavage for blunt trauma in pregnant women. *Am J Obstet Gynecol* 1977;**129**(5):479–81.

25. Katz V, Balderston K, DeFreest M. Perimortem cesarean delivery: were our assumptions correct? *Am J Obstet Gynecol* 2005;**192**(6):1916–20; discussion 20–1.

26. Katz VL, Dotters DJ, Droegemueller W. Perimortem cesarean delivery. *Obstet Gynecol* 1986;**68**(4):571–6.

27. Whitten M, Irvine LM. Postmortem and perimortem caesarean section: what are the indications? *J R Soc Med* 2000;**93**:6–9.

28. Sugrue M, Kolkman KA. Trauma during pregnancy. *Aust J Rural Health* 1999;**7**:82–4.

29. Schiff MA, Holt VL. The injury severity score in pregnant trauma patients: predicting placental abruption and fetal death. *J Trauma* 2002;**53**(5):946–9.

30. Schiff MA, Holt VL. Pregnancy outcomes following hospitalization for motor vehicle crashes in Washington state from 1989 to 2001. *Am J Epidemiol* 2005;**161**(6):503–10.

31. Johnson HC, Pring DW. Car seatbelts in pregnancy: the practice and knowledge of pregnant women remain causes for concern. *BJOG* 2000;**107**(5):644–7.

32. McGwin G, Jr., Russell SR, Rux RL, et al. Knowledge, beliefs, and practices concerning seat belt use during pregnancy. *J Trauma* 2004;**56**(3):670–5.

33. Metz TD, Abbott JT. Uterine trauma in pregnancy after motor vehicle crashes with airbag deployment: a 30-case series. *J Trauma* 2006;**61**(3):658–61.

Geriatric trauma

Phillip D. Levy and Michael Stern

Introduction

Over the past half-century, there has been a steady increase in the proportion of individuals living beyond the age of 65 in the United States. This trend is expected to continue such that, by 2040, nearly 1 out of every 5 Americans will be in the geriatric age range (i.e., aged 65 or older).[1–3] A considerable portion of this demographic shift is due to growth among the subset of elderly who are > 85 years of age.[4] Such improvements in longevity can be attributed to both advances in health care and a burgeoning societal focus on maintenance of wellness through exercise, diet modification, and smoking cessation. As a result, the elderly are not only living longer but are also living better, increasing their exposure to potentially injurious activity (e.g., jogging, skiing, and bicycling) and high-energy mechanical forces (e.g., motor vehicle collisions and pedestrian-related accidents).[3,4]

Trauma registry data reflect this population trend, with a consistent increase in the number of emergency department (ED) visits for traumatic events in the elderly over the past 20 years.[5,6] It is expected that this will continue, with a projection for geriatric patients to represent 40% of all trauma encounters by 2050.[7] From a societal perspective, this is important because elderly trauma victims are at greater risk for adverse outcome, account for more healthcare expenditures (nearly 30% overall), and are more likely to suffer long-term functional decline than their younger counterparts.[7–14] Trauma is in fact, the fifth leading cause of mortality among geriatric patients, with an age-specific case-fatality rate that ranges from 15% to 30% (vs. from 4% to 8% for those < 65 years of age).[4,8,12,15] On the whole, elderly patients account for almost one third of annual trauma related deaths in the United States.[1,16–18]

Clinical anatomy and pathophysiology

Although age 65 is traditionally regarded as the age at which one becomes "elderly," there is evidence to suggest that risk of poor outcome from trauma begins to rise as early as age 40.[6,19] Mortality in particular, increases significantly after age 56, with a 6% rise in the odds of death per year after age 65 and a doubling in risk by age 75.[2,20–22] Much of this is due to anatomic changes associated with senescence, which place the aging patient at greater risk for injury from traumatic events, and physiologic alterations that decrease their ability to respond to resulting systemic insults. Each organ is affected in specific ways, tends to age independently, and, in general, follows a functional decline of roughly 1% per year after the age of 30. In an interrelated fashion, a combination of these changes predisposes an elderly person to injury. Older individuals may have decreased peripheral vision, hearing, balance and coordination, and delayed reaction times, thereby increasing their risk of trauma. As well they may have decreased cognitive ability, memory, and judgment. Often, postural instability or changes, such as kyphosis, may make hazards or warning signs difficult to see. For instance, the crossing rate of traffic signals, which is equal to 4 ft/s, may be too fast for weak, arthritic, or disabled individuals.[13]

Comorbid disease states and pre-existing medical conditions (PMC), which are present in approximately 35–45% of those who are 65 or older, 65% of those ≥ 75 years, and 90% of those ≥ 85 years, strongly contribute by increasing the possibility of a traumatic event (especially vehicular collisions), diminishing available physiological reserve, and worsening the degree of injury.[15,23–30] These interactions may be a direct consequence of the underlying

Trauma: A Comprehensive Emergency Medicine Approach, eds. Eric Legome and Lee W. Shockley. Published by Cambridge University Press. © Cambridge University Press 2011.

Table 22.1 Combination of variables predictive of death in the elderly

Anatomic variables	Severe thoracic or abdominal injury (AIS > 3)	Moderate to severe head injury (AIS ≥ 3)
Physiologic variables	Hypotension on arrival (SBP < 90 mmHg)	Evidence of profound shock (base deficit ≤ −12)

AIS, Abbreviated Injury Scale; SBP, systolic blood pressure.

condition (i.e., related to auditory, visual, neuromuscular, cardiovascular, or pulmonary impairments) or indirectly due to medication side effects. Certain medications including psychotropics (i.e., antidepressants, neuroleptics, and sedatives), antihypertensives (i.e., beta-blockers, calcium channel blockers, angiotensin-converting enzyme [ACE] inhibitors, and diuretics), hypoglycemic agents, and anticoagulants/antiplatelet agents are especially problematic.[1,31] These drugs can affect the vestibular system, cause profound sedation or disorientation, blunt the tachycardic response, lower blood sugar, and produce postural hypotension. Concurrent therapy with four or more chronic medications has been shown to increase an elderly person's risk for falls.[32,33]

Neurological

Changes in brain anatomy can cause unique patterns of intracranial injuries in the elderly patient (Table 22.1). The dura mater is firmly adherent to the calveria, therefore epidural hematomas are extremely uncommon. In contrast, normal age-related cerebral atrophy causes tension and stretching of the bridging veins; shear stresses can lead to tearing of the veins and subsequent acute subdural hematomas, which are more prevalent in geriatric head trauma patients. Age-related cerebral atrophy allows for more intracranial space and therefore greater accumulation of blood or edema leading to delays in the onset of neurologic dysfunction. This atrophy also causes increased mobility of the brain within the skull which can lead to cerebral contusions due to coup or contrecoup impact. An age-related decline in cerebrovascular autoregulation may exacerbate the effect of such injuries and be associated with the increased rate of adverse outcomes seen in elderly patients with head trauma.[34]

Hypersensitivity to central nervous system-mediated medications, such as benzodiazepines, antidepressants, and antihistamines is more common with aging. As a result, side effects, such as delirium, agitation, somnolence, depression, and even worsening dementia are frequently seen in the elderly. Such medication-related events can confuse the clinical presentation and may incorrectly be interpreted as injury-related decompensation. They ultimately may be implicated in the cause of the traumatic event, further obfuscating the clinical scenario.

Cardiovascular

Cardiac functional reserve is diminished with age. Progressive stiffening of the myocardium can lead to decreased pumping efficacy causing a lower maximal cardiac output. By example, an 80 year old without any significant coronary artery disease has, on average, 50% of the maximal cardiac output compared to a 20 year old. Cardiac index ([stroke volume × heart rate]/body surface area) is the physiologic variable that differs most between elderly and younger patients and carries the most clinical significance during trauma resuscitation.[35] The existence of underlying systolic cardiac dysfunction with a reduced ejection fraction is an important factor and may limit the ability of the elderly to mount a compensatory increase in stroke volume in the face of increased metabolic needs associated with trauma. The elderly also have a blunted inotropic and chronotropic response to trauma-induced pain, anxiety, or hypovolemia, due in large part to diminished myocardial sensitivity to endogenous and exogenous catecholamines and a progressive fibrosis of the cardiac conduction system. Evidence of poor perfusion in the elderly trauma patient, therefore, may not necessarily reflect a hemorrhagic etiology and instead may be caused by the profound cardiac changes associated with aging. The presence of hypoperfusion, even if transient, can be especially problematic for elderly patients, especially those with coronary artery disease, resulting in an increased risk of cardiac ischemia and its associated consequences. This may be difficult to recognize however, based on blood pressure alone as there is an age-related increase in peripheral vascular resistance. Reduced vascular elasticity and compliance caused by atherosclerosis may also produce a relative increase in blood pressure and coincidentally, enhance the risk of arterial injury, particularly to the aorta. As a result, a "normal" blood pressure may actually represent relative hypotension in an older patient.

Responses to certain medications are also altered with aging, resulting in potentially significant consequences. In particular, the elderly appear to have an age-related decrease in response to cardiac medications, including calcium channel blockers and parasympathetic agonists and antagonists. These changes may contribute to the absent tachycardic response often seen in elderly patients who develop hypotension.[36,37]

Pulmonary

Pulmonary changes as a result of aging are numerous and include a decline in lung elasticity and thus recoil, leading to a decreased mechanical compliance and an increase in work of breathing. In addition, there exists an almost linear, age-dependent decline in PaO_2 of 2–3 mmHg per decade after the age of 20 years old as a result of alveolar surface area loss and decreased diffusion capacity.[38] As a result, an 80-year-old patient can have a baseline PaO_2 of between 78 and 92 mmHg. In addition, bronchial ciliary function declines with age, affecting the ability to clear mucus secretions. All of these changes result in an increased residual volume and concomitant decreased vital capacity, as well as an increased risk of aspiration and infection. Elderly patients may also have an increased anterior-posterior diameter of the thorax that can lead to a severe loss of intrathoracic volume and bone cage compliance.[39] This, coupled with the high prevalence of osteoporosis leads to a higher incidence of rib and sternal fractures with fewer pulmonary contusion injuries.[40]

Renal

Changes in renal function due to aging include a decrease in approximately one third of the renal mass and, therefore, functioning nephrons and renovascular bed, resulting in an age-related decline in creatinine clearance. Because muscle mass is the primary source of creatinine and declines commensurately in the elderly, a serum creatinine level is often misinterpreted as "normal" when, in fact, it may actually reflect a significant reduction in renal function. In addition, aging causes a narrowing of the renal arteries and a reduction in renal blood flow, contributing to a decline in the glomerular

filtration rate (GFR). Diminished GFR and creatinine clearance greatly affect drug elimination by the kidneys. Drugs with narrow therapeutic windows, such as digoxin and the aminoglycosides, need to be administered with diminished renal function in mind in order to avoid potential toxicity. Dosage adjustment for many medications is required using the Cockroft and Gault formula, and a heightened awareness must be maintained regarding medication choice (including intravenous contrast dye) because of the potential for drug-related complications.[41,42]

Box 22.1 Cockcroft and Gault formula

Estimating creatinine clearance (ml/min)

Cockcroft and Gault equation

CrCl = (140 − age) × IBW/(Scr × 72) (× 0.85 for females)

IBW, ideal body weight in (kg).

Hepatic

In addition, to renal elimination, hepatic metabolism is an important factor in drug clearance. Aging is associated with decreased hepatic blood flow, which can alter the clearance of drugs that undergo rapid first-pass hepatic metabolism, such as beta-blockers, calcium channel blockers, and narcotics, thereby increasing their potential toxicity. An age-related decline in functional hepatocyte number and enzyme activity affects the clearance of other drugs, such as phenytoin. Also, aging affects the non-synthetic hepatic biotransformation reactions (oxidative and hydrolytic) more readily than synthetic enzymatic reactions, such as conjugation. Therefore, diazepam is more likely to cause increased sedation because it undergoes oxidative metabolism, unlike lorazepam, which is conjugated by the liver.[43]

Musculoskeletal

The musculoskeletal changes of aging can have a profound effect on the elderly trauma patient. The decrease in bone mass and disruption in its micro-architecture associated with age-related osteopenia and osteoporosis increase the risk of fracture. Overall, impaired strength, mobility, and bone density place the elderly at an increased risk for falls. Their relative inability to withstand the mechanical and kinetic forces of trauma can have devastating orthopedic consequences.

In addition to their direct effects on skeletal injury, a decline in muscle mass and lean body weight as well as an increase in fat can impact drug absorption and clearance. Drugs such as aminoglycosides, procainamide, digoxin, and coumadin are distributed primarily in lean tissues and consequently have reduced distribution volumes and increased serum concentrations. Therefore, dosages often need to be adjusted downward to avoid toxicity. Other drugs, such as phenytoin, benzodiazepines, and barbiturates, have increased volumes of distribution in the elderly, as a result of their higher proportion of adipose tissue. This effectively prolongs their duration of action, leading to potential side effects such as increased sedation.[43]

Dermatological

The effects of aging on skin are numerous and result in a decline of virtually all skin functions. A decrease in melanocytes, cutaneous nerves, subcutaneous fat, sweat glands, epidermal/dermal contact, and collagen matrix composition can cause impaired thermal regulation, a reduced sensitivity to touch and pain, impaired defenses against microorganisms, and diminish tensile strength. This increases the potential for traumatic injury, especially burns and skin avulsions/tears. Intrinsic wound repair is also impaired with a delay of 20–60% in the rate of healing and a decline in all four phases of the healing continuum (i.e., hemostasis, inflammation, proliferation, and resolution).[44] As a result, both the risk of dermal injury and the likelihood of complications such as hypothermia and infection are increased with age.

Sensory

The visual and auditory changes of aging increase the risk of trauma in the elderly. Increased lens size and permeability and decreased lens flexibility can cause presbyopia and reduced visual acuity, as well as increased glare, impaired darkness adaption, and cataracts. With regard to hearing, decreased elasticity of the tympanum, impaired articulation of ossicles, and loss of auditory cortex neurons can cause high-frequency hearing loss and impaired functional capacity. Each of these changes confers an increased trauma risk for the elderly person.

Box 22.2 Overview of anatomic and physiologic factors that contribute to injuries and adverse outcome among elderly trauma victims

Anatomic	Physiologic
Airway	
• Floppy epiglottis	
• Temporomandibular joint (TMJ) arthritis	
• Cervical spine arthritis	
Pulmonary	**Pulmonary**
• ↑ Chest wall rigidity	• ↑ Work of breathing
• ↑ Mechanical compliance	• ↓ Diffusion capacity
• ↓ Lung elasticity	• ↓ Residual volume
• ↓ Alveolar surface area	• ↓ Vital capacity
• ↓ Mucociliary function	
• ↑ Thoracic anteroposterior (AP) diameter	
• ↓ Intrathoracic volume	
• ↓ Thoracic cage compliance	
Cardiovascular	**Cardiovascular**
• Myocardial stiffening	• ↓ Cardiac output
• Conduction defects	• ↓ Sensitivity to catecholamines
	• ↓ Inotropic/chronotropic response
	• ↑ Peripheral vascular resistance
	• ↓ Baroreceptor response
Neurological	**Neurological**
• Cerebral atrophy	• ↓ Cerebrovascular autoregulation
• Stretching of bridging veins	• ↓ Central thermoregulation
Hepato-renal	**Hepato-renal**
• ↓ Hepatic and renal blood flow	• ↓ Creatinine clearance
• ↓ Nephron and hepatocyte mass	• ↓ GFR
• Renal artery stenosis	• Alteration in RAAS axis
	• Altered pharmacokinetics and pharmacodynamics

Musculoskeletal
- ↓ Muscle mass
- ↓ Lean body weight
- ↑ Fat
- ↓ Bone mass and density
- Kyphosis

Musculoskeletal
- ↓ Peripheral thermoregulation

Dermatological
- ↓ Melanocytes
- ↓ Cutaneous nerves
- ↓ Subcutaneous fat
- ↓ Sweat glands
- ↓ Epidermal/ dermal contact

Dermatological
- ↓ Sensitivity to touch and pain
- ↓ Infection defense
- ↓ Wound healing

Sensory
- ↓ Lens flexibility
- ↑ Lens size and permeability
- Cataracts
- ↓ Tympanic elasticity
- Impaired articulation of ossicles
- ↓ Auditory cortex neurons

Sensory
- ↓ Visual acuity
- ↓ Darkness adaption
- ↑ Glare
- High frequency hearing loss
- Impaired functional hearing capacity

Prehospital

In general, most prehospital trauma algorithms can be applied to the elderly with little change. Caution, however, should be exercised with regard to aggressive fluid resuscitation and opioid analgesic administration for those with known cardiovascular or renal disease, as these interventions may precipitate hemodynamic decompensation. Because some elderly patients (particularly those who reside in nursing homes) have diminished speech and cognitive function, a comprehensive history may not be readily available. Prehospital personnel, therefore, should make every effort to obtain information regarding PMCs and current pharmaceutical therapy from existing documents, pill bottles, caregivers, knowledgeable family members, or friends/neighbors who may be familiar with the individual's health status. If the incident occurred at the patient's home, prehospital personnel should also appraise the safety of the living situation and make note of factors that render the location potentially hazardous for return.

Once the patient and their injuries have been adequately assessed and stabilized, the prehospital provider must decide what level of hospital-based care is required. Appropriate triage of the injured elderly can profoundly impact outcome with clear survival advantages for those seriously injured who are treated at designated trauma centers.[45–47] There is evidence to suggest that older trauma patients are less likely to receive trauma center care, particularly when injury severity is perceived to be low.[48–51] This may be due to over-reliance on physiologic criteria (i.e., hypotension and tachycardia), which are often absent in geriatric trauma victims leading to an under-recognition of the true risk associated with seemingly minor injuries.[52–54] Some hospitals have begun to include age as a stand-alone criterion for trauma team activation which has resulted in a substantial mortality benefit.[55] It may be best for prehospital providers too.

Box 22.3 Essentials in prehospital care of the elderly

- In general, most prehospital trauma algorithms can be applied to the elderly with little change.
- Caution should be exercised with regard to aggressive fluid resuscitation and opioid analgesic administration.
- Physiologic criteria (i.e., hypotension and tachycardia) may not be present in seriously injured elderly patients.
- Adopt a rule-out (i.e., consider level of injury to be significant until proven otherwise) rather than a rule-in philosophy for all geriatric trauma patients and consider a low-threshold for triage to trauma centers.

Emergency department evaluation and management

Presentation

While age itself is an independent contributor to the disproportionate mortality which exists among elderly trauma patients, injury severity appears to be a critical factor.[10,16,23,28,29,56–59] In general, the extent of injury is reflective of the causal mechanism but for similar events, severity tends to be more significant among older patients. This is particularly evident for trauma related to falls and pedestrian-struck incidents where the elderly are 3–4 times more likely to die from their injuries and account for nearly 50% of the overall associated mortality.[1,3,60–63]

Falls are responsible for the majority (~60%) of elderly traumatic events, most of which occur at a standing height.[64] The overall risk for geriatric patients is significant, with 30–40% of those living in the community and 50% of those who reside in a long-term care facility experiencing at least 1 fall after age 65.[31,65] Though high-level falls (i.e., > 15 ft) are less common, they are more likely to result in injury, especially pelvic and femur fractures and lead to a dramatic increase in mortality (25% vs. 11%).[1,60]

Motor vehicle-related incidents (i.e., automobile collisions and pedestrian-struck events) are the second most common cause of trauma in the elderly and are responsible for some of the most devastating injuries.[1,3,56] With the exception of a predisposition towards sternal fractures, injury patterns do not differ dramatically for elderly individuals involved in a collision.[52] On the other hand, older pedestrians who have been struck by a motor vehicle are at increased risk for severe trauma to the head and chest, spinal injuries, and fractures of the pelvis and tibia.[61,63] Elderly patients struck as pedestrians also have an in-hospital mortality which exceeds 25% and are responsible for nearly 40% of all fatalities which occur at cross-walks.[3,61]

Thermal injuries in the elderly account for 13% of all burn unit admissions in the United States.[1] Though less common than other causes of trauma in the elderly, burns are associated with extensive tissue damage and significant morbidity as many of these individuals do not have the reflexes, muscle strength, or motor coordination to move away from the inflicting source until significant injury has occurred. Additionally, the process of wound healing is altered in the elderly increasing potential exposure to nosocomial infection and prolonging the time to recovery.[44] Consequently, mortality for these individuals is high, approaching 50% overall and 100% when a body surface area of ≥ 50% is involved.[1]

Though uncommon in many settings, penetrating trauma is responsible for 5–10% of all traumatic events that occur in the elderly (vs. 25–45% in younger patients).[66] While injuries are generally similar in location and severity to other age groups, wounds are more likely to be self-inflicted with a firearm among the elderly, particularly if the individual is a white male.[67] Despite comparable severity, penetrating trauma in the geriatric population is associated with prolonged intensive care unit (ICU) and hospital stays.[66,68] This is thought to be related to the disproportionate presence of comorbid conditions and resulting complications, but other factors related to the normal physiology of aging may be involved.

Though prior investigation has suggested an increased risk of death for elderly penetrating trauma victims,[10,69] recent studies have found no difference in severity-matched mortality for young vs. old patients.[66,68]

Box 22.4 Essentials of geriatric trauma presentations

- In general, the extent of injury is reflective of the causal mechanism but for similar events, severity tends to be more significant among older patients vs. younger.
- This is particularly evident for trauma related to falls and pedestrian-struck incidents.
- Falls are responsible for the majority of elderly traumatic events, followed by motor vehicle-related injuries.
- Pedestrian-struck injuries are particulary devastating with very high mortality and morbidity.
- Burns are associated with extensive tissue damage and significant morbidity (approaching 50% overall and 100% when a body surface area of ≥ 50% is involved).

Initial evaluation and management

Adherence to usual protocols during the initial evaluation and resuscitation of a geriatric trauma patient is appropriate. Signs and symptoms of respiratory difficulty should take precedence over other, potentially distracting injuries. Due to baseline physiological alterations, older patients are prone to develop hypoxia and supplemental oxygen should be administered upon presentation. More extensive airway management and breathing support, however, may be complicated by edentulousness, nasopharyngeal fragility, or arthritis, both cervical and temporomandibular. For patients who require mechanical ventilation, care must be taken to avoid overzealous manipulation of the oropharynx and hyperextension of the neck. If present, broken dentures should be removed as they increase the risk of further injury and foreign body aspiration but intact dentures will enhance facial seal during bag-valve-mask (BVM) respirations and should be left in place until definitive airway control is achieved. If medication is required to facilitate intubation, a 20–40% dose reduction should be considered for sedatives (i.e., benzodiazepines, barbiturates, etomidate, and propofol) to minimize the risk of cardiovascular decompensation, but adjustment of neuromuscular blocking agents is not necessary.[70]

Blunting of the ventilatory response to hypoxia and hypercarbia may be present and patients with subtle insufficiency can rapidly progress to respiratory failure. Pneumothorax, hemothorax, and pulmonary contusion should all be considered early in the evaluation of an elderly patient with thoracic trauma. Rib fractures may also cause dyspnea and are especially common in elderly trauma patients (estimated incidence: ~60%).[71] When present, rib fractures are a marker for more severe polytrauma and portend a far worse prognosis, increasing the risk of death and pneumonia by 19% and 27% (i.e., relative risk [RR] = 1.19 and 1.27), respectively for each additional rib involved.[72–76] Intubation and mechanical ventilation can assist the work of breathing and improve lung aeration and should be considered early on for those with significant hypoventilation due to their injuries.

Once the airway and breathing have been stabilized, circulatory assessment should be initiated. It is critical to remember that in the elderly, the degree of physiologic compromise cannot be accurately predicted by derangement from "normal" hemodynamic parameters (i.e., heart rate < 100 beats/min and a systolic blood pressure > 100 mmHg). This may be due to age-related changes of the cardiovascular system, which include a reduction in maximal heart rate (estimated by subtracting age from 220), decrease in cardiac index (~1% per year after age 30) and an overall increase in vascular resistance, and increased sensitivity to pharmacological therapy, especially beta-blockers and calcium channel blockers.[55,77] Significant hypoperfusion, therefore, may be present in a seemingly stable patient and investigation to identify occult reduction in tissue oxygen delivery should be considered. Initial assessment by blood gas (arterial or venous) can provide important laboratory data to estimate adequacy of perfusion (i.e., base deficit and serum lactic acid level) and should be stongly considered in all moderate to severe geriatric trauma patients. Impaired perfusion as indicated by a base deficit ≤ -6 mEq/L or a lactic acid concentration ≥ 2.4 mmol/L has been shown to correlate with greater trauma severity and an elevated risk of death.[78–82] The sensitivity of these markers, however, is more limited than the specificity and values within the normal range should be interpreted with caution. Repeat analysis within an hour of arrival therefore may be useful to help identify subtle or evolving hypoperfusion. Worsening of the base deficit or failure to clear lactic acid,[81,83] on serial measurement are particularly ominous signs and should be considered indicative of insufficient resuscitation or developing complications (i.e., blood loss or ischemia).[84]

Given the difficulty associated with cardiovascular evaluation in the elderly, early initiation of advanced hemodynamic monitoring is recommended for those with evidence of moderate or severe injury. Such an approach enables delineation of cardiac output and systemic vascular resistance resulting in the ability to optimize perfusion through targeted resuscitation using crystalloid fluids, vasopressors, and inotropes. Management in this manner has been shown to reduce mortality and multiorgan system failure for elderly trauma patients.[18,53,85,86] While pulmonary artery catheterization (PAC) is the time-honored method, there is ample evidence to suggest equivalent diagnostic and therapeutic yield from the use of non-invasive, thoracic bioimpedance technology with the benefit of lower associated cost and risk.[87–90] Such monitoring, however, is beyond the scope of usual ED practice and requires equipment typically reserved for an advanced critical-care setting. Limited bedside echocardiography in the ED may be a useful adjunct to hemodynamic monitoring (particularly for those patients with low cardiac output and elevated preload), providing rapid information with regard to the presence or absence of a pericardial effusion and a gross estimation of ejection fraction (i.e., normal vs. mild, moderate, or severe dysfunction).

> **Box 22.5 Essentials of initial evaluation in the geriatric patient**
>
> - Airway management and breathing support may be complicated by edentulousness, nasopharyngeal fragility, or arthritis.
> - A 20–40% dose reduction should be considered for intubation sedatives (i.e., benzodiazepines, barbiturates, etomidate, and propofol) to minimize the risk of cardiovascular decompensation; adjustment of neuromuscular-blocking agents is not necessary.
> - Rib fractures may also cause dyspnea and are especially common in elderly trauma patients.
> - Multiple rib fractures are a marker for more severe polytrauma and portend a worse prognosis.
> - In the elderly, the degree of physiologic compromise cannot be accurately predicted by

387

Box 22.5 (*cont.*)

derangement from "normal" hemodynamic parameters.

• Blood gas (arterial or venous) may provide laboratory data to estimate adequacy of perfusion (i.e., base deficit and serum lactic acid level) and should be considered in all moderate to severe geriatric trauma patients.

Secondary survey

In elderly trauma patients, closed head injury is relatively common and severe (i.e., Abbreviated Injury Scale [AIS] > 3).[53] Traumatic brain injury and intracranial hemorrhage occur with greater frequency in individuals older than 65 years who sustain closed head trauma (incidence of 12.5% vs. 7.9% in the National Emergency X-Radiography Utilization Study [NEXUS] II) and are associated with poorer outcome, particularly for those in whom the presenting Glasgow Coma Scale (GCS) score is ≤ 8 (in-hospital mortality 70–100%).[2,91–93] The vast majority (~75%) of these events are related to low-level falls,[94,95] which may result in only minor external injury. This can be deceiving however, and studies have shown limited applicability of typical "low-risk" criteria for potential intracranial injury (i.e., absence of loss of consciousness, lack of significant facial or cranial injury, and a GCS of 15) in the elderly.[94,96] Physiological factors such as dural adherence to the skull, bridging vessel fragility, and cerebral atrophy increase the likelihood of vascular disruption and permit mass effect accommodation leading to a greater risk of occult intracranial hemorrhage (especially subdural hematoma) from lower level trauma. Pharmaceutical therapy with anticoagulant or antiplatelet medications further enhances this risk and may be associated with a precipitous clinical deterioration.[97–101] As such, liberal use of computed tomography (CT) is recommended for elderly individuals with closed head trauma. For those patients on anticoagulation, rapid reversal using vitamin K, fresh frozen plasma, and possibly activated factor 7 should also be strongly considered.

Cervical spine injuries are also more common in the elderly occurring twice as frequently as in non-elderly patients (4.59% vs. 2.19% – NEXUS data).[102] In particular, there is a predilection towards injury at C1–C2 in older individuals, with a specific increase in the prevalence of odontoid fractures (RR [95% confidence interval] = 8.11 [5.37–12.3]).[102,103] Most of these injuries are caused by minor falls which may lead to under appreciation of the potential for injury. Incorporation of clinical decision rules for risk stratification in the elderly however, is somewhat complex. The Canadian Cervical Spine Rule includes age ≥ 65 as an independent, "high-risk" criterion, thus mandating radiographic assessment for all older trauma patients.[104] Conversely, the NEXUS Low-risk Criteria (which do not consider age) have been validated in a geriatric cohort, with estimation by study investigators that routine application could lead to a 14% reduction in cervical spine imaging for those aged 65 or older.[102] While it is difficult to say which approach is ideal, it is clear that radiographic study of the cervical spine will be necessary for the majority of geriatric trauma patients. Computed tomography is rapidly emerging as the modality of choice for initial evaluation of potential cervical spine injury in those with high-risk mechanisms, suspicious clinical findings, or anatomical variants likely to limit plain film interpretation, regardless of age.[105–107] Given the near ubiquitous presence of cervical osteophytosis and arthritis in the elderly and the elevated risk of injury, primary evaluation with CT, if practical, is recommended for all geriatric patients with cervical spine trauma. Concurrent performance with CT scanning of the brain for those with associated head trauma will maximize efficiency and cost-effectiveness.[108] Although spinal cord injury itself is rare, the elderly are at increased risk for development of central cord compression due to a high prevalence of underlying spondylosis and a common occurrence of fall-related cervical hyperextension. Classic signs and symptoms include upper motor neuron weakness (arms > legs, distal > proximal) with variable sensory deficit. When present, prompt neurosurgical consultation should be obtained and an emergent magnetic resonance imaging (MRI) should be considered.

Vertebral fractures of the thoracic and lumbar regions are also relatively common in the elderly and may be present in close to 40% of those with identified injuries of the cervical spine.[103] Osteoporosis, particularly among older females, increases the risk, especially for development of anterior wedge compression fractures. Though such fractures are unlikely to result in significant neurological complications, they can be a source of debilitating pain. While region-specific, plain film radiographs are sufficient for initial evaluation of those with point tenderness, subsequent investigation with CT should be performed for those with evidence of bony abnormalities or pain out of proportion to physical exam findings. Computed tomography, however, lacks sufficient sensitivity to definitively rule-out occult fractures and MRI or bone scanning may ultimately be required. Given the high prevalence of concurrent injury, with trauma below the neck complete spine X-rays should be obtained in all patients with cervical spine fractures, even in the absence of physical exam findings.

Thoracic trauma is a source of significant morbidity and mortality for the geriatric population.[72] Rib fractures, in particular, occur with increased frequency and result in an increased incidence of pulmonary complications.[76] Initial evaluation with a single view, AP chest radiograph is appropriate but may not clearly delineate subtle rib injuries, underlying lung contusion or small pneumothoraces. Computed tomography can enhance identification of such conditions and should be considered in those with a non-diagnostic CXR and significant discomfort or respiratory difficulty. Adequate pain control is essential and can have a profound impact on ventilatory status.[73] Epidural analgesia may be the most effective method,[73,109] but is difficult to initiate in the immediate treatment period. Opioid medications, therefore, should be administered with a low threshold for intubation if respiratory distress develops. Intercostal nerve blocks using bupivacaine are an effective alternative and can improve both pain and respiratory mechanics. In the patient with an isolated rib fracture, oral medication is probably appropriate; however, with multiple fractures, titrated intravenous sedation should be used.

Abdominal trauma in the elderly results in injury patterns similar to younger patients and can be approached in a manner generally analogous. Prompt recognition of hemodynamic instability, is particularly critical in older individuals, however, as they do not have the physiological reserve to withstand large volume blood loss. When identified as unstable, immediate evaluation by ultrasound or diagnostic peritoneal lavage (DPL) should be undertaken with a plan for possible surgical exploration or transfer if positive. Prior to operative intervention, early transfusion of packed red blood cells (PRBC) should be initiated and alternative causes of hypotension such as myocardial ischemia, pneumothorax, or cardiac tamponade should be ruled-out. Patients who remain unstable despite initial resuscitation (i.e., transfusion of 2 units of PRBC) should be targeted for surgical exploration. For stable patients, initial screening with ultrasound is reasonable, but negative results should be interpreted with caution, particularly for those with significant abdominal pain. A normal initial ultrasound can be followed by serial sonography and physical examination or CT scanning, based on underlying concerns. Those with abnormalities identified on ultrasound or suspicious clinical findings should be further evaluated using CT with inclusion of comprehensive organ injury grading to help guide treatment. While early reports suggested a higher failure rate for non-operative management of solid organ injuries in patients ≥ 55, recent evidence has shown outcome to be independent of age.[110] Consequently, non-operative management has emerged as the standard approach to care for hemodynamically stable, elderly patients with blunt hepatic or splenic injuries, regardless of grade.[73]

Declining muscle mass and bone density render the elderly highly susceptible to extremity fractures, particularly those that involve the wrist, hip, proximal femur, or humerus.[111,112] Primary intervention in the ED should be directed at injury identification with immobilization and reduction of gross deformities. Prompt diagnosis of hip fractures is especially important as outcome depends in part on the timing of operative fixation (goal in absence of comorbid medical conditions ≤ 24 hours).[73,113–115] Of note, occult hip fractures may be present in close to 5% of elderly individuals with initial negative radiographs.[116] Patients with persistent significant hip pain or inability to ambulate, therefore, should undergo subsequent evaluation, either by CT with fine cuts or MRI (preferred). Similar symptoms may be caused by injuries to the bony pelvis. While pelvic fractures in those ≤ 65 tend to be less severe than younger patients, the elderly are more likely to suffer from complications such as hemorrhage, have higher rates of angiography and ICU admission and are at increased risk of death.[117–119] Injury patterns differ as well, with a greater frequency of lateral (vs. anterior) compression fractures among older individuals.[117,119] Though in general geriatric patients are not thought to be disproportionately vulnerable to pelvic fractures, those with significant osteoporosis are at risk for a specific injury known as a sacral insufficiency fracture.[120] Although infrequent, it should be suspected in those with persistent low back

389

pain or sacral tenderness after seemingly minor trauma and is best diagnosed by CT or isotope bone scan.[120] Treatment of this condition, however, is generally conservative and a delay in diagnosis is unlikely to have any untoward consequences.

Additional considerations

The potential for contribution of a PMC to the patient's traumatic event should be considered. Because of the high rate of cardiac disease in the elderly, an electrocardiogram should be obtained in all elderly trauma patients with more than minimal or isolated mechanism (i.e., humeral fracure) to assess for potential ischemia or arrhythmias. Laboratory tests may reveal important findings such as electrolyte abnormalities, anemia, thrombocytopenia, or clotting disorders. Accurate depiction of renal function should also be sought, and can be achieved most effectively through calculation of creatinine clearance. For those with identified renal dysfunction, premedication (i.e., theophylline, bicarbonate, ascorbic acid or N-acetylcysteine) should be initiated (if time permits) to potentially help prevent contrast-induced nephropathy[121] and routine use of non-steroidal anti-inflammatory agents should be avoided, due to their effect on prostaglandin-mediated renal blood flow. A blood or breath alcohol level may be useful, especially for patients with altered mental status or apparent intentional injury.[122]

The goal of resuscitation for elderly trauma patients is survival to hospital discharge with intact neurological function. Because this may be achievable in > 50% of those who are severely injured,[123] initial aggressive resuscitation is warranted regardless of age, provided such an effort is not in contradiction with existing advanced directives. Most of the time, however, advanced directives are not applicable or known in the acute trauma situation. Although patient level factors such as underlying pulmonary disease and immunosuppression contribute, additional morbidity can be minimized through adherence to strict sterile technique when performing invasive procedures (especially central venous access and chest tube placement) and simple maneuvers such as elevation of the head of the bed (~30°) for those who are intubated. While expeditious management is essential to improve outcomes, it should be noted that geriatric trauma patients are more than twice as likely to develop nosocomial infections and more than five times as likely to die as a result of related complications.[124–126]

Based on a study of 76 304 elderly patients in the National Trauma Databank®, certain injuries are highly predictive (> 95% probability of death).[82]

While ongoing resuscitative efforts in such patients may be futile, the decision to withdraw care in the ED can be problematic. Such a pronouncement, therefore, should be deferred to the attending trauma surgeon with involvement of a palliative care or geriatric specialist and family members (if available).[2] If practicing at an institution where such services are not available, it is reasonable to discuss prognosis with family and assess their wishes prior to intervention or transfer.

Documentation

Other than documentation of advanced directives (i.e., present and reviewed or absent), there are few issues specific to the geriatric population. As with other patients, it is important to note a comprehensive history including PMCs and medications and indicate a consideration of how they may impact management. The ED chart should also contain information regarding procedures and who performed them as well as preventative measures which have been initiated. Inclusion of a listing of outstanding and reviewed radiographic and laboratory studies should also be done.

Disposition

The disposition of an elderly trauma patient should be determined on a case by case basis, yet certain guidelines should prevail. Admission is required for virtually all elderly patients who sustain multiple injuries. With less severe injuries, admission may still be warranted to search for potential causes of the trauma such as antecedent infection, metabolic derangement, intoxication, seizure, or ischemic event. As a general rule, when in doubt, err on the side of prudence and consider admission at least for a period of observation. High morbidity and mortality are seen in the elderly, particularly in the first 24 hours of admission and so a low threshold for utilization of an ICU setting should be incorporated.[127] Overall, these patients have longer hospital stays, incur higher overall hospital charges, require longer periods of rehabilitation, and have higher complication rates with poorer subsequent outcomes.[16,127–129]

Despite lack of data from a prospective randomized trial, evidence strongly favors the transfer to a designated trauma center for severely injured elderly trauma patients.[130,131] Patients with injuries requiring surgical or neurosurgical intensive care or burn care necessitate transfer to the appropriate center once best attempts at adequate stabilization have occurred. As well, patients requiring repeated or special surgical expertise should be considered for transfer. Attempts at delineating all injuries at the transferring hospital should be avoided if they will not change management or will delay transfer time to a designated trauma center for definitive care.[1] Additionally, studies are often repeated at the receiving facility, increasing risk of unnecessary radiation exposure and the total cost of care.[132]

Lower extremity orthopedic injuries confer a particularly high risk for elderly patients, and admission should therefore be strongly considered. The impact of joint or extremity immobilization on the patient's overall functional status must be considered. Arm slings, crutches, canes, and walkers can all contribute to gait instability, have not been shown to reduce the risk of falls, and may necessitate the need for admission.[133] If warranted, appropriate training in the use of any assist device is recommended.

The decision to discharge an elderly trauma patient needs to be made with a number of caveats in mind. If an isolated minor injury is sustained (usually from a fall) that yields a negative workup/evaluation, the patient can be considered a candidate for discharge. However, any patient who has an abnormal mental status, exhibits generalized weakness or profound fatigue after the event, has any gait instability, or reports recent recurrent falls is a poor candidate for discharge. Observation should be considered for minor head trauma patients on anticoagulant or antiplatelet medication. A referral for thorough falls assessment by a geriatric specialist may be warranted but this can be arranged through discussion with the patient's internist.

Once discharge has been decided, the emergency physician must assure timely and appropriate follow up. A multidisciplinary team approach may be indicated, including family members, the primary care physician, visiting nurse services, social work, and surgical and rehabilitation specialists. When necessary, adjustments in potentially dangerous chronic medications should be made, as well as arrangement of a home safety assessment to help prevent future falls. It is important to be aware that morbidity extends beyond the initial sustained injuries. Restricted activity and mobility, deconditioning, fear, social isolation, and loss of independence may be part of the long-term sequelae of a traumatic injury for an elderly patient.

References

1. Aschkenasy MT, Rothenhaus TC. Trauma and falls in the elderly. *Emerg Med Clin North Am* 2006;**24**(2):413–32.

2. Chang TT, Schecter WP. Injury in the elderly and end-of-life decisions. *Surg Clin North Am* 2007;**87**(1):229–45.

3. Pudelek B. Geriatric trauma: special needs for a special population. *AACN Clin Issues* 2002;**13**(1):61–72.

4. McMahon DJ, Shapiro MB, Kauder DR. The injured elderly in the trauma intensive care unit. *Surg Clin North Am* 2000;**80**(3):1005–19.

5. Clark DE, Chu MK. Increasing importance of the elderly in a trauma system. *Am J Emerg Med* 2002;**20**(2):108–11.

6. Hannan EL, Waller CH, Farrell LS, Rosati C. Elderly trauma inpatients in New York state: 1994–1998. *J Trauma* 2004;**56**(6):1297–304.

7. MacKenzie EJ, Morris JA, Jr., Smith GS, Fahey M. Acute hospital costs of trauma in the United States: implications for regionalized systems of care. *J Trauma* 1990;**30**(9):1096–101; discussion 101–3.

8. Champion HR, Copes WS, Buyer D, et al. Major trauma in geriatric patients. *Am J Public Health* 1989;**79**(9):1278–82.

9. DeMaria EJ, Merriam MA, Casanova LA, Gann DS, Kenney PR. Do DRG payments adequately reimburse the costs of trauma care in geriatric patients? *J Trauma* 1988;**28**(8):1244–9.

10. Finelli FC, Jonsson J, Champion HR, Morelli S, Fouty WJ. A case control study for major trauma in geriatric patients. *J Trauma* 1989;**29**(5):541–8.

11. MacKenzie EJ, Siegel JH, Shapiro S, Moody M, Smith RT. Functional recovery and medical costs of trauma: an analysis by type and severity of injury. *J Trauma* 1988;**28**(3):281–97.

12. McGwin G, Jr., Melton SM, May AK, Rue LW. Long-term survival in the elderly after trauma. *J Trauma* 2000;**49**(3):470–6.

13. Schwab CW, Kauder DR. Trauma in the geriatric patient. *Arch Surg* 1992;**127**(6):701–6.

14. Grossman M, Scaff DW, Miller D, et al. Functional outcomes in octogenarian trauma. *J Trauma* 2003;**55**(1):26–32.

15. McMahon DJ, Schwab CW, Kauder D. Comorbidity and the elderly trauma patient. *World J Surg* 1996;**20**(8):1113–19; discussion 19–20.

16. Ferrera PC, Bartfield JM, D'Andrea CC. Outcomes of admitted geriatric trauma victims. *Am J Emerg Med* 2000;**18**(5):575–80.

17. Koval KJ, Meek R, Schemitsch E, et al. An AOA critical issue. Geriatric trauma: young ideas. *J Bone Joint Surg Am* 2003;**85-A**(7):1380–8.

18. Lonner JH, Koval KJ. Polytrauma in the elderly. *Clin Orthop Relat Res* 1995;**318**:136–43.

19. Morris JA, Jr., MacKenzie EJ, Damiano AM, Bass SM. Mortality in trauma patients: the interaction between host factors and severity. *J Trauma* 1990;**30**(12):1476–82.

20. Grossman MD, Miller D, Scaff DW, Arcona S. When is an elder old? Effect of preexisting conditions on mortality in geriatric trauma. *J Trauma* 2002;**52**(2):242–6.

21. Kuhne CA, Ruchholtz S, Kaiser GM, Nast-Kolb D. Mortality in severely injured elderly trauma patients – when does age become a risk factor? *World J Surg* 2005;**29**(11):1476–82.

22. Taylor MD, Tracy JK, Meyer W, Pasquale M, Napolitano LM. Trauma in the elderly: intensive care unit resource use and outcome. *J Trauma* 2002;**53**(3):407–14.

23. Bergeron E, Lavoie A, Moore L, Clas D, Rossignol M. Comorbidity and age are both independent predictors of length of hospitalization in trauma patients. *Can J Surg* 2005;**48**(5):361–6.

24. Hollis S, Lecky F, Yates DW, Woodford M. The effect of pre-existing medical conditions and age on mortality after injury. *J Trauma* 2006;**61**(5):1255–60.

25. McGwin G, Jr., Sims RV, Pulley L, Roseman JM. Relations among chronic medical conditions, medications, and automobile crashes in the elderly: a population-based case-control study. *Am J Epidemiol* 2000;**152**(5):424–31.

26. Milzman DP, Boulanger BR, Rodriguez A, et al. Pre-existing disease in trauma patients: a predictor of fate independent of age and injury severity score. *J Trauma* 1992;**32**(2):236–43; discussion 43–4.

27. McGwin G, Jr., MacLennan PA, Fife JB, Davis GG, Rue LW, 3rd. Preexisting conditions and mortality in older trauma patients. *J Trauma* 2004;**56**(6):1291–6.

28. Pickering SA, Esberger D, Moran CG. The outcome following major trauma in the elderly. Predictors of survival. *Injury* 1999;**30**(10):703–6.

29. Richmond TS, Kauder D, Strumpf N, Meredith T. Characteristics and outcomes of serious traumatic injury in older adults. *J Am Geriatr Soc* 2002;**50**(2):215–22.

30. Rehm CG, Ross SE. Elderly drivers involved in road crashes: a profile. *Am Surg* 1995;**61**(5):435–7.

31. Tinetti ME, Baker DI, McAvay G, et al. A multifactorial intervention to reduce the risk of falling among elderly people living in the community. *N Engl J Med* 1994;**331**(13):821–7.

32. Robbins AS, Rubenstein LZ, Josephson KR, et al. Predictors of falls among elderly people. Results of two population-based studies. *Arch Intern Med* 1989;**149**(7):1628–33.

33. Tinetti ME, Williams TF, Mayewski R. Fall risk index for elderly patients based on number of chronic disabilities. *Am J Med* 1986;**80**(3):429–34.

34. Czosnyka M, Balestreri M, Steiner L, et al. Age, intracranial pressure, autoregulation, and outcome after brain trauma. *J Neurosurg* 2005;**102**(3):450–4.

35. McKinley BA, Marvin RG, Cocanour CS, et al. Blunt trauma resuscitation: the old can respond. *Arch Surg* 2000;**135**(6):688–93; discussion 94–5.

36. Demarest GB, Osler TM, Clevenger FW. Injuries in the elderly: evaluation and initial response. *Geriatrics* 1990;**45**(8):36–8, 41–2.

37. Cheitlin M, Zipes D. Cardiovascular disease in the elderly. In Braunwald E, Zipes D, Libby P (eds), *Heart Disease: A Textbook of Cardiovascular Medicine*, 6th edn. Philadelphia, PA: WB Saunders, 2001: pp. 2019–37.

38. Pontoppidan H, Geffin B, Lowenstein E. Acute respiratory failure in the adult. *N Engl J Med* 1972;**287**(14):690–8.

39. Brandstetter RD, Kazemi H. Aging and the respiratory system. *Med Clin North Am* 1983;**67**(2):419–31.

40. Martin RE, Teberian G. Multiple trauma and the elderly patient. *Emerg Med Clin North Am* 1990;**8**(2):411–20.

41. Montamat SC, Cusack BJ, Vestal RE. Management of drug therapy in the elderly. *N Engl J Med* 1989;**321**(5):303–9.

42. Podrazik PM, Schwartz JB. Cardiovascular pharmacology of aging. *Cardiol Clin* 1999;**17**(1):17–34.

43. Evans R, Ireland G, Morely J, Sheahan S. Pharmacology and aging. In Sanders A (ed.), *Emergency Care of the Elder Person*. St. Louis, MO: Beverly Cracom Publications, 1996: pp. 29–41.

44. Gosain A, DiPietro LA. Aging and wound healing. *World J Surg* 2004;**28**(3):321–6.

45. MacKenzie EJ, Rivara FP, Jurkovich GJ, et al. A national evaluation of the effect of trauma-center care on mortality. *N Engl J Med* 2006;**354**(4):366–78.

46. Pracht EE, Langland-Orban B, Tepas JJ, 3rd, Celso BG, Flint L. Analysis of trends in the Florida Trauma System (1991–2003): changes in mortality after establishment of new centers. *Surgery* 2006;**140**(1):34–43.

47. Tepas JJ, 3rd, Veldenz HC, Lottenberg L, et al. Elderly injury: a profile of trauma experience in the Sunshine (Retirement) State. *J Trauma* 2000;**48**(4):581–4; discussion 4–6.

48. Zimmer-Gembeck MJ, Southard PA, Hedges JR, et al. Triage in an established trauma system. *J Trauma* 1995;**39**(5):922–8.

49. Lane P, Sorondo B, Kelly JJ. Geriatric trauma patients-are they receiving trauma center care? *Acad Emerg Med* 2003;**10**(3):244–50.

50. Scheetz LJ. Effectiveness of prehospital trauma triage guidelines for the identification of major trauma in elderly motor vehicle crash victims. *J Emerg Nurs* 2003;**29**(2):109–15.

51. Scheetz LJ. Trauma center versus non-trauma center admissions in adult trauma victims by age and gender. *Prehosp Emerg Care* 2004;**8**(3):268–72.

52. Ma MH, MacKenzie EJ, Alcorta R, Kelen GD. Compliance with prehospital triage protocols for major trauma patients. *J Trauma* 1999;**46**(1):168–75.

53. Demetriades D, Karaiskakis M, Velmahos G, et al. Effect on outcome of early intensive management of geriatric trauma patients. *Br J Surg* 2002;**89**(10):1319–22.

54. Scheetz LJ. Relationship of age, injury severity, injury type, comorbid conditions, level of care, and survival among older motor vehicle trauma patients. *Res Nurs Health* 2005;**28**(3):198–209.

55. Demetriades D, Sava J, Alo K, et al. Old age as a criterion for trauma team activation. *J Trauma* 2001;**51**(4):754–6; discussion 6–7.

56. Hui T, Avital I, Soukiasian H, Margulies DR, Shabot MM. Intensive care unit outcome of vehicle-related injury in elderly trauma patients. *Am Surg* 2002;**68**(12):1111–14.

57. Knudson MM, Lieberman J, Morris JA, Jr., Cushing BM, Stubbs HA. Mortality factors in geriatric blunt trauma patients. *Arch Surg* 1994;**129**(4):448–53.

58. Shabot MM, Johnson CL. Outcome from critical care in the "oldest old" trauma patients. *J Trauma* 1995;**39**(2):254–9; discussion 9–60.

59. Tornetta P, 3rd, Mostafavi H, Riina J, et al. Morbidity and mortality in elderly trauma patients. *J Trauma* 1999;**46**(4):702–6.

60. Demetriades D, Murray J, Brown C, et al. High-level falls: type and severity of injuries and survival outcome according to age. *J Trauma* 2005;**58**(2):342–5.

61. Demetriades D, Murray J, Martin M, et al. Pedestrians injured by automobiles: relationship of age to injury type and severity. *J Am Coll Surg* 2004;**199**(3):382–7.

62. Kong LB, Lekawa M, Navarro RA, et al. Pedestrian-motor vehicle trauma: an analysis of injury profiles by age. *J Am Coll Surg* 1996;**182**(1):17–23.

63. Sklar DP, Demarest GB, McFeeley P. Increased pedestrian mortality among the elderly. *Am J Emerg Med* 1989;**7**(4):387–90.

64. Spaite DW, Criss EA, Valenzuela TD, Meislin HW, Ross J. Geriatric injury: an analysis of prehospital demographics, mechanisms, and patterns. *Ann Emerg Med* 1990;**19**(12):1418–21.

65. Graafmans WC, Ooms ME, Hofstee HM, et al. Falls in the elderly: a prospective study of risk factors and risk profiles. *Am J Epidemiol* 1996;**143**(11):1129–36.

66. Nagy KK, Smith RF, Roberts RR, et al. Prognosis of penetrating trauma in elderly patients: a comparison with younger patients. *J Trauma* 2000;**49**(2):190–3; discussion 3–4.

67. Crandall M, Luchette F, Esposito TJ, et al. Attempted suicide and the elderly trauma patient: risk factors and outcomes. *J Trauma* 2007;**62**(4):1021–7; discussion 7–8.

68. Roth BJ, Velmahos GC, Oder DB, et al. Penetrating trauma in patients older than 55 years: a case-control study. *Injury* 2001;**32**(7):551–4.

69. Champion HR, Copes WS, Sacco WJ, et al. The Major Trauma Outcome Study: establishing national norms for trauma care. *J Trauma* 1990;**30**(11):1356–65.

70. Milzman DP, Rothenhaus TC. Resuscitation of the geriatric patient. *Emerg Med Clin North Am* 1996;**14**(1):233–44.

71. Cameron P, Dziukas L, Hadj A, Clark P, Hooper S. Rib fractures in major trauma. *Aust N Z J Surg* 1996;**66**(8):530–4.

72. Alexander JQ, Gutierrez CJ, Mariano MC, et al. Blunt chest trauma in the elderly patient: how cardiopulmonary disease affects outcome. *Am Surg* 2000;**66**(9):855–7.

73. Victorino GP, Chong TJ, Pal JD. Trauma in the elderly patient. *Arch Surg* 2003;**138**(10):1093–8.

74. Bergeron E, Lavoie A, Clas D, et al. Elderly trauma patients with rib fractures are at greater risk of death and pneumonia. *J Trauma* 2003;**54**(3):478–85.

75. Stawicki SP, Grossman MD, Hoey BA, Miller DL, Reed JF, 3rd. Rib fractures in the elderly: a marker of injury severity. *J Am Geriatr Soc* 2004;**52**(5):805–8.

76. Bulger EM, Arneson MA, Mock CN, Jurkovich GJ. Rib fractures in the elderly. *J Trauma* 2000;**48**(6):1040–6; discussion 6–7.

77. Jacobs DG, Plaisier BR, Barie PS, et al. Practice management guidelines for geriatric trauma: the EAST

393

Practice Management Guidelines Work Group. *J Trauma* 2003;**54**(2):391–416.

78. Rixen D, Raum M, Bouillon B, Lefering R, Neugebauer E. Base deficit development and its prognostic significance in posttrauma critical illness: an analysis by the trauma registry of the Deutsche Gesellschaft fur unfallchirurgie. *Shock* 2001;**15**(2):83–9.

79. Davis JW, Kaups KL. Base deficit in the elderly: a marker of severe injury and death. *J Trauma* 1998; **45**(5):873–7.

80. Zehtabchi S, Baron BJ. Utility of base deficit for identifying major injury in elder trauma patients. *Acad Emerg Med* 2007;**14**(9):829–31.

81. Schulman AM, Claridge JA, Young JS. Young versus old: factors affecting mortality after blunt traumatic injury. *Am Surg* 2002;**68**(11):942–7; discussion 7–8.

82. Nirula R, Gentilello LM. Futility of resuscitation criteria for the "young" old and the "old" old trauma patient: a National Trauma Data Bank analysis. *J Trauma* 2004;**57**(1):37–41.

83. McNelis J, Marini CP, Jurkiewicz A, et al. Prolonged lactate clearance is associated with increased mortality in the surgical intensive care unit. *Am J Surg* 2001; **182**(5):481–5.

84. Tisherman SA, Barie P, Bokhari F, et al. Clinical practice guideline: end-points of resuscitation. *J Trauma* 2004;**57**(4):898–912.

85. Scalea TM, Simon HM, Duncan AO, et al. Geriatric blunt multiple trauma: improved survival with early invasive monitoring. *J Trauma* 1990;**30**(2):129–34; discussion 34–6.

86. Friese RS, Shafi S, Gentilello LM. Pulmonary artery catheter use is associated with reduced mortality in severely injured patients: a National Trauma Data Bank analysis of 53 312 patients. *Crit Care Med* 2006;**34**(6):1597–601.

87. Shoemaker WC, Wo CC, Chien LC, et al. Evaluation of invasive and noninvasive hemodynamic monitoring in trauma patients. *J Trauma* 2006;**61**(4):844–53; discussion 53–4.

88. Brown CV, Shoemaker WC, Wo CC, Chan L, Demetriades D. Is noninvasive hemodynamic monitoring appropriate for the elderly critically injured patient? *J Trauma* 2005;**58**(1):102–7.

89. Velmahos GC, Wo CC, Demetriades D, Shoemaker WC. Early continuous noninvasive haemodynamic monitoring after severe blunt trauma. *Injury* 1999; **30**(3):209–14.

90. Asensio JA, Demetriades D, Berne TV, Shoemaker WC. Invasive and noninvasive monitoring for early recognition and treatment of shock in high-risk trauma and surgical patients. *Surg Clin North Am* 1996;**76**(4):985–97.

91. Rathlev NK, Medzon R, Lowery D, et al. Intracranial pathology in elders with blunt head trauma. *Acad Emerg Med* 2006;**13**(3):302–7.

92. Kilaru S, Garb J, Emhoff T, et al. Long-term functional status and mortality of elderly patients with severe closed head injuries. *J Trauma* 1996;**41**(6):957–63.

93. Masson F, Thicoipe M, Aye P, et al. Epidemiology of severe brain injuries: a prospective population-based study. *J Trauma* 2001;**51**(3):481–9.

94. Nagurney JT, Borczuk P, Thomas SH. Elderly patients with closed head trauma after a fall: mechanisms and outcomes. *J Emerg Med* 1998;**16**(5):709–13.

95. Nagurney JT, Borczuk P, Thomas SH. Elder patients with closed head trauma: a comparison with nonelder patients. *Acad Emerg Med* 1998;**5**(7):678–84.

96. Mack LR, Chan SB, Silva JC, Hogan TM. The use of head computed tomography in elderly patients sustaining minor head trauma. *J Emerg Med* 2003; **24**(2):157–62.

97. Reynolds FD, Dietz PA, Higgins D, Whitaker TS. Time to deterioration of the elderly, anticoagulated, minor head injury patient who presents without evidence of neurologic abnormality. *J Trauma* 2003; **54**(3):492–6.

98. Cohen DB, Rinker C, Wilberger JE. Traumatic brain injury in anticoagulated patients. *J Trauma* 2006;**60** (3):553–7.

99. Ivascu FA, Janczyk RJ, Junn FS, et al. Treatment of trauma patients with intracranial hemorrhage on preinjury warfarin. *J Trauma* 2006;**61**(2):318–21.

100. Li J, Brown J, Levine M. Mild head injury, anticoagulants, and risk of intracranial injury. *Lancet* 2001;**357**(9258):771–2.

101. Ohm C, Mina A, Howells G, Bair H, Bendick P. Effects of antiplatelet agents on outcomes for elderly patients with traumatic intracranial hemorrhage. *J Trauma* 2005;**58**(3):518–22.

102. Touger M, Gennis P, Nathanson N, et al. Validity of a decision rule to reduce cervical spine radiography in elderly patients with blunt trauma. *Ann Emerg Med* 2002;**40**(3):287–93.

103. Lomoschitz FM, Blackmore CC, Mirza SK, Mann FA. Cervical spine injuries in patients 65 years old and older: epidemiologic analysis regarding the effects of age and injury mechanism on distribution, type, and stability of injuries. *AJR Am J Roentgenol* 2002;**178** (3):573–7.

104. Stiell IG, Wells GA, Vandemheen KL, et al. The Canadian C-spine Rule for radiography in alert and stable trauma patients. *JAMA* 2001;**286**(15):1841–8.

105. Gale SC, Gracias VH, Reilly PM, Schwab CW. The inefficiency of plain radiography to evaluate the cervical spine after blunt trauma. *J Trauma* 2005;**59**(5):1121–5.

106. Holmes JF, Akkinepalli R. Computed tomography versus plain radiography to screen for cervical spine injury: a meta-analysis. *J Trauma* 2005;**58**(5):902–5.

107. American College of Radiology. *Appropriateness Criteria: Suspected Spine Trauma.* Available from http://www.acr.org.

108. Grogan EL, Morris JA, Jr., Dittus RS, et al. Cervical spine evaluation in urban trauma centers: lowering institutional costs and complications through helical CT scan. *J Am Coll Surg* 2005;**200**(2):160–5.

109. Bulger EM, Edwards T, Klotz P, Jurkovich GJ. Epidural analgesia improves outcome after multiple rib fractures. *Surgery* 2004;**136**(2):426–30.

110. Gibson DE, Canfield CM, Levy PD. Selective nonoperative management of blunt abdominal trauma. *J Emerg Med* 2006;**31**(2):215–21.

111. Johansen A, Harding K, Evans R, Stone M. Trauma in elderly people: what proportion of fractures are a consequence of bone fragility? *Arch Gerontol Geriatr* 1999;**29**(3):215–21.

112. Cummings SR, Melton LJ. Epidemiology and outcomes of osteoporotic fractures. *Lancet* 2002; **359**(9319):1761–7.

113. Zuckerman JD, Sakales SR, Fabian DR, Frankel VH. Hip fractures in geriatric patients. Results of an interdisciplinary hospital care program. *Clin Orthop Relat Res* 1992;**274**:213–25.

114. Grimes JP, Gregory PM, Noveck H, Butler MS, Carson JL. The effects of time-to-surgery on mortality and morbidity in patients following hip fracture. *Am J Med* 2002;**112**(9):702–9.

115. Kenzora JE, McCarthy RE, Lowell JD, Sledge CB. Hip fracture mortality. Relation to age, treatment, preoperative illness, time of surgery, and complications. *Clin Orthop Relat Res* 1984;**186**:45–56.

116. Dominguez S, Liu P, Roberts C, Mandell M, Richman PB. Prevalence of traumatic hip and pelvic fractures in patients with suspected hip fracture and negative initial standard radiographs–a study of emergency department patients. *Acad Emerg Med* 2005;**12**(4):366–9.

117. Henry SM, Pollak AN, Jones AL, Boswell S, Scalea TM. Pelvic fracture in geriatric patients: a distinct clinical entity. *J Trauma* 2002;**53**(1):15–20.

118. Alost T, Waldrop RD. Profile of geriatric pelvic fractures presenting to the emergency department. *Am J Emerg Med* 1997;**15**(6):576–8.

119. O'Brien DP, Luchette FA, Pereira SJ, et al. Pelvic fracture in the elderly is associated with increased mortality. *Surgery* 2002;**132**(4):710–14; discussion 14–15.

120. Blake SP, Connors AM. Sacral insufficiency fracture. *Br J Radiol* 2004;**77**(922):891–6.

121. Sinert R, Doty CI. Evidence-based emergency medicine review. Prevention of contrast-induced nephropathy in the emergency department. *Ann Emerg Med* 2007;**50** (3):335–45, 45 e1–2.

122. Sorock GS, Chen LH, Gonzalgo SR, Baker SP. Alcohol-drinking history and fatal injury in older adults. *Alcohol* 2006;**40**(3):193–9.

123. van Aalst JA, Morris JA, Jr., Yates HK, Miller RS, Bass SM. Severely injured geriatric patients return to independent living: a study of factors influencing function and independence. *J Trauma* 1991;**31** (8):1096–101; discussion 101–2.

124. Hoover L, Bochicchio GV, Napolitano LM, et al. Systemic inflammatory response syndrome and nosocomial infection in trauma. *J Trauma* 2006;**61** (2):310–16; discussion 16–17.

125. Bochicchio GV, Joshi M, Knorr KM, Scalea TM. Impact of nosocomial infections in trauma: does age make a difference? *J Trauma* 2001;**50**(4):612–17; discussion 17–19.

126. El-Masri MM, Hammad TA, McLeskey SW, Joshi M, Korniewicz DM. Predictors of nosocomial bloodstream infections among critically ill adult trauma patients. *Infect Control Hosp Epidemiol* 2004;**25**(8):656–63.

127. Zietlow SP, Capizzi PJ, Bannon MP, Farnell MB. Multisystem geriatric trauma. *J Trauma* 1994;**37** (6):985–8.

128. DeMaria EJ. Evaluation and treatment of the elderly trauma victim. *Clin Geriatr Med* 1993;**9**(2):461–71.

129. Gomberg BF, Gruen GS, Smith WR, Spott M. Outcomes in acute orthopaedic trauma: a review of 130 506 patients by age. *Injury* 1999;**30**(6):431–7.

130. McConnell KJ, Newgard CD, Mullins RJ, Arthur M, Hedges JR. Mortality benefit of transfer to Level I versus Level II trauma centers for head-injured patients. *Health Serv Res* 2005;**40**(2):435–57.

131. Sampalis JS, Denis R, Frechette P, et al. Direct transport to tertiary trauma centers versus transfer from lower level facilities: impact on mortality and morbidity among patients with major trauma. *J Trauma* 1997;**43**(2):288–95; discussion 95–6.

132. Thomas SH, Orf J, Peterson C, Wedel SK. Frequency and costs of laboratory and radiograph repetition in trauma patients undergoing interfacility transfer. *Am J Emerg Med* 2000;**18**(2):156–8.

133. American Geriatrics Society, British Geriatrics Society, and American Academy of Orthopaedic Surgeons Panel on Falls Prevention. Guideline for the prevention of falls in older persons. *J Am Geriatr Soc* 2001;**49** (5):664–72.

Medical concerns in trauma patients

23

Phillip D. Levy

Introduction

Patient outcome subsequent to a traumatic event is largely influenced by the location and degree of injury, the timing of medical intervention, and the quality of care delivered.[1,2] Host factors such as age, gender, and pre-injury health status also contribute to the clinical course and are important determinants of morbidity and mortality.[1–10] The presence of underlying chronic illness is particularly consequential, dramatically increasing the incidence of in-hospital complications and death, even when other variables are taken into account. The effect of pre-existing disease is strongest for those with less severe injuries (Injury Severity Score [ISS] ≤ 20). This is probably due to the fact that in the immediate setting death is usually due to the trauma itself; however, during the hospital course, the ability to recover may be dependent on the comorbid conditions of the injured individual.[4,6,8,10] Related medication use, particularly antihypertensive, antiplatelet, and anticoagulant agents, may enhance the risk of poor outcome associated with pre-existing medical conditions (PMCs) through both direct activity (i.e., intended pharmaceutical effects) and indirect activity (e.g., drug–drug interactions).

Box 23.1 Essentials of medical concerns in the trauma patient

- The presence of underlying chronic illness in the trauma patient is a consequential modifier of outcome, dramatically increasing the incidence of in-hospital complications and death, even when other variables are taken into account.
- The effect of pre-existing disease is strongest for those with less severe injuries.

- Related medication use, particularly antihypertensive, antiplatelet, and anticoagulant agents, may enhance the risk of poor outcome associated with PMCs.

Clinical anatomy and pathophysiology

The frequency of PMCs in those with traumatic injury is not entirely certain, but appears to range from 5% to 32%, depending on the data source (i.e., single institution vs. multicenter registry).[6,7,9,10] This is particularly important, however, as the risk of prolonged hospital stay and death increases three- to sixfold when one or more PMCs are present.[1,3,5–16] Specific conditions that constitute a PMC have been inconsistent in prior studies; some present data on specific disease states and others use broader illness categories. It is clear, however, that involvement of certain organ systems (cardiac, pulmonary, hepatic, renal, and endocrine [especially diabetes mellitus]) and the presence of one general ailment (e.g., malignancy) portend greater risk.[1,3,5–8,10–13,16] Representative prevalence estimates for major illness categories and their corresponding odds-ratios for mortality from a study by Hollis et al. ($n = 65\ 743$) are presented in Table 23.1.[10]

Reasons as to why PMCs are associated with greater risk are complex but reflect the systemic effects of these conditions as much as (if not more than) the organ-specific contributions. It is important to recognize that, to differing degrees, all of these conditions limit functional reserve, making it difficult for the body to respond appropriately to increased stress. For instance, an individual with a history of coronary artery disease may experience decreased cardiac perfusion as a result of

Trauma: A Comprehensive Emergency Medicine Approach, eds. Eric Legome and Lee W. Shockley. Published by Cambridge University Press. © Cambridge University Press 2011.

Table 23.1 Pre-existing medical conditions with significant effect on mortality from trauma*

Condition	Prevalence (%)	OR[†]	95%CI
Cardiovascular disease	29.8	7.0	5.1–9.6
Respiratory	19.0	5.6	4.9–8.1
Endocrine	9.0	4.5	3.1–6.5
Musculoskeletal	8.3	3.3	2.2–5.1
Neurological	4.7	5.0	2.8–9.1
Alcoholism	3.2	10.2	5.0–20.7
Dementia	2.3	5.9	3.6–9.7
Psychosis	2.3	4.9	2.0–12.0
Gastrointestinal	1.9	5.2	2.5–10.6
Malignancy	1.7	7.3	4.0–13.3
Renal	0.9	22.4	11.6–43.3
Hematological	0.6	5.3	1.8–15.6

*Data based on a study of 65 743 subjects in a UK Trauma Registry.[10]
†Adjusted for age, gender, and Injury Severity Score (ISS).
CI, confidence intervals; OR, odds ratio.

exsanguination from an extremity injury leading to development of angina or myocardial infarction. Another with the same condition may not be able to mount an increase in cardiac output resulting in hypotension. Similarly, a patient with renal failure may develop pulmonary edema from a small fluid bolus while one with asthma or emphysema may develop a pneumothorax from use of seemingly normal tidal volumes during mechanical ventilation. While such examples are unlikely to fully explain the variability in outcomes associated with PMCs, they do highlight their potential clinical significance. A summary of sequelae associated with selected medical conditions can be found in Table 23.2.[10]

Obesity (defined as a body mass index [BMI] ≥ 30 kg/m^2) is an important co-factor which dramatically increases the risk of trauma related morbidity and mortality.[17–21] This correlation appears to involve more than an association between obesity and other PMCs and may be due in part to an interaction between body habitus and injury pattern, with obese patients displaying a greater likelihood of chest trauma and lower extremity fractures and a diminished frequency of head and intra-abdominal injuries (possibly due to protection from

a "cushion effect").[18,19,21–23] The impact of chest trauma on pulmonary function and ventilation may be especially prominent among those who are obese due to the existence of a baseline reduction in lung capacity. This may be further exacerbated by anatomical issues related to obesity which predispose to difficult airway management and increase the risk of aspiration such as glottic obstruction from submental adiposity, mobility limitations due to posterior cervical fat accumulation, and obscuration of anterior neck landmarks from the presence of excess subcutaneous tissue. A higher incidence of pulmonary complications has been suggested as one cause of poor outcome in obese patients, with several published reports showing a substantial increase in the mean number of ventilator days for those who are intubated and an overall prolongation of both intensive care unit (ICU) and total hospital length of stay.[18–21,23,24] Obese patients also appear to be at risk for development of multiorgan system failure with worse outcomes.[17–19,21,25,26] It has been suggested that the disparate progression to overwhelming systemic infection witnessed in obese trauma patients may be bimodal in origin, with early (< 72 hours) development occurring secondary to a general proinflammatory state associated with obesity itself[21] and late onset due to hospital-acquired infections (e.g., ventilator-associated pneumonias and catheter-related septicemia),[17,27,28] but the exact etiology is unclear.

Box 23.2 Effect of obesity of trauma patients

- Obesity increases morbity and mortality in trauma patients; this may be due in part to an interaction between body habitus and injury pattern.
- Obese patients have a greater likelihood of chest trauma and lower extremity fractures and a diminished frequency of head and intra-abdominal injuries (possibly due to protection from a "cushion effect").
- The impact of chest trauma on pulmonary function and ventilation may be especially prominent among those who are obese.
- Obese patients also appear to be at risk for development of multiorgan system failure with worse outcomes.
- This multiorgan system failure may be bimodal in origin, with early (< 72 hours) development occurring secondary to a general proinflammatory state associated with obesity itself[21] and late onset due to hospital-acquired infections.

Table 23.2 Organ specific and systemic sequelae of selected pre-existing medical conditions

Category	Condition	Organ-specific sequelae	Systemic sequelae
Cardiovascular	Coronary artery disease	Angina Myocardial infarction Dysrhythmia Left ventricular dysfunction	Hypoperfusion Syncope
	Hypertension	Cardiomyopathy Nephropathy Encephalopathy Retinopathy	Atherosclerosis Aneurysms
	Heart failure	Dyspnea Hepatic congestion Peripheral edema/ascites	Hypoxia Hypotension Hypoperfusion Fatigue
Respiratory	Asthma/COPD	Dyspnea Tachypnea Alveolar distention	Hypoxia Hypercarbia Respiratory alkalosis
Endocrine	Diabetes mellitus	Hyperglycemia Hypoglycemia	Altered mentation Metabolic acidosis Electrolyte imbalance Poor wound healing
	Hyper or hypothyroidism	Palpable neck mass Distorted airway	Tachy or bradycardia Hyper or hypothermia Altered mentation Myxedema
	Adrenal insufficiency		Hypoglycemia Refractory hypotension Hyperkalemia with hyponatremia
Gastrointestinal	Hepatitis	Hepatomegaly RUQ pain	Jaundice Fever
	Cirrhosis	RUQ pain	Coagulopathy Ascites Malnutrition Prolonged drug half-life
	Peptic ulcer disease/ gastritis	Pain Hematemesis	Anemia Hypotension
	Diverticulosis or inflammatory bowel disease	Pain Abscess Hematochezia	Anemia Fever/sepsis
Renal	Chronic kidney disease	Oliguria or anuria	Anemia Uremia Hypervolemia Hyperkalemia and other electrolyte abnormalities
Neurological	CVA	Regional motor/sensory deficits Aphasia	Malnutrition Ambulatory difficulties Cognitive difficulties
	Seizures	Tonic/clonic movement Absence-type behavior Post-ictal state ($\pm$ focal weakness [i.e., Todd's paralysis])	Tachycardia Secondary injury Airway obstruction Metabolic acidosis Rhabdomyolysis

Table 23.2 (cont.)

Category	Condition	Organ-specific sequelae	Systemic sequelae
	Dementia or psychosis	Altered mentation	Agitation Tachycardia
Malignancy	Numerous	Site dependent	CNS or bone metastases Thromboemboli Effusions (pericardial or pleural) Effects from radiation or chemotherapy
Hematological	Immunosuppression	Local wound infections	Sepsis
	Coagulopathy Thrombocytopenia	Excessive wound bleeding Uncontrollable hematomas	Internal hemorrhage
	Hypercoagulation		Thromboemboli

COPD, chronic obstructive pulmonary disease; CNS, central nervous system; CVA, cerebrovascular accident; RUQ, right upper quadrant pain.

Prehospital

While prehospital trauma care is largely focused on performance of the primary survey and initiation of resuscitative efforts for those with critical injury, some attention should be directed to the ascertainment of information regarding medical history. Reasons for this are twofold. The presence of certain PMCs (immunosuppression, cardiac disease, respiratory disease, insulin-dependent diabetes, cirrhosis, morbid obesity, and coagulopathy) has been used as secondary criterion for consideration of transport to a trauma center.[29,30] Given the high risk for delayed adverse outcome, this may be especially important for those with PMCs who appear to have less severe injury. Second, for certain patients (i.e., those with closed head injury, deteriorating mental status, or major distracting injury) this information may only be available at the point of initial contact, when the patient is still lucid or when family, friends, or coworkers are present. The absence of such information upon arrival to the emergency department (ED) could result in suboptimal initial care.

Emergency department evaluation and management

Although the issue of associated medical concerns may seem extraneous to the initial resuscitation of the trauma patient, failure to recognize their potential consequences can be disastrous. As such, it is important that the emergency physician attempts, given constraints, to access available resources (Emergency Medical Services, medical records, family) to obtain a comprehensive patient history. For patients in whom a medical history cannot be obtained, the potential for precipitation of the traumatic event by an underlying PMC should be considered and investigated upon completion of stabilization measures. Episodes without a clear cause such as those involving a single person motor vehicle collision or an un-witnessed fall with facial injury are particularly concerning and should prompt consideration of a hypoglycemic, cardiac, or neurological event.

Integral to the management of a patient with known or suspected PMCs is an appreciation of the implications of pharmaceutical therapy. Patients with hypertension or underlying heart disease are likely to be on medications (e.g., alpha-blockers, beta-blockers, or calcium channel blockers) which may affect their ability to develop an appropriate cardiovascular response to hypovolemia. This could mask early signs of shock and may lead to precipitous deterioration in the presence of subtle yet ongoing blood loss. The regular use of anticoagulant medications (i.e., warfarin or low-molecular-weight heparins), significantly enhances the probability of post-traumatic bleeding. Antiplatelet agents also theoretically may increase risk. The incidence of potentially fatal ICH remains higher even for those with seemingly minor injuries, up to 10% mortality with a Glasgow Coma

Scale (GCS) score of 15, up to 20% mortality with a GCS of 14, and up to 35% mortality with a GCS of 13.[33,35] This is particularly important for patients with closed head trauma on warfarin, in whom a higher frequency of intracranial hemorrhage (ICH) and an increased risk for mortality (2–5 times greater) exists.[31–38] A list of these and other potentially important medication-related complications for trauma patients is provided in Table 23.3.

A proactive approach to the treatment of trauma patients with PMCs in the ED can be life saving. The strongest evidence exists for certain measures, including: early reversal (i.e., < 4 hours) of anticoagulation for patients with evidence of intracranial or other significant hemorrhage using vitamin K (10 mg by intravenous [IV] infusion) and fresh frozen plasma (2 universal donor units initially, followed by 2 type-specific units with subsequent administration of 1–2 type specific units until the INR is within hemostatic range [< 1.6]);[34,35,37] rapid platelet transfusion (5–10 units) for patients with major hemorrhage (especially ICH) and a history of aspirin, clopidogrel, or ticlodipine use; and initiation of IV insulin therapy for those with diabetes and a serum glucose $\geq$ 200 mg/dl.[39–43] More aggressive glycemic control (target range: 80–110 mg/dl) using a continuous insulin infusion has been shown in some non-trauma studies to be efficacious for patients admitted to surgical and medical intensive care units and may ultimately be found useful in those with traumatic injuries of a critical nature.[44–46]

Other important interventions to consider include the administration of anticonvulsant medications to individuals with a known seizure disorder and subtherapeutic levels, use of IV vasodilators for patients with uncontrolled hypertension (particularly in the presence of traumatic ICH, depending on coronary perfusion pressure), and initiation of packed red blood cell transfusions, IV vasopressors, inotropes or anti-arrhythmics for patients with cardiovascular disease who develop circulatory compromise. While perioperative use of beta-blockers in high-risk patients undergoing non-cardiac surgery has been shown to reduce the incidence of cardiovascular events (i.e., mortality, non-fatal myocardial infarction, and non-fatal cardiac arrest) by 56% (relative risk [RR] = 0.44, 95% confidence interval [CI]: 0.20–0.97),[47–49] there have been no trials conducted in the setting of trauma. Given this, and the demonstration in a large meta-analysis of

Table 23.3 Potentially important medication-related complications for trauma patients

Medications	Potential complications
Antiplatelet and anticoagulant agents	
Aspirin	Local bleeding or hematoma
Ticlodipine	Internal or intracranial hemorrhage
Clopidogrel	Delayed hematoma expansion
Coumadin	
Low-molecular-weight heparins	
Catecholamine and calcium inhibitors	
Beta- and alpha/beta-blockers	Relative bradycardia
Calcium channel blockers	Hypotension
Angiotensin-aldosterone antagonists	
Angiotensin-converting enzyme inhibitors	Hypotension
Angiotensin II receptor blockers	Renal insufficiency/failure
Aldosterone receptor blockers	Hyperkalemia
Oral diabetic agents	
Sulfonylureas	Hypoglycemia
Biguanides (i.e., metformin)	Lactic acidosis
	Renal failure (with intravenous contrast dye)
Anti-inflammatory agents	
Steroids	Adrenal insufficiency
Non-steroidals	Infections
	Renal failure

potential adverse outcomes associated with beta-blocker use in surgical settings (RR for bradycardia needing treatment = 2.27, 95% CI: 1.53–3.36 and RR for hypotension needing treatment = 1.27, 95% CI: 1.04–1.56),[49] routine administration for cardio-protective purposes in trauma patients is not recommended.

Box 23.3 Specific treatments for trauma patients with comorbid conditions

- Early reversal (i.e., < 4 hours) of anticoagulation for patients with evidence of intracranial or other significant hemorrhage using vitamin K and fresh frozen plasma.
- Rapid platelet transfusion for patients with major hemorrhage (especially ICH) and aspirin, clopidogrel, or ticlodipine use.
- Intravenous insulin therapy for those with diabetes and a serum glucose ≥ 200 mg/dl.
- Administration of anticonvulsant medications to individuals with a known seizure disorder and subtherapeutic levels.
- Initiation of packed red blood cell transfusions, IV vasopressors, inotropes, or anti-arrhythmics for patients with cardiovascular disease who develop circulatory compromise.

Secondary considerations

Though typically not performed in the ED, guided resuscitation of trauma patients using hemodynamic monitoring (both invasive and non-invasive) has been shown to confer a mortality benefit, especially for those who have higher ISS (≥ 25) or severe shock on presentation and those who are > 60 years of age.[50–56] Degree of injury severity therefore is a common indication for hemodynamic monitoring, which is most often performed invasively using a pulmonary artery catheter (PAC). Study of the National Trauma Data Bank®, however, has shown that PAC use is also more likely when PMCs (particularly cardiac) are present.[52] This may be related to the increased risk of poor outcome associated with PMCs and the inherent difficulty associated with management of such patients. Several studies have demonstrated that care of these individuals can be improved through PAC use, largely because they permit earlier identification of hypoperfusion than conventional measures (i.e., blood pressure and heart rate) and enable targeted intervention using objective cardiovascular end-points.[50,52,53,55,57] Placement of a PAC, however, may not be possible in many EDs and has potential for serious complications. Additionally, PAC insertion invariably requires admission to an ICU setting. Its use for strictly diagnostic purposes (e.g., detection of occult hypoperfusion) or in those who clearly have less severe injuries is not recommended. Given the challenges associated with PAC use, it is reasonable to defer the decision to perform invasive hemodynamic monitoring to the admitting surgical service.

Non-invasive methods of hemodynamic assessment are a viable alternative and offer certain advantages over PAC placement including ease of use, increased safety, and lower cost.[51,54–56,58] Of the technologies which are available, bioelectrical thoracic impedance appears to be the most promising, yielding measures of cardiac function (i.e., cardiac output and index) which correlate well ($r = 0.91$) with those determined invasively by thermo-dilution.[55,56] When combined with measurement of peripheral tissue oxygen delivery using transcutaneous sensors, a comprehensive, low-risk, non-invasive approach can be employed, which enables prompt identification of and response to post-traumatic circulatory deficits.[55,56] Of importance to the emergency physician, these devices are easy to use and provide readily interpretable results. Although not in widespread use in most EDs, acceptance will be dependent on large studies showing their effectiveness on management.

Documentation

When PMCs are recognized, it is important that they be documented along with an assessment of their potential implications on trauma management. If there is a discrepancy between what is recommended for response to a known PMC and the treatment which is actually being provided, reasons should be noted. When disagreements arise between the physicians in management, it is important to document why deviations may have occurred through terms such as "deferral to the admitting service," while avoiding use of the medical record as a means to air grievances. It should also be noted when information regarding medical history is not available and when new conditions have been discovered in the course of routine laboratory or radiographic evaluation. For the latter, it is important to acknowledge the potential need for further treatment or workup but that this responsibilty will be carried by the admitting service. Likewise, when studies are outstanding it should be noted which service will assume responsibility for following through with their results.

Disposition

It is reasonable to consider the presence of PMCs in a patient with less severe injuries as an indication to admit to the hospital for observation, particularly for individuals with closed head trauma and anticoagulation use with a significantly elevated International Normalized Ratio (INR) (no absolute standard cut-off exists). For those with more severe injuries, the existence of PMCs (especially cardiac) should be taken as an indication for

401

admission to a monitored setting, with use of the ICU for any patient in whom: (1) physical examination may be unreliable due to prior neurological or vascular deficit; and (2) hemodynamic stability may be compromised by underlying cardiovascular pathophysiology or pharmacology. The existence of PMCs should also prompt consideration of transfer to a higher level of care if the current facility does not have in-house intensivists, trauma surgeons, neurosurgeons, and cardiologists (depending on the underlying concern).

References

1. Wardle TD. Co-morbid factors in trauma patients. *Br Med Bull* 1999;**55**(4):744–56.

2. Bochicchio GV, Joshi M, Bochicchio K, et al. Incidence and impact of risk factors in critically ill trauma patients. *World J Surg* 2006;**30**(1):114–18.

3. MacKenzie EJ, Morris JA, Jr., Edelstein SL. Effect of pre-existing disease on length of hospital stay in trauma patients. *J Trauma* 1989;**29**(6):757–64; discussion 64–5.

4. Morris JA, Jr., MacKenzie EJ, Damiano AM, Bass SM. Mortality in trauma patients: the interaction between host factors and severity. *J Trauma* 1990;**30**(12):1476–82.

5. Morris JA, Jr., MacKenzie EJ, Edelstein SL. The effect of preexisting conditions on mortality in trauma patients. *JAMA* 1990;**263**(14):1942–6.

6. Milzman DP, Boulanger BR, Rodriguez A, et al. Pre-existing disease in trauma patients: a predictor of fate independent of age and injury severity score. *J Trauma* 1992;**32**(2):236–43; discussion 43–4.

7. Sacco WJ, Copes WS, Bain LW, Jr., et al. Effect of preinjury illness on trauma patient survival outcome. *J Trauma* 1993;**35**(4):538–42; discussion 42–3.

8. McGwin G, Jr., MacLennan PA, Fife JB, Davis GG, Rue LW, 3rd. Preexisting conditions and mortality in older trauma patients. *J Trauma* 2004;**56**(6):1291–6.

9. Bergeron E, Lavoie A, Moore L, Clas D, Rossignol M. Comorbidity and age are both independent predictors of length of hospitalization in trauma patients. *Can J Surg* 2005;**48**(5):361–6.

10. Hollis S, Lecky F, Yates DW, Woodford M. The effect of pre-existing medical conditions and age on mortality after injury. *J Trauma* 2006;**61**(5):1255–60.

11. Boulanger BR, Gann DS. Management of the trauma victim with pre-existing endocrine disease. *Crit Care Clin* 1994;**10**(3):537–54.

12. Cachecho R, Millham FH, Wedel SK. Management of the trauma patient with pre-existing renal disease. *Crit Care Clin* 1994;**10**(3):523–36.

13. Lorelli DR, Kralovich KA, Seguin C. The impact of pre-existing end-stage renal disease on survival in acutely injured trauma patients. *Am Surg* 2001;**67**(7):693–6.

14. O'Brien GM, Criner GJ. Chronic pulmonary disease in the trauma patient. *Crit Care Clin* 1994;**10**(3):507–22.

15. Wilson RF. Pre-existing peripheral arterial disease in trauma. *Crit Care Clin* 1994;**10**(3):567–93.

16. Wilson RF. Trauma in patients with pre-existing cardiac disease. *Crit Care Clin* 1994;**10**(3):461–506.

17. Bochicchio GV, Joshi M, Bochicchio K, et al. Impact of obesity in the critically ill trauma patient: a prospective study. *J Am Coll Surg* 2006;**203**(4):533–8.

18. Brown CV, Neville AL, Rhee P, et al. The impact of obesity on the outcomes of 1153 critically injured blunt trauma patients. *J Trauma* 2005;**59**(5):1048–51; discussion 51.

19. Neville AL, Brown CV, Weng J, Demetriades D, Velmahos GC. Obesity is an independent risk factor of mortality in severely injured blunt trauma patients. *Arch Surg* 2004;**139**(9):983–7.

20. Duane TM, Dechert T, Aboutanos MB, Malhotra AK, Ivatury RR. Obesity and outcomes after blunt trauma. *J Trauma* 2006;**61**(5):1218–21.

21. Ciesla DJ, Moore EE, Johnson JL, et al. Obesity increases risk of organ failure after severe trauma. *J Am Coll Surg* 2006;**203**(4):539–45.

22. Boulanger BR, Milzman D, Mitchell K, Rodriguez A. Body habitus as a predictor of injury pattern after blunt trauma. *J Trauma* 1992;**33**(2):228–32.

23. Brown CV, Rhee P, Neville AL, et al. Obesity and traumatic brain injury. *J Trauma* 2006;**61**(3):572–6.

24. Reiff DA, Hipp G, McGwin G, Jr., et al. Body mass index affects the need for and the duration of mechanical ventilation after thoracic trauma. *J Trauma* 2007;**62**(6):1432–5.

25. Belzberg H, Wo CC, Demetriades D, Shoemaker WC. Effects of age and obesity on hemodynamics, tissue oxygenation, and outcome after trauma. *J Trauma* 2007;**62**(5):1192–200.

26. Brown CV, Velmahos GC. The consequences of obesity on trauma, emergency surgery, and surgical critical care. *World J Emerg Surg* 2006;**1**:27.

27. Bochicchio GV, Napolitano LM, Joshi M, et al. Persistent systemic inflammatory response syndrome is predictive of nosocomial infection in trauma. *J Trauma* 2002;**53**(2):245–50; discussion 50–1.

28. Hoover L, Bochicchio GV, Napolitano LM, et al. Systemic inflammatory response syndrome and nosocomial infection in trauma. *J Trauma* 2006;**61**(2):310–16; discussion 16–17.

29. American College of Surgeons Committee on Trauma. *Resources for Optimal Care of the Injured Patient 1999.* Chicago, IL: American College of Surgeons, 1999.

30. Mackersie R. History of trauma field triage development and the American College of

Surgeons criteria. *Prehosp Emerg Care* 2006;
10:287–94.

31. Lavoie A, Ratte S, Clas D, et al. Preinjury warfarin use among elderly patients with closed head injuries in a trauma center. *J Trauma* 2004;**56**(4):802–7.

32. Bair H, Ivascu F, Janczyk R, et al. Nurse driven protocol for head injured patients on warfarin. *J Trauma Nurs* 2005;**12**(4):120–6.

33. Cohen DB, Rinker C, Wilberger JE. Traumatic brain injury in anticoagulated patients. *J Trauma* 2006;**60**(3):553–7.

34. Ivascu FA, Howells GA, Junn FS, et al. Rapid warfarin reversal in anticoagulated patients with traumatic intracranial hemorrhage reduces hemorrhage progression and mortality. *J Trauma* 2005;**59**(5):1131–7; discussion 7–9.

35. Ivascu FA, Janczyk RJ, Junn FS, et al. Treatment of trauma patients with intracranial hemorrhage on preinjury warfarin. *J Trauma* 2006;**61**(2):318–21.

36. Li J, Brown J, Levine M. Mild head injury, anticoagulants, and risk of intracranial injury. *Lancet* 2001;**357**(9258):771–2.

37. Mina AA, Bair HA, Howells GA, Bendick PJ. Complications of preinjury warfarin use in the trauma patient. *J Trauma* 2003;**54**(5):842–7.

38. Mina AA, Knipfer JF, Park DY, et al. Intracranial complications of preinjury anticoagulation in trauma patients with head injury. *J Trauma* 2002;**53**(4):668–72.

39. Bochicchio GV, Salzano L, Joshi M, Bochicchio K, Scalea TM. Admission preoperative glucose is predictive of morbidity and mortality in trauma patients who require immediate operative intervention. *Am Surg* 2005;**71**(2):171–4.

40. Bochicchio GV, Sung J, Joshi M, et al. Persistent hyperglycemia is predictive of outcome in critically ill trauma patients. *J Trauma* 2005;**58**(5):921–4.

41. Gale SC, Sicoutris C, Reilly PM, Schwab CW, Gracias VH. Poor glycemic control is associated with increased mortality in critically ill trauma patients. *Am Surg* 2007;**73**(5):454–60.

42. Sung J, Bochicchio GV, Joshi M, et al. Admission hyperglycemia is predictive of outcome in critically ill trauma patients. *J Trauma* 2005;**59**(1):80–3.

43. Yendamuri S, Fulda GJ, Tinkoff GH. Admission hyperglycemia as a prognostic indicator in trauma. *J Trauma* 2003;**55**(1):33–8.

44. van den Berghe G, Wouters P, Weekers F, et al. Intensive insulin therapy in the critically ill patients. *N Engl J Med* 2001;**345**(19):1359–67.

45. Van den Berghe G, Wilmer A, Hermans G, et al. Intensive insulin therapy in the medical ICU. *N Engl J Med* 2006;**354**(5):449–61.

46. Vanhorebeek I, Ingels C, Van den Berghe G. Intensive insulin therapy in high-risk cardiac surgery patients: evidence from the Leuven randomized study. *Semin Thorac Cardiovasc Surg* 2006;**18**(4):309–16.

47. Auerbach AD, Goldman L. Beta-blockers and reduction of cardiac events in noncardiac surgery: clinical applications. *JAMA* 2002;**287**(11):1445–7.

48. Auerbach AD, Goldman L. Beta-blockers and reduction of cardiac events in noncardiac surgery: scientific review. *JAMA* 2002;**287**(11):1435–44.

49. Devereaux PJ, Beattie WS, Choi PT, et al. How strong is the evidence for the use of perioperative beta blockers in non-cardiac surgery? Systematic review and meta-analysis of randomised controlled trials. *BMJ* 2005;**331**(7512):313–21.

50. Asensio JA, Demetriades D, Berne TV, Shoemaker WC. Invasive and noninvasive monitoring for early recognition and treatment of shock in high-risk trauma and surgical patients. *Surg Clin North Am* 1996;**76**(4):985–97.

51. Brown CV, Shoemaker WC, Wo CC, Chan L, Demetriades D. Is noninvasive hemodynamic monitoring appropriate for the elderly critically injured patient? *J Trauma* 2005;**58**(1):102–7.

52. Friese RS, Shafi S, Gentilello LM. Pulmonary artery catheter use is associated with reduced mortality in severely injured patients: a National Trauma Data Bank analysis of 53312 patients. *Crit Care Med* 2006;**34**(6):1597–601.

53. Scalea TM, Simon HM, Duncan AO, et al. Geriatric blunt multiple trauma: improved survival with early invasive monitoring. *J Trauma* 1990;**30**(2):129–34; discussion 34–6.

54. Shoemaker WC, Wo CC, Bishop MH, et al. Noninvasive physiologic monitoring of high-risk surgical patients. *Arch Surg* 1996;**131**(7):732–7.

55. Shoemaker WC, Wo CC, Chien LC, et al. Evaluation of invasive and noninvasive hemodynamic monitoring in trauma patients. *J Trauma* 2006;**61**(4):844–53; discussion 53–4.

56. Velmahos GC, Wo CC, Demetriades D, Shoemaker WC. Early continuous noninvasive haemodynamic monitoring after severe blunt trauma. *Injury* 1999;**30**(3):209–14.

57. Parks JK, Elliott AC, Gentilello LM, Shafi S. Systemic hypotension is a late marker of shock after trauma: a validation study of Advanced Trauma Life Support® principles in a large national sample. *Am J Surg* 2006;**192**(6):727–31.

58. Shoemaker WC. New approaches to trauma management using severity of illness and outcome prediction based on noninvasive hemodynamic monitoring. *Surg Clin North Am* 2002;**82**(1):245–55.

Sexual assault

24

Kristin E. Harkin, Elizabeth Borock, and Andrew Amaranto

Introduction

Sexual assault is non-consensual sexual contact or behavior. Different jurisdictions have different definitions, but share a common theme of an unwilling or incompetent participant. Sexual assault is often underreported in the United States. The US Department of Justice statistics indicate that on average every 2.5 minutes a sexual assault occurs in the United States.[1]

Most medical institutions follow protocols for the evaluation and treatment of the sexual assault victim. In order to be consistent, efficient, and legally sound it is important to adhere to these protocols. This chapter is not a substitute for, but an adjunct to understanding these protocols in general and managing the patient who presents with a history or concern for sexual assault. Specifically rape, as defined by the American College of Emergency Physicians, is forced, non-consensual sexual intercourse (vaginal, anal, or oral).

A systematic approach to evaluating the patient helps complete the exam in as gentle and expeditious a manner as possible. Physical injuries may span the spectrum of occult or absent to severe and life threatening. Sexual assault may or may not cause physical injuries. A negative examination does not imply that a sexual assault did not occur.

The medical and emotional needs of a sexual assault patient must be handled in tandem. The examination of a sexual assault patient is comprehensive and includes a complete physical exam, forensic exam, pregnancy assessment and prevention, sexually transmitted disease prevention, and psychological support. The evaluation of a sexual assault patient is a challenge in a busy emergency department (ED); confidentiality and privacy are essential. A solid protocol must be established for handling of forensic evidence to meet the requirements of the criminal justice system.

Box 24.1 Components of the Examination of the Sexual Assault Patient

- Complete physical exam – including complete genitourinary (GU) exam
- Forensic exam – rape kit and drug-facilitated kit (up to 96 hours)
- Pregnancy assessment and prevention
- Sexually transmitted disease prevention
- Psychological support

Clinical anatomy and pathophysiology

Anogenital injury

Although sexual assault may be violent, a significant number of patients who present after assault do not have detectable anogenital injury. Slaughter and Brown, in a 1992 study using colposcopy, found anogenital trauma in 68% (213/311) of rape victims.[2] The frequency of injury by anatomic sites was posterior fourchette (70%), labia minora (53%), hymen (29%), and fossa navicularis (25%).[3] Jones et al. in 2003 studied 766 adolescent and adult female victims of sexual assault, and found that persons over the age of 17 had no discernable pattern of anogenital injuries.[4] This study concluded that adolescent girls were more likely to suffer injuries at the fossa navicularis, hymen, posterior fourchette, and labia minora.[4] These findings were further corroborated by a study by Adams et al. in 2001 using colposcopic photography to evaluate female rape victims ages 14–19 years of age.[5] Sixty four percent of the subjects had anogenital injury: 36% had tears of the posterior fourchette, 32% had erythema of the labia minora,

---

and 28% had erythema of the fossa navicularis.[5] Colposcopy detects injuries not visible to the naked eye, and has replaced toluidine dye for most exams.

Prehospital

Although the basics of trauma evaluation are paramount, other considerations must take place. The main difference with the sexual assault patient is that it is essential to preserve the forensic evidence and maintain the chain of custody of that evidence, as failure to do so may result in that evidence being thrown out of court. Items, such as clothing that the patient is not wearing, should be placed in paper bags and not disturbed. Until the examination patients should be encouraged to not engage in any activity that may damage evidence such as urinating, defecating, vomiting, douching, removing/inserting a tampon, bathing, gargling, brushing teeth, smoking, eating, drinking, chewing gum, changing clothes, or taking medications.

Emergency department evaluation and management

The triage nurse should be alerted upon arrival of the patient so that he or she may be triaged quickly, assessed for stability, and then led to a private area if the patient is hemodynamically stable.

Certain hospitals in the United States have been designated as specialty centers for rape victims. For example, in New York state, the department of health has designated certain hospitals as SAFE Centers, or Sexual Assault Forensic Examination Centers. They have to provide, in addition to the appropriate basic medical management services, enhanced social services, specially trained examiners, data collections, collaboration and data sharing with the state, a quality assurance (QA) program, improved physical accommodations, and continuing education for the staff. Several other states, including New Jersey and Nebraska, have similar programs, yet as of 2008 there does not exist a standard at the federal level. However, the authors again stress that a properly prepared emergency physician can manage all aspects of these cases without the help of additional services. Upon arrival of a sexual assault patient to the ED, the attending should be alerted, and the appropriate staff members involved. Best practices support the provision of a rape victim advocate. This advocate on-call should optimally be available within 30 minutes of notification. They should be trained to provide emotional support during the rape exam, essential information regarding follow-up care, and should remain with the patient until safe discharge. At some sites, the ED social worker acts as an advocate for the patient during the exam. The sexual assault examination is optimally performed early in the course; whether or not it is done by the ED physician or a special sexual assault examiner the emergency physician must perform an initial evaluation of the patient, treat any acute injuries, and if medically feasible, preserve evidence including clothing and debris. Ideally, for example, a victim of sexual assault undresses over roll-paper in order to capture debris and DNA evidence on clothing, and items of clothing are placed in paper bags for further forensic evaluation. If undressing of the patient can be deferred until the sexual assault examiner or similar arrives, then this should be encouraged. The patient should not eat or drink anything before evidentiary oral swabs are obtained. The first urine should be saved for analysis in suspected cases of drug facilitated sexual assault. Recent sexual assault is usually defined as within 72 hours. However, the collection of evidence may be performed up to 96 hours with the advancement of DNA analysis.

Initial evaluation

The evaluation should proceed in the usual step-wise approach for any trauma patient. The patient's condition and stability will guide the rapidity and focus of the evaluation. In addition to assuring an adequate airway the mouth and oropharynx should be examined for any evidence of injury. If suction is necessary, all secretions should optimally be kept and labeled for forensic analysis. Special attention should be made for signs of strangulation. Observe the neck for any disruption of anatomy or superficial abrasions and palpate for evidence of airway injury, ensuring that the trachea is midline and that there is no crepitus. Note hoarseness or stridor which may be a clue to laryngeal injury.

Assess the patient's respiratory status. Sexual assaults often involve the involuntary ingestion of a sedative–hypnotic drugs which have the potential for respiratory suppression and apnea. Fully inspect the patient's thorax and axilla for any evidence of penetrating trauma and treat appropriately.

The initial assessment of the patient's circulatory status hinges on the presence and degree of shock. Special considerations in the sexual assault victim are occult abdominal hemorrhage and perineal hemorrhage. Toxic ingestion should be considered based on the clinical picture. Interventions for hypotensive patients should be directed at the underlying cause.

Ascertain if the patient has an abnormal mental status or if there is a history of loss of consciousness. This may indicate the use of a drug-facilitated assault, the presence of an occult head injury, or cerebral hypoxia.

Common presentations

Severe

Strangulation injuries can cause direct insult to the airway, esophagus, or carotid arteries. Of note is laryngotracheal and hyoid injuries. Hoarseness, stridor, or significant anterior throat pain, swelling or ecchymosis should prompt indirect laryngoscopy or computed tomography (CT) scan. Otolaryngology consultation should also be considered. Rarely it may cause an injury to the cervical spine. Although there is no evidence that routinely immobilizing the cervical spine in strangulation cases is necessary, it is reasonable to immobilize high risk or any neurologically impaired patients. The voluntary or involuntary consumption of any drug including alcohol that leads to impairment can facilitate a sexual assault. A common life-threatening co-ingestion of alcohol and sedative–hypnotics can induce respiratory failure complicated by vomiting. A rapidly changing mental status with severe depression cycling with agitation can be consistent with gamma hydroxybutyrate (GHB), another common drug used to facilitate sexual assault.

Moderate

The most common types of non-life-threatening injuries specific to sexual assault are oral, genital, and anorectal. For the purposes of forensic collection the victim should not eat or drink or rinse their mouth until after an exam of the mouth and throat has been completed. Forced oral penetration can produce a recognizable pattern of injury, and the exam should focus on the frenulum, buccal mucosa, soft and hard palate, as well as the posterior pharynx. Forced penile entry can cause tears in both the lingual and labial frenulum, abrasions to the buccal surfaces, and petechia to the soft palate. If the history of the assault includes oral ejaculation, specimens should be collected with moist sterile swabbing along all buccal mucosa.

All female patients should be evaluated in the lithotomy position with an initial close inspection of the legs, inner thighs, external genitalia, perineum, and anus. A Wood's light exam will help identify dried secretions that can be collected with a damp sterile swab. The most common site of laceration in forced penetration is the posterior fourchette. Victims of forced penetration tend not to tilt their hips anteriorly during intercourse and thus sustain abrasions or lacerations along the posterior vagina and labia minora. Speculum examination should be performed to look for introital or cervical injury *The majority of victims of forced vaginal penetration will have a normal pelvic exam without evidence of trauma*. The literature describes colposcopy as being valuable in augmenting the genital exam. If the emergency physician or other examiner is untrained in this procedure but it is available, gynecologic consultation should be obtained.[6]

Anal and rectal injuries are common injuries that victims are often reluctant to include in the history, and an anal exam looking for evidence of trauma is part of the complete examination. Gross visualization will reveal evidence of most injuries. If there is any concern for penetration, anoscopy lubricated with warm water should be perfomed. Similar attention to swabbing the perianal region and collection of debris should be maintained for the anorectal exam.

Minor

A recent study of nearly 1000 victims of sexual assault found that general bodily injuries (commonly abrasions and bruises), were twice as common as genital–anal injuries.[7] Examination and documentation of minor abrasions on the extremities, chest, and abdomen may be the only evidence of an assault. A thorough exam of a fully undressed patient is essential.

Occult injuries

A thorough and well-documented exam will benefit the patient in the acute setting as well as in future legal proceedings. One reason for this complete exam is to identify injuries that may not be readily apparent. There are several typical injury patterns that should be evaluated for in all victims as shown in Table 24.1.

Table 24.1 Typical injury patterns

Scalp	Bald spots where hair may have been pulled
Eye	Subconjuctival hemorrhages
Neck	Evidence of minor strangulation injuries
Extremities	Presence of restraint injuries
Hands and feet	Broken nails

Acute interventions

The unique acute intervention specific for the sexual assault victim is the involvement of a patient advocate as early as possible in your evaluation. Many hospitals have a designated nurse or social worker on call 24 hours a day to respond to incidents of sexual assault, and it is incumbent on the practitioner to know how to access the workplace-specific protocols. The advocate can be indispensable in helping with acute crisis intervention.

Secondary evaluation

The major components of the secondary evaluation are: (1) forensic examination; (2) evaluation and treatment for sexually transmitted disease exposure; and (3) evaluation and treatment for pregnancy risk. Forensic examination functions include thorough documentation of pertinent history and physical findings and the proper collection and handling of evidence.

Evidentiary examination

Special considerations

In a case in which the patient is unconscious, or unable to consent as a result of mental impairment or disability, a Health Care Proxy may consent to the exam. If no Health Care Proxy has been named, this decision must be left to the discretion of the physician caring for the individual. If it appears a patient is temporarily incapacitated, as a result of drugs or alcohol, the exam and consent should be postponed until the patient is alert enough to adequately comprehend the proposed procedure and its implications.

Critically injured patient

In the case of a critical trauma patient, the designated examiner may collect evidence for the sexual assault forensic examination ("rape kit"), and perform a focused evaluation of sexual assault-related injuries if this exam does not interfere with lifesaving procedures. Otherwise, a comprehensive sexual assault exam may be deferred until a more acceptable time, understanding that some evidence may be lost. (i.e., povidone iodine preparation for a Foley catheter). A thorough examination of the anogenital region should be performed as part of the secondary survey; any injuries should be documented on the patient chart. Photographs of severe injuries during the initial resuscitation period provide significant supportive evidence, though they should be taken only if the clinical scenario allows, and submitted to law enforcement only after the patient is able to consent.

Intoxicated patient

In the case of an intoxicated patient with a concern for a sexual assault, one should postpone the evidentiary exam until the patient is able to consent. If possible, maintain evidence such as clothing and debris. The patient's first urine specimen should be saved in the case of a possible drug-facilitated sexual assault (DFSA). A specialized DFSA kit is available in most states and consists of two gray-topped serum tubes and a urine container. If labs are drawn prior to the evaluation for sexual assault, the two serum tubes may be collected at this time but only if the kit is able to remain in the custody of the examiner or appropriate lock box (thus maintaining the chain of custody).

Stable ambulatory patient

Step 1: patient education and consent

Patients should hear a summary of the events which constitute the forensic exam prior to initiation, and to know that they have the right at any time to refuse any steps in the exam. Patients in most states must also be informed that they have a choice regarding reporting the assault to law enforcement. There are some states where healthcare providers are mandated reporters. It is essential that providers are familiar with state and local laws. Furthermore, there are some forms of sexual assault which must be reported under federal guidelines. A rape kit may be collected whether the patient chooses to report the assault or not, and stored for several months (facility-dependent) in case a victim decides to prosecute later. Specialized sexual assault charts found at many facilities include a form for patient consent. For facilities without such charts examiners may obtain informed consent using the forms or guidelines specific to their hospital.

Step 2: interview

Examiners should tailor the interview to patient level of communication skill, provide a medical interpreter as necessary, and conduct all interactions in a private setting. Clinicians must adopt a non-judgmental, supportive approach, and should have the rape advocate present for emotional support (provided the patient consents to his or her presence). If a designated rape advocate is unavailable, a social worker or nurse may be able to fill this role. It is generally accepted that the interview of adult patients should be conducted without the presence of family or friends. Open-ended, non-leading questions with time for a patient to speak freely is key.

Medical and forensic history
Pertinent medical history:

- past medical history/past surgical history
- medications
- use of contraceptives
- current pregnancy status
- allergies
- immunizations
- last consensual intercourse
  (Note: Gravida/Para and history of sexually transmitted infections is not considered pertinent to the exam.)

Assault-related history:

- date and time of assault
- location where assault occurred (general – i.e., woods, park)
- loss of consciousness
- possible identity of suspect
- number and gender of perpetrators.
- use of force, threats of force, weapons, or coercion (many states have mandatory reporting laws for use of a deadly weapon)
- use of drugs and/or alcohol – voluntary or suspected
- type or means of assault (oral, vaginal, anal – include if forced to perform oral sex or if oral sex was performed on patient)
- occurrence of penetration of any body part with a penis, body part, or other object

- means of restraint (tied or pinned down against a part of the patient's body)
- other violent acts – attempted choking, punching, slapping, spitting, etc
- was the patient bitten or did the patient bite the perpetrator
- does the patient know if the perpetrator ejaculated – if so, where

Intervening variables –– Inquire if patient has showered, changed clothing or underwear, and taken anything by mouth. Also document if the patient has urinated, defecated, vomited, douched, removed or inserted a tampon, brushed teeth or hair, or smoked. This may corroborate forensic findings or lack thereof.

Assess for mental health intervention –– Survivors may express profound depression or suicidality as a result of the assault, and may require urgent psychiatric consultation and/or admission. If this is the case, a 1 : 1 guard must be assigned to the patient for the duration of his or her stay in the ED or until psychiatrically cleared.

Step 3: laboratory testing

Pregnancy test –– Baseline laboratory tests if human immunodeficiency virus (HIV) post-exposure prophylaxis (PEP) initiated:

- complete blood count (CBC), basic metabolic panel, hepatic panel, beta human chorionic gonadotrophin (hCG)

Other labs (may be acquired in ED or within week if reliable for follow up):

- hepatitis B virus (HBV) serology
- hepatitis C (HCV) serology
- HIV (if proper pre- and post-test counseling available, and consent obtained)
  (Note: many facilities now have rapid HIV testing available [consider if patient able to accept immediate results])

Labs in case of suspected drug-facilitated sexual assault:

- two grey-topped serum tubes
- urine sample (**not** a clean catch i.e., no prep)
  (Part of standardized DFSA kit; subject to chain of custody requirements)

Step 4: sexual assault evidence collection kit (rape kit)

General considerations and evidence integrity --Although minor variation may exist among different jurisdictions, most contain similar articles and forms and require similar steps. The examiner must prevent cross-contamination of evidence by changing gloves whenever cross-contamination could occur. Proper collection, preservation, and maintenance of the chain of custody of evidence is imperative. All samples or clothing must be completely dry prior to packaging and storage. A fan may aid in air drying both collected swabbings as well as wet clothes. Mold and mildew destroys DNA evidence. In the absence of an included fan, wet clothes should be air dried, ideally with the aid of a fan obtained separately. Each paper bag with evidence should be labeled for contents, and sealed with initials inscribed across tape. Storage duration is variable per jurisdiction (Figure 24.1).

Rape kit

Step 1: oral swab and smear

This step should precede oral administration of medications if possible to preserve DNA evidence. Discussion of HIV PEP should be prioritized to ensure timely administration. The HIV PEP would be best administered just after Step 1 (Figure 24.2).

Step 2: trace evidence/undressing (consider over roll-paper)

Enables capture of debris (i.e., grass, further evidence). Place down paper over which patient

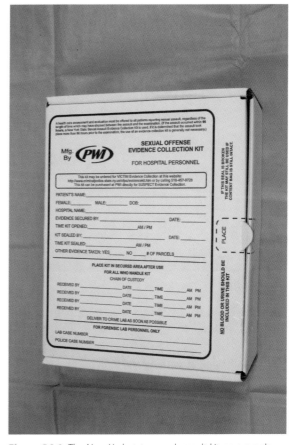

Figure 24.1 The New York state sexual assault kit: an example of a rape kit.

Figure 24.2 The New York state sexual assault kit: oral swabs from kit.

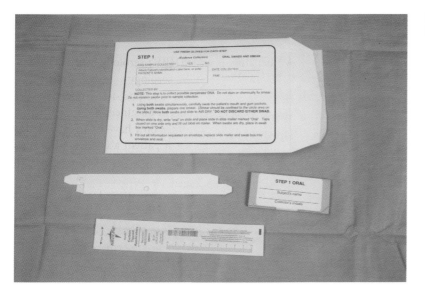

409

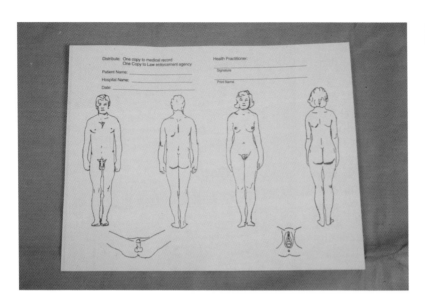

Figure 24.3 The New York state sexual assault kit: body diagram from kit.

undresses in a labeled paper bag. The patient may then step into gown.

Step 3: packaging of clothing and underwear

Each item of clothing is placed in a labeled, sealed paper bag. Some jurisdictions request a separate bag for each item of clothing. Initials of the examiner are inscribed over tape to indicate proper sealing. Underwear is placed in prelabeled envelope within the kit.

Note: clothing must be dried completely prior to packaging in order to prevent mold and mildew, which may compromise DNA collection.

Step 4: debris collection

Foreign material found on the patient's body should be acquired with forceps and placed in a paper towel provided in the exam kit, or if indicated, additional paper towels. Each paper towel should then be labeled to reflect anatomic area where debris was discovered, (i.e., "R shoulder" written on the outside of the paper towel before being placed in the envelope).

Step 5: focused examination for injuries

The focused examination discussed here assumes a primary evaluation has been completed. Abrasions, lacerations, orthopedic deformities, ecchymoses, bite marks, patterned injuries (shape of belt, thumbprints used to restrain during attack, outline of objects used as weapon) must all be documented. The exam should focus on breasts (often the site of bite injuries), lower lumbar spine (patient dragged), periorbital petechiae or subconjunctival hemorrhages (strangled), or neck (overt signs of strangulation). The mouth, arms, wrists, legs, and thighs may also show signs of injury. All findings must be documented on body diagram (Figure 24.3). Each injury should optimally be measured with measuring tape, and documented on chart, (i.e., 3.5 × 1.5 cm ecchymosis).

Box 24.2 Common areas of non-genital injury during sexual assault

- Breasts
- Lower lumbar spine
- Periorbital petechiae or subconjunctival hemorrhages
- Neck
- Mouth
- Extremities

Step 6: dried secretions and bite marks

Dried semen, saliva, or other fluids should be collected with a slightly moistened cotton swab, air-dried using the collection box, then labeled by anatomic location and packaged. A Wood's lamp may help illuminate where semen is located. However, not all semen illuminates in this manner, and what is illuminated with the Wood's lamp may not necessarily be semen. Nevertheless, these specimens are important to collect. Each sample should be collected and packaged separately.

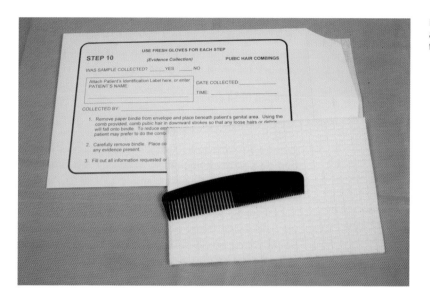

Figure 24.4 The New York state sexual assault kit: hair-combing equipment from kit.

Step 7: fingernail scrapings

Skin, blood, and debris may be found under fingernails. Use the wooden fingernail scrapers to collect possible evidence into paper envelopes in kit. Label each envelope R or L, respectively. Nail clippings may also be used in place of fingernail scrapings.

Step 8: pulled head hairs

Twenty five hairs from five different areas, including the cuticle, must be collected for adequate DNA analysis and comparisons. Patients may collect strands of hair themselves, or if this step is too traumatic, patients may defer, and realize that if more DNA is needed at a later time, that law enforcement or the prosecution may collect samples in the future. Although controversial, hair samples may be used to detect the presence of drugs used by an assailant in a case of drug-facilitated sexual assault. It can take up to 4 weeks for the presence of toxins to appear in hair samples, and will not specify time of use or administration. In addition, fine or lightly pigmented hair will not retain exposed toxins as strongly as heavily pigmented hair. The advantage of hair samples is that toxins remain in hair far longer than in urine or blood and can be tested at a later date.

Step 9: pubic hair combings

At this time, the patient may be placed in lithotomy position for the next few steps. Combing of pubic hair is performed in order to collect possible stray hairs from the assailant. Place the paper towel in the kit under a patient's buttocks for efficient collection (Figure 24.4).

Step 10: pulled pubic hairs

Instructions in most kits suggest that 15 complete pubic hairs should be collected for adequate DNA typing. This step however, is controversial, and many experts feel this is not necessary. As with pulled head hairs, DNA from the patient may be collected later, and in a less traumatic fashion.

Step 11: anal swabs and smears

Two cotton swabs are used simultaneously to collect secretions from the perianal region, and then used to make two slides. Both swabs are then air-dried before being placed in the collection box.

Step 12: vaginal or penile swabs and smears

When the vaginal exam is performed, the speculum is moistened with tap water only as lubricants may affect test results. Four cotton swabs (not moistened) are used to collect semen from the vaginal vault or periurethral/penile area. Two swabs are used simultaneously to collect and prepare slides, then placed in collection box to air-dry prior to packaging. This step is then repeated with the other cotton swabs. Anoscopy may be performed in the same manner, if indicated. Then, the examiner may perform a colposcopic evaluation, if available (see below).

Step 13: oral brushing

Oral brushing collects the patients own DNA (replacing prior use of blood sample). The brush is used to scrape both sides of patient's cheeks, and then placed in a collection box for air-drying prior to packaging.

Colposcopy

Colposcopy is a diagnostic test using a lighted magnifying device to examine the cervix, vagina and vulva. If trained in the use of colposcopy, the examiner may now visualize the genital structures for injuries not apparent to the naked eye. According to a frequently cited study published by Slaughter and Brown, the magnification of a colposcope (5–30%) may detect up to 87% more injuries.[2] A later study evaluated 311 sexual assault victims as compared to 75 persons who had consensual intercourse, and found that the victims of sexual assault had a higher incidence of injury, and multiple injuries, than controls.[3] The authors did not, however, control for time since event, use of lubrication, condom use, and other important variables. Although colposcopy is an excellent tool for detecting injury, controversy exists surrounding its use as injury may also be detected after consensual intercourse.[8]

Drug-facilitated sexual assault

The legal definition of DFSA is sexual assault facilitated by an offender's use of an "anesthesia-type" drug which, when administered to the victim, rendered the victim "physically incapacitated or helpless" and thus incapable of giving or not giving consent.[9]

Studies determining the prevalence of DFSA include both cases in which patients were surreptitiously drugged as well as cases in which intended use of alcohol or drugs led to a condition of increased susceptibility to assault. The Department of Justice estimates that over 35% of sexual assaults are perpetrated by offenders under the influence of alcohol, other drugs, or both.[10] One multicenter study looking at victims of sexual assault found that of DFSA patients who presented for examination, approximately 4.3% of the DFSAs examined were surreptitiously drugged and 35.4% of the DFSAs involved voluntarily used illicit drugs. A common scenario suggestive of DFSA is a patient who is amnestic to events of the prior evening, though recalls having only one or two drinks, and wakes up in a foreign place

without underwear or in some other unusual situation. Assume sexual assault in such patients, and a consideration for both a rape kit as well as a DFSA kit (see below) should be completed.

Common DFSA drugs

Common DFSA drugs (often referred to as "date-rape drugs") include gamma hydroxybutyrate (GHB), gamma butyrolactone (GBL), benzodiazepines such as flunitrazepam (Rohypnol®), ketamine hydochloride, methylenedioxymethamphetamine (MDMA), lysergic acid diethylamide (LSD), and alcohol.

The drug GHB was designated as a Federal Schedule 1 drug as of March 2000. It is a colorless, odorless liquid which acts as a central nervous system (CNS) depressant and causes a dissociative mental state. Its effects are enhanced by alcohol. It is often homemade in clandestine labs, and costs $5–10 per dose.

The drug GBL is an industrial degreaser, which is converted to GHB *in vivo*. It typically causes nausea and vomiting, and a dissociative mental state. Overdose may lead to respiratory depression or arrest. Low doses of GHB and GBL cause an increase in libido, euphoria, passivity, amnesia, and have been associated with sexual assault. In higher doses, these drugs have a sedative effect. Laboratory detection of both GHB and GBL is via targeted analysis with gas chromatography and mass spectrometry. Because of its rapid metabolism, plasma samples should optimally be collected < 6–8 hours after ingestion and urine samples collected within 10–12 hours. Urine and plasma may exhibit endogenous levels of GHB (< 1 mg/dl) in urine, (< 4 mg/L) in blood/plasma).[11] Flunitrazepam is a benzodiazepine manufactured by Hoffman-La Roche, available only outside of the United States. It is marketed as a sleep aid, and because of its reputation for use in DFSA, now comes in a new formula which contains blue dye. Flunitrazepam binds to the CNS GABA receptor, is much more potent than diazepam, and causes anterograde amnesia.[12] Because of its potency and use for DFSA, it is being considered for designation as a Schedule 1 drug of abuse.

Ketamine is a dissociative anesthetic chemical similar to phencyclidine (PCP). It can be smoked, injected, or insulated. Although it can be ingested orally, a very large amount must be used to cause a dissociative state. It has a short duration of action dependent on dosage and method of administration. Methylenedioxymethamphetamine (MDMA), often referred to as ecstasy, is a CNS stimulant which causes adrenergic symptoms including an increase in heart rate, blood pressure, and temperature. It often has a strong positive emotional experience for the user such as euphoria and increased feeling of intimacy, and may cause short-term memory loss. Lysergic acid diethylamide (LSD) is a hallucinogen, which has seen resurgence after a long period of decline in the 1980s and 1990s. Its time of onset is 30–60 minutes, and duration of effects lasts up to 12 hours. It causes impaired judgment.

Alcohol is the most commonly detected drug in urine specimens of sexually assaulted patients. It acts as a CNS depressant and enhances the effects of many other drugs.

For a variety of reasons, sexually assaulted patients may delay their presentation to the ED. This delay inevitably leads to a lower likelihood of detection of DFSA drugs in the serum or urine. Hair analysis is an additional method of detecting drugs days to weeks and months after sexual assault. Mechanisms by which drugs are deposited in hair remain unknown, and prosecution of sexual assault offenders based on hair analysis remains controversial. Furthermore, most hospital labs do not routinely analyze for "date-rape" drugs, though more private labs nationwide are doing so. The decision whether to analyze DFSA kits is that of the District Attorney. Patients should be informed of this during the exam.

DFSA kit

In case of suspected DFSA, serum and urine may be collected for toxicologic testing. Most DFSA kits contain a urine specimen cup and 2 gray-topped serum tubes which may be collected up to 96 hours after sexual assault (variability between states). Toxins may be detected in urine for up to 96 hours and in serum for up to 24 hours depending on the nature of toxin and amount ingested. Of note: DFSA kits are processed through a forensic laboratory, not the hospital.

Box 24.3 Pearls for ED evaluation and management of a sexually assaulted patient

- Early involvement of a patient advocate
- Keep and label first urine for forensic analysis
- Recognize patterns of injury
- Do not miss occult injuries
- A normal genital exam does not exclude forced penetration
- Carefully preserve evidence and chain of custody

Treatment
Post-exposure prophylaxis
Sexually transmitted infections

Following sexual assault, patients with exposure should be offered to be treated empirically for *Chlamydia*, Gonorrhea, Trichomonas, and Hepatitis B.

- *Chlamydia*: Azithromycin 1 g (2 g will also cover gonorrhea), or doxycycline 100 mg BID × 7 days
- Gonorrhea: Ceftriaxone 125 mg IM (considerable resistance to ciprofloxacin in some communities)
- Trichomonas: Flagyl 2 g PO × 1 dose
- HBV: Hepatitis B immune globulin (if no previous immunization); hepatitis B vaccine with follow-up vaccine. If previously vaccinated, check titers.

It is reasonable for tetanus toxoid to be updated for those whose immunizations are not current (Figure 24.5).

HIV PEP

Although no prospective studies have been performed to determine efficacy of non-occupational post-exposure prophylaxis (nPEP), studies evaluating efficacy of nPEP in newborns to reduce mother-to-child transmission of HIV, and studies examining the efficacy of occupational PEP, conceptually support the use of nPEP in cases of sexual assault.[13–16] A recent study by Roland et al. documented seroconversion at 3 months in 7 of 702 individuals who initiated PEP.[17] The authors of this study propose that some may have resulted from ongoing exposures and others from failure of PEP to prevent HIV infection.[17]

Recommendations

The Centers for Disease Control and Prevention (CDC) recommends a 28-day course of highly active antiretroviral therapy (HAART) for patients who have had high-risk non-occupational exposure to blood, genital secretions, or other potentially infected body fluids of HIV-infected persons (Figure 24.5) if she or he presents within 72 hours of exposure. Although the CDC makes no official recommendation for patients with similar exposure to persons of unknown serostatus, it may be reasonable to assume a perpetrator's seropositivity in the case of sexual assault based on local prevalence and risk. Most states recommend a triple-drug regimen to be administered

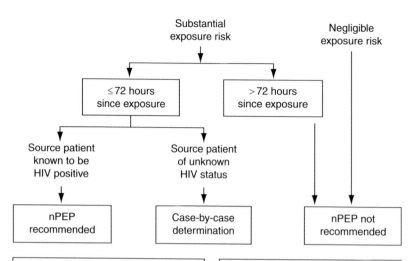

Figure 24.5 Algorithm for evaluation and treatment of possible non-occupational human immunodeficiency virus (HIV) exposures. nPEP, non-occupational post-exposure prophylaxis. (From Centers for Disease Control and Prevention. Antiretroviral post-exposure prophylaxis after sexual, injection-drug use, or other non-occupational exposure to HIV in the United States: recommendations from the US Department of Health and Human Services. *MMWR* 2005;54.)

Substantial risk for HIV exposure	Negligible risk for HIV exposure
Exposure of vagina, rectum, eye, mouth, or other mucus membrane, non-intact skin, or percutaneous contact	*Exposure of* vagina, rectum, eye, mouth, or other mucus membrane, intact or non-intact skin, or percutaneous contact
With blood, semen, vaginal secretions, rectal secretions, breast milk, or any body fluid that is visibly contaminated with blood	*With* urine, nasal secretions, saliva, sweat, or tears if not visibly contaminated with blood
When the source is known to be HIV-infected	*Regardless* of the known or suspected HIV status of the source

up to 72 hours after sexual assault. Animal studies have shown that antiretrovirals are less effective when used after 72 hours.[18]

Recommended triple drug regimen

Clinical trials have revealed the increased efficacy of dual nucleoside reverse transcriptase inhibitors (NRTIs) combined with a nucleotide analog reverse transcriptase inhibitor (NNRTI) for a more potent regimen:[19]

- Zidovudine (AZT): 300 mg BID (NRTI)
- Lamivudine (3TC): 150 mg BID (NRTI)
  (Note: Combivir (AZT + 3TC) one tablet BID is an efficient, though more expensive, alternative)
- Tenofovir: 300 mg each day (NNRTI)

Starter packs

A 3–5 day supply of nPEP should be optimally be supplied to all sexual assault victim patients in order to increase the likelihood of compliance.

Adverse effects

Initial concerns about the potential toxicity of antiretroviral therapy have been tempered by data provided over time by healthcare workers taking PEP. Of 492 healthcare workers reported to the occupational PEP registry, 63% took at least 3 medications. Seventy six percent reported adverse effects, including nausea (57%) and fatigue or malaise (38%). Only 8% of these workers had laboratory abnormalities, all of which resolved by the end of treatment.[20] Because of a significant number of severe adverse reactions in patients who had taken nevirapine-containing regimens for occupational or non-occupational exposures, most agree that it should not be used for nPEP.[21]

HIV testing

All at risk patients should be tested for HIV antibodies at baseline, 4–6 weeks, 3 months, and 6 months to determine if seroconversion occurred. If rapid testing is available in the ED, it is beneficial in order to prevent treatment of the patient who may have pre-existing unkown HIV positivity. The HIV test results should be recorded separately from other findings documented on the sexual assault chart in order to ensure patient's confidentiality in the event medical records are released for legal proceedings. Follow-up appointments must be arranged to monitor liver, renal, and hematologic function. While some protocols initiate this testing in the ED, medication can be started and testing can be done in early follow up unless there is a medical concern otherwise.

Emergency contraception

Plan B:

- Levonorgestrel 0.75 mg PO Q 12 × 2 doses (May give both tablets at once if reliability questionable; studies show comparable efficacy)

Alternative – Ovral:

- Ethinylestradiol 100 mcg + levonorgestrel 0.5 mg × 2 tablets PO Q 12 × 2 doses

Studies have proven increased efficacy and superior tolerability of Plan B when compared with Ovral.[22] Side effects may be further ameliorated with administration of an antiemetic such as metoclopramide 10 mg 30 minutes prior to administration of emergency contraception.[23] It is important to provide emergency contraception as soon after sexual assault as possible as efficacy wanes with time. A number of studies support the use of emergency contraception up to 120 hours after unprotected intercourse.[24] Although the evidentiary exam (rape kit) is not performed for patients presenting more than 96 hours after sexual assault, it is important to consider providing emergency contraception.

Documentation

Documentation should only include a description of the findings, not inferences or conclusions. Some facilities have specialized sexual assault charts which help ensure a thorough, focused assessment, and which include consent forms for the exam and photography. The only medical issues documented in the forensic evaluation aspect of the medical record should be acute findings that potentially relate to the assault or pre-existing medical factors that could influence interpretation of findings.

It is best to document the history of present illness in the patient's own words. For example, use phrases such as: "Patient states" and then use quotation marks for direct quotes, or use language such as: "Patient describes," "Patient recalls," "Patient reports," or "Patient states that." When describing the patient's overall appearance, document specifics, such as, patient is lying in the fetal position, crying, and looking down at the floor. Every attempt should be made to maintain objectivity when documenting the physical exam. In any given circumstance the physician's ultimate duty is to document truthfully what he or she sees. Finally, do not use language that implies judgment on the part of the examiner, such as "patient alleges."

Law enforcement

Where permitted by law, patients, rather than health-care providers, should make the decision whether or not to report a sexual assault to law enforcement. Patients should be provided with information about the possible benefits and consequences of reporting so that they can make an informed decision. Different jurisdictions have different policies regarding reporting and, furthermore, different circumstances are subject to specific reporting laws (see below). Patients should be told about mandatory reporting obligations and procedures that will be used.

Patients should be told that delays in reporting may negatively affect the ability of the criminal justice system to investigate and prosecute a case.

Sexual assault reporting laws

Many states have mandatory reporting laws for specific victims including children, the elderly, or a vulnerable adult who has been a victim of a crime. Few states require mandatory reporting of sexual assault in a competent adult, except in certain outstanding cases, such as with the use of a deadly weapon.

At the time of this writing, California is the only state that explicitly requires medical personnel to report the treatment of a competent adult sexual assault victim (California Penal Code 11160). Kentucky mandates reporting of rape to the Kentucky Cabinet for Family and Children if the crime also constitutes domestic violence (KRS 209.030). Massachusetts requires that medical personnel who treat a rape victim report the case without identifying information to the Criminal History Systems Board.[25]

Many states have mandatory reporting laws in the case of certain types of crimes and therefore may affect the competent adult sexual assault victim. For example, many states require that the following types of injuries are reported: injuries caused by firearms, stab wounds or non-accidental wounds inflicted by a sharp-pointed object, injury caused by a deadly weapon, and burns. Sexual assault examiners must be familiar with the reporting laws in their state. A helpful website is: http://www.ipba.net/pubs/RapeandSexualAssaultReportingLaws.pdf.

Forensic photography

Consent must be obtained prior to any photo documentation. Each injury should be photographed separately, making sure there is a label in the photograph frame. The label should show the date, the patient's initials and medical record number, and should have a ruler edge to illustrate size when held adjacent to the injury. (Note: the cotton-swab wrappers contained in some rape kits have a ruler on the side; you may use these for labels.) For the best image, it is recommended that the label or ruler is positioned parallel to the length of the injury, and that blue or green surgical drapes are placed under the body part being photographed. If possible, capture the patient's face in the photograph of injury, for identification purposes.

Disposition

Transfers

If a nearby hospital is a designated center for sexual assault forensic examination and the patient is stable and amenable, one may consider transferring the patient if there is a minimal possibility that evaluation, treatment, or evidence collection will be compromised.

Consultations

Many hospitals have an on-call panel of rape advocates and social service support. They should be utilized with the patient's consent. If there is no one trained in the ED to examine sexually assaulted patients, there is no designated forensic examiner on call, and a transfer is not possible, one may consider consulting the gynecologist on call for assistance. If there is a suspicion of a DFSA, one may contact the local poison control center for guidance. Finally, for patients where one is concerned about suicidal ideation, a psychiatric assessment for risk should be performed by the emergency physician or the psychiatric consult on call.

Discharges

Patients may be discharged if they are clinically stable, sober, have a safe place to go to, and if there is no concern of their ability to follow up. If there is a concern that a patient will be lost to follow up, then it is reasonable to consider hospitalization or keeping the patient in the ED until safe discharge planning is arranged. All follow-up counseling should be arranged prior to discharge. This includes the follow up of labs sent to the hospital laboratory (crime lab. studies are generally not available to the patient), the continuation of medical therapy, arrangements for the repeat evaluation of indicated lab. studies, psychosocial services and counseling, and law enforcement if they were contacted. As with any patient, all discharge instructions must be clearly documented for the patient in a language that the patient comprehends. Patients must be provided with suitable clothing if their clothes were taken during the exam.

Forensic kits

All kits should be labeled and sealed accordingly. Each institution should have protocols describing the storage of forensic kits and photo-documents if the police have not been notified. If the police do respond and take a report, the kit and photographs may be released to them, if the patient consents. It is of the utmost importance, that the chain of evidence is maintained and documented meticulously. For example: date, time, your name, "I handed contents of sealed rape kit to officer X, badge number Y."

References

1. Rape, Abuse, and Incest National Network (RAINN) calculation based on Maston, C., Klaus, P, *National Criminal Victimization Survey, 2005*. Bureau of Justice Statistics: US Department of Justice, 2006.

2. Slaughter L, Brown CRV. Colposcopy to establish physical finding in rape victims. *Am J Obstet Gynecol* 1992;**166**:83–6.

3. Slaughter L, Brown CRV, Crowley S, Peck R. Patterns of genital injury in female sexual assault victims. *Am J Obstet Gynecol* 1997;**175**:609–16.

4. Jones J, Dunnuck C, Rossman L, Wynn B, Genco M. Adolescent Foley catheter technique for visualizing

hymenal injuries in adolescent sexual assault. *Acad Emerg Med* 2003;**10**:1001–4.

5. Adams JA, Girardin B, Faugno D. Adolescent sexual assault: Documentation of acute injuries using photo-colposcopy. *J Pediatr Adolesc Gynecol* 2001;**14**:175–80.

6. Lenahan LC, Ernst A, Johnson B. Colposcopy in evaluation of the adult sexual assault victim. *Am J Emerg Med* 1998;**16**:183–4.

7. Sugar N, Fine D, Eckert L. Physical injury after sexual assault: findings of a large case series. *Am J Ob Gyn* 2004;**190**:1.

8. Sommers MS. Using colposcopy in the rape exam: health care, forensic, and criminal justice issues. *J Forensic Nurs* 2005;**1**(1):28–34.

9. Negrusz A, Juhascik M, Gaensslen RE. *Estimate of the Incidence of Drug-facilitated Sexual assault in the US.* Washington, DC: US Department of Justice 2005.

10. Maston C, Klaus P. *National Criminal Victimization Survey, 2005.* Washington, DC: US Department of Justice, 2006.

11. Yeatman DT, Reid K. A study of urinary endogenous gamma-hydroxybutyrate (GHB) levels. *J Anal Toxicol* 2003;**27**(1):40–2.

12. Waltzman ML. Flunitrazepam: a review of "roofies." *Pediatr Emerg Care* 1999;**15**(1):59–60.

13. Taha TE, Kumwenda NI, Gibbons A, et al. Short postexposure prophylaxis in newborn babies to reduce mother-to-child transmission of HIV-1: NVAZ randomized clinical trial. *Lancet* 2003;**362**:1171–7.

14. Roland M. Postexposure prophylaxis after sexual exposure to HIV. *Curr Opin Infect Dis* 2007;**20**:39–46.

15. Speight CG MC, Kuria E, Kilonzo N, Onchwari P, Taegtmeyer M. Providing post-exposure prophylaxis as part of comprehensive post-rape care – Thika District Hospital, Kenya. In XV International AIDS Conference. July 11–16, 2004. Bangkok, Thailand, 2004.

16. Roland, M. *HIV Post-exposure Prophylaxis Following Non-Occupational Exposures. Background Paper for WHO Expert Consultation for the Development of Policy and Guidelines on Occupational and Non-Occupational HIV Post-Exposure Prophylaxis.* Geneva,

Switzerland, September 3–5, 2005. Available from http://hivinsite.ucsf.edu/pdf/p01-kb-new/kbr-07-02-07-roland.pdf.

17. Roland ME, Neilands TB, Krone MR, et al. Seroconversion following nonoccupational postexposure prophylaxis against HIV. *Clin Infect Dis* 2005;**41**:1507–13.

18. Pullium JK, Adams DR, Jackson E, et al. Pig-tailed macaques infected with human immunodeficiency virus (HIV) type 2GB122 or simian/HIV89.6p express virus in semen during primary infection: new model for genital tract shedding and transmission. *J Infect Dis* 2001;**183**(7):1023–30.

19. Hammer S, Kubin C. Antiretroviral agents. In Cohen J, Powderly WG (eds), *Infectious Diseases*, 2nd edn. Barcelona, Spain: Elsevier Ltd, 2004: pp. 1871–93.

20. Centers for Disease Control and Prevention. Antiretroviral postexposure prophylaxis after sexual, injection drug use, or other non-occupational exposure to HIV in the United States: recommendations from the US Department of Health and Human Services. *MMWR Recomm Rep* 2005;**54**:RR-2.

21. Centers for Disease Control and Prevention. Serious adverse events attributed to nevirapine regimens for postexposure prophylaxis after HIV exposures world wide, 1997–2000. *MMWR Recomm Rep* 2001; **49**:1153–6.

22. WHO Task Force on Postovulatory Methods of Fertility Regulation. Randomized controlled trial of levonorgestrel versus the Yuzpe regimen of combined oral contraceptives for emergency contraception. *Lancet* 1998;**352**:428–33.

23. Ragan RE, Rock RW, Buck HW. Metoclopramide pretreatment attenuates emergency contraception-associated nausea. *Am J Obstetr Gynecol* 2003;**188** (2):330–3.

24. Ellertson C, Evans M, Ferden S, et al. Extending the time limit for starting the Yuzpe regimen of emergency contraception to 120 hours. *Obstetr Gynecol* 2003;**101**:1168–71.

25. Scalzo T. Rape and sexual assault reporting laws. *APRI* 2007;**1**(3):1–4.

25

Injury prevention

Salvatore Pardo

Introduction

Historically, accidents have not been perceived as preventable events. In a 1949 paper entitled "The epidemiology of accidents," John E. Gordon, pioneer of injury prevention, placed injury control within the public health framework. Gordon identified that the death rate from accidents in 1949 remained essentially unchanged from the same rate 40 years earlier.[1] While, over the early part of the century, great advancements had been made in understanding and controlling infectious, neoplastic, and congenital disease, little progress had been made in accident prevention. Gordon hypothesized that the same biologic laws that govern in the epidemiology of medicine could also operate in respect to injury. He compared two important events with mass casualties: The epidemic of typhoid fever in 1934 and the Coconut Grove nightclub fire of 1942. The former was attributed to untreated drinking water and the latter was attributed to inadequacies of fire codes. He asserted that these examples could be each traced back to a single preventable cause. This revelation led to the introduction of the concept of injury prevention. Gordon essentially asserted that, like the medical epidemic of typhoid fever, accidental injuries could be preventable.

Gordon proposed that, like the medical disease processes, there is a host, an agent, and an environment involved in each accident.[1] The host can be described by their age, gender, race, or genetics. The environment can be described in physical, biological, or socioeconomic terms. An accident evolves as a disturbance. This can occur either through the principal action of the agent, because of the host, or as a function of the environment. Most often, however, it is through some combination of all three. These are the fundamental factors in causation. Using this basic theorem, the science of injury prevention has evolved over the past half century.

> **Box 25.1   Essentials of injury prevention science**
> - Like the medical disease processes, there is a host, an agent, and an environment involved in each accident/injury.
> - The host can be described by their age, gender, race, or genetics. The environment can be described in physical, biological, or socioeconomic terms.
> - An accident/injury can be due to a single factor; however, it is most often through some combination of the host, agent, and environment.
> - These are the fundamental factors in causation.

Theory of injury prevention

William Haddon, Jr. is best known for being the first administrator of the National Highway Safety Bureau. As a disciple of Gordon's concepts, his goal was to change the focus of highway safety and consequently reduce the number of deaths that resulted from motor vehicle accidents.[2] He re-examined the view of accidents as "chance" events. In fact, he influenced the change in language from "motor vehicle accident" to the more recently accepted phrase "motor vehicle collision."

He developed a conceptual model called the Haddon matrix. This tool is used amongst epidemiologists to understand the concepts of injury prevention and to develop ideas to prevent injury. Within each matrix, there is a pre-event phase, an event phase, and post-event phase. These are represented by the rows of the matrix. The factors, represented by the columns of the matrix, refer to the interacting

Trauma: A Comprehensive Emergency Medicine Approach, eds. Eric Legome and Lee W. Shockley. Published by Cambridge University Press. © Cambridge University Press 2011.

Table 25.1 Haddon's matrix of motor vehicle collisions[4]

Phase	Host	Vehicle	Physical environment	Social environment
Pre-event	Driver ability, driver training	Maintenance of brakes, vehicle inspection programs, installation of child restraint, child restraint checking programs	Adequate roadway markings, correct installation of child restraint, right child restraint for child's height and weight	Attitudes to drink driving/speed/use of child restraints for every car trip
Event	Human tolerances to crash forces, wearing of seat belt, having child in a correctly fitting child restraint	Crash worthiness of the vehicle (e.g., crush space), crash worthiness of child restraint (e.g., head extrusion)	Presence of fixed object near roadway, presence of unsecured object within the vehicle	Enforcement of mandatory seatbelt and child restraint use
Post-event	Crash victims general health status	Petrol tanks designed to minimize likelihood of post-crash fire	Availability of effective and timely emergency response	Public support for trauma care and rehabilitation

factors that contribute to the injury process. The four factors are the host, the agent, the physical environment, and the social environment.

In the event of motor vehicle collision, the rows are defined as the pre-collision, collision, and post-collision phases. The columns are defined as the host (driver), the agent (automobile), the physical environment (road), and the social environment (attitude). The pre-collision phase involves the prevention of the etiologic agent from reaching the host. For the host, this may involve the education or experience of the driver. The collision phase involves the interaction of the etiologic agents and the host. For the agent, this may involve the crash worthiness of the vehicle itself or the integrity of the seat belts and other restraint devices. The post-collision phase involves the maximizing salvage once the damage has been done.[3] In reference to the physical environment, this includes the development of an emergent trauma care system (Table 25.1).[4]

The Haddon matrix has been used frequently in the development of safety measures. By filling in the different cells of the matrix, a complete strategy to combat any injury can be formulated. One needs to clearly identify the problem to be addressed and carefully assign when the pre-event, event, and post-event phases begin and end. Haddon also organized 10 countermeasure strategies to address injury control.[5–7] As seen in Table 25.2, an example of his countermeasures are shown as applied to child injury prevention.[8] These models can be used in understanding public heath issues from the perspective of risk factor

identification. Further, they allow the drafting of preventive strategies. In doing so, they provide both public health practitioners and researchers a framework within which to examine problems systematically and take action.[4,8]

In an article in 1998, Carol Runyan expanded on Haddon's methodology.[5] She realized that, when making decisions about policy, there are certain values that guide the process. She proposed that by using the principals of policy analysis there could be a concrete articulation of these values. As a result, she created an additional dimension in Haddon's matrix incorporating the use of value criteria. The suggested criteria include, but are not limited to: effectiveness, cost, freedom, equity, stigmatization, feasibility, and the preferences of the affected community or individual.[4] The decision maker must determine the relative weights to be placed on each value to determine the worth of any intervention. Overall, this third dimension creates an opportunity to brainstorm, organize, evaluate, and explain the assessment process. The application of the third dimension of Haddon's matrix should facilitate the decision-making process.

Behavioral theory

Historically, due to the unparalleled success of passive or structural strategy, such as childhood immunization and fluoridation of water in public health measures, the application of behavioral science to injury prevention has been de-emphasized.[9] That is, it is

Table 25.2 Countermeasure strategies for childhood injury[8]

Countermeasure	Example
1. Prevent the creation of the hazard	Banning the sale of unsafe nursery products such as baby walkers
2. Reduce the amount of the hazard	Package medicines in smaller, safer amounts
3. Prevent the release of hazards that already exist	Medicine containers that are child resistant
4. Modify the rate or spatial distribution of the hazard from its source	Use properly fitted child restraints
5. Separate by time or space the hazard from that which can be protected	Do not install children's playgrounds near unfenced/unprotected bodies of water
6. Separate the hazard and what is to be protected by a material barrier	Install isolation fencing on all four sides of a swimming pool
7. Modify relevant basic qualities of the hazard	Change the spaces between the bars in a cot to prevent child strangulation
8. Make what is to be protected more resistant to damage from the hazard	All children learn to swim
9. Move rapidly to detect and evaluate the damage that has occurred and counter its continuation and extension	All parents and caregivers learn cardiopulmonary resuscitation (CPR) and provide efficient emergency services
10. Stabilize, repair, and rehabilitate the damage or injured person	Develop rehabilitation plans at an early stage of treatment

easier to change engineering than behavior. It is the integration of active and passive strategies (behavior and engineering), however, which are leading to the greatest change in public health and injury prevention.

There are several behavioral models applied to injury prevention including, the health-belief model, the theory of reasoned action, the stages of change model, and applied behavioral analysis.[9] In the health-belief model, preventive behaviors are thought to be a function of one's beliefs of susceptibility to the problem. Also involved in this model are one's understanding of the severity of the health problem, and the cost of adopting the preventative behavior. Peterson et al. studied the beliefs and practices of 198 parents with children between 8 and 17 years of age.[10] They discovered that the majority of parents were not initially worried about accidental injuries to their children. The study then educated parents on their child's susceptibility to injury while increasing their competency to intervene. After the interventions, parents then believed that their actions could be effective and they were more competent to implement these preventative measures.

In the theory of reasoned action, one's intention to perform a behavior predicts actual behavior.[11] This intention is a function of community attitudes, education, and social norms. This theory was used to develop a survey of parents' beliefs and practices regarding the use of car safety seats. The survey revealed that parents' attitudes regarding the effectiveness of car seats were the single best predictor of parents implementing their use. As a result, marketing was then directed at educating parents and caretakers in the value of car seats as an important means of injury prevention.

A more recent model has been developed called the stages of change. The theory is based on the premise that change occurs in defined stages and people differ in their willingness to advance among these stages. The steps to change are: precontemplative, contemplative, preparation, action, and maintenance. The model incorporates the notion of relapsing and describes the cyclical nature of relapse and progression during the maintenance phase. Depending on which stage the individual is in, the individual or group wishing to intervene and end a harmful behavior selects the most appropriate strategy. Examples of this model are found in strategies developed to stop smoking as well as to avoid abusive relationships.

Applied behavioral analysis seeks to understand and modify behavior by addressing the "ABCs" (**A**ntecedents, **B**ehavior, **C**onsequences) of behavior. Understanding the ABCs can help shape the behavior and the environment. Application of behavioral analysis has helped to increase the use of safety belts, bicycle helmets, and child restraints, reduce vehicular speeding and impaired driving, improve pedestrian and occupational safety, and modify many other risky behaviors.

Ultimately, many of these behavioral science theories have been integrated to develop a consensus of the factors that appear to account for most of the variation in behaviors directly affecting injury prevention: (1) intentions; (2) environmental barriers; (3) skills; (4) outcome expectancies or attitude; (5) social norms; (6) self-standards; (7) emotional reactions; and (8) self-efficacy. From this model, Fishbein and Ajzen then concluded that in order for a person to perform a behavior, one or more of the following must be present:[11–13]

1. The person forms a strong positive intention or makes a commitment to perform the behavior.
2. There are no environmental barriers that make it impossible to perform the behavior.
3. The person possesses the skills necessary to perform the behavior.
4. The person believes that the advantages of performing the behavior outweigh the disadvantages.
5. The person perceives more normative pressure to perform the behavior than to not perform it.
6. The person perceives that performance of the behavior is consistent with his or her self-image or values.
7. The person's emotional reaction to performing the behavior is more positive than negative.
8. The person perceives that he or she has the capabilities to perform the behavior under different circumstances.

The first three factors are viewed as necessary to produce a given behavior, and the remaining five are simply modifying variables. From a hypothetical example, we can apply this to one specific injury control behavior; the testing of the home smoke alarm. If the homeowner is committed to test the device, has access to it, and has the skills to test it, there is a high probability that he or she will perform the behavior. These chances will increase as more of the eight factors are present.[11–13]

Injury prevention can also be effectively implemented at the community level. Several efforts have been developed which focus on the active participation of social communities to decrease traumatic injuries. One example of a successful organization in injury control is the Injury Free Coalition for Kids®. It is one of the country's fastest growing and most effective injury-prevention programs. It is a national program of the Robert Wood Johnson Foundation comprised of hospital-based, community-oriented programs, whose efforts are anchored in research, education, and advocacy. Currently, the coalition includes 40 sites located in 37 cities, each housed in the trauma centers of their participating institutions. The implementation of playground renovations, a Safety City, which teaches children the proper way to cross the street, window guard legislation, community dance and sports programs, and free bicycle helmets are some of the specific components of the program. With the inception of this program in central Harlem in 1988, major traumatic injuries requiring hospital admission decreased by 55% in the subsequent 10 years. In the same period, violent injuries decreased by 46% in this neighborhood while they doubled in the neighboring community.[14] Utilizing these statistics, the Northern Manhattan Injury Surveillance System has validated these results were for the appropriate and targeted groups.[15]

Box 25.2   Behavioral models applied to injury prevention

Model	Overview
Health-belief model	Preventive behaviors are thought to be a function of one's beliefs of susceptibility to the problem. Includes one's understanding of the severity of the health problem, and the cost of adopting the preventative behavior
Theory of reasoned action	One's intention to perform a behavior predicts actual behavior. This intention is a function of community attitudes, education, and social norms.
Stages of change model	The theory is based on the premise that change occurs in defined stages and people differ in their willingness to advance among these stages. Depending on which stage the individual is in, the individual or group wishing to intervene and end a harmful behavior selects the most appropriate strategy.
Applied behavioral analysis	Seeks to understand and modify behavior by addressing the "ABCs" (Antecedents, Behavior, Consequences) of behavior.

Motor vehicle safety

Motor vehicle collisions are among the leading contributors to death and injury each year in the United States.[16–19] Over 40 000 lives are lost annually, and countless others sustain significant injuries. Trauma due to motor vehicle collisions puts a significant strain on our healthcare system with costs estimated at approximately $230 billion in the year 2000.[20] Injuries to occupants of motor vehicles are generally attributable to several key factors including the speed and size of the vehicle, and the amount of protection that the occupant had from the impact.[21] A significant number of these deaths could be reduced with proper adherence to established legislation and appropriate safety measures.

Combating impaired driving has been a daunting challenge for law enforcement agencies and legislators in every state across the United States. On a national level, it continues to be the leading cause of motor vehicle crashes and related deaths.[21] Driving under the Influence (DUI) laws and zero-tolerance laws for teenagers are critical in remedying this nationwide problem. With implementation of legislation that specifically targets those individuals who drink and drive, there has been an estimated 30% decrease in alcohol-related motor vehicle deaths.[21] Currently, all 50 states and the District of Columbia have established laws that make it illegal for persons aged 21 years or older to drive with a blood alcohol concentration (BAC) of 0.08 g/dl or more.[1] The National Highway Traffic Safety Administration's (NHTSA's) zero-tolerance laws make it illegal for drivers under the legal drinking age to operate a motor vehicle with any amount of alcohol in their blood. Zero-tolerance laws were established in the late 1990s to tackle the increased relative risk that these inexperienced drivers face, particularly when operating motor vehicles under the influence of alcohol or drugs. Approximately one-third of adolescent motor vehicle deaths are associated with driving while intoxicated.[22]

The emergency department (ED) serves as an excellent place for physicians to identify individuals with alcohol-related problems. Patients with alcoholism generally have repeated ED visits due to trauma and are therefore ideal targets for injury prevention counseling.[19] Alcoholism screening coupled with interventions by emergency physicians may act as the support needed to help those with alcohol-related problems receive additional social support and affect behavioral change.[23]

Another important measure of protecting ourselves from serious and debilitating injuries is wearing seat belts. Despite the simplicity and proven effectiveness of this intervention, studies have shown that adults and children alike do not fully comply with seat belt laws.[24] Motor vehicle safety reached an important milestone with the requirement of standard seat belts in the 1960s. This developed from the understanding that most serious injuries from motor vehicle collisions occur from the body's direct impact with the automobile's interior automotive parts, i.e., steering wheel, after the vehicle's initial collision.[17] A recent ED study demonstrated that in motor vehicle crashes where seat belts were not worn, there was a three times greater likelihood of fatalities. In addition, alcohol use was closely associated with patients who did not use seat belts.[20] Further studies investigated the effectiveness of seat belts with and without airbag deployment. When driver and passenger airbags are deployed in conjunction with seat belt use, the risk of death is reduced by approximately 50%, whereas a risk reduction of only 13% has been observed in cases where airbags were deployed without seat belt use.[16] More stringent enforcement of seat belt regulations has proven to be an effective measure for preventing fatal motor vehicle crashes. With the inception of the "Click It or Ticket" campaign, a significant increase in seat belt use has been observed in recent years. Seat belt use nationwide was 81% in 2006, up from 71% in 2000, as measured by NHTSA's National Occupant Protection Use Survey (NOPUS).[25]

Speed is another significant contributor to injuries acquired from motor vehicle crashes. As speed increases, kinetic energy increases exponentially ($KE = 1/2 \ MV^2$). In 1974 the national speed limit was set at 55 mph to conserve fuel; however, it had the additional effect of decreased motor vehicle collision fatalities.[16,17] Upon repeal of the national maximum speed limit in 1995, 32 states raised their speed limits to at least 70 mph.[3] States that increased their speed limits saw an increase in motor vehicle mortalities compared to states that maintained the 55 mph speed limit.[16,17]

Additional technological advances in car safety include collapsible steering columns, shatterproof glass, and side airbags. Although these improvements continually enhance overall motor vehicle safety, it is still equally important to educate drivers and passengers about precautionary techniques and defensive driving skills. With the combined efforts of education, legislation, and new technology, it is possible to prevent some of the potentially dangerous scenarios.

Head injury prevention

Traumatic brain injury is one of the most serious and debilitating injuries. As a result preventive interventions have focused on increasing the use of helmets, particularly when motorcycles or bicycles are involved.[18] Motorcyclists face a tremendous risk on the road; they generally experience a fatality rate 20 times greater than drivers and passengers of other motor vehicles.[16] The use of a helmet can reduce the risk of serious head injuries by up to 85%.[18] Additional factors, such as decreasing the motorcyclist's speed at impact, may also influence this level of risk reduction.[26] The primary challenge to reducing this risk has been the acceptance of helmet use by motorcyclists. As of June 2006, only 20 states and the District of Columbia had established laws mandating the use of helmets by all motorcyclists. An additional 26 states have established laws that mandate helmet use only by certain individuals, such as young, inexperienced riders.[4] The average rate of helmet use in states without current legislation is between 30% and 50%. This number rises to almost 100% in states where helmet laws are in effect.[16]

Likewise bicyclists encounter a risk of head injury; however, the majority of injuries result from falls, not collisions.[27] Despite 600 000 bicyclists sustaining injuries annually, 30 states do not have mandatory helmet laws.[4,27] The leading cause of head trauma among children is attributable to bicycle injuries.[28,29] With bicycling remaining among the top outdoor leisure activities in both adults and children, bicycle helmet use, regardless of established law, is prudent.[27,28] Analogous to motorcyclists, the challenge

has been persuading cyclists to wear their safety helmets on a consistent basis. By combining proper education with legislation mandating helmet use, the associated risk of mortality and morbidity of bicycle injuries should be reduced.[16,27] Additionally, physicians assume integral roles in influencing the behavior of their patients. By educating parents and children on the use of helmets, physicians can contribute to injury prevention.[16] In response to the bicycling deaths of two children, Howard County, Maryland, became the first US jurisdiction to mandate use of bicycle helmets for children. Pre-legislation and post-legislation helmet use was observed in Howard County and two control counties: Montgomery (which sponsored a community education program) and Baltimore County (no helmet activities). Pre-legislation crude helmet use rates for children were 4% (95% confidence interval [CI] 0–10%) for Howard, 8% (95% CI 3–13%) for Montgomery, and 19% (95% CI 5–33%) for Baltimore. Post-legislation rates were 47% (95% CI 32–62%), 19% (95% CI 11–27%), and 4% (95% CI 0–11%), respectively. The rate of bicycle helmet use by Howard County children is now the highest documented for US children.[30]

Residential injury prevention

Burns are the fourth leading cause of accidental death in the United States.[17,31] Residential fires are responsible for three quarters of all fire-related deaths, and most of these deaths are attributable to asphyxiation as the primary cause of injury.[17,33] By taking appropriate safety measures in the home, public health measures have made great strides in the prevention of potentially life-threatening burns and asphyxiation from smoke inhalation.[17,32] The main areas of concentration in residential injury prevention include residential fires, water scalding, and clothing ignition.

Careless smoking is a significant contributor to residential fires.[32,33] Approximately 65% of residential fires are started by cigarettes.[33] Direct fire prevention efforts through the establishment of "fire-safe" cigarettes (cigarettes with a reduced propensity to burn when left unattended) continue to be investigated, but research has not been actively pursued by the cigarette industry.[17,31–33] Currently, the most effective preventive measures are the proper installation and maintenance of smoke detectors in the home. The use of smoke detectors has been effectively increased through strict legislation, as well as educational efforts.[17] With smoke detectors, the risk of mortality in residential fires is lowered by approximately 80%.[17,32]

Another potentially injurious situation involves clothing ignition. Young children and the elderly are the most vulnerable segment of the population to this risk.[17,32] Children are more prone to play with fire and lighting devices. The elderly are generally less mobile, and have more physical impairments, which drastically reduce their ability to navigate dangerous situations.[33] Clothing ignition can result from various external factors, including unintentional contact with household appliances or lighting devices. Efforts were made to prevent these injuries with the development of fire retardant clothing. Legislation first was initiated to increase use of these materials in children's clothing through the Children's Sleepwear Standard Law in the 1970s. However, the regulations were eventually eased by the Consumer Product Safety Commission, with a resultant decreased adherence to these standards.[17]

Conclusion

The theory of injury prevention is relatively young. Over the past 60 years, there have been great efforts to create a safer environment. Through the work of Haddon and other injury prevention experts, a tangible, clear method can be used to develop and implement strategies to combat preventable injury.

References

1. Gordon J. The epidemiology of accidents. *Am J Public Health* 1949;**39**:504–15.

2. O'Neill B. Accidents. Highway safety and William Haddon, Jr. In *Contingencies* Jan/Feb 2002, pp. 30–2. Available from http://www.contingencies.org/janfeb02/crashes.pdf.

3. Haddon W. The changing approach to the epidemiology, prevention, and amelioration of trauma: the transition to approaches etiologically rather than descriptively based. *Am J Public Health* 1968;**58**:1431–8.

4. State of Queensland. Haddon's matrix. *Queensland Health, Australia*. April 4, 2007. Available from http://www.health.qld.gov.au/chipp/what_is/matrix.asp.

5. Runyan C. Using the Haddon matrix: introducing the third dimension. *Inj Prev* 1998;**4**:302–7.

6. Runyan C. Introduction: back to the future-revisiting Haddon's conceptualization of injury epidemiology and prevention. *Epidemiol Rev* 2003;**25**:60–4.

7. Haddon W. Energy damage and the 10 countermeasure strategies. *J Trauma* 1973;**13**:321–31.

8. State of Queensland. Haddon's countermeasures. *Queensland Health, Australia*. April 4, 2007. Available from http://www.health.qld.gov.au/chipp/what_is/countermeasures.asp.

9. Geilen AC, Sleet D. Application of behavior-change theories and methods to injury prevention. *Epidemiol Rev* 2003;**25**:65–76.

10. Peterson L, Farmer J, Kashani JH. Parental injury prevention endeavors: a function of health beliefs? *Health Psychol* 1990;**9**:177–91.

11. Fishbein M, Ajzen I. *Belief, Attitude, Intention, and Behavior: An Introduction to Theory and Research*. Reading, MA: Addison Wesley Publishing Company, 1975.

12. Fishbein M. Developing effective behavior change interventions: some lessons learned from behavioral research. In Backer TE, David SL, Soucy G (eds), *Reviewing the Behavioral Science Knowledge Base on Technology Transfer* (Research Monograph no. 155). Bethesda, MD: National Institute on Drug Abuse, 1995: pp. 246–61.

13. Fishbein M, Triandis HC, Kanfer FH, et al. Factors influencing behavior and behavior change. In Baum A, Revenson TA, Singer JE (eds), *Handbook of Health Physiology*. Mahwah, NJ: Lawrence Erlbaum Associates, 2001: pp. 3–17.

14. Durkin MS, Kuhn L, Davidson L, Laraque D, Barlow B. Epidemiology and prevention of severe assault and gun injuries to children in an urban community. *J Trauma* 1996;**41**:667–73.

15. Durkin MS, Davidson LL, Kuhn L, O'Connor P, Barlow, B. Low income neighborhoods and the risk of severe pediatric injury: a small area analysis in Northern Manhattan. *Am J Public Health* 1994;**84**:587–92.

16. Broderick J, McKenna D. Injury control. *Trauma Manag* 2001;**42**:623–30.

17. Maier R, Mock C. Injury prevention. *Trauma* 2000;**4**(3):41–55.

18. Rivara F, Grossman D, Cummings P. Injury prevention: first of two parts. *N Engl J Med* 1997;**337**(8):543–8.

19. Feury K. Injury prevention: where are the resources? *Orthop Nurs* 2003;**22**(2):124–30.

20. Allen S, Zhu S, Sauter C, et al. A comprehensive statewide analysis of seatbelt non-use with injury and hospital admissions: new data, old problem. *Acad Emerg Med* 2006;**13**:427–34.

21. National Highway Traffic Safety Administration. *Traffic Safety Facts. 2006 Traffic Safety Annual*

Assessment Alcohol-Related Fatalities. Research Note DOT HS 810 821, August 2007, pp 1–6. Available from http://www-nrd.nhtsa.dot.gov/Pubs/810821.pdf.

22. Margolis LH, Foss RD, Tolbert WG. Alcohol and motor vehicle–related deaths of children as passengers, pedestrians, and bicyclists. *JAMA* 2000;**283**:2245–8.

23. Crawford MJ, Patton R, Touquet R, et al. Screening and referral for brief intervention of alcohol-misusing patients in an emergency department: a pragmatic randomized controlled trial. *Lancet* 2004;**364**:1334–9.

24. Glassbrenner D. *Safety Belt Use in 2005: Use Rates in the States and Territories. Publication No. DOT HS 809 970.* Available from http://www-nrd.nhtsa.dot.gov/pdf/nrd-30/NCSA/RNotes/2005/809970.pdf.

25. National Highway Traffic Safety Administration. *Traffic Safety Facts, April 2007.* Available from http://www-nrd.nhtsa.dot.gov/Pubs/810690.pdf.

26. Liu B, Ivers R, Norton R, et al. Helmets for preventing injury in motorcycle riders. *Cochrane Database System Rev* 2003;**4**:CD004333.

27. Rosenkranz K, Sheridan R. Trauma to adult bicyclists: a growing problem in the urban environment. *Injury* 2003;**34**:825–9.

28. Ortega H, Shields B, Smith G. Bicycle-related injuries to children and parental attitudes regarding bicycle safety. *Clin Pediatr* 2004;**43**(3):251–9.

29. Sosin DM, Sacks JJ, Webb KW. Pediatric head injuries and deaths from bicycling in the United States. *Pediatrics* 1996;**98**(5):868–70.

30. Coté TR, Sacks JJ, Lambert-Huber DA, et al. Bicycle helmet use among Maryland children: effect of legislation and education. *Pediatrics* 1992;**89**(6):1216–20.

31. Mallonee S, Istre GR, Rosenberg M, et al. Surveillance and prevention of residential-fire injuries. *N Engl J Med* 1996;**335**(1):27–31.

32. Rivara F, Grossman D, Cummings P. Injury prevention: second of two parts. *N Engl J Med* 1997;**337**(9):613–18.

33. Warda L, Tenenbein M, Moffatt M. House fire injury prevention update part I: a review of risk factors for fatal and non-fatal house fire injury. *Inj Prev* 1999;**5**:145–50.

Chapter

26

Rural trauma care

Neil Waldman and David Dreitlein

Introduction

Only 8% of rural American residents have access to Level I or II trauma centers within 45 minutes, compared to 73% of suburban residents and 89% of urban residents. Of the 46.7 million Americans without access within an hour of a Level I or II trauma center, the majority reside in rural areas.[1]

Far from regional trauma centers where emergency physicians, trauma surgeons and specialty consultants both train and practice, rural emergency physicians must use their skills to manage and stabilize trauma patients, often without any assistance from physician colleagues or consultants. Advanced Trauma Life Support (ATLS®) -trained practitioners at rural trauma centers improve outcomes for trauma patients and are associated with risk-adjusted survival.[2,3] According to one study, the majority of non-standard care rendered in the rural emergency department (ED) leading to preventable mortality is related to airway and chest injury management.[4] Although no definitive proof exists, it is not hard to postulate that these injuries and their complications could be prevented through the use of ATLS® training at minimum or, even better, emergency medicine boarded physicians in rural areas. Accomplishing these goals of providing this level of care to rural parts of the country remains problematic. Statistics from the early 2000s revealed that nationwide only 42% of all practicing emergency physicians are residency trained and only 50% are board certified.[5] Most trained and board certified physicians practice in urban areas. While there has been an increase in the staffing of rural EDs with emergency trained physicians, the need still remains. In a 2005 study of the Upper Midwest, the number of American Board of Emergency Medicine (ABEM) -certified emergency

physicians and residency trained emergency physicians in the urban vs. rural setting was 65.2% vs. 30.8% boarded and 48.3% vs. 12.3% emergency medicine trained.[6] This is compared to West Virginia where only 12% are board certified and only 7.5% are residency trained.[7]

Technology has also started to help minimize the care gap between urban and rural areas. One of the best examples of this is the widespread availability of computed tomography (CT) scanning and digital imaging combined with off-site radiologists. This has also changed the ability of properly trained rural practitioners to manage trauma at their facility. Telemedicine may also make it possible for patients in rural areas to benefit from the expertise of specialists "seeing" the patient from hundreds of miles away.

Determining your local environment

To practice in a rural environment one must be knowledgeable regarding the abilities of the hospital and community to provide care. Time spent learning these variables prior to needing them will be rewarded by easier and more efficient practice when they are required. Specific areas of knowledge include the following.

1. *Local Emergency Medical Services (EMS)*: How many ambulance crews are available in your community and how many are advanced life support (ALS) vs. basic life support (BLS)? Will a transfer crew be made from these same crews? Many rural areas have single paramedic coverage. Often numbers of ambulances are limited and transport times are long. Transport of a patient to a tertiary care hospital could drain local resources and may limit the ability to respond to other emergencies in the community.

Trauma: A Comprehensive Emergency Medicine Approach, eds. Eric Legome and Lee W. Shockley. Published by Cambridge University Press. © Cambridge University Press 2011.

Table 26.1 State of Colorado trauma center transfer criteria[9]

Mandatory transfer to tertiary trauma center from rural trauma designated hospital	Possible care at rural trauma designated hospital in conjunction with mandatory tertiary trauma center consultation
Critically injured age 0–5 years	High-risk mechanism as defined by local regional trauma counsel protocol
Bilateral pulmonary contusions with non-traditional ventilation	Critically injured age 6–12 years
Multisystem trauma with pre-existing coagulopathy	Significant head/spinal cord injuries with deficit
Aortic tears	Bilateral femur or posterior pelvic fracture plus chest or abdominal injury
Liver injuries requiring emergency surgery and liver packing or vena cava injury	Mechanical ventilation over 4 days
Coma for more than 6 hours or with focal neurologic deficit	Life-threatening complications such as acute renal failure or coagulopathy
	Persistent in-hospital physiologic compromise
	Hemodynamically stable children with documented visceral injury requiring blood or fluids > 40 cc/kg
	Penetrating injuries to head, neck, torso or proximal extremities

2. *Air ambulance/helicopter or fixed-wing services*: What is the availability of air ambulance services, and how do they interface with the hospital and the prehospital services? If a patient is to be flown out of a hospital is it necessary to transport the patient first by ground to the airport or can helicopters land at the hospital? Consider air transport services in nearby states as well as your own. Learn how to dispatch these services; is a phone call made to the receiving hospital, a regional dispatch center, or to the transport agency itself? If helicopter resources are limited, it is also feasible to transport more than one patient in a single helicopter? A recent study showed no adverse outcomes from helicopter crews transporting multiple patients.[8] If the helicopter is occupied on a non-emergent mission, can they divert for a sicker patient at your facility?

3. *Transport efficiencies*: How long does it take to get to the nearest trauma center by ground ambulance and how long is the flight time for the air ambulance? Does your ground transportation have unbroken communication throughout the journey? Do you have a helicopter landing pad near the ED or do patients have to be transported to the airport? If the helicopter is unavailable, is a fixed-wing aircraft acceptable?

4. *Hospital surgical capabilities*: How many operating rooms are staffed during and after business hours and are they often busy? In what time frame are the on call personnel (both physician and other staff) available?

5. *Backup and ancillary support*: What ancillary and specialty backup services are on call and what is their availability? Is there a way to get hold of backup physicians by more than one means, i.e., pager and cell phone? What types of injuries can your facility treat?

6. *Pre-existing protocols*: What are the specific protocols for your institution regarding the types of trauma your facility can treat vs. those requiring transfer to other facilities? This will often relate to the trauma center designation of your facility and the organized trauma system for the state or region (e.g., see Table 26.1 for Colorado state's requirements for trauma center transfer[9]).

Who to keep and who to transfer

Prehospital decisions

The physician in the rural ED is often involved in decisions with local EMS crews about whether a helicopter from a tertiary trauma center should be launched immediately to the scene of a major trauma, or should the EMS crew transport to the closest ED for evaluation and initial stabilization. A study of 459 major trauma victims demonstrated that rural scene times are slightly longer and transport times are significantly longer than urban ones. Rural trauma victims are also seven times more likely to die before arrival of EMS.[10] Patients transferred from a referral non-trauma center hospital took almost six times as long to reach definitive care as those transported directly from the scene.[11] Recent literature is conflicted regarding outcomes of "on-scene" helicopter transport vs. ground ambulance bringing patients to a trauma center.[12–15] Presumably, an advantage of a helicopter would be the ability to bypass a non-trauma designated hospital and go directly to a trauma center. It would seem that any benefit of survival is only for a subset of severely injured patients.[15,16] In the end these decisions must be made by the paramedics using pre-established protocols, their clinical judgment, and consultation with their base station physician. Multiple examples exist in both the authors' hospital and many other rural hospitals of common concerns that arise in these settings. Examples include a case where transport to the local hospital is delayed in order to wait for the tertiary care scene helicopter to provide transport to a referral center; a critically ill patient with a head injury and exsanguinating leg amputation waits with the local EMS ambulance crew on scene for over 30 minutes for the helicopter to arrive. The local hospital is only 15 minutes away and the patient expires while in transport to the Level II trauma center which has a neurosurgeon on call. In another example, the loud and crowded helicopter environment prevents a tension pneumothorax from being diagnosed and the patient expires. In another example, an unhelmeted motorcyclist strikes a deer and is thrown. Paramedics find a responsive but confused patient with abdominal pain. The helicopter transport time is 30 minutes while the nearest hospital is 10 minutes away. The crew opts to transport the patient to the rural hospital suspecting an intra-abdominal hemorrhage, easily

managed by the ED physician and general surgeon. Upon arrival the patient becomes progressively obtunded and the head CT shows epidural hematoma; CT of the chest and abdomen are negative. The tertiary care hospital is contacted at that time and begins the procedure for air transport, unfortunately in the 60 minutes it takes to get to the referral hospital the patient dies of uncal herniation.

These cases illustrate the rural reality where there is no one single correct answer and they present a real dilemma. Helicopter crews, under good conditions, can place chest tubes or provide needle decompression of chests, rapid sequence intubate, and institute blood transfusions. However, a local surgeon/emergency physician may be able to stop uncontrolled exsanguinations, and local EDs may have more personnel and may provide a more controlled environment to help with critical procedures.

The authors recommend that in cases of critically injured and unstable patients (as determined by either prehospital regional trauma protocol or consultation with base station physician), that consideration be given to *both* dispatching the tertiary care center helicopter for a scene flight and to have the local rescue crew begin rapid transport to the closest rural ED. If the helicopter arrives before the rescue crew arrives at the hospital, then a rendezvous could occur somewhere in the middle. If the patient arrives at the ED, stabilization begins and rapid assessment of life-threatening injuries occurs. The patient can then be put into the awaiting helicopter for transfer to tertiary trauma center. A 3.5 year study comparing trauma patients directly admitted to a Level I trauma center with those first stabilized at an outlying hospital, found no adverse effect to mortality.[17] In the authors' experience, a frequent pitfall in transporting patients, is once the helicopter is dispatched for a scene flight, the ambulance crew waits for the helicopter to arrive on the scene and loses the ability of the local hospital to provide life-saving stabilization (Table 26.2[18,19]).

Which patients need referral to a higher level of care?

There are ATLS® guidelines about when a patient needs to be transferred to a tertiary care hospital.[20] These guidelines are, however, very conservative and assume that the rural trauma designated hospital or outlying clinic has very limited to no capabilities nor trained emergency staff. With increasing CT scan

Table 26.2 Considerations in hospital vs. ground transport[18,19]

Consider helicopter scene flight	Consider transport to closest rural emergency department
Remote location of more then 10 miles from the nearest appropriate trauma center and/or difficult access by road*	Hospital with ability to provide care is less then 10 miles away with easy access by road
Prolonged extrication time	Patient's condition is felt to be amenable to initial stabilization at closest hospital (tension pneumothorax, loss of airway, uncontrolled hemorrhage, Class IIII shock) even if definitive care will require eventual transport and associated delay
Severe isolated head trauma	

availability at rural hospitals and as trained emergency physicians begin to become more common in the rural setting, many trauma patients can be cared for in consultation with a general surgeon in the rural trauma designated hospital without need for transfer. Some select critically injured and high-risk patients can be managed at a Level III rural trauma facility, with consultation to a higher level trauma center.[9] The combination of performing a CT scan in a rural hospital with remote CT interpretation, and management by a local surgeon is a formula that is currently evolving and needs to be better delineated. Although the benefits of establishing a system have been generally accepted, until recently they were not well proven.[21–30]

A recent study compared of 4087 adult patients discharged alive and 1104 adult patients who died in the hospital and were treated at either a Level I trauma center or treated at a non-trauma center, showed a risk of death that was 25% lower in the group treated at the level one trauma center after adjustment for differences in the case mix. The relative differences in risk were primarily among more severely injured patients.[25]

The organized trauma system will specify which subset of trauma patient it mandates to be transferred to a tertiary trauma center by their criteria (see Table 26.1 above).

Recent literature also supports that head injuries not requiring immediate neurosurgical intervention could be managed outside a tertiary trauma center. Head injured patients with normal initial head CT scan could be kept at the rural hospital or referred for outpatient follow up. However, which physician will admit and observe these patients may be problematic. Recent literature suggests that the admitting physician need not be a neurosurgeon or even the trauma

surgeon. A national trauma data bank chart review of 213 357 patients with reported head injury showed that 95% were managed non-operatively. The authors of this study state that the "trauma surgeon or other healthcare provider can appropriately monitor patients for neurologic decline and effect early transfer."[27,28] At the other extreme, patients with severe head injuries will need transfer to a hospital with appropriate neurosurgical capability. Patients with subdural hematomas, epidural hematomas, or neurological deterioration also can present a dilemma to a rural ED physician. Often these patients are quite unstable, yet they may require neurosurgical intervention to be stabilized. Transfer in these patients should not be delayed for unstable vital signs. Emergent craniotomy is generally beyond the scope of the emergency physician unless specifically trained.[29]

The rural trauma system

A rural trauma designated hospital receiving a trauma patient should be pre-notified. Each organized trauma system will have its own rules as to trauma activation procedures. If a trauma patient does not meet criteria for emergent surgical intervention in the ED upon arrival, the emergency physician will generally initiate the evaluation for possible life-threatening traumatic injuries. Most rural trauma hospitals will have a CT scanner available and electronic radiology, allowing extensive trauma workups to be done at that rural location. However, a high degree of clinical suspicion and vigilance must be maintained for those patients thought to be at risk for deterioration as extensive imaging may delay transport to a tertiary care center if critical injuries are discovered.

The scope of practice for an emergency physician in a rural setting may be somewhat different than an urban environment. For example, fracture reduction and tendon repair by the emergency physician, rather than the orthopedist, is often common practice. Plastic surgeons may not be immediately available, and therefore rural emergency physicians may often practice complex wound closure techniques. This is also true of other complex procedures. The rural trauma hospital should have policies in place to address the responsibilities and obligations of the admitting physician. Complex trauma patients admitted for observation may be best managed by a surgeon rather than a family practitioner or internist. The rural trauma hospital must have plans in place to handle unexpected deterioration of patients admitted for observation.

Transfer of patients to closest facility

In many cases rural ambulances, because of limited resources, must transport all trauma patients to the closest healthcare facility. This may even be a rural clinic without any inpatient resources. Many patients will subsequently require transport to a secondary facility. Federal law (Emergency Medicine Treatment and Labor Act [EMTALA]) has specified conditions under which this transfer must occur. Typically, once the ambulance has brought the patient to the ED or rural clinic, the physician or other healthcare provider needs to perform a medical screening exam, and stabilize the patient within the capabilities of the facility. At a rural trauma-designated hospital this may include imaging or invasive studies looking for intra-abdominal injuries that could be corrected there. Waiting for responses from on-call physicians or for records/X-rays to be copied are not acceptable reasons to unduly delay transfer in the unstable patient. The transport itself can be problematic with the limited resources of rural ambulance services. Rural ambulance services will often only transport patients for medically indicated reasons.

How stable do they need to be to transfer?

The overriding question is whether the patients' injuries require treatment at a facility with a higher level of care than can currently be provided. The rural hospital has an obligation to provide as much care as necessary and possible without delaying transfer. Perhaps the most challenging cases are those with multiple life-threatening injuries, some

of which can be treated at the rural trauma designated facility and some requiring transfer. Prioritizing the treatment of these injuries and the decision of when to transfer must be made in conjunction with the local general surgeon and the receiving specialty surgeon.

Choosing the mode of transfer

While intuitively helicopter or fixed transport is faster than ground ambulance, adding in warm-up time, shut-down time, landing, and patient loading, ground ambulance may be faster in selected cases. Facilities should review their emergent transfer times by different modes to understand the quickest modes of transport. Those times may also change due to local conditions such as weather and traffic. Other considerations could include the degree of availability of the local ambulance vs. helicopter and the medical crew configuration and training. The cost may also play a role. While the transferring vehicle (helicopter or ambulance) is en route, the rural facility should attempt to perform as many important tests and stabilizing procedures as possible. In some settings information, including radiologic images and laboratory studies, may be transmitted electronically to the receiving hospital prior to the arrival of the patients. An example of utilizing this strategy would be a case where your facility receives a multiple traumatized unconscious intubated head injury patient without a neurosurgeon at your facility. A tertiary care helicopter is put en route and the rural facility immediately performs standard trauma stabilization followed by a CT scan of the head and neck, and possibly additional exams, while the helicopter is en route to the facility. This is then transmitted to the waiting neurosurgeon or general surgeon at the receiving hospital enabling the patient to have rapid operative intervention upon arrival. See Figure 26.1 for a summary algorithm.

Who will accept the patient?

The transferring physician must contact a receiving physician and document the acceptance of the care of the patient. This includes documentation that a physician will accept responsibility for the care of the patient upon their arrival and that the receiving facility has the capacity to care for the patient. Federal EMTALA rules require documentation that the patient is willing or requests to be transferred,

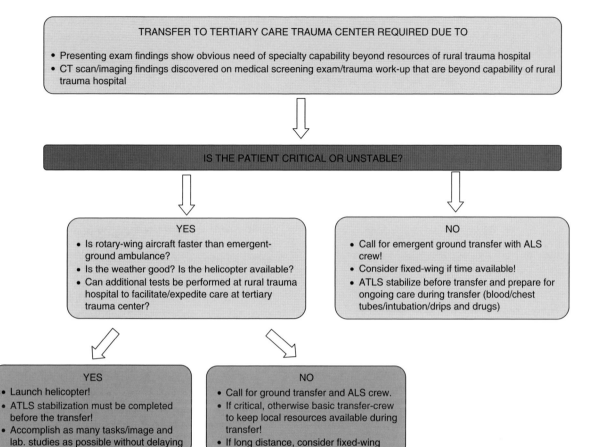

Figure 26.1 Choosing the mode of transfer: summary algorithm. ALS, advanced life support; ATLS, advanced trauma life support; CT, computed tomography.

or requires transfer and is unable to consent. The necessity of the transfer should be documented.

Who will arrange the transfer?

It is the responsibility of the transferring physician, in consultation with the receiving hospital, to arrange the mode of transportation for the transfer and to find an accepting physician. Some large tertiary care centers have administrative staff that will arrange transport and accepting physicians for referring physicians. It is also the responsibility of the transferring physician to arrange for the on-going care of the patient until they arrive at the receiving facility; EMS physician advisors should have transfer order protocols developed. It is the responsibility of the transferring physician to ensure that copies of charts, laboratory results, imaging studies, and procedure documentation are sent to the receiving facility.

Things to do awaiting transfer

One study reviewing ATLS® protocols prior to transfer found the most frequent deviations included: inadequate cervical spine immobilization (32%); failure to document neurological status (47%); and failure to place nasogastric tube (72%) (Table 26.3).[30]

Challenges for the future

While the level of trauma care provided to people living in rural areas has improved over the years, there still continues to be a substantial gap between the trauma services in an urban area vs. rural area. Fortunately, as the number of specialty trained emergency physicians increases, rural areas are beginning to see a greater number of hospitals able to provide improved trauma services. Additionally telemedicine has the potential to allow rural hospitals to provide

Table 26.3 Evaluation and potential management prior to transfer

Immediate stabilization by emergency personnel or surgeon prior to impending transport

Trauma assessment

Adequate IV access

Chest tubes/pericardiocentesis

Initial fluid/blood resuscitation

Stabilization of the spine

Stabilize unstable pelvic fractures with a sheet or external fixator

Stop external life-threatening hemorrhage

Endotracheal intubation as needed and confirm placement

Pain medication as appropriate

Thirty minutes until transport

Laboratory tests

Portable radiographs (chest X-ray/cervical spine/pelvis/ etc., as indicated)

Antibiotics, tetanus, medications/drips as indicated in consultation with receiving specialist

Urinary and nasogastric catheterization as required

Reduce and stabilize long bone fractures

Consider fasciotomy for circumferential burns (if respiratory or circulatory compromise)

Sixty minutes until transport

CT scanning if indicated

Extremity radiographs if indicated

Wound care

Address coagulopathy (FFP, platelets, calcium if possible)

CT, computed tomography; FFP, fresh frozen plasma; IV, intravenous.

increased access to specialty consultants who in the past have been limited to major urban centers.

However, even with these advances, many challenges remain. Even to the well-trained physician, providing trauma care in a rural setting can be quite difficult with the inherent limitations of less personnel and backup services. The rural emergency physician continues to be faced with difficult decisions as to which patients to transfer, at what time transfer is appropriate, and what should be done for the patient prior to transfer. These are questions for which there is often gray areas. The rural emergency physician may be called upon to provide a wide array of procedures. Many residency programs are beginning to appreciate these unique challenges as well as the large unmet need and are starting to focus a portion of their training on this setting.

Inevitably there will continue to be a gap between the ability of the rural hospital and tertiary facilities to manage specialty trauma care. However, that gap can be minimized through recognition of the problem, improved training in trauma care, and the technological developments. We can be hopeful that morbidity from this devastating disease will continue to decrease for all citizens, regardless of the geographic area in which they live.

References

1. Branas CC, MacKenzie EJ, Williams JC, et al. Access to trauma centers in the United States. *JAMA* 2005; **293**(21):2626–33.

2. Hedges JR, Adams AL, Gunnels MD. ATLS® practices and survival at rural Level III trauma hospitals, 1995–1999. *Prehosp Emerg Care* 2002;**6**(3):299–305.

3. Olsen CJ, Arthur M, Mullins RJ, et al. Influence of trauma system implementation on process of care delivered to seriously injured patients in rural trauma centers. *Surgery* 2001;**130**(2): 273–9.

4. Esposito TJ, Sanddal ND, Hansen JD, Reynolds S. Analysis of preventable trauma deaths and inappropriate trauma care in a rural state. *J Trauma* 1995;**39**(5):955–62.

5. Moorhead JC, Gallery ME, Hirshkorn C, et al. A study of the workforce in emergency medicine: 1999. *Ann Emerg Med* 2002;**40**(1):3–15.

6. Wadman MC, Muelleman RL, Hall D, Tran TP, Walker RA. Qualification discrepancies between urban and rural emergency department physicians. *J Emerg Med* 2005;**28**(3):273–6.

7. McGirr J, Williams JM, Prescott JE. Physicians in rural West Virginia emergency departments: residency training and board certification status. *Acad Emerg Med* 1998;**5**(4):333–6.

8. Tortella BJ, Lavery RF, Corriere C, Bell RA, Mann KJ. The impact of multiple patient transport on patient care in helicopter emergency medicine services. *Air Med J* 1996;**15**(3):108–10.

9. Colorado Board of Health. *Minutes, November 16, 2005. Designation of Trauma Facilities. Colorado Department of Public Health and Environment, Health Facilities and Emergency Services.* Available from

http://www.cdphe.state.co.us/op/bh/minutes/2005minutes/bhnovember05final.pdf.

10. Grossman DC, Kim A, MacDonald SC, et al. Urban-rural differences in prehospital care of major trauma. *J Trauma* 1997;**42**(4):723–9.

11. Falcone RE, Herron H, Werman H, Bonta. Air medical transport of the injured patient:scene versus referring hospital. *Air Med J* 1998;**17**(4):161–5.

12. Brathwaite CE, Rosko M, McDowell R, et al. A critical analysis of on-scene helicopter transport on survival in a statewide trauma system. *J Trauma* 1998;**45**(1):140–4.

13. Kerr WA, Kerns TJ, Bissell RA. Differences in mortality rates among trauma patients transported by helicopter and ambulance in Maryland. *Prehospital Disaster Med* 1999;**14**(3):159–64.

14. Cummings G, O'Keefe G. Scene disposition and mode of transport following rural trauma: a prospective cohort study comparing patient cost. *J Emerg Med* 2000;**18**(3):349–54.

15. Cunningham P, RutledgeR, Baker CC, Clancy TV. A comparison of the association of helicopter and ground ambulance transport with the outcome of injury in trauma patients transported from the scene. *J Trauma* 1997;**43**(6):940–6.

16. Thomas SH, Biddinger PD. Helicopter trauma transport: an overview of recent outcomes and triage literature. *Curr Opin Anaesthesiol* 2003;**16**(2):153–8.

17. Rogers FB, Osler TM, Shackford SR, Cohen M, Camp L, Lesage M. Study of the outcome of patients transferred to a Level I hospital after stabilization at an outlying hospital in a rural setting. *J Trauma* 1999;**46**(2):328–33.

18. Diaz MA, Hendey GW, Bivins HG. When is helicopter faster? A comparison of helicopter and ground ambulance times. *J Trauma* 2005;**58**(1):148–53.

19. Lerner EB, Billittier AJ, Sikora J, Moscati RM. Use of a geographic information system to determine appropriate means of trauma patient transport. *Acad Emerg Med* 1999;**6**(11):1127–33.

20. American College of Surgeons Committee on Trauma. *Advanced Trauma Life Support for Doctors, ATLS®, Student Manual*, 7th edn. Chicago, IL: American College of Surgeons, 2004: p. 162.

21. Nathens AB, Jurkovich GJ, Rivara FP, Maier RV. Effectiveness of state trauma systems in reducing injury-related mortality: a national evaluation. *J Trauma* 2000;**48**(1):25–30.

22. Clay Mann N, Mullins RJ, Hedges JR, et al. Mortality among seriously injured patients treated in remote rural trauma centers before and after implementation of a statewide trauma system. *Med Care* 2001;**39**(7):643–53.

23. Barringer ML, Thomason MH, Kilgo P, Spallone L. Improving outcomes in a regional trauma system: impact of a Level II trauma center. *Am J Surg* 2006;**192**(5):685–9.

24. Mullins RJ, Hedges JR, Rowland DJ, et al. Survival of seriously injured patients first treated in rural hospitals. *J Trauma* 2002;**52**(6):1019–29.

25. Esposito TJ, Sanddal TL, Reynolds SA, Sanddal ND. Effect of a voluntary trauma system on preventable death and inappropriate care in a rural state. *J Trauma* 2003;**54**(4):663–9.

26. MacKenzie EJ, Rivara FP, Jurkovich GJ, et al. A national evaluation of the effect of trauma-center care on mortality. *N Engl J Med* 2006;**354**(4):366–78.

27. Esposito TJ, Reed RL, Gamelli RL, Luchette FA. Neurosurgical coverage: essential, desired, or irrelevant for good patient care and trauma center status. *Ann Surg* 2005;**242**(3):364–70.

28. Esposito TJ, Luchette FA, Gamelli RL. Do we need neurosurgical coverage in the trauma center? *Adv Surg* 2006;**40**:213–21.

29. Rinker CF, McMurry FG, Groeneweg VR, et al. Emergency craniotomy in a rural Level II trauma center. *J Trauma* 1998;**44**(6):984–9.

30. Martin GD, Cogbill TH, Landercasper J, Strutt PJ. Prospective analysis of rural interhospital transfer of injured patients to a referral trauma center. *J Trauma* 1990;**30**(8):1014–19.

27

Pain management

Knox H. Todd and Christine Preblick

Introduction

Pain is the most frequent reason for seeking emergency treatment. As a presenting complaint, pain accounts for over 70% of visits to US emergency departments (ED).[1–3] Although it is commonly believed that injury and trauma are responsible for the majority of ED visits associated with pain, this impression is misleading. In a recent multicenter study of adults presenting to EDs in the USA and Canada with moderate to severe pain, two thirds of presentations resulted from medical, rather than traumatic, conditions.[4] Nonetheless, trauma is a major cause of pain among ED patients, accounting for approximately 25 million patient visits annually in the United States.

Suboptimal treatment of pain due to trauma remains a persistent concern in ED and prehospital settings. Notwithstanding the clinician's duty to provide compassionate care, pain that is not managed appropriately causes an increase in oxygen requirements and a potential for venous thrombosis due to decreased movement.[5,6] Failure to recognize and treat pain may also result in dissatisfaction with medical care, hostility toward the physician, unscheduled returns to the ED, delayed complete return to full function, and, potentially, an increased risk of litigation.[7–12] A variety of factors are felt to give provenance to pain undertreatment (Table 27.1).

Beyond the acute setting, undertreatment of pain may contribute to the development of chronic pain syndromes. Rivara et al., in a recent multicenter study, reported that almost two thirds of trauma patients report continued pain related to their initial injury 12 months after the inciting event.[13] The authors suggest that aggressive interventions to control pain during the acute phase are needed to prevent chronic pain. Studies of pain and disability after acute hip fracture support this argument.[14]

Pathophysiology

Nociception refers to the sensory detection of tissue damage or potential damage, while pain is a much more complex experience, involving sensory, psychological, and cognitive components. The physiologic mechanisms underlying pain can broadly be classified as nociceptive or neuropathic. Nociceptive pain results from the activation of primary peripheral nociceptors (A-delta and C fibers) in response to noxious stimuli, such as tissue trauma and inflammation. Somatic nociceptive pain may involve superficial structures (e.g., skin and subcutaneous tissue) and is perceived as sharp and well localized; when deeper structures (e.g., joints, tendons, and bones) are involved, pain may be more diffuse or radiating, with an aching or cramping quality. Visceral nociceptive pain arises from the internal organs in response to organ distention, ischemia, or inflammation and is characterized by poor localization and a deep aching quality. Neuropathic pain results from aberrant signal processing in the peripheral or central nervous system. Although neuropathic pain may possess a variety of sensory qualities, it is more often described as burning, tingling, or shooting.

Tissue damage causes the release of many inflammatory chemicals, including bradykinin, serotonin, histamine, acetylcholine, and prostaglandins among others. Prolonged noxious stimulation can lead to peripheral and central sensitization, and alterations in pain processing. Hyperalgesia, a lower threshold to painful stimuli, occurs as a result of these mechanisms, and can be primary (at the site of the injury) or

Trauma: A Comprehensive Emergency Medicine Approach, eds. Eric Legome and Lee W. Shockley. Published by Cambridge University Press. © Cambridge University Press 2011.

Table 27.1 Barriers to emergency department analgesia

Patient factors

Fears of side effects

Fears of addiction

Hemodynamic instability

Altered mental status

Physician factors

Concerns about side effects

Fear of addiction

Fear of obscuring diagnosis

Lack of knowledge about pain management

System factors

Lack of educational emphasis on pain management

Inadequate pain assessment

Sociocultural barriers, including ethnic bias

Inadequate quality improvement mechanisms

Lack of emergency department pain research, particularly among geriatric and pediatric populations

secondary (at sites surrounding the injury). Allodynia, in which normally innocuous stimuli are perceived as painful, can result from neuroplastic changes in both primary nociceptors and the central nervous system. Left untreated, these changes in pain processing can result in chronic pain states.

Pain assessment

Pain is inherently subjective and inevitably complex. Patients experience pain and suffering as individuals; clinicians assess it only indirectly. The emergency provider's task is to use a commonly understood vocabulary and classification system in assessing pain so that our findings can be communicated consistently. Only by quantifying the pain experience in meaningful ways can we move beyond practices that are influenced by myth and opinion toward a scientific approach to our many questions regarding the pain experience. This challenge is at the root of our difficulties in treating pain, and not only in the ED setting. Issues surrounding pain assessment should have primacy in our attempts to understand our patients' pain experiences.

EDs employ a number of pain assessment tools. Viewing pain as the "fifth vital sign," as encouraged by The Joint Commission, has fostered the widespread use of such tools. For those without cognitive impairment, pain intensity is routinely assessed with either an 11-point numerical rating scale (NRS) or a graphical rating scale (GRS). The NRS is sensitive to the short-term changes in pain intensity associated with emergency care and is the most commonly employed pain assessment instrument.[15,16] The GRS or picture scales are particularly useful for populations with limited literacy, including children.[17,18] The visual analog scale (VAS) is used by some EDs; however, this instrument is more commonly employed in research settings. There is no demonstrated advantage in using a VAS over an NRS in the ED settings; both are reliable and valid measures of pain intensity.[19] In fact, certain patient populations find the NRS easier to complete, therefore it is preferred over the VAS for routine use.[15,20] Among non-verbal patients, including infants or those with cognitive impairment or dementia, a number of observational pain scales are available for use. They use graded indicators such as breathing, movements, crying and other verbalizations as well as consolability and facial expressions to derive numerical indications of pain intensity. Both the FLACC (Face, Legs, Activity, Cry, Consolability) observational scale for use in very young children, and the PAINAD (Pain Assessment in Advanced Dementia) scale for use in the setting of advanced dementia are used in some EDs; however, adequate observational pain assessments are more the exception than the rule.[21,22]

No matter the specific pain scale used, assessments should be repeated after therapeutic interventions and at the time of ED discharge. Despite efforts to promote pain intensity as an outcome measure with which to judge the quality of ED pain practice, the finding that pain intensity is measured only once in most EDs may mirror medicine's traditional view of pain as a diagnostic indicator rather than an outcome deserving of attention in its own right.

A number of studies support the importance of education and standardized pain assessment in improving the quality of pain practice. After finding that only 38% of trauma patients in 1 center received ED analgesics, Silka et al. instituted verbal pain scores and pain management education with resultant increases in documented pain assessments and analgesic administration.[23,24] More recently, Decosterd et al. implemented pain management guidelines in a Swiss ED, tying pain scores to explicit treatment

435

recommendations and found improvements in pain assessment, analgesic administration, pain relief, and patient satisfaction.[25]

Pain treatment

The assessment and treatment of acute traumatic pain should optimally begin in the prehospital setting. Although many studies have documented oligoanalgesia in the prehospital setting, it is encouraging that more prehospital research is addressing pain treatment in this setting.[26–29] Importantly, the National Association of EMS Physicians (NAEMSP) has developed a position paper to guide Emergency Medical Services (EMS) directors in developing and implementing prehospital analgesic protocols.[30] A brief overview is listed in Box 27.1.

Box 27.1 The NAEMSP position statement

- The National Association of EMS Physicians (NAEMSP) believes that the relief of pain and suffering of patients must be a priority for every Emergency Medical Services (EMS) system. Adequate analgesia is an important step in achieving this goal.
- NAEMSP believes that every EMS system should have a clinical care protocol to address prehospital pain management. Adequate training and education of prehospital personnel and EMS physicians should support this pain management protocol.
- NAEMSP recommends that prehospital pain management protocols should include the following components:
  a. Mandatory assessment of both the presence and severity of pain.
  b. Use of reliable tools for the assessment of pain.
  c. Indications and contraindications for prehospital pain management.
  d. Non-pharmacologic interventions for pain management.
  e. Pharmacologic interventions for pain management.
  f. Mandatory patient monitoring and documentation before and after analgesic administration.
  g. Transferral of relevant patient care information to receiving medical personnel.
  h. Quality improvement and close medical oversight to ensure appropriate use of prehospital pain management.

In the ED, non-pharmacologic therapies should be used for all patients with traumatic pain when possible. Cold therapy (ice packs), immobilization, and elevation of injured extremities are low-cost interventions that are immediately available. Perhaps most importantly, ED personnel should reassure the patient that pain treatment is important and that effective analgesic interventions are available. Such reassurance helps to alleviate the anxiety that invariably accompanies and complicates traumatic pain. In fact, in one study of patient satisfaction with pain treatment, having staff stress the importance of pain treatment was a stronger predictor of satisfaction than analgesic administration itself.[31]

Nurse-initiated analgesic protocols are currently underutilized in the ED and hold the promise of decreasing the time interval between patient presentation and analgesic administration as well as increasing patient satisfaction. Analgesic protocols have been implemented at triage and include both opioid and non-opioid therapies.[32]

Analgesics for traumatic pain

A wide variety of analgesics are available to the emergency physician, including acetaminophen, nonsteroidal anti-inflammatory drugs (NSAIDs), and opioids. In general, the anxiety associated with traumatic pain should be managed by controlling pain primarily. The coadministration of anxiolytics should be avoided. Anxiolytics, such as the benzodiazepines, may cause excessive sedation while leaving the underlying cause of anxiety untreated. If anxiolytics are used, they should be reserved for patients in whom anxiety is felt to be a primary cause of their symptoms. One of the most important features of pain and its treatment is the tremendous interindividual variability in pain experience and the response to analgesics. For a given amount of tissue injury, patients may complain of mild, moderate, or severe pain and this variability in pain experience is the norm. It is important to tailor a pharmacologic regimen to each individual patient. For mild pain, simple analgesics will often be all that is required. In contrast, moderate or severe pain may demand a more multifaceted approach to analgesia. We now know that pain is an extremely complex process involving many different classes of mediators and receptors. For this reason, the concept of multimodal analgesia is a crucial one in pain medicine. Multi-modal analgesia is the combining of different classes of drugs to improve pain relief while minimizing the potential for side effects due to reduced reliance on one agent.[33]

Specific analgesics

Acetaminophen

Acetaminophen is indicated for mild to moderate pain and has an excellent side effect profile. Its mechanism of action is not well defined; however, it likely involves prostaglandin synthesis in the central nervous system. It has both analgesic and antipyretic properties, with minimal anti-inflammatory effects. It is commonly coadministered with opioids and can be administered by the oral or rectal route. An intravenous form of acetaminophen is used in Europe and may be available in the future for US physicians.

Acetaminophen is the most frequently used analgesic in the United States and, unless contraindications exist, it should be included in most multimodal analgesic regimens. Although acetaminophen has a high toxic to therapeutic ratio, hepatotoxicity can result from overdose or chronic high dosing. Chronic alcoholics and others with liver disease are at the most risk for hepatotoxicity. However, this must be balanced with the potential for adverse side effects with non-steriodals and opioids in the alcohol abusing population. Short-term administration of acetominophen may be preferable.

Non-steroidal anti-inflammatory drugs

Non-steroidal anti-inflammatory drugs have analgesic, antipyretic and anti-inflammatory properties. They inhibit cyclooxygenase (COX), the enzyme responsible for prostaglandin synthesis. Prostaglandin inhibition largely explains their side effect profile, including nephrotoxicity caused by decreases in prostaglandin-maintained renal perfusion, as well as gastroduodenal ulcer formation, due to decreases in prostaglandin-mediated gastrointestinal mucosal perfusion and mucus production. Both side effects are more common in the elderly and those with renal insufficiency or a history of peptic ulcer disease. Non-steroidal anti-inflammatory drugs also cause platelet dysfunction, limiting their use in the setting of acute hemorrhage.

Ketorolac is the only available parenteral NSAID in the United States and it is widely used by emergency physicians. Reports of renal failure and gastrointestinal bleeding with prolonged administration have limited its use. Its onset of action is similar to less expensive oral NSAIDs; therefore, in the patient able to take oral medications, it may be hard to justify its utility as a first-line agent.

Cyclooxygenase exists in two forms. The COX-1 isoenzyme is widely distributed and is responsible for many homeostatic functions, including maintaining renal perfusion and mucosal integrity of the gastrointestinal tract. The COX-2 isoenzyme is induced by tissue injury and serves to enhance inflammation and pain. Selective COX-2 inhibitors have been developed with the goal of reducing NSAID gastrointestinal side effects; however, there is little evidence that they reduce gastrointestinal symptoms or bleeding and they have been associated with thrombotic cardiovascular complications. There is little to support their use in the ED. Two COX-2 drugs, valdecoxib (Bextra®) and rofecoxib (Vioxx®) were withdrawn from the market in the last several years due mainly to cardiovascular concerns.

All NSAIDs have a therapeutic ceiling whereby, unlike opioids, higher doses do not lead to increased analgesia. Non-steroidal anti-inflammatory drugs are appropriate for mild to moderate pain and are often prescribed in combination with opioids.

Opioids

Opioids are the mainstay for treating moderate to severe traumatic pain.[34] Importantly, opioids exhibit no therapeutic ceiling and can be titrated to effect or dose-limiting sedation. Morphine, hydromorphone, and fentanyl are the most commonly used parenteral opioids; while oxycodone and hydrocodone, usually combined with acetaminophen or ibuprofen, are the most frequently prescribed oral opioids. Common opioid side effects include nausea, constipation, pruritis, urinary retention, and dose-dependent respiratory depression.

Morphine is the standard comparison analgesic for opioids. Nausea and pruritis are common side effects of morphine and other opioids. Morphine causes histamine release from mast cells and the resulting rash and pruritis are often attributed to an allergic response; however, most often this is a non-allergic phenomenon.

Hydromorphone is derived from morphine, has fewer active metabolites, and may cause less histamine release and gastrointestinal side effects. It is preferred to morphine for patients with hepatic and renal disease because of its lack of active metabolites that can accumulate with reduced hepatic or renal clearance.

Fentanyl is a synthetic opioid with a rapid onset and short duration of action.[35] It causes less histamine release and hypotension than morphine and is the opioid of choice for patients with potential hemodynamic instability or for those requiring procedural analgesia. Alfentanil, sufentanil, and remifentanil are synthetic opioids that, given their even shorter durations of action, might be preferred for procedural analgesia; however, currently their use in the ED is uncommon.

Meperidine was a commonly used synthetic opioid. Its metabolite, normeperidine, has a long half-life and may cause neurotoxicity and seizures, particularly in the setting of renal insufficiency, thus its use in the ED is decreasing.

Codeine, hydrocodone, and oxycodone, in combination with acetaminophen or ibuprofen, are the most commonly prescribed oral opioids. Codeine requires demethylation to morphine for analgesic activity and a significant proportion of the population lacks the ability to metabolize it to the active agent. These codeine non-responders cannot be predicted in advance, thus hydrocodone and oxycodone are more rational choices for treatment. In addition, clinical experience suggests that nausea and constipation are more frequent with codeine than with equianalgesic doses of other opioids.[36]

Tramadol is a weak opioid agonist that also inhibits the reuptake of serotonin and norepinephine. It is an unscheduled analgesic with low potential for abuse or respiratory depression and is available as monotherapy or in combination with acetaminophen (Table 27.2).[37]

The role of local and regional anesthetics

Local and regional anesthetics block the conduction of pain impulses in peripheral nerves, preventing nociceptive input from reaching the central nervous system. For patients with localized traumatic injuries, these techniques allow analgesia without sedation.

Table 27.2 Opioid equianalgesic dosing: dose (mg) equianalgesic to 10 mg SC/IV morphine

Drug (Trade name)	SC/IV	PO/PR	PO : SC/IV ratio
Morphine	10	30	3 : 1
Hydromorphone (Dilaudid)	1.5	7.5	5 : 1
Meperidine (Demerol)	100	300	3 : 1
Fentanyl	100 mcg	NA	NA
Hydrocodone (in Lortab, Vicodin, others)	NA	30	NA
Oxycodone (Roxicodone, also in Percocet, Percodan, others)	NA	30	NA

IV, intravenously; NA, not applicable; PO, by oral; PR, by rectal; SC, subcutaneously.

Topical

Local anesthetics can be applied directly to mucosal surfaces and to the skin.[38,39] Many small lacerations can be anesthetized by this technique, avoiding the use of needles. For the oral mucosa, 1–4% lidocaine jelly can be applied directly; however, care must be taken to limit the total dose of anesthetic as mucosal absorption may occur rapidly. For intact skin, a variety of local anesthetic preparations are available, including EMLA cream, the acronym standing for eutectic mixture of local anesthesics (prilocaine/lidocaine); ELA-Max (4% lidocaine in a liposomal matrix); or lidocaine administered by iontophoresis or jet injectors.[40–43] Local anesthetics can be used in combination with vasoconstrictors for non-intact skin anesthesia. Such preparations include TAC (tetracaine, adrenaline, and cocaine), LET (lidocaine, epinephrine, and tetracaine) and MAC (Marcaine, adrenaline, and cocaine).[44,45]

Local infiltration

Injections of subcutaneous lidocaine or bupivacaine, with or without vasoconstrictors, allow for the painless suturing of wounds. In order to lessen the pain of anesthetic injection, small needles (27–30 gauge) should be used, the anesthetic should be injected slowly, buffering agents may be added to the anesthetic, and injections should be made from within the laceration rather than through intact skin.[46–48]

Peripheral nerve blocks

A variety of peripheral nerve blocks are commonly performed in the ED. Advantages of nerve blocks over local infiltration include less pain, less tissue distortion, and, in some cases, less total anesthetic dose.[49] Most peripheral nerve blocks are performed using only anatomic landmarks; however, nerve stimulators may be useful for some blocks and ultrasound localization for needle placement is becoming more common.

Digital blocks for finger and toe injuries are preferred to local infiltration. The blocks are best performed by inserting a small needle (27 gauge) into the proximal dorsal web space of the digit and, after raising a subcutaneous wheal, injecting 1.0–1.5 ml of local anesthetic. The procedure is then repeated on the other side of the digit. While common practice has been to avoid vasoconstrictors in the digits, the preponderance of recent evidence suggests that in the patient with normal vasculature, it is safe.

The ulnar, median, and/or radial nerves can be blocked at the level of the wrist, allowing laceration repair, fracture reduction, or foreign body removal. These blocks are relatively simple and safe, but require familiarity with wrist anatomy.[50] Similarly, ankle blocks provide analgesia and allow for procedures on the foot. Selective blocks of individual nerves can be performed and blocking all five nerves (posterior tibial, sural, saphenous, superficial, and deep peroneal) provides complete anesthesia below the ankle.

Femoral nerve blocks provide partial pain relief for hip fractures, femoral shaft fractures, superficial anterior thigh injuries, and patellar injuries. The block is relatively simple to perform using local landmarks; nerve stimulator and ultrasound-guided blocks are being performed with increasing frequency.[51]

Intercostal nerve blocks may be indicated for multiple rib fractures, and have also been shown to improve peak expiratory flow rates and oxygenation.[52] They also decrease pain with chest tube thoracostomy. Pneumothorax is a complication in approximately 1.4% of intercostals blocks; the incidence increases in patients with obstructive lung disease.[53] A chest radiograph is not routinely indicated after the procedure; however, an expiratory chest radiograph may be obtained an hour after the procedure at the clinician's discretion or if the patient develops clinical symptoms consistent with a pneumothorax.

Table 27.3 Additional nerve blocks

Nerve block	Indication
Interscalene brachial plexus block	Shoulder or elbow injuries
Axillary brachial plexus block	Forearm and hand injuries
Lumbar plexus block	Femur fractures, thigh injuries
Sciatic nerve block	Tibia/fibula fracture, ankle/foot fracture, injuries of the posterior thigh or lower leg
Popliteal nerve block	Tibia/fibula fracture, ankle/foot fracture, injuries below the knee

A variety of additional nerve blocks may be used that require additional training and it may be appropriate to consult an anesthesiologist to perform these. The blocks and their indications are listed in Table 27.3.

Intravenous regional anesthesia (Bier block)

Bier blocks are indicated for injuries of the forearm or leg and the most common use is for upper extremity fracture reductions in children. The procedure has an excellent safety record and is relatively easy to perform.[54] Briefly, the procedure involves exsanguinating a limb using a compressive device, inflating a double tourniquet on the proximal extremity, and then injecting lidocaine intravenously into the now isolated limb. Rare complications are related to inappropriate management of the double cuff, leading to systemic toxicity from the local anesthetic.

Epidural anesthesia

Epidural anesthesia is rarely performed in the ED, but may be contemplated for multiple rib fractures (thoracic epidural) and anorectal or lower-limb crush injuries (lumbar epidural).[55,56] Epidural anesthesia should only be used for conditions that are extremely painful and are expected to remain painful for at least 48–96 hours. Over this period, other methods of analgesia may be instituted allowing the epidural to be discontinued. Coagulopathy and hemodynamic instability are contraindications to the procedure.

Conclusion

Relieving pain and reducing suffering are primary responsibilities of emergency medicine and much can be done to improve the care of trauma patients in pain. Emergency physicians and nurses have refined their approach to the problem of pain over time and analgesic practices continue to improve. Our specialty should continue to define high standards for emergency medicine pain practice and engage in ongoing quality improvement initiatives to achieve this goal.

References

1. Johnston CC, Gagnon AJ, Fullerton L, et al. One-week survey of pain intensity on admission to and discharge from the emergency department: a pilot study. *J Emerg Med* 1998;**16**:377–82.

2. Tanabe P, Buschmann M. A prospective study of ED pain management practices and the patient's perspective. *J Emerg Nurs* 1999;**25**:171–7.

3. Cordell WH, Keene KK, Giles BK, et al. The high prevalence of pain in emergency medical care. *Am J Emerg Med* 2002;**20**:165–9.

4. Todd KH, Ducharme J, Choiniere M, et al. Pain in the emergency department: results of the Pain and Emergency Medicine Initiative (PEMI) Multicenter Study. *J Pain* 2007;**8**(6):460–6.

5. Gureje O, Von Korff M, Simon GE, et al. Persistent pain and well-being: a World Health Organization study in primary care. *JAMA* 1998;**280**:147–51.

6. Anderson FA, Jr., Spencer FA. Risk factors for venous thromboembolism. *Circulation* 2003;**107** (23 Suppl. 1):I9–16.

7. Furrow BR. Pain management and provider liability: no more excuses. *J Law Med Ethics* 2001;**29**:28–51.

8. Stalnikowicz R, Mahamid R, Kaspi S, et al. Undertreatment of acute pain in the emergency department: a challenge. *Int J Qual Health Care* 2005;**17**(2):173–6.

9. Pines JM, Perron AD. Oligoanalgesia in ED patients with isolated extremity injury without documented fracture. *Am J Emerg Med* 2005;**23**(4):580.

10. Neighbor ML, Honner M, Kohn MD. Factors affecting emergency department opioid administration to severely injured patients. *Acad Emerg Med* 2004;**11**(12):1290–6.

11. Fosnocht DE, Swanson ER, Barton ED. Changing attitudes about pain and pain control in emergency medicine. *Emerg Med Clin North Am* 2005;**23**(2):297–306.

12. Rupp T, Delaney KA. Inadequate analgesia in emergency medicine. *Ann Emerg Med* 2004;**43**(4):494–503.

13. Rivara FP, MacKenzie EJ, Jurkovich GJ, et al. Prevalence of pain in patients 1 year after major trauma. *Arch Surg* 2008;**143**(3):282–7.

14. Morrison RS, Magaziner J, McLaughlin MA, et al. The impact of post-operative pain on outcomes following hip fracture. *Pain* 2003;**103**(3):303–11.

15. Paice J, Cohen F. Validity of a verbally administered numeric rating scale to measure cancer pain intensity. *Cancer Nurs* 1997;**20**:88–93.

16. Farrar JT, Cleary J, Rauck R, et al. Oral transmucosal fentanyl citrate: randomized, double-blinded, placebo-controlled trial for treatment of breakthrough pain in cancer patients. *J Natl Cancer Inst* 1998;**90**:611–16.

17. Breyer JE, Knott CB. Construct validity estimation for the African-American and Hispanic versions of the Oucher Scale. *J Pediatr Nurs* 1998;**13**:20–31.

18. Bellamy N, Campbell J, Syrotuik J. Comparative study of self-rating pain scale in osteoarthritis patients. *Curr Med Res Opin* 1999;**15**:113–19.

19. Todd KH. Pain assessment instruments for use in the emergency department. *Emerg Med Clin N Amer* 2005;**23**(2):285–95.

20. Stahmer SA, Shofer FS, Marino A, Shepherd S, Abbuhl S. Do quantitative changes in pain intensity correlate with pain relief and satisfaction. *Acad Emerg Med* 1998;**5**:851–7.

21. Merkel S, Vopepl-Lewis T, Shayevitz JR, et al. The FLACC: a behavioral scale for scoring postoperative pain in young children. *Pediatr Nurse* 1997;**23**(3):209–97.

22. Warden V, Hurley AC, Volicer L. Development and psychometric evaluation of the pain assessment in advanced dementia (PAINAD) scale. *J Am Med Dir Assoc* 2003;**4**:9–15.

23. Silka PA, Roth MM, Geiderman JM. Patterns of analgesic use in trauma patients in the ED. *Am J Emerg Med* 2002;**20**:298–302.

24. Silka PA, Roth MM, Moreno G, et al. Pain scores improve analgesic administration patterns for trauma patients in the emergency department. *Acad Emerg Med* 2004;**11**:264–70.

25. Decosterd I, Hugli O, Tamches E, et al. Oligoanalgesia in the emergency department: short-term beneficial effects of an education program on acute pain. *Ann Emerg Med* 2007;**50**(4):462–71.

26. Hennes H, Kim MK, Pirrallo RG, et al. Prehospital pain management: a comparison of providers' perceptions and practices. *Prehosp Emerg Care* 2005;**9**(1):32–9.

27. McEachin CC, McDermott JT, Swor R, et al. Few emergency medical services patients with lower-extremity fractures receive prehospital analgesia. *Prehosp Emerg Care* 2002;**6**(4):406–10.

28. Swor R, McEachin CM, Seguin D, et al. Prehospital pain management in children suffering traumatic injury. *Prehosp Emerg Care* 2005;**9**(1):40–3.

29. Ricard-Hibon A, Belpomme V, Chollet C, et al. Compliance with a morphine protocol and effect on pain relief in out-of-hospital patients. *J Emerg Med* 2008;**34**(3):305–10.

30. Alonso-Serra H, Wesley K. National Association of EMS Physicians position paper: prehospital pain management. *Prehosp Emerg Care* 2003;**7**:483–8.

31. Todd KH, Sloan EP, Chen C, Eder S, Wamstad K. Survery of pain etiology, management practices and patient satisfaction in two urban emergency departments. *CJEM* 2002;**4**(4):252–6.

32. Seguin D. A nurse-initiated pain management advanced triage protocol for ED patients with an extremityinjury at a level 1 trauma center. *J Emerg Nursing* 2004;**30**(4):330–5.

33. Innes GD, Zed PF. Basic pharmacology and advances in emergency medicine. *Emerg Med Clin N Am* 2005;**23**:433–65.

34. McQuay H, Moore A, Justins D. Treating acute pain in hospital. *BMJ* 1997;**314**:1531–5.

35. Walsh M, Smith GA, Yount RA. Continuous intravenous infusion fentanyl for sedation and analgesia of the multiple trauma patient. *Ann Emerg Med* 1991;**20**:913–15.

36. Turturro MA, Paris PM, Yealy DM, et al. Hydrocodone vs. codeine in acute musculoskeletal pain. *Ann Emerg Med* 1991;**20**(10):1100–3.

37. Hewitt DJ, Todd KH, Xiang J, Jordan DM, Rosenthan NR. Tramadol/acetaminophen or hydrocodone/acetaminophen for the treatment of ankle sprain: a randomized, placebo-controlled trial. *Ann Emerg Med* 2007;**49**(4):468–80.

38. Singer AJ, Stark MJ. Pretreatment of lacerations with lidocaine, epinephrine, and tetracaine at triage: a randomized double-blind trial. *Acad Emerg Med* 2002;**7**:751–6.

39. Priestly S, Kelly AM, Chow L. Application of topical local anesthetic at triage reduces treatment time for children with lacerations: a randomized controlled trial. *Ann Emerg Med* 2003;**42**:34–40.

40. Rogers TL, Ostrow CL. The use of EMLA cream to decrease venipuncture pain in children. *J Pediatr Nurs* 2004;**19**:33–9.

41. Eichenfield LF, Funk A, Fallon-Friedlander S, et al. A clinical study to evaluate the efficacy of ELA-Max (4% liposomal lidocaine) as compared with eutectic mixture of local anesthetics cream for pain reduction of venipuncture in children. *Pediatrics* 2002;**109**:1093–9.

42. Wallace MS, Ridgeway B, Jun E, et al. Topical delivery of lidocaine in healthy volunteers by electorporation, electroincorporation, or iontophoresis: an evaluation of skin anesthesia. *Reg Anesth Pain Med* 2001;**26**:229–38.

43. Peter DJ, Scott JP, Watkins HC, Frasure HE. Subcutaneous lidocaine delivered by jet-injector for pain control before IV catheterization in the ED: the patients' perception and preference. *Am J Emerg Med* 2002;**20**:562–6.

44. Ernst AA, Marvez-Valls E, Nick TG, et al. LAT (lidocaine-adrenaline-tetracaine) versus TAC (tetracaine-adrenaline-cocaine) for topical anesthesia in face and scalp lacerations. *Am J Emerg Med* 1995;**13**:151–4.

45. Kuhn M, Rossi SO, Plummer JL, Raftos J. Topical anaesthesia for minor lacerations: MAC versus TAC. *Med J Aust* 1996;**164**:277–80.

46. Scarfone RJ, Jasani M, Gracely EJ. Pain of local anesthetics: rate of administration and buffering. *Ann Emerg Med* 1998;**31**:36–40.

47. Christophe RA, Buchanan L, Begalla K, et al. Pain reduction in local anesthetic administration through pH buffering. *Ann Emerg Med* 1988; **17**:117–20.

48. Bartfield JM, Sokaris SJ, Raccio-Robak N. Local anesthesia for lacerations: pain of infiltration inside vs outside the wound. *Acad Emerg Med* 1998;**5**:100–5.

49. Crystal CS, Blankenship RB. Local anesthetics and peripheral nerve blocks in the emergency department. *Emerg Med Clin N Am* 2005;**23**:477–502.

50. Thompson WL, Malchow RJ. Peripheral nerve blocks and anesthesia of the hand. *Mil Med* 2002;**167**:478–82.

51. Stella J, Ellis R, Sprivulis P. Nerve stimulator-assisted femoral nerve block in the emergency department. *Emerg Med* 2000;**12**:322–5.

52. Osinowo OA, Zahrani M, Softah A. Effect of intercostal nerve block with 0.5% bupivacaine on peak expiratory flow rate and arterial oxygen saturation in rib fractures. *J Trauma* 2004;**56**:345–7.

53. Shanti CM, Carlin AM, Tyburski JG. Incidence of pneumothorax from intercostal nerve block for analgesia in rib fractures. *J Trauma* 2001;**41**:536–9.

54. Brill S, Middleton W, Brill G, Fisher A. Bier's block: 100 years old and still going strong! *Acta Anaesthesiol Scand* 2004;**48**:117–22.

55. Bulger EM, Edwards T, Klotz P, et al. Epidural analgesia improves outcome after multiple rib fractures. *Surgery* 2004;**13**:426–30.

56. Karmakar MK, Ho AM. Acute pain management of patients with multiple fractured ribs. *J Trauma* 2003;**54**:615–25.

441

David T. Schwartz, Nancy Kwon, and Alexander Baxter

Accidental and intentional injuries are among the top 15 leading causes of death in the United States, with trauma being the leading cause of death among children and young adults.[1] For the trauma patient, initial diagnosis and management often relies on the results of plain radiographs. Conventional radiography ("plain radiography") can be performed quickly and easily, is inexpensive, and may provide an immediate diagnosis.

General principles

Plain radiographs are ordered based on mechanism of injury, suspicion of injury, patient complaint, physical examination, and patient condition. In the multitrauma victim, the routine trauma series historically consisted of an anteroposterior (AP) portable chest, cross-table lateral cervical spine, and AP pelvis radiographs. However, a number of experts have questioned this dogma, and management based on mechanism and patient complaints have led to protocols calling for additional or fewer radiographs depending on the individual circumstances.

X-rays

X-rays are high-energy photons produced by the interaction of charged particles with matter. X rays and gamma rays have similar properties, but different origins.[2] X-rays are emitted from processes outside the nucleus, while gamma rays originate inside the nucleus. X-rays are generally lower in energy and therefore less penetrating than gamma rays. X-ray machines are used daily in the trauma setting. X-rays are the single largest source of man-made radiation exposure because of their widespread use. A few millimeters of lead can stop medical X-rays.[3]

The main risk to patients receiving X-ray evaluation is cancer induced by radiation exposure, such as leukemia, thyroid cancer, breast cancer, lung cancer, and gastrointestinal cancer.[3] However, for a single radiographic study, this is not truly a clinically significant risk.

Radiation dosage

Units used for measuring radiation exposure

X-ray and gamma-ray exposure are measured in units of roentgen (R). The roentgen (R) refers to the amount of ionization present in the air. One roentgen of gamma- or X-ray exposure produces approximately 1 rad (0.01 gray) tissue dose. Another unit of measuring gamma ray intensity in the air is "air dose or absorbed dose rate in the air" in grays per hour (Gy/h) units. This unit is used to express gamma ray intensity in the air from radioactive materials in the earth and in the atmosphere.[4]

Units used for measuring radiation dose

When ionizing radiation interacts with the human body, it transmits its energy to the tissues. The amount of energy absorbed per unit weight of the organ or tissue is called absorbed dose and is expressed in units of gray (Gy). One gray dose is equivalent to one joule radiation energy absorbed per kilogram of organ or tissue. Rad is the old and still used unit of absorbed dose. One gray is equivalent to 100 rads:[4]

$$1 \text{ Gy} = 100 \text{ rads.}$$

Different types of ionizing radiation are not equally harmful in the same doses. Alpha particles are more harmful than beta particles, gamma rays and X-rays for a given absorbed dose. To account for this difference, radiation dose is expressed as *equivalent dose* in units of sievert (Sv). The dose in Sv is equal

Trauma: A Comprehensive Emergency Medicine Approach, eds. Eric Legome and Lee W. Shockley. Published by Cambridge University Press. © Cambridge University Press 2011.

Table 28.1 Recommended radiation weighting factors[4]

Type and energy range	Radiation weighting factor (WF)
Gamma rays and X-rays	1
Beta particles	1
Neutrons, energy < 10 keV	5
> 10–100 keV	10
> 100 keV to 2 MeV	20
> 2–20 MeV	10
> 20 MeV	5

Table 28.2 Estimated radiation dose to the ovaries/pelvic uterus[8]

Type of radiographic examination	Dose (mrad)
Low-dose group	
Head	< 1
Cervical spine	< 1
Thoracic spine	< 1
Chest	< 1
Extremities	< 1
High-dose group	
Lumbar spine	204–1260
Pelvis	190–357
Hip	124–450
Intravenous pyelogram	503–880
Urethrocystogram	1500
KUB (kidney, ureter, bladder)	200–503

to "absorbed dose" multiplied by a "radiation weighting factor" – W_R (Table 28.1).[4]

Equivalent dose is often referred to simply as "dose" in everyday use of radiation terminology. The old unit of "equivalent dose" or "dose" was "rem":

Dose in Sv = absorbed dose in Gy × radiation weighting factor (W_R)

Dose in rem = dose in rad × W_R

1 Sv = 100 rem

1 rem = 10 mSv (millisievert = one thousandth of a sievert)

1 Gy air dose is equivalent to 0.7 Sv tissue dose

1 R (roentgen) exposure is approximately equivalent to 10 mSv tissue dose.[4]

What effects do different doses of radiation have on people?

The recommended threshold limit values (TLV) is an average annual dose of 0.05 Sv (50 mSv).

The effects of acute exposures of large doses of radiation vary with the dose:

10 Sv – Risk of death within days or weeks

1 Sv – Risk of cancer later in life (5/100)

100 mSv – Risk of cancer later in life (5/1000)

50 mSv – TLV for annual dose for radiation workers in any 1 year

20 mSv – TLV for annual average dose, averaged over 5 years.[4]

What are the limits of exposure to radiation?

The TLVs published by the American Conference of Governmental Industrial Hygienists (ACGIH) are guidelines for occupational exposure limits:

20 mSv – TLV for average annual dose for radiation workers, averaged over 5 years

1 mSv – Recommended annual dose limit for general public (International Commission on Radiological Protection [ICRP]).[4]

What are the effects of radiation exposure to the pregnant patient?

Sensitivity to radiation is greatest during intrauterine development. However, the risk to the fetus of 1 rad (1000 mrad) exposure, approximately 0.003%, is less than the spontaneous risk of malformations, abortions, or genetic disease.[5–8] Research reveals that higher doses of radiation (10 rad) are associated with a small increase in the number of childhood cancers.[8–11] When intrauterine radiation doses increase to 15 rad, there is approximately a 6% chance that the fetus could experience severe mental retardation, a 3% chance of developing childhood cancer, and a 15% chance of having a small head.[12] Table 28.2 lists the quantity of radiation exposure to the female gonads.[8]

Providing information on radiation exposure from diagnostic radiographs is difficult. The individual amount of fetal dosage may vary by a factor of 50 or more, depending on the equipment used, technique, number of radiographs done in a complete study, maternal size, and fetal–uterine size.

Diagnostic radiographic studies should be performed with regard for fetal protection, but necessary diagnostic studies should not be withheld. When possible, fetal irradiation should be minimized by limiting the scope of the examination, using technical means such as shielding, and using alternative imaging if available (e.g., ultrasound). The National Council on Radiation Protection states that the risk is negligible at 5 rad or less, and the risk of malformation is significantly increased at doses above 15 rad.[13]

Use of radiographic imaging in trauma patients

Trauma in emergency department (ED) patients spans a broad spectrum of injuries from life-threatening major trauma to minor injuries of limited morbidity. In some instances, the injury initially appears minor even though more significant injuries are present but occult. For this reason, a low threshold should be maintained in ordering imaging studies in trauma patients. At the same time, clinical judgment must be exercised to avoid excessive use of imaging studies when the likelihood of injury is low; excessive use contributes to unnecessary cost, treatment time, and radiation exposure.

Common areas of potentially missed injury include the extremities in proximity to joints, as well as injuries to the head, neck, abdomen, and chest. Certain patient populations are at higher risk for clinically inapparent serious injuries. These include the elderly, young children, patients with altered mentation due to head injury, intoxication, or underlying cognitive disorders, and patients with pre-existing medical conditions that increase the risk of injury, such as coagulopathies and osseous disorders. Another common cause for diagnostic error is distraction from consideration of a second injury due to the presence of a more obvious injury.

For a number of specific injuries, clinical decision rules have been developed to aid clinical management. Examples include the Ottawa Ankle and Knee Rules, the National Emergency X-Radiography Utilization Study (NEXUS) and Canadian Cervical Spine Rule, and head injury rules developed in Canada and in New Orleans.[14-19] Many other rules have been proposed or are in development. Before being used clinically, however, a rule must be prospectively validated. In addition, the rule's impact on clinical practice should be assessed by an implementation study that demonstrates that the rule confers advantages over routine clinical practice.[20-22] Above all, decision rules must be applied in light of the patient's clinical presentation and using sound clinical judgment. For most clinical circumstances, decision rules do not exist and management must be based on a careful and complete clinical evaluation focusing first on potentially life- or limb-threatening injuries as well as on serious injuries that can potentially be missed.

In a major trauma victim who is hemodynamically stable, computed tomography (CT) – particularly multidetector CT (MDCT), when readily available from the ED – has assumed a major role in trauma management. This is particularly true for major abdominal, thoracic, spine, and head injuries. However, conventional radiography still plays an important role in major trauma victims as an initial screening tool during resuscitation, in patients who are too unstable to be transported to CT, and when CT is not readily available.

The basic radiographic series in a major blunt trauma victim includes portable AP radiographs of the chest and pelvis, and a cross-table lateral view of the cervical spine – the three view "*trauma series*." The goal of the trauma series is to quickly identify major life-threatening injuries that need immediate treatment while the patient is in the resuscitation area. It is performed after initial assessment and stabilization of the airway, breathing, and circulation. Once these vital functions are stabilized, the trauma series radiographs are performed in conjunction with the secondary survey.

When MDCT is readily available, radiographs of the cervical spine and pelvis may be omitted. Chest radiography should still be performed prior to CT because it can rapidly identify major thoracic injuries and also plays a role in the decision to obtain a chest CT. If a major blunt trauma victim is not immediately undergoing CT due to hemodynamic instability or the unavailability of CT, pelvis and cervical spine radiographs should be obtained to identify injuries that may benefit from stabilization in the resuscitation area, e.g., mechanically unstable pelvic or cervical spine injuries.

In a non-major trauma victim or a patient with localized trauma, the three-view trauma series should be used selectively based on the clinical suspicion of injury. For example, in a patient with isolated blunt head trauma, pelvic radiography can be omitted.

445

A patient with relatively minor trauma can be cleared based on the clinical examination and radiography can be safely omitted. Nonetheless, as noted earlier, a low threshold should be maintained for ordering radiographs to avoid missing an injury. This is particularly true for the cervical spine.

Initial imaging evaluation of the major trauma victim should optimally include bedside sonographic evaluation of the abdomen (focused abdominal sonography in trauma [FAST]) looking for hemoperitoneum or pericardium effusion that could contribute to hemodynamic compromise. Sonography of the chest may be used to detect a pneumothorax that may not be evident on a supine portable chest radiograph.[23,24]

Radiograph interpretation

Accurate radiograph interpretation entails both a targeted review in which common injury patterns are sought and a systematic review in which each tissue density is examined in all regions of the image.[3] After an **overall review** looking for obvious findings, the **technical adequacy** of the radiographic series is assessed, i.e., whether positioning and exposure are correct.

Next, a **targeted review** is performed. Sites of common injury and injuries suspected based on the clinical examination are sought. The radiographs are then examined for injuries that have subtle radiographic manifestations which can easily be missed. This is particularly important when there are serious consequences if the diagnosis and treatment are delayed.

Finally, a **systematic review** of the radiographs is performed to assure that all pertinent findings are identified. For chest radiography, a systematic approach entails examining first the bones, then soft tissues (heart, mediastinum, and diaphragm), the lungs, and finally any inserted tubes or lines. For skeletal radiographs, an "ABCS" approach is useful. First, evaluate the osseous *alignment*. Then, the *bones* are examined for signs of a fracture. Next, the *cartilage* (spaces between the bones) is examined for widening, which is indicative of ligamentous injury. Finally, *soft tissue* clues to an injury, such as swelling or a joint effusion are sought, which can serve as an indirect indicator of a fracture.

Chest radiography

The chest radiograph plays an essential role in patients with blunt and penetrating chest trauma. It can reliably identify life-threatening injuries and is therefore obtained soon after the initial assessment and stabilization of major trauma victims. Chest radiography can detect a pneumothorax, hemothorax, pulmonary contusions, rib fractures, hemomediastinum (potential aortic injury), and diaphragm rupture (Box 28.1). Chest radiography assists in patient care by determining the need for tube thoracostomy (a pneumothorax or large hemothorax) or chest CT, particularly CT aortography, when there are findings suggestive of an aortic injury. In some circumstances, treatment should proceed before radiography, such as when a tension pneumothorax or massive hemothorax causes respiratory compromise and hemodynamic instability. On the other hand, chest radiography can miss significant pathology such as a large pneumothorax, and chest CT is often warranted in major trauma victims to detect such occult thoracic pathology.

Box 28.1 Thoracic injuries detected on chest radiography

- Pneumothorax, hemothorax, pulmonary contusion
- Pneumomediastinum, subcutaneous air
- Hemomediastinum (indicative of aortic injury)
- Rib fractures, flail chest, clavicle, scapular or proximal humeral fractures
- Vertebral fractures
- Diaphragmatic injury

Many thoracic injuries are evident on clinical examination; for example, rib fractures, a flail chest, pneumothorax, or hemothorax – radiography serves to confirm the clinical diagnosis. Other injuries, however, produce no characteristic clinical findings, such as an aortic tear or diaphragmatic rupture, and chest radiography may provide essential information about the presence of these injuries.[25]

The **technique** of chest radiography in major trauma patients is often suboptimal and major injuries can thereby be missed. Initial chest radiography is performed using portable equipment and AP technique. AP chest radiographs are prone to various distortions and shortcomings in comparison to the standard posteroanterior (PA) technique. The AP radiographs are often technically suboptimal with rotated positioning, an incomplete level of inspiration, and over- or underpenetration. On AP chest radiographs, particularly with supine positioning and poor inspiration, the heart often appears enlarged and the mediastinum widened and indistinct (Figure 28.1a). These distortions can usually be corrected by obtaining an upright radiograph with the patient taking a full inspiration, when this is feasible (Figure 28.1b).[26–28]

Box 28.2 Shortcoming of AP chest radiography

- Suboptimal technique: poor inspiration, rotation, under or over-penetration
- Heart and mediastinum widened and indistinct
- Pneumothorax (anterior) and hemothorax (posterior) difficult to detect
- Superimposed monitor leads, backboards
- Upright rather than supine radiograph should be obtained whenever possible
- Portable chest radiography – suboptimal and correct technique – is shown in Figure 21.1.

Hemothorax, pneumothorax, and pulmonary contusion

Using the supine AP radiographic technique, a hemothorax or pneumothorax, even when large, may be difficult or impossible to detect. This is because extrapleural air collects anteriorly and extrapleural blood collects posteriorly and do not form margins parallel to the X-ray beam (Figure 28.2a). On a supine chest radiograph, signs of a ***pneumothorax*** include inferior and medial displacement of the diaphragm (deep sulcus sign) and subcutaneous emphysema (Figure 28.2b).[29] An upright AP radiograph, if it can be obtained, will more readily detect a pneumothorax or hemothorax. A CT scan is the most accurate, and often used as the gold standard.[30–34]

Tension pneumothorax (extrapleural area under pressure in the thoracic cavity) is a clinical diagnosis – hypotension associated with unilateral absent breath sound and contralateral tracheal deviation. There are, however, certain radiographic findings that suggest this diagnosis. These include a pneumothorax along with a shift of the trachea or mediastinum to the opposite side and depression of the diaphragm.

Both a hemothorax and pulmonary contusion cause increased opacity of the thorax. A massive ***hemothorax*** will result in a homogeneous increased opacity of the hemithorax, which often obscures the margin of the hemi-diaphragm – a "silhouette sign"

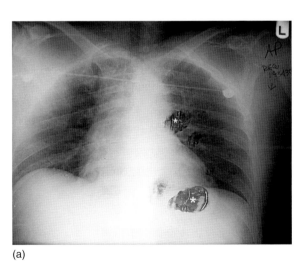

(a)

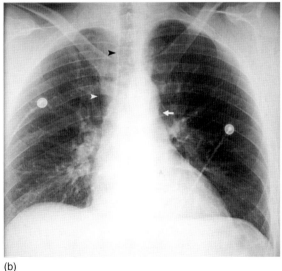

(b)

Figure 28.1 Portable chest radiography: suboptimal and correct technique. (a) Suboptimal anteroposterior (AP) supine chest radiograph. The mediastinum is markedly widened (11 cm) and indistinct. However, the radiographic technique is suboptimal – incomplete inspiration and rotated positioning – which accounts for these findings. A normal right paratracheal stripe can be seen despite the suboptimal radiographic technique (*arrowheads*). The trachea is displaced to the right. Although this finding is associated with aortic injury, the patient was positioned with rightward rotation, which accounts for the tracheal deviation (asterisks – defects in X-ray film). There were no other clinical or radiographic signs of thoracic trauma such as rib fractures, pulmonary contusion, or hemothorax, which makes an aortic injury less likely. Repeat radiograph with upright positioning and full inspiration. The mediastinum now appears normal, although not as well delineated as on a PA radiograph. Normal features that can be identified include the aorticopulmonary window (*white arrow*) and the right paratracheal stripe (*black arrowhead*). The mediastinal width is < 6 cm. Measurement of mediastinal width should not include the superior vena cava (*white arrowhead*). (From Schwartz DT. *Emergency Radiology: Case Studies*. New York: McGraw-Hill, 2008, with permission.)

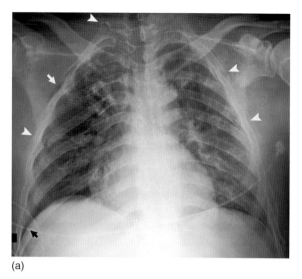

(a)

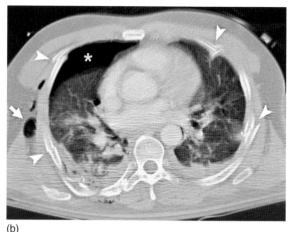

(b)

Figure 28.2 Bilateral flail chest, pulmonary contusions and occult pneumothorax. A 40-year-old man sustained bilateral rib fractures. The examination revealed crepitus and paradoxical chest wall motion on the right consistent with a flail chest. (a) The chest radiograph revealed multiple bilateral rib fractures and patchy pulmonary opacities due to pulmonary contusions. A pneumothorax was not visible. However, there was subcutaneous emphysema on the right suggestive of a pneumothorax (*white arrow*). In addition, the right costophrenic sulcus was widened (*black arrow*) – known as the "deep sulcus sign." (b) Chest computed tomography (CT) confirmed the bilateral flail chest (*arrowheads*) and pulmonary contusions. A pneumothorax (*asterisk*) was not visible on the chest radiograph because of its anterior location. Subcutaneous emphysema (*arrow*) and small bilateral hemothoraces were also present. (From Schwartz DT. *Emergency Radiology: Case Studies*. New York: McGraw-Hill, 2008, with permission.)

(Figure 28.3a). A massive ***pulmonary contusion*** also causes increased opacity of the lung, but typically causes inhomogeneous opacification due to remaining aerated portions of the lung (an air-bronchogram or air alveologram) (Figure 28.2a). Pulmonary contusions often progress over several hours and may not be evident on the initial chest radiograph. Chest CT is more accurate at detecting these injuries (Figure 28.2b and 28.3c).

Aortic injury

Detection of signs of an aortic injury is one of the most critical roles of chest radiography because this is a potentially fatal disorder that often does not produce characteristic clinical findings (Box 28.3).[25] However, owing to the frequently suboptimal radiographic technique, chest CT is often needed to detect signs of aortic injury.

On chest radiography, widening of the mediastinum and indistinct mediastinal contours are the key findings (Figure 28.3b). These findings are due to blood in the mediastinum that originates from torn smaller branch vessels and not from the aortic injury itself. Therefore, while a sensitive finding, it is non-specific because it may occur without an aortic injury.

The specificity is only about 10–30%; however, due to the critical nature of aortic injury, further investigation must be performed. Other radiographic signs of mediastinal blood (hemomediastinum) include: widening of the right paratracheal stripe, rightward deviation of the trachea or a naso-gastric tube, displacement of the left paraspinal line, superior extension of the left paraspinal line towards the apex of the lung forming a left apical pleural cap, and obliteration (opacification) of the aorticopulmonary window located between the inferior margin of the aortic knob and superior margin of the left main pulmonary artery.[35,36]

> **Box 28.3 Chest radiographic signs suggestive of an aortic injury (hemomediastinum)**
>
> - Wide mediastinum
> - Indistinct mediastinal contour
> - Widened right paratracheal stripe
> - Left paraspinal line displaced to the left and visible superior to the aortic knob
> - Left apical pleural cap
> - Leftward deviation of the trachea or a nasogastric tube, depression of the left mainstem bronchus
> - Obliteration of the aorticopulmonary window

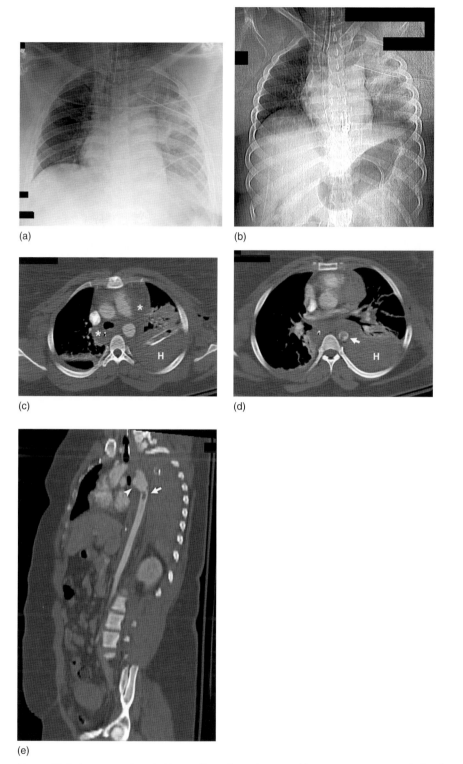

(a)

(b)

(c)

(d)

(e)

Figure 28.3 Acute traumatic aortic injury and hemothorax. A 30-year-old woman was in a motor vehicle collision. On arrival to the emergency department, she was intubated due to respiratory distress. A thoracostomy tube was inserted because the breath sounds were diminished on the left. (a) The chest radiograph revealed homogeneous opacification of the left hemithorax and obliteration of the left hemidiaphragm consistent with a large hemothorax. The mediastinum is markedly widened. This is partly obscured by the left hemothorax, which is better seen on the computed tomography (CT) scout radiograph (b). Other signs of hemomediastinum include rightward deviation of the trachea and widening of the right paratracheal stripe. (c–e) Chest CT angiography confirmed the hemomediastinum (*asterisks*) (c) responsible for the mediastinal widening, and the left hemothorax (H) (c, d). A left pulmonary contusion is also present. An aortic intimal flap (*arrows*) (d, e) and pseudoaneurysm (contained hematoma) (*arrowhead*) (e) is seen on the axial and coronal images. (From Schwartz DT. *Emergency Radiology: Case Studies*. New York: McGraw-Hill, 2008, with permission.)

449

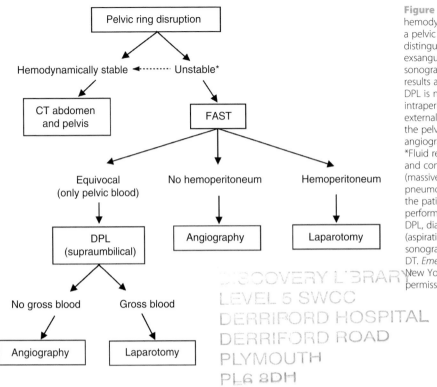

Figure 28.4 Management of a hemodynamically unstable patient with a pelvic fracture. The goal is to distinguish intra-abdominal from pelvic exsanguination. Bedside abdominal sonography is performed first. If the results are equivocal, supraumbilical DPL is needed looking for gross intraperitoneal blood on aspiration. An external fixator can be applied to stabilize the pelvis during or after laparotomy, angiography, or computed tomography. *Fluid resuscitation, bind pelvis in sheet and consider thoracic causes of shock (massive hemothorax, tension pneumothorax, cardiac tamponade). If the patient becomes stable, CT can be performed. CT, computed tomography; DPL, diagnostic peritoneal lavage (aspiration); FAST, focused acute sonography in trauma. (From Schwartz DT. *Emergency Radiology: Case Studies.* New York: McGraw-Hill, 2008, with permission.)

When there are signs of hemomediastinum, the patient should proceed as quickly as possible to a definitive diagnostic test – MDCT aortography, catheter aortography, or transesophageal echocardiography (TEE).[37–45] The chest radiograph, when correctly performed and accurately interpreted, is a highly sensitive test with a high negative predictive value. However, because the chest radiograph is often suboptimal, or may appear "normal" in up to 7% of cases of such injury, when the clinical suspicion of aortic injury is high (e.g., there are other signs of major thoracic trauma or a high-energy deceleration mechanism of injury), CT aortography is indicated.[46–51]

Diaphragmatic rupture

Diaphragmatic rupture is a second injury that does not produce characteristic clinical findings and may not be detected on chest radiography. In blunt trauma victims, it occurs in association with a major impact to the abdomen, and usually is seen on the left side. On radiography, there may be herniation of the stomach or bowel into the left hemithorax or simply an indistinct contour of the left hemidiaphragm. However, you may have a completely normal radiograph in up to 30%.[52] An MDCT scan or laparoscopy/thoracoscopy may be used to detect small diaphragmatic tears, especially those due to penetrating trauma, which are not initially associated with herniation of abdominal contents into the chest.

Pelvic radiography

Because pelvic fractures can cause significant morbidity and mortality in victims of major blunt trauma, an AP pelvic radiograph is included in the radiographic "trauma series." Rapid detection of a pelvic fracture alters trauma management in several ways.[53]

First, major pelvic fractures can be a source of significant blood loss. In a hemodynamically **unstable** patient with a pelvic fracture, the site of blood loss may either be the abdomen or pelvis. Treatment differs substantially. Intra-abdominal exsanguination requires laparotomy, whereas pelvic exsanguinations may be treated with angiography and embolization or, if laparotomy is being performed, with intra-abdominal packing (Figure 28.4).

An unstable pelvic fracture can generally be detected on physical examination. The examiner gently compresses the iliac crests to detect abnormal mobility. However, even without obvious clinical instability, pelvic imaging is advisable in the major blunt trauma victim.

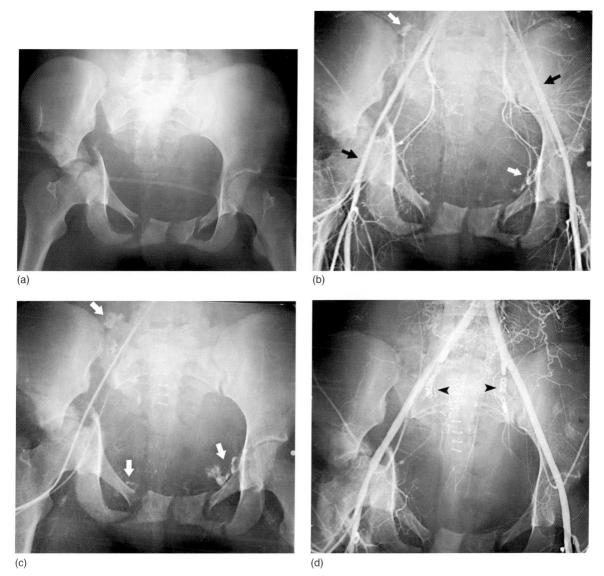

Figure 28.5 Mixed pelvic injury – "pelvic smash" in a hemodynamically unstable patient. A complex pelvic fracture occurred in a young woman who fell two storeys (a). She was hemodynamically unstable on arrival in the emergency department – blood pressure 80/50 mmHg and pulse 130 beats/min. Rapid fluid resuscitation was initiated without improvement in her vital signs. A focused acute sonography in trauma (FAST) found no blood in the hepatorenal fossa (Morison's pouch). The splenorenal fossa was poorly visualized, and free-fluid appeared to be present in the pelvis (retrovesicle recess). Due to the equivocal FAST, a supraumbilical diagnostic peritoneal lavage (DPL) was performed which did not detect gross intraperitoneal blood on aspiration. The pelvis was stabilized by external compression using a bed sheet. The patient was taken immediately to angiography, which revealed bilateral active arterial extravasation (*white arrows* in b and c). This was treated with coil embolization of both hypogastric (internal iliac) arteries (*black arrowheads* in d). (The external iliac arteries and femoral arteries are indicated by the *black arrows* in b). The patient survived. (From Schwartz DT. *Emergency Radiology: Case Studies*. New York: McGraw-Hill, 2008, with permission.)

If the patient is hemodynamically stable and will be undergoing MDCT of the abdomen and pelvis, a pelvic radiograph may be omitted because pelvic fractures can be better detected on CT.[54] However, a standard AP pelvic radiograph may be useful in providing an overview of the anatomy of a pelvic fracture (Figure 28.5).

In addition, the technique of CT may be altered in the presence of a major pelvic fracture due to a possible associated bladder injury. For instance, lateral compression anterior pelvic injuries are associated with extraperitoneal bladder rupture. In such cases, the CT technique is altered to include a *CT*

451

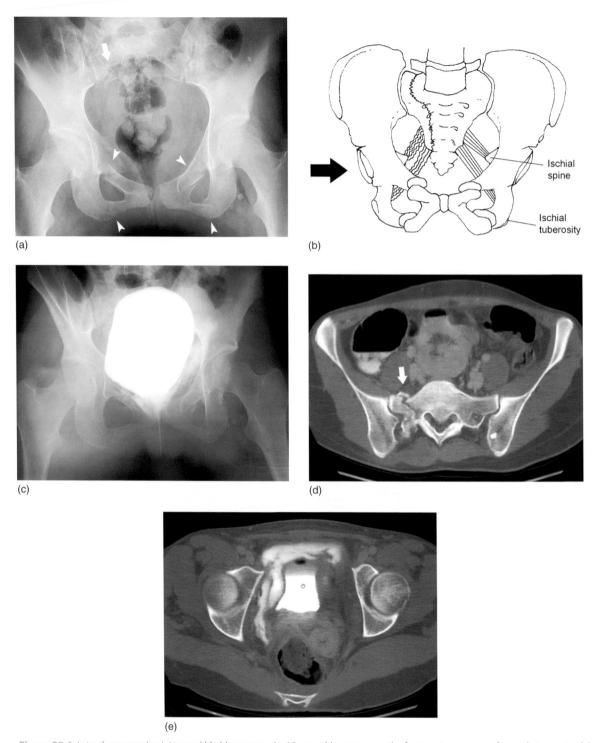

(a)

(b)

Ischial spine

Ischial tuberosity

(c)

(d)

(e)

Figure 28.6 Lateral compression injury and bladder rupture. An 18-year-old woman was the front-seat passenger of a car that was struck by another motor vehicle to the passenger side. She complained of lower back pain. She was hemodynamically stable and had no overt signs of trauma on examination. (a and b) Lateral compression injury in this patient causes both anterior and posterior injuries: bilateral pubic rami fractures (*arrowheads*) and a right sacral wing fracture (*arrow*). (c) Extraperitoneal bladder rupture – retrograde cystogram. Retrograde cystogram showing extravasation of contrast into the perivesical tissues. The bladder is otherwise intact. Postvoid radiograph shows contrast in the pelvic soft tissues. (d and e) Abdominopelvic computed tomography (CT). (d) The impacted fracture of the right sacral wing (*arrow*) was confirmed by CT. (e) A CT of extraperitoneal bladder rupture. Extravasated contrast surrounds the bladder. (The tip of the Foley catheter is seen within the bladder.) No contrast was seen within the peritoneal cavity, which excluded an intraperitoneal bladder rupture. (From Schwartz DT. *Emergency Radiology: Case Studies.* New York: McGraw-Hill, 2008, with permission.)

cystogram (delayed pelvic slices obtained with the bladder distended with water-soluble contrast) to detect a bladder rupture (Figure 28.6c).[55,56]

In a non-major trauma victim, pelvic radiography can be ordered selectively.[57] Pelvic radiography is indicated in patients with significant pelvic pain, tenderness, or instability. The elderly and patients with underlying bone disorders such as Paget disease are at higher risk of a pelvic fracture following minor trauma, such as a fall from standing, and the physician should have a lower threshold for ordering pelvic radiographs.

The standard radiograph of the pelvis is an AP view. This is a good screening test for pelvic fractures, although non-displaced or minimally displaced fractures may be missed by this single view. In addition, the anatomy of a complex pelvic fracture generally requires additional views. In the past, angled AP views were used to assess displacement of pelvic ring disruption. These included an inlet view (caudal angulation of the X-ray beam) and outlet view (cranial angulation of the X-ray beam). Oblique views of the pelvis (Judet views) were used to assess acetabulum fractures. However CT, particularly with two- and three-dimensional reformatted images, has largely replaced these supplementary radiographic views. In the ED, CT or supplementary radiographic views are used to detect a fracture not visible on the standard AP view and could be useful in a patient with excessive pain despite negative radiographs.

Cervical spine radiography

The cervical spine has a high priority in trauma care because the consequences of spinal cord injury can be devastating. The relative lack of mechanical support in comparison to the other spinal segments accounts for this vulnerability. A low threshold should therefore be maintained for imaging the cervical spine. The overall incidence of cervical spine injury among ED patients having cervical spine radiographs is < 3%.[58] Among patients admitted to a trauma service, the incidence of cervical spine injury is in the range of 5% to 10%.[59]

Prior to the ready availability of MDCT for acute trauma patients, a cross-table lateral cervical spine radiograph was one of the three views of the "trauma series" obtained during the initial trauma evaluation. Currently, in trauma centers with ready access to MDCT, CT rather than cervical spine radiographs

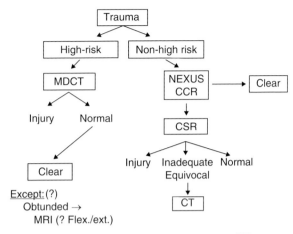

Figure 28.7 Cervical spine trauma imaging strategy. CCR, Canadian Cervical Spine Rule; CSR, cervical spine radiographs; CT, computed tomography; Flex./ext., flexion/extension; MDCT, multidetector CT; MRI, magnetic resonance imaging; NEXUS, National Emergency X-Radiography Utilization Study.

are commonly obtained in major trauma victims (Figure 28.7). The ability to generate high-quality sagittal and coronal reformatted images is essential to this imaging strategy because axial images alone can miss certain injuries.

A MDCT scan is also used in non-high-risk patients who are undergoing another CT, particularly head CT, and in elderly patients. In patients who are undergoing head CT, the addition of a cervical spine CT takes considerably less time than plain radiography and the costs to the hospital are similar. These benefits of CT must be balanced against the increased charges to the patient (charges for CT are up to 10 times greater than radiography), and the increased radiation exposure (14 times greater for CT), an especially significant issue for younger patients.[60] Computed tomography is useful in the elderly because they often have degenerative changes which put them at greater risk of injury following minor trauma such as a fall from standing. In addition, cervical spine radiographs can be difficult to interpret due to degenerative changes.

In centers with ready access to MDCT, a single cross-table lateral view may still be obtained in the major trauma victim who is hemodynamically unstable. The role of such a single lateral view is not to "clear" the cervical spine, but is instead used to identify major unstable injuries that may need more rigorous stabilization or notification of a spine surgeon while other aspects of trauma care are ongoing.

The three-view (lateral, AP, and odontoid views) or five-view (addition of right and left oblique views) cervical spine series was formerly the principal cervical spine imaging study and is currently still used in non-high-risk trauma victims – i.e., those without other major injuries or a high energy mechanism of injury. Nonetheless, because non-high-risk patients are considerably more common in ED practice than high-risk patients, cervical spine radiography is still the most commonly ordered imaging study. In one large prospective series of over 4000 patients, 11% had CT as the initial imaging study based on the severity of injury, of which 9% had a cervical spine injury. The remaining nearly 90% of patients underwent radiography.[59]

Among non-high-risk patients, the frequency of injury is exceedingly low – as low as 0.2% (7/3685 patients).[59] More selective use of radiography in such patients is therefore warranted. Selective use of radiography is based on a careful clinical examination and an appreciation of the fact that, despite the very low incidence of injury among non-high-risk patients, unstable injuries do rarely occur. Common reasons that cervical spine injuries are missed should also be kept in mind. These include an inadequate clinical examination, inadequate radiographs, missed subtle radiographic findings, altered mental status or intoxication, advanced age, and a high energy mechanism of injury despite a lack of clinically apparent injury.[61]

Cervical spine trauma imaging strategy

High-risk patients include those who have had a severe mechanism of injury or other significant injuries or neurological deficits referable to the spinal cord or a spinal nerve root.

In high-risk patients who are hemodynamically unstable and cannot undergo CT, an initial cross-table lateral view of the cervical spine should be obtained, if possible, to detect grossly displaced and mechanically unstable injuries.

Non-high-risk patients who may also undergo CT as the initial imaging test include patients undergoing another CT, most often of the head, and the elderly with degenerative spondylosis.

Magnetic resonance imaging (MRI) is indicated in patients who have neurological deficits referable to the spinal cord or a nerve root. It can detect spinal cord injury, and intervertebral disk herniation, epidural hematoma, and vascular injury. An MRI may also be used to detect ligamentous injuries.

Clinical decision making for cervical spine radiography

The NEXUS Low-risk Criteria (LRC) and the Canadian Cervical Spine Rule (CCR) are two validated clinical decision rules used to determine whether to obtain cervical spine radiographs in trauma victims, i.e., when the patient can be clinically cleared without radiography.[18,19] The rules share certain similarities, but differ considerably in others. The NEXUS LRC is simpler – a patient can be clinically cleared without radiography if none of five criteria are present (Box 28.4). It is based on the principle that radiography can be omitted if the patient has no midline cervical tenderness so long as there are no other features that could interfere with pain perception – intoxication, altered mental status (e.g., due to head trauma), or another painful distracting injury. In the presence of a focal neurological deficit, radiography is also indicated, although CT and MRI are the definitive imaging studies in such cases.

Box 28.4   NEXUS Low-risk Criteria

Radiography is not recommended if a patient meets all of the following criteria
- No tenderness at the posterior midline of the cervical spine
- No focal neurologic deficit
- Normal level of alertness
- No evidence of intoxication
- Absence of clinically apparent pain that might distract the patient from the pain of a cervical spine injury

---

The CCR is more complicated and consists of nine criteria that are arranged in three steps (Figure 28.8). First, three high-risk features are assessed: dangerous mechanism of injury, extremity paresthesias, and age > 65 years. If any are present, radiography is indicated. Second, the patient is assessed for the presence of five low-risk features. If no low-risk feature is present, radiography is indicated. If any of the five low-risk features is present, the third step is to assess the ability of the patient to rotate his or her neck 45° to the left and right. If the patient is able to rotate his or her neck, the cervical spine can be cleared without radiography.

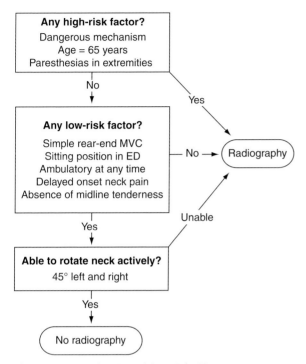

Any high-risk factor?

Dangerous mechanism
Age = 65 years
Paresthesias in extremities

No

Yes

Any low-risk factor?

Simple rear-end MVC
Sitting position in ED
Ambulatory at any time
Delayed onset neck pain
Absence of midline tenderness

No → Radiography

Yes

Unable

Able to rotate neck actively?
45° left and right

Yes

No radiography

Figure 28.8 Canadian Cervical Spine Rule. ED, emergency department; MVC, motor vehicle collision.

The criteria used in NEXUS are not precisely defined, and the use of each criterion is left to the judgment of the examining clinician. This is both its strength and its weakness. It avoids creating a long, cumbersome, and potentially incomplete list defining each criterion. On the other hand, clinicians may vary in their assessment of each criterion. In addition, the NEXUS rule is based largely on a single clinical finding – midline neck tenderness; other potentially important factors such as the severity of the injury forces and age of the patient are not included.

The CCR uses more clinical factors in deciding to obtain or omit cervical spine radiography. This adds to its complexity but makes it a potentially more precise instrument. For example, a low-suspicion patient with midline neck tenderness may not need radiography if one of the five low-risk features are present and the patient is able to rotate his or her neck. On the other hand, the CCR mandates radiography for all patients over age 65 years, whereas the NEXUS Criteria are valid in elderly patients.

One potential approach would be to use the one that fits the situation best. For instance, in a low-risk patient who exhibits midline neck tenderness, the CCR can be used to avoid radiography when other low-risk features are present and the patient is able to perform neck rotation. For the elderly, in which the CCR mandates radiography, a NEXUS evaluation could be used, so long as the examiner recognizes that the elderly have a higher incidence of cervical spine injury (twice that of younger patients) and can sustain injury from relatively minor mechanisms of injury, such as a fall from standing. This approach has not been validated, however.

In summary, the use of clinical decision rules can obviate the need for radiography. The NEXUS and CCR are the two main validated rules. Conventional radiography is still appropriate for the low-risk patient. In high-risk patients, e.g., other major injuries, high energy mechanism of injury, or advanced age, MDCT is generally the initial study. Because the sensitivity of radiography is as low as 90%, i.e., radiography is normal or has non-specific findings on 10% of injuries, conventional radiography is inadequate to exclude an injury in high-risk patients.[62] Flexion–extension views, sometimes advocated as a way to improve sensitivity and rule out ligamentous injury, are unproven and provide minimal or no benefit in the acute setting. They cannot be recommended.[63,64] In addition, inadequate cervical spine radiographs are common in major trauma victims, and routine use of CT in this population eliminates this problem.

Interpretation of cervical spine radiographs

Although the frequency of cervical spine injury in patients imaged with radiography is exceedingly low, interpretation of the radiographs must be careful and complete to avoid missing an injury. Common injury patterns as well as injuries with subtle radiographic findings should be sought.[65] In addition, radiographic findings that can mimic injuries should be correctly identified such as congenital variants, degenerative changes, and developmental findings in children.

The lateral view: The "ABCS" mnemonic device works well for the lateral radiograph (Figures 28.9a and b; and Table 28.3). First, the technical *adequacy* of the radiograph is assessed. All seven vertebrae should be visible, including the C7 vertebra and the C7–T1 interface. If not seen, the radiographs can be repeated with greater traction on the arms to lower the shoulders, a swimmer's view or CT should be obtained (Figure 28.10).

The *alignment* of the vertebra is then assessed. There should be four smooth lordotic curves – the

455

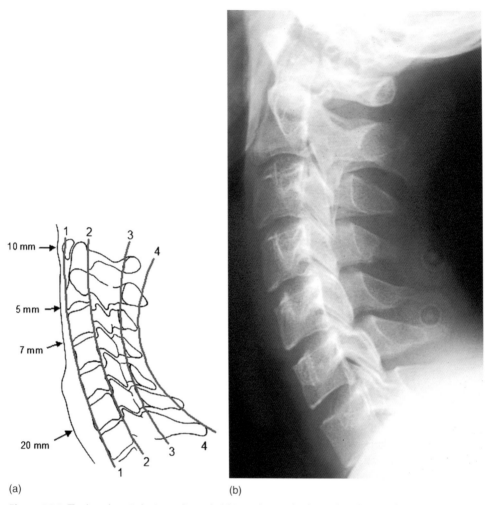

(a)

(b)

Figure 28.9 The lateral cervical spine radiograph. (a) Lateral cervical radiograph with lines of alignment and prevertebral soft tissues. (b) Normal lateral cervical radiograph. (From Schwartz DT. *Emergency Radiology: Case Studies*. New York: McGraw-Hill, 2008, with permission.)

anterior and posterior aspects of the vertebral bodies, the spinolaminar junctions, and the tips of the spinous processes (see Figure 28.9a).

Next, each **bone** is examined for a fracture or deformity. The **cartilage** is then assessed – the spaces between the vertebral bodies, laminae, and spinous processes should be uniform. Finally, the prevertebral **soft tissues** are examined. Swelling can be an important clue to an injury, particularly for the cervicocranium. In the lower cervical spine, the esophagus is interposed within the prevertebral soft tissues and swelling is rarely seen.

After an "ABCS" review of the lateral view, each vertebral segment should be re-examined to avoid missing an isolated injury at one level (Figure 28.11).

Open mouth view: The second most important view is the open mouth view – an AP view of the cervicocranium. Cervicocranial injuries may only be visible on this view. Key injuries to identify are fractures through the base of the dens and widening of the lateral masses of C1 relative to the superior articular surfaces of C2 – the key sign of a Jefferson burst fracture of C1 (Figures 28.12 and 28.13).

The AP view: It is less likely to identify an injury on the AP view that is not visible on the lateral view. The vertebral bodies and uncinate processes are seen. The lateral masses form a continuous skeletal structure having an undulating lateral contour. The facet joints should not be visible because they lie in an oblique plane relative to the X-ray beam.

Table 28.3 How to read a lateral cervical spine radiograph

Systematic approach

Two steps: (1) overall review ("ABCS"); then (2) examine each individual vertebra

Targeted approach

Look for specific injury patterns and easily missed injuries

Overall review – "ABCS"

Adequacy

All seven vertebrae seen

No rotation (lateral masses superimposed)

Alignment

Four smooth lordotic curves

Bones

Fractures of vertebral bodies, lateral masses, laminae, spinous processes

Cartilage

Intervertebral disk spaces, interspinous process distances

Soft tissues

Prevertebral soft tissues (especially C1–C3)

Extremity radiography

Radiography plays a major role in patients with extremity trauma, particularly fractures and dislocations. However, the initial diagnosis must be based on a thorough clinical examination. Radiography serves to confirm the clinical diagnosis and to define its anatomy. In some cases, a clinically suspected fracture may not be visible radiographically – an "occult" fracture. In these cases, the patient must be treated as though a fracture were present with adequate immobilization and follow up. This is most important when a delay in fracture diagnosis can result in permanent disability.

Two key examples of fractures that have considerable morbidity if inadequately treated are scaphoid fractures and femoral neck fractures. A scaphoid fracture is characteristically associated with tenderness in the anatomical snuff-box and may be complicated by avascular necrosis. A proximal femoral fracture, particularly in an older individual with osteoporosis, may also be radiographically occult. The patient may present with hip pain after relatively minor trauma such as a fall from standing. If misdiagnosed on the initial visit, a non-displaced fracture may become displaced necessitating more extensive surgery

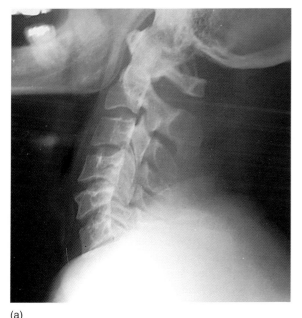
(a)

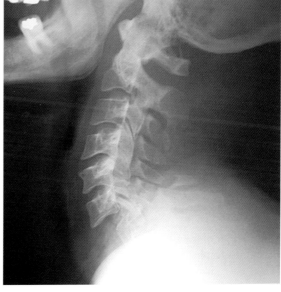
(b)

Figure 28.10 All seven cervical vertebrae must be seen in the lateral cervical spine radiograph. (a) With inadequate visualization, a C6–C7 "hyperextension fracture/dislocation" is missed in a patient who presented with quadriparesis after a fall. (b) In addition to the marked anterior vertebral body displacement, there are multiple posterior element fractures of C5–C7 due to compressive forces. (From Schwartz DT. *Emergency Radiology: Case Studies.* New York: McGraw-Hill, 2008, with permission.)

457

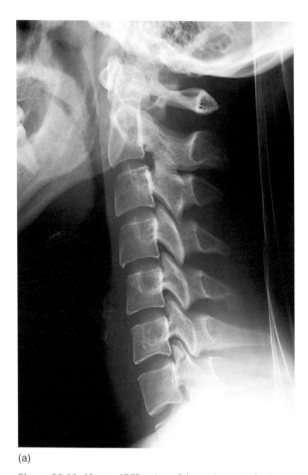

(a)

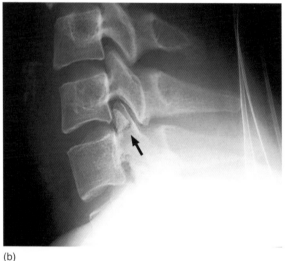

(b)

Figure 28.11 After an ABCS review of the entire cervical spine, each vertebra should be examined individually to avoid missing a subtle injury. Without such a step-wise examination, the facet fracture of C7, not easily seen, could have been missed (*arrow*). (From Schwartz DT. *Emergency Radiology: Case Studies.* New York: McGraw-Hill, 2008, with permission.)

(hemi-arthroplasty) rather than simple screw fixation. Although the physical examination and radiograph are useful, no clear constellation of physical or radiographic findings allows the clinician to rule out a fracture when there is persistent severe pain or inability to ambulate. In one study of ED patients with negative radiographs but clinical suspicion, 4.4% had fractures diagnosed by MRI. At this point, CT does not seem to be sensitive enough to exclude an occult fracture of the hip.[66]

A number of fractures and dislocations often have subtle radiographic findings that can easily be missed (Table 28.4).[3] In some cases, the diagnosis is made by ordering additional (supplementary) radiographic views or other imaging (CT or MRI). Additional imaging is ordered when the clinical examination suggests a fracture or dislocation and the radiographs are equivocal or normal.

In some patients with extremity trauma, soft tissue injuries – neurovascular, ligamentous, and musculotendonous – can be of greater significance than the skeletal injury. Diagnosis rests on clinical examination and knowledge of the soft tissue injuries commonly associated with particular fractures and dislocations. Soft tissue injuries may truly be limb threatening such as a popliteal artery injury associated with a knee dislocation.[67] In some cases, specific imaging studies are needed. Finally, neurovascular status must always be assessed before any manipulation is performed and pre- and post-manipulation findings should be documented.

Radiographic views: At least two views in perpendicular planes should be obtained to adequately assess an injury. This typically includes a frontal view (AP or PA) and a lateral view. In some cases, a lateral view cannot be obtained, such as the shoulder, hip, and

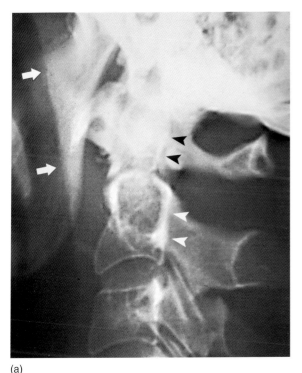
(a)

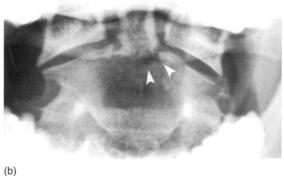
(b)

Figure 28.12 Type 2 odontoid fracture. A 26-year-old woman pedestrian was struck on her leg by a motor vehicle and knocked to the ground. She had a displaced tibial fracture, but denied having neck pain. Her neurological examination was normal. On the lateral view (a), the posterior cortex of the C2 vertebral body (*white arrowheads*) is not continuous with the posterior cortex of the dens (*black arrowheads*). The prevertebral soft tissues are nearly normal, although there is loss of the normal concavity superior to C1 and anterior to the base of the dens (*arrows*). The open mouth view (b) clearly shows the fracture through the base of the dens (*arrowheads*). (From Schwartz DT. *Emergency Radiology: Case Studies*. New York: McGraw-Hill, 2008, with permission.)

pelvis, and an oblique view or a view in an orthogonal (right angle) plane such as an axial view (e.g., the shoulder) is obtained (Figure 28.14).

In regions of complex anatomy, a third or sometimes a fourth view is routinely obtained. Examples include a pronation oblique view of the wrist or hand, a mortise view of the ankle, and an internal oblique view of the foot. The views included in a standard radiographic series may vary between hospitals and clinicians and should be familiar with the views considered standard at their institution.

In some cases, additional or ***supplementary views*** may be needed to detect a fracture. Supplementary views are ordered when an injury is suspected on clinical examination, but the standard radiographs are normal or equivocal. Examples include the scaphoid view of the wrist (PA view with the wrist in ulnar deviation), axillary view of the shoulder looking for a posterior dislocation, oblique (Judet) views of the pelvis looking for an acetabular fracture, oblique

views of the knee looking for a tibial plateau fracture, an axial ("sunrise") view of the patella looking for a vertical fracture of the patella, and an axial view of the calcaneus (Figures 28.15 and 28.16).[68,69] Increasingly, CT or MRI has replaced supplementary views in many cases (Figure 28.17).[70]

Radiograph interpretation: The first step is to identify the views obtained and determine whether they have been properly performed. Technically inadequate radiographs can mask injuries and should be repeated with correct positioning if a suspected injury is potentially obscured (Figure 28.18).

A ***systematic "ABCS" approach*** works well for extremity radiographs, particularly in regions of complex anatomy, such as the wrist. It directs attention to the radiographic signs of skeletal injury – abnormalities in alignment, bones, cartilage (joint spaces), and soft tissues (see Table 28.4).

The most obvious radiographic sign of a fracture is interruption or deformity of the osseous cortex or

459

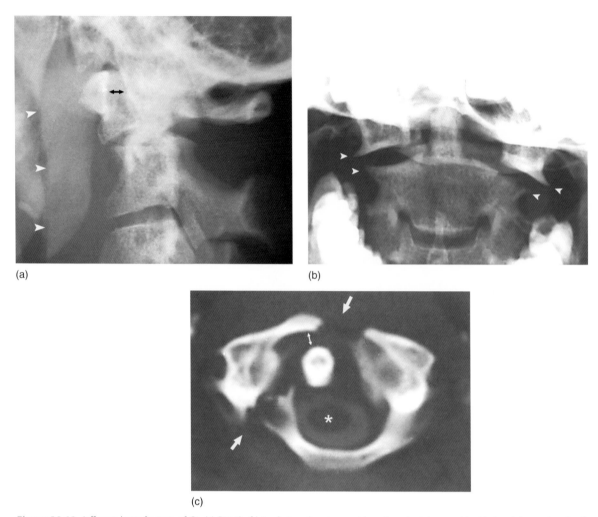

(a)

(b)

(c)

Figure 28.13 Jefferson burst fracture of C1. (a) Detail of lateral view showing a widened predental space (*double-headed arrow*) and soft tissue swelling (*arrowheads*). (b) Open mouth view. The lateral masses of C1 are displaced laterally with respect to the superior articular facets of C2 (*arrowheads*). (c) CT myelogram. There are anterior and posterior fractures of C1 (*arrows*). The predental space is widened (*double-headed arrow*). The spinal cord (*asterisk*) is seen within the spinal canal. (From Schwartz DT. *Emergency Radiology: Case Studies*. New York: McGraw-Hill, 2008, with permission.)

trabeculae. Alteration in the alignment between bones also serves as a clue to a fracture or dislocation. The joint spaces (cartilage) should be examined for widening or malalignment which is indicative of a fracture, dislocation, or ligmentous injury. Soft tissue clues of a fracture include swelling or a joint effusion, which can sometimes be more radiographically conspicuous than the fracture itself. For example, the elbow fat pad sign, indicative of a hemarthrosis, is often associated with a radial head fracture in an adult and a supracondylar fracture of the distal humerus in a child (Figure 28.18c). A lipohemarthrosis of the knee seen in the suprapatellar bursa on a cross-table lateral view is a clue to an intra-articular fracture, e.g., tibial plateau fracture. This fracture can be confirmed on a supplementary oblique view or CT.

A complimentary **targeted approach** should also be used for skeletal radiograph interpretation. It is both efficient and effective and is based on knowledge of the radiographic manifestations of various injuries. First, common sites of injury are examined, particularly injuries suspected based on the clinical examination. Next, injuries that can have subtle radiographic findings that can be easily missed are sought.

Table 28.4 Easily missed fractures and dislocations. Common injuries that present with subtle clinical and radiographic findings. Fractures are usually non-displaced or minimally displaced. Additional radiographic views are sometimes needed to visualize these injuries. Some of these fractures can have particularly serious consequences if missed (*)[3]

Shoulder	Posterior dislocation*
	Concomitant proximal humeral fracture and posterior dislocation*
	Distal clavicle fracture or A–C separation
Elbow	Adult – radial head fracture
	Child – supracondylar, lateral condylar, and medial epicondylar fractures*
Forearm	Monteggia and Galeazzi fracture–dislocations*
Wrist	Distal radius fracture
	Carpal fractures: scaphoid*, triquetrum, etc.
	Dislocations/instability: perilunate, lunate, scapholunate dissociation*
	Metacarpal base fractures
Hand	Tendon and ligament injuries*; phalangeal avulsion fractures
Pelvis	Isolated pubic ramus fracture, iliac wing fracture, avulsions (ischial tuberosity, iliac spine)
	Acetabular fractures*
	Posterior pelvic ring fractures (sacral wing fractures)
Hip	Femoral neck fracture (elderly, osteoporosis)*
	Intertrochanteric fracture*
	Pubic ramus fracture or other pelvic fracture
Knee	Tibial plateau fracture (lateral plateau)*
	Patella fractures (vertical or oblique)
	Osteochondral fractures and ligament or meniscal injuries*
Ankle	Lateral malleolus fracture
	Ligament tears and instability, tibio-fibular syndesmosis tear*
	Fifth metatarsal base, navicular and other midfoot fractures
Foot	Calcaneus and talus (hindfoot) fractures*
	Tarso-metatarsal fracture–dislocation (Lisfranc)*

Fractures in children

   Growth plate fractures (Salter–Harris)*

   Torus (buckle) fractures, and acute plastic bowing

Missed fractures in the multiple trauma victim (requires complete secondary survey)*

Indications for radiography in extremity trauma

Radiographs are needed whenever a fracture or dislocation is suspected based on the clinical examination (Table 28.5). Radiographs are not needed in patients with relatively minor sprains, strains or contusions or when the findings would not change management. Nonetheless, it can be difficult to definitely distinguish minor from more significant injuries solely based on the clinical examination. This is particularly true for injuries in proximity to the joints – fractures of the shafts (diaphyses) of the long bones are usually more clinically obvious. In a

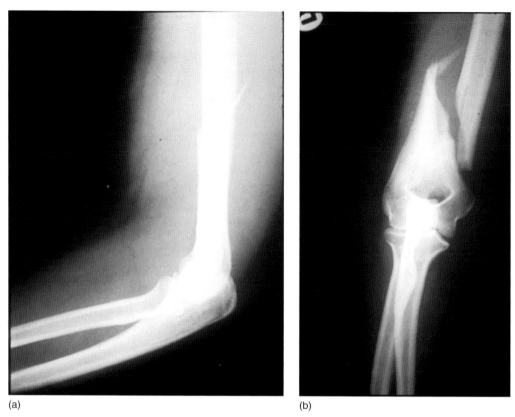

(a)   (b)

Figure 28.14 At least two views are needed to define an injury. (a) On the lateral view, the distal humeral shaft fracture is barely visible. (b) The fracture is obvious on the anteroposterior (AP) view.

few instances, clinical decision rules have been developed and validated to assist in deciding to obtain or omit radiography, e.g., the Ottawa Ankle (Table 28.6) and Mid-foot Rules and a number of knee rules.[14–17]

Although application of these rules does result in a limited but significant reduction in radiograph ordering, the majority of radiographs will still be negative for an injury. For example, traditionally only about 15% of ankle radiographs will show an injury. Using the Ottawa Ankle Rules, only 20% of radiographs will show an injury.[22] This demonstrates that in order to avoid missing an injury particularly in proximity to a joint, a large proportion of radiographs will be negative.

Radiopaque foreign bodies – penetrating trauma

Radiography can be used to detect, localize, and estimate the trajectory of metallic objects that have

caused penetrating injuries – both impalement (e.g., by a knife blade) and projectile injuries (e.g., gunshot wounds). To assess impalement by a metallic object at least two views in perpendicular planes are needed to localize the object (Figure 28.19). Radiographs can also assist in estimating local tissue damage and in planning surgical removal of the object. More precise determination of associated soft tissue injury can be made using CT, which can directly visualize nearby soft tissue structures. However, streak artifacts emanating from the metallic object may obscure the CT images.

For projectile injuries, most often bullets, radiography can localize the resting place of the projectile. Two views in perpendicular planes are necessary. However, for bullet wounds, it is difficult to determine the trajectory of the bullet and the injured vital organs. Placing a radiopaque marker on the entry wound and drawing a line from the entry site to the resting place of the bullet does not always reflect the trajectory of the bullet. A bullet often follows a non-

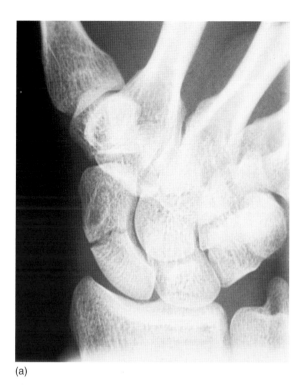
(a)

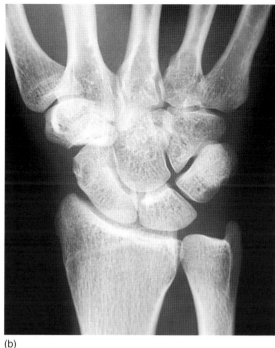
(b)

Figure 28.15 Supplementary views are sometimes needed to detect a fracture. (a) The scaphoid view (PA view with the wrist in ulnar deviation) reveals fractures through the mid portion of the scaphoid. (b) The posteroanterior (PA) view of the wrist is normal in this patient who had fallen on his outstretched hand and had tenderness in the "anatomical snuff box." (From Schwartz DT. *Emergency Radiology: Case Studies.* New York: McGraw-Hill, 2008, with permission.)

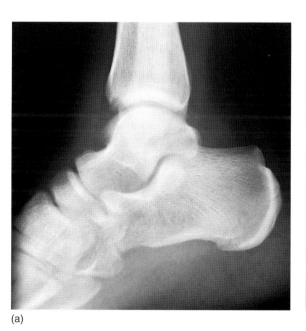
(a)

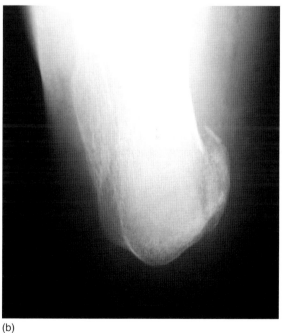
(b)

Figure 28.16 A patient who had jumped from a fence and complained of heel pain. (a) A fracture is not evident on the lateral view. Anteroposterior (AP) and oblique views of the foot and ankle also did not disclose an injury. (b) An axial calcaneus view revealed a longitudinal fracture of the posterior tuberosity of the calcaneus. (From Schwartz DT. *Emergency Radiology: Case Studies.* New York: McGraw-Hill, 2008, with permission.)

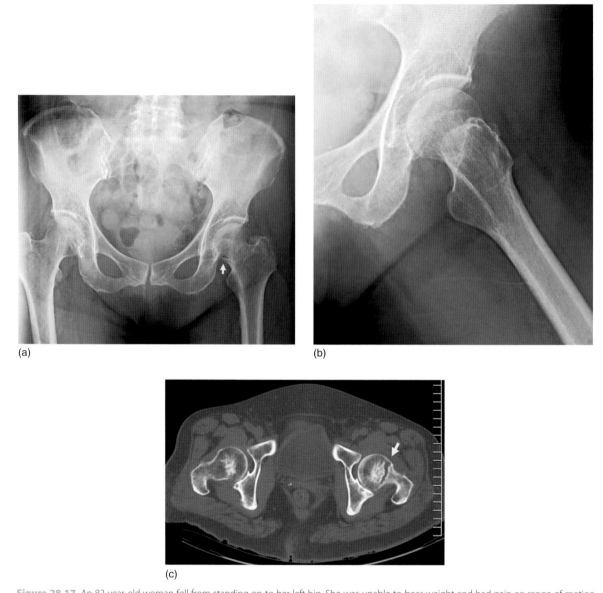

Figure 28.17 An 82-year-old woman fell from standing on to her left hip. She was unable to bear weight and had pain on range of motion of the hip. The initial radiographs did not clearly show a fracture although there was a questionable cortical irregularity on the anteroposterior (AP) view of the pelvis (a, *arrow*). The frog-leg view was normal (b). Multidetector computed tomography (MDCT) clearly demonstrated the subcapital femoral neck fracture (c, *arrow*).

linear path, changing direction as it moves through the body. The bullet may even enter the circulation and be transported far from the site of injury.

For gunshot wounds to the torso (chest or abdomen), radiography determines the resting location of the bullet. Management of gunshot wounds to the abdomen generally entails exploratory surgery.

Advanced imaging such as CT is usually not indicated preoperatively. On the other hand, MDCT has an increasing role in *stable* patients with gunshot wounds to the chest, particularly those with transmediastinal injuries.[71] For gunshot wounds to the extremities, radiography is used to localize the bullet as well as assess skeletal injuries. Angiography is indicated if

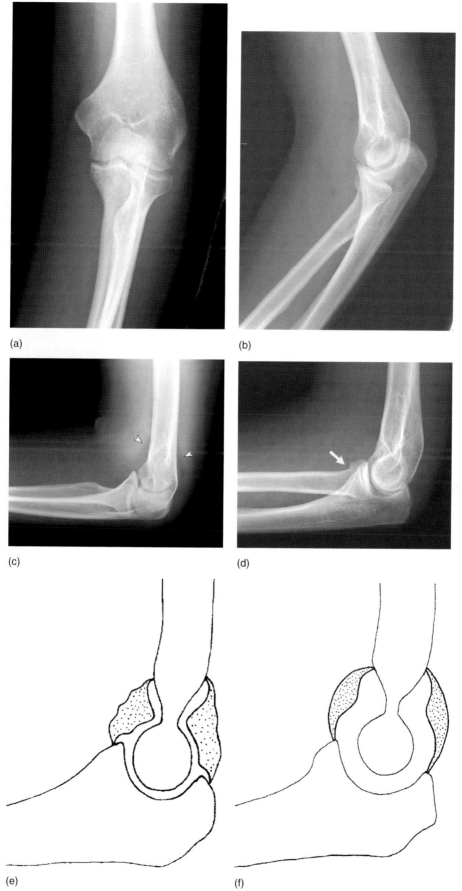

(a)

(b)

(c)

(d)

(e)

(f)

For caption, see p. 466.

465

Table 28.5 Standard and supplementary views of the extremities

	Standard views	Supplementary views
Shoulder	AP views: External rotation Internal rotation	Y view (usually standard for trauma) Axillary view
Clavicle	AP Angled AP (15º)	
Elbow	AP Lateral	Oblique views (2), Capitellum view Olecranon view (axial)
Wrist	PA Lateral Pronation oblique	Scaphoid view (ulnar deviation PA) Supination oblique Carpal tunnel view (axial)
Hand	PA Lateral Pronation oblique	Supination oblique (ball catcher view)
Finger	PA Lateral Pronation oblique	
Pelvis	AP	CT Judet views (oblique of acetabulum) Inlet and outlet views
Hip	AP (pelvis) "Frog-leg" or external oblique	Cross-table (groin) lateral
Knee	AP Lateral	Oblique views (2) Axial "sunrise" patellar view Intercondylar notch view
Ankle	AP Lateral Mortise (15º internal oblique)	Oblique views (2)
Foot	AP Lateral Internal oblique	Calcaneus axial view External oblique

Views that are standard vary from institution to institution. Supplementary views are oblique views, axial views (third perpendicular plane), altered positioning (scaphoid view). Obtain supplementary views when: (1) a fracture is suspected on physical examination but not seen on the standard views; or (2) to better define a questionable abnormality seen on the standard views. CT, computed tomography; AP, anteroposterior; PA, posteroanterior.

Table 28.6 Ottawa Ankle Rules

Radiographs of the ankle are only required if there is bony pain in the malleolar zone and any one of the following:

Bone tenderness along the distal 6 cm of the posterior edge of the tibia or tip of the medial malleolus

Bone tenderness along the distal 6 cm of the posterior edge of the fibula or tip of the lateral malleolus

An inability to bear weight for four steps both immediately after the injury and in the emergency department

vascular injury is suspected. For gunshot wounds to the head or spine, radiography can localize the projectile and assess skeletal injury whereas CT is used to more precisely assess neurological (brain and spinal cord) as well as skeletal injury.[72–75]

Summary

Plain radiography plays an important role in the evaluation of the majority of trauma patients. However, the use of radiography must be judicious in order to attain maximal efficiency, optimal information retrieval, minimal cost, and minimal risk. Although additional imaging modalities, such as CT, MRI, and ultrasound, have modified the application of plain radiographs in many instances, clinicians must have a firm understanding of the use of plain radiography.

Caption for Figure 28.18 Poor positioning of the patient can obscure an injury. (a and b) The initial anteroposterior (AP) and lateral views are normal, although the lateral view is inadequate because the elbow is not flexed to 90°. (c) On the repeat lateral, the elbow is in 90° of flexion and the anterior and posterior fat pads are visible, an indirect sign of a fracture. However, the fracture is not visible because the view is again not correctly positioned – it is oblique rather than a true lateral view (the distal humeral article surfaces [capitellum and trochlea] are not superimposed). (d) The lateral view was again repeated, this time correctly positioned and a radial head fracture is visible. (e and f) Genesis of the elbow fat pad signs. Normally on a lateral view, the posterior fat pad is not visible and the anterior fat pad is only slightly visible. With a joint effusion (hemarthrosis in the setting of trauma with an intra-articular fracture), the fat pads are displaced outwards and are now visible on the radiograph. This is a soft tissue clue to the presence of a fracture and is sometimes more evident than the fracture itself. (Copyright D. T. Schwartz, MD.)

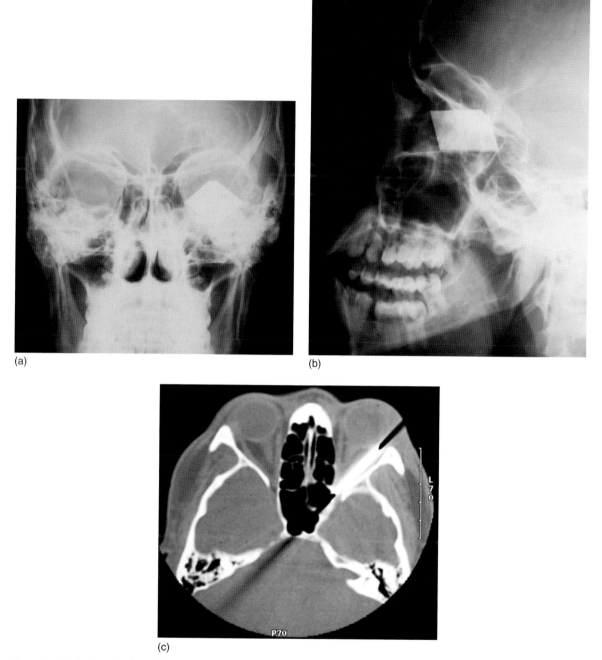

(a)

(b)

(c)

Figure 28.19 Radiographs (a and b) show foreign body in skull in perpendicular planes. A computed tomography (CT) image of face (c) shows a more precise localization and can show associated soft tissue injury.

References

1. Miniño AM, Heron MP, Smith BL. *Deaths: Final Data for 2004. National Vital Statistics Reports.* Hyattsville, MD: National Center for Health Statistics. 2006.

Available from http://www.cdc.gov/nchs/products/pubs/pubd/hestats/finaldeaths04/finaldeaths04.htm.

2. US Environmental Protection Agency. *Ionizing Radiation Fact Sheet Series: No. 1.* Available from

http://www.epa.gov/rpdweb00/docs/ionize/402-f-98-009.htm.

3. Schwartz DT, Reisdorff EJ (eds.). *Emergency Radiology*. New York: McGraw-Hill, 2000.

4. Canadian Centre for Occupational Health and Safety. *Radiation – Quantities and Units of Ionizing Radiation. June 19, 2007.* Available from http://www.ccohs.ca/oshanswers/phys_agents/ionizing.html.

5. Grande CM, Stene JK. Mechanisms of injury: etiologies of trauma. In Stene JK, Grande CM (eds), *Trauma Anesthesia*. Baltimore, MD: Lippincott, Williams and Wilkins, 1990: pp. 37–63.

6. Mono J, Holienberg RD, Harvey JT. Occult transorbital intracranial penetrating injuries. *Ann Emerg Med* 1988;**15**:589–91.

7. Brent RL. The effects of embryonic and fetal exposure to X-ray, microwaves, and ultrasound. *Clin Perinatol* 1986;**13**:615.

8. Neufeld, JDG. Trauma in pregnancy. In Marx J, Walls R, Hockberger R (eds), *Rosen's Emergency Medicine: Concepts and Clinical Practice*, 6th edn. Philadelphia, PA: Mosby, 2006: pp. 316–28.

9. National Council on Radiation Protection and Measurements. *Medical Radiation Exposure of Pregnant and Potentially Pregnant Women, No. 54.* Washington, DC: National Council on Radiation Protection and Measurements, 1979.

10. Harvey EB, Boice JD, Jr., Honeyman M, et al. Prenatal X-ray exposure and childhood cancer in twins. *N Engl J Med* 1985;**312**:541–5.

11. Ornoy A, Patlas N, Schwartz L. The effects of in utero diagnostic X-irradiation on the development of preschool-age children. *Isr J Med Sci* 1996;**32**:112–15.

12. Wagner LK, Lester RG, Saldana LR. *Exposure of the Pregnant Patient to Diagnostic Radiations: A Guide to Medical Management*. Philadelphia, PA: JB Lippincott, 1985.

13. National Council on Radiation Protection and Measurements. *Medical Radiation Exposure of Potentially Pregnant Women, No. 54.* Bethesda, MD: National Council on Radiation Protection and Measurements, 1977.

14. Stiell IG, McKnight RD, Greenberg GH, et al. Implementation of the Ottawa ankle rules. *JAMA* 1994;**271**:827–32.

15. Stiell IG, Greenberg GH, Wells GA, et al. Prospective validation of a decision rule for the use of radiography in acute knee injuries. *JAMA* 1996;**275**:611–15.

16. Bauer SJ, Hollander JE, Fuchs SH, Thode HC. A clinical decision rule in the evaluation of acute knee injuries. *J Emerg Med* 1995;**13**:611–15.

17. Weber JE, Jackson RE, Peacock WF, et al. Clinical decision rules discriminate between fractures and nonfractures in acute isolated knee trauma. *Ann Emerg Med* 1995;**26**:429–33.

18. Hoffman JR, Mower WR, Wolfson AB, et al. Validity of a set of clinical criteria to rule out injury to the cervical spine in patients with blunt trauma. *New Engl J Med* 2000;**343**:94–9.

19. Stiell IG, Wells GA, Vandemheen KL, et al. The Canadian C-Spine Rule for radiography in alert and stable trauma patients. *JAMA* 2001;**286**:1841–8.

20. Stiell IG, Wells GA. Methodologic standards for the development of clinical decision rules in emergency medicine. *Ann Emerg Med* 1999;**33**:437–47.

21. McGinn TG, Guyatt GH, Wyer PC, et al. Users' guides to the medical literature: how to use articles about clinical decision rules. *JAMA* 2000;**284**:79–84.

22. Stiell IG, Wells G, Laupacis A, et al. A multicenter trial to introduce clinical decision rules for the use of radiography in acute ankle injuries. *BMJ* 1995;**311**:594–7.

23. Blaivas M, Lyon M, Duggal S. A prospective comparison of supine chest radiography and bedside ultrasound for the diagnosis of traumatic pneumothorax. *Acad Emerg Med* 2005;**12**:844–9.

24. Kirkpatrick AW, Sirois M, Laupland KB, et al. Hand-held thoracic sonography for detecting post-traumatic pneumothoraces: the Extended Focused Assessment with Sonography for Trauma (EFAST). *J Trauma* 2004;**57**:288–95.

25. Schwartz DT. *Emergency Radiology: Case Studies*. New York: McGraw-Hill, 2008: pp. 93–104.

26. Ho RT, Blackmore CC, Bloch RD, et al. Can we rely on mediastinal widening on chest radiography to identify subjects with aortic injury? *Emerg Radiol* 2002;**9**:183–7.

27. Cook AD, Klein JS, Rogers FB, et al. Chest radiographs of limited utility in the diagnosis of blunt traumatic aortic laceration. *J Trauma* 2001;**50**:843–7.

28. Mirvis SE, Bidwell JK, Buddemeyer EU, et al. Value of chest radiography in excluding traumatic aortic rupture. *Radiology* 1987;**163**:487–93.

29. Kong A. The deep sulcus sign. *Radiology* 2003;**228**:415–16.

30. Ball CG; Kirkpatrick AW, Laupland KB, et al. Incidence, risk factors and outcomes for occult pneumothoraces in victims of major trauma. *J Trauma* 2005;**59**:917–25.

31. Ball CG; Kirkpatrick AW; Fox DL; et al. Are occult pneumothoraces truly occult or simply missed? *J Trauma* 2006;**60**:294–9.

32. Gilligan P, Hegarty D, Hassan TB. The point of the needle. Occult pneumothorax: a review. *Emerg Med J* 2003;**20**:293–6.

33. Henderson SO, Shoenberger JM. Anterior pneumothorax and a negative chest X-ray. *J Emerg Med* 2004;**26**:231–2.

34. Kikuchi N, Satoh H, Ohtsuka M, et al. Anterior pneumothorax. *J Emerg Med* 2005;**29**:485–6.

35. Mirvis SE. Value of chest radiography in excluding traumatic aortic rupture. *Radiology* 1987;**163**:487–93.

36. Kram HB. Diagnosis of traumatic thoracic aortic rupture: a 10-year retrospective analysis. *Ann Thorac Surg* 1989;**47**:282–6.

37. Rivas LA, Fishman JE, Múnera F, Bajayo DE. Multislice CT in thoracic trauma. *Radiol Clin North Am* 2003;**41**:599–616.

38. Mirvis SE. Thoracic vascular injury. *Radiol Clin North Am* 2006;**44**:181–97.

39. Alkadhi H, Wildermuth S, Desbiolles L, et al. Vascular emergencies of the thorax after blunt and iatrogenic trauma: multidetector row and three-dimensional imaging. *Radiographics* 2004;**24**:1239–55.

40. Malloy PC, Richard HM. Thoracic angiography and intervention in trauma. *Radiol Clin North Am* 2006;**44**:239–49.

41. Dyer DS, Moore EE, Ilke DN, et al. Thoracic aortic injury: how predictive is mechanism and is chest computed tomography a reliable screening tool? A prospective study of 1516 patients. *J Trauma* 2000;**48**:673–83.

42. Gavant ML, Flick P, Menke P, Gold RE. CT aortography of thoracic aortic rupture. *AJR Am J Roentgenol* 1996;**166**:955–61.

43. Bruckner BA, DiBardino DJ, Cumbie TC, et al. Critical evaluation of chest computed tomography scans for blunt descending thoracic aortic injury. *Ann Thorac Surg* 2006;**81**:1339–46.

44. Smith MD, Cassidy JM, Souther S, et al. Transesophageal echocardiography in the diagnosis of traumatic rupture of the aorta. *New Engl J Med* 1995;**332**:356–62.

45. Minard G, Schurr MJ, Croce MA, et al. A prospective analysis of transesophageal echocardiography in the diagnosis of traumatic disruption of the aorta. *J Trauma* 1996;**40**:225–30.

46. White CS, Mirvis SE, Templeton PA. Subtle chest radiographic abnormalities in patients with traumatic aortic rupture. *Emerg Radiol* 1994;**1**:72–7.

47. Woodring JH. The normal mediastinum in blunt traumatic rupture of the thoracic aorta and brachiocephalic arteries. *J Emerg Med* 1990;**8**:467–76.

48. Lee FT, Katzberg RW, Gutierrez OH, et al. Re-evaluation of plain radiographic findings in the diagnosis of aortic rupture: the role of inspiration and positioning on mediastinal width. *J Emerg Med* 1993;**11**:289–96.

49. Savitt DL. Traumatic aortic rupture: delayed presentation with a normal chest radiograph. *Am J Emerg Med* 1999;**17**:285–7.

50. Fabian TC, Richardson JD, Croce MA, et al. Prospective study of blunt aortic injury: multicenter trial of the AAST. *J Trauma* 1997;**42**:374–80.

51. Hunt JP, Baker CC, Lentz CW, et al. Thoracic aorta injuries: management and outcome of 144 patients. *J Trauma* 1996;**40**:547–55.

52. Gelman R. Diaphragmatic rupture due to blunt trauma: sensitivity of plain chest radiographs. *AJR Am J Roentgenol* 1991;**156**:51–7.

53. Hammel J, Legome E. Pelvic fracture. *J Emerg Med* 2006;**30**:87–92.

54. Guillamondegui OD, Pryor JP, Gracias VH, et al. Pelvic radiography in blunt trauma resuscitation: a diminishing role. *J Trauma* 2002;**53**:1043–7.

55. Morgan DE, Nallamala LK, Kenney PJ, et al. CT cystography: radiographic and clinical predictors of bladder rupture. *AJR Am J Roentgenol* 2000;**174**:89–95.

56. Quagliano PV, Delair SM, Malhotra AK. Diagnosis of blunt bladder injury: a prospective comparative study of computed tomography cystography and conventional retrograde cystography. *J Trauma* 2006;**61**:410–22.

57. Niedens BA, Gross EA. Validation of a decision instrument to limit pelvic radiography in blunt trauma. *Acad Emerg Med* 2003;**10**:475–6.

58. Hoffman JR, Mower WR, Wolfson AB, et al. Validity of a set of clinical criteria to rule out injury to the cervical spine in patients with blunt trauma. *New Engl J Med* 2000;**343**:94–9.

59. Hanson JA, Blackmore CC, Mann FA, Wilson AJ. Cervical spine injury: a clinical decision rule to identify high-risk patients for helical CT screening. *AJR Am J Roentgenol* 2000;**174**:713–17.

60. Rybicki F, Nawfel RD, Judy PF, et al. Skin and thyroid dosimetry in cervical spine screening: two methods for evaluation and a comparison between a helical CT and radiographic trauma series. *AJR Am J Roentgenol* 2002;**179**:933–7.

61. Davis JW, Phreaner DL, Hoyt DB, et al. The etiology of missed cervical spine injuries. *J Trauma* 1993; **34**:342–6.

62. Mower WR, Oh JY, Zucker MI, Hoffman JR. Occult and secondary injuries missed by plain radiography of

469

the cervical spine in blunt trauma patients. *Emerg Radiol* 2001;**8**:200–6.

63. Daffner RH, Hackney DB. ACR Appropriateness criteria on suspected spine trauma. *J Am Coll Radiol* 2007;**4**:762–75.

64. Pitt E, Thakore S. Role of flexion/extension radiography in neck injuries in adults. *Emerg Med J* 2004;**21**:587–8.

65. Schwartz DT. *Emergency Radiology: Case Studies.* New York: McGraw-Hill, 2008: pp. 359–72.

66. Dominguez S, Liu P, Roberts C, et al. Prevalence of traumatic hip and pelvic fractures in patients with suspected hip fracture and negative initial standard radiographs – a study of emergency department patients. *Acad Emerg Med* 2005;**12**:366–9. [Float1]

67. Perron AD, Brady WJ, Sing RF. Vascular injury associated with knee dislocation. *Am J Emerg Med* 2001;**19**:583–8.

68. Perron AD, Brady WJ, Keats TE, Hersh RE. Scaphoid fractures. *Am J Emerg Med* 2001;**19**:310–16.

69. Perron AD, Jones RL. Posterior shoulder dislocation: avoiding a missed diagnosis. *Am J Emerg Med* 2000;**18**:189–91.

70. Perron AD, Miller MD, Brady WJ. Radiographically occult hip fracture. *Am J Emerg Med* 2002;**20**:234–7.

71. Shanmuganathan K, Matsumoto J. Imaging of penetrating chest trauma. *Radiol Clin North Am* 2006;**44**:225–38.

72. Wilson AJ. Gunshot injuries: what does a radiologist need to know. *Radiographics* 1999;**19**:1358–68.

73. Hollerman JJ, Fackler ML, Coldwell DM, Ben-Menachem Y. Gunshot wounds. I. Bullets, ballistics, and mechanisms of injury. *AJR Am J Roentgenol* 1990;**155**:685–90.

74. Hollerman JJ, Fackler ML, Coldwell DM, et al. Gunshot wounds. II. Radiology. *AJR Am J Roentgenol* 1990;**155**:691–702.

75. Phillips CD. Emergent radiologic evaluation of the gunshot wound victim. *Radiol Clin North Am* 1992;**30**:307–24.

Ultrasound

John L. Kendall and Brandon H. Backlund

Introduction

Trauma ultrasound is used to detect fluid or abnormalities within anatomic spaces that would otherwise require invasive testing such as diagnostic peritoneal lavage (DPL), expensive imaging such as computed tomography (CT), or potentially delayed methods such as clinical observation. This becomes particularly useful in the evaluation of patients with blunt or penetrating trauma to the chest or abdomen.

This chapter will discuss the clinical applications, techniques, and use of the standard focused abdominal sonography in trauma (FAST) exam, as well as expanded applications for those with more advanced skills.

Principles of ultrasound

Basic familiarity with the sonographic appearance of different tissues will allow the sonographer to characterize tissue as either solid organ, fluid-filled, bowel, or bone.

Ultrasound works by emitting high-frequency sound waves, which are transmitted through tissues. At the interface between tissues of differing densities, some of the sound waves are reflected, and these reflected signals are captured by the transducer to generate an image. Sound waves interact in characteristic ways with different tissue types. Tissues having molecules that are organized and relatively close together transmit sound waves better than those that are disorganized or farther apart. For example, solid parenchymal organs provide good ultrasound images since they are compact and have some fluid density. The liver and spleen are typical of organs with excellent transmission properties. When visualized by ultrasound they have a uniform, mid-level echogenic pattern with defined borders.

Gases have unique properties that make ultrasound imaging through them difficult. Molecules in gases are randomly placed, so sound waves are reflected in different directions. When encountering gas during scanning, images are typically poorly defined, since the transducer sees a random array of signals. Consequently, ultrasound protocols avoid gas-filled areas such as bowel and lung.

Fluid densities form ideal sonographic imaging environments, because the molecules have uniformity and they allow for easy transmission of sound waves to and from deeper tissue. A fluid-filled structure is thought of as an *acoustic window* since it can be used to visualize deeper structures. For instance, the bladder is often used in scanning, because the urine provides a uniform fluid density that allows most of the signal to penetrate to deeper structures (e.g., uterus); additionally, the full bladder displaces bowel allowing for clearer visualization.

Another commonly encountered tissue is bone. Most of the sound striking bone is reflected and cannot penetrate deeper. Therefore, scanning over a bony structure, such as a rib, produces a shadow, or anechoic area, on the ultrasound image deep to the bone. Moving the transducer away from the bone allows the signal to reach deeper structures. However, just because bone is dense does not mean it is excluded from all clinical applications for ultrasound. In musculoskeletal ultrasound, the near field cortex can be visualized in order to identify fractures or other abnormalities of the bone.

Equipment

Most trauma ultrasound exams are performed with compact or cart-based systems using a 3.5 MHz transducer. While most aspects of the exam can be

Trauma: A Comprehensive Emergency Medicine Approach, eds. Eric Legome and Lee W. Shockley. Published by Cambridge University Press. © Cambridge University Press 2011.

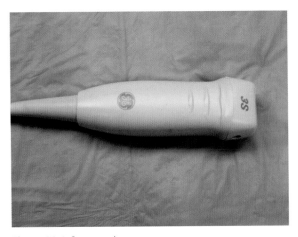

Figure 29.1 Sector probe.

Table 29.1 Ultrasound probes

Probe type	Frequency	Common uses
Curvilinear	Low (2–5 MHz)	General abdominal
		Obstetrics
Sector/ phased array	Low (2–5 MHz)	Echocardiography
		Intercostal, subxiphoid views of FAST
Linear	High (5–14 MHz)	Vascular access
		Nerve blocks
		Pleural ultrasound
		Foreign body localization

FAST, focused abdominal sonography in trauma.

done with a curvilinear abdominal transducer, the tighter the radius of the probe and the smaller the footprint, or size of the transducer head, the easier it is to perform the upper quadrant, cardiac, and thoracic views of trauma ultrasound. A smaller footprint can facilitate imaging between and around the ribs. This can be in the form of a tight-curved abdominal transducer or alternatively, a phased-array transducer commonly used for echocardiographic exams (Figure 29.1).

Most current machines have multifrequency transducers with frequency and depth controls allowing adjustment for a variety of applications and for differences in body habitus. Higher-frequency sound waves provide better resolution of small structures or structures that are very close together, but are attenuated (weakened) more rapidly as they pass through tissues. By contrast, lower-frequency sound penetrates more deeply into tissues, but image resolution is poorer. Therefore, lower frequencies are used to visualize deeper or larger structures, such as the heart or aorta, whereas higher frequencies are used for small, superficial structures, such as blood vessels and nerves. For this reason, in larger adults, a lower frequency (2 MHz) may be preferable, whereas in children and smaller statured adults, a higher frequency (5 MHz) may provide better imaging. If available, some physicians prefer a phased array transducer for the cardiac and abdominal imaging and a linear probe (with better near field resolution) for the detection of pneumothorax and for sonographic procedural guidance (Table 29.1; Figures 29.2 and 29.3).

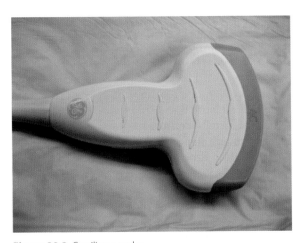

Figure 29.2 Curvilinear probe.

Clinician training for trauma ultrasound

Training in emergency bedside ultrasound, including the FAST exam, has become a required part of the emergency medicine residency core curriculum.[1] However, the addition of this component to standard residency training is relatively new; many practicing emergency physicians may have received little or no training in the FAST exam during residency. Consequently, there is considerable interest in determining the best method of learning the technique, attaining proficiency, and measuring proficiency. This process can be divided into three phases: the training phase, the experiential phase, and the independent phase.[2]

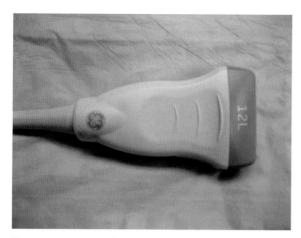

Figure 29.3 Linear probe.

The training phase should consist of both a didactic component and a practical, "hands-on" component, in order for the clinician to understand the theory behind the exam, as well as afford the opportunity to practice the required psychomotor skills on human models. Recruitment of patients receiving chronic ambulatory peritoneal dialysis as models for the practical sessions can be helpful in illustrating the findings of a positive FAST exam (dialysate fluid has a similar appearance to hemoperitoneum). A single training session of no more than 8 hours devoted to the FAST exam is generally considered sufficient to learn the theory and technique.[3–5]

During the experiential phase, the clinician performs the FAST exam on patients in the clinical setting, with a quality control mechanism in place evaluating image quality and correct interpretation of the study. This may be achieved by a variety of methods, including supervision/proctoring by an appropriately qualified second clinician, use of predetermined "gold standard" confirmatory testing (e.g., CT scan, DPL, laparotomy, observation, etc.), and review of static or video images. This phase may correlate to a "provisional privileges" status for the purposes of credentialing within a hospital or institution.

There is some debate as to the number of FAST exams that a clinician needs to perform before sufficient competency can be attained to perform the exam independently. Some have suggested that proficiency can be attained after performing as few as 10 exams,[3] but there is evidence that an examiner's accuracy improves significantly after performing somewhere in the range of 20–30 exams.[6–10] The American College of Emergency Physicians (ACEP) endorses a minimum of 25 exams performed as a threshold for competence and credentialing, recommending that 25–50 exams be documented and evaluated before the clinician should be considered independently qualified to perform the FAST exam, with the further stipulation that some discretionary percentage of positive studies must be included in that number.[4]

Once the requisite number of FAST exams has been performed, the clinician may be qualified and granted departmental privileges to perform the exam independently, subject to standard quality assurance review processes. As the level of experience progresses, an examiner's confidence in the exam increases, often decreasing the need for confirmatory alternative imaging modalities.[2,7] The examiner will also frequently be able to make more sophisticated interpretations of the FAST exam, such as increased sensitivity at detecting smaller amounts of fluid, improved skill at distinguishing normal variants from pathologic findings, greater accuracy in estimating free fluid volume, and possibly detecting solid organ injury in the absence of hemoperitoneum. Even at this stage, it is recommended that clinicians continue to engage in ultrasound-specific continuing medical education activities throughout their practice, to maintain their skills and keep abreast of advancements in the field.

Ultrasound compared to other diagnostic and imaging modalities

The diagnostic approach to the traumatically injured patient typically involves a variety of diagnostic tests, including plain radiographs, DPL, ultrasound, CT, and clinical observation with serial examination. Each test has advantages and disadvantages and the integration of each in the management of trauma is influenced by many factors, including the nature of the trauma and the stability of the patient.

Patients with blunt abdominal trauma present a distinct challenge to physicians. The workup for blunt abdominal trauma primarily focuses on the detection of free intraperitoneal fluid, usually correlated with an injury to a solid viscus. The physical exam for significant injuries is notoriously unreliable with error rates reported to be as high as 45%,[11] and accuracy rates approaching 65%.[12] Diagnostic peritoneal lavage has a long history in the evaluation of patients with blunt abdominal trauma, but it is invasive, time-consuming, not specific for organ injury, and sometimes overly sensitive, resulting in non-therapeutic laparotomies. Computed tomography scan comprises the majority of diagnostic imaging in blunt abdominal trauma; however, it is expensive, requires contrast, is time-consuming, and requires that the patient be stable. Ultrasound offers many advantages for rapid information accrual compared with DPL and CT. It is sensitive for hemoperitoneum, non-invasive, can be performed quickly and simultaneously with other resuscitative measures, and provides immediate information at the patient's bedside. Ultrasound has not replaced CT or DPL, but has assumed a primary role in the early bedside assessment of blunt trauma.

While detecting intraperitoneal fluid is of some importance, the more critical issue is whether a laparotomy is indicated. In the past, this question was often answered by the results of a DPL. A positive DPL by either initial aspiration or subsequent cell counts was an indication for an exploratory laparotomy. While looking for a non-invasive, less time-consuming alternative to DPL, a number of studies have assessed the ability of ultrasound as an adjunct in making this decision.[13–18] All of these studies report favorable results when comparing sensitivity and specificity of ultrasound to DPL. Many trauma centers, therefore, have abandoned the use of DPL in the blunt trauma patient in favor of ultrasonography or more commonly, ultrasonography in conjunction with CT scan.

There are a few exceptions to the generalization that ultrasound can entirely replace DPL. These include the unstable hypotensive patient with blunt trauma and a negative ultrasound, and patients with penetrating abdominal trauma. While it has been suggested that a negative ultrasound for peritoneal fluid in the hemodynamically unstable patient is reliable enough to prompt a search for an extraperitoneal source of instability,[19] in some emergency departments (EDs), DPL will still be the study of last resort after a thorough consideration for other sources of shock. As well, the negative results of an ultrasound exam in a patient with an abdominal stab wound cannot exclude small bowel or diaphragmatic injuries, so it is useful solely in the case of a positive study.

Detecting hemoperitoneum or predicting the need for laparotomy are significant diagnostic end-points for the emergency physician, but it is also important to determine the extent of specific organ injury. This has become even more relevant as surgeons manage the majority of splenic and liver injuries non-operatively. In most centers indications for laparotomy are currently based on clinical status along with CT grading of organ injury. Enthusiasm for a similar role for ultrasound has been present for some time.[20] Despite the early interest, investigators have failed to establish a definitive role for ultrasound in specific organ injury detection. Not only is ultrasound not accurate for evaluating retroperitoneal hemorrhage or bowel injuries, but it also cannot be relied upon to grade the severity of organ injury, detect active bleeding, or isolate injury to a single organ. These limitations of ultrasound are in competition with the fact that access, speed, and accuracy of CT scanning has increased significantly in recent years. Therefore, in trauma centers, where timely access to high-speed CT scanners is available, there is little evidence for ultrasound replacing CT scan in the diagnostic evaluation of the stable blunt abdominal trauma patients.

Unfortunately, unlimited access to abdominal CT scanning is not always available. Trauma centers may be presented with multiple stable patients requiring CT scanning; ultrasound may assist prioritization of scanning order. Furthermore, patients may present with blunt abdominal trauma to hospitals where there is limited or no access to a CT scanner. A positive ultrasound exam in this setting can be used to mobilize a CT technologist from home, alert a trauma surgeon on call, or initiate immediate transport to a trauma center.

Bedside vs. consultative ultrasound exam

The FAST is a bedside examination, and should be performed in the ED, concurrent with or in close proximity to the initial assessment of the trauma patient. Therefore, in most institutions, it is performed by a physician on the trauma team. The FAST exam was developed, taught, and propagated by surgeons and emergency physicians. Consequently, the views, sequence of transducer positions, and findings are not taught nor described by historical imaging specialties. In fact, to date no ICD code exists that describes the FAST exam, since it comprises both abdominal and cardiac views. As such, in some institutions, in order to obtain a complete FAST exam, sonographers from the Departments of Radiology and Cardiology would need to be consulted. Lastly, and probably most importantly, time is of the essence in the evaluation of the

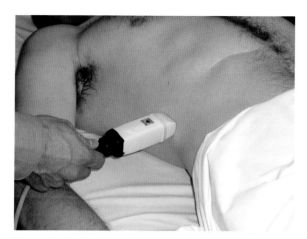

Figure 29.4 Right upper quadrant transducer position for the focused acute sonography in trauma (FAST) exam.

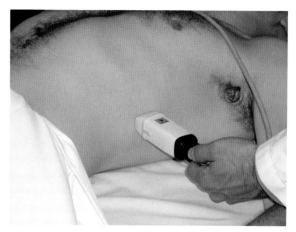

Figure 29.5 Left upper quadrant transducer position for the focused acute sonography in trauma (FAST) exam.

trauma patient, and a consultative study typically cannot be supplied in a clinically useful time-frame by the majority of best staffed radiology departments or echocardiography laboratories.

Technique

The basic FAST exam includes four views:[21]

1. Perihepatic (right upper quadrant)
2. Perisplenic (left quadrant)
3. Pelvic (pouch of Douglas or retrovesicular)
4. Pericardial (cardiac).

Perihepatic

The right upper quadrant view, also known as the Morison's pouch or perihepatic view, is considered the classic image of trauma ultrasound. It allows for visualization of free fluid in the potential space (Morison's pouch) between the liver and right kidney. In addition, fluid above and below the diaphragm in the costophrenic angle or subdiaphragmatic space can be seen. The transducer is initially placed in a coronal orientation in the mid-axillary line directly over an intercostal space of one of the lower ribs (Figure 29.4). Once Morison's pouch is visualized, the transducer should be angled in all directions to fully visualize the potential spaces of the right upper quadrant.

Perisplenic

The left upper quadrant view is also known as the perisplenic or, less accurately, the splenorenal view. It can be challenging to obtain because the spleen does

not provide as large a sonographic window as the liver and the examiner frequently needs to reach across the patient in order to access the left upper quadrant. Ideal placement of the transducer in the left upper quadrant differs from the perihepatic view in that it is generally oriented more cephalad and posterior (Figure 29.5). The transducer should be angled to see the anterior, posterior, superior, and inferior portions of the perisplenic space.

Pelvic

The pelvic view is an important, and potentially under-appreciated, window for detecting free peritoneal fluid. Since it is one of the most dependent and easily visualized portions of the peritoneal cavity, fluid collections may be seen here before being detected in other areas.[22] As well, it is away from the chest and upper abdomen, so images can be obtained simultaneously with the evaluation and resuscitation of the trauma patient. The key to the pelvic view is scanning through a moderately full bladder to facilitate visualization of the underlying and adjacent structures, so imaging should be done before placement of a Foley catheter or spontaneous voiding. The transducer can then be angled side-to-side, superiorly, and inferiorly to gain a full appreciation of the retrovesicular space (Figure 29.6).

Pericardial

The subxiphoid approach is the most commonly used and convenient way to visualize cardiac structures and the pericardial space. The four-chamber subxiphoid

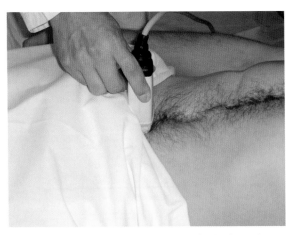

Figure 29.6 Suprapubic transducer position for the focused acute sonography in trauma (FAST) exam.

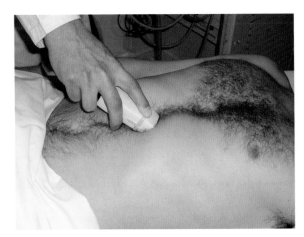

Figure 29.7 Subxiphoid transducer position for the focused acute sonography in trauma (FAST) exam.

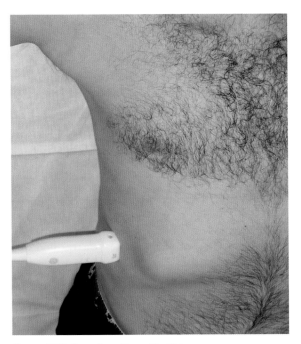

Figure 29.8 Paracolic gutter positioning.

view is performed with the transducer oriented transversely in the subcostal region and almost parallel to the skin of the anterior torso as it is pointed to a location just to the left of the sternum towards the patient's head (Figure 29.7). The subxiphoid view may not be obtainable in all patients, so other cardiac views such as the left parasternal may need to be obtained to rule out traumatic pericardial effusion, especially in those with large anterior pericardial fat pads.[23]

Extended views

Paracolic gutters

The paracolic gutters are additional sonographic views that can help roughly quantify the amount of peritoneal fluid present. These views are obtained by placing the transducer in either upper quadrant in a coronal plane and then sliding it caudally from the inferior pole of the kidney. In general, peritoneal fluid will accumulate earliest in the perihepatic, perisplenic, or pelvic areas, the three areas that comprise the "core" abdominal views of the FAST. As the amount of fluid increases, it will eventually be visible in the paracolic gutters; as such, the presence of fluid in these areas suggests a larger intra-abdominal fluid volume (Figure 29.8).

Costrophrenic angle or pleural base

The sonographic evaluation of the pleural space for fluid is an adaptation of the right and left upper quadrant views described in the standard FAST exam. The transducer is initially placed in position to obtain a right or left upper quadrant view. It is then angled or moved superiorly to visualize the diaphragm and pleural space. The region immediately above the diaphragm should be imaged to detect fluid. When pleural fluid is present, an anechoic space appears above the diaphragm (Figure 29.9).

Anterior thorax (pneumothorax)

Evaluation of the anterior pleura for the presence of pneumothorax or normal lung can be done with a number of transducers, although a high-frequency,

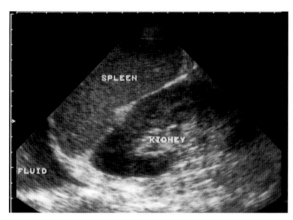

Figure 29.9 Ultrasound image demonstrating fluid in the costophrenic angle.

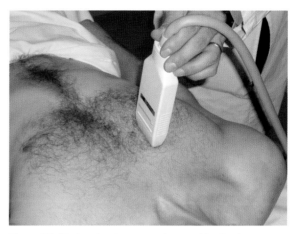

Figure 29.10 Anterior thorax transducer position for the evaluation of pneumothorax.

linear model set to a shallow depth of penetration (4–6 cm) is preferable. The transducer is placed longitudinally in the midclavicular line over the third or fourth intercostal space (Figure 29.10).

Order

While there is no current standard for the order in which the views of the FAST exam are obtained, arguments have been made for starting with certain windows. For instance, the right upper quadrant view is a common starting point since it is one of the most sensitive and specific locations for detecting hemoperitoneum and many physicians routinely scan from the patient's right side.[24–26] Alternatively, the pelvic view may be the first view obtained, as it is one of the most dependent portions of the peritoneal cavity so smaller fluid collections may be detected here before other locations.[24] As well, placement of a urinary catheter to decompress the bladder essentially eliminates the sonographic window to the pelvis, so there is a priority on obtaining this window before the Foley is placed. Another approach is to scan the left upper quadrant first, but this is usually advocated by institutions that have a protocol of scanning from the patient's left side. Finally, the subxiphoid approach is often proposed as a starting point for the FAST exam so that potentially life-threatening cardiac injuries can be quickly identified. In addition, intracardiac blood can be used as a reference point of an anechoic fluid collection to facilitate adjustment of the overall gain and time gain compensation (TGC). Consequently, there is no standard order for performing the FAST exam and in many instances the order will

be dictated by the patient's clinical presentation and institutional preferences.

Free peritoneal fluid

Fluid (blood) in the trauma patient is usually detected in the dependent areas of the peritoneal cavity including the hepatorenal space (Morison's pouch), the perisplenic space, the pelvis, and the paracolic gutters (Figure 29.11). In general, free fluid appears anechoic (black) and is defined by the borders of the potential spaces it occupies. As an example, free fluid in Morison's pouch will be bounded by Glisson's capsule of the liver anterolaterally and Gerota's fascia of the kidney posteromedially (Figure 29.11). There are a number of variables that affect the appearance and location of fluid within the peritoneal cavity. These include the site of origin of the bleeding, the rate of accumulation, time since the injury, and movement of fluid within the peritoneal cavity.

Minimum amount of fluid

The ability to detect free intraperitoneal fluid by ultrasound was first illustrated in a cadaver study in 1970 that demonstrated that as little as 100 cc of instilled peritoneal fluid was detectable by ultrasound when the body was placed in a hand–knee position and scanned from the abdomen.[27] Additional studies have been done since, including one finding that as little as 10 ml of fluid could be consistently visualized in the pouch of Douglas.[22] The minimal amount of fluid detected by ultrasound depends on a number of factors, most notably, the location of the fluid and

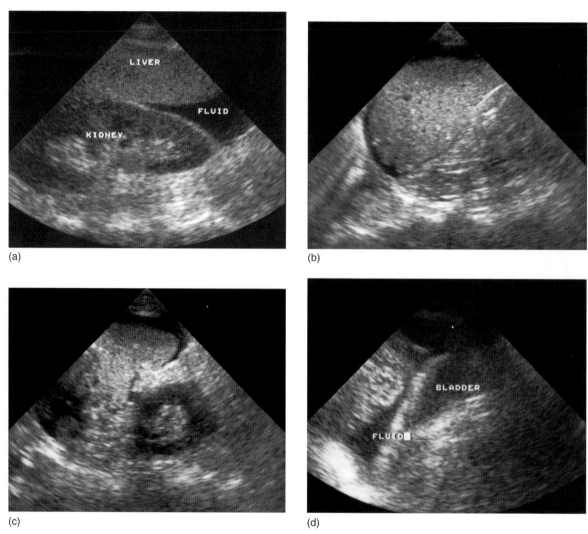

(a)

(b)

(c)

(d)

Figure 29.11 (a) Ultrasound image of blood in Morison's pouch. (b) Fluid visualized in the left subdiaphragmatic space. (c) Fluid seen at the inferior aspect of the spleen. (d) Sagittal orientation of male pelvis demonstrating fluid at the superior aspect of the bladder.

positioning of the patient. Most studies that have assessed the ability of ultrasound to detect minimal volumes of peritoneal fluid have focused on Morison's pouch using a saline infusion model.[22,28] In one study using DPL as a model for intraperitoneal fluid, the mean volume detected in Morison's pouch was 619 ml (standard deviation, 173 ml). Only 10% of the sonographers could detect fluid volumes of 400 ml or less.[28] Using a similar DPL model, another study assessed the minimum volume detected using the pelvic view.[29] They determined that the average minimum detectable volume was 157 ml by one participant and 129 ml by an independent reviewer, thus suggesting that the pelvic view may be more sensitive

than Morison's pouch for small volumes of peritoneal fluid.

Patient positioning has also been studied as a factor in detecting peritoneal fluid. For instance, one study found that the optimal position for detecting minimal volumes of fluid in a cadaver model was right lateral decubitus or facing downward while being supported on both hands and knees.[27] Since neither of these positions is practical for scanning the trauma patient, other positioning has been investigated. For example, a small amount (5°) of Trendelenburg positioning has been shown to statistically increase the sensitivity for detecting peritoneal fluid in the right upper quadrant.[30]

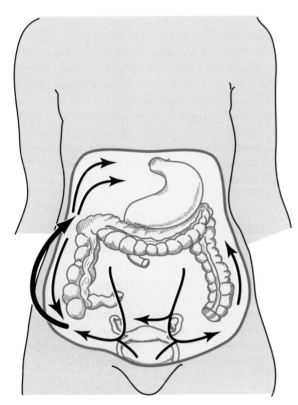

Figure 29.12 Fluid flow patterns.

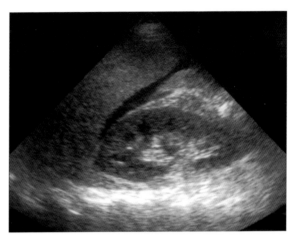

Figure 29.13 Echogenic clot seen in conjunction with free fluid in Morison's pouch.

Lastly, attempts have been made to correlate the width of the fluid stripe in Morison's pouch with intraperitoneal fluid volumes. In a DPL model, a mean stripe width of 1.1 cm was found after 1 L of saline had been instilled.[28] Other studies have proposed that fluid can be seen at similar or even smaller volumes,[31] but how the authors of these studies derived their results is largely unknown and, therefore, unsubstantiated.

Fluid flow patterns

Fluid in the peritoneal cavity collects and spreads in a predictable manner. One study found that in the supine position, the pelvis is the most dependent portion of the peritoneal cavity and that the right paracolic gutter is the main communication between the upper and lower abdominal compartments.[32] Measured flow patterns have shown that fluid tracking up the right paracolic gutter preferentially collects in Morison's pouch before progressing to the right subphrenic space. Interestingly, the phrenicocolic ligament restricts similar flow between the left paracolic gutter to the left upper quadrant, so fluid in the supramesocolic space actually spreads across the midline into the right upper

quadrant. Clinical studies support these findings as the majority of peritoneal fluid collections are detected in the perihepatic region (Figure 29.12).[24,33]

Echogenic hemorrhage and clot

Most fresh peritoneal hemorrhage will appear anechoic, however, as clot forms and organizes, it becomes more echogenic. Clotted blood has a mid-level echo pattern that has some sonographic similarities to tissue, such as the spleen or liver parenchyma (Figure 29.13).

Collections of clotted blood can be found in patients scanned after a prolonged delay or large volumes of peritoneal bleeding. The ability to differentiate clotted peritoneal blood from normal parenchyma can at times be difficult, but in most cases, thorough inspection of the area in question will demonstrate that an anechoic stripe, representing free peritoneal fluid, borders the clotted blood.

Management based on ultrasound and clinical picture

Peritoneal free fluid in the unstable patient

The finding of free peritoneal fluid in the unstable traumatized patient suggests the findings of intraperitoneal injury necessitating immediate operative intervention. The decision to operate will depend on the patient's other injuries, the amount and location of free peritoneal fluid, and whether the vital signs stabilize after resuscitation. Large peritoneal fluid collections associated with unstable vital signs usually mandate laparotomy.[34,35]

Peritoneal free fluid in the stable patient

A patient with stable vital signs, but an ultrasound that demonstrates peritoneal fluid is a candidate for non-operative management. Therefore, regardless of whether any other ultrasound findings such as specific organ injury are present, a CT of the abdomen and pelvis should be performed. This form of management utilizes the strength of the CT scan for determining the source of hemoperitoneum; thus, it can usually differentiate between lesions that are operable vs. those that can be managed non-operatively.

No free fluid in the unstable patient

Ultrasound is extremely sensitive for hemoperitoneum in the hypotensive patient.[36] However, the patient with unstable vital signs and a negative ultrasound remains problematic, since hemoperitoneum remains a lethal, albeit remote, possibility. A few options exist for this diagnostic dilemma. Some have suggested a repeat ultrasound, potentially by a more experienced operator.[37] Others opt for an immediate DPL, which is generally more sensitive than ultrasound. However, a negative ultrasound suggests that the source of hypotension is outside the peritoneum. Diagnostic efforts to identify alternative injuries should focus on other common causes, including retroperitoneal injuries and neurogenic shock. In one study of 47 hypotensive trauma patients with a negative ultrasound, none required a laparotomy for acute control of hemorrhage.[19] The primary cause of hypotension in these patients was extraperitoneal, such as retroperitoneal hemorrhage caused by pelvic fractures or neurogenic shock. If you have a hypotensive patient with a negative ultrasound, a laparotomy, while still a possible need, will be much less likely to be therapeutic. The editors suggest another rapid repeat ultrasound within 5–20 minutes, although the absolute timing is not literature based and dependent on the clinical situation. If clearly negative and all views well visualized, a search for another cause is warranted. If all areas are not completely visualized or inconclusive, a DPL is recommended (unless another obvious source for the hypotension is present).

No free fluid in the stable patient

The finding of no free fluid in a hemodynamically stable patient does not "clear" that patient of injury. Patients may still have encapsulated solid organ injury, mesenteric or bowel injury, retroperitoneal hemorrhage, or delayed intraperitoneal injury. Patients who are at higher risk include those with lower rib, lumbar spine, or pelvic fractures. Prior to discharge, every patient should have a repeat clinical exam and any new findings of abdominal pain, tenderness, distracting injury, or laboratory abnormalities should prompt further diagnostic evaluation, most commonly a CT scan. In this case, management of the patient will be influenced largely by the mechanism of trauma, suspicion of occult injury, and the presence of other injuries.

Indeterminate findings

Certain patients will have indeterminate ultrasound exams. Anatomic defects (pectus excavatum), acquired pathology (open wounds, subcutaneous air), difficult habitus (obesity), and poor acoustic windows (evacuated bladder) are situations that may result in an indeterminate ultrasound exam.[38] These patients should receive further clinical, radiographic, or alternative diagnostic evaluation based on mechanism and clinical findings.

Solid organ injury

The sonographic appearance of specific organ injury varies. The ultrasound appearance of parenchymal damage in the liver or spleen can appear as anechoic or echogenic distortion of the normal architecture and manifestations of injury can include subcapsular fluid collections and intraperitoneal fluid (Figure 29.14).

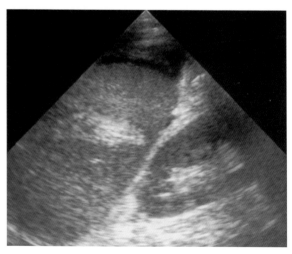

Figure 29.14 Splenic injury visualized sonographically as a discrete area of increased echogenicity.

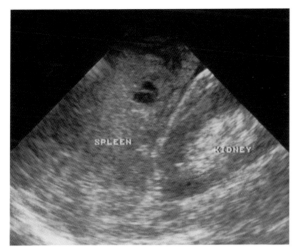

Figure 29.15 Splenic injury manifested as hypoechoic sonographic pattern.

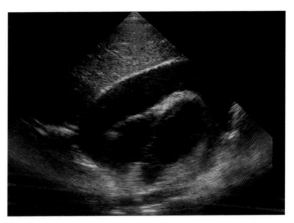

Figure 29.16 Pericardial fluid outlining the cardiac structures.

The most common pattern of parenchymal injury identified by ultrasonography in patients with blunt abdominal trauma is a discrete region of increased echoes followed by a diffuse hyperechoic pattern (Figure 29.15).

The clinical utility of positive and negative sonographic examinations for specific organ injuries is limited. Some studies have inferred that a negative exam, in certain patients, is sufficient to change medical decision making.[39,40] Each of these studies recommended that ultrasound be the initial diagnostic modality for evaluating patients with renal trauma. If a stable, normotensive patient has a normal renal ultrasound, no hematuria, and no other significant injuries, then their evaluation was complete. There have been no similar recommendations for the ultrasound evaluation of other organs.

A positive result, on the other hand, may direct certain aspects of the diagnostic evaluation. For instance, in most series, a positive ultrasound exam in a hemodynamically stable patient is an indication for additional diagnostic testing. Commonly this is a CT scan of the abdomen and pelvis, which provides specific information regarding the extent and severity of the organ injuries. Another benefit is that CT scanning can determine whether there are injuries to other organs.

The identification of solid organ injury in the hemodynamically unstable patient provides very little useful information. If a specific etiology for the hypotension is not identified, yet the patient has free intraperitoneal fluid, invariably the patient will undergo laparotomy or occasionally an urgent angiogram. Knowing that a specific organ injury exists does not change the approach, technique, or decision making in hemodynamically unstable patients. Another important issue is that ultrasound is poor at identifying injuries to multiple organs, so there is no assurance that an injury identified sonographically is the primary or only etiology of the instability. As a result, there are no widely recognized algorithms that include the presence or absence of specific organ injury identified by ultrasound into clinical decision making.

Pericardial effusion

Hemorrhage can accumulate quickly in the potential space between the visceral and parietal pericardium and create hypotension due to a cascade of increasing intrapericardial pressure leading to a lack of right heart filling followed by decreased left ventricular stroke volume. Fluid in the pericardial space appears as an anechoic stripe that conforms to the outline of the cardiac structures (Figure 29.16). In most cases, the fluid should have the same anechoic character as blood within the cardiac chambers. From the subxiphoid orientation, fluid will initially be seen between the right side of the heart and the liver, which is the most dependent area visualized (Figure 29.17). In the parasternal orientation, fluid may also be seen anteriorly and superior to the right ventricle or posteriorly as it outlines the free wall of the left atria and ventricle (Figure 29.18).

Cardiac tamponade

After determining that a pericardial effusion is present, the next step is to determine whether there is

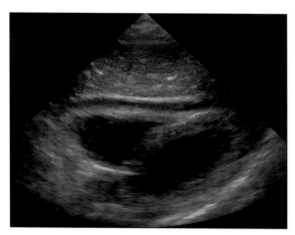

Figure 29.17 Ultrasound image taken from the subxiphoid transducer position demonstrating fluid in the pericardial space.

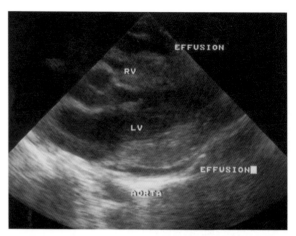

Figure 29.18 Parasternal long axis view of the heart showing fluid in the pericardial space.

sonographic evidence of cardiac tamponade. The pathophysiology of tamponade is characterized by increasing pericardial pressure that eventually exceeds atrial and ventricular pressures, thus inhibiting cardiac filling. As pericardial pressure increases, there is sequential collapse of the right atrium and subsequently the right ventricle Although the right atrial collapse occurs sooner than right ventricular collapse, this finding is less specific for diagnosing tamponade.[41] Another potentially helpful sonographic finding is bowing of the interventricular septum into the left ventricle. This late finding is very specific for tamponade.[42]

An additional means of assessing for elevated central venous pressure is to image the inferior vena cava. One method is the "sniff test," in which the patient is instructed to inhale quickly through his or her nose while the examiner simultaneously visualizes the inferior vena cava. Two studies have shown that incomplete collapse (< 40%) of the inferior vena cava correlates well with elevated central venous pressure measurements.[43,44]

Pleural fluid

The detection of hemothorax in a supine trauma patient can be problematic as the supine portable chest radiograph is insensitive for small fluid collections. Ultrasound, on the other hand, has been estimated to detect as little as 20 ml of pleural fluid.[45] Ultrasound may be useful for the detection of hemothorax in both blunt and penetrating thoracic trauma; however, this is an evolving standard that has

not yet been widely accepted.[46–48] Pleural fluid detected during trauma ultrasound should be interpreted in the clinical context of the effusion. Patients with decreased breath sounds, evidence of chest trauma, hypoxemia, hypotension, or other findings suggestive of tension hemothorax, may be aided by the sonographic findings of fluid in the pleural space. Decompression and evacuation procedures should then proceed. However, an ultrasound exam that does not demonstrate pleural fluid should not be interpreted as eliminating traumatic pleural effusion from the differential, especially in the patient with blunt chest trauma.[48]

Pneumothorax

The use of ultrasound to evaluate for pneumothorax in trauma decision making is evolving. At this time, it is an adjunctive technique that may identify pneumothorax earlier than chest radiography, especially in the supine patient or those with small pneumothoraces. Several studies provide support for the use of ultrasound to detect or exclude pneumothorax in the trauma patient.[49,50] In one study, a single ultrasound exam of the anterior thorax was 95% sensitive and 100% specific for pneumothoraces that were detected by chest radiography.[49] A second study found similar results,[50] adding weight to this conclusion. Standard radiographs for the detection of pneumothorax may be limited by patient position. Air that collects anteriorly or inferiorly, rather than in the apices, may be difficult to appreciate on a supine chest radiograph. Several studies suggest, in fact, that ultrasound

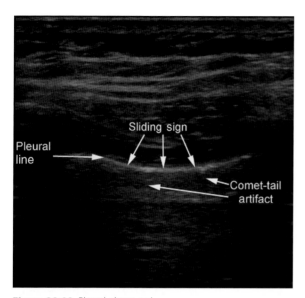

Figure 29.19 Pleural ultrasound.

exceeds plain X-ray in its ability to detect pneumo-thorax, and nearly matches that of chest CT. Using chest CT as a gold standard, or air rush from chest tube in patients suspected of having tension pneumo-thorax where obtaining a chest CT would not be feasible, the sensitivity and specificity of ultrasound for pneumothorax as compared to CT approaches 100%.[51–54] Ultrasound findings that suggest pneumo-thorax include the absence of a *sliding sign* or *comet tail* artifact (Figure 29.19). These findings should be followed by clinical correlation of breath sounds and chest radiography. Ultrasound is probably most useful in its negative predictive value. In other words, if the ultrasound exam performed by an experienced sonographer is interpreted as negative for pneumo-thorax, the diagnosis can be excluded or considered less likely.

Testicular

Testicular fracture and testicular infarction are the principal concerns in patients presenting with either blunt or penetrating testicular trauma. A testicular fracture occurs when the integrity of the tunica albu-ginea is disrupted. The pathophysiology of testicular rupture is similar to that of a ruptured optic globe. If struck with sufficient force the internal pressure within the testicle exceeds that of the structural resist-ance integrity of the tunica albuginea, with leakage of its internal contents. Sonographically the perimeter of the testicle is often non-contiguous and irregular,

with a hemorrhagic region at the area of the fracture. A hematocele may be present and can be difficult to distinguish from testicular tissue. A hematocele in the patient with acute scrotal trauma may be an indirect indicator of a testicular fracture, much like free fluid in the trauma exam may represent a solid organ injury. Testicular fracture and its associated findings represent a surgical emergency, as testicular function and fertility may be lost if the testicle is not repaired. The suspicion of a testicular fracture should prompt expeditious urologic and potentially further radio-logical evaluation.

Obstetric patients

The use of ultrasound for the diagnostic evaluation of the pregnant blunt trauma patient has the benefits of not exposing the mother and fetus to ionizing radi-ation and invasive procedures while also being able to assess for peritoneal fluid and fetal viability.[55–57] The primary application of trauma ultrasound in the preg-nant patient is no different than that in the non-pregnant patient, which is the non-invasive evaluation of the peritoneal and thoracic cavities for blood. While the peritoneal anatomy will change in preg-nancy, especially in the late second and third trimes-ters, the FAST exam technique is the same and fluid is still readily identifiable in the standard potential spaces.

Another useful application of ultrasound in the pregnant trauma patient is the assessment of fetal gestational age and fetal cardiac activity. In later preg-nancy, the easiest estimation of gestational age is obtained by measuring the biparietal diameter. This has increased utility as the pregnancy is in the second trimester. Although there is some institutional vari-ation, fetuses > 24 weeks gestational age are con-sidered "viable." Fetal cardiac activity should be assessed for presence and rate as bradycardia is a marker of fetal distress caused by poor perfusion or hypoxia. Blood may be shunted away from the fetus before the mother exhibits obvious signs of hypotension.

Pediatric patients

One of the primary roles of emergency sonography of pediatric patients is blunt abdominal trauma. While the finding of peritoneal fluid is a similar primary goal for adult and pediatric patients, results have been somewhat discouraging for the latter.[58–63] This is surprising, since one of the limitations of sonography, obesity, is encountered much less commonly in pediatric patients. Although the sensitivity is reported to be lower in pediatric patients, the specificity is still excellent (95% [93–97%]).[64]

Even more discouraging have been the pediatric studies citing the accuracy of ultrasound in the evaluation of solid organ injury. Little useful information can be gleaned from an ultrasound to evaluate the solid organs; CT is far superior in this regard.

The role of ultrasound in pediatric blunt abdominal trauma is limited by the non-operative management of solid organ injuries in children. While ultrasound may detect free peritoneal fluid, this information has little impact on management since CT and clinical observation will determine the course of action in pediatric patients with splenic and liver injuries. An exception to this is the hypotensive patient with blunt abdominal trauma; in this population the sensitivity and specificity of FAST have been shown to be as high as 100%.[65]

Ultrasound-guided procedures

Vascular access

Ultrasound may be useful to facilitate vascular access in the trauma patient. It can be used to guide both peripheral and central venous access. For patients in whom peripheral access cannot be obtained, ultrasound can be used to localize venous structures for cannulation, such as the deep brachial, basilic, or cephalic veins. This problem is most commonly encountered secondary to obesity, edema, intravenous drug use, peripheral vasoconstriction, or hypovolemia.

It has been clearly demonstrated that the use of ultrasound to guide the insertion of central venous catheters increases the likelihood of first-pass success, decreases the total number of attempts before successful placement, and decreases the frequency of complications, including arterial puncture, pneumothorax, and catheter malposition.[66] This technique is valuable when surface landmarks are obscured (e.g., obesity or edema), or in the setting of hypovolemia, where traditional, landmark-based approaches are more likely to fail or require multiple attempts.

Localization of foreign bodies

Ultrasound may be used to detect soft tissue foreign bodies, and if a foreign body is known to exist in a

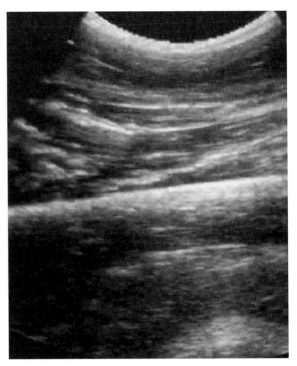

Figure 29.20 Solid line in middle of field represents the anterior humeral cortex.

wound, ultrasound may aid in its localization and removal. A linear probe should be used, with the depth range adjusted to the suspected depth of the foreign body. For irregular surfaces, small body parts, very painful areas, or superficial wounds, a water bath may be used to improve the ultrasound image;[67] the body part may be immersed in water, and the ultrasound probe placed in the water directed at the area of interest (all modern ultrasound transducers are watertight). Using this technique, it is not necessary to directly make contact with the skin over the area of interest, as the interposed water itself acts as a conducting medium. This may be particularly useful for evaluation of wounds on the hands and feet, common locations for foreign bodies.

Generally, plain X-ray is superior to ultrasound for identification of radiopaque soft tissue foreign bodies.[68] However, ultrasound has been demonstrated to have some utility at detecting radiolucent soft tissue foreign bodies, particularly those made of wood. Estimates of the sensitivity and specificity of ultrasound for the detection of soft tissue foreign bodies are highly variable. In general, ultrasound can be used as an additional tool, but may not be

Table 29.2 Glossary of commonly used terms

Acoustic window	Structure that is used to visualize deeper structures, e.g., bladder
Anechoic	Structure or tissue that does not reflect ultrasound signals; appearance is dark/black on ultrasound display
Artifact	A display phenomenon not truly representing anatomic features of structure(s) being imaged
Comet-tail artifact	Tapered vertical bright stripe originating from the pleural line; seen in normal pleural ultrasound
Echogenic	Structure or tissue that reflects ultrasound signals; appearance ranges from grey to white on ultrasound display
Far field	Portion of ultrasound image towards the bottom of the screen; corresponds to tissues farthest from the ultrasound transducer
Near field	Portion of ultrasound image at the top of the screen; corresponds to tissues closest to the ultrasound transducer
Probe	See **Transducer**
Shadow	Area of darkness seen behind structures or tissues that are very dense and strongly reflect ultrasound signals (e.g., gallstones, bone)
Sliding sign	Bright granular-appearing moving line seen along pleural line in normal pleural ultrasound; represents sliding of apposed visceral and parietal pleura during respiration
Transducer	Synonym for probe; portion of ultrasound machine that is applied to patient's body; both transmits and receives ultrasound signal. Many different transducer shapes and frequency ranges are available for various applications

sufficiently reliable to be used as the only modality, to screen for soft tissue foreign bodies.[67–71]

Fracture identification

It has been shown that ultrasound can be used to identify bony fractures, particularly of the long bones.[72,73] However, given the usual ready availability of plain X-ray in most EDs, the only real advantage would be to rapidly identify long bone fractures as the cause of hypotension when the clinical exam may be unclear, or to rapidly triage multiple patients in mass casualty situations when they have displaced fractures not clinically evident. Ultrasound is most likely to offer advantages for this application in remote areas where plain radiographs cannot be easily obtained or potentially in field triage of disasters or military conflicts (Figure 29.20).

Triage of multiple patients or disaster situations

Ultrasound has qualities, such as being quick, non-invasive, portable, and sensitive, that make it an ideal imaging modality for the evaluation of large numbers of traumatically injured patients. In trauma centers it is not unusual to experience the simultaneous presentation of multiple, potentially critically injured patients. The impact of decisions regarding patient priority for the operating room, CT scan, or procedural intervention is magnified when resources are stretched to their limits. One study demonstrated that the results of a FAST exam could be used to determine patient priority for operative intervention.[74] Others have incorporated an ultrasound exam into the evaluation of patients sustaining injuries on the battlefield and during a natural disaster.[75,76] See Table 29.2 for a glossary of commonly used terms.

References

1. Accreditation Council for Graduate Medical Education. *Emergency Medicine Guidelines.* Available from http://www.acgme.org/acWebsite/RRC_110/110_guidelines.asp.
2. Salen PN, Melanson SW, Heller MB. The focused abdominal sonography for trauma (FAST) examination: considerations and recommendations for training physicians in the use of a new clinical tool. *Acad Emerg Med* 2000;7:162–8.
3. Shackford SR, Rogers FB, Osler TM, et al. Focused abdominal sonogram for trauma: the learning curve of nonradiologist clinicians in detecting hemoperitoneum. *J Trauma* 1999;46:553–64.
4. American College of Emergency Physicians. ACEP emergency ultrasound guidelines-2001. *Ann Emerg Med* 2001;38:470–81.
5. Thomas B, Falcone RE, Vasquez D, et al. Ultrasound evaluation of blunt abdominal trauma: program

implementation, initial experience, and learning curve. *J Trauma* 1997;**42**:384–90.

6. Staren ED, Knudson MM, Rozycki GS, et al. An evaluation of the American College of Surgeons' ultrasound education program. *Am J Surg* 2006;**191**:489–96.

7. Ma OJ, Gaddis G, Steele MT, et al. Prospective analysis of the effect of physician experience with the FAST examination in reducing the use of CT scans. *Emerg Med Australs* 2005;**17**:24–30.

8. Jang T, Aubin C, Naunheim R. Minimum training for right upper quadrant ultrasonography. *Am J Emerg Med* 2004;**22**:439–43.

9. Jang T, Sineff S, Naunheim R, Aubin C. Residents should not independently perform focused abdominal sonography for trauma after 10 training examinations. *J Ultrasound Med* 2004;**23**:793–7.

10. Gracias VH, Frankel HL, Gupta R, et al. Defining the learning curve for the focused abdominal sonogram for trauma (FAST) examination: implications for credentialing. *Am Surg* 2001;**67**:364–7.

11. Olsen WR, Hildreth DH. Abdominal paracentesis and peritoneal lavage in blunt abdominal trauma. *J Trauma* 1971;**11**:824–9.

12. Powell DC, Bivins BA, Bell RM. Diagnostic peritoneal lavage. *Surg Gynecol Obstet* 1982;**155**:257–63.

13. Gruessner R, Mentges B, Duber C, et al. Sonography versus peritoneal lavage in blunt abdominal trauma. *J Trauma* 1989;**29**:242–4.

14. Bode PJ, Niezen RA, van Vugt AB, Schipper J. Abdominal ultrasound as a reliable indicator for conclusive laparotomy in blunt abdominal trauma. *J Trauma* 1993;**34**:27–31.

15. Glaser K, Tschmelitsch J, Klingler P, et al. Ultrasonography in the management of blunt abdominal and thoracic trauma. *Arch Surg* 1994;**129**:743–7.

16. McKenney M, Lentz K, Nunez D, et al. Can ultrasound replace diagnostic peritoneal lavage in the assessment of blunt trauma? *J Trauma* 1994;**37**:439–41.

17. Lentz KA, McKenney MG, Nunez DB, Jr., Martin L. Evaluating blunt abdominal trauma:role for ultrasonography. *J Ultrasound Med* 1996; **15**:447–51.

18. Porter RS, Nester BA, Dalsey WC, et al. Use of ultrasound to determine need for laparotomy in trauma patients. *Ann Emerg Med* 1997; **29**:323–30.

19. Wherrett LJ, Boulanger BR, McLellan BA, et al. Hypotension after blunt abdominal trauma: the role of emergent abdominal sonography in surgical triage. *J Trauma* 1996;**41**:815–20.

20. Asher WM, Parvin S, Virgillo RW, Haber K. Echographic evaluation of splenic injury after blunt trauma. *Radiology* 1976;**118**:411–15.

21. Scalea TM, Rodriguez A, Chiu WC, et al. Focused assessment with sonography for trauma (FAST): results from an international consensus conference. *J Trauma* 1999;**46**:466–72.

22. Forsby J, Henriksson L. Detectability of intraperitoneal fluid by ultrasonography. an experimental investigation. *Acta Radiol Diagn (Stockh)* 1984; **25**:375–8.

23. Blaivas M, DeBehnke D, Phelan MB. Potential errors in the diagnosis of pericardial effusion on trauma ultrasound for penetrating injuries. *Acad Emerg Med* 2000;**7**:1261–6.

24. Ma OJ, Kefer MP, Mateer JR, Thoma B. Evaluation of hemoperitoneum using a single- vs multiple-view ultrasonographic examination. *Acad Emerg Med* 1995;**2**:581–6.

25. Rozycki GS, Ochsner MG, Feliciano DV, et al. Early detection of hemoperitoneum by ultrasound examination of the right upper quadrant: a multicenter study. *J Trauma* 1998;**45**:878–83.

26. Jehle D, Guarino J, Karamanoukian H. Emergency department ultrasound in the evaluation of blunt abdominal trauma. *Am J Emerg Med* 1993;**11**:342–6.

27. Goldberg BB, Goodman GA, Clearfield HR. Evaluation of ascites by ultrasound. *Radiology* 1970;**96**:15–22.

28. Branney SW, Wolfe RE, Moore EE, et al. Quantitative sensitivity of ultrasound in detecting free intraperitoneal fluid. *J Trauma* 1995;**39**:375–80.

29. Von Kuenssberg Jehle D, Stiller G, Wagner D. Sensitivity in detecting free intraperitoneal fluid with the pelvic views of the FAST exam. *Am J Emerg Med* 2003;**21**:476–8.

30. Abrams BJ, Sukumvanich P, Seibel R, et al. Ultrasound for the detection of intraperitoneal fluid: the role of Trendelenburg positioning. *Am J Emerg Med* 1999;**17**:117–20.

31. Goletti O, Ghiselli G, Lippolis PV, et al. The role of ultrasonography in blunt abdominal trauma: results in 250 consecutive cases. *J Trauma* 1994;**36**:178–81.

32. Meyers MA. The spread and localization of acute intraperitoneal effusions. *Radiology* 1970;**95**:547–54.

33. Hahn DD, Offerman SR, Holmes JF. Clinical importance of intraperitoneal fluid in patients with blunt intra-abdominal injury. *Am J Emerg Med* 2002;**20**:595–600.

34. Ma OJ, Kefer MP, Stevison KF, Mateer JR. Operative versus nonoperative management of blunt abdominal trauma: role of ultrasound-measured intraperitoneal fluid levels. *Am J Emerg Med* 2001;**19**:284–6.

35. McKenney KL, McKenney MG, Cohn SM, et al. Hemoperitoneum score helps determine need for therapeutic laparotomy. *J Trauma* 2001;**50**:650–6.

36. Rozycki GS, Ballard RB, Feliciano DV, et al. Surgeon-performed ultrasound for the assessment of truncal injuries: lessons learned from 1540 patients. *Ann Surg* 1998;**228**:557–67.

37. Forster R, Pillasch J, Zielke A, et al. Ultrasonography in blunt abdominal trauma: influence of the investigators' experience. *J Trauma* 1993;**34**:264–9.

38. Boulanger BR, Brenneman FD, Kirkpatrick AW, et al. The indeterminate abdominal sonogram in multisystem blunt trauma. *J Trauma* 1998; **45**:52–6.

39. Furtschegger A, Egender G, Jakse G. The value of sonography in the diagnosis and follow-up of patients with blunt renal trauma. *Br J Urol* 1988;**62**:110–16.

40. Rosales A, Arango O, Coronado J, et al. The use of ultrasonography as the initial diagnostic exploration in blunt renal trauma. *Urol Int* 1992;**48**:134–7.

41. Singh S, Wann LS, Schuchard GH, et al. Right ventricular and right atrial collapse in patients with cardiac tamponade–a combined echocardiographic and hemodynamic study. *Circulation* 1984;**70**:966–71.

42. Reddy PS, Curtiss EI, Uretsky BF. Spectrum of hemodynamic changes in cardiac tamponade. *Am J Cardiol* 1990;**66**:1487–91.

43. Moreno FL, Hagan AD, Holmen JR, et al. Evaluation of size and dynamics of the inferior vena cava as an index of right-sided cardiac function. *Am J Cardiol* 1984;**53**:579–85.

44. Kircher BJ, Himelman RB, Schiller NB. Noninvasive estimation of right atrial pressure from the inspiratory collapse of the inferior vena cava. *Am J Cardiol* 1990;**66**:493–6.

45. Rothlin MA, Naf R, Amgwerd M, et al. Ultrasound in blunt abdominal and thoracic trauma. *J Trauma* 1993;**34**:488–95.

46. Sisley AC, Rozycki GS, Ballard RB, et al. Rapid detection of traumatic effusion using surgeon-performed ultrasonography. *J Trauma* 1998;**44**:291–7.

47. Ma OJ, Mateer JR. Trauma ultrasound examination versus chest radiography in the detection of hemothorax. *Ann Emerg Med* 1997;**29**:312–16.

48. Abboud PA, Kendall J. Emergency department ultrasound for hemothorax after blunt traumatic injury. *J Emerg Med* 2003;**25**:181–4.

49. Dulchavsky SA, Schwarz KL, Kirkpatrick AW, et al. Prospective evaluation of thoracic ultrasound in the detection of pneumothorax. *J Trauma* 2001; **50**:201–5.

50. Knudtson JL, Dort JM, Helmer SD, Smith RS. Surgeon-performed ultrasound for pneumothorax in the trauma suite. *J Trauma* 2004;**56**:527–30.

51. Rowan KR, Kirkpatrick AW, Liu D, et al. Traumatic pneumothorax detection with thoracic US: correlation with chest radiography and CT-initial experience. *Radiology* 2002;**225**(1):210–14.

52. Blaivas M, Lyon M, Duggal S. A prospective comparison of supine chest radiography and bedside ultrasound for the diagnosis of traumatic pneumothorax. *Acad Emerg Med* 2005;**12**(9):844–9.

53. Soldati G, Testa A, Sher S, et al. Occult traumatic pneumothorax: diagnostic accuracy of lung ultrasonography in the emergency department. *Chest* 2008;**133**(1):204–11.

54. Zhang M, Liu ZH, Yang JX, et al. Rapid detection of pneumothorax by ultrasonography in patients with multiple trauma. *Crit Care* 2006;**10**(4):R112.

55. Bochicchio GV, Haan J, Scalea TM. Surgeon-performed focused assessment with sonography for trauma as an early screening tool for pregnancy after trauma. *J Trauma* 2002;**52**:1125–8.

56. Ma OJ, Mateer JR, DeBehnke DJ. Use of ultrasonography for the evaluation of pregnant trauma patients. *J Trauma* 1996;**40**:665–8.

57. Goodwin H, Holmes JF, Wisner DH. Abdominal ultrasound examination in pregnant blunt trauma patients. *J Trauma* 2001;**50**:689–93.

58. Thourani VH, Pettitt BJ, Schmidt JA, et al. Validation of surgeon-performed emergency abdominal ultrasonography in pediatric trauma patients. *J Pediatr Surg* 1998;**33**:322–8.

59. Partrick DA, Bensard DD, Moore EE, et al. Ultrasound is an effective triage tool to evaluate blunt abdominal trauma in the pediatric population. *J Trauma* 1998;**45**:57–63.

60. Coley BD, Mutabagani KH, Martin LC, et al. Focused abdominal sonography for trauma (FAST) in children with blunt abdominal trauma. *J Trauma* 2000;**48**:902–6.

61. Emery KH, McAneney CM, Racadio JM, et al. Absent peritoneal fluid on screening trauma ultrasonography in children: a prospective comparison with computed tomography. *J Pediatr Surg* 2001;**36**:565–9.

62. Holmes JF, Brant WE, Bond WF, et al. Emergency department ultrasonography in the evaluation of hypotensive and normotensive children with blunt abdominal trauma. *J Pediatr Surg* 2001;**36**:968–73.

63. Ong AW, McKenney MG, McKenney KA, et al. Predicting the need for laparotomy in pediatric trauma patients on the basis of the ultrasound score. *J Trauma* 2003;**54**:503–8.

64. Holmes JF, Gladman A, Chang CH. Performance of abdominal ultrasonography in pediatric blunt trauma patients: a meta-analysis. *J Ped Surg* 2007;**42**:1588–94.

65. Holmes JF, Brant WE, Bond WF, Sokolove PE, Kuppermann N. Emergency department ultrasonography in the evaluation of hypotensive and normotensive children with blunt abdominal trauma. *J Pediatr Surg* 2001;**36**(7):968–73.

66. Hind D, Calvert N, McWilliams R, et al. Ultrasonic locating devices for central venous cannulation: meta-analysis. *BMJ* 2003;**327**:361–70.

67. Blaivas M, Lyon M, Brannam L, et al. Water bath evaluation technique for emergency ultrasound of painful superficial structures. *Am J Emerg Med* 2004;**22**(7):589–93.

68. Manthey D, Storrow A, Milbourn J, Wagner B. Ultrasound versus radiography in the detection of soft-tissue foreign bodies. *Ann Emerg Med* 1996;**28**(1):7–9.

69. Schlager D, Sanders A, Wiggins D, Boren W. Ultrasound for the detection of foreign bodies. *Ann of Emerg Med* 1991;**20**(2):189–91.

70. Hill R, Conron R, Greissinger P, Heller M. Ultrasound for the detection of foreign bodies in human tissue. *Ann Emerg Med* 1997;**29**(3):353–6.

71. Orlinsky M, Knittel P, Feit T, Chan L, Mandavia D. The comparative accuracy of radiolucent foreign body detection using ultrasonography. *Am J Emerg Med* 2000;**18**(4):401–3.

72. Marshburn TH, Legome E, Sargsyan A, et al. Goal-directed ultrasound in the detection of long-bone fractures. *J Trauma* 2004;**57**:329–32.

73. Tayal VS, Antoniazzi J, Pariyadath M, Norton HJ. Prospective use of ultrasound imaging to detect bony hand injuries in adults. *J Ultrasound Med* 2007;**26**:1143–8.

74. Blaivas M. Triage in the trauma bay with the focused abdominal sonography for trauma (FAST) examination. *J Emerg Med* 2001;**21**:41–4.

75. Miletic D, Fuckar Z, Mraovic B, et al. Ultrasonography in the evaluation of hemoperitoneum in war casualties. *Mil Med* 1999;**164**:600–2.

76. Sarkisian AE, Khondkarian RA, Amirbekian NM, et al. Sonographic screening of mass casualties for abdominal and renal injuries following the 1988 Armenian earthquake. *J Trauma* 1991;**31**:247–50.

Chapter 30

Computed tomography

Sassan Naderi and Mark Bernstein

Introduction

Computed tomography (CT) has become the primary imaging tool in the evaluation of the hemodynamically stable trauma patient. Since its inception in the 1970s, CT has challenged nearly all previously held gold standards in the assessment of the acutely injured patient. Computed tomography began as a non-invasive tool to look for intracranial hemorrhage; a role previously performed by angiography which looked at cerebrovacular displacement as a marker of mass effect. Non-invasive intracranial imaging was now possible to diagnose and exclude hemorrhage and herniation.

By the early 1980s, emergency CT had revolutionized the assessment of traumatic brain injury. Advancement in CT technology allowed greater data acquisition at greater speed and by the mid 1980s leading trauma centers began scanning patients to evaluate for blunt abdominal injuries. Early experience found CT to be highly sensitive, specific, and accurate for diagnosing traumatic injury. Computed tomography dramatically reduced the need for exploratory laparotomy and eliminated the use of radionuclide imaging and abdominal aortography for diagnosis.[1] While CT's role in trauma looked promising, further progress was necessary before comprehensive imaging of the polytrauma patient could be performed in a single visit to the CT suite.

A technological leap for CT came in the late 1980s with the introduction of helical, or spiral, CT. Helical CT was made possible with the advent of the slip-ring gantry design. This technology permitted non-stop X-ray tube and detector rotation while the patient traveled through the CT gantry in one continuous motion generating a helical "volume" of image data. Volumetric acquisition permitted the off-axial evaluation of image information with multiplanar reformations and three-dimensional (3D) reconstructions. Unmatched speed of acquisition and advances in computer technology markedly dropped scan times and provided greater coverage in a single breath hold. Faster microprocessors enabled prompt image reconstruction, so the acutely injured patient could be imaged in a relatively brief period of time. Helical CT quickly became the preferred method to evaluate the thorax and abdomen, as well as vascular structures, particularly the aorta.

By 1998, the multidetector era arrived with the creation of the four-detector CT scanners, collecting four slices of data in a single revolution. One of the hallmarks of the multidetector CT (MDCT) is its rapid acquisition of image data. Total body scanning times have been reduced to < 30 seconds. The advantage of rapid scanning allows one to scan multiple body parts in the polytrauma patient, making larger patient coverage possible in a single breath hold with improved spatial and temporal resolution.

Greater spatial resolution with submillimeter slice thickness allows exquisite multiplanar reconstructions and 3D reconstructions. Three-dimensional images from volume-acquired datasets provide additional information with enhanced diagnostic accuracy, and allow one to better visualize complex injuries such as facial and pelvic fractures. The improved temporal resolution allows reduction in intravenous (IV) contrast material because scan time is reduced. Moreover, power injectors for IV contrast material and faster scanning techniques can optimize the delivery of contrast and more precisely separate arterial and venous phase imaging. The result is dynamic imaging which has stimulated the evolution of CT angiography in trauma.

Trauma: A Comprehensive Emergency Medicine Approach, eds. Eric Legome and Lee W. Shockley. Published by Cambridge University Press. © Cambridge University Press 2011.

The subsequent advance of MDCT technology has brought forth the newest "extreme" MDCT scanners with 32-, 40-, 64-, and 128-detectors; 256- and 320-detectors are in development. While the increased number of detectors is correlated with increased dose efficiency, the actual radiation dose required to stimulate the multiple detectors, however, is increased by about 27% within the plane of the image as compared with single slice CT.[2] Newer scanners contain several features that work in real time to adjust the dose depending on the thickness and tissue type presented to the scanner. Thus, scanning through the air-filled lungs would require less radiation than scanning through the same patient's much denser shoulders.

The era of extreme MDCT scanning has changed the way we image patients. Technology that had strictly been one of depicting anatomy has become one now able to display function. Extreme MDCT scanners boast greater anatomical coverage with unparalleled temporal resolution allowing assessment of organ perfusion and even gated cardiac motion with quantitative measurements. Cerebral perfusion studies on brain-injured patients may be able to predict prognosis. "Cardiac contusion," a potentially significant injury that has long escaped an imaging diagnosis, may one day be identified and quantified by MDCT. The future of MDCT technology in evaluating the multitrauma patient is only beginning to be realized (Table 30.1).

Role of CT

Widespread availability of MDCT has revolutionized the screening of blunt and penetrating trauma victims. Computed tomography evaluation provides important information for the evaluation and management of the multitrauma patient. Precise localization and extent of organ injury and presence of hemorrhage can be determined with increasing confidence. Contrast-enhanced MDCT can indicate the presence of vascular injury including active arterial extravasation or traumatic pseudoaneurysm formation. Injuries such as high-grade hepatic or splenic lacerations that previously would have mandated surgical exploration may now be managed by observation with close monitoring utilizing repeat CT evaluation or angiographic assessment for potential intervention. Multidetector CT also plays a major role in the follow up of the trauma patient, determining injury resolution or progression and identifying potential complications.

Table 30.1 Basic computed tomography (CT) terminology

Terminology	Definition
Source/detectors	Source is the production unit of the scanner that produces the radiation that passes through the subject. After passing through the patient this radiation is then picked up by the detector. The variation in the radiation returning to the detector then allows for the reconstruction of a three-dimensional image. In helical CT the X-ray sources are attached to a freely rotating gantry. Multislice CT scanners contain multiple detector rings (4, 8, 16, 32, 40, and 64 detector rings) with increasing rotation speeds
Dose efficiency	The fraction of primary X-rays reaching the patient that contribute to the image. This is made of two components: geometric efficiency (amount of X-rays leaving the patient and interacting with active detector areas) and absorption efficiency (fraction of actually-captured X-rays interacting with active detector areas)
Volumetric acquisition	Acquiring data about three-dimensional space. This is in contrast to planar acquisition which describes data acquired about two-dimensional space
Collimation	Slice thickness
Hounsfield units	The scale used to describe the radiodensity (attenuation) of an object. The Hounsfield unit (HU) scale defines the radiodensity of distilled water at standard pressure and temperature (STP) as 0 HU, while the radiodensity of air at STP is defined as −1000 HU and ranges to high-density bone at +1000 HU

While history and clinical examination are crucial to evaluate hemodynamic status, determine life- and limb-threatening trauma, and assess mechanisms and patterns of injury, internal injuries may escape detection. A decreased level of consciousness or distracting injury may limit clinical assessment in the multitrauma patient. Contrast-enhanced MDCT is therefore extremely beneficial for injury screening in the hemodynamically stable blunt or penetrating trauma patient with concern for underlying injury.

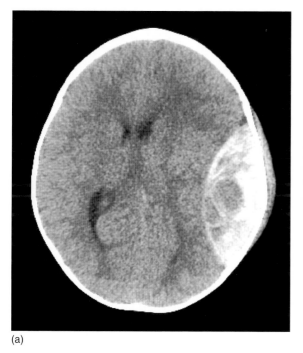
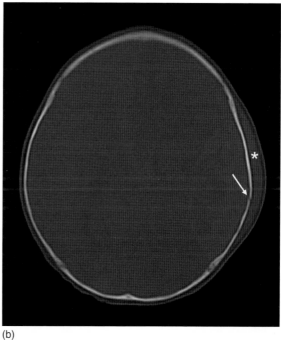

(a)   (b)

Figure 30.1 Epidural hematoma. Pediatric trauma after falling from window sill shows large left biconvex mixed density epidural hematoma (EDH): (a) The mixed density represents both clotted and unclotted blood, implying ongoing bleeding. Overlying skull fracture shown in (b) (arrow). Note the EDH occurs at the impact site as shown by the subgaleal hematoma (*).

Craniocerebral trauma

In the United States there are almost 8 million incidents per year of head trauma, with 500 000 considered severe. The majority of deaths from motor vehicle collisions and falls occur secondary to head trauma. Alcohol further increases the risk of traumatic brain injury. Fortunately, however, the routine use of seat belts, airbags, and helmets has brought about a decline in the incidence of these injuries.[3]

The primary goal in managing severe head injury patients is to preserve life and neurologic function. The secondary goal is to identify and treat intracranial lesions that will negatively affect outcome. Consequently, patients presenting to the emergency department (ED) with acute neurological deficits or a significant history of head trauma require imaging. Three imaging modalities exist: skull radiographs, CT, and magnetic resonance imaging (MRI). Computed tomography, the most practical and cost-effective imaging, is the method of choice for rapid, accurate evaluation of intracranial trauma.

Non-contrast CT is excellent for detection of traumatic intracranial pathology, including epidural hematoma (Figure 30.1), subdural hematoma (Figure 30.2), subarachnoid hemorrhage (Figure 30.3), cerebral contusion (Figure 30.4), diffuse axonal injury (Figure 30.5), cerebral edema (Figure 30.6), herniation (Figure 30.7), and infarction.

Scalp

The scalp and galea are separated from the skull by loose connective tissue. This potential subgaleal space provides an area for hemorrhage and pus accumulation. Subgaleal hematomas and scalp contusions are useful in localizing the point of contact with the calvarium, defining coup vs. contrecoup injuries, and delineating the vector forces that may help identify subtle skull injuries (see Figures 30.1a and 30.2b). Subgaleal hematomas in particular may be a sign of both skull fracture and epidural hematoma since blood from the epidural space may decompress out through the skull.

Skull and skull base fractures

Bone windows with application of a dedicated sharp bone algorithm aid in the detection of subtle skull fractures. Even with ideal technique, small, linear non-displaced fractures may be missed because of volume averaging (Figure 30.8).

491

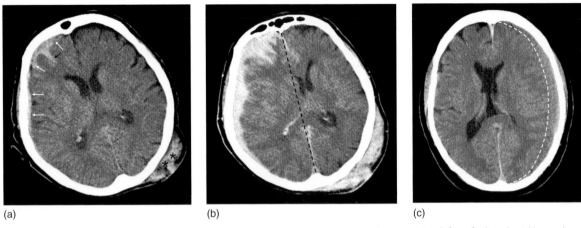

(a)   (b)   (c)

Figure 30.2 Subdural hematoma: (a) Thin right frontoparietal subdural hematoma (SDH) (white arrows) with foci of subarachnoid hemorrhage anteriorly (black arrow). Impact site subgaleal hematoma is contre-coup (*); (b) Follow-up CT 3 hours later shows marked interval expansion of right SDH now causing subfalcine herniation, seen as midline shift (dotted black line); (c) Different patient shows a subacute SDH with hemorrhage now isodense to underlying brain (dotted white line) evident by loss of sulci on the ipsilateral side and contralateral midline shift.

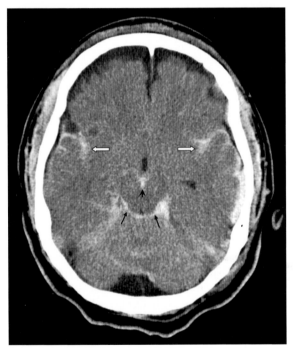

Figure 30.3 Traumatic subarachnoid hemorrhage. CT image of the brain shows high density blood in the basal cisterns (black arrows), interpeduncular fossa (arrowhead), and within the Sylvian fissures (white arrows), representing subarachnoid blood.

Skull fracture patterns can be described as linear/curvilinear, stellate, or eggshell. If the skin is interrupted and the dura is lacerated, the fracture is described as "open" since there is communication between the brain and the outside world. Stellate fractures consist of a central defect with curved and linear fractures radiating from the center. This is seen when a small diameter object, such as a bullet, impacts the skull. Longer curvilinear fractures occur when a cylindrical object with a large diameter, such as a baseball bat, impacts the skull. A simple linear fracture may be seen when the skull impacts a flat object. Eggshell fracture describes multiple calvarial fractures held together only by the overlying scalp. Basilar skull fractures are of particular significance because of potential cranial nerve damage and vascular injury. Following routine CT head depicting a skull base fracture where the fracture extends across the carotid canal, or where there is blood in the sphenoid sinus, a dedicated high-resolution submillimeter skull base CT angiogram (CTA), will help to demonstrate bony impingement and assess vascular integrity (Figure 30.9).

Brain

Technological advances have made CT a cost-effective and convenient mode for intracranial imaging. As such, many intracranial injuries are now diagnosed that may have been missed in previous years. The decision to image a patient should be based on both the patient risk factors for intracranial injury and the mechanism of injury. Patient risk factors that may make one prone to intracranial injury involve both structural and hematologic factors. Structurally, patients will be at greater risk if there is cerebral volume loss. Characteristics that may alert the clinician that a patient may be at such risk include the elderly, history of stroke, craniotomy or dementia, or chronic alcohol abuse. Additionally, an intracerebral

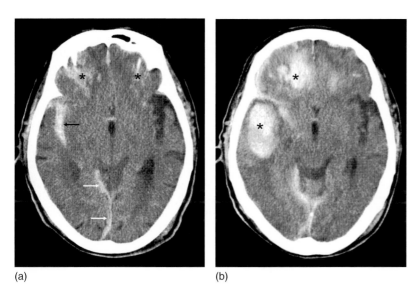

Figure 30.4 Cerebral contusions. 81 year old man after falling down stairs: (a) Initial CT head shows subarachnoid hemorrhage (black arrow) in the right Sylvian fissure, and small foci of hyperdense hemorrhage, representing cerebral contusions (*) within the inferior frontal lobes. A small subdural hematoma (white arrows) layers on the tentorium; (b) Follow-up CT head 12 hours later shows marked blossoming of cerebral contusions in the inferior frontal lobes and right temporal lobe (*).

(a)   (b)

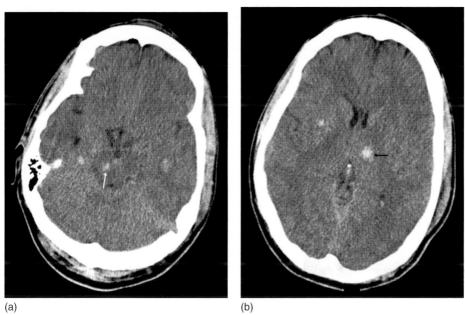

(a)   (b)

Figure 30.5 Diffuse axonal injury. 36 year old male after motor vehicle crash with petechial hemorrhages within the brainstem (white arrow in A), and left thalamus (black arrow in B).

mass, whether oncologic, infectious, or vascular, may make a patient more prone to hemorrhage. Other hematologic risk factors involve bleeding diatheses including use of anticoagulants. Obvious signs of serious injury should alert the clinician to pursue imaging, although significant brain injury sometimes is associated with seemingly minor external injuries. Likewise, acute intracerebral bleeds may have little or no acute clinical sequelae acutely. In 2000, Haydel et al. performed a two-phase study to identify patients with minor head trauma that would require a CT scan of the brain.[4] In the first phase they identified risk factors in patients with positive CT scans. These included headache, vomiting, age over 60, intoxication, memory deficits seizure, or signs of trauma above the clavicles. In the second phase they performed a CT scan on 909 patients with minor head injury. They found that of the 6.9% with positive CT scans, 100% had at least one of these findings.[4] Later, in 2001,

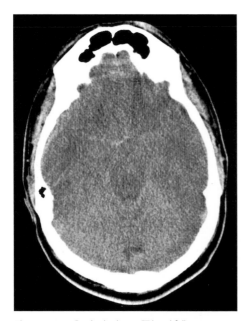

Figure 30.6 Cerebral edema. CT head following motor vehicle crash with complete effacement of sulci and cisterns with loss of gray-white matter differentiation. Findings represent diffuse cerebral edema.

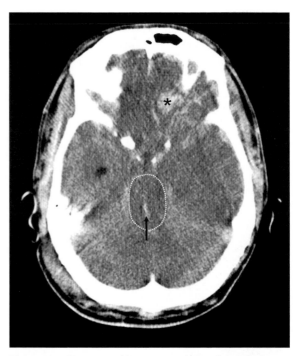

Figure 30.7 Transtentorial herniation and Duret hemorrhage. Pedestrian struck with cerebral edema as seen by sulcal effacement and loss of gray-white interface. Inferior frontal lobe contusions (*) present with compression and elongation of the brainstem (dotted white oval). Note the Duret hemorrhage within the brainstem (black arrow). Patient did not survive.

Steill et al. published the Canadian CT Head Rule for patients with minor head injury.[5] They evaluated over 3000 patients with minor head injuries, defined as Glasgow Coma Scale (GCS) score of 13–15, and derived medium- and high-risk criteria to determine those patients who benefited from CT imaging. Five high-risk factors were identified: (1) failure to reach GCS 15 within 2 hours; (2) suspected open skull fracture; (3) any sign of basal skull fracture; (4) more than 2 episodes of vomiting; and (5) age > 65 years. Two medium-risk factors were identified: (1) more than 30 minutes of retrograde amnesia; and (2) dangerous mechanism of injury. The presence of high-risk factors were 100% sensitive for determining neurological intervention; this required only 32% of their total patient population presenting with head trauma as necessitating head CT. The presence of medium risk factors were 98% sensitive and 50% specific for detecting clinically important brain injury. These factors required 54% of study patients to undergo head CTs. One major criticism of these rules is that they require patients with a GCS of < 15 initially to wait 2 hours to see if they reach 15.

Epidural hematoma

Epidural hematomas (EDHs) occur in 1–5% of significant head injuries. More than 90% of adult patients with EDHs have associated skull fractures. This is not necessarily true in the pediatric population, probably because of the elasticity of the developing skull. The epidural space is a potential space that expands when the dura is stripped from the calvarium usually secondary to hemorrhage from a skull fracture that may also tear an underlying artery or vein; hence EDHs may be arterial or venous. Most commonly, the skull fracture is of the temporal bone and the lacerated dura contains the branches of the middle meningeal artery. The EDH then forms as a result of the vessel bleeding into this potential space. This expanding hemorrhagic mass will extend to the margins of the cranial sutures where the dura is tightly adherent. As such, EDHs are typically biconvex, forming a lenticular mass toward the brain. On CT this appears as a high attenuation lens-shaped extra-axial collection bound by the cranial sutures (see Figure 30.1a). Epidural hematomas may cross the midline, unlike subdural collections.

Subdural hematoma

The subdural space is a potential space between the inner layer of the dura and the arachnoid membrane.

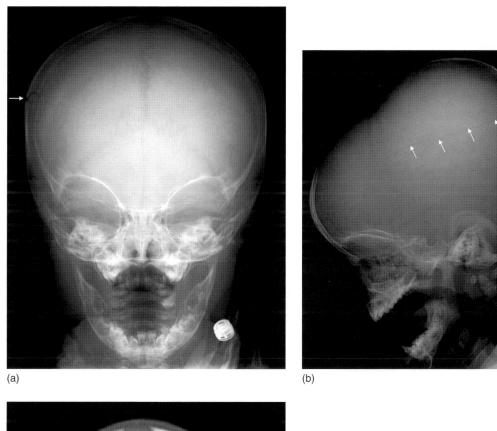

(a)

(b)

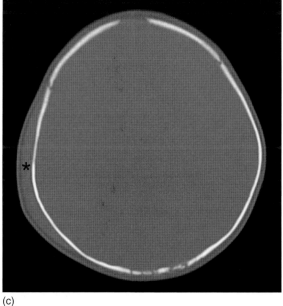

(c)

Figure 30.8 Skull fracture missed on CT. 8 month old girl with linear skull fracture (arrows in a and b) after fall from crib; (c) Subsequently performed CT head failed to identify this fracture, as the fracture lies in the plane of scan acquisition. Subgaleal hematoma (*) marks the impact site.

Usually a subdural hematoma (SDH) results from tearing of the bridging cortical veins following a sudden deceleration as the brain continues inertial momentum within the skull. Prognosis of SDH may be related more to the concurrent cerebral injury than to the SDH itself, and relates directly to the promptness of diagnosis and intervention with mortality ranging from 30% to 90%.[6] On CT, the SDH

495

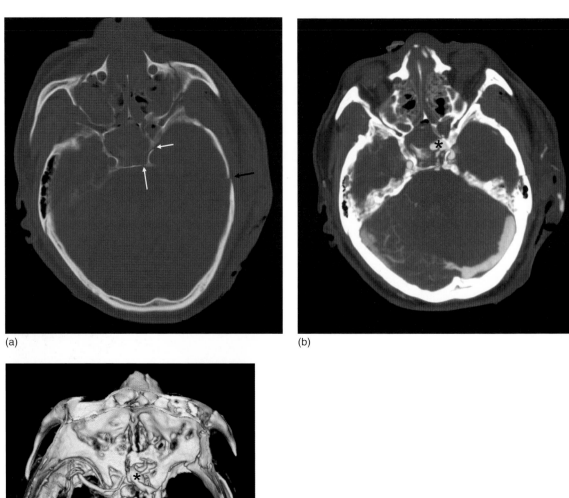

(a)

(b)

(c)

Figure 30.9 Skull base fractures. 58 year old man after fall from ladder striking metal object and sustaining multiple facial fractures and intracranial injuries: (a) CT head in bone windows shows fractures of the sphenoid sinus walls (white arrows), with complete opacification within the sinus raising suspicion for carotid vascular injury. Depressed left temporal calvarial fracture (black arrow); (b) Thick slab maximum intensity projection (MIP) CT angiogram through the head shows extravasation of contrast material from the left internal carotid through the sphenoid fractures into the sinus (*); (c) 3D CTA reconstruction shows large pool of extravasating contrast material from vascular injury (*). Note there are no branching vessels in the left hemisphere consistent with massive traumatic cerebral ischemia. Patient did not survive his injuries.

appears as a high attenuation crescent, concave toward the brain, along the inner table of the skull (see Figure 30.2a). Unlike EDHs, SDHs usually have no associated skull fracture, are often "contrecoup" in location, and are limited in spread by the dural folds of the falx and tentorium. Thus, subdural collections will not cross the midline. The CT findings will change over time as the hyperdense acute SDH progresses to an isodense/hypodense subacute SDH after about 3 days and finally to a hypodense chronic SDH between 3–20 days later, as the hemoglobin is reabsorbed (see Figure 30.2c).

Subarachnoid hemorrhage

Subarachnoid hemorrhage (SAH) is the most common type of traumatic intracerebral bleed. Computed tomography findings of traumatic SAH are typically linear hyperdensities in the subarachnoid space seen between sulci and layering in cisterns (see Figure 30.3). Posttraumatic SAH may result from a SDH with a tear in the arachnoid membrane, an intraparenchymal hematoma with leakage into the ventricular system, or most commonly be secondary to direct injury to the cortical vessels in the subarachnoid space.

Cerebral contusion

Contusions are intracerebral hematomas with progressive surrounding edema secondary to traumatic injury. The mechanical forces of the injury are transmitted to the brain, damaging capillaries and venules. These injuries occur most commonly at the crests or crowns of gyri, especially along the inferior frontal lobes and anterior temporal poles where the brain strikes the rough adjacent bone of the anterior and middle cranial fossae (see Figure 30.4). Forces transmitted through the calvarium to the cortical surface are termed "coup." Impact of the cerebrum against the point opposite the site of contact is termed a "contrecoup" contusion. The CT appearance is a localized mixture of tissue densities, including the spectrum from dense blood clots to lower density cerebral edema.

Diffuse axonal (shear) injury

Diffuse axonal injury (DAI) is a common and devastating intracerebral injury resulting from acceleration–deceleration forces. There is often no impact injury, rather the consequence of sudden rotational forces with differing behaviors of gray and white matter. These forces are transmitted through the brain causing widespread axonal shearing and disruption along white matter tracts, the major cause of unconsciousness and persistent vegetative state. These result in the triad of microscopic diffuse axonal damage at gray/white matter interface and deep gray matter, focal lesions within the corpus callosum, and focal lesions within the brainstem. Computed tomography cannot directly demonstrate the presence of DAI, as such; the latter two findings along with punctate hemorrhages from vessels in close proximity to the axon bundles provide the major CT markers for these injuries (see Figure 30.5a and b).

Cerebral edema and herniation

Mechanisms leading to cerebral edema are hyperemic swelling and true cerebral edema. Hyperemia is secondary to the brain's loss of autoregulation leading to vasodilatation and engorgement of the brain with blood. True brain edema from blunt trauma results from disruption of the blood/brain barrier leading to interstitial water accumulation. Both types may be recognized on CT by obliteration of the cerebrospinal fluid (CSF) spaces of the sulci, loss of the basal cisterns, and effacement of the lateral ventricles (see Figure 30.6). Hyperemic edema can be distinguished from true edema by increased CT attenuation, corresponding to the increased blood contained in the brain.

Mass effect from intracranial hemorrhage or edema may be associated with elevated intracranial pressure and subsequent displacement of brain parenchyma leading to herniation. The brain does not respond well to sudden changes in intracranial volume and pressure and is often unable to compensate. This leads to devastating neurological compromise including infarction and death. Subfalcine herniation represents shift of midline structures under the falx cerebri. On CT, subfalcine herniation is seen as midline shift, often with ventricular effacement on the ipsilateral side of an intracranial hematoma with subsequent entrapment of the contralateral lateral ventricle (see Figure 30.2b). Transtentorial and tonsillar herniation occur when the cerebrum pushes down through the tentorium cerebelli and foramen magnum, respectively. The resulting pressure on the brainstem causes respiratory and cardiac arrest. Computed tomography demonstrates obliteration of basal cisterns and lateral compression of the brainstem. Duret hemorrhage, small areas of midbrain bleeding, with blood in the mesencephalon and upper pons may be seen (see Figure 30.7). The result is usually fatal.

Craniofacial trauma

Facial fractures can be divided into solitary injuries, complex injuries, or transfacial injuries.

Solitary injuries

Solitary injuries are simple fractures that involve a single bony wall.

Orbital blow-out fractures

Orbital blowout fractures are among the most common facial injuries. These fractures result from blunt impact to the orbit causing an acute rise in intraorbital pressure.

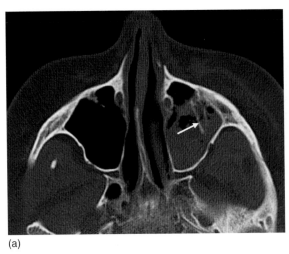

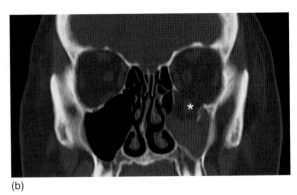

(a)   (b)

Figure 30.10 Orbital floor blow-out fracture: (a) Transverse CT image through the maxillary sinuses in patient status post altercation shows a free fragment of bone (white arrow) and hemorrhage in the left maxillary sinus; (b) Coronal CT reformation shows a large orbital floor defect with herniation of orbital fat, bone, and inferior rectus muscle (*) into the left maxillary sinus below.

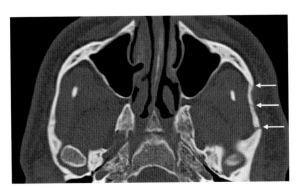

Figure 30.11 Zygomatic arch fracture. 29 year old following altercation shows a comminuted and mildly depressed zygomatic arch fracture (white arrows).

This rise in pressure is then transmitted to the bony walls, where the orbital floor and/or medial orbital wall are fractured. Computed tomography diagnosis of an orbital floor fracture requires coronal imaging (reconstructions, not direct coronal acquisition) to properly characterize the fracture and distinguish causes of diplopia, if present. These causes could include muscle entrapment by bone, injury to the oculomotor nerve or direct inferior rectus muscle injury. Indirect signs of orbital floor fractures include air fluid levels in the sinuses, free bone fragment within the maxillary sinus, and orbital emphysema (Figure 30.10).

Zygomatic arch fractures

Zygomatic arch fractures usually result from a focused blow and may displace inward (Figure 30.11)

or outward. The degree of displacement as seen on CT is important when determining operative repair. When inwardly displaced, these fractures are repaired because of possible impingement of the mandibular coronoid process, leading to limitation of mandibular range of motion and to repair cosmetic deformity.

Frontal sinus fractures

Frontal sinus fractures usually result from a direct high-energy blow to the supraorbital region, and involve the anterior table with or without posterior table fracture (Figure 30.12). Displaced posterior table fractures are important to identify since these may lacerate the dura with connection between the frontal sinus and the intracranial compartment. Complications include meningitis, encephalitis, brain abscess, and cavernous sinus thrombosis. Computed tomography is often important to demonstrate posterior table fracture along with potential underlying brain injury.

Nasal bones

Nasal fractures are among the most common facial injuries, comprising 50% of facial fractures. Isolated trauma to the nose may be non-displaced, displaced or depressed (Figure 30.13). Imaging is usually to search for associated fracture, but may aid the surgeon if planning operative fixation. However, if clinical diagnosis of isolated nasal fracture is made, CT scan in the ED is not an indicated test.

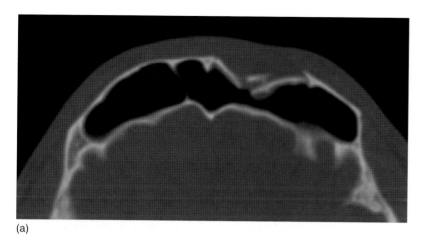

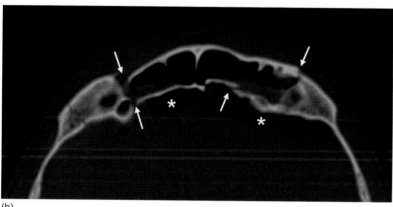

(b)

Figure 30.12 Frontal sinus fractures:
(a) Fracture isolated to the anterior table
of the frontal sinus. Posterior wall remains
intact; (b) Greater force is required to
fracture both anterior and posterior tables
of the frontal sinus (white arrows). Note
the extensive pneumocephalus as a result
of sinus air reaching the intracranial
contents (*).

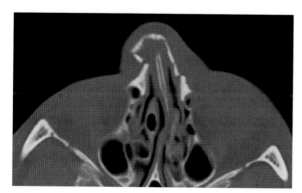

Figure 30.13 Nasal bone fractures. Following assault,
comminuted nasal bones are seen displaced to the right, consistent
with impact from right-handed assailant.

Complex fractures
Naso-orbital-ethmoid

Anatomically, the naso-orbtial ethmoid (NOE) region
refers to the inter-orbital space, where the nasal bones
meet the medial orbital wall and inferomedial extension

of the frontal bones. Deep to this region lie the cribriform
plate and crista galli. The NOE fractures are always comminuted involving two of the four struts. The essence of
these fractures is involvement of the nasal bone and
frontal process of the maxilla anchoring the medial
canthal ligament. The classic clinical finding is free movement of the frontal process of the maxilla with telecanthus
(abnormally widened distance between the medial canthi
of the eyes). Because the cribriform plate is located just
posteriorly, there is a high incidence of dural tears, intracranial hemorrhage, pneumocephalus and intracranial
infection. Cerebrospinal fluid rhinorrhea may develop
in 40% of these patients. Because of the complex anatomic
relationships in this region, these injuries require open
reduction and internal fixation. A CT scan is used both to
diagnose, define the full extent of the injury, and help plan
operative repair (Figure 30.14).

Zygomaticomaxillary

Zygomaticomaxillary complex (ZMC) fractures were
previously referred to as "tripod fractures." These injuries

499

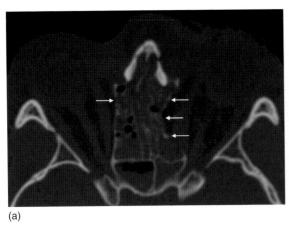

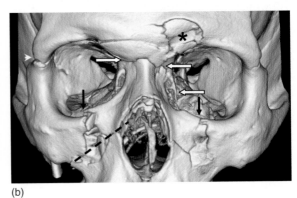

(a)   (b)

Figure 30.14 Naso-orbital-ethmoid (NOE) fractures: (a) Transverse CT image in a 39-year-old male status post motor vehicle crash shows fractures of the nasal bones with telescoping and comminution of the blood filled ethmoid air cells (arrows); (b) 3D CT reconstruction of same patient shows comminuted NOE fractures between the orbits (white arrows) with hallmark fractures through the inferior orbital rims bilaterally (vertical black arrows). Additional fractures include the right lateral orbital wall (white arrowhead), the frontal sinus (*), and a right hemi-Le Fort I (dashed line).

represent a disjunction of the zygoma from its four, not three, osseous connections making it a free moving piece of bone. These injuries involve a fracture though the lateral orbital wall and rim (zygomaticofrontal suture), a fracture through the anterolateral maxilla (zygomatico-maxillary suture), a fracture through the orbital floor (sphenoid suture), and a fracture through the zygomatic arch (zygomaticotemporal suture). Computed tomography clearly details the depression, rotation, and comminution of ZMCs fractures (Figure 30.15).

Transfacial

Le Fort

The Le Fort fracture classification system was described in the pre-CT era to aid limited plain film evaluation for surgical planning. Three progressive levels of fractures were described (Figure 30.16). The advent of CT, and particularly MDCT, has demonstrated that such severe facial trauma usually result in a constellation of facial fractures that do not neatly fit into the Le Fort classification system; as such the Le Fort system may be an oversimplification. The Le Fort classification is best applied to each half of the facial skeleton separately and allows for improved communication between physicians describing these complex facial injuries. The characteristic feature of all Le Fort fractures is the involvement of the pterygoid plates.

Le Fort I fractures involves a horizontally oriented fracture line through the inferior portion of the midface extending across the inferior portions of the maxillary antra, involving all the walls of the maxillae, as well as the inferior nasal cavity. The fracture continues posteriorly through the pterygoid plates leading to a floating palate on clinical examination. As such, Le Fort I releases the palate and maxillary ridge from its attachments. Current high resolution MDCT is able to give a thorough evaluation of this injury, despite its in-line nature, through reformatting techniques for the generation of high-quality coronal, sagittal, and 3D images (Figures 30.17 and 30.18).

Le Fort II is the most commonly encountered pattern of the Le Fort fractures. This pattern leads to a pyramidal shape of disconnected facial structures by including disruption of the orbits and upper nasal cavity structures. Thus the fracture lines are superiorly centered at the nasal bridge and frontonasal complex and descend into a triangle involving the medial orbital walls, and orbital floors and continue inferolaterally to involve the maxillary antra and pterygoid plates posteriorly. Here the hard palate does not float but serves as the base of the detached pyramidal midface unit (Figure 30.19).

Le Fort III, also called craniofacial disjunction, is the most severe of the Le Fort midface fractures. It involves a complete disruption between the facial skeleton from the skull base. It differs from the Le Fort II in its involvement of the lateral orbital walls and zygomatic arches. Thus, the entire facial skeleton is separated from the anterior skull base and the zygomas are separated from the temporal bones on each side (see Figures 30.18 and 30.19).

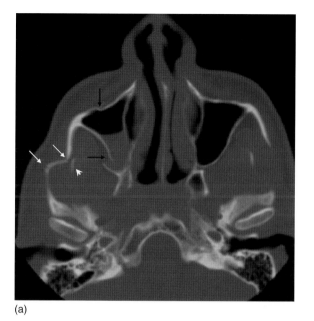

(a)

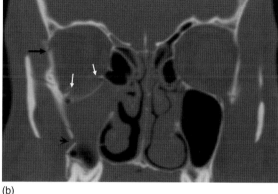

(b)

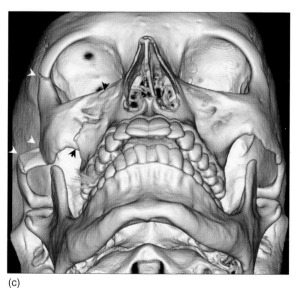

(c)

Figure 30.15 Zygomaticomaxillary complex (ZMC) fractures: (a) Transverse CT image shows comminuted, depressed, zygomatic arch fracture (white arrows) nearly impinging upon the coronoid process of the mandible (arrowhead). Fractures of the anterior and lateral walls of the maxillary sinus (black arrows) are also part of the fracture pattern; (b) Coronal reformation shows right orbital floor fractures (short white arrows) and right lateral orbital wall fracture (black arrow). Lateral maxillary wall fracture again identified (black arrowhead); (c) 3D CT Water's view reconstruction shows depressed right ZMC fracture (arrowheads) and proximity to the mandibular coronoid process.

Mandible

Mandibular fractures involve more than one site in the majority of cases. Fractures are described by anatomic region: symphyseal, body, angle, ramus, coronoid process, and condylar or subcondylar. The most frequent fracture site is in the condylar or subcondylar region. Computed tomography imaging is the modality of choice for mandibular injury evaluation. High-resolution transaxial images are used for multiplanar reformatting and panoramic and 3D reconstructions to identify and display the extent of injury (Figure 30.20).

Spine trauma

Cervical spine

Introduction

The patient's mental status and severity of injuries, and potentially mechanism of injury, may be used to stratify the patient's likelihood of having sustained cervical spine injury. Special consideration maybe given to trauma patients with extremes of age, a significant mechanism of injury, signs and symptoms of spinal injury, a distracting injury with unreliable

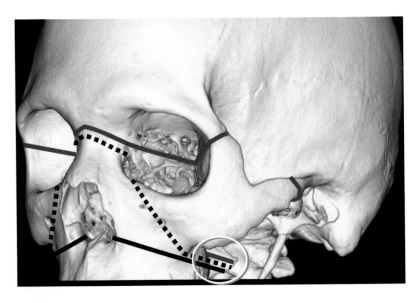

Figure 30.16 Le Fort fracture patterns. 3D CT with overlays. Le Fort I fracture pattern (solid black lines crosses the maxillae horizontally, extending through the pterygoid plates posteriorly (white oval). Le Fort II fracture pattern (dashed black lines) crosses the nasal bridge and descends obliquely across the maxillae, reaching the pterygoid plates posteriorly. Le Fort III fracture pattern (solid dark red lines) is horizontal across the nasal bridge and orbits, also fracturing the zygomatic arches and pterygoid plates.

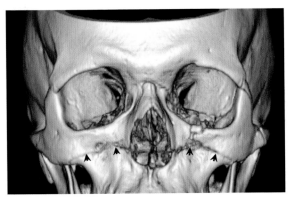

Figure 30.17 Bilateral Le Fort I fractures. 3D CT reconstruction of 24-year-old after motorcycle crash with bilateral transverse fractures of the maxillae (arrowheads). Fractures extend through the pterygoid plates bilaterally (not shown).

information regarding the mechanism of their injury, and unreliable mental status after trauma. These variables have been studied in depth and published as the National Emergency X-Radiography Utilization Study (NEXUS), Canadian, and British (a combination of the two) rules. Cervical spine rules that stratify patients into possible or no risk of unstable cervical spine injury.[7,8]

Until recently anteroposterior (AP), open-mouth odontoid, and lateral X-ray images of the spine were the initial imaging modality for trauma patients with suspected cervical spine injuries. Downsides of this approach were fair accuracy for some patients, extensive time to complete radiographs, and the need to reimage many patients. Plain film sensitivity for cervical spine fracture has been reported as low as 65%,[9] with

specificity in high-risk patients < 75%.[10] These numbers are variable depending on the gold standard and whether or not minor stable fractures are included. Computed tomography is rapid and provides excellent bony detail without the superimposition of overlapping structures that plagues plain film interpretation. Nunez et al. first compared screening the entire cervical spine with helical CT to plain radiographs and found 98% sensitivity for CT fracture detection using all imaging studies and medical records as the gold standard.[11] In an evaluation of over 600 blunt trauma patients with single-slice helical CT, Hanson et al. reported a 95% sensitivity, 93% specificity, and an overall accuracy of 93%.[12] Ptak et al. screened 676 polytrauma patients for cervical spine injury and found 98% sensitivity, 100% specificity, accuracy of 99.9%, and positive and negative predictive values of 100% and 99.8%, respectively.[13]

Early studies with single-slice helical CT encountered difficulty with the diagnosis of undisplaced transversely oriented fractures, such as the type II odontoid, as well as purely ligamentous injuries. These limitations highlight the importance of reviewing the sagittal and coronal reformations of the cervical spine in every case before excluding injury. With the addition of high-resolution multiplanar reformations, the radiologic features indicative of instability or ligament disruption also apply to CT and include wide interspinous distance, wide facet joints, wide interpedicular distance, subluxation, and dislocation.[14]

Consequently, as the technology of CT has evolved to become a faster and more accurate tool, it has become the

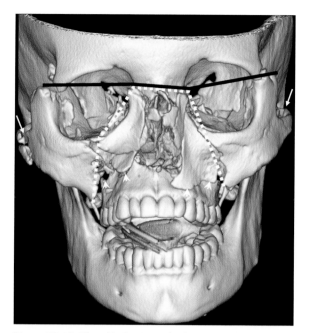

Figure 30.18 Bilateral Le Fort I, II, and III fractures. 3D CT reconstruction of a 26 year old female pedestrian following a motor vehicle strike. Transverse fractures across the maxillae (white arrowheads) represent the bilateral Le Fort I pattern. Pyramidal fracture across the maxillary walls, inferior orbital rims, and crossing the nasal bridge (white dotted line) represents the bilateral Le Fort II pattern. Fractures across both zygomaticofrontal sutures and lateral orbital walls extending medially across the nasal bridge (solid black line), along with bilateral zygomatic arch fractures (white arrows) represent bilateral Le Fort III pattern. Bilateral pterygoid plate fractures are not shown.

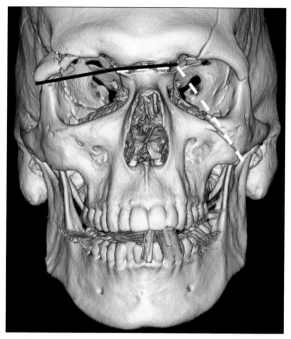

Figure 30.19 Left hemi-Le Fort II and right hemi-Le Fort III fractures. 3D CT reconstruction of construction worker status post fall. Oblique fracture across the left maxilla and crossing the nasal bridge is characteristic of a Le Fort II fracture pattern (dashed white line). The transverse fracture from nasal bridge across the right orbit and through the right lateral orbital wall is consistent with a Le Fort III pattern (solid black line). The necessary fractures through the right zygomatic arch and both pterygoid plates are present, but not shown.

initial imaging modality of choice for the trauma patient at greater risk of injury.[10,15] Since 2006, the American College of Radiology has advocated screening for cervical spine injury with high resolution CT imaging with sagittal and coronal reformations rather than with plain radiographs.[16] This must be balanced by the excess cost and radiation, and while there is general agreement about high-risk patients the recommendation for CT as initial screening for low risk remains controversial. Improved fracture pattern classification and differentiation between stable and unstable fractures is possible with CT.

Fractures

The greatest benefit of CT lies in diagnosing injuries that are difficult to visualize with plain radiographs: atlanto-occipital subluxation, occipital condyle fracture, odontoid fractures, atlantoaxial rotary subluxation, unilateral facet dislocation, and pedicolaminar fracture (also referred to as traumatic isolation of the articular pillar).

The craniocervical junction is anatomically unique with respect to the remainder of the spine and thus has

fracture patterns that do not follow the classic patterns seen elsewhere, and the vast majority are unstable. Atlanto-occipital subluxations appear as prevertebral soft tissue swelling, increased distance (> 12 mm) from the skull base inferior tip of the clivus (known as the basion) to the tip of the odontoid with separation between occipital condyles and the condylar fossae of the atlas (Figure 30.21).

Occipital condyle fractures are seen almost exclusively on CT. These fractures are classified into three types. Type 1 represents an undisplaced fracture isolated to the condyle (Figure 30.22). Type 2 spans from the occipital bone into the condyle. Type 3 is an unstable fracture involving avulsion and displacement of the condyle fracture fragment secondary to the forces applied by the alar ligaments.

Atlantoaxial rotary subluxation results in asymmetry of the lateral masses of C1 relative to the articular pillar of C2, protrusion of the articular mass of C1 into the spinal canal, exaggeration of the tilt of C1, and ability to visualize the disarticulated inferior surface of the lateral mass of C1 on 3D CT imaging (Figure 30.23).

503

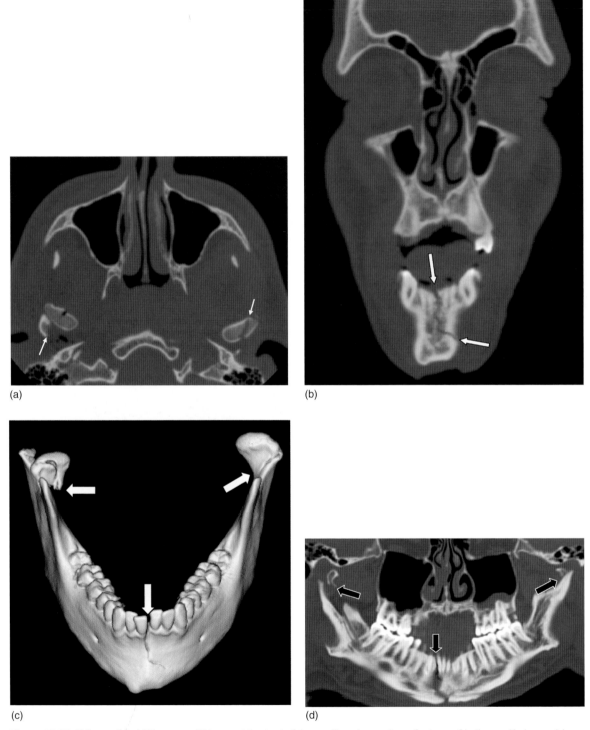

(a)

(b)

(c)

(d)

Figure 30.20 Flail mandible: (a) Transverse CT image at the level of the maxillary sinuses shows fractures of both mandibular condyles (white arrows), displaced on the right, and undisplaced on the left; (b) Coronal reformation through the anterior face shows a symphyseal mandibular fracture (white arrows), undisplaced; (c) 3D CT reconstruction of the mandible shows symphyseal fracture and bilateral condylar fractures (white arrows) representing a flail mandible fracture pattern; (d) Panoramic reconstruction of a different patient with a flail mandible (black arrows).

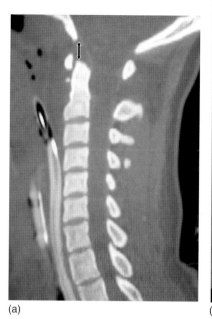

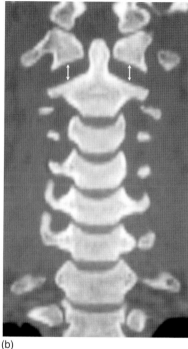

(a) (b)

Figure 30.21 Atlanto-occipital subluxation: (a) Sagittal CT reformation of the cervical spine shows increased distance (> 12 mm) between the basion and the tip of the dens (black double arrow); (b) Coronal CT reformation shows increased distance between the lateral masses of C1 and C2 (white arrows), confirming a two level (skull base/C1 and C1/C2) distraction injury.

Other fractures at the C1–C2 level include the Jefferson burst fracture (Figure 30.24), odontoid fracture (Figure 30.25), hangman fracture (Figure 30.26), and extension teardrop fracture (Figure 30.27).

Fractures from C3 through C7 are classically stratified by mechanism. Hyperflexion injuries include the unstable hyperflexion teardrop (Figure 30.28), bilateral interfacetal dislocation (BID) (Figure 30.29), anterior subluxation (also referred to as hyperflexion sprain) (Figure 30.30), and stable simple wedge compression fracture. Hyperextension mechanisms are responsible for the unstable hyperextension dislocation (Figure 30.31) and fused spine fractures (Figure 30.32). Rotational mechanisms produce the unilateral interfacetal dislocation (UID) (Figure 30.33) and pedicolaminar fracture (Figure 30.34).

Computed tomography has limited sensitivity for soft tissue injury without bony malalignment. This is particularly a problem in unconscious or altered patients who are unable to complain about pain or limited range of motion of the neck. In such scenarios, MRI of the cervical spine can be used to exclude such injuries,[17] and is recommended by the American College of Radiology if the patient has not become awake and alert by 48 hours.[16]

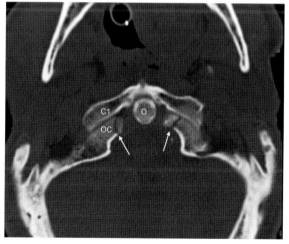

Figure 30.22 Bilateral occipital condyle fractures. Transverse CT image at the craniocervical junction shows undisplaced fractures (arrows) of both occipital condyles (OC). Note the intimate relationship between the occipital condyles and the C1 ring, and between the odontoid (O) and C1 anterior arch.

There is evidence, however, to suggest that even in such cases MDCT may be accurate enough to negate the need for MRI. Tomycz et al. identified 180 post-traumatic comatose patients in whom concomitant CT and MRI were performed.[18] Cervical spine MRI

505

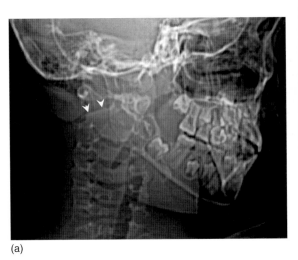

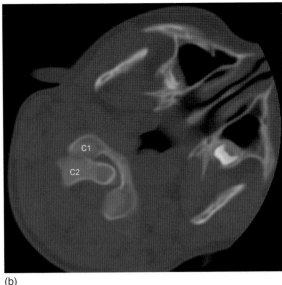

(a)

(b)

Figure 30.23 Atlantoaxial rotatory subluxation: (a) Scout view from CT shows AP view of the cervical spine while head is turned to the left. The right side of the C1/C2 articulation is bare (arrowheads), revealing that this is not simply physiologic rotation; (b) Transverse CT image at the C1/C2 level shows patient's head turned to the left. There is marked subluxation at the right C1/C2 articulation, where both articular surfaces are visible (C1, C2) and translated.

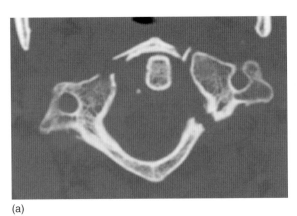

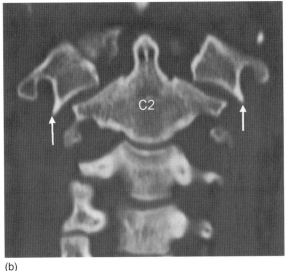

(a)

(b)

Figure 30.24 Jefferson fracture: (a) Transverse CT image of C1 ring shows three fractures with displacement; (b) Coronal CT reformation shows lateral displacement of the C1 articular masses (arrows). The lateral corners of C1 should line up exactly with the lateral margins of C2.

identified 38 patients with acute traumatic findings not identified on CT. However, none of these patients had an unstable injury and no patient required surgery or developed evidence of delayed instability. They concluded that MRI is unlikely to uncover unstable cervical spine injuries in patients who are obtunded or comatose when cervical spine CT is normal.

Thoracic and lumbar spine
Plain radiography vs. CT

Anteroposterior and lateral radiographs are still the initial method of investigating the thoracic and lumbar spine. However, CT has become an indispensable adjunct to plain radiography. Indication for CT

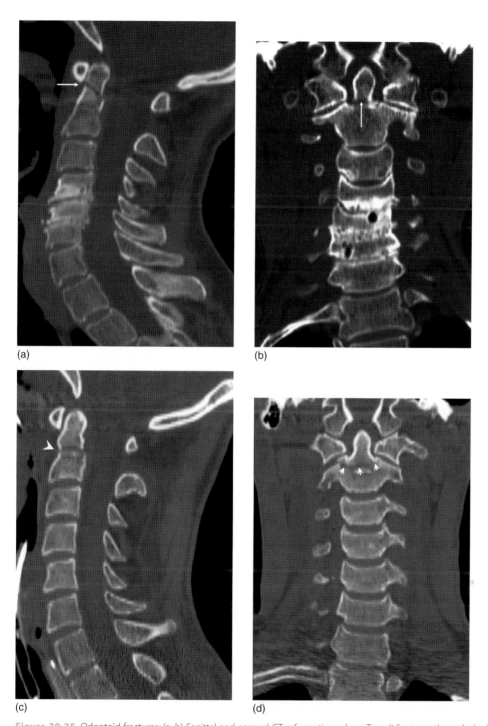

Figure 30.25 Odontoid fractures: (a, b) Sagittal and coronal CT reformations show Type II fractures through the base of odontoid (arrows); (c, d) Sagittal and coronal reformations show Type III fractures which extend into the C2 vertebral body (arrowheads).

includes the presence or suspicion of vertebral fracture on X-ray or a discrepancy between neurological physical findings and radiographic findings.

Neurologic deficits occur in over 40% of thoracolumbar injuries.[19] One approach with patients demonstrating physical exam or neurological findings

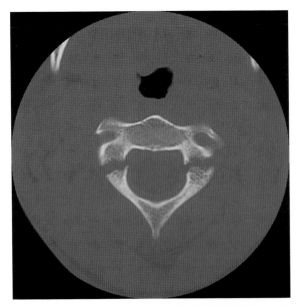

Figure 30.26 Hangman fracture. Transaxial CT image through C2 shows bilateral fractures through the pars interarticularis.

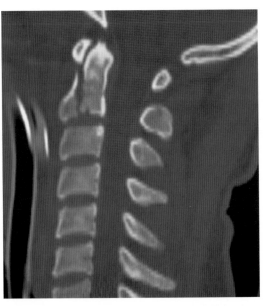

Figure 30.27 Extension teardrop fracture. Sagittal CT shows vertical fracture through the C2 body involving only the anterior column, hence a stable injury. Note the vertical height of the fracture is greater than its transverse dimension, typical of the extension teardrop.

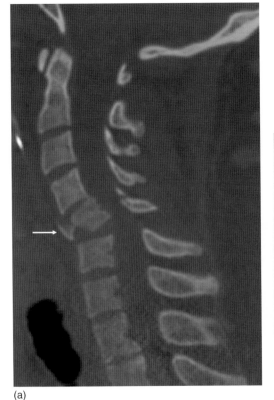

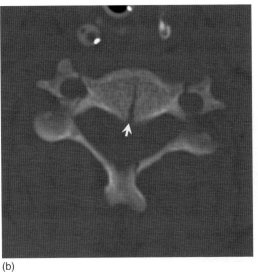

(a)   (b)

Figure 30.28 Hyperflexion teardrop fracture: (a) Mid-sagittal plane CT reformation of the cervical spine shows the small anterior inferior corner fracture of C5 (arrow), representing the teardrop fragment. The larger C5 fragment is retropulsed into the spinal canal, typically causing an anterior cord syndrome; (b) Transverse CT image through C5 vertebral body shows hallmark mid-sagittal fracture (arrowhead). Associated fractures through the left lamina and both vertebral artery foramina are present. The latter place the vertebral arteries at risk of injury and could be screened with CTA.

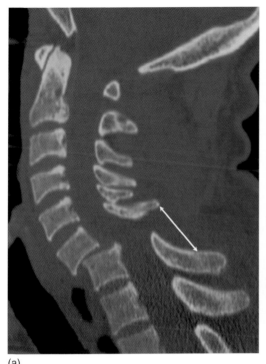
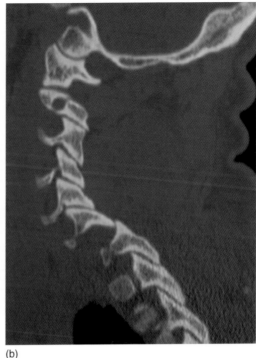

(a)   (b)

Figure 30.29 Bilateral interfacetal dislocation (BID): (a) Mid-sagittal CT reformation shows anterior translation of C6 on C7 of approximately 50% and interspinous widening (double arrow); (b) Parasagittal reformation illustrates the jumped facets.

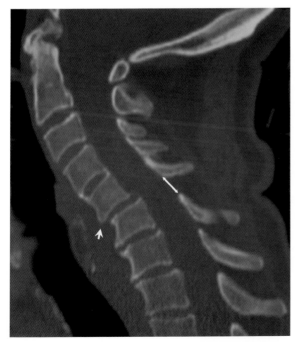

Figure 30.30 Anterior subluxation. Sagittal CT reformation shows widening of C5/6 interspinous distance (double headed arrow) and anterior translation of C5 on C6 (arrowhead). These features are consistent with a hyperflexion mechanism of injury.

suggesting thoracolumbar injury, is to undergo CT imaging directly without initial plain film evaluation.

Advantages of CT are the ability to rapidly obtain optimal transaxial assessment of vertebral injuries which are then reconstructed to provide high quality sagittal and coronal views. This gives more accurate assessment of bony and soft tissue injury as well as relaying information regarding the stability of injury without requiring the movement of the patient. In patients with exam findings indicating neurological injury or potential ligamentous laxity, MRI may be indicated. Magnetic resonance imaging can evaluate spinal cord injury, ligamentous disruption, EDH, and traumatic intervertebral disk herniation.

Fracture patterns

Fractures of the thoracolumbar spine have been classified as either major of minor. Minor injuries include isolated fractures of the transverse process or spinous process. These are fractures that do not violate the bony ring that surrounds the spinal cord. Major injuries have been classified into the anterior compression fracture, the burst fracture, the flexion–distraction injury, and fracture–dislocations.

509

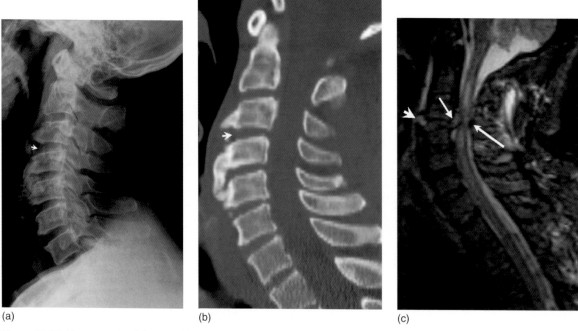

(a) (b) (c)

Figure 30.31 Hyperextension dislocation: (a) Crosstable lateral cervical spine radiograph reveals slight anterior disc space widening at C3/4 (arrowhead). This is the only clue to this highly unstable injury; (b) Mid-sagittal CT reformation is just as subtle as the radiograph with slight C3/4 widening anteriorly (arrowhead). Due to neurological deficit (central cord syndrome), MRI was performed; (c) Sagittal MRI T2 weighted sequence reveals an unstable injury with disruption of the anterior longitudinal ligament (arrowhead), posterior disc herniation (short arrow), buckling of the ligamentum flavum (long arrow) and high signal edema in the pinched spinal cord.

Figure 30.32 Fused spine hyperextension fracture. Mid-sagittal: (a) and parasagittal; (b) CT reformations show a fused cervical spine with bony bridging. Hyperextension has caused fracture at C7 (arrowheads).

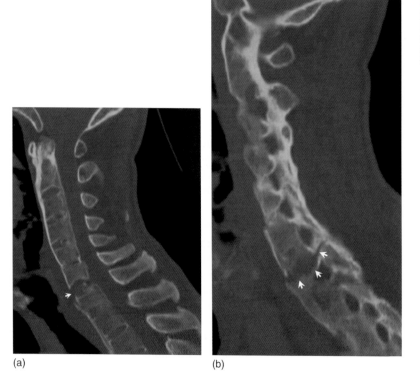

(a) (b)

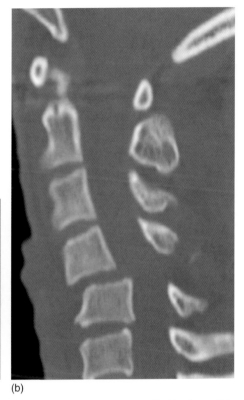

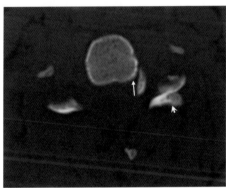

(a)   (b)

Figure 30.33 Unilateral interfacetal dislocation (UID): (a) Transverse CT image shows vertebral body translation (arrow) and reversal of left sided facets (the "reverse hamburger bun" sign; arrowhead); (b) Mid-sagittal CT image shows anterior translation of C4 on C5 by approximately 25% (less than the 50% expected for BID), and focal kyphosis.

Anterior compression (stable): The most common type of thoracolumbar fracture is the simple compression fracture. This results from hyperflexion, frequently from a motor vehicle collision, and accounts for 48% of thoracolumbar fractures. Eighty percent of these fractures heal without intervention.[20] The decision to do a CT of the lumbar spine should be made when symptoms alert the clinician to the potential for serious or unstable injury that has not been visualized on plain X-ray. Such symptoms include acute onset of thoracic back pain accompanied by weakness, autonomic dysfunction, significant reflex abnormality, bladder/bowel symptoms, ataxia, spasticity, or sensory loss. Computed tomography images reveal impaction of the anterior superior aspect of the vertebral body, typically with a rim of surrounding hematoma (Figure 30.35). It is imperative to closely review the CT scan for signs of a posterior vertebral body fracture that would reclassify a stable compression injury as an unstable burst fracture.

Burst fractures (generally considered unstable) account for 14% of spinal injuries.[21] They most commonly involve the thoracolumbar junction and typically result from an axial-loading mechanism, such as a fall from height. Fragments of the posterior aspect of the vertebral body may cause posterior buckling or may show retropulsion into the spinal canal (Figure 30.36). Neurological deficits are seen in half of the cases.[22] Computed tomography is particularly helpful in the evaluation of the fragments that may lie in the spinal canal. However, because the spinal canal is widest at the lumbar spine, CT findings may appear worse than the neurologic deficits.

Flexion–distraction injuries (unstable): Best known is the Chance Type Burst fracture shown in Figure 30.37.[23]

Fracture dislocations (unstable) represent 16% of all spinal fractures.[24] Combinations of compression, tension, rotation, and shear forces lead to this type of devastating injury. Often there is displacement or subluxation of one vertebral body with respect to another (Figure 30.38a). Most of these injuries are secondary to direct force to the dorsal aspect of the spine. Computed tomography is optimal in evaluation of vertebral body displacement, spinal canal involvement, and facet injury. Sagittal reformations allow assessment of the

511

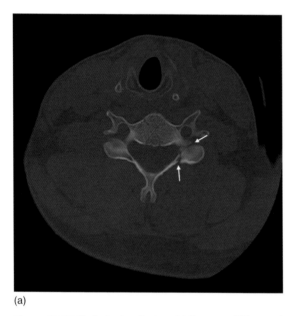

(a)

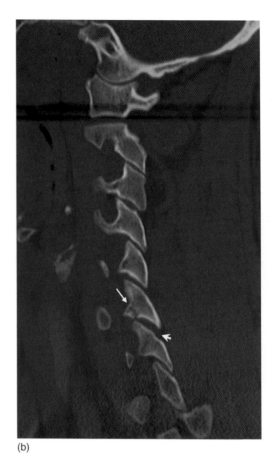

(b)

Figure 30.34 Pedicolaminar fracture: (a) Transverse CT image shows fractures through the left pedicle and lamina (arrows); (b) Parasagittal CT reformation shows fracture (arrow) and slight facet joint widening (arrowhead).

degree of vertebral body displacement and canal compromise (Figure 30.38b and c).

Chest and major vessels

Introduction: blunt vs. penetrating

Multidetector CT is the test of choice for screening high-risk patients with thoracic trauma. While the chest radiograph is often the initial study performed, it suffers from limitations including portable technique, magnification artifact, and overlapping lines and backboard. Computed tomography overcomes these limitations with improved sensitivity, specificity, and accuracy.

About 4–7% of admissions to major trauma centers are due to penetrating thoracic injuries.[25] Multidetector CT is playing an increasingly important role in the early assessment of penetrating trauma. Visualization of the bullet or stab trajectory may be useful to direct further angiographic or surgical evaluation and

treatment. The bullet course is more easily identified because of a greater cavity often lined with bone and metal fragments or air (Figure 30.39). However, even low-energy knife tracks can be identified as a hemorrhagic cavitation especially if the wound entry site is known so optimal MDCT windows can be used.

Transmediastinal gunshot wounds have a prehospital mortality of up to 86–92%.[25] Up to 60% of those who arrive alive to the ED are stable for imaging. Multidetector CT is optimal for visualization of wounds that penetrate the great vessels, pericardium, thoracic esophagus, trachea, or spine. This is because of the ability of the MDCT to give 3D information about areas in question (volumetric data) at peak contrast enhancement while minimizing motion artifact. It is optimal for screening before traditional angiography, bronchoscopy, or barium swallow is initiated. Such traditional workups may be unnecessary if the MDCT demonstrates that the wound track does not traverse the

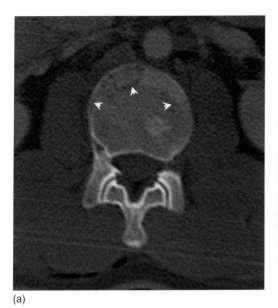
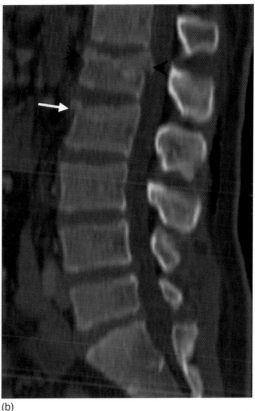

(a)   (b)

Figure 30.35 Compression fracture: (a) Transverse CT image shows subtle fractures across the anterior L2 vertebral body (arrowheads); (b) Mid-sagittal CT image of the lumbar spine demonstrates the L2 compression fracture (arrow). Note that the posterior cortex is intact, unlike the L1 burst fracture (black arrowheads).

mediastinum. However, any question of mediastinal violation must be pursued since occult injuries to mediastinal structures are associated with high mortality.[26] As such, patients with transmediastinal gunshot wounds who are hemodynamically stable may benefit from MDCT to exclude a mediastinal injury. If the CT cannot rule out the course of bullet though the mediastinum, further evaluation is necessary.

Patients suffering from blunt thoracic trauma with a high-energy mechanism may benefit from direct evaluation of mediastinal, pulmonary, and pleural injuries using a contrast-enhanced CT scan. In general, patients with obvious injuries or multiple trauma benefit the most. Computed tomography for mechanism alone is less useful and should be balanced with suspicion of injury and other findings.

Aorta

Chest radiography remains the initial screening study for assessment of traumatic aortic injury (TAI).

Abnormal mediastinal contour is a sensitive marker, but not specific and may be normal in around 7% of patients with significant injury. This may happen when a traumatic pseudoaneurysm is not accompanied by mediastinal hemorrhage, and the pseudoaneurysm is either small or is situated in such a way that it does not alter the mediastinal contour.[27] Technological advancements in CT scanning and the development of MDCT have enabled rapid high quality images of the aorta, allowing it to replace aortography as the initial test of choice, Use of single-slice CT to detect blunt aortic trauma has been reported to have a sensitivity of 96% and specificity of 98%.[28] Data from multidetector scanners improves diagnostic confidence by reducing artifact from cardiac motion and aortic pulsations.

Twenty percent of patients that survive to the ED with deceleration injuries to the aorta suffer from partial tears to the intima or media.[29] If the adventitia remains intact, arterial blood pressure and/or pressure from the vasovasorum may force blood between the layers and

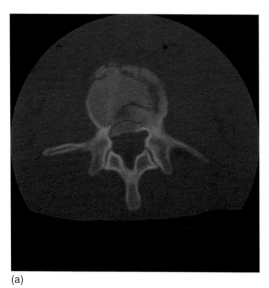

(a)

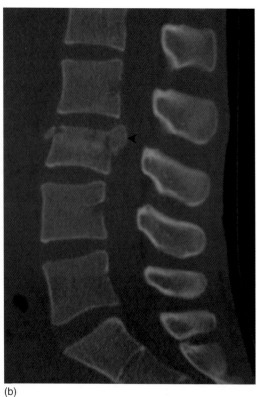

(b)

Figure 30.36 Burst fracture: Transverse (a) and mid-sagittal; (b) CT images of L3 demonstrate comminution of the vertebral body with retropulsion of the posterior cortex into the canal (arrowhead). The dashed line in (a) represents the normal arc of the posterior cortex. The burst fracture involves both the anterior and middle columns and may disrupt the facet joints or the lamina of the posterior column.

form a pseudoaneurysm. Computed tomography findings include a saccular outpouching demarcated from the aortic lumen, typically in the anterior aspect of the proximal descending aorta (Figure 30.40). Complications of these aortic pseudoaneurysms serve as secondary signs of TAI on CT. These include luminal compression by the dissected intimal or medial layers. This may decrease downstream blood flow, resulting in aortic pseudocoarctation (Figure 30.41). Another sign of TAI on CT is the presence of an intimal flap projecting into the aortic lumen (Figure 30.40). Visualization of this flap is possible in low-contrast windows, since high-density vascular contrast can obscure the low-attenuation intimal flaps.[30] There may be visible thrombus formation at the site of the pseudoaneurysm. The suspicion for TAI may also be heightened by findings on CT of a periaortic hemorrhage, usually presenting as a mediastinal hematoma adjacent to the aortic arch. This hemorrhage most likely arises from small veins around the aorta, since direct hemorrhage from the aorta often leads to exsanguination of the patient. When large enough, this

hematoma, may lead to rightward displacement of the trachea and esophagus. This hematoma, however, is not diagnostic of an aortic rupture, but is often found in conjunction with one. Rarely, the hematoma may arise from the injured aorta itself and present with active extravasation, a sign that is diagnostic of rupture and carries a very high mortality (Figure 30.42). Multidetector CT can also impact TAI management. It is able to provide the multiplanar reformats, volume rendering, and information about the surface contour of the aorta. This detailed information about the anatomy of the injury will help to determine whether the patient will benefit most from a thoracotomy, stent-graft placement, or observation with blood pressure control.[31]

Complete aortic rupture is a rare finding as most of these patients die in the prehospital setting. Computed tomography findings associated with aortic rupture include a sleeve of subadventitial contrast medium with a ruptured isthmus. Indirect signs include hemomediastinum with hemorrhage surrounding the aorta and hemothorax.[32]

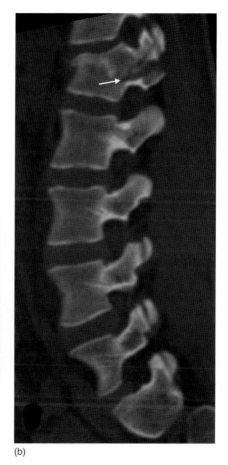

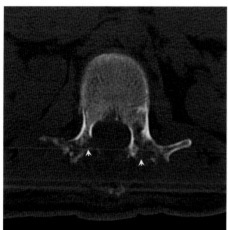

(a)   (b)

Figure 30.37 Chance-type fracture: (a) Transverse CT image depicts the "dissolving pedicle" sign (arrowheads). The lucency through the pedicles represents the loss of bone in the horizontal fracture plane. (b) Mid-sagittal CT demonstrates the horizontal fracture through the pedicle (arrow). Compression deformity of the vertebral body supports the flexion mechanism. This fracture involves the posterior and middle columns, and may propagate into the anterior column; hence it is unstable.

Traumatic aortic dissection is an uncommon finding in the setting of blunt thoracic trauma. Only 11% of traumatic aortic tears are reported to result in aortic dissection.[33] The hallmark CT sign of traumatic aortic rupture involves the identification of the intimal flap, separating the true lumen and false lumen (Figure 30.43). Accuracy of CT in identifying aortic dissection approaches 100%.[34]

With penetrating trauma, the role of CT is more to determine whether the mediastinum is involved. Following the course of the projectile helps to determine if this is true. The most consistent, though indirect, sign of aortic involvement is perivascular hemorrhage. However, there may be direct signs of injury, such as, irregular vascular contours, luminal narrowing or irregularity, pseudoaneurysms, dissection, and active bleeding.[31]

Pericardium and heart
Pneumopericardium
Pneumopericardium may result from prolonged positive pressure ventilation, traumatic disruption of the trachea, or tension pneumothorax. Computed tomography can demonstrate pneumopericardium, distinguish it from pneumomediastinum, and show evidence suggestive of tamponade or "tension" pneumopericardium (Figure 30.44). Elevated intrapericardial pressure leads to cardiac tamponade manifest by flattened right heart, and distension of the inferior vena cava (IVC), hepatic, and renal veins.

Hemopericardium
Hemopericardium typically results from blunt crush injuries or penetrating injuries to the heart. Sonographic

515

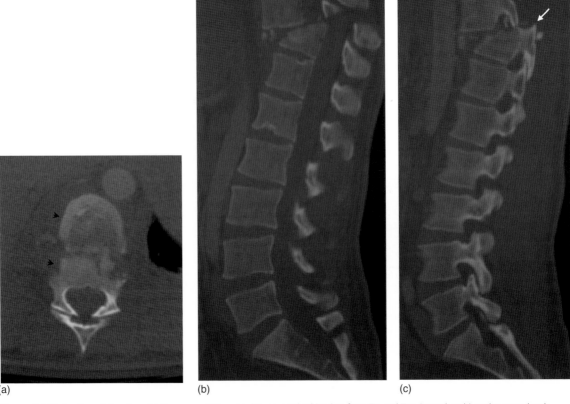

(a) (b) (c)

Figure 30.38 Fracture dislocation: (a) Transverse CT image shows vertebral bodies from T9 and T10 (arrowheads) at the same level; (b, c) Mid-sagittal and para-sagittal CT reformations, respectively, reveal jumped facets (arrow) indicating dislocation. There is anterior translation of T11 on T12 with multiple fracture fragments characteristic of this highly unstable injury.

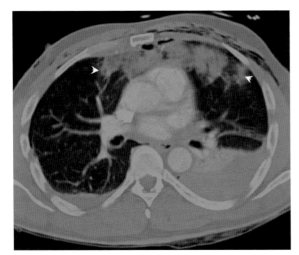

Figure 30.39 Transthoracic gunshot wound (GSW). Transverse CT image at the level of the aortic root shows the path a bullet (between arrowheads) made of hemorrhage and air just anterior to the heart and origin of the great vessels.

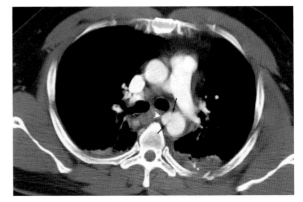

Figure 30.40 Traumatic aortic injury – pseudoaneurysm. Transverse contrast enhanced CT image shows classic aortic pseudoaneurysm (arrowhead) at the proximal descending aorta. This is the location of the ligamentum arteriosum, on CT found just beyond the carina, at the level of the left main pulmonary artery. Note the presence of intimal flaps (arrows).

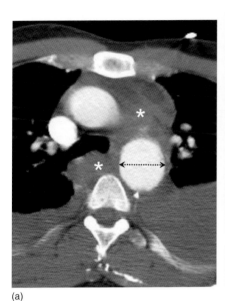
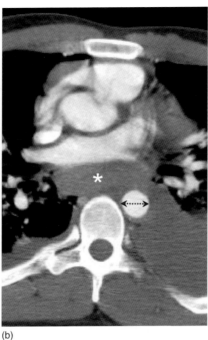

(a)   (b)

Figure 30.41 Traumatic aortic injury – pseudocoarctation: (a) Proximal and (b) distal transverse contrast enhanced CT images of the mediastinum show a relative larger diameter proximal descending thoracic aorta (a) compared to a much smaller diameter (b) distally (double headed dotted arrows). Note the extensive mediastinal hematoma (*) and bilateral hemothoraces.

bedside evaluation of the heart permits rapid detection of pericardial fluid. The presence of hemopericardium should generally necessitate operative intervention bypassing CT altogether. Computed tomography is also very sensitive for diagnosing intrapericardial fluid. Hemorrhage is indicated when the fluid is of high attenuation around 40 Hounsfield units (HU) in the acute setting (Figure 30.45). Cardiac tamponade is indicated on CT as with tension pneumopericardium by distension of the IVC, hepatic, and renal veins.

Pneumomediastinum

Pneumomediastinum may represent disruption of the tracheobronchial tree or esophagus. The most common source of pneumomediastinum is air from ruptured alveoli entering the pulmonary interstitium and dissecting centrally around the airway into the mediastinum. Computed tomography is more sensitive than radiography for the presence of mediastinal air. Pneumomediastinum may appear as retrosternal lucency with streaks of mediastinal fat (Figure 30.46).

Esophageal rupture

Esophageal rupture occurs in < 1% of patients with blunt trauma. Though not well studied, CT is probably a

sensitive mode of imaging because of the ability to detect small quantities of air adjacent to the torn esophagus as well as peri-esophageal hematomas. The gold standard remains an esophagram with water-soluble contrast material.

Tracheobronchial rupture

Tracheaobronchial rupture is an uncommon injury with a 78% early mortality. Sixty to eighty percent occur within 2.5 cm of the carina,[35] with a right-sided predominance.[36] Computed tomography is more sensitive than chest radiograph in providing precise early diagnosis. Diagnostic CT signs include visualization of discontinuity of the airway (Figure 30.47), deformity of the tracheal rings, continuity of intraluminar and extraluminar air, and abnormal positioning or abnormal shape of the endotracheal tube balloon.

Chest wall
Rib fractures and flail chest

Injuries to the ribs, clavicle, and scapula should alert the physician of potentially more significant injuries. In children the more compliant chest wall may allow

517

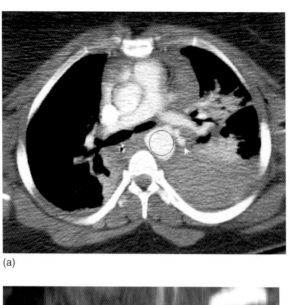

(a)

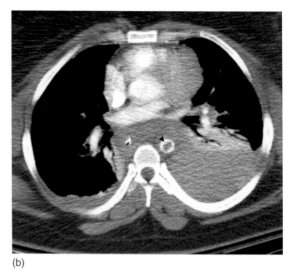

(b)

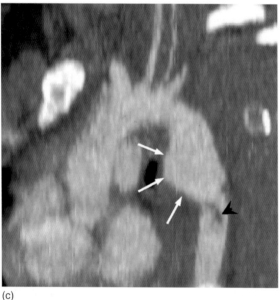

(c)

Figure 30.42 Traumatic aortic injury – multiple signs: (a) Transverse contrast enhanced CT image shows an abnormal contour to the proximal descending thoracic aorta (dotted circle) with focus of active arterial extravasation (white arrowhead) into the mediastinum; (b, c) CT image distal to A and oblique sagittal reformation, respectively, show intraluminal thrombus (black arrowhead) at the distal margin of an aortic pseudoaneurysm (arrows).

transmission of force and injury without imparting fractures. Rib fractures are the most common skeletal injuries in blunt trauma, occurring in up to 50% of patients.[37] Upper-rib fractures (first through third) are associated with high-velocity traumas and may be associated with injury to the brachial plexus and subclavian vessels. Lower rib fractures (8th through 11th) may be clues to potential intra-abdominal injuries, most often of the liver and spleen. Holmes et al. found that in 301 patients with isolated left lower rib injury, 3% had splenic injuries.[38] Two fractures in

three or more adjacent ribs may lead to a focal area of chest wall instability referred to as a flail chest (Figure 30.48). This is seen in 5–13% of patients with chest wall trauma.[39]

Sternum

Fractures of the sternum occur in 3–8% of significant blunt chest trauma patients.[40] Sternal fractures typically occur in the manubrium or body. Routine portable AP chest radiographs miss the majority of sternal fractures, though more are picked up on true lateral. Although

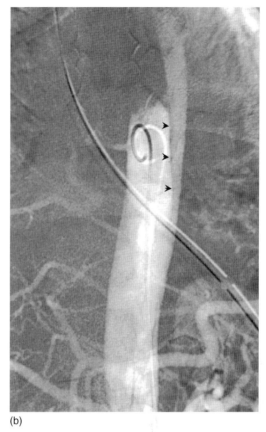

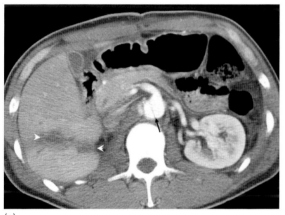

(a)   (b)

Figure 30.43 Traumatic aortic dissection: (a) Transverse contrast enhanced CT image shows an aortic intimal flap (arrow) in a patient following a gunshot wound. Note the liver laceration (between white arrowheads); (b) Angiographic image shows dual aortic lumen separated by intimal flap (black arrowheads) consistent with dissection.

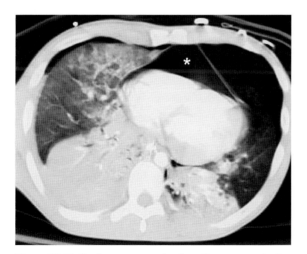

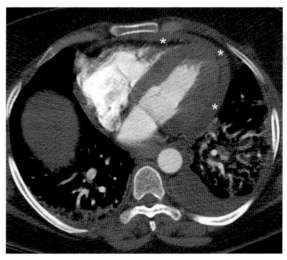

Figure 30.44 Tension pneumopericardium. Transverse contrast enhanced CT image shows bilateral pneumothoraces with lung contusions and consolidation. Air within the pericardial space (*) flattens the underlying right ventricle, suggestive of "tension" pneumopericardium.

Figure 30.45 Hemopericardium. Transverse contrast enhanced CT image in a patient stabbed into the left ventricle shows high density pericardial fluid, consistent with blood (*).

519

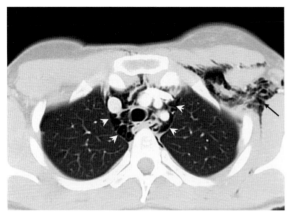

Figure 30.46 Pneumomediastinum. Transverse CT image shows abnormal air within the superior mediastinum surrounding the great vessels (white arrowheads). Subcutaneous air is present deep to the left pectoralis muscle (black arrow).

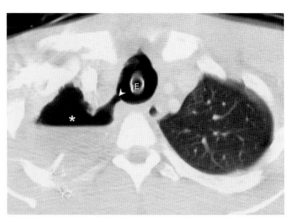

Figure 30.47 Tracheal injury. Transverse CT image in lung windows shows endotracheal tube (E) and its surrounding inflated balloon bridging a right posterolateral tracheal defect (arrowhead) caused by a gunshot wound. Note right hemopneumothorax (*).

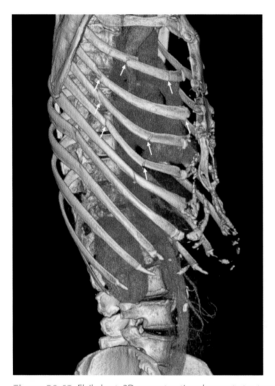

Figure 30.48 Flail chest. 3D reconstruction demonstrates two fractures in each of the right 2nd through 5th ribs (arrows) consistent with a flail chest.

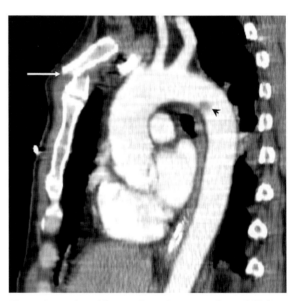

Figure 30.49 Sternal fracture. Sagittal contrast enhanced CT chest reformation shows a displaced sternal fracture (white arrow). Note the concomitant aortic injury seen as focal thrombus on an underlying intimal tear (black arrowhead).

and coronal planes (Figure 30.49). Computed tomography can also detect secondary signs of sternal fracture such as retrosternal hematomas (Figure 30.50), and coexisting mediastinal injury or thoracic spine fracture.

Sternoclavicular dislocation

Sternoclavicular dislocations are most often anterior, i.e., the clavicle is displaced anterior to the sternum. These dislocations are often benign but may indicate

usually performed for other indications, routine CT can detect most sternal fractures, with the exception of non-displaced axial fractures. Axial fractures are best detected using multiplanar reconstructed images in the sagittal

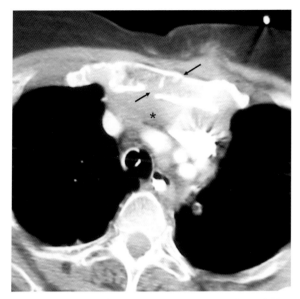

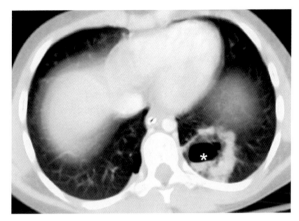

Figure 30.51 Pulmonary laceration. Transverse CT image shows large air and blood filled cavity at the left lung base consistent with a pulmonary laceration (*) with surrounding lung contusion. Small right hemopneumothorax is also present.

Figure 30.50 Sternal fracture. Transverse contrast enhanced CT image shows oblique sternal fracture (arrow) and retrosternal hematoma (*).

a significant mechanism of injury. Up to two thirds have other chest injuries such as pneumothorax, hemothorax, pulmonary contusions, and rib fractures.[41] When the proximal clavicle is posteriorly dislocated relative to the manubrium, there is a higher incidence of injury to the great vessels, trachea, superior mediastinal nerves, and esophagus. These injuries are most efficiently diagnosed using contrast-enhanced MDCT of the chest.

Lung

Pulmonary laceration

Pulmonary laceration may result from shearing of the lung secondary to compression of the chest wall or direct puncture by fractured ribs. Computed tomography is superior to plain radiography in detection of pulmonary lacerations.[42] Initial plain radiographic assessment of pulmonary laceration may be obscured by surrounding contusion and may not become evident for days.[43] On CT, lacerations appear ovoid or round secondary to the elastic recoil of the lung tissue. They may be lucent (air filled), opacified (blood filled), or, most commonly, present with an air–blood level (Figure 30.51). Likewise, complications of pulmonary lacerations are best evaluated by CT. These include abscess formation, enlargement of the laceration, and formation of bronchopulmonary fistulae.

Pneumothorax

Pneumothorax is an air collection in the pleural space either from a leak in the proximal or distal airway or from penetrating trauma. Computed tomography is much more sensitive in detecting pneumothorax than chest radiograph; up to 50% of pneumothoraces seen on CT are not evident on chest X-ray.[42,44] Air in the pleural space will vary in appearance depending on patient position and size of the pneumothorax. In the supine patient large amounts of air may collect in the ventral pleural space making it undetectable on plain chest radiograph (Figure 30.52).

Hemothorax and effusion

Pleural fluid after trauma is usually due to hemorrhage and appears in up to 50% of patients following thoracic trauma.[45] Hemothorax may remain undetectable on an upright chest radiograph until at least 200 cc have collected in the pleural space. Computed tomography is highly sensitive in detecting even a small hemothorax. In addition, the use of the Hounsfield unit for measurement of fluid density may help to identify the origin of the fluid (Table 30.2). In the multitrauma patient other sources of fluid should be considered including chylothorax, bilothorax, and urothorax. Likewise, once determined that the effusion is blood, CT may identify secondary signs to identify the source of bleeding. Blood from venous origin is low pressure and self-limited while blood from arterial trauma may exert a mass effect. Additionally, CT may identify active bleeding usually as a focus of high density (within 10 HU of the nearest artery) (Figure 30.53).[43]

Pulmonary contusion

Pulmonary contusion is the most common non-penetrating lung injury in blunt trauma,[46] and carries a mortality of 10–25%.[47] Injury to the alveoli allows leakage of blood resulting in radiologic "ground glass" opacification and areas of consolidation indicating pulmonary contusion (Figure 30.54). These radiographic findings may be delayed for up to 6 hours. Unlike other airspace diseases, pulmonary contusions have non-segmental distributions that cross pulmonary fissures. They tend to occur adjacent to solid structures such as ribs, sternum, or vertebral bodies and reflect the site of blunt trauma. However, fracture of these adjacent structures is often absent, especially

in children. Clearing of contusions begins 48–72 hours after injury but complete resolution may take as long as 2 weeks. Failure to resolve reflects possible superimposition of another process such as pneumonia, aspiration, atelectasis, or acute respiratory distress syndrome (ARDS). Computed tomography is much more sensitive than chest radiographs in detecting and quantifying pulmonary contusions. A study using anesthetized canines with autopsy as the gold standard showed that chest radiographs detected 38% of pulmonary contusions, while CT demonstrated 100%.[48] Beyond detection, CT is a powerful tool in quantifying pulmonary contusions, which may be a prognostic aid. Miller et al. performed volume reconstructions of chest CTs in 49 patients with isolated chest contusions.[49] They found that contusion volume was an independent predictor of morbidity and mortality. Patients with > 20% contusion volume developed ARDS 82% of the time, compared with 22% in those with < 20% contusion.[49]

Diaphragm injury

Diaphragm injury may result from blunt or penetrating trauma. Blunt diaphragm rupture (BDR) occurs in only 0.16–5.0% of blunt trauma, of these over 90% are due to motor vehicle collisions.[50] Left hemidiaphragm is reportedly injured 40% more often than the right. This is not true in pediatrics where left- and right-sided injuries manifest at equal rates.[51] On the left, diaphragmatic

Table 30.2 Hounsfield units (HU)

Tissue/substances	HU
Air	−1000
Fat	−120
Water	0
Blood	35–55
Muscle	+40
Contrast	+130

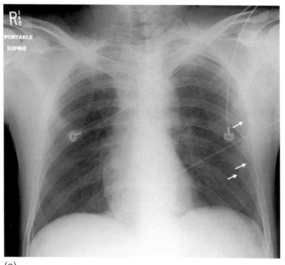

(a)

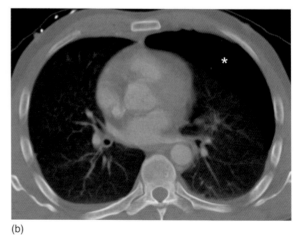

(b)

Figure 30.52 Pneumothorax: (a) Supine portable AP chest in the trauma bay shows left sided rib fractures (arrows). No discernable pneumothorax is evident; (b) Transverse CT image reveals moderate left pneumothorax (*).

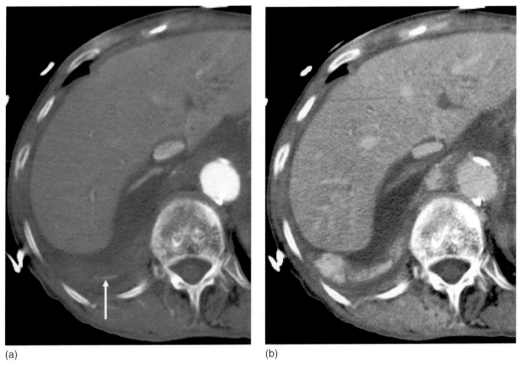

(a)   (b)

Figure 30.53 Actively bleeding hemothorax: (a) initial and (b) delayed phase CT images of the right lower thorax/upper abdomen show a hyperdense pleural collection. Contrast blush in (a) (arrow) increases on delayed imaging, (b) consistent with active arterial extravasation from an injured intercostal artery.

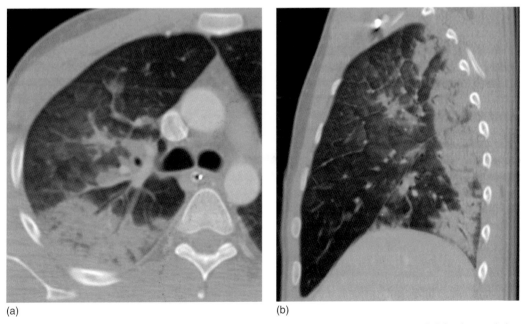

(a)   (b)

Figure 30.54 Pulmonary contusion: (a) transverse CT image and (b) parasagittal reformation show ill-defined ground glass densities and areas of consolidation representing alveolar hemorrhage.

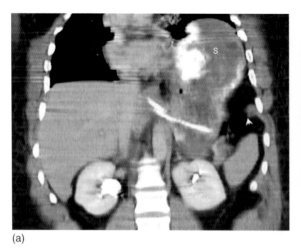
(a)

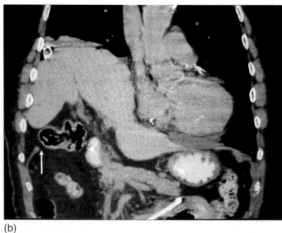
(b)

Figure 30.55 Blunt diaphragm injury: (a) Coronal contrast enhanced CT image shows left hemidiaphragm rupture with intrathoracic stomach (S) and adjacent omental fat. The free edge of the diaphragm is seen (arrowhead); (b) Coronal CT reformation shows a right hemidiaphragm rupture with herniation of liver and hepatic flexure into the chest. The diaphragm defect and retraction of the free edge is seen (arrow).

rupture leads to herniation of abdominal viscera into the pleural space while on the right, this is typically blocked by the liver. Diagnosis by imaging of the diaphragm is challenging, initial chest radiographs may be normal in up to 50% of cases. Up to 7.2% of diaphragmatic injuries that are missed initially result in delayed complications.[52] Studies of helical CT reveal sensitivities for detection of BDR ranging from 71% to 100%.[53] The advent of MDCT has improved this by improving multiplanar reformatting. To further increase sensitivity of CT for diaphragmatic injury, high-resolution thin-slice acquisition with sagittal and coronal reformations are recommended. Computed tomography signs of diaphragm injury, explained below, include direct visualization of the injury, segmental diaphragm non-visualization, intrathoracic herniation of viscera, the collar sign, the dependent viscera sign, diaphragm thickening, and peridiaphragmatic active contrast extravasation.[54] With direct visualization of diaphragmatic injury, images demonstrate the free edge of the defect, which may appear thickened due to muscle retraction or hemorrhage (Figure 30.55). This is in contrast to segmental non-visualization whereby a portion of the diaphragm is absent. Segmental non-visualization must be used with caution if other signs are not present as it may appear as a normal variant in some individuals. Visualization of herniated abdominal contents within the chest has a sensitivity of up to 90% when limited to the left,[55] where typically the stomach and colon herniated (Figure 30.56). Injuries that decrease intrathoracic pressure (such as a large hemothorax or positive pressure ventilation) may

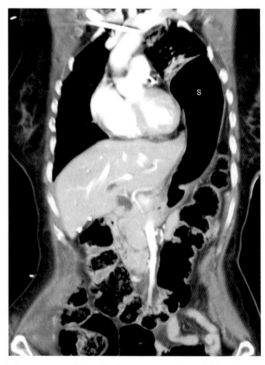

Figure 30.56 Blunt diaphragm injury. Coronal CT reformation shows left hemidiaphragm rupture with herniation of stomach (S) into the left chest.

prevent intrathoracic herniation. The collar sign, or the image created by the free edges of the ruptured diaphragm as it constricts the organ herniating through it, carries a sensitivity of up to 85% and a specificity of up to 100% (Figure 30.57).[55] The dependent viscera sign is seen in the supine patient whose upper abdominal contents are in abnormal contact with the posterior chest wall secondary to a torn diaphragm (Figures 30.57 and 30.58). Of note, this sign may be hindered by the presence of a large pleural effusion or hemothorax. An abnormally thickened diaphragm may signify the presence of an intramuscular hematoma, edema, or muscle retraction. A major limitation of this sign is that hemorrhage of structures adjacent to the diaphragm may mimic intradiaphragmatic hemorrhage. Likewise, the final sign of diaphragmatic injury, active contrast extravasation should not be used as a sole indicator of diaphragmatic injury as active hemorrhage from adjacent sites may mimic diaphragmatic injury.

The accuracy of CT in diagnosis of penetrating diaphragm injury (PDI) is not well defined. Though CT signs of BDR may be applied to PDI, they are less helpful because of the relatively smaller size of the defect. In addition to the CT signs for BDR, visualization of the wound tract may help in diagnosing PDI. A wound tract that extends along both sides of the diaphragm has a sensitivity of 36% and specificity of 100% without demonstrating the actual defect (Figure 30.59).

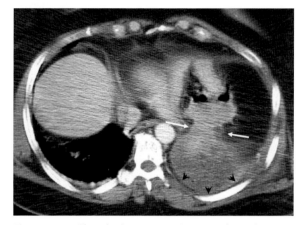

Figure 30.57 Blunt diaphragm injury. Contrast enhanced transverse CT image shows constriction of the stomach, or collar sign, (between arrows) as it crosses the left hemidiaphragm defect. Note that the fundus of the stomach lies dependently on the posterior lower ribs (the dependent viscera sign; arrowheads).

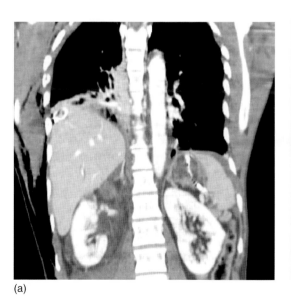

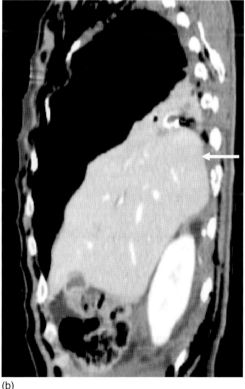

(a) (b)

Figure 30.58 Blunt diaphragm injury: (a) Coronal and (b) sagittal CT reformations show large right hemidiaphragm rupture with herniation of liver into the right chest cavity. Sagittal images best demonstrate the dependent viscera sign with upper liver lying upon the posterior ribs (arrow), no longer subtended by the diaphragm.

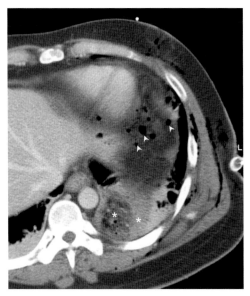

Figure 30.59 Penetrating diaphragm injury. Transverse contrast enhanced CT image in patient following gunshot wound shows gas and hemorrhage above (*) and below (arrowheads) the injured left hemidiaphragm.

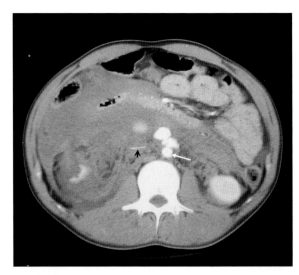

Figure 30.60 Abdominal aortic active bleeding. Transverse contrast enhanced CT image through the midabdomen in a patient stabbed through the aorta shows a small caliber aorta (arrow) with active contrast extravasation anteriorly surrounded by massive retroperitoneal hematoma. Note the flattened IVC (arrowhead).

Abdomen

Introduction

In the trauma patient with multisystem injury or altered mental status, physical examination is not a sensitive diagnostic modality to evaluate for or exclude serious intra-abdominal injury. Clinical findings are unreliable in up to 50% of patients with traumatic intra-abdominal injury and unreliable up to 85% of the time if the patient has sustained head trauma or has an altered mental status.[56]

Patients that have sustained penetrating abdominal injury and remain hemodynamically stable may undergo CT to evaluate both the intraperitoneal and retroperitoneal cavities as well as to evaluate the wound tract.[57]

Imaging options

Focused abdominal sonography for trauma

Of the imaging modalities available, ultrasound and CT are the modalities most commonly used to evaluate intra-abdominal injuries sustained by the trauma patient. Focused abdominal sonography in trauma (FAST) gives immediate information regarding free intraperitoneal fluid. It is mostly useful for the unstable patient. The stable patient, with or without free fluid, can be further imaged by CT.

Computed tomography

Computed tomography offers a thorough evaluation of the entire abdomen including information about the retroperitoneum, injury to the solid and hollow viscera, and detection of active bleeding via extravasation of IV contrast.[58,59]

The retroperitoneum may be the site of occult blood loss. Retroperitoneal hematomas most often result from blunt trauma; most commonly caused by renal and pelvic injury. Because of the ability and high accuracy of MDCT to rapidly evaluate the intraperitoneal and retroperitoneal spaces, as well as the skeletal system, it is the ideal screening tool for the hemodynamically stable patient.

Vascular injury
Abdominal aorta and branches

Penetrating trauma to the abdominal aorta is rare and often lethal secondary to exsanguination of the patient.[60] These patients are rarely stable for CT unless the bleeding is contained. Prognosis of the patient that has sustained penetrating trauma to the abdominal aorta is better if the injury is below the renal arteries (Figure 30.60).

Vena cava and branches

In the setting of blunt abdominal trauma, IVC injury is relatively uncommon. Signs of caval injury include retroperitoneal hematoma surrounding the IVC, irregular vessel contour, and contrast extravasation (Figure 30.61).[61] Retrohepatic IVC injury is associated with a 50% mortality.[62] Signs of retrohepatic IVC injury on CT include liver laceration extending into the porta hepatis and retrohepatic IVC and irregular contour of the retrohepatic IVC.

Solid organ injury

Liver

The role of CT in evaluation of blunt hepatic injury is threefold: establish diagnosis, guide management, and monitor injury progression.

Traumatic liver injury presents as capsular disruption, intraparenchymal laceration (Figure 30.62), fracture, or subcapsular or intraparenchymal hematoma.

In the past, CT was used to dictate the need for early surgical intervention in hemodynamically stable patients. Likewise, hepatic injury grading systems have been made on CT findings to guide surgical vs. non-operative management of the injury. There is now a general consensus that the majority of hemodynamically stable patients with blunt liver trauma can be successfully managed without surgery regardless of the grade (severity) of the injury.[63] Even the presence of significant hemoperitoneum (considered an indicator of severe liver injury) has not been shown to correlate to the success or failure of non-surgical management. Computed tomography does play a more active role in the evaluation of the hemodynamically stable patient when there is pooling,[64] or active extravasation of contrast (Figure 30.62). In this case, the decision to take the patient to

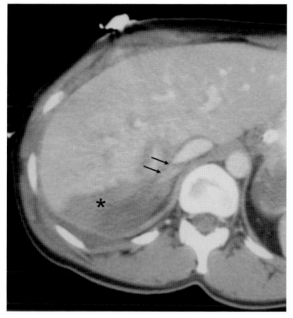

Figure 30.61 Inferior vena cava injury. Transverse contrast enhanced CT through the upper abdomen shows contrast extravasation from the IVC (arrows) and adjacent right hepatic injury (*).

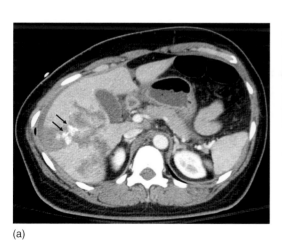

(a)

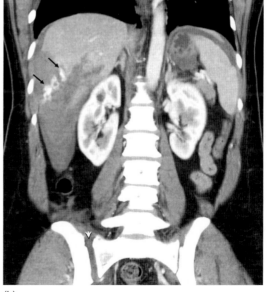

(b)

Figure 30.62 Hepatic lacerations with active bleeding: (a) Transverse and (b) coronal contrast enhanced CT images shows multiple irregular low density hepatic lacerations with focus of active contrast extravasation (arrows). Note widening of the right sacroiliac joint (arrowhead).

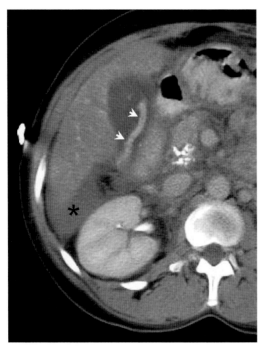

Figure 30.63 Gallbladder rupture. Transverse CT image shows collapsed gallbladder (arrowheads) with surrounding bile. Hemorrhage present in Morrison's pouch (*).

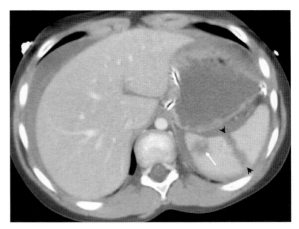

Figure 30.64 Splenic fracture. Contrast enhanced transverse CT image shows fracture through the spleen (arrowheads) and smaller laceration (arrow). Perisplenic and perihepatic hemoperitoneum are present.

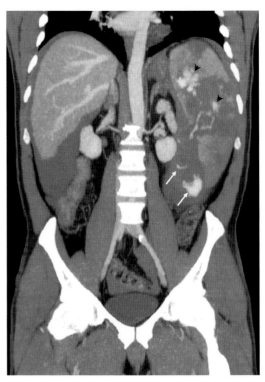

Figure 30.66 Splenic lacerations and active bleeding. Coronal contrast enhanced CT image shows extensive laceration through the mid-portion of the spleen with multiple foci of active contrast extravasation, also referred to as "splenic blush", both within the spleen (arrowheads) and into the peritoneum (arrows).

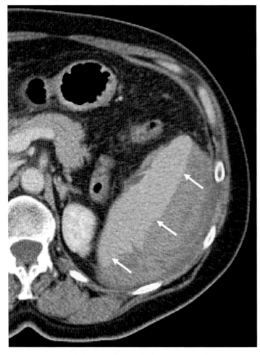

Figure 30.65 Splenic subcapsular hematoma. Contrast enhanced transverse CT image shows subcapsular hemorrhage applying mass effect and compressing the underlying splenic parenchyma (arrows).

angiography is common, even in the stable patient. In these cases, despite the patient being stable, there is a high likelihood that conservative management will fail.

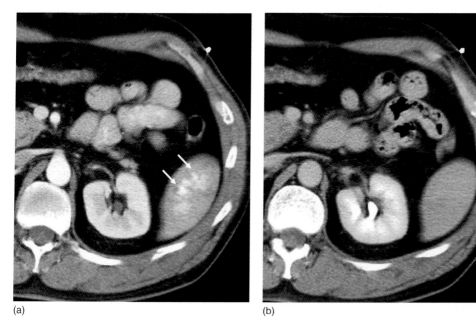

(a)   (b)

Figure 30.67 Splenic pseudoaneurysms: Transverse contrast enhanced CT images in portal venous phase (a) show abnormal collections of contrast in the lower pole of the spleen (arrows). Imaging in the excretory phase (b) shows the disappearance of these collections consistent with splenic pseudoaneurysms. No hemoperitoneum was present in this patient.

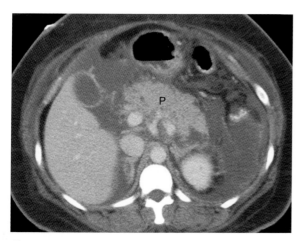

Figure 30.68 Pancreatic contusion. Contrast enhanced transverse CT image shows diffuse pancreatic swelling (P) with retroperitoneal hemorrhage.

The major role of CT with respect to blunt hepatic trauma in the hemodynamically stable patient is to monitor progression.[65] Delayed complications include abscess that occur secondary to devascularization or large hematomas.

Biliary tract

Blunt abdominal trauma may rarely result in injury to the biliary tract, including the gallbladder, the

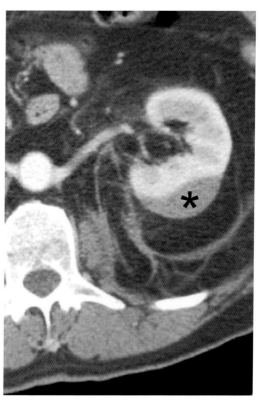

Figure 30.69 Subcapsular hematoma. Transverse contrast enhanced CT image of the left kidney shows hemorrhage within the renal capsule (*) compressing the underlying renal parenchyma representing a subcapsular hematoma.

529

intrahepatic bile ducts, and the extrahepatic bile ducts. The most common location of biliary injury is the gallbladder. Biliary tract injuries are highly associated with additional injuries, most notably the liver, spleen, and duodenum.[66] Computed tomography imaging of this system is often overshadowed by injuries to adjacent organs. Findings that are helpful include collapsed gallbladder, which may indicate gallbladder perforation or avulsion (Figure 30.63). Likewise, thickened gallbladder wall and/or pericholecystic fluid may indicate gallbladder wall injury. Dense layering of fluid within the gallbladder lumen may indicate intraluminal hemorrhage.

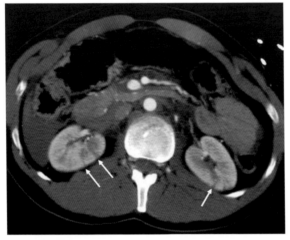

Figure 30.70 Minor renal lacerations. Contrast enhanced transverse CT image shows small renal cortical lacerations bilaterally (arrows).

Spleen

The spleen is the most frequently injured abdominal organ in blunt trauma. Contrast-enhanced CT is up to 98% accurate for detecting splenic injuries.[67,68] Typical findings include capsular disruption, laceration or fracture (Figure 30.64), perisplenic/intrasplenic and subcapsular hematoma (Figure 30.65), active extravasation (Figure 30.66), and intrasplenic pseudoaneurysm (Figure 30.67). While CT may aid in determination of which patients may benefit from early surgical intervention, the initial management is similar to liver trauma, with hemodynamic stability taking precedence. In those who are managed non-operatively, CT becomes essential in follow-up monitoring. Computed tomography signs that may indicate failure of non-operative management include intrasplenic or perisplenic contrast collections, or pseudoaneurysm, referred to as the splenic blush (Figure 30.66).[69] Presence of splenic blush is being used as an indication for embolization or surgery.[70] Splenic pseudoaneurysms may not be present at admission and appear 1–3 days later, highlighting the importance of CT monitoring as part of non-operative management (Figure 30.67).

Pancreas

Pancreatic and biliary injuries are often subtle and, thus, may be overlooked in the multisystem trauma patient. Pancreatic injuries are relatively uncommon, occurring in < 2% of blunt abdominal

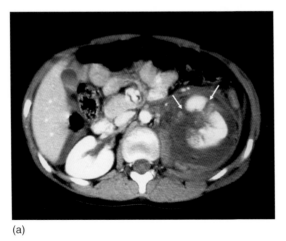

(a)

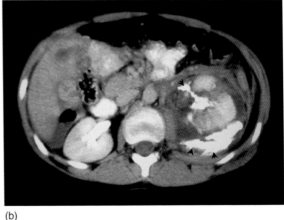

(b)

Figure 30.71 Major renal lacerations: (a) Transverse contrast enhanced CT image in portal venous phase shows left renal lacerations extending from cortex through medulla (arrows). Note perinephric fluid; (b) Transverse contrast enhanced CT image in delayed excretory phase shows extensive contrast extravasation and accumulation (arrowheads) from the renal collecting system representing a urine leak.

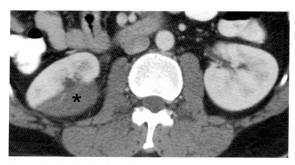

Figure 30.72 Renal infarct. Contrast enhanced transverse CT image of the kidneys in a blunt trauma patient shows segmental nonperfusion (*) in the right kidney representing a traumatic infarct.

trauma.[71] But early diagnosis is crucial, since delayed complications such as hematoma, fistula, and abscess may occur in up to 20% of cases and lead to significant mortality.

Since concomitant injuries to the liver, stomach, spleen, and duodenum occur in over 90% of patients with pancreatic injuries, laboratory and clinical findings are consequently non-specific and unreliable.[72]

Direct CT signs of pancreatic injury include pancreatic laceration, transaction, and comminution. Other signs of pancreatic injury include focal

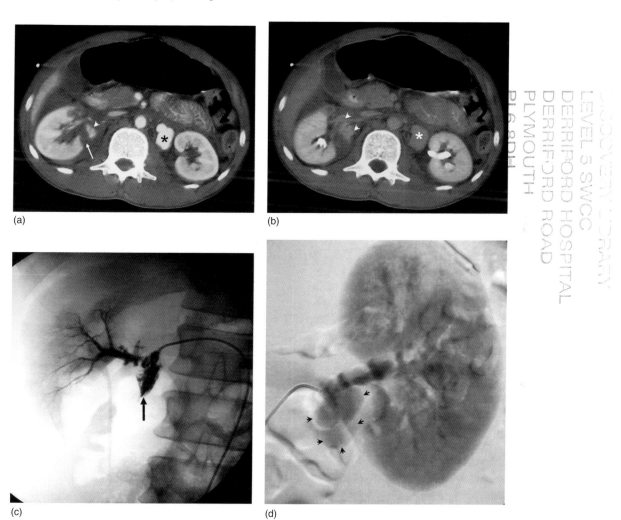

(a)

(b)

(c)

(d)

Figure 30.73 Renal vascular injuries: (a) Transverse contrast enhanced CT image in portal venous phase shows right renal laceration (arrow) and contrast blush (arrowhead). Abnormal lobulated contrast collection lies just medial of the left kidney (*). Shock bowel is present; (b) Transverse contrast enhanced delayed excretory phase CT image shows accumulation of contrast on the right (arrowheads) representing active hemorrhage. On the left, the lobulated contrast collection (*) has washed out, representing a pseudoaneurysm; (c) Right renal angiogram confirms active arterial extravasation from the main right renal artery (black arrow); (d) Left renal angiogram confirms the presence of a large renal artery pseudoaneurysm (black arrowheads).

Table 30.3 Renal injury based on computed tomography (CT) findings

Category of renal injury	Description	Comment
Category 1	Minor cortical contusion, subcapsular hematoma (see Figure 30.69), minor lacerations (see Figure 30.70) with limited perinephric hematoma and small cortical infarct	Constitute 75–85% of all renal injuries and are generally managed conservatively
Category 2	All major renal lacerations extending to the medulla (see Figure 30.71a and b) and segmental renal infarcts (see Figure 30.72)	Comprise about 10% of renal injuries
Category 3	Multiple renal lacerations and vascular injury (see Figure 30.73a–d) including the renal pedicle	Comprise about 5% of all injuries. Catastrophic Require surgical exploration and nephrectomy
Category 4	Injuries involving ureteropelvic region	Caused by sudden deceleration, creating tension at the renal pedicle. One third do not have hematuria. Clinical assessment is important in making the decision to image

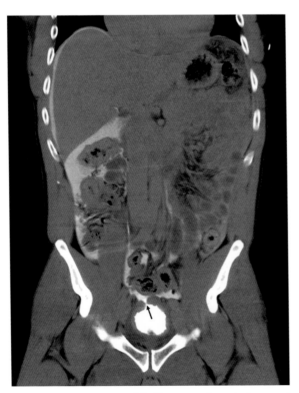

Figure 30.74 Intraperitoneal bladder rupture. Coronal reformatted CT cystogram shows defect through the dome of the bladder (arrow) with intrtaperitoneal leak of contrast material outlining bowel loops and surrounding the liver.

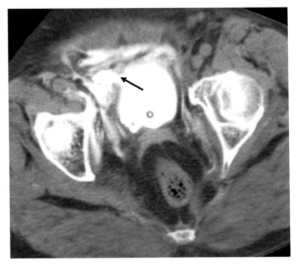

Figure 30.75 Extraperitoneal bladder rupture. Transverse CT cystogram image shows right lateral bladder wall defect (arrow) with contrast spilling into the extraperitoneal spaces.

enlargement of the pancreas and peripancreatic fluid (Figure 30.68). Peripancreatic fat stranding, hemorrhage, and fluid between the splenic vein and pancreas are secondary signs indicative of injury.

Because CT will not always illustrate direct signs of pancreatic trauma, endoscopic retrograde cholangiopancreatography (ERCP) remains an important tool to establish diagnosis and direct appropriate surgical

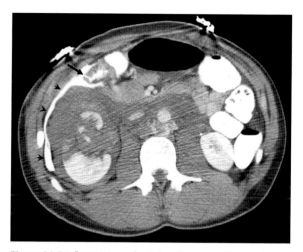

Figure 30.76 Penetrating colon injury. Transverse CT image from a triple contrast (IV, oral and rectal) study performed following abdominal gunshot wound. Image shows disruption of right colon (black arrow) with leak of rectal contrast (arrowheads). Major right renal injury with active hemorrhage and active arterial extravasation between the vertebral body and abdominal aorta.

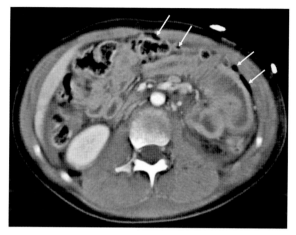

Figure 30.77 Blunt bowel injury. Transverse contrast enhanced CT image shows foci of free air (arrows) and bowel wall thickening. Patient sustained a Chance fracture (not shown) and surgery confirmed focal bowel perforation.

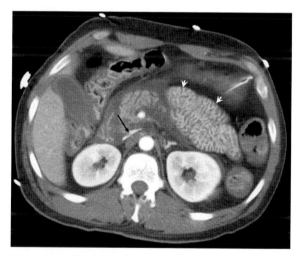

Figure 30.78 Shock bowel. Transverse contrast enhanced CT image shows bowel wall hyperenhancement (arrowheads) in the setting of a flat IVC (arrow) and small aorta. Signs are compatible with shock bowel and hypoperfusion complex. Bowel changes are reversible with fluid management. Pancreatic injury with peripancreatic hemorrhage is also present.

repair when the CT suggests injury to the pancreas. Likewise, in situations with mild duct injury, stent placement may obviate the need for surgical repair.[73]

Kidney

About 8–10% of traumatic abdominal injuries involve the kidneys.[74] Hematuria is present in over 95% of patients with traumatic renal injury. However, over 30% of patients with ureteropelvic junction injury have no hematuria.[75] As such, recommendations have been made to do diagnostic imaging of patients with penetrating abdominal or flank trauma and any hematuria, blunt abdominal or flank trauma and gross hematuria, or with possibility of direct renal injury (lower rib fractures, flank hematoma, thoracolumbar spine, or transverse process injury).[76] Computed tomography can provide diagnostic information necessary to differentiate patients that have injuries that need immediate intervention from those than can be observed (Figures 30.69–30.73). There are four categories of classifications for traumatic renal injuries based on CT findings (Table 30.3).[76,77]

Anterior penetrating injuries affecting the kidneys are usually associated with other intra-abdominal injuries and thus warrant surgical exploration. Stab wounds to the flank or back may undergo contrast-enhanced CT to assess the extent of injury and possibly obviate the need for surgery.[78]

Bladder

Seventy percent of patients with traumatic bladder injury also sustain pelvic fractures. Likewise, 5–10% of patients with pelvic fractures suffer from urinary bladder rupture. As such, patients with pelvic fractures and gross hematuria should undergo cystography or CT cystography after urethral injury has been excluded. Computed tomography cystogram is

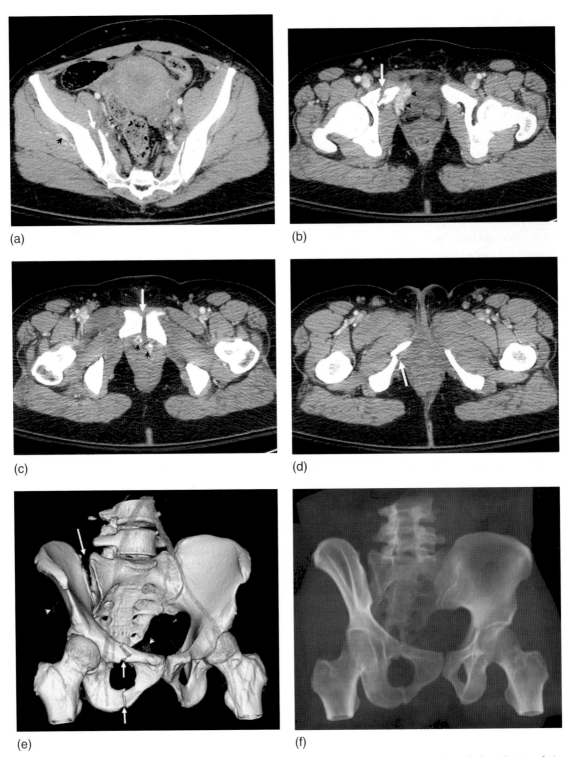

(a)

(b)

(c)

(d)

(e)

(f)

Figure 30.79 Pelvic fractures with active hemorrhage: (a-d) Transverse contrast enhanced CT images through the pelvis in soft tissue windows show widening of the right sacroiliac joint (arrow in a), sagittally oriented fractures of the right superior and inferior pubic rami (arrows in b and d, respectively), and slight widening of the pubic symphysis (arrow in c). 3D Judet CT reconstructions in traditional (e) and virtual radiograph, or transparent bone (f), filters aid in surgical planning. Arrows highlight fractures. Fracture pattern represents an anterior-posterior compression (APC) pelvic injury. Note multiple foci of active bleeding (arrowheads).

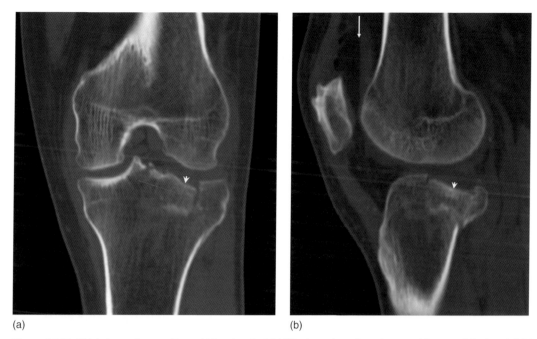

(a)   (b)

Figure 30.80 Tibial plateau fracture: Coronal (a) and sagittal (b) CT reformations show depressed fracture of the lateral tibial plateau (arrowheads). Note lipohemarthrosis seen as fat/blood interface in the suprapatellar joint space (arrow).

accomplished by instilling at least 350 cc of 1 : 20 dilution of contrast material to water into the bladder through a Foley catheter. This is the minimum needed to distend the detrussor muscle and initiate contraction, decreasing the likelihood of false negatives.

Bladder rupture can be classified into either intraperitoneal rupture, where the dome is injured, usually from blunt trauma to a full bladder, or extraperitoneal rupture. These can be distinguished by CT. Intraperitoneal rupture results in free contrast spillage into the peritoneum (Figure 30.74). Dense urinary contrast may obscure other intraperitoneal injuries. In comparison, extraperitoneal bladder rupture creates streaky intrafascial patterns (Figure 30.75). Contrast can extend to the perineum and scrotum.

Bowel and mesentery

Computed tomography has become the primary modality for imaging of patients suspected to have injury to hollow organs or mesentery.[79] Signs of bowel and mesenteric injury include bowel discontinuity, oral contrast leak (Figure 30.76), free air (Figure 30.77), intramural air, and bowel wall thickening.

Oral contrast material within the peritoneum is 100% specific for bowel perforation. Extraluminal free air is not diagnostic of bowel perforation, since barotraumas and mechanical ventilation can result in air below the diaphragm. In the setting of penetrating trauma, extraluminal air alternatively may be introduced from abdominal wall violation. Retroperitoneal free air is, however, sensitive for duodenal perforation. Circumferential bowel wall thickening has a greater sensitivity for transmural injuries than extravastion of oral contrast material or pneumoperitoneum.[80,81]

Bowel wall hyperenhancement may represent hypoperfusion complex/shock bowel (Figure 30.78),[82] or perforation in children.[83] Retroperitoneal hematomas occur with duodenal trauma and are often accompanied by bowel wall thickening. In distinction, hemoperitoneum often indicates blood from solid organs. In the absence of solid organ injury, isolated hemoperitoneum may be a sign of mesenteric or bowel laceration.[84] However, intra-abdominal fluid may not be blood, but rather leakage of bowel contents, pancreatic juice, urine, or ascites. This may mask the presence of intraperitoneal blood. The use of Hounsfield units may help distinguish.

Mesenteric infiltration or stranding may be associated with mesenteric injury and, when associated with bowel wall thickening, is indicative of bowel wall injury.[85] Isolated bowel wall injury is more common when the bowel injury is along the mesenteric border. Isolated hematoma within the mesentery usually indicates a laceration.

Lower extremity

Pelvis and acetabulum

Pelvic fractures are common sequelae of high-energy injuries. Classification systems exist that take into account the direction of force and severity of injury. Since most clinically pertinent injuries can be diagnosed using AP radiographs of the pelvis, classification systems base their fracture pattern on these films. Computed tomography delineates the pelvic and acetabular injuries with greater precision and provides details, including active hemorrhage, helpful in the management of the patient with multiple traumatic injuries (Figure 30.79).

Tibial plateau

Tibial plateau fractures often result from a valgus stress mechanism. The tibial cartilage is 3 mm thick, as such any tibial depression > 3 mm is significant. Since these fractures are sometimes subtle, CT is a great diagnostic tool following plain radiography, to diagnose the injury when still suspected by clinical examination or subtle radiographic signs, as well as define the extent of the fracture (Figure 30.80).

References

1. Wing VW, Federle MP, Morris JA, Jr., Jeffrey RB, Bluth R. The clinical impact of CT for blunt abdominal trauma. *AJR Am J Roentgenol* 1985;**145**(6):1191–4.

2. Thomton FJ, Paulson EK, Yoshizumi TT, Frush DP, Nelson RC. Single versus multi-detector row CT: comparison of radiation doses and dose profiles. *Acad Radiol* 2003;**10**(4):379–85.

3. Sosin DM, Sniezek JE, Waxweiler RJ. Trends in death associated with traumatic brain injury, 1979 through 1992. Success and failure. *JAMA* 1995;**273**(22):1778–80.

4. Haydel MJ, Preston, CA, Mills TJ, et al. Indications for computed tomography in patients with minor head injury. *N Engl J Med* 2000;**343**(2):100–5.

5. Stiell IG, Wells GA, Vandemheen K, et al. The Canadian CT Head Rule for patients with minor head injury. *Lancet* 2001;**357**(9266):1391–6.

6. Seelig JM, Becker DP, Miller JD, et al. Traumatic acute subdural hematoma: major mortality reduction in comatose patients treated within 4 hours. *N Engl J Med* 1981;**304**(25):1511–18.

7. Stiell IG, Clement CM, McKnight RD, et al. The Canadian C-spine Rule versus the NEXUS Low-risk Criteria in patients with trauma. *N Engl J Med* 2003;**349**(26):2510–18.

8. British Trauma Society. Guidelines for the initial management and assessment of spinal injury, 2002. *Injury* 2003;**34**(6):405–25.

9. Schenarts PJ, Kaiser DJ, Carrillo Y, Eddy V, Morris JA, Jr. Prospective comparison of admission computed tomographic scan and plain films of the upper cervical spine in trauma patients with altered mental status. *J Trauma* 2001;**51**(4):663–8; discussion 8–9.

10. Holmes JF, Akkinepalli R. Computed tomography versus plain radiography to screen for cervical spine injury: a meta-analysis. *J Trauma* 2005;**58**(5):902–5.

11. Nuñez DB, Jr., Zuluaga A, Fuentes-Bernardo DA, Rivas LA, Becerra JL. Cervical spine trauma: how much more do we learn by routinely using helical CT? *Radiographics* 1996;**16**(6):1307–18; discussion 18–21.

12. Hanson JA, Blackmore CC, Mann FA, Wilson AJ. Cervical spine injury: a clinical decision rule to identify high-risk patients for helical CT screening. *AJR Am J Roentgenol* 2000;**174**:713–17.

13. Ptak T, Kihiczak D, Lawrason JN. Screening for cervical spine trauma with helical CT: experience with 676 cases. *Emerg Radiol* 2001;**8**(6):315–19.

14. Hogan GJ, Mirvis SE, Shanmuganathan K, Scalea TM. Exclusion of unstable cervical spine injury in obtunded patients with blunt trauma: is MR imaging needed when multi-detector row CT findings are normal? *Radiology* 2005;**237**(1):106–13.

15. Brown CV, Antevil JL, Sise MJ, Sack DI. Spiral computed tomography for the diagnosis of cervical, thoracic, and lumbar spine fractures: its time has come. *J Trauma* 2005;**58**(5):890–5; discussion 5–6.

16. Daffner RH, Hackney DB. ACR Appropriateness Criteria on suspected spine trauma. *J Am Coll Radiol* 2007;**4**(11):762–75.

17. Tins BJ, Cassar-Pullicino VN. Imaging of acute cervical spine injuries: review and outlook. *Clin Radiol* 2004;**59**(10):865–80.

18. Tomycz ND, Chew BG, Chang YF, et al. MRI is unnecessary to clear the cervical spine in obtunded/comatose trauma patients: the four-year experience of a Level I trauma center. *J Trauma* 2008;**64**(5):1258–63.

19. Brant-Zawadzki M, Jeffrey RB, Jr., Minagi H, Pitts LH. High resolution CT of thoracolumbar fractures. *AJR Am J Roentgenol* 1982;**138**(4):699–704.

20. Ferguson RL, Allen BL, Jr. A mechanistic classification of thoracolumbar spine fractures. *Clin Orthop Relat Res* 1984;**189**:77–88.

21. Denis F. Spinal instability as defined by the three-column spine concept in acute spinal trauma. *Clin Orthop Relat Res* 1984;**189**:65–76.

22. Guerra J, Jr., Garfin SR, Resnick D. Vertebral burst fractures: CT analysis of the retropulsed fragment. *Radiology* 1984;**153**(3):769–72.

23. Bernstein MP, Mirvis SE, Shanmuganathan K. Chance-type fractures of the thoracolumbar spine: imaging analysis in 53 patients. *AJR Am J Roentgenol* 2006;**187**(4):859–68.

24. Denis F. The three column spine and its significance in the classification of acute thoracolumbar spinal injuries. *Spine* 1983;**8**(8):817–31.

25. von Oppell UO, Bautz P, De Groot M. Penetrating thoracic injuries: what we have learnt. *Thorac Cardiovasc Surg* 2000;**48**(01):55–61.

26. Gasparri MG, Lorelli DR, Kralovich KA, Patton JH, Jr. Physical examination plus chest radiography in penetrating periclavicular trauma: the appropriate trigger for angiography. *J Trauma* 2000;**49**(6):1029–33.

27. Woodring JH. The normal mediastinum in blunt traumatic rupture of the thoracic aorta and brachiocephalic arteries. *J Emerg Med* 1990;**8**(4): 467–76.

28. Mirvis SE, Shanmuganathan K, Buell J, Rodriguez A. Use of spiral computed tomography for the assessment of blunt trauma patients with potential aortic injury. *J Trauma* 1998;**45**(5):922–30.

29. Wintermark M, Wicky S, Schnyder P. Imaging of acute traumatic injuries of the thoracic aorta. *Eur Radiol* 2002;**12**(2):431–42.

30. Mirvis SE, Shanmuganathan K. Diagnosis of blunt traumatic aortic injury 2007: still a nemesis. *Eur J Radiol* 2007;**64**(1):27–40.

31. Mirvis SE. Thoracic vascular injury. *Radiol Clin North Am* 2006;**44**(2):181–97, vii.

32. Alkadhi H, Wildermuth S, Desbiolles L, et al. Vascular emergencies of the thorax after blunt and iatrogenic trauma: multi-detector row CT and three-dimensional imaging. *Radiographics* 2004; **24**(5):1239–55.

33. Fisher RG, Hadlock F. Laceration of the thoracic aorta and brachiocephalic arteries by blunt trauma. Report of 54 cases and review of the literature. *Radiol Clin North Am* 1981;**19**(1):91–110.

34. Yoshida S, Akiba H, Tamakawa M, et al. Thoracic involvement of type A aortic dissection and intramural hematoma: diagnostic accuracy–comparison of emergency helical CT and surgical findings. *Radiology* 2003;**228**(2):430–5.

35. Maltby JD. The post-trauma chest film. *Crit Rev Diagn Imaging* 1980;**14**(1):1–36.

36. Henry C. Thoracic trauma: triage of the chest radiograph. Eighty-seventh American Roentgen Ray Society Meeting, Miami Beach, FL, May 1, 1987.

37. DeLuca SA, Rhea JT, O'Malley TO. Radiographic evaluation of rib fractures. *AJR Am J Roentgenol* 1982;**138**(1):91–2.

38. Holmes JF, Ngyuen H, Jacoby RC, et al. Do all patients with left costal margin injuries require radiographic evaluation for intraabdominal injury? *Ann Emerg Med* 2005;**46**(3):232–6.

39. LoCicero J, 3rd, Mattox KL. Epidemiology of chest trauma. *Surg Clin North Am* 1989;**69**(1):15–19.

40. Athanassiadi K, Gerazounis M, Moustardas M, Metaxas E. Sternal fractures: retrospective analysis of 100 cases. *World J Surg* 2002;**26**(10):1243–6.

41. de Jong KP, Sukul DM. Anterior sternoclavicular dislocation: a long-term follow-up study. *J Orthop Trauma* 1990;**4**(4):420–3.

42. Trupka A, Waydhas C, Hallfeldt KK, et al. Value of thoracic computed tomography in the first assessment of severely injured patients with blunt chest trauma: results of a prospective study. *J Trauma* 1997; **43**(3):405–11; discussion 11–12.

43. Miller LA. Chest wall, lung, and pleural space trauma. *Radiol Clin North Am* 2006;**44**(2):213–24.

44. Wagner RB, Crawford WO, Jr., Schimpf PP. Classification of parenchymal injuries of the lung. *Radiology* 1988;**167**(1):77–82.

45. Stark P. *Radiology of Thoracic Trauma*. Boston: Andover Medical Publishers, 1993.

46. Cohn SM. Pulmonary contusion: review of the clinical entity. *J Trauma* 1997;**42**(5):973–9.

47. Hoff SJ, Shotts SD, Eddy VA, Morris JA, Jr. Outcome of isolated pulmonary contusion in blunt trauma patients. *Am Surg* 1994;**60**(2):138–42.

48. Schild HH, Strunk H, Weber W, et al. Pulmonary contusion: CT vs plain radiograms. *J Comput Assist Tomogr* 1989;**13**(3):417–20.

49. Miller PR, Croce MA, Bee TK, et al. ARDS after pulmonary contusion: accurate measurement of contusion volume identifies high-risk patients. *J Trauma* 2001;**51**(2):223–8; discussion 29–30.

537

50. Mihos P, Potaris K, Gakidis J, et al. Traumatic rupture of the diaphragm: experience with 65 patients. *Injury* 2003;**34**(3):169–72.

51. Shanmuganathan K, Killeen K, Mirvis SE, White CS. Imaging of diaphragmatic injuries. *J Thorac Imaging* 2000;**15**(2):104–11.

52. Patselas TN, Gallagher EG. The diagnostic dilemma of diaphragm injury. *Am Surg* 2002;**68**(7):633–9.

53. Killeen KL, Mirvis SE, Shanmuganathan K. Helical CT of diaphragmatic rupture caused by blunt trauma. *AJR Am J Roentgenol* 1999; **173**(6):1611–16.

54. Sliker CW. Imaging of diaphragm injuries. *Radiol Clin North Am* 2006;**44**(2):199–211, vii.

55. Nchimi A, Szapiro D, Ghaye B, et al. Helical CT of blunt diaphragmatic rupture. *AJR Am J Roentgenol* 2005;**184**(1):24–30.

56. Schurink GW, Bode PJ, van Luijt PA, van Vugt AB. The value of physical examination in the diagnosis of patients with blunt abdominal trauma: a retrospective study. *Injury* 1997;**28**(4):261–5.

57. Shanmuganathan K, Chiu WC, Killeen KL, Hogan GJ, Scalea TM. Penetrating torso trauma: triple-contrast helical CT in peritoneal violation and organ injury–a prospective study in 200 patients. *Radiology* 2004; **231**(3):775–84.

58. Becker CD, Mentha G, Terrier F. Blunt abdominal trauma in adults: role of CT in the diagnosis and management of visceral injuries. Part 1: liver and spleen. *Eur Radiol* 1998;**8**(4):553–62.

59. Hewett JJ, Freed KS, Sheafor DH, Vaslef SN, Kliewer MA. Blunt abdominal trauma in adults: role of CT in the diagnosis and management of visceral injuries. Part 2: Gastrointestinal tract and retroperitoneal organs. *Eur Radiol* 1998;**8**(5):772–80.

60. Bernstein MP, Mirvis SE. Penetrating trauma to the abdominal aorta: CT demonstration of active bleeding. *Emerg Radiol* 2001;**8**(1):43–7.

61. Hewett JJ, Freed KS, Sheafor DH, et al. The spectrum of abdominal venous CT findings in blunt trauma. *AJR Am J Roentgenol* 2001;**176**(4):955–8.

62. Sheafor DH, Foti TM, Vaslef SN, Nelson RC. Fat in the inferior vena cava associated with caval injury. *AJR Am J Roentgenol* 1998;**171**(1):181–2.

63. Croce MA, Fabian TC, Menke PG, et al. Nonoperative management of blunt hepatic trauma is the treatment of choice for hemodynamically stable patients. Results of a prospective trial. *Ann Surg* 1995;**221**(6):744–53; discussion 3–5.

64. Fang JF, Chen RJ, Wong YC, et al. Classification and treatment of pooling of contrast material on computed tomographic scan of blunt hepatic trauma. *J Trauma* 2000;**49**(6):1083–8.

65. Hagiwara A, Yukioka T, Ohta S, et al. Nonsurgical management of patients with blunt hepatic injury: efficacy of transcatheter arterial embolization. *AJR Am J Roentgenol* 1997;**169**(4):1151–6.

66. Chen X, Talner LB, Jurkovich GJ. Gallbladder avulsion due to blunt trauma. *AJR Am J Roentgenol* 2001;**177**(4):822.

67. Brasel KJ, DeLisle CM, Olson CJ, Borgstrom DC. Splenic injury: trends in evaluation and management. *J Trauma* 1998;**44**(2):283–6.

68. Federle MP, Griffiths B, Minagi H, Jeffrey RB, Jr. Splenic trauma: evaluation with CT. *Radiology* 1987;**162**(1):69–71.

69. Gavant ML, Schurr M, Flick PA, et al. Predicting clinical outcome of nonsurgical management of blunt splenic injury: using CT to reveal abnormalities of splenic vasculature. *AJR Am J Roentgenol* 1997;**168**(1):207–12.

70. Shanmuganathan K, Mirvis SE, Boyd-Kranis R, Takada T, Scalea TM. Nonsurgical management of blunt splenic injury: use of CT criteria to select patients for splenic arteriography and potential endovascular therapy. *Radiology* 2000;**217**(1):75–82.

71. Fischer JH, Carpenter KD, O'Keefe GE. CT diagnosis of an isolated blunt pancreatic injury. *AJR Am J Roentgenol* 1996;**167**(5):1152.

72. Madiba TE, Mokoena TR. Favourable prognosis after surgical drainage of gunshot, stab or blunt trauma of the pancreas. *Br J Surg* 1995;**82**(9):1236–9.

73. Kim HS, Lee DK, Kim IW, et al. The role of endoscopic retrograde pancreatography in the treatment of traumatic pancreatic duct injury. *Gastrointest Endosc* 2001;**54**(1):49–55.

74. McAninch JW, Renal injuries. In Gillenwater JY (ed.), *Adult and Pediatric Urology*, 3rd edn. St. Louis, MO: Mosby, 1995: pp. 539–53.

75. Boone TB, Gilling PJ, Husmann DA. Ureteropelvic junction disruption following blunt abdominal trauma. *J Urol* 1993;**150**(1):33–6.

76. Kawashima A, Sandler CM, Corl FM, et al. Imaging of renal trauma: a comprehensive review. *Radiographics* 2001;**21**(3):557–74.

77. Federle MP. Evaluation of renal trauma. In Pollack HM (ed.), *Clinical Urography*. Philadelphia, PA: WB Saunders, 1989: pp. 1422–94.

78. Federle MP, Brown TR, McAninch JW. Penetrating renal trauma: CT evaluation. *J Comput Assist Tomogr* 1987;**11**(6):1026–30.

79. Brody JM, Leighton DB, Murphy BL, et al. CT of blunt trauma bowel and mesenteric injury: typical findings and pitfalls in diagnosis.

Radiographics 2000;**20**(6):1525–36; discussion 36–7.

80. Levine CD, Gonzales RN, Wachsberg RH, Ghanekar D. CT findings of bowel and mesenteric injury. *J Comput Assist Tomogr* 1997;**21**(6):974–9.

81. Strouse PJ, Close BJ, Marshall KW, Cywes R. CT of bowel and mesenteric trauma in children. *Radiographics* 1999;**19**(5): 1237–50.

82. Taylor GA, Fallat ME, Eichelberger MR. Hypovolemic shock in children: abdominal CT manifestations. *Radiology* 1987;**164**(2):479–81.

83. Sivit CJ, Eichelberger MR, Taylor GA. CT in children with rupture of the bowel caused by blunt trauma: diagnostic efficacy and comparison with hypoperfusion complex. *AJR Am J Roentgenol* 1994;**163**(5):1195–8.

84. Levine CD, Patel UJ, Wachsberg RH et al. CT in patients with blunt abdominal trauma: clinical significance of intraperitoneal fluid detected on a scan with otherwise normal findings. *AJR Am J Roentgenol* 1995;**164**(6):1381–5.

85. Dowe MF, Shanmuganathan K, Mirvis SE, Steiner RC, Cooper C. CT findings of mesenteric injury after blunt trauma: implications for surgical intervention. *AJR Am J Roentgenol* 1997;**168**(2):425–8.

Chapter 31

Angiography and interventional radiology

Stephen J. Wolf, Giustino Albanese, and Charles Ray, Jr.

Introduction

The role of interventional radiology (IR) in the evaluation and management of traumatic injuries has dramatically changed over the past 20 years. Diagnostic studies used to account for a majority of procedures, with aortic angiography being the most frequently performed study. Since the mid 1990s, computed tomography (CT) technology has greatly advanced allowing for greater vascular resolution and resulting in a decrease in the need for some diagnostic procedures (e.g., aortic angiogram).[1] However, there has been an expansion in the therapeutic interventions capable within the angiograhic suite (e.g., transcatheter embolization, endovascular stenting). The significant advantages of performing certain procedures in IR vs. the operating room (e.g., general anesthesia not required, less risk of morbidity and mortality, quicker recovery time) can be substantial in a critically ill multisystem trauma patient. Interventional radiology has evolved considerably becoming a more integral part of the multidisciplinary approach to trauma.

General principles

The most important consideration regarding the need for treatment of trauma patients with vascular injuries is that of hemodynamic stability. If the patient is stable, there is time for a comprehensive laboratory and non-invasive imaging analysis, which allows for a step-wise and planned approach to treatment. Hemodynamic instability often makes angiography the first imaging modality performed, due to the emergent conditions and the ability to render vascular treatment simultaneous with diagnosis.

Interventional procedures are used in the immediate trauma setting to stop active bleeding and reverse hemodynamic instability in patients whose vasculature has been compromised. The major risk of embolization is ischemia, which may result in loss of function of the end-organ supplied by the artery undergoing embolization. If the distal organ has a unique and vital function, such as the brain or heart, therapies other than embolization (e.g., stenting) are performed. A stent or graft allows for cessation of bleeding while maintaining distal perfusion. In tissues with abundant physiologic reserve, such as the liver and spleen, partial embolization allows minimal tissue infarction without long-term detrimental effects.

Contraindications to angiography are considered relative, especially in emergent circumstances where there may be no other techniques available. They include renal insufficiency, coagulopathy, and contrast allergies. Patients with renal insufficiency may be at higher risk for contrast-induced nephropathy (CIN), which is defined by a 25–50% increase of creatinine or an absolute increase of creatinine of 0.5–1.0 mg/dl. Contrast-induced nephropathy usually occurs 48–72 hours after contrast administration. Although CIN is transient in most patients with normal renal function, risk of renal failure makes management of reversible risk factors important in overall outcomes. Among risk factors, renal vasoconstriction secondary to decreased intravascular volume is the most important. Aggressive saline bolus hydration or volume repletion in patients whose hemodynamic status and cardiac function allows, should be performed prior to and after the procedure. Sodium bicarbonate with or without N-acetyl-cysteine may also be used, although research remains unclear as to any additional benefit over the administration of intravenous (IV) saline alone. Ongoing research into partial dopamine agonists such as fenoldopam may also provide additional CIN protection in the future, although again current evidence is lacking. Finally, the use of non-ionic contrast agents should be

Trauma: A Comprehensive Emergency Medicine Approach, eds. Eric Legome and Lee W. Shockley. Published by Cambridge University Press. © Cambridge University Press 2011.

considered when serum creatinine levels are above 1.5 or glomerular filtration rate (GFR) is < 60, and the use of low osmolarity contrast agents should be considered when serum creatinine levels are above 2.0 mg/dl.

Coagulopathy, whether intrinsic to a patient's disease process or acquired (e.g., dilutional or hypothermic), should be addressed prior to invasive procedures whenever possible. Elevated prothrombin time (PT), international normalized ratio (INR), and thrombocytopenia should be corrected as soon as possible but may be corrected even after the procedure has begun. Additionally, if the serum creatinine is significantly elevated or the patient has renal failure, consideration should be given to obtaining a bleeding time. Theoretically, empiric DDAVP (0.3 mcg/kg IVPB over 30 minutes) improves platelet function in the setting of acquired trauma-related coagulopathy, and could be considered. Keeping the patient in a supine position with the sheath left in place after the procedure for several hours or longer may provide enough time for improvement of the patient's clotting parameters, and significantly decrease the risk of access site bleeding. Coagulopathy may also cause a change in the plan for therapeutic embolization; the anatomic approach and agent used (e.g., some agents such as coils require superimposed thrombosis to function appropriately) should be considered with this concern in mind.

Premedication should be considered for any patient with a history of an allergic reaction to contrast. This may include oral or IV steroids and diphenhydramine for mild skin reactions, to adequate preparation for anaphylactic reactions, including a nearby, well-stocked, crash cart. In the case of a previously documented anaphylactoid reaction, consideration should be given to use of other non-iodinated contrast agents such as carbon dioxide or gadolinium, although these also have their own technical limitations.

Box 31.1 Essentials of angiography and IR in trauma

- Advances and widespread use of CT has led to a decrease in angiography for diagnostic procedures in trauma; however, there has been a significant expansion in the use for therapeutic interventions such as transcatheter embolization and endovascular stenting.

- Interventional procedures are used in the immediate trauma setting to stop active bleeding and reverse hemodynamic instability in patients whose vasculature has been compromised.

- The major risk of embolization is ischemia, which may result in loss of function of the end-organ supplied by the artery undergoing embolization.

- If the distal organ has a unique and vital function, such as the brain or heart, therapies other than embolization (e.g., stenting) are performed to allow bleeding cessation while maintaining distal perfusion.

- Contraindications to angiography are considered relative, especially in emergent circumstances where there may be no other techniques available. They include renal insufficiency, coagulopathy, and contrast allergies.

Priniciples of radiation safety

Once the decision has been made to proceed with radiologic examination of the trauma patient, the foremost goal is to obtain the necessary information to treat and keep the patient alive while keeping the radiation dose As Low As Reasonably Achievable (ALARA). This is based on both short-term and long-term retrospective evaluation of radiation effects in people directly exposed. This includes radiologists and patients in clinical settings to those exposed at Hiroshima and Chernobyl who developed acute radiation syndrome (ARS). Although the life-threatening changes of ARS affecting rapidly reproducing tissues such as skin, blood, and the immune system are usually reserved for history books and movies, prolonged fluoroscopy necessitated by challenging cases has led to skin and deep soft tissue non-healing ulceration and necrosis not amenable to treatment. Additionally, long-term radiation associated carcinogenic risk is not thought to have a triggering threshold (e.g., there may be no completely "safe" radiation dose), thus making ALARA the best long-term policy.

There are standard rules used in the angiographic suite to minimize exposure to radiation:

- Positioning to the area of interest should be done visually, not with fluoroscopy.
- The radiation source is kept distant from the patient's skin by raising the table while the image intensifier is brought next to the patient.

- The image is "coned down" to the areas of interest only, improving image clarity, while minimizing radiation scatter and exposure to areas that are not of clinical interest.
- The position of the patient or fluoroscope should be adjusted during the procedure so that no one area of skin bears the brunt of the radiation dose.
- Each fluoroscopic image functions as a frame in a film, causing radiation doses to rapidly rise with "beam-on" time. Reduction in the number of frames per second, also known as pulsed fluoroscopy, and intermittent use of fluoroscopy limited to when a dynamic change is expected, help reduce overall actual "beam-on" time and significantly decrease the dose of radiation to which these patients are exposed.

Pregnant patients are of particular interest when considering radiation doses. Lead shielding to the abdomen and pelvis should be used to reduce fetal exposure whenever possible; however, a radiation dose to the fetus will be delivered even with this protection. It is important to remember that in most angiography suites, the radiation dose comes from BELOW the patient. In such a setting, placement of a lead shield on top of a pregnant patient rather than underneath actually INCREASES radiation dose to the fetus. Uncontrolled trials of *in utero* exposure suggests that first-trimester exposure, particularly during organogenesis, may increase risk of birth defects, with childhood leukemia being the only proven increased risk after 20 weeks gestation. However, if regulatory radiation limits are observed, fatal childhood cancer risk is limited to 1 in 3300.[2,3]

The key is that ALARA is a relative standard to *primum non nocere*. Skin necrosis, cancer, and fetal exposure are treatment-associated morbidities to be minimized while addressing the patient's primary peril, the traumatic injury.

General principles of equipment

Arterial access is achieved using vascular catheters and guidewires not unlike those used in the ED. The main difference is the size; catheters used for embolizations are usually submillimeter in diameter, and wires may be as small as 0.010 inches in diameter. These smaller devices allow access to very small arteries, expanding the number of possible treatment approaches.

Embolic technique is used in the trauma setting to produce hemodynamic stability by occluding vessels that are actively bleeding, allowing temporary, or sometimes permanent, occlusion at the site of hemorrhage. This technique is reserved for instances where some tissue loss can be tolerated without significant long-term sequelae, since some distal ischemia and infarction may occur.

The original embolic material used was autologous clot. Historically, a clot was formed by drawing blood from the patient and allowing it to clot in a bowl on the angiography sterile table. The clot was then loaded into a syringe and injected into the bleeding vessel, with occlusion lasting hours to days. Lack of control and reliability, along with variable clinical results, led to development of additional synthetic embolic media which have since replaced autologous clots.

Gelfoam® (Upjohn, Kalamazoo, MI, USA) is a key embolic agent for trauma patients, in large part due to its adaptability and ease of use. It is a compressible material that can be injected through the catheter, which causes a temporary mechanical occlusion of the vessel into which it is injected for a period of 3–12 weeks. The most commonly used form is a sponge, which can either be cut into small cubes and injected directly into the catheter, or pushed to and fro through a three-way stopcock to form a slurry. Although drawbacks to Gelfoam® exist – difficulty in directing the embolization, clumping of the agent, non-radioopacity, the risk of unrecognized non-target embolization – it remains the workhorse embolic agent used for trauma embolization.

Coils consist of a metal scaffold onto which small fibrils are attached. They are available in a variety of sizes, and are most commonly used for precise occlusion of arterial aneurysms and arteriovenous malformations. When the anatomy of the target is well known, they offer the most precise embolic agent placement. However, since occlusion is permanent, their use is limited in the trauma population. In addition, coils by themselves do not cause vascular occlusion; rather, the fibrils elicit a thrombogenic response, which in turn causes mechanical occlusion by clot formation.

Stents and stent grafts are used when maintaining circulation distal to the vessel is of the highest importance, such as in the brain or heart. There is as of yet no investigational proof of how long stents and stent grafts actually remain patent. A stent is a scaffold that, when placed endoluminally, provides support to keep a vessel open. Although widely used in the vascular system, the use of many stents is considered off-label since the US Food and Drug Administration (FDA) approval for many stents is for biliary tract and pulmonary airways use. There are two broad categories of stent: those placed and expanded by a balloon (usually used in short arteries where precise placement is mandatory), and self-expanding stents (often used for longer arteries and veins with varying diameters over their course, and in superficial vessels where external compression may lead to stent occlusion). Drawbacks to the use of stents include expense ($500.00 or more per stent), interference with subsequent surgical interventions, and the need for anticoagulation and/or antiplatelet therapy, which may be contraindicated in trauma patients who are at high risk for bleeding.

A stent graft is a metal stent with a synthetic membrane (e.g., Gore-Tex®, Dacron®) on the outside and/or inside of the metal stent. Unlike bare metal stents, a stent graft allows isolation of a mural defect from the main vessel lumen by forming a seal, allowing the blood to bypass the defect without hemorrhage or clot formation. A stent graft must be fully apposed to the vessel wall to completely occlude the vessel injury. They remain quite expensive, but indications such as aortic aneurysm, transjugular intrahepatic portosystemic shunt (TIPS), and trauma may overcome the price differential. Stent grafts are particularly useful in the setting of a proximal injury to an artery that cannot be safely sacrificed without the risk of infarction of the distal outflow organ. Once again, long-term outcomes are not available.

Major roles of IR

Aortic and great vessels trauma

Blunt trauma is the leading cause of thoracic aortic and great vessel injuries. Thoracic aortic injuries are associated with other traumatic injuries, vascular and non-vascular, which bode poorly for patient survival.

The two most likely outcomes from injury to the thoracic aorta are a complete vessel wall tear resulting in death via either exanguination or cardiac tamponade, or an incomplete tear resulting in pseudoaneurysm formation, typically occurring at the level of the ligamentum arteriosum (just distal to the origin of the left subclavian artery). Pseudoaneurysms are unstable,

with a $> 90\%$ rupture rate within the first month post-injury.[4] Helical CT scanning has largely supplanted angiography as the diagnostic modality of choice, with diagnostic angiography usually reserved for cases in which there is any doubt on radiographs or CT imaging.[5,6] In general, treatment for aortic injury has been surgical, with significant risk (~10%) of cord ischemia due to exclusion of collateral vessel supply to the anterior spinal artery. Endovascular repair with stent grafts is still being developed, but is becoming more commonplace now that thoracic devices are commercially available.[5,7,8]

The role of angiography in the treatment of acute injury to cervico-cerebral vessels is based on the zone of injury and the type of injury. Endovascular interventions, typically diagnostic angiography and/or embolization or stent placement, may include primary endovascular treatment, adjunct treatment to medical or surgical treatment, or diagnosis only. Location of the injury, described by Zones 1–3 defines ease of surgical access. Injuries to Zones 1 (below the clavicle) and 3 (above the angle of the mandible) are surgically challenging and are associated with undesired operative comorbidities. Endovascular options include embolization of bleeding or severely injured vessels, and stent or stent/graft placement.[9] The latter therapy is limited to instances in which large vessels that supply vital end-organs are injured; long-term results of endovascular stents or stent/grafts in the great vessels of the mediastinum are lacking.

One commonly used injury scale defines injury to the cervical carotid and vertebral arteries, from minor intimal injury (Grade 1) with a high likelihood of healing with conservative treatment (anticoagulation/antiplatelet therapy only), to dissection (Grade II), pseudoaneurysm formation (Grade III), vessel occlusion (Grade IV), transaction (Grade V), and arteriovenous (AV) fistula formation (Grade VI).[10] Effectiveness of endovascular treatments for cervical arterial injuries has been demonstrated in numerous small series, although long-term vessel patency has not yet been evaluated.[9,11–16] The choice of endovascular treatment is based on the size of the injured vessel, the need for permanent vs. temporary occlusion, and whether sacrifice of arterial flow to distal tissue is acceptable. Lower grade injuries (I and II) are typically treated with conservative treatment, as serial evaluation of this patient population demonstrates initially high Glasgow Coma Scale (GCS) scores, minimal complications from conservative treatment, and often spontaneous healing.[17] Injuries typically amenable to endovascular therapy include transections with active contrast extravasation (embolization therapy), flow-limiting dissections (stent placement), or pseudoaneurysm/AV fistula formation (stent or stent/graft placement). Although excellent immediate responses are noted with stent placement, long-term results suggest significant vessel restenosis and occlusion rates (up to 45%).[16] Due to this, treatment algorithms currently trend towards much more conservative therapies, even with high-grade injuries.

Hepatic trauma

The excellent diagnostic accuracy of CT of the abdomen for the presence and extent of solid organ injuries leaves little role for angiography in the diagnostic workup of either blunt or penetrating hepatic injuries.[18] However, selected angiography followed by transcatheter embolization of injured vessels can be extremely effective in the management of ongoing hemorrhage.[19,20]

The role of IR as a therapeutic option in hepatic trauma depends on the hemodynamic status of the patient. Unstable patients classically undergo immediate laparotomy in attempts to achieve hemorrhage control by means of direct surgical repair or partial resection.[19,21] When bleeding cannot be controlled or the patient's hemodynamic status will not allow for a more extensive surgical repair, the perihepatic bed may be packed to temporarily control hemorrhage with the intent to reoperate following continued resuscitation, i.e., damage control surgery. In this situation, interim angiography and embolization may be of assistance in trying to achieve definitive hemorrhage control.[19,22] Findings of active extravasation, pseudoaneurysm, or fistula on angiography are often amenable to transcatheter embolization.

Hemodynamically stable patients with hepatic injuries are managed non-operatively, even with high-grade injuries; recent data suggests that up to 80% of these injuries are managed in this way.[20,23] The presence of significant active extravasation of CT contrast material or other clinical or radiographic signs suggesting ongoing hemorrhage are indications for immediate angiography.[19,24,25] Targeted transcatheter embolization in this setting results in successful hemorrhage control in up to 100% of patients undergoing angiography.[19,20,23,26] Hemodynamically stable patients without obvious ongoing hemorrhage are

observed for complications such as a worsening hemodynamic status.[21] Delayed or persistent hemorrhage of the hepatic injuries, as suggested by a drop in a patient's hematocrit and usually confirmed by repeat CT of the abdomen, would also prompt the use of angiography and transcatheter embolization.[19,20,23]

Complications of angiography and transcatheter embolization include rare instances of hepatic ischemia, which is minimized by the liver's duplicate circulation. Unlike the remainder of the liver, the biliary tree is supplied solely by the hepatic artery. There is, therefore, a risk of biliary duct ischemia following hepatic arterial embolization that may lead to biliary duct strictures or the formation of intrahepatic bilomas.

Splenic trauma

Angiographic evaluation and management of splenic trauma is similar to that of hepatic trauma. When suspected, hemodynamic instability dictates immediate operative intervention, while stability affords the time for evaluation with CT of the abdomen to identify and grade potential splenic injuries. Given the recognized benefits of splenic salvage, including minimizing morbidity from non-therapeutic laparotomies, reducing transfusion requirements, and preserving immunologic splenic function, all but the highest grade injuries in hemodynamically unstable patients are considered for non-operative management.[27–29] Recent studies suggest that up to 89% of blunt splenic injuries are managed non-operatively, with up to 25% of those undergoing angiographic evaluation with embolization rather than splenectomy for persistent or latent bleeding, or radiologic evidence of pseudoaneurysm formation at some point in their hospital stay.[27,29,30] This management approach reduces the operative intervention rate by 13–16% without a change in mortality.[27,30] Distinct indications for splenic angiography and potential transcatheter embolization in hemodynamically stable patients include evidence of bleeding, as indicated by either extravasation of contrast on CT scan or a persistently dropping hematocrit on serial testing, or evidence of pseudoaneurysm formation on imaging studies.

Although non-operative management utilizing angiographic embolization yields similar mortality rates to splenectomy, some studies suggest a two to fourfold increase in complication rates in management strategies designed to maximize splenic preservation.[27,31–33] These complications include splenic

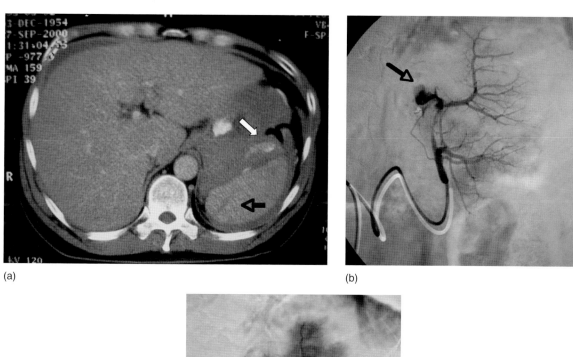

(a)

(b)

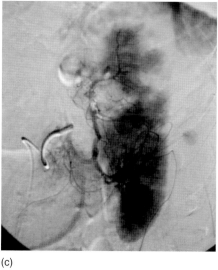

(c)

Figure 31.1 A 45-year-old male, unrestrained driver in a T-bone motor vehicle accident. The patient had free fluid on an ultrasound examination, but was hemodynamically stable. (a) Contrast-enhanced computed tomography (CT) scan demonstrates a splenic laceration (black arrow) with contrast extravasation into a subcapsular hematoma (white arrow). (b) Digital subtraction angiogram of the distal splenic artery demonstrates active contrast extravasation from the upper pole branch (arrow). The upper pole branch was embolized via a 3 Fr catheter, using Gelfoam® slurry and microcoils. (c) Digital subtraction angiogram following selective embolization, demonstrating segmental occlusion of multiple intraparenchymal branches and cessation of contrast extravasation. Note the normal filling of the lower pole branch, demonstrating the benefit of performing selective embolization procedures.

ischemia, splenic artery pseudoaneurysm formation or recurrence, splenic abscess, and rebleeding. Many of these complications can be treated with a repeat IR procedure, and still prevent the patient from undergoing splenectomy. The failure rate for splenic embolization is reported to be as high as 33% in unselected populations, and failures are particularly noted in patients with high-grade injuries (Grades IV and V).[27,28,32–34] These limitations underscore the importance of appropriate patient selection for the procedure and close patient observation. Figure 31.1 illustrates the management of a splenic laceration with angiography and transcatheter embolization.

Renal trauma

The majority of renal trauma is managed non-operatively, with only 5–10% of patients undergoing

545

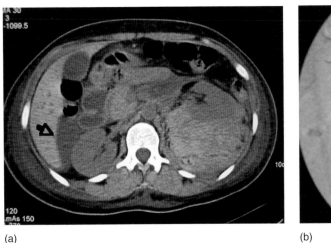

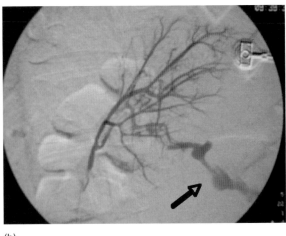

(a)

(b)

Figure 31.2 A 23-year-old woman presenting with acute renal failure. She underwent a percutaneous renal biopsy, after which her hematocrit level immediately dropped by 10 points. The patient was hemodynamically stable. (a) Non-contrast computed tomography (CT) scan demonstrates a very large pararenal retroperitoneal hematoma (white arrow), as well as free intraperitoneal fluid in Morison's pouch (black arrow). (b) Digital subtraction angiography of the left renal artery demonstrates severe active contrast extravasation from a segmental lower pole renal arterial branch (arrow). The bleeding vessel was successfully embolized to stasis.

surgical intervention.[35–37] Renal injuries are best diagnosed and graded with a CT scan of the abdomen with arterial and delayed contrast phase imaging. Management algorithms are typically based on the grade or severity of the injury.[37–39] Grade I and II injuries seldom require more than simple observation, while Grade V injuries involving the renal pedicle or avulsion of the hilum require operative repair or nephrectomy.[39,40] However, Grade III and IV injuries, depending on the presentation and findings, may be best managed by endovascular means. The role of IR in these patients can involve endovascular stenting of major renal vessels, super-selective embolization of distal vasculature to gain hemorrhage control, or in the delayed setting, percutaneous drainage of urinomas.[35,37,38,40]

Although rare, major renal vascular injuries often require nephrectomy due to significant hemorrhage, large retroperitoneal hematoma formation, or complete thrombosis resulting in severe organ ischemia.[39] Organ ischemia may result in impaired renal function in as little as an hour.[35,37] Intimal flaps, vessel dissections, pseudoaneurysms, and varying degrees of thrombosis are indications for consideration of endovascular stenting. Early studies suggest this approach has a higher rate of renal tissue salvage and a lower incidence of post-injury renovascular hypertension than open surgical repair or non-operative management alone.[38,40]

In the presence of significant renal parenchymal hemorrhage, continuous hematuria, pseudoaneurysm, or AV fistula formation, microcatheter angiography and super-selective embolization is often a therapeutic option for Grade III and IV renal injuries.[35,37] Super-selective distal embolization is performed since the kidney is an end-organ with poor collateral circulation, making distal ischemia a significant concern. By performing the embolization as distally as possible, more normal renal tissue is preserved. Success rates for endovascular treatment in this setting have ranged from 61% to 100%.[40] Complications include rare renal artery dissection, pseudoaneurysm formation, or abscess. An average of 10–15% of the distal renal parenchyma undergoes infarction with super-selective embolization, however this seldom effects overall renal function.[36] Figure 31.2 illustrates an iatrogenic renal injury managed by microcatheter angiography and super-selective embolization.

Pelvic trauma

Pelvic trauma is associated with high mortality rates. Studies indicate up to 85% of victims with major pelvic trauma die before even making it to the hospital if there is associated abdominal aortic trauma, and even once in hospital, mortality rates are as high as 43% without aortic trauma.[41–43] Although some patients die due to severe concomitant injuries, many patients die from exsanguination associated with their pelvic fractures. Hemorrhage may arise from hemorrhagic cancellous bone, venous structures, and arterial injury. Improved survival rates are thought associated with effective tamponade by an intact retroperitoneum, prompt stabilization of pelvic fractures, and interventional treatment of vascular injuries.[41,42] Factors exacerbating hemorrhage include hypothermia and dilutional coagulopathy secondary to massive transfusion.[44] Pelvic arterial injuries are generally very difficult to treat surgically, and therefore endovascular techniques have evolved into a front-line therapy.

Most commonly, injury to the pelvis is secondary to blunt trauma following motor vehicle collisions. Three injury patterns may be responsible for the injuries leading to vascular injury; the pelvic girdle may be compressed laterally, anteroposteriorly, or there may be vertical shear. Each of these mechanisms in isolation or in combination may shear vessels, avulse bone fragments and their associated vessels, or create loose bone fragments injuring vessels. Of these patterns, vertical shear is most often associated with the need for embolization therapy (reported in up to 20–28% of cases).[41,42] This may relate to the large potential volume that is created by the injury and the likelihood of a large internal iliac branch vessel, such as the superior gluteal or internal pudendal artery, being injured. Once concomitant injuries that may be causing hemodynamic instability are excluded, persistent hemodynamic instability requires emergent angiographic evaluation of the pelvic vasculature.

Evaluation begins with a pelvic arteriogram to evaluate for free extravasation of contrast, pseudoaneurysm, or large AV fistula. Selective catheterization of branches of the internal iliac artery is then performed to localize the injured vessel. The embolic agent of choice in this region is Gelfoam®, allowing temporary occlusion for 3–12 weeks. This temporary occlusion allows time for the artery to heal itself, and decreases the risk of long-term sequelae from pelvic embolization (e.g., buttock ischemia, impotence). Due to the extensive nature of collateral vessels in the pelvis, there is minimal risk of distal tissue necrosis. Endografts may be considered if a large vessel is injured, particularly if there is injury to the infrarenal aorta, but for the most part pelvic trauma resulting in hemodynamic instability usually results in an embolization procedure.

Resolution of bleeding is evidenced by near immediate hemodynamic stabilization and documented with a completion angiogram to exclude bleeding from collateral vascular pathways. Accidental distal lower extremity embolization may be clinically silent or may require emergent revascularization. This slight risk (~1%) is accepted given the high morbidity and mortality of prolonged hemodynamic instability associated with pelvic vascular injuries. Figure 31.3 illustrate endovascular management of an unstable pelvic fracture.

Peripheral vessel trauma

Angiography in the IR suite for the diagnosis and management of extremity vascular trauma represents the largest portion of diagnostic angiograms performed in trauma patients. While most angiograms performed in other organ systems result in an endovascular intervention, only 15% of angiograms performed for peripheral trauma result in therapy.[1]

Computed tomographic angiography (CTA) has improved markedly over the past several years. The resolution of CTA approaches that of catheter angiography, and the ability to reconstruct images in multiple planes is a distinct advantage to using CTA in the trauma population. Although 64-slice scanners afford the greatest sensitivity and specificity, 16-slice scanners have been used successfully to this end. By using CTA, the optimal treatment for many patients may be planned without further vascular imaging. This fact, coupled with the limited utility of catheter-directed endovascular treatments, makes CTA the initial vascular imaging modality of choice. Catheter angiography is usually reserved for cases in which an intervention can be performed.

Angiographic evaluation can identify complete transaction, lacerations, thrombosis, intimal injuries, or pseudoaneurysms of arterial vessels. Although complete transections are usually managed by open repair, the remainder of these injuries can often be repaired endovascularly. Thrombectomy or catheter directed lytic therapy can be employed when significant thrombus is identified. Endovascular angioplasty or stenting is a therapeutic option for some lacerations and intimal injuries. Long-term patency rates of stents and stent-grafts in the distal circulation are unknown. Finally, selected embolization may be used for uncontrolled vascular hemorrhage, pseudoaneurysms, or fistula formation. Due to the great collateral circulation in the extremities, distal tissues can tolerate a longer ischemic times than other end-organs; in general, there are fewer distal complications from endovascular intervention.

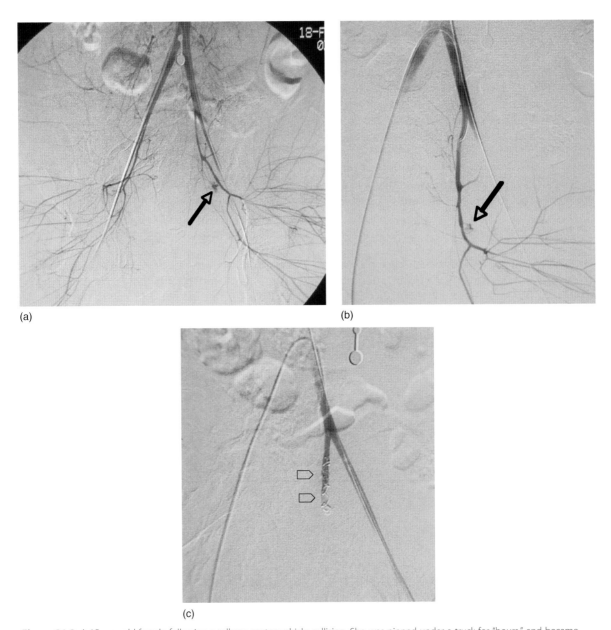

(a)

(b)

(c)

Figure 31.3 A 15-year-old female following a rollover motor vehicle collision. She was pinned under a truck for "hours," and became hemodynamically unstable as soon as the truck was moved. She was transported by air and arrived in the emergency department with a systolic blood pressure of < 60 mmHg and a core body temperature of 27°C. She was transferred directly to the interventional radiology (IR) suite for embolization. (a) Digital subtraction pelvic angiogram demonstrates gross contrast extravasation from the left internal iliac artery distribution (arrow). Notice how attenuated the pelvic vessels are, secondary to the severe hypotension. (b) Selective digital subtraction angiography of the left internal iliac artery demonstrating contrast extravasation from the proximal internal iliac artery (arrow). The entire internal iliac artery on the left was embolized with Gelfoam® and coils. (c) Post-embolization angiography demonstrating complete occlusion of the left internal iliac artery. Notice the artifact from the endovascular coils (arrowheads).

Conclusion

With significant advancements in technology, CTA has supplanted many, but not all, of the diagnostic indications for IR. However, a substantial broadening of the therapeutic indications of angiography and endovascular procedures in trauma patients over the past 20 years has established IR's continued critical role in the management of these patients.

Box 31.2 Major roles for IR in trauma

Area	Common interventions
Aorta and great vessels	Mostly supplanted in diagnosis of aortic injury by CT; still used for diagnostic uncertainty. Increasingly used for endovascular stenting. For great vessels/neck injury endovascular therapy includes treatment of transections with active contrast extravasation (embolization therapy), flow-limiting dissections (stent placement), or pseudoaneurysm/AV fistula formation (stent or stent/graft placement).
Spleen	Embolization rather than splenectomy for persistent or latent bleeding, contrast blush on CT, or radiologic evidence of pseudoaneurysm formation during hospital stay.
Pelvis	Embolization and occasional endografts of pelvic vessels, especially branches of the internal iliac after fracture.
Kidney	Endovascular stenting of major renal vessels, super-selective embolization of distal vasculature to gain hemorrhage control, or in the delayed setting percutaneous drainage of urinomas.
Liver	Selected angiography followed by transcatheter embolization of injured vessels for management of ongoing hemorrhage. May be used as an interim step after operative procedure for both diagnostic and therapeutic reasons.
Peripheral vascular	Decreased due to multidetector CT, but still used diagnostically. Used therapeutically for endovascular stenting, thrombectomy, and lytic therapy, and embolization of hemorrhage, fistula, or pseudoaneurysm.

References

1. Pryor JP, Braslow B, Reilly PM, et al. The evolving role of interventional radiology in trauma care. *J Trauma* 2005;**59**(1):102–4.

2. Doll R, Wakeford R. Risk of childhood cancer from fetal irradiation. *Br J Radiol* 1997;**70**:130–9.

3. Bushberg JT, Jr. Radiology biology. In Bushberg JT, Jr. (ed). *The Essential Physics of Medical Imaging*, 2nd edn. Philadelphia, PA: Lippincott, Williams, and Wilkins, 2001: pp. 813–64.

4. Coady MA, Rizzo JA, Goldstein LJ, Elefteriades JA. Natural history, pathogenesis, and etiology of thoracic aortic aneurysms and dissections. *Cardiol Clin* 1999;**17**(4):615–35.

5. Demetriades D, Velmahos GC, Scalea TM, et al. Diagnosis and treatment of blunt thoracic aortic injuries: changing perspectives. *J Trauma* 2008;**64**(6):1415–18.

6. Gavant ML. Helical CT grading of traumatic aortic injuries. Impact on clinical guidelines for medical and surgical management. *Radiol Clin North Am* 1999;**37**(3):553–74, vi.

7. Yamane BH, Tefera G, Hoch JR, Turnipseed WD, Acher CW. Blunt thoracic aortic injury: open or stent graft repair? *Surgery* 2008;**144**(4):575–80.

8. Xenos ES, Abedi NN, Davenport DL, et al. Meta-analysis of endovascular vs open repair for traumatic descending thoracic aortic rupture. *J Vasc Surg* 2008;**48**(5):1343–51.

9. Ray CE, Jr., Spalding SC, Cothren CC, et al. State of the art: noninvasive imaging and management of neurovascular trauma. *World J Emerg Surg* 2007;**2**:1.

10. Biffl WL, Moore EE, Offner PJ, et al. Blunt carotid arterial injuries: implications of a new grading scale. *J Trauma* 1999;**47**(5):845–53.

11. Redekop G, Marotta T, Weill A. Treatment of traumatic aneurysms and arteriovenous fistulas of the skull base by using endovascular stents. *J Neurosurg* 2001;**95**(3):412–19.

12. Duane TM, Parker F, Stokes GK, Parent FN, Britt LD. Endovascular carotid stenting after trauma. *J Trauma* 2002;**52**(1):149–53.

13. Malek AM, Higashida RT, Phatouros CC, et al. Endovascular management of extracranial carotid artery dissection achieved using stent angioplasty. *AJNR Am J Neuroradiol* 2000;**21**(7):1280–92.

14. Castellan L, Casasco A, Toso V, Bernardi L. Stenting of the extracranial internal carotid artery for dissecting aneurysm. *Ital J Neurol Sci* 1999;**20**(4):251–3.

15. Duke BJ, Ryu RK, Coldwell DM, Brega KE. Treatment of blunt injury to the carotid artery by using

endovascular stents: an early experience. *J Neurosurg* 1997;**87**(6):825–9.

16. Cothren CC, Moore EE, Ray CE, Jr., et al. Carotid artery stents for blunt cerebrovascular injury: risks exceed benefits. *Arch Surg* 2005;**140**(5):480–5.

17. Biffl WL, Ray CE, Jr., Moore EE, et al. Treatment-related outcomes from blunt cerebrovascular injuries: importance of routine follow-up arteriography. *Ann Surg* 2002;**235**(5):699–706.

18. Peitzman AB, Makaroun MS, Slasky BS, Ritter P. Prospective study of computed tomography in initial management of blunt abdominal trauma. *J Trauma* 1986;**26**(7):585–92.

19. Lee SK, Carrillo EH. Advances and changes in the management of liver injuries. *Am Surg* 2007;**73**(3):201–6.

20. Hagiwara A, Yukioka T, Ohta S, et al. Nonsurgical management of patients with blunt hepatic injury: efficacy of transcatheter arterial embolization. *AJR Am J Roentgenol* 1997;**169**(4):1151–6.

21. Pachter HL, Liang HG, Hofstetter SR. Liver and biliary tract trauma. In Mattox KL, Feliciano DV, Moore EE (eds), *Trauma*, 4th edn. New York: McGraw-Hill, 1999: pp. 633–82.

22. Kushimoto S, Arai M, Aiboshi J, et al. The role of interventional radiology in patients requiring damage control laparotomy. *J Trauma* 2003;**54**(1):171–6.

23. David RJ, Franklin GA, Lukan JK, et al. Evolution in the management of hepatic trauma: a 25-year perspective. *Ann Surg* 2000;**232**(3):324–30.

24. Moore EE, Cogbill TH, Malangoni MA, et al. Organ injury scaling. *Surg Clin North Am* 1995;**75**(2):293–303.

25. Hagiwara A, Murata A, Matsuda T, Matsuda H, Shimazaki S. The efficacy and limitations of transarterial embolization for severe hepatic injury. *J Trauma* 2002;**52**(6):1091–6.

26. Monnin V, Sengel C, Thony F, et al. Place of arterial embolization in severe blunt hepatic trauma: a multidisciplinary approach. *Cardiovasc Intervent Radiol* 2008;**31**(5):875–82.

27. Smith HE, Biffl WL, Majercik SD, et al. Splenic artery embolization: have we gone too far? *J Trauma* 2006;**61**(3):541–4.

28. Duchesne JC, Simmons JD, Schmieg RE, Jr., McSwain NE, Jr., Bellows CF. Proximal splenic angioembolization does not improve outcomes in treating blunt splenic injuries compared with splenectomy: a cohort analysis. *J Trauma* 2008;**65**(6):1346–51.

29. Peitzman AB, Heil B, Rivera L, et al. Blunt splenic injury in adults: Multi-institutional Study of the Eastern Association for the Surgery of Trauma. *J Trauma* 2000;**49**(2):177–87.

30. Wei B, Hemmila MR, Arbabi S, Taheri PA, Wahl WL. Angioembolization reduces operative intervention for blunt splenic injury. *J Trauma* 2008;**64**(6):1472–7.

31. Cooney R, Ku J, Cherry R, et al. Limitations of splenic angioembolization in treating blunt splenic injury. *J Trauma* 2005;**59**(4):926–32.

32. Ekeh AP, McCarthy MC, Woods RJ, Haley E. Complications arising from splenic embolization after blunt splenic trauma. *Am J Surg* 2005;**189**(3):335–9.

33. Kaseje N, Agarwal S, Burch M, et al. Short-term outcomes of splenectomy avoidance in trauma patients. *Am J Surg* 2008;**196**(2):213–17.

34. Gaarder C, Dormagen JB, Eken T, et al. Nonoperative management of splenic injuries: improved results with angioembolization. *J Trauma* 2006;**61**(1):192–8.

35. Mansi MK, Alkhudair WK. Conservative management with percutaneous intervention of major blunt renal injuries. *Am J Emerg Med* 1997;**15**(7):633–7.

36. Chatziioannou A, Brountzos E, Primetis E, et al. Effects of superselective embolization for renal vascular injuries on renal parenchyma and function. *Eur J Vasc Endovasc Surg* 2004;**28**(2):201–6.

37. Dinkel HP, Danuser H, Triller J. Blunt renal trauma: minimally invasive management with microcatheter embolization experience in nine patients. *Radiology* 2002;**223**(3):723–30.

38. Bruce LM, Croce MA, Santaniello JM, et al. Blunt renal artery injury: incidence, diagnosis, and management. *Am Surg* 2001;**67**(6):550–4.

39. Knudson MM, Harrison PB, Hoyt DB, et al. Outcome after major renovascular injuries: a Western Trauma Association multicenter report. *J Trauma* 2000 December;**49**(6):1116–22.

40. Breyer BN, McAninch JW, Elliott SP, Master VA. Minimally invasive endovascular techniques to treat acute renal hemorrhage. *J Urol* 2008;**179**(6):2248–52.

41. Cook RE, Keating JF, Gillespie I. The role of angiography in the management of haemorrhage from major fractures of the pelvis. *J Bone Joint Surg Br* 2002;**84**(2):178–82.

42. Ben-Menachem Y, Coldwell DM, Young JW, Burgess AR. Hemorrhage associated with pelvic fractures: causes, diagnosis, and emergent management. *AJR Am J Roentgenol* 1991;**157**(5):1005–14.

43. Parmley LF, Mattingly TW, Manion WC, Jahnke EJ, Jr. Nonpenetrating traumatic injury of the aorta. *Circulation* 1958;**17**(6):1086–101.

44. Rutledge RSG. Bleeding and coagulation problems in trauma. In Moore EE, Mattox K, Feliciano D (eds). *Trauma*, 2nd edn. Norwalk, CT: Appleton and Lange, 1991: pp. 891–908.

Chapter

32

Anesthesia

Maria E. Moreira

Introduction

Alleviation of pain is a priority for patients presenting with traumatic injuries. However, pain management is not only important for the patient's satisfaction; pain causes negative physiologic effects such as impeding pulmonary function, altering hemodynamic values and cardiovascular function, and modifying stress response to injury.[1] Patients experiencing pain are more likely to be immobile thereby increasing the risk for thromboembolism.[1] Adequate pain management reduces morbidity of trauma patients and improves short- and long-term outcomes.[2–6] Also, removing the distraction of pain may allow patients to give a more accurate and detailed history. This may also help patients make better medical decisions and allow the physician to obtain a more accurate assessment and diagnosis.[7]

There are various methods of pain control available to the physician. The use of each method will be dependent on the presenting injury. The main objective is to allow for the tolerance of unpleasant procedures while maintaining cardiorespiratory function and limiting adverse effects. In turn, treating pain and anxiety will lead to the following: decreased patient suffering; facilitating medical interventions; increased patient and family satisfaction; improved patient care; and improved patient outcome.[8–11]

General principles

Local anesthetics block the conduction of neural impulses between the peripheral and central nervous systems. These agents bind to closed sodium channels on the nerve preventing activation and cellular depolarization thereby inhibiting the propagation of a nerve impulse.[12]

Topical and local anesthesia is the practice of providing the anesthetic agent directly at the wound site. Various topical agents are available for use on mucous membranes, intact skin, or lacerations. Table 32.1 lists the different topical anesthetics, indicated use (mucous membrane vs. intact skin vs. laceration), and adverse effects.[13,14] One of the major drawbacks to the use of topical anesthetics in the emergency department (ED) is the slow onset of action of some of these agents. A way of ameliorating this problem is the prompt administration of the anesthetic very early in the course, such as at triage.[15] See Table 32.1 for an overview of topical and local anesthesia.[13,14]

Local anesthetics are often used for simple uncomplicated wounds. Local infiltration is quick and has the added benefit of providing local hemostasis when an epinephrine combination is used. Techniques to decrease pain of injection include: injecting subcutaneously through open wounds rather than through intact skin, using small needles (e.g., 27–30-gauge needle, using warm solutions, slow rates of infiltration, pretreating with a topical anesthetic, and buffering lidocaine solution with sodium bicarbonate in a 1 to 10 solution (1 ml of bicarbonate added to 10 mg of lidocaine).[16–20] Table 32.2 lists various choices for local infiltrative anesthesia.

There are two main contraindications to local anesthesia. One is when the wound is of a size that the amount of local agent required to achieve anesthesia would put the patient at risk for systemic toxicity. The second, a relative contraindication, would be where distortion of tissues may hinder precise anatomic alignment of such tissues (e.g., vermillion border).

Complications of local anesthetic administration are mostly related to effects on the central nervous system and cardiovascular system. Multiple central

Table 32.1 Overview of topical and local anesthesia[13,14]

Anesthetic product	Type of wound	Methods	Onset/duration	Effectiveness	Complications
TAC* (0.5% tetracaine, 1 : 2000 epinephrine, and 11.8% cocaine)	Laceration	2–5 ml (1 ml per cm of laceration) applied to wound with cotton or gauze for 10–30 min	Onset: effective 10–30 min after application Duration: not established	May be as effective as lidocaine for lacerations on face and scalp	Rare severe toxicity, including seizures, respiratory arrest, and sudden cardiac death
LET (4% lidocaine, 1 : 2000 epinephrine, and 0.5% tetracaine)	Laceration	1–3 ml directly applied to wound for 15–30 min	Onset: 20–30 min Duration: not established	Similar to TAC for face and scalp lacerations; less effective on extremities	No severe adverse effects reported
EMLA (2.5% lidocaine and 2.5% prilocaine)	Intact skin	Thick layer (1–2 g per 10 cm²) applied to intact skin with covering patch of Tegaderm	Onset: must be left on for 1–2 hours	Variable, depending on duration of application	Contact dermatitis, methemoglobinemia (very rare)
Tetracaine (0.25–1.00%)	Mucus membranes	Topical placement on mucosa	Duration: 0.5–2.0 hours Onset: 3–8 min Duration: 30–60 min	Effective and potent topical agent	Severe cardiovascular toxicity in overdose, methemoglobinemia (very rare)
Lidocaine (2–10%)	Mucus membranes	Topical placement on mucosa	Onset: 2–5 min Duration: 15–45 min	Effective topical agent	Serious toxicity (CNS, CV) with misuse
Cocaine* (4%)	Mucus membranes	Topical placement on mucosa	Onset: 2–5 min Duration: 30–45 min	Effective, but potentially toxic	Susceptibility to abuse, CNS excitement, seizures, hyperthermia, HTN, MI, tachycardia, ventricular arrhythmias

*Must be treated as a controlled substance.
CNS, central nervous system; CV; cardiovascular; HTN, hypertension; MI, myocardial infarction.

nervous system (CNS) effects have been described including: lightheadedness, tongue numbness, metallic taste, restlessness, peri-oral paresthesias, slurred speech, excitability, drowsiness, and seizures. Seizures can be treated with benzodiazepines. Cardiac effects have included palpitations, cardiac dysrhythmias,

Table 32.2 Types of local anesthesia

Anesthetic	Onset of action	Duration of action	Maximum dose
Lidocaine	4–7 min	0.5–1.5 hours	5 mg/kg
Lidocaine with epinephrine	4–7 min	3.5 hours	7 mg/kg
Bupivacaine	10–15 min	2–4 hours	2.5 mg/kg
Bupivacaine with epinephrine	10–15 min	3–7 hours	3.5 mg/kg
Procaine	2–5 min	15–45 min	7 mg/kg

hypertension, hypotension, and cardiovascular collapse.[21] Hypoxia, hypercarbia, and acidosis worsen toxicity of local anesthetics.[21]

Patients can have allergic reactions to anesthetics, presenting with a rash or upper airway involvement. The reactions are usually due to the para-aminobenzoic acid in ester anesthetics and to the preservative methylparaben in amide anesthetics.[21] Esters are responsible for most of the true allergic reactions. If a patient is allergic to an anesthetic, a preservative free agent from another class should be used. Another option, although less effective, is to use benzyl alcohol or diphenhydramine. Use of diphenhydramine, however, can cause severe pain on injection, prolonged analgesia, and prolonged rebound hyperesthesia.[22] Diphenhydramine can also cause local irritation and necrosis of the skin when used in areas supplied by end arteries.[23]

Basic and advanced anesthesia techniques

Regional anesthesia is based on the principal of blocking the nerve supply to the injured area. The anesthetic is injected in proximity to the nerve rather than locally at the site of injury. Therefore, knowledge of anatomy and nerve innervation is essential for the proper performance of these blocks. This is the preferred method of achieving anesthesia in the following situations: when wanting to avoid local tissue distortion; when toxic doses of local anesthetic would be required; or in areas where local infiltration would be very painful (e.g., plantar surface of the foot). Regional blocks tend to be less painful than local subcutaneous injection. Blocks are specifically useful in trauma patients with multiple injuries as it avoids the hemodynamic and sedating effects of systemic analgesics.

Regional blocks should not be performed on uncooperative patients or on those who cannot communicate pain. It is important that the patient be able to detect the presence of severe pain or radiculopathy on injection, as these are indicators of intraneural infiltration. Intraneural injection can lead to an ischemic nerve due to the high pressures created within the nerve. Other contraindications to performance of a regional block include infection over the site of needle insertion, distortion of anatomic landmarks, or presence of allergy to the anesthetic.

Facial trauma is present in approximately 80% of trauma patients with 20% having multiple facial fractures.[24] Table 32.3 outlines the different facial blocks available for pain management along with the portions of the face innervated by these blocks.

In the setting of chest trauma, analgesia helps to improve respiratory function.[25,26] Adequate analgesia allows for deep breathing by decreasing inspiratory pain. Patients will be able to cough preventing atelectasis, hypoxemia, and the associated morbidity and mortality. The patient with good pain control will also be more likely to sit up and move around thereby decreasing the above mentioned complications. Intrapleural anesthesia and intercostal nerve blocks are options for pain control in the setting of chest trauma (Table 32.4).

Hematoma block, peripheral nerve blocks, and Bier blocks are options available for pain management during fracture reduction, relocations, and wound management. Other common and highly useful blocks described below include digital and regional blocks of the hand and wrist or foot and ankle, brachial plexus blocks, and intra-articular blocks. The choice of anesthesia will depend on type of injury, time required for repair, and physician experience and preference (Tables 32.5–32.10).[27,28]

Ultrasound-guided hematoma block has been described.[29] A 5.0–10 MHz transducer is used and provides the best images when the transducer is placed sagitally over the long axis of the bone. The fracture site is placed in the middle of the image and the needle is placed into the hematoma by entering the skin along the middle of the transducer.

Table 32.3 Types of facial blocks

Nerve	Innervation	Procedure
Supraperiosteal block	Anesthesia to a single tooth	Insert needle into mucobuccal fold with bevel facing the bone. Deposit 1–2 ml of anesthetic at the apex of the tooth, close to the periosteum
Infraorbital nerve block	Anesthesia to skin of lower eyelid, nose, and upper lip	Infraorbital foramen located in line with pupil on inferior border of the infraorbital ridge. Hold one finger over inferior border of infraorbital rim inserting needle in the labial mucosa opposite the apex of the 1st premolar tooth. Advance needle superiorly until palpated near the foramen; 2–3 ml of anesthetic is deposited at this site
Inferior alveolar nerve block	Sensation to ipsilateral mandibular teeth and the lower lip and chin	Palpate retro-molar fossa with index finger or thumb identifying the coronoid notch. Hold syringe parallel to occlusal surface of teeth with barrel of syringe between 1st and 2nd premolars on the opposite side of the mandible.

Table 32.3 (*cont.*)

Nerve	Innervation	Procedure
		Can facilitate this angle by bending 25-gauge needle about 30°. Puncture is made in the pterygomandibular triangle 1 cm above the occlusal surface of the molars. Advance needle until feel bone. Withdraw needle slightly and inject 1–2 ml of solution
Mental nerve block	Innervates skin and mucosa of the ipsilateral lip, with mild midline crossover	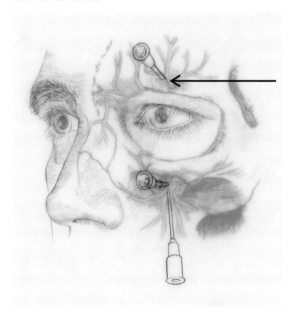 Mental foramen is 1 cm inferior and anterior to the 2nd premolar. For midline lip anesthesia need to anesthetize both mental nerves
Supraorbital nerve	Innervates the forehead and the scalp	With the patient looking straight ahead, the supraorbital notch is in line with the pupil and palpated along the

Table 32.3 (*cont.*)

Nerve	Innervation	Procedure
		superior orbital rim. The nerve is found 0.5–1.0 cm medial to the notch. Place 1–3 ml of anesthetic in the area of the supraorbital block. A line of anesthetic solution can also be placed along the orbital rim from medial to lateral
Field block of the ear	Type of regional anesthesia Small nerves blocked *en masse* with local anesthetic placed in the subcutaneous tissue forming a barrier proximal to the field of interest	Provides anesthesia to the entire ear, except the concha and external auditory canal which are possible complications

Figures 32.1–32.4 from Burton J, Miner J. *Emergency Sedation and Pain Management*. Cambridge: Cambridge University Press, 2008.

Femoral nerve block is an anesthesia choice in the setting of femur fractures and hip fractures. When performing the block, clinicians need to be careful to avoid infiltration of the femoral artery or vein. Ultrasound can be used to assist. Performing aspiration prior to injection of anesthetic is useful in preventing this complication. The femoral nerve block has been reported to provide quicker relief of pain than systemic intravenous (IV) morphine (5–10 mg/hour) (Table 32.11).[30]

Bier block is a type of regional anesthesia used for extremity trauma providing anesthesia, muscle relaxation, and a bloodless field. When local anesthetic is injected into the venous system, the anesthetic diffuses through distal vessels into the nerve endings producing subsequent anesthesia. In order for this diffusion of anesthetic to occur, a high concentration of anesthetic needs to be present in the venous system.[31] In order for this to not cause toxicity, a

Table 32.4 Anesthesia for pulmonary/rib injury

Intrapleural anesthesia

Procedure

- If chest tube in place inject anesthetic through chest tube

- Then clamp tube for 10–15 min to allow anesthetic to diffuse in patients not requiring a chest tube

- Position patient in the lateral position with affected side up

- Place 16-gauge Tuohy needle or spinal needle 8–10 cm from the posterior midline in the 8th intercostal space

- Angle the needle at 30–40° to the skin and aim medially, bevel up directed above the rib

- Once penetrating the posterior intercostal membrane, remove stylet, attaching a well-wetted air-filled glass syringe to the needle

- Advance needle until entering the pleural space (plunger will be drawn down the syringe due to the negative pressure created during inspiration)

- Remove syringe and introduce an epidural catheter 5–6 cm into the pleural space

- Remove needle and obtain chest X-ray for catheter placement

- Secure the catheter

- Most common anesthetic used = 20 ml of 0.5% bupivacaine

- Level of anesthesia can extend from T2 to T12

Contraindication

- Patients who will need multiple abdominal exams to rule out an injury

Relative contraindication

- Would need to rule-out intra-abdominal injury before performing the block. The reason is that intrapleural anesthesia can create a level of anesthesia below the umbilicus

Intercostal nerve block

Procedure

- Position patient sitting upright leaning over a Mayo stand

- Palpate rib and follow it posteriorly to the posterior midaxillary line

- With the index finger retract skin superiorly at the inferior border of the rib

- Insert the needle at the tip of the finger directed cephalad at an 80° angle

- Advance the needle until it contacts the rib

- Once traction is removed, the needle will move perpendicular to the chest wall

- Walk the needle off the inferior edge of the rib

- Advance the needle about 3 mm

- Perform aspiration and inject 2–5 ml of anesthetic

- Move needle in and out while injecting to ensure penetration of the compartment between the internal and external intercostal muscles

- Repeat the above technique with two ribs above and two below to ensure blockage of overlapping nerves

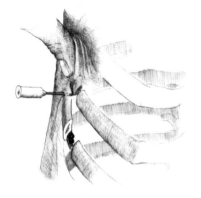

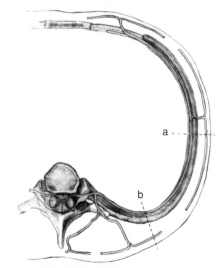

Figure 32.6 Intercostal block. On the left: Retraction of the skin cephalad from the lower edge of the rib exposes the site of entry. The needle is inserted at an 80° angle, tip cephalad, until contact is made with the lower rib edge. When the skin is released, the needle is allowed to slide caudad to the lower-most rib border. The needle is advanced 3 mm, aspiration

Caption for Figure 32.6 (cont.)
is attempted, and 2–5 ml of anesthetic is injected as the needle is inserted and withdrawn 1 mm in each direction. On the right: a cross-section of the chest shows the relevant branching of a typical intercostal nerve. Blocks are commonly performed at (a) the mid-axillary line and (b) the posterior axillary line.

Contraindications

- Infection over the injection site
- Flail chest

Complications

- Pneumothorax

Pearl

- Dosage of drug is one-tenth of the maximum for peripheral blocks secondary to the high vascularity in the area of intercostal blocks

Table 32.5 Hematoma block

Procedure

- Prep. the skin
- Insert needle into the area of the fracture
- Aspirate blood to confirm placement
- Inject anesthetic (about 10 ml into the hematoma and another 5 ml around the site)
- Anesthesia occurs in 5 mins, lasting for several hours

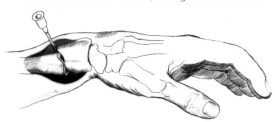

Figure 32.7 Hematoma block. After careful palpation for the fracture edge, the needle is inserted with care taken to avoid vessels. (From Burton J, Miner J. Emergency Sedation and Pain Management. Cambridge: Cambridge University Press, 2008.)

Contraindications

- Dirty skin
- Open fracture
- Small children

proximal tourniquet must kept inflated for at least 20–30 minutes after injection. The preferred anesthetic is lidocaine 3 mg/kg injected as a 0.5% solution. This solution can be made by combining 1% lidocaine with equal parts of sterile saline in a 50 ml syringe. Mohr reported this type of anesthesia to be useful for procedures involving the extremities lasting < 60 minutes.[32]

Absolute contraindications to the Bier block include allergy to the anesthetic and uncontrolled hypertension. This block also cannot be performed when a procedure requires the continuous monitoring of a pulse such as is required with supracondylar fractures. Table 32.12 gives an overall description of the block.

A recent review of 1816 Bier blocks reported 9 complications: 1 medication error, 3 improper cuff inflation errors, and 5 errors of inadequate anesthesia.[32] Other possible complications include: systemic toxicity of the local anesthetic secondary to inadequate tourniquet application; hematoma at the puncture site; engorgement of the extremity; ecchymoses and subcutaneous hemorrhage, and thrombophlebitis at the IV site. Engorgement is more common in patients with arteriosclerosis. The calcified vessels in these patients prevent the proper function of the tourniquet. The outcome is that arterial blood continues to enter the distal extremity while venous blood is unable to escape resulting in engorgment.

Emergency physicians should be familiar with penile blocks; clinical scenarios requiring penile anesthesia can present to the ED. Trauma-related injuries such as lacerations require appropriate anesthesia for proper management. Table 32.13 describes one option for penile anesthesia.[33]

There are occasions in which, often secondary to the patient's anxiety, a form of regional anesthesia may not be adequate. In these situations, procedural sedation and analgesia (PSA) provides for anxiolysis, sedation, amnesia, and analgesia. The ideal agent has a rapid onset of action with a short duration of action and minimal adverse effects. The purpose of procedural sedation is to provide for the tolerance of unpleasant procedures while maintaining cardiopulmonary function and the ability to respond to verbal commands and tactile stimuli.[34]

Controversy exists over the need for fasting prior to procedural sedation. The American Society of Anesthesiologists (ASA) recommends a 2-hour fasting period for clear liquids and 6 hours for solids and other fluids. However, this is based on consensus opinion alone.[35] Several studies have shown no increase in gastric volume or acidity when clear

Table 32.6 Digital nerve blocks of the hand

Various procedures for digital block

Dorsal approach

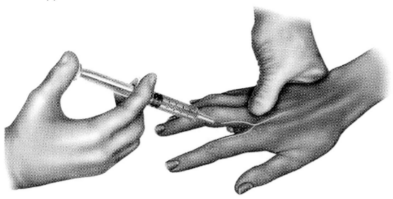

Insert a 27-gauge needle at the web space distal to the knuckle and lateral to the bone. Inject 1 ml of anesthetic subcutaneously and then advance needle to the point see tenting of skin on palmar aspect of hand. Then withdraw the needle 1 mm and inject 1.5 ml of anesthetic. Repeat on other side. This approach blocks all four nerves. This is the preferred approach. Since dorsal skin is thinner, the dorsal approach is less painful than the volar approach

Volar approach

Insert needle over the center of the metacarpal head on the volar side of the digit injecting anesthetic as needle is advanced to the bone. When at bone, needle withdrawn 3–4 mm and angled to each side of digit. Total anesthetic used is about 5 ml

Thecal approach

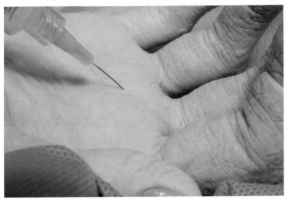

Uses tendon sheath to distribute anesthesia. At level of distal palmar crease puncture skin at 45° angle until "pop" occurs as the needle enters the sheath. Inject 2–3 ml of anesthesia. If the needle hits bone, withdraw 3–5 mm before injecting

liquids were administered up to 2 hours before elective surgery. There was no excess risk for the development of aspiration.[36,37] One prospective observational study of 1014 children noted no difference with airway complications, emesis, or other adverse events between patients classified by their preprocedural fasting status. Among the 509 patients that did not meet preprocedural fasting guidelines for elective procedures, there were no episodes of aspiration documented.[38] Also there are no reported cases of aspiration during ED PSA in the medical literature to date.

Table 32.7 Regional nerve blocks of the hand

Nerve	Innervation	Procedure
Radial nerve block	• Lateral dorsum of the hand	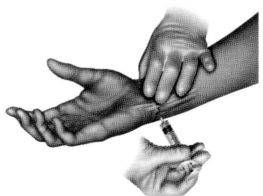

(a)

(b)

• Place 3 ml of anesthetic lateral to the radial artery at the level of the radial styloid

	• Lateral aspect of the forearm	• Also inject anesthetic dorsally along the wrist up to the dorsal midline
Ulnar nerve block	• Small finger and ulnar half of the ring finger	

Table 32.7 (cont.)

Nerve	Innervation	Procedure
	• Ulnar aspect of the hand	• Inject at the level of the proximal palmar crease on the ulnar side of the wrist • Advance the needle 1.0–1.5 cm under the flexor carpi ulnaris • Administer anesthetic subcutaneously from the lateral border of the flexor carpi ulnaris tendon to the dorsal midline to anesthetize cutaneous nerves branching off the ulnar nerve
Median nerve block	• Index, middle, and radial portion of the ring fingers	

(a)

(b)

	• Palmar aspect of the thumb and lateral palm	• Inject 1 cm ulnar to the flexor carpi radialis tendon • In patients with a palmaris longus inject between this tendon and the flexor carpi radialis tendon • Inject anesthetic after penetrating the deep fascia of the flexor retinaculum

A clinical policy developed by the American College of Emergency Physicians provided a Level C recommendation for fasting prior to procedural sedation stating "Recent food intake is not a contraindication for administering procedural sedation and analgesia, but should be considered in choosing the timing and target level of sedation."[39] Green et al. have also suggested a consensus-based

Table 32.8 Brachial plexus nerve block[27]

Indications

- Upper extremity

dislocations

fractures

abscesses

- Requirement for anesthesia proximal to forearm (not obtained with median, ulnar, and radial nerve blocks)

Procedure

- Use ultrasound to localize the brachial plexus by orienting the linear transducer transversely in the supraclavicular fossa
- Brachial plexus looks like a group of hypoechoic nodules lying lateral to the subclavian artery
- Inject 30 ml of anesthetic under direct visualization adjacent to the brachial plexus using a 27-gauge or 22-gauge non-cutting spinal needle

Complications

- Pneumothorax
- Arterial puncture
- Recurrent laryngeal or phrenic nerve paralysis
- Permanent neurologic dysfunction (rare)

Table 32.9 Intra-articular anesthesia[28]

Indications

- Shoulder dislocations

Procedure

- Aspirate blood from joint
- Inject 10–20 cc of anesthetic into the joint through the lateral sulcus, aiming slightly caudad (Anterior approach also acceptable)
- Takes 15–20 min for anesthetic to take effect

clinical practice advisory.[40] The advisory takes into account the limitations of published evidence and expert consensus. This advisory consists of four steps. The first step is to assess patient risk for aspiration: factors placing patients at risk are listed in Table 32.14. The second step is to assess the timing and nature of recent oral intake in the 3 hours before sedation and analgesia. The third step is to assess the urgency of the procedure, and the fourth step is to determine the prudent limit of targeted depth and length of procedural sedation.[40]

Presedation evaluation for possible complications and monitoring during the procedure are important components of procedural sedation. Presedation evaluation includes the evaluation for possibility of a difficult intubation or difficulty with ventilation, current medications taken which may interact with the analgesics, and medical problems that may have an effect on the pharmacology of the drugs used. Patients are assigned an ASA Class (Table 32.15) based on medical history. Their risk

increases from minimal to low with Classes I and II, to high or very high with Classes IV or V. Significant relationship between aspiration during general anesthesia and the ASA physical status has been noted. Patients in Classes III and IV are at increased risk of aspiration as compared to Classes I and II.[41] This has not been well studied in procedural sedation, however.

During procedural sedation, the patient should be monitored for hypoxia and other potential side effects of the analgesics used. Ideally one person should be responsible for the procedure, and one person should be available to have the sole responsibility of monitoring the patient and instituting bag–mask ventilation and cardiopulmonary resuscitation if necessary.[42] Physicians need to have the skills to rescue a patient from any airway or hemodynamic compromise due to the sedation.

The Bispectral Index (BIS) can be used to measure the electrophysical state of the brain during anesthesia. This is an analog electroencephalogram (EEG) monitor describing the level of sedation on a 100-point scale with a score of 1 being no EEG activity and a score of 100 being an alert state. This scale, however, has been found to be imprecise and is not commonly used in the ED.[43]

Pulse oximetry is often used during procedural sedation to monitor for respiratory depression and associated hypoxia. However, end-tidal carbon dioxide ($ETCO_2$) monitoring might be a better monitoring tool because it is not affected by the use of supplemental oxygen. However, the clinical significance of changes in $ETCO_2$ during procedural sedation are not clear.[43] In one prospective, observational study on children undergoing sedation with propofol, capnography detected apnea before clinical examination or oximetry in all occurrences and first detected airway obstruction in 6 of the 10 occurrences.[44]

Table 32.10 Lower extremity anesthesia

Nerve	Innervation	Procedure
Posterior tibial nerve block	Sensation to most of the volar aspect of the foot and toes	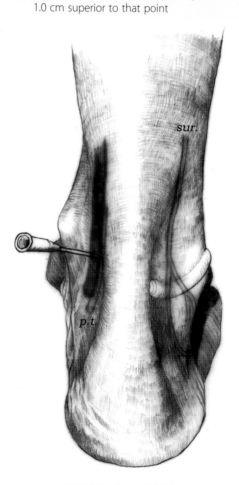

- Nerve located between medial malleolus and Achilles tendon
- Palpate posterior tibial artery and provide anesthetic 0.5–1.0 cm superior to that point

| Sural nerve block | Sensation to lateral border of foot, both volar and dorsal aspects | |

The above figure was taken from Burton J, Miner J. *Emergency Sedation and Pain Management*. Cambridge: Cambridge University Press, 2008.

563

Table 32.10 (*cont.*)

Nerve	Innervation	Procedure
		• Nerve located on lateral aspect of ankle between the Achilles tendon and the lateral malleolus
		• Superficial nerve
		• Blocked at level 1 cm above the lateral malleolus
		• Inject 3–5 ml of anesthesia subcutaneously between the Achilles tendon and the lateral malleolus
Superficial peroneal nerve block	Sensation to large portion of dorsal aspect of the foot	 • Anesthetic administered superficially between extensor hallucis longus tendon and the lateral malleolus • Blocked using 4–10 ml of anesthetic in a band between the landmarks
Deep peroneal nerve block	Sensation to web space between big and second toes	

Table 32.10 (*cont.*)

Nerve	Innervation	Procedure

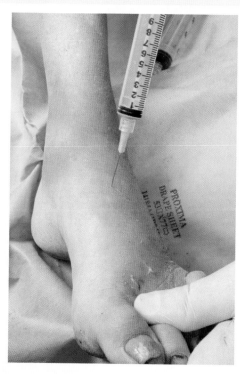

- Blocked between the anterior tibial tendon and the extensor hallucis longus, 1 cm above the base of the medial malleolus

- Can palpate tendons by:

  having patient dorsiflex the big toe and foot

  needle directed 30° laterally and under the extensor hallucis tendon until striking the tibia

- Needle then withdrawn 1 mm and 1 ml of anesthetic administered

Saphenous nerve block	Sensation to medial aspect of the foot near the arch	

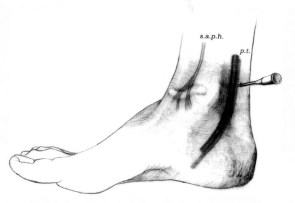

- Blocked between the medial malleolus and the anterior tibial tendon

- Blocked with 3–5 ml of anesthetic injected subcutaneously between landmarks

The above figure was taken from Burton J, Miner J. *Emergency Sedation and Pain Management*. Cambridge: Cambridge University Press, 2008.

Table 32.11 Femoral nerve block anesthesia

Procedure

- Palpate femoral artery 1–2 cm distal to inguinal ligament

- Keep non-dominant hand on artery at all times to maintain landmarks

- Insert needle at a 90° angle 1–2 cm lateral to the location of the artery raising a subcutaneous wheal of anesthetic

- Advance needle until a paresthesia is elicited or the needle pulsates laterally

- Paresthesia elicited:

  inject 10–20 ml of anesthetic

- Paresthesia not elicited

  inject 10–20 ml of anesthetic in a fan-like distribution lateral to artery attempting to anesthetize the nerve

- onset of anesthesia 15–30 min, duration 3–8 hours

Complications

- Nerve injury

- Hematoma from perforating the femoral artery

Pearl

- Always aspirate before injection to reduce risk of intravascular injection

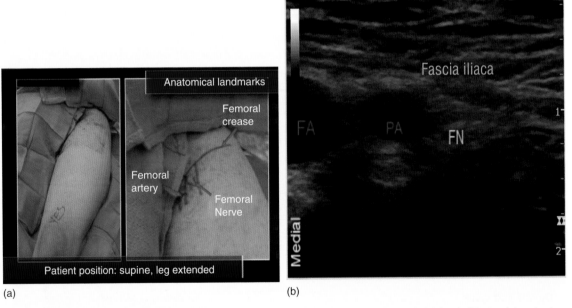

(a)   (b)

Figure 32.18 (a and b) Anatomy and landmarks for femoral nerve anesthesia. (Courtesy of New York School of Regional Anesthesia, with permission.)

The importance of monitoring after the completion of the procedure has been evaluated by Newman et al.[45] A prospectively collected database of 1367 pediatric patients demonstrated that the highest risk of serious adverse events occurred within 25 minutes of receiving the last dose of IV medications.[45] During the procedure and while monitoring after the procedure, reversal agents should be readily

Table 32.12 Bier block procedure

Single cuff system

- 20 g catheter or butterfly needle placed in superficial vein as close to injury site as possible:

  needs to be at least 10 cm distal to tourniquet used on extremity to avoid injection of anesthetic proximal to tourniquet

- Pneumatic tourniquet placed proximal to the injured site

- Exsanguinations of extremity (two techniques):

  elevate the extremity for at least 3 min

  wrap the extremity in a distal to proximal direction with an elastic bandage

- Inflate pneumatic tourniquet to 250 mmHg (50 mmHg above systolic pressure in a child):

  if wrap used for exsanguinations it should be removed after pneumatic tourniquet is inflated

- Slowly inject anesthetic (anesthesia should be obtained in 10–20 min)

- Perform the procedure

- Once procedure completed, deflate tourniquet and cycle to prevent bolus effect of lidocaine that may still be in the intravascular space:

  tourniquet time should not exceed 90 min

  do not deflate cuff until it has been inflated for at least 30 min (this allows for adequate tissue fixation of lidocaine)

- If mini-dose of 1.5 mg/kg of lidocaine has been used can deflate after a 20 min cut-off

- Mini-dose is as effective as 3 mg/kg and is the recommended dose in the emergency department:

  alternate between deflating cuff for 5 s and re-inflation for 1–2 min

  repeat above cycle 3 or 4 times

  anesthesia should resolve 5–10 min after cuff is removed

Double cuff system

- Used with longer-lasting procedures secondary to presence of pain at the cuff site after 20–30 min

- Proximal cuff is inflated at the beginning of the procedure and anesthesia is obtained under the distal cuff

- When patient complains of pain at the proximal cuff, the distal cuff is inflated and then the proximal cuff is deflated

- Do not deflate the proximal cuff until the distal cuff has been inflated:

  this is important to prevent diffusion of anesthetic into the general circulation

Table 32.13 Dorsal penile nerve block[33]

Indications

- Reduction of phimosis or paraphimosis

- Laceration repair

Procedure

- At base of penis raise skin wheals at 2 o'clock and 10 o'clock positions using a 27-gauge needle

- Then insert needle through center of each wheal towards center of shaft to depth of about 0.5 cm

- Aspirate to make sure needle not in blood vessel and inject about 2 cc of anesthetic (without epinephrine) on each side

Contraindications

- Infection at site of injection

- Suspected testicular torsion

Complications

- Infection

- Bleeding and hematoma

- Failure to achieve adequate anesthesia

available. When using opioids, the opioid antagonist naloxone should be available; when using benzodiazepines, flumazenil should be available. These drugs, however, should only be used to prevent major complications. If used, they need to be followed by an observation period as the duration of effects of the sedatives will frequently exceed the duration of the effects of the reversal agent.

There are many drugs available for procedural sedation and often a combination of drugs is used (Table 32.16).[46–66] The clinician should be familiar with the properties of each drug as well as its potential side effects. Some drugs when combined, such as benzodiazepines and opioids, can pose a

Table 32.14 Risk factors for aspiration in moderate sedation

- Potential for difficult or prolonged assisted ventilation should an airway complication occur
- Conditions predisposing to esophageal reflux
- Extremes of age (> 70 or < 6 months)
- Severe systemic disease with definite functional limitation
- Other physical findings the clinician judges to put the patient at high risk for aspiration (i.e., altered mental status)

Table 32.15 American Society of Anesthesiologists (ASA) classification

Class	Description
I	Normal, healthy
II	Mild systemic disease without functional limitations
III	Severe systemic disease with functional limitations
IV	Severe systemic disease which is a constant threat to life
V	Moribund patient who may not survive without the procedure

greater risk of respiratory depression. When these drugs are used together, the opioid should be given first. The benzodiazepine dose can then be titrated to effect.[46]

New drugs becoming available for procedural sedation include dexmedetomidine, alfentanil, and remifentanil. Dexmedetomidine is an alpha-2 agonist with dose-dependent sedation. The benefit of this drug is that it does not cause respiratory depression. Remifentanil and alfentanil are ultra-short-acting opioids, providing a period of analgesia of about 5–10 minutes. These drugs may be useful for very brief painful procedures.[43]

Though airway complications are a known side effect of the use of sedating medications, the rate of these complications remain as low as 1.4% for ketamine[43,67] and 5.0–9.4% for propofol.[68–71] In all these studies, serious complications such as aspiration, anoxia with neurologic impairment, and death were extremely rare.

Other reported adverse effects associated with procedural sedation include apnea, hypoxia, stridor, laryngospasm, bronchospasm, cardiovascular instability, paradoxic reactions, emergence reactions, emesis, and aspiration.[72,73] Children have been reported to demonstrate motor imbalance, agitation, and restlessness at home after undergoing procedural sedation.[74] However, most studies report the rate of major adverse events (i.e., respiratory compromise, hypotension, laryngospasm, dysrhythmias) after procedural sedation to be < 1%.[72]

Special populations

Infants, the elderly, and pregnant patients are subgroups of patients requiring special consideration. Infants and the elderly have increased sensitivity to most drugs requiring that doses be adjusted

accordingly.[75] The elderly often have other medical problems that can pose further risks from anesthetic medications. Benzodiazepines and barbiturates in patients with chronic obstructive pulmonary disease (COPD) can lead to excessive respiratory depression.[76] Patients with cirrhosis will have a prolonged duration of action of barbiturates and hepatically metabolized benzodiazepines. A history of coronary artery disease (CAD) or congestive heart failure (CHF) in a patient should warrant consideration of the hemodynamic effects of many of the procedural sedation drugs. Other anesthetic options, such as local or regional anesthesia, should be considered to avoid these hemodynamic effects.

When providing procedural sedation for the pregnant patient, consideration should be given to the effects of drugs on both the mother and the fetus. Consideration has to be given to the possible teratogenesis from medications used for sedation. Using the smallest effective dose of a drug may help to avoid teratogenic effects. Other options such as regional nerve blocks may be better options for pain management in these patients if the condition lends itself to that type of pain control.

Less invasive methods of pain management have been described in the pediatric population. Oral sucrose has been shown to reduce signs of distress due to minor, painful procedures in neonates.[72] In a Cochrane Collaboration systematic review of pain management in neonates, sucrose was found to be safe and effective for reducing pain caused by a single, painful event such as a heel lance or venipuncture.[77]

Psychological approaches and techniques have been used in children and have been shown to reduce anxiety and alter pain perception.[43] Examples of these

Table 32.16 Procedural sedation medications[46-66]

Drug	Properties	Pharmacokinetics	Dosing	Side effects	Benefits
Ketamine	Sedation	IV: onset 2 min; duration 10–15 min	IV: 1–2 mg/kg	Laryngospasm	Low incidence of respiratory or hemodynamic depression
	Analgesia	IM: onset 5 min; duration 20–30 min	IM: 4 mg/kg	Increased salivary and bronchial secretions; increase in BP and HR; increased ICP	
	Amnesia			Pregnancy: Category B	
Propofol	Sedation	Onset: 30–60 s	1.0–1.5 mg/kg IV; repeat 0.5 mg doses every 3–5 min	Respiratory depression, hypotension (more prevalent with rapid infusion and adjunct use of opioids)	Antiemetic; anticonvulsant properties
	Amnesia	Duration: 2–5 min		Dysrhythmias, heart block, and cardiac arrest have occurred in presence of metabolic acidosis	
				Pregnancy: Category B	
Ketofol	Sedation Analgesia Amnesia	Duration: 5–45 min	0.75 ml/kg of ketamine + 0.75 ml/kg of propofol		Sympathomimetic properties of ketamine can mitigate propofol-induced hypotension Propofol might counteract nausea and psychic recovery effects of ketamine
Etomidate	Sedation	Onset: < 1 min	0.1–0.2 mg/kg IV; slowly over 30–60 s	Myoclonus, vomiting, adrenal insufficiency, emergence delirium	Favorable hemodynamic profile; no histamine release
		Duration: 3–5 min		Pregnancy: Category C	
Chloral hydrate	Sedation	Onset: 40 min	25–100 mg/kg per dose PO/PR	Resedation; paradoxical hyperactivity	No cardiac or respiratory adverse effects
		Duration: 4–8 h		Caution used in patients with neurodevelopmental disorders: increased incidence of side effects and decreased efficiency	
				Safety not established in pregnancy	
Pentobarbital	Sedation	Onset: 6 min	2–5 mg/kg IV; 3–5 mg/kg IM, PR	Paradoxical excitation can occur; hypotension; respiratory depression	

Table 32.16 (cont.)

Drug	Properties	Pharmacokinetics	Dosing	Side effects	Benefits
		Duration: variable (most alert within 30–60 min)			
Benzodiazepine	Sedation	Onset: 2–3 min	Up to 0.1 mg/kg IV; 0.2–0.5 mg/kg PO, IM, PR	Strong respiratory depressant	Rapid onset and short duration
Midazolam (Versed)	Amnesia	Duration: 30–60 min		Pregnancy: Category D	
	Anxiolysis				
Opiate	Sedation	Onset: 2–3 min	1–2 mcg/kg	Strong respiratory depressant	Rapid onset and short duration
Fentanyl	Analgesia	Duration: 30–60 min		Glottic and chest rigidity with rapid infusion and doses above 15 mcg/kg (can be reversed with naloxone)	
	Anxiolysis			Pregnancy: Category C	
Nitrous oxide (50% concentration)	Sedation	Onset: 1–2 min	30–50% mixture with O_2	Emesis, nausea, dizziness, euphoria, and dysphoria	
	Analgesia	Duration: effects gone within 5 min of cessation of administration			
	Amnesia				
	Anxiolysis				

BP, blood pressure: HR, heart rate; ICP, intracranial pressure; IM, intramuscularly; IV, intravenously; PO, by oral; PR, by rectal.

techniques include breathing exercises as a form of distraction, imagery, filmed modeling, and reinforcement and incentives.[78] These methods can serve to ameliorate the patient's anxiety.

Conclusion

Pain management is an important aspect of emergency care. In order to appropriately treat patients, clinicians must be aware of the different options available for pain control, including the risks and benefits of each option. In trauma patients, particular attention needs to be given to hemodynamic alterations produced by medications used for sedation and analgesia. In such patients, local or regional anesthesia may present a better option. As clinicians, we should attempt to

provide the best analgesia possible both because of its medical and psychological benefits to the patient.

References

1. Lewis KS, Whipple JK, Micheal KA, Quebbeman EJ. Effect of analgesic treatment on the physiological consequences of acute pain. *Am J Hosp Pharm* 1994;**51** (12):1539–54.

2. Gregoretti C, Decaroli D, Miletto A, et al. Regional anesthesia in trauma patients. *Anesthesiol Clin* 2007;**25**:99–116.

3. Bulger EM, Edwards T, Klotz PRN, et al. Epidural analgesia improves outcome after multiple rib fractures. *Surgery* 2004;**2**:246–30.

4. Osinowo OA, Zahrani M, Softah A. Effect of intercostals nerve block with 0.5% bupivacaine on peak expiratory

flow rate and arterial oxygen saturation in rib fractures. *J Trauma* 2004;**56**(2):345–7.

5. Davidson EM, Ginosar Y, Avidan A. Pain management and regional anesthesia in the trauma patient. *Curr Opin Anaesthesiol* 2005;**18**:169–74.

6. Cohen SP, Christo PJ, Moroz L. Pain management in trauma patients. *Am J Phys Med Rehabil* 2004;**83**:142–61.

7. Heins A. Focus on: effective acute pain management. *ACEP News*. Available from http://www.acep.org/.

8. American Academy of Pediatrics and American Pain Society. The assessment and management of acute pain in infants, children, and adolescents. *Pediatrics* 2001;**108**: 793–7.

9. Mace SE, Murphy M. Pain management and procedural sedation: definitions and clinical emergency department management. In Mace SE, Ducharme J, Murphy M (eds), *Pain Management and Sedation: Emergency Department Management*. New York: McGraw Hill, 2006: pp. 7–14.

10. American Academy of Pediatrics and Canadian Paediatric Society. Prevention and management of pain and stress in the neonate. *Pediatrics* 2000;**105**:454–61.

11. Anand KJ. Clinical importance of pain and stress in preterm neonates. *Biol Neonate* 1998;**73**:1–9.

12. Tetzlaff JE. The pharmacology of local anesthetics. *Anesthesiol Clin N Am* 2000;**18**(2):217–33.

13. Kundu S, Achar S. Principles of office anesthesia. Part II. Topical anesthesia. *Am Fam Physician* 2002;**66**:99–102.

14. Jacobsen S. Errors in emergency practice. *Emerg Med* 1987;**19**:109.

15. Singer AJ, Stark MJ. Pretreatment of lacerations with lidocaine, epinephrine, and tetracaine at triage: a randomized double-blind trial. *Acad Emerg Med* 2000;**7**(7):751–6.

16. Kelly AM, Cohen M, Richards D. Minimizing the pain of local infiltration anesthesia for wounds by injection into the wound edges. *J Emerg Med* 1994;**12**:593–5.

17. Bartfield JM, Sokaris SJ, Raccio-Robak N. Local anesthesia for lacerations: pain of infiltration inside vs. outside the wound. *Acad Emerg Med* 1998;**5**:100–4.

18. Bartfield JM, Gennis P, Barbera J, et al. Buffered versus plain lidocaine as a local anesthetic for simple laceration repair. *Ann Emerg Med* 1990;**19**(12):1387–9.

19. Brogan GX, Jr., Giarrusso E, Hollander JE, et al. Comparison of plain, warmed, and buffered lidocaine

for anesthesia of traumatic wounds. *Ann Emerg Med* 1995;**26**(2):121–5.

20. Bartfield JM, Lee FS, Raccio-Robak N, et al. Topical tetracaine attenuates the pain of infiltration of buffered lidocaine. *Acad Emerg Med* 1996;**3**:1001–5.

21. Crystal CS, McArthur TJ, Harrison B. Anesthetic and procedural sedation techniques for wound management. *Emerg Med Clin N Am* 2007;**25**:41–71.

22. Xia Y, Chen E, Tibbits DL, et al. Comparison of effects of lidocaine hydrochloride, buffered lidocaine, diphenhydramine, and normal saline after intradermal injection. *J Clin Anesth* 2002;**14**(5):339–43.

23. Dire DJ, Hogan DE. Double-blinded comparison of diphenhydramine versus lidocaine as a local anesthetic. *Ann Emerg Med* 1993;**22**(9):1419–22.

24. Thaller SR, Beal SL. Maxillofacial trauma: a potentially fatal injury. *Ann Plast Surg* 1991;**27**:281–3.

25. Karmakar MK, Ho AMH. Acute pain management of patients with multiple fractured ribs. *J Trauma* 2003;**54**:612–15.

26. Karmakar MK, Critchley LAH, Ho AMH, et al. Continuous thoracic paravertebral infusion of bupivacaine for pain management in patients with multiple fractured ribs. *Chest* 2003;**123**:424–31.

27. Stone MB, Price DD, Wand R. Ultrasound-guided supraclavicular block for the treatment of upper extremity fractures, dislocations, and abscesses in the ED. *Am J Emerg Med* 2007;**25**:472–5.

28. Ufberg J, McNamara R. Management of common dislocations. In Roberts JR, Hedges JR, Custalow C (eds), *Clinical Procedures in Emergency Medicine*, 4th edn. Philadelphia, PA: WB Saunders, 2004: pp. 946–88.

29. Crystal CS, Miller MA, Young SE. Ultrasound guided hematoma block: a novel use of ultrasound in the traumatized patient. *J Trauma* 2007; **62**(2):532–3.

30. Fletcher AK, Rigby AS, Heyes FL. Three-in-one femoral nerve block as analgesia for fractured neck of femur in the emergency department: a randomized, controlled trial. *Ann Emerg Med* 2003;**41**:227–33.

31. New York School of Regional Anesthesia (NYSORA). *Intravenous Regional Block (Bier Block)*. Available from http://www.nysora.com/techniques/bier_block.

32. Mohr B. Safety and effectiveness of intravenous regional anesthesia (Bier block) for outpatient management of forearm trauma. *CJEM* 2006; **8**(4):247–50.

33. Shlamovitz GZ. *Nerve Block, Dorsal Penile*. Available from http://emedicine.medscape.com/article.

34. Gross JB, Bailey PL, Connis RT, et al. Practice guidelines for sedation and analgesia by nonanesthesiologist. *Anesthesiology* 2002;**96**:1004–17

35. American Society of Anesthesiologists. Practice guidelines for preoperative fasting and the use of pharmacologic agents to reduce the risk of pulmonary aspiration: application to healthy people undergoing elective procedures. *Anesthesiology* 1999;**90**:896–905.

36. Green SM, Krauss B. Pulmonary aspiration risk during emergency department procedural sedation – an examination of the role of fasting and sedation depth. *Acad Emerg Med* 2002;**9**:35–42.

37. Engelhardt T, Webster NR. Pulmonary aspiration of gastric contents in anaesthesia. *Br J Anaesth* 1999;**83**:453–60,

38. Agrawal E, Manzi SF, Gupta R, et al. Preprocedural fasting state and adverse events in children undergoing procedural sedation and analgesia in a pediatric emergency department. *Ann Emerg Med* 2003;**42**:636–46.

39. Godwin SA, Caro DA, Wolf SJ, et al. Clinical policy: procedural sedation and analgesia in the emergency department. *Ann Emerg Med* 2005;**45**:177–96.

40. Green SM, Roback MG, Miner JR, et al. Fasting and emergency department procedural sedation and analgesia: a consensus-based clinical practice advisory. *Ann Emerg Med* 2007;**49**(4):454–61.

41. Borland LM, Sereika SM, Woelfel SK, et al. Pulmonary aspiration in pediatric patients during general anesthesia: incidence and outcome. *J Clin Anesth* 1998;**10**:95–102.

42. Hertzog JH, Havidich JE. Non-anesthesiologist-provided pediatric procedural sedation: an update. *Curr Opin Anaesthesiol* 2007;**20**:365–72.

43. Miner JR, Krauss B. Procedural sedation and analgesia research: state of the art. *Acad Emerg Med* 2007;**14**:170–8.

44. Anderson JL, Junkins E, Pribble C, Guenther E. Capnography and depth of sedation during propofol sedation in children. *Ann Emerg Med* 2007;**49**(1):9–13

45. Newman DH, Azer MM, Pitetti RD, et al. When is a patient safe for discharge after procedural sedation? The timing of adverse effect events in 1367 pediatric procedural sedations. *Ann Emerg Med* 2003;**42**:627–35.

46. Bell GD, McCloy RF, Charlton JE, et al. Recommendations for standards of sedation and patient monitoring during gastrointestinal endoscopy. *Gut* 1991;**32**:823–7.

47. Green SM, Nakamura R, Johnson NE. Ketamine sedation for pediatric procedures: part 1, a prospective series. *Ann Emerg Med* 1990;**19**:1024–32.

48. Green SM, Rothrock SG, Lynch EL, et al. Intramuscular ketamine for pediatric sedation in the emergency department: safety profile in 1022 cases. *Ann Emerg Med* 1998;**31**:688–97.

49. Green SM, Klooster M, Harris T, et al. Ketamine sedation for pediatric gastroenterology procedures. *J Pediatr Gastroenterol Nutr* 2001;**32**:26–33.

50. Guenther-Skokan E, Pribble C, Bassett K, et al. Use of propofol sedation in a pediatric emergency department: a prospective study. *Clin Pediatr* 2001;**40**:663–71.

51. Parke TJ, Stevens JE, Rice AS, et al. Metabolic acidosis and fatal myocardial failure after propofol infusion in children: five case reports. *BMJ* 1992;**305**:613–16.

52. Rothermel LK. Newer pharmacologic agents for procedural sedation of children in the emergency department – etomidate and propofol. *Curr Opin Pediatr* 2003;**15**:200–3.

53. Schenarts C, Burton J, Riker R. Adrenocortical dysfunction following etomidate induction in emergency department patients. *Acad Emerg Med* 2001;**8**:1–7.

54. Absalom A, Pledger D, Kong A. Adrenocortical function in critically ill patients 24 hours after a single dose of etomidate. *Anaesthesia* 1999;**54**:861–7.

55. Allolio B, Stuttmann R, Leonhard U, et al. Adrenocortical suppression by a single induction dose of etomidate. *Klin Wochenschr* 1984;**62**:1014–17.

56. Allolio B, Dorr H, Stuttmann R, et al. Effect of a single bolus of etomidate upon eight major corticosteroid hormones and plasma ACTH. *Clin Endocrinol (Oxf)* 1985;**22**:281–6.

57. Wonsiewicz MJ, Morriss JM. *Goodman and Gillman's The Pharmacological Basis of Therapeutics*, 10th edn. New York: McGraw-Hill, 2001.

58. Guldner G, Schultz J, Sexton P, et al. Etomidate for rapid-sequence intubation in young children: hemodynamic effects and adverse events. *Acad Emerg Med* 2003;**10**:134–9.

59. Sokolove PE, Price DD, Okada P. The safety of etomidate for emergency rapid sequence intubation of pediatric patients. *Pediatr Emerg Care* 2000;**16**:18–21.

60. Malviya S, Voepel-Lewis T, Prochaska G, et al. Prolonged recovery and delayed side effects of sedation for diagnostic imaging studies in children. *Pediatrics* 2000;**104**:E42.

61. Cote CJ, Karl HW, Notterman DA, et al. Adverse sedation events in pediatrics: analysis of medications used for sedation. *Pediatrics* 2000;**106**:633–44.

62. Marti-Bonmati L, Ronchera-Oms CL, Casillas C, et al. Randomized double-blind clinical trial of intermediate- versus high-dose chloral hydrate for

neuroimaging of children. *Neuroradiology* 1995;**37**:687–91.

63. Malviya S, Voepel-Lewis T, Tait AR, et al. Pentobarbital vs chloral hydrate for sedation of children undergoing MRI: efficacy and recovery characteristics. *Pediatr Anesth* 2004; **14**:589–95.

64. D'Agostino J, Terndrup TE. Chloral hydrate versus midazolam for sedation of children for neuroimaging: a randomized clinical trial. *Pediatr Emerg Care* 2000;**16**:1–4.

65. Chudnofsky CR, Wright SW, Dronen SC, et al. The safety of fentanyl use in the emergency department. *Ann Emerg Med* 1989;**18**(6):635–9.

66. Parbrook GD. The levels of nitrous oxide analgesia. *Br J Anaesth* 1967;**39**:974–82.

67. Green SM, Krauss B. Clinical practice guideline for emergency department ketamine dissociative sedation in children. *Ann Emerg Med* 2004;**44**: 460–71.

68. Miner JR, Biros M, Krieg S, et al. Randomized clinical trial of propofol versus methohexital for procedural sedation during fracture and dislocation reduction in the emergency department. *Acad Emerg Med* 2003;**10**:931–7.

69. Miner JR, Biros MH, Seigel T, Ross K. The utility of the bispectral index in procedural sedation with propofol in the emergency department. *Acad Emerg Med* 2005;**12**:190–6.

70. Burton JH, Miner JR, Shipley ER, et al. Propofol for emergency department procedural sedation and analgesia: a tale of three centers. *Acad Emerg Med* 2006;**13**:24–30.

71. Swanson ER, Seaberg DC, Mathias S. The use of propofol for sedation in the emergency department. *Acad Emerg Med* 1996;**3**:234–8.

72. American College of Emergency Physicians. Clinical policy for procedural sedation and analgesia in the emergency department. *Ann Emerg Med* 1998;**31**: 663–77.

73. Miller MA, Levy P, Patel MM. Procedural sedation and analgesia in the emergency department: what are the risks? *Emerg Med Clin N Am* 2005;**23**:551–72.

74. Malviya S, Voepel-Lewis T, Prochaska G, et al. Prolonged recovery and delayed side effects of sedation for diagnostic imaging studies in children. *Pediatrics* 2000;**105**:E42.

75. Cepeda MS, Farrar JT, Baumgarten M, et al. Side effects of opioids during short-term administration: effect of age, gender, and race. *Clin Pharmacol Ther* 2003;**74**:102–12.

76. Gross JB, Zebrowski ME, Carel WD, et al. Time course of ventilatory depression after thiopental and midazolam in normal subjects and in patients with chronic obstructive pulmonary disease. *Anesthesiology* 1983;**58**:540–4.

77. Stevens B, Yamada J, Ohlsson A. Sucrose for analgesia in newborn infants undergoing painful procedures. *Cochrane Database Syst Rev* 2004;**3**:CD001069.

78. Powers SW. Empirically supported treatments in pediatric psychology: procedure-related pain. *J Pediatr Psychol* 1999;**24**(2):131–45.

33

Fluid and blood component therapy administration

Ugo A. Ezenkwele and Spiros G. Frangos

Introduction

Most emergency physicians and trauma surgeons resuscitate injured patients according to a standardized approach, which includes a primary survey, a resuscitation phase, and a secondary survey. During the primary survey, airway protection, ventilatory support, and hemodynamic stabilization are addressed. Volume resuscitation remains an integral part of therapy in patients with hemorrhagic shock, serving to improve oxygen delivery and preserve normal cellular metabolism.

The optimal fluid choice and strategy for resuscitation remain controversial. Crystalloid, blood products, and a variety of adjunct colloid plasma expanders serve as options. The ideal resuscitation fluid should have certain characteristics:

- rapidly restore plasma volume
- enhance microcirculation
- optimize oxygen delivery
- lack significant undesirable side effects, e.g., immune response suppression
- be readily stored and transportable
- be inexpensive.

Box 33.1 Essentials of blood, fluid, and component therapy

- The mainstay of therapy in fluid resuscitation is expansion of plasma volume and increasing oxygen delivery to vital organs so as to maintain viability without increasing bleeding prior to surgical hemostasis.
- Indications for transfusion in the trauma setting include acute blood loss, i.e., any patient with uncontrolled bleeding or a predicted volume loss of 1500 ml or an inability to respond to crystalloid resuscitation.

- Before transfusion, the blood should be typed and cross-matched. If the clinical situation is urgent, the blood can be typed and screened (takes 15 minutes). If the situation is critical, type O-negative blood can be given.
- If type O-negative blood is unavailable, then O-positive blood can be given.
- Alternatives to blood transfusion include the use of hemoglobin substitutes and perfluorocarbons, stimulation of endogenous production of red blood cells (RBCs) with the use of erythropoietin, reduction of blood loss through use of antifibrinolytics, hemostatic agents, and cell salvage.

General principles of fluid resuscitation

During the second half of the twentieth century, aggressive fluid administration was encouraged in order to replace the lost circulating volume in patients with hemorrhagic shock.

The timing, amount, and end-points as well as the type of fluid continue to be debated. The main questions revolve around whether fluid administration should be given early, or delayed until definitive control of the hemorrhage is gained, and whether or not the fluid should be given in large or smaller amounts. While the most common strategies employ large volume isotonic fluid, underlying research strongly supporting this in humans does not exist. The majority of animal studies support that for large blood loss, some fluid is better than minimal or none, but for non-major hemorrhage, less fluid or delayed resuscitation is associated with lower mortality. Large volume fluid resuscitation also comes with downsides. Crystalloid appears to improve hemodynamic indices in the short term, but clotting factor dilution contributes

Trauma: A Comprehensive Emergency Medicine Approach, eds. Eric Legome and Lee W. Shockley. Published by Cambridge University Press. © Cambridge University Press 2011.

to blood loss exacerbation.[1] Similarly, aggressive volume prior to control of surgical bleeding may increase intravascular pressure and disrupt established clot amplifying bleeding.

There have been few human studies evaluating permissive hypotension in trauma. While the first study clearly showed a trend toward improvement with delayed resuscitation, the other was unable to find a difference.[2–5] While there are criticisms of both studies, some methodological, some due to insufficient number of patients, ultimately there will remain questions until a large randomized study is performed with significant power to provide a definitive answer. In the meantime, many emergency physicians and trauma surgeons tend to lean toward moderate resuscitation with a goal toward keeping the systolic blood pressure around 90–100 mmHg. The one caveat is the patient with a significant brain injury where it is imperative to maintain a blood pressure above 90 systolic to avoid increased morbidity and mortality.

Controversy over the use of crystalloid vs. colloid solutions persists despite a large number of clinical trials that have examined the issue.[6–9] Although not fully settled, the most common current therapy is isotonic crystalloid solutions as the initial fluid of choice. The classical axiom dictates that three times the volume of lost blood in isotonic crystalloid is required to replace the volume of lost blood. Only a portion of the volume of crystalloid will remain intravascular; however, complete equilibration requires multiple hours. This ratio has since been questioned as being too conservative and may actually be as high as 7 : 1 or even 10 : 1 as a result of the decreased colloid osmotic pressure and serum protein losses from hemorrhage and ensuing capillary leaks.[10,11] Crystalloids also cause endothelial and RBC swelling, impair microcirculation, and decrease the surface area for tissue oxygen exchange.[6] Of the two commonly used isotonic crystalloid solutions (lactated Ringer's [LR] and normal saline [NS]), the Advanced Trauma Life Support® (ATLS®) course recommends the use of LR as the resuscitation solution of choice secondary to its reduced chloride load; hyperchloremic metabolic acidosis is a common consequence of NS infusion. Although the chloride load may not seem impressively different (Table 33.1), the hyperchloremia and acidosis become more obvious and problematic with increasing resuscitation volumes. Unfortunately, LR also has its own drawbacks,

Table 33.1 Constituents of commonly used isotonic solutions

	Lactated Ringer's (mEq)	Normal saline (mEq)
NA	130	154
K	4	
Ca	3	
Cl	109	154
HCO$_3$	28	

mEq, milliequivalents.

including neutrophil activation.[12,13] As the detrimental immunologic effects of currently available resuscitative fluids continue to be identified,[14–16] a search for newer solutions and recommendations for the initial fluid resuscitation may be warranted.

Hypertonic crystalloid solutions have a greater ability to expand blood volume and to more rapidly elevate blood pressure with a smaller infusion volume and shorter time period. Recent systematic reviews, however, have not demonstrated a significant benefit over isotonic solutions.[17,18]

Crystalloids primarily fill the interstitial space, and consequently tissue edema is expected and remains an important consideration, especially in the brain-injured. Unfortunately, it is not clear that other volume expanders, while theoretically better, provide improved outcomes.[19,20]

Artificial and natural colloid solutions are currently used as a complementary mode of therapy. They are more efficient than crystalloids in expanding plasma volume and achieve similar resuscitation endpoints faster and with much smaller volumes. There are four basic types of colloids: natural human albumin and three synthetic alternatives – dextrans, gelatins, and starches.[21]

Albumin, the prototypical colloid, is synthesized in the liver and is responsible for 80% of the plasma oncotic pressure. Its osmotic pressure is similar to the oncotic pressure of the plasma.[22] Although crystalloid and blood products are used initially in trauma resuscitation, there may be a role for albumin in the long-term intensive care of the trauma patient.[23] A recent meta-analysis which includes trials with trauma patients suggests that albumin may reduce morbidity in the critically ill.[24] Disadvantages of albumin include its short supply, high cost, and the small risk of transmission of infectious particles (e.g., prions) or viruses.

Of the synthetic colloids, dextran and gelatins are less common in the resuscitation of trauma patients. Although dextran has plasma-expanding properties, it also has powerful anticoagulant effects that limits it's role in trauma resuscitation. Gelatins, e.g., Haemaccel®, Gelofuscine®, are mostly unavailable in North America, and their modest and short-lived effectiveness in expanding plasma volume has limited their use.[25]

On the other hand, hydroxyethyl starch (HES) – specifically the high-molecular-weight hetastarch and pentastarch – is an attractive option. The colloid osmotic pressure of 10% pentastarch is 2 times that of the oncotic pressure of plasma and expands plasma volume 1.5 times the infused volume.[26] Besides its effectiveness in volume expansion, HES is readily available, has a large supply, carries negligible risk of transmitting infectious disease, has a long shelf life, and is less expensive than albumin. Although promising at moderate doses,[27] its use in injured patients has not caught on because of its dose-dependent effect on coagulopathy.[28]

Basic and advanced treatment principles

Red cell antigens and antibodies

Blood type is inherited and is determined by specific antigens and antibodies found in the blood. Over 300 antigens on RBC membranes have been identified, including the ABO and Rh systems (Table 33.2).

Once the decision to transfuse has been made, the patient's blood should be typed and screened. A Type and Screen is a laboratory testing technique used to identify ABO blood group antigens (type) and to detect atypical serum antibodies that may have formed (screen). This testing precedes the cross-matching (also known as compatibility testing), where donor red cells are mixed with recipient plasma in a tube to rule out agglutination, or the clumping of cells. Were red cell agglutination (hemagglutination) to occur *in vivo*, the resulting hemolysis would lead to a severe transfusion reaction. The direct hemagglutination technique is simple and inexpensive, does not require sophisticated equipment, and is sensitive and specific. The indirect agglutination test is used to cross-match blood and seeks immunogenic antigens that are not present on screening tests. The process takes longer (about an hour) and may delay blood transfusion.

Table 33.2 ABO blood types*

Blood type	RBC membrane antigens	Serum antibodies
A	A	Anti-B
B	B	Anti-A
AB	A and B	Neither
O	Neither A nor B	Anti- A and Anti-B

*Of note, universal donor for red blood cells (RBC) is type O; Universal recipient for RBC is type AB; however, the opposite is true for plasma. The universal plasma donor is type AB; the universal plasma recipient is type O.

Packed red blood cells

Packed red blood cells (PRBCs) are excellent volume expanders as they are maintained in the intravascular space for prolonged periods. Red blood cells are the main transport mechanism for oxygen.[29] Packed RBCs are processed from whole blood through centrifugation (removing 80% of the plasma) and the addition of preservatives (citrate–phosphate–dextrose, adenosine, glucose, or mannitol).[29] The resultant product may then be leukocyte-reduced, irradiated, washed, or frozen depending on hospital and patient needs.[29] Common teaching is that after 1 unit (approximately 300 ml) of PRBCs, a patient's hematocrit will increase by about 3 percentage points.[30] This has not been well studied, although a single retrospective study has found that it will increase by 1.9% ± 1.2%, which shows that it has clear variability.[30]

Packed red blood cell transfusion in the trauma setting is performed on patients with significant acute blood loss suggested by hemodynamic instability. In a life-threatening situation, type O-negative blood should be given, and trauma centers should have at least two units readily available. Although a case can be made for using O-positive blood (more readily available) for women beyond childbearing age and men, many trauma centers choose to avoid potential errors by relying solely on type O-negative blood in these circumstances. The blood of all patients who sustain severe trauma should be typed and screened for ABO classification; cross-matching can then be performed if blood transfusion becomes necessary. Time to transfusion should be minimized if the clinical situation dictates. However, if time is available,

Table 33.3 Special blood preparations

Special blood preparations	Indication
Leukocyte reduction	• To decrease the frequency of recurrent febrile non-hemolytic transfusion reactions
	• To reduce the incidence of HLA alloimmunization
	• To reduce the risk of transfusion-transmissible CMV
	• Does not prevent GVHD
	• May cause hypotension particularly in patients on ACE inhibitors
Irradiation	• Patient are at risk for GVHD
	• Fetuses receiving intrauterine transfusions
	• Selected immunocompromised patients
	• Donated blood from a blood relative
	• Recipients who have undergone marrow or peripheral blood progenitor cell transplantation
	• Recipients of cellular components whose donor is selected for HLA compatibility
Washed cells	• IgA-deficient patients
	• Anaphylactoid reactions to plasma components

ACE, angiotensin-converting enzyme; CMV, cytomegalovirus; GVHD, graft-vs.-host disease; HLA, human leukocyte antigen; IgA, immunoglobulin A.

then properly treated blood (i.e., leukocyte-reduced, irradiated, washed or frozen, etc.) may need to be administered as it may reduce allergic reactions, post-transfusion fever, and alloimmunization in select patients (Table 33.3).

Ideally, most stored PRBCs should be used within 21 days; by 42 days, they should be discarded since longer storage times result in a diminished capacity of the cells to release their oxygen molecules.[31] Although RBCs are an essential requirement for oxygen transport, the potential adverse reactions of allogeneic transfusions, including infections and immunologic risks, should be considered.

Platelets

The level of platelet decline following hemorrhage is difficult to predict. Certain patients are able to maintain normal or near-normal counts despite ongoing blood loss by mobilizing platelets from the spleen and marrow. Most patients, however, approach the critical platelet count of 50 000/μL (microliter) after losing 2 blood volumes. A declining platelet count usually requires intervention much later than the deficit of plasma factors, i.e., fresh frozen plasma (FFP) is usually required prior to platelets.[32]

Although the absolute platelet count can be readily determined, there are no practical methods to rapidly assess the function of native platelets or to assure the viability and activity of transfused platelets. Platelet function assays do exist but are too cumbersome to use in the setting of acute hemorrhage. Ease of platelet transfusion depends on storage and availability. Platelets must be kept in the blood bank where stringent storage requirements (20–24°C on a shaker or rotator) must be adhered to. Coordination between the trauma service and the blood bank is required to make these concentrates readily available.

Hemorrhaging patients with platelet counts under 40 000–50 000 μL should be transfused. A patient with a platelet count of < 10 000μL despite hemorrhage control also warrant a transfusion. Patients who were on antiplatelet medications (e.g., aspirin or clopidogrel) prior to injury may also benefit from platelet transfusion despite normal or near-normal counts. It would be reasonable to assume patients with uremia, alcoholism, and chronic malnutrition have reduced platelet function. In the setting of severe hemorrhage, early transfusion is reasonable.

Fresh frozen plasma

Fresh frozen plasma is generated by removing platelets and cells from whole blood then freezing and storing the remaining plasma. A single unit of FFP (about 250 ml) contains 400–500 mg of fibrinogen and 1 unit of each clotting factor.[32] Clotting factors are lost during massive hemorrhage while remaining levels dip further as a result of dilution from large volumes of crystalloid and colloid resuscitation fluid. A transfusion of 15 ml/kg of FFP should increase clotting factors by 20%;[32] clinically, this translates into a transfusion of 4 units of FFP in a 70 kg adult.

Severely injured trauma patients require and benefit from FFP well before losing one blood volume.[32] Hemodynamic instability necessitating significant PRBC transfusion should prompt physicians to order and transfuse FFP in these patients. While different protocols exist, the greater the hemorrhage and the likehood of ongoing bleeding should prompt earlier use of FFP. If the clinical situation permits, the use of FFP may be guided by abnormal coagulation tests, notably prothrombin time (PT) and activated partial thromboplastin time (PTT) followed by the international normalized ratio (INR). Abnormally elevated tests – generally 1.5 times greater than control – indicate a need for FFP to control hemorrhage.

Bleeding trauma patients who on warfarin therapy should be transfused factors empirically. While in certain situations it may be lifesaving, it must also be tempered with a knowledge of why the person is anticoagulated and the potential downsides of full reversal. For example, a patient with a mechanical heart valve and a minor injury with no ongoing hemorrhage would not benefit from reversal. Trauma patients with liver failure, disseminated intravascular coagulation (DIC), and specific coagulation factor deficiencies may also benefit from early FFP.

Units of FFP take 20–30 minutes to thaw (each one is a 250 g frozen block of plasma in a plastic bag at −30 to −80°C). Therefore transfusion services supporting trauma centers often maintain thawed plasma (which can be kept for up to 5 days). Since FFP is blood-type specific, there may be a delay as the blood bank performs the blood typing, processes the order, and transports the plasma.

Cryoprecipitate

Cryoprecipitate is the insoluble protein fraction of FFP that is separated out during centrifugation. Rich in fibrinogen, factor VIII, factor XIII, fibronectin, and von Willebrand factor (vWF), it has a limited role in the acute trauma setting. In trauma patients who are known hemophiliacs, who have von Willebrand disease, or who have low fibrinogen levels (< 100 mg/dl), cryoprecipitate may be indicated.[32]

Given the complexities of these cases and the immediate resources available, a consultation with the blood bank to decide on whether cryoprecipitate or other specific factors should be given can be extremely useful.

A unit of cryoprecipitate contains 0.25 g of fibrinogen (much greater concentration than FFP). However, provided the replacement volume is sufficient, FFP should be able to ensure hemostatic concentrations of all coagulation factors including fibrinogen; cryoprecipitate supplementation is therefore not routinely necessary.

Process of transfusion

Informed consent is preferred prior to any transfusion; however, in a hemodynamically unstable trauma patient who is unable to provide consent, blood products should not be withheld. Once products arrive from the blood bank and are ready to be administered, correct patient identification procedures must be stringent. Often these practices are dictated by institutional policy and clinical situation. Typically, hospital policy mandates that blood be checked by two licensed professionals, at least one of whom is a registered nurse.[33] The verification includes patient name, hospital number, transfusion number, ABO group and Rh type, donor number, expiration date, and volume of blood. The information on the blood tag is compared with that on the blood bag itself and to the patient's name band and blood bank identification band. Because of the risk of contamination, the blood should be hung within 15 minutes of arrival to the patient unit.[31] If it cannot be hung within that time period, it should be returned to the blood bank.

Two large-bore peripheral intravenous cannulas (16 gauge or larger) are generally adequate for the purposes of trauma resuscitation. If peripheral veins are difficult to access, an introducer catheter should be placed in the femoral or subclavian vein using the Seldinger technique. Rapid infusing systems can infuse fluids at rates reaching 1000 ml over 5 minutes and can be used if blood loss is expected to be high *and* aggressive resuscitation is being practiced. In-line fluid warming allows for resuscitation fluids to be warmed to at least body temperature prior to infusion.

With the exception of NS, no medications or intravenous fluids should be added to or mixed with blood products. The calcium in LR will interact with the anticoagulant, citrate, and cause the blood to clot. All blood products must be administered using a filter specified for that product. The in-line filter should be primed with either saline or the blood product.[33,34]

Vital signs should be taken immediately prior to transfusion. Any temperature elevation should be noted. A pre-existing low-grade fever is not a contraindication to transfusion. The trauma team must remain vigilant, however, because escalation of the fever during the transfusion would require careful evaluation and may make treatment decisions more difficult.

Monitoring resuscitation

In the early hours after injury, basic non-invasive hemodynamic parameters, such as heart rate, blood pressure, capillary refill, and urine output, are often adequate to guide the progress of resuscitation. Invasive monitoring may be useful to guide the resuscitation in the elderly and in those patients with underlying cardiopulmonary or renal disease. A central line (e.g., triple lumen catheter, introducer) helps to monitor central venous pressure. A pulmonary artery catheter may provide additional benefit in select patients, however it is rarely performed in the emergency department (ED) and is mainly used in the intensive care unit (ICU) or operating room (OR) setting. Various additional monitoring techniques, such as esophageal Doppler monitoring, thoracic electrical impedance, transpulmonary cardiac output, pulse contour analysis, and lithium dilution cardiac output continue to be explored. Each has certain advantages and disadvantages, but experience is limited, especially in the ED, and the instrumentation and techniques are not yet widely available.

Massive transfusion protocols

Massive blood loss is defined as the loss of 1 blood volume (80 ml/kg or about 5 L in a 70 kg male) within a 24 hour period. Acute massive hemorrhage is accompanied by the need for rapid, large volume transfusion and is associated with mortality as high as 70%. The consequences of uncontrolled hemorrhage include the triad of death – acidosis, hypothermia, and coagulopathy.[35]

Relatively few institutions have a massive transfusion protocol, and it is not an institutional requirement in the United States.[36] Nonetheless, such protocols offer a systematic means for the administration of blood products in an emergency setting. These are often comprised of three main components: early transfusion requirements (while surgical control

of bleeding is attained), anticipation of further transfusion needs, and the role of laboratory support.

In the early stages, blood is typically ordered in amounts of 4–8 units of PRBCs, 4–6 units of FFP, and an apheresis platelet pack equivalent to 6–11 units. Once a blood type is established, the delay between order and issue of type-specific PRBCs and thawed plasma, the latter of which is maintained in the blood bank, should be minimal.

Although massive resuscitation may be life-saving, it may contribute to multiple adverse sequelae, including hypothermia, dilutional thrombocytopenia, coagulopathy, decreased blood viscosity, and the dislodgement of hemostatic plugs its blood pressure is raised to normal or supranormal levels,[36] all of which may further contribute to bleeding leading to a vicious cycle. Intra-abdominal hypertension and abdominal compartment syndrome also have been associated with massive resuscitation and may occur in the presence or absence of an intra-abdominal injury.

Other methods for trauma resuscitation are practiced. The concept of delayed resuscitation suggests that fluid be withheld until surgical bleeding is controlled, while permissive hypotension allows for a "less aggressive" fluid resuscitation with the goal of a blood pressure below normotension.[2–5] Advocates of these methods believe that in penetrating trauma, blood pressure must be kept low (systolic blood pressure 80–90 mmHg) until surgical control of bleeding is obtained. By diluting clotting factors and "popping" formed clot, the hemorrhage is merely made worse. More research is needed before such modalities may be fully recommended for routine practice.

Special situations

There are a number of alternatives to blood transfusion that are directly applicable to the trauma patient in the acute setting, including the use of hemoglobin substitutes, perfluorocarbons, and cell salvage techniques. Reducing the amount of acute blood loss through the use of antifibrinolytics and hemostatic agents can be a vital adjunct.

Hemoglobin substitutes and perfluorocarbons may offer an alternative to the oxygen-carrying capacity of PRBCs.[37,38] Hemoglobin-based oxygen carriers have been under investigation for some time, especially from sources such as human blood, bovine blood, and recombinant technology. Unfortunately,

579

the data is limited. Human hemoglobin oxygen carriers are prepared from outdated RBCs which can be difficult to obtain, limiting its availability. Bovine blood, although widely available from slaughterhouses, has issues with antigencity and hypersensitivity. Recombinant technology has the advantage of genetic code modification that can produce a hemoglobin with the most desirable properties and fewest adverse effects: Polyheme®, Hemopure®, HemAssist®, Hemolink® are several examples. Although initially promising, a meta-analysis of the effectiveness of hemoglobin-based oxygen carriers, published in 2008, found excess mortality and myocardial infarction significantly associated with their use and significantly dampened enthusiasm for their use.[39]

Perfluorocarbons are created by replacing the hydrogen atoms of hydrocarbons with fluorine atoms,[38] and they have a high affinity for oxygen. They have a stable shelf life and a long intravascular half-life and should be easy and inexpensive to produce. Although promising, recent studies have demonstrated their toxicity to the reticuloendothelial system.[40] Consequently, much further investigation is warranted.

Cell salvage is a cost effective strategy to reduce transfusion requirements in the trauma patient.[41] A recent trial found that cell salvage reduced exposure to allogeneic transfusions in the perioperative and post-operative setting for orthopedic and cardiac patients, respectively.[42] However, no randomized controlled trials of cell salvage in the multitrauma patient have been conducted. If useful, it more likely is helpful in the OR than the ED.

Antifibrinolytic and hemostatic agents may also have a place in reducing blood loss in the acutely bleeding trauma patient. Aprotinin, a selective antifibrinolytic agent has been studied in patients with trauma and traumatic brain injury.[43] However, due to methodological issues and small trial sizes, there is insufficient evidence to support or refute a role for aprotinin in trauma.

Recombinant activated coagulation factor VII (rFVIIa) is a hemostatic agent originally approved for use in hemophilia patients with inhibitors to other factors. There has been substantial recent interest in its use to treat bleeding in the injured and it is undergoing extensive evaluation in this population.[44–46] A recent randomized controlled trial of activated factor VIIa[47] showed a significant reduction in RBC transfusion following blunt trauma and a similar trend following penetrating trauma. Concerns for thromboembolic events, including pulmonary embolism, myocardial infarction, and stroke following drug administration persist; these safety concerns need to be addressed in further studies before the drug can be recommended for general use.

The stimulation of endogenous RBC production with erythropoietin analogs in the ICU has been shown to reduce transfusion requirements,[48] an important goal that contributes to reduced infection rates and potentially improved mortality.[49]

Complications and adverse reactions

Infectious risks from RBC transfusion include the transmission of human immunodeficiency virus (HIV) (1 in 1.8 million), hepatitis B (1 in 220 000), hepatitis C (1 in 1.6 million) virus, human T-cell lymphocyte virus (HTLV), West Nile virus and, at least theoretically, variant Creutzfeldt–Jacob disease.[50,51]

Immunologic complications include febrile reactions (1 in 200 units transfused), simple allergic reactions (1 in 333 units transfused), transfusion-related acute lung injury (1 in 5000 units transfused) and acute hemolytic reactions (non-fatal, 1 in 6000–33 000 units transfused; fatal, 1 in 250 000–600 000 units transfused).[34] Other potential adverse reactions include the immune suppression induced by transfused RBCs, which increases the risk of nosocomial infections (Table 33.4).[52]

Special populations
Geriatric patients

As the proportion of the elderly population continues to increase, trauma centers will see more patients who are in their seventies, eighties, and even nineties. Many of these patients will have sustained serious injuries requiring aggressive critical care. Basic principles of fluid resuscitation in the injured elderly are similar to younger patients. However, there are important pitfalls that must be considered. The physiologic changes associated with aging, as well as the presence of comorbid conditions, make their assessment and monitoring more challenging. These patients have less physiologic reserve, and early invasive monitoring in these patients may be warranted to optimize resuscitation.

Table 33.4 Transfusion reactions[52]

Transfusion reaction	Features	Management
Febrile non-hemolytic transfusion reaction	• Most common adverse reaction (about 1% of transfusions) • Frequently in patients previously alloimmunized by transfusion or pregnancy • Fever and dyspnea 1–6 hours after transfusion • No lasting sequelae	• Stop transfusion • Manage as acute hemolytic reaction (because they are initially indistinguishable) • Acetaminophen for fever • Patients with previous severe reactions may benefit from leukocyte-reduced transfusions
Bacterial infection	• Bacterial growth during storage • Highest with platelet transfusion (stored near room temperature) • Risk of severe bacterial infection and sepsis: 1 in 50 000 platelet transfusions; 1 in 500 000 RBC transfusions	• Infectious workup, including cultures • Antibiotics
Other infectious agents	• Transmission of infectious disease: HIV, HTLV, hepatitis, and syphilis, CMV, *Babesia*, *Bartonella*, *Borrelia*, *Brucella*, Colorado tick fever, *Leishmania*, *Parvovirus*, plasmodia, rickettsia, *Toxoplasma*, and certain trypanosomes • Greatly reduced by careful donor selection criteria and blood screening	• Treat as appropriate for the individual infection
Acute hemolytic reaction	• True medical emergency • Can occur within minutes • Rapid hemolysis of donor cells by host antibodies • Usually related to ABO blood group incompatibility • Most severe: group A red cells being given to a patient with group O type blood • Symptoms: fever and chills, sometimes with back pain and hemoglobinuria • Acute hemoglobinuric renal failure	• Immediately stop transfusion • Hydrate; diuretics • Cardiorespiratory support
Anaphylactic reaction	• True medical emergency • 1 per 30 000–50 000 transfusions • Most common in selective IgA deficiency	• Stop transfusion • Antihistamines • Corticosteroids • Epinephrine • Cardiopulmonary support
Transfusion-associated acute lung injury (TRALI)	• Acute respiratory distress; often with fever, non-cardiogenic pulmonary edema, and hypotension • 1 in 2000 transfusions • Mortality rate < 10% • Most recover fully within 96 hours	• Oxygen • Cardiopulmonary support

Table 33.4 (*cont.*)

Transfusion reaction	Features	Management
Volume overload	• Edema, dyspnea, and orthopnea	• Slow rate of transfusion
	• Often in patients with pre-existing impaired cardiac function	• Diuretics
	• Sometimes called TACO (transfusion associated circulatory overload)	• Cardiopulmonary support
Iron overload	• Each unit of RBCs contains ~250 mg of elemental iron	• Chelation
	• Liver, heart, kidneys, and pancreas damage	
	• Significant if more than 12–20 units of RBCs transfused	
Delayed hemolytic reaction	• 3–21 days after transfusion	• Specific treatment is usually not required
	• Subclinical to life-threatening reactions	
	• Fever, low hemoglobin, jaundice, and urobilinogenuria	
Transfusion-associated graft-vs.-host disease (GVHD)	• Immune attack by transfused cells against the recipient	• Supportive treatment
	• Exceedingly rare complication of blood transfusion	
	• Only in severely immunosuppressed patients (congenital immune deficiencies or hematologic malignancies on chemotherapy)	
	• Almost uniformly fatal	
	• Prevented by transfusing irradiating blood products	
Post-transfusion purpura (PTP)	• Rare syndrome	• High dose immune globulin (IVIG) may promptly correct the thrombocytopenia
	• Sudden and self-limited thrombocytopenia, 7–10 days after transfusion	
	• History of sensitization by either pregnancy or transfusion	
Hypothermia	• Most common in large volume transfusion given rapidly	• Blood warming
		• Active external and core rewarming techniques
Hypocalcemia	• Citrate "toxicity"	• Ionized calcium measurement or ECG monitoring
	• Seen in severe liver disease or liver hypoperfusion	• Intravenous calcium gluconate or calcium chloride
	• Rapid, large-volume transfusion, especially via central intravenous access	
	• Ventricular arrhythmias	

CMV, cytomegalovirus; ECG, electrocardiogram; HIV, human immunodeficiency virus; HTLV, human T-lymphotropic virus; IgA, immunoglobulin A; RBC, red blood cell.

Pediatric patients

In regards to hemorrhage and resuscitation, children present a unique population for a number of reasons. They have an increased physiologic reserve and so manifestations of shock may be delayed despite blood loss. Their vital signs vary with age, while their height and weight determine their fluid resuscitation volumes and medication dosages.

When hemorrhagic shock is suspected in a child, a fluid bolus of 20 cc/kg is indicated. If there is little or no response, a second bolus is given. Packed RBCs (10 cc/kg) should be considered if the hemodynamic instability persists. All fluid and blood products should ideally be warmed prior to administration.

Pregnancy

Pregnancy induces a number of hemodynamic and hematologic changes that are amplified with its progression. The RBC mass increases while the plasma volume rises preferentially, leading to a decreased hematocrit. Heart rate also increases, as does cardiac output, while peripheral vascular resistance drops. As a result of the increased blood volume, an injured pregnant patient may lose a significant amount of blood before signs of maternal hypovolemia and shock develop. If blood products are required and the Rh-type of the mother is unknown, it is important to use Rh-negative components to avoid sensitization. These women should also be treated with Rh immune globulin to minimize the risk of Rh sensitization attributable to fetomaternal transfusion. Patients with minimal trauma or very early in pregnancy can probably be treated with a 50 mcg dose, although those with significant trauma should generally receive 300 mcg, the more common dose. Unless a spinal injury is suspected, an injured pregnant woman should be maintained on her left side at 10–15° to relieve pressure on the inferior vena cava by the gravid uterus; i.e., the supine hypotension syndrome, which may compromise venous return. Adequate resuscitation for the mother should result in restoration of an appropriate placental blood flow in the fetus.

Obese patients

Obesity is increasingly a public health problem. The blood volume of obese individuals must be estimated based on ideal body weight rather than on actual body weight to prevent overestimating resuscitation needs. These patients may also harbor weight-related comorbidities such as diabetes mellitus, coronary artery disease, congestive heart failure, and sleep apnea which may further challenge the clinician.

Burns

Patients who sustain 20% or more second- and third-degree body surface area (BSA) burns require aggressive fluid resuscitation using isotonic crystalloid solutions. There are several burn resuscitation protocols. A common one is the Parkland formula where initial resuscitation uses 4 ml of LR/kg/%BSA burn as a guide for fluid requirements in the first 24 hours post-burn. One-half of the calculated 24-hour fluid requirement is given during the first 8 hours, while the rest over the next 16. The actual total volume of fluid infused is guided by the response to resuscitation as evidenced by vital signs, urine output, mental status, and resolution of metabolic acidosis.

Head injuries

Traumatic brain injury is a leading cause of death and disability. After the initial injury, a rim of brain tissue surrounding the injured region becomes very susceptible to additional cellular neuronal injury as a result of local edema and inflammation. This secondary brain injury is often attributable to hypotension and hypoxia, which are associated independently with significant increases in morbidity and mortality.[53] It is therefore important to maintain high cerebral perfusion pressures (CPP) by supporting an adequate mean arterial blood pressure. Further, avoidance of hypoxemia is extremely important. The primary objective of fluid resuscitation in these patients is to minimize secondary brain injury related to hypotension; pharmacologic support in the form of vasopressors may additionally be indicated. The goal is to maintain a CPP in the 50–70 mmHg range while avoiding hypotonic solutions that may worsen brain edema.[54]

In brain-injured patients, where dilutional hypo-osmolarity contributes to cerebral edema and may impact mortality,[53] there is evidence that hypertonic saline reduces intracranial pressure and may play an important management role.[55] Although hypertonic saline resuscitation of brain-injured patients may increase survival, neurological outcomes may not be improved,[19] and therefore more studies are needed to elicit clear and consistent indications for its use or lack thereof.

Appropriate volumes of crystalloid and ratios of blood products remain controversial for the severely injured. Earlier use of platelets and FFP in ratios more even to packed cells during massive transfusions may be more appropriate,[56] although most resuscitations currently use PRBCs and crystalloid preferentially in the early period and add plasma and platelets only in a second phase. Recent military experience suggests survival may be optimized with a 1 : 1 : 1 ratio of PRBCs, FFP, and platelets, a strategy which reduces crystalloid volumes and replaces what was lost. Having a massive transfusion protocol in place appears to reduce the odds of mortality and overall product consumption.[57]

The search for the best approach continues. Hemodynamically unstable blunt trauma victims with little response to an immediate crystalloid bolus deserve early and aggressive use of products. Unstable penetrating trauma patients requiring surgery should not receive large volumes of crystalloid in attempts at normotension; once surgical bleeding is controlled, a more aggressive resuscitation strategy may be instituted. Continued studies in humans will hopefully explore the heterogeneous nature of the trauma patient and allow the physician to know which patient responds best to the various types of resuscitation protocols and parameters.

References

1. Thompson RCC. Physiological 0.9% saline in the fluid resuscitation of trauma. *J R Army Med Corps* 2005;**151**(3):146–51.

2. Stern SA. Low-volume fluid resuscitation for presumed hemorrhagic shock: helpful or harmful? *Curr Opin Crit Care* 2001;7(6):422–30.

3. Holmes JF, Sakles JC, Lewis G, Wisner DH. Effects of delaying fluid resuscitation on an injury to the systemic arterial vasculature. *Acad Emerg Med* 2002;**9**(4):267–74.

4. Dutton RP, Mackenzie CF, Scalea TM. Hypotensive resuscitation during active hemorrhage: impact on in-hospital mortality. *J Trauma* 2002;**52**(6):1141–6.

5. Bickell WH, Wall MJ, Jr., Pepe PE, et al. Immediate versus delayed fluid resuscitation for hypotensive patients with penetrating torso injuries. *N Engl J Med* 1994;**331**(17):1105–9.

6. Roberts I, Alderson P, Bunn F, et al. Colloids versus crystalloids for fluid resuscitation in critically ill patients. *Cochrane Database Syst Rev* 2004;**4**: CD000567.

7. Rizoli SB. Crystalloids and colloids in trauma resuscitation: a brief overview of the current debate. *J Trauma* 2003;**54**(5 Suppl.):S82–8.

8. Alderson P, Schierhout G, Roberts I, Bunn F. Colloids versus crystalloids for fluid resuscitation in critically ill patients. *Cochrane Database Syst Rev* 2000;**2**: CD000567.

9. Choi PT, Yip G, Quinonez LG, Cook DJ. Crystalloids vs. colloids in fluid resuscitation: a systematic review. *Crit Care Med* 1999;**27**(1):200–10.

10. Tisherman SA. Trauma fluid resuscitation in 2010. *J Trauma* 2003;**54**(5 Suppl.):S231–4.

11. Mizushima Y, Tohira H, Mizobata Y, Matsuoka T, Yokota J. Fluid resuscitation of trauma patients: how fast is the optimal rate? *Am J Emerg Med* 2005;**23**(7):833–7.

12. Koustova E, Stanton K, Gushchin V, et al. Effects of lactated Ringer's solutions on human leukocytes. *J Trauma* 2002;**52**(5):872–8.

13. Rhee P, Burris D, Kaufmann C, et al. Lactated Ringer's solution resuscitation causes neutrophil activation after hemorrhagic shock. *J Trauma* 1998;**44**(2):313–19.

14. Rhee P, Koustova E, Alam HB. Searching for the optimal resuscitation method: recommendations for the initial fluid resuscitation of combat casualties. *J Trauma* 2003;**54**(5 Suppl.):S52–62.

15. Rhee P, Wang D, Ruff P, et al. Human neutrophil activation and increased adhesion by various resuscitation fluids. *Crit Care Med* 2000;**28**(1):74–8.

16. Deb S, Martin B, Sun L, et al. Resuscitation with lactated Ringer's solution in rats with hemorrhagic shock induces immediate apoptosis. *J Trauma* 1999;**46**(4):582–8; discussion 8–9.

17. Bunn F, Roberts I, Tasker R, Akpa E. Hypertonic versus near isotonic crystalloid for fluid resuscitation in critically ill patients. *Cochrane Database Syst Rev* 2004;**3**:CD002045.

18. Perel P, Roberts I. Colloids versus crystalloids for fluid resuscitation in critically ill patients. *Cochrane Database Syst Rev* 2007;**4**:CD000567.

19. Cooper DJ, Myles PS, McDermott FT, et al. Prehospital hypertonic saline resuscitation of patients with hypotension and severe traumatic brain injury: a randomized controlled trial. *JAMA* 2004;**291**(11):1350–7.

20. Myburgh J, Cooper DJ, Finfer S, et al. Saline or albumin for fluid resuscitation in patients with traumatic brain injury. *N Engl J Med* 2007;**357**(9):874–84.

21. Bellomo R. Fluid resuscitation: colloids vs. crystalloids. *Blood Purif* 2002;**20**(3):239–42.

22. Mendez CM, McClain CJ, Marsano LS. Albumin therapy in clinical practice. *Nutr Clin Pract* 2005;**20**(3):314–20.

23. Finfer S, Bellomo R, Boyce N, et al. A comparison of albumin and saline for fluid resuscitation in the intensive care unit. *N Engl J Med* 2004;**350**(22): 2247–56.

24. Vincent J-L, Navickis RJ, Wilkes MM. Morbidity in hospitalized patients receiving human albumin: a meta-analysis of randomized, controlled trials. *Crit Care Med* 2004;**32**(10):2029–38.

25. Whitfield C. Gelatin colloids in the resuscitation of trauma. *J R Army Med Corps* 2006;**152**(4):197–201.

26. Boldt J, Heesen M, Müller M, Pabsdorf M, Hempelmann G. The effects of albumin versus hydroxyethyl starch solution on cardiorespiratory and circulatory variables in critically ill patients. *Anesth Analg* 1996;**83**(2):254–61.

27. Via D, Kaufmann C, Anderson D, Stanton K, Rhee P. Effect of hydroxyethyl starch on coagulopathy in a swine model of hemorrhagic shock resuscitation. *J Trauma* 2001;**50**(6):1076–82.

28. Brummel-Ziedins K, Whelihan MF, Ziedins EG, Mann KG. The resuscitative fluid you choose may potentiate bleeding. *J Trauma* 2006;**61**(6):1350–8.

29. Smith MJ, Stiefel MF, Magge S, et al. Packed red blood cell transfusion increases local cerebral oxygenation. *Crit Care Med* 2005;**33**(5):1104–8.

30. Elzik ME, Dirschl DR, Dahners LE. Correlation of transfusion volume to change in hematocrit. *Am J Hematol* 2006;**81**(2):145–6.

31. Zallen G, Offner PJ, Moore EE, et al. Age of transfused blood is an independent risk factor for postinjury multiple organ failure. *Am J Surg* 1999;**178**(6):570–2.

32. Ketchum L, Hess JR, Hiippala S. Indications for early fresh frozen plasma, cryoprecipitate, and platelet transfusion in trauma. *J Trauma* 2006;**60**(6 Suppl.): S51–8.

33. Simmons P. A primer for nurses who administer blood products. *Medsurg Nurs* 2003;**12**(3):184–90; quiz 91–2.

34. Richards NM, Giuliano KK. Transfusion practices in critical care. *Am J Nurs* 2002;(Suppl.):16–22.

35. Hess JR, Zimrin AB. Massive blood transfusion for trauma. *Curr Opin Hematol* 2005;**12**(6):488–92.

36. Malone DL, Hess JR, Fingerhut A. Massive transfusion practices around the globe and a suggestion for a common massive transfusion protocol. *J Trauma* 2006;**60**(6 Suppl.):S91–6.

37. Standl T. Haemoglobin-based erythrocyte transfusion substitutes. *Expert Opin Biol Ther* 2001;**1**(5):831–43.

38. Lowe KC. Perfluorinated blood substitutes and artificial oxygen carriers. *Blood Rev* 1999;**13**(3):171–84.

39. Levien LJ, Hodgson RE, James MF. Hemoglobin-based blood substitutes and risk of myocardial infarction and death. *JAMA* 2008;**300**(11):1295; author reply 98–9.

40. Palaparthy R, Wang H, Gulati A. Current aspects in pharmacology of modified hemoglobins. *Adv Drug Deliv Rev* 2000;**40**(3):185–98.

41. Crotty B. Recycling blood: sharing the benefits of cell salvage. *Appl Health Econ Health Policy* 2006;**5**(1): 5–10.

42. Huët C, Salmi LR, Fergusson D, et al. A meta-analysis of the effectiveness of cell salvage to minimize perioperative allogeneic blood transfusion in cardiac and orthopedic surgery. International Study of Perioperative Transfusion (ISPOT) Investigators. *Anesth Analg* 1999;**89**(4):861–9.

43. Coats T, Roberts I, Shakur H. Antifibrinolytic drugs for acute traumatic injury. *Cochrane Database Syst Rev* 2004;**4**:CD004896.

44. Harrison TD, Laskosky J, Jazaeri O, Pasquale MD, Cipolle M. "Low-dose" recombinant activated factor VII results in less blood and blood product use in traumatic hemorrhage. *J Trauma* 2005;**59**(1):150–4.

45. Holcomb JB, Jenkins D, Rhee P, et al. Damage control resuscitation: directly addressing the early coagulopathy of trauma. *J Trauma* 2007;**62**(2):307–10.

46. Martinowitz U, Kenet G, Segal E, et al. Recombinant activated factor VII for adjunctive hemorrhage control in trauma. *J Trauma* 2001;**51**(3):431–8; discussion 8–9.

47. Boffard KD, Riou B, Warren B, et al. Recombinant factor VIIa as adjunctive therapy for bleeding control in severely injured trauma patients: two parallel randomized, placebo-controlled, double-blind clinical trials. *J Trauma* 2005;**59**(1):8–15; discussion 15–18.

48. Corwin HL, Gettinger A, Pearl RG, et al. Efficacy of recombinant human erythropoietin in critically ill patients: a randomized controlled trial. *JAMA* 2002;**288**(22):2827–35.

49. Hébert PC, Wells G, Blajchman MA, et al. A multicenter, randomized, controlled clinical trial of transfusion requirements in critical care. Transfusion Requirements in Critical Care Investigators, Canadian Critical Care Trials Group. *N Engl J Med* 1999;**340**(6):409–17.

50. Baggaley RF, Boily MC, White RG, Alary M. Risk of HIV-1 transmission for parenteral exposure and blood transfusion: a systematic review and meta-analysis. *AIDS* 2006;**20**(6):805–12.

51. Shorr AF, Jackson WL. Transfusion practice and nosocomial infection: assessing the evidence. *Curr Opin Crit Care* 2005;**11**(5):468–72.

52. AABB, America's Blood Centers, American Red Cross. *Circular of Information for the Use of Human Blood and Blood Components.* Available from http://www.aabb.org/AABBContent/Templates/.

53. Jeremitsky E, Omert L, Dunham CM, Protetch J, Rodriguez A. Harbingers of poor outcome the day after severe brain injury: hypothermia, hypoxia, and hypoperfusion. *J Trauma* 2003;**54**(2):312–19.

54. White H, Cook D, Venkatesh B. The use of hypertonic saline for treating intracranial hypertension after traumatic brain injury. *Anesth Analg* 2006;**102** (6):1836–46.

55. Munar F, Ferrer AM, de Nadal M, et al. Cerebral hemodynamic effects of 7.2% hypertonic saline in patients with head injury and raised intracranial pressure. *J Neurotrauma* 2000;**17**(1):41–51.

56. Ketchum L, Hess JR, Hiippala S. Indications for early fresh frozen plasma, cryoprecipitate, and platelet transfusion in trauma. *J Trauma* 2006;**60**(6 Suppl.): S51–8.

57. Cotton BA, Gunter OL, Isbell J, et al. Damage control hematology: the impact of a trauma exsanguination protocol on survival and blood product utilization. *J Trauma* 2008;**64**(5):1177–82; discussion 82–3.

Chapter 34

Trauma procedure I

Mari Siegel and Elizabeth L. Mitchell

Introduction

Emergency physicians must be familiar with the techniques for performing and interpreting diagnostic procedures in trauma. Further, they must take the responsibility for understanding the indications and contraindications. Deferring a procedure to a trauma surgeon or subspecialist is often not feasible, given the critical and dynamic nature of major trauma. Frequently these procedures are extremely time-critical and may have both diagnostic and therapeutic benefits.

Pericardiocentesis

Indications and contraindications

The primary role of pericardiocentesis in the emergency department (ED) is as a therapeutic tool to treat pericardial tamponade in a hemodynamically unstable patient or a patient in PEA (pulseless electrical activity). Pericardiocentesis has a limited role in trauma as a diagnostic tool. Echocardiography, where available, is the diagnostic procedure of choice for pericardial tamponade. However, in a hemodynamically unstable patient in whom pericardial effusion is suspected and emergency echocardiography is not immediately available, emergent pericardiocentesis can be both diagnostic and life saving.

Pericardiocentesis is insensitive in trauma, with a false negative rate in diagnosing cardiac tamponade of between 20 and 40%. A positive test relies on aspirating blood, and in trauma, the blood may clot leading to a negative aspirate.[1,2]

Pericardiocentesis is performed electively and most safely with fluoroscopic or ultrasound (US) guidance. In the trauma setting, however, when the role of pericardiocentesis is to diagnose and relieve cardiac tamponade, the procedure is emergent and is performed blindly or with bedside US or electrocardiographic (ECG) assistance.

Pericardiocentesis is generally used for the hypotensive patient in whom the need for emergent thoracotomy is unclear or when a small aspiration of blood may temporize the hemodynamic status and allow for transfer to the operating room (OR). Pericardiocentesis is contraindicated when a patient requires an emergency thoracotomy. Complications of pericardiocentesis include injury of nearby structures, including pneumothorax, laceration of the coronary vessels, myocardial laceration, and hemothorax. Dysrhythmias may complicate the procedure when the needle contacts the epicardium. Several studies have shown the complication rate from blind and ECG-guided pericardiocentesis is higher than with US guidance.[3-5]

Box 34.1   Pericardiocentesis equipment

Necessary	Optional
• 3–5 inch (7–13 cm) 18-gauge needle with an obturator	• Guidewire and catheter for Seldinger placement
• 10–30 cc syringe (depending on amount of fluid expected)	• ECG machine with "alligator clip lead"
	• Bedside US (highly recommended)
	• Nasogastric tube (if distended abdomen)

The equipment needed for pericardiocentesis includes a 3–5 inch (7–13 cm) 18-gauge needle with an obturator, and a large syringe. Optional equipment

---

Trauma: A Comprehensive Emergency Medicine Approach, eds. Eric Legome and Lee W. Shockley. Published by Cambridge University Press. © Cambridge University Press 2011.

includes guidewire and catheter for Seldinger placement as well as an ECG machine with "alligator clip lead" or a bedside US. Some would recommend premedicating the patient with atropine to prevent vasovagal reactions, although this is unproven. The patient should be positioned at a 45° head up angle rather than supine to bring the heart closer to the anterior chest wall. A nasogastric tube should be inserted if the patient has a distended abdomen and time permits.

Procedure

As mentioned there are three main methods for performing pericardiocentesis commonly used in the ED: (1) ECG guidance; (2) US guidance; or (3) blindly based on surface landmarks. If time allows, ECG guidance may be combined with US guidance, although the benefit of the combined procedures are not well documented.

Electrocardiographic guidance of pericardiocentesis is performed by attaching an alligator clip to any precordial ECG lead (V1–V6), usually V1 or V5. This allows continuous monitoring for disturbances in the QRS morphology and a "current of injury" during the procedure. When using US, the area of the pericardium with the largest fluid collection can be marked ahead of time. This area may then be aspirated with direct observation of the needle entering the pericaridium. On US the needle appears as a hyperechoic long thin structure with reverberation artifact. Since it may be difficult to perform this in real time, another option is to insert the needle at the area of maximal fluid after it is found on US but without following the needle's progress on US.

There are two approaches to needle insertion in pericardiocentesis. The classic approach is in the subxyphoid area, but this has been challenged recently by studies of US-guided pericardiocentesis that show that the pericardial fluid collections are best approached in the intercostal space near the apex of the heart.[6,7] Needle entry in the parasternal area in the 5th intercostal space is safer than the subxyphoid approach, causing fewer complications and is successful more often. Without echocardiography using the subxyphoid approach, the needle is inserted at a 30–45° angle between the xyphoid process and left costal border, aiming at the left shoulder (Figure 34.1). In the parasternal approach, the needle is inserted at a 90° angle in the 5th intercostal space at the sternal border. The obturator is only removed after the skin

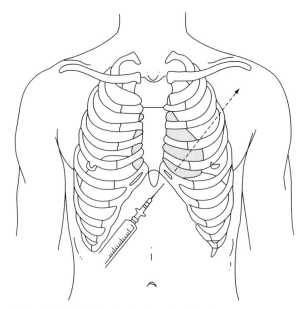

Figure 34.1 Traditional technique of pericardiocentesis.

has been punctured, preventing the needle lumen from becoming obstructed. A syringe is attached after the obturator is removed. The needle is advanced until fluid is returned. Aspiration of fluid usually occurs 6–8 cm below the skin in adults and 5 cm in children.

An additional technique used after fluid is aspirated, involves inserting a guidewire through the needle, placing a catheter over the guidewire, and leaving the capped catheter in place for repeated aspirations as necessary.

If ECG monitoring is used, the needle is connected to one of the V leads of the ECG machine via alligator clips prior to advancement into the pericardium. The ECG machine should be continuously recording the V lead that is attached to the pericardial needle as the needle is advanced. If the needle touches the epicardium, the ECG machine will record a wide complex PVC with ST elevation, a "current of injury" pattern; i.e., ST elevation, or ventricular dysrhythmias. Contact of the needle with the atrium can cause atrial arrhythmias, PR prolongation, or AV dissociation. If these findings are noted on ECG, the needle should be withdrawn until the abnormality resolves.

Complications

Complications rates are significantly improved by using US guidance. Complications of pericardiocentesis include myocardial laceration, coronary artery laceration, pneumothorax, air embolism, arrhythmias, PR prolongation, or AV dissociation, and infection.

The physiologic changes that occur with the reversal of tamponade and restoration of right ventricular stroke volume can lead to right ventricular overload, circulatory collapse, and flash pulmonary edema. Although these consequences of pericardiocentesis are rare, some authors recommend a drainage rate of no more than 50 ml/min.[8]

Diagnostic peritoneal lavage

Indications and contraindications

Diagnostic peritoneal lavage (DPL) emerged as a diagnostic tool in abdominal trauma in 1965 and remained a mainstay in trauma management until recently. In recent years, emergency US and high-definition computed tomography (CT) scanning have largely replaced DPL in the initial evaluation of the abdomen in trauma. Ultrasound provides sensitive and specific evaluation of peritoneal and cardiac injury by diagnosing free fluid in the abdomen and pericardial effusion or tamponade.[9] Computed tomography technology continues to advance, and its ability to diagnose intra-abdominal pathology continues to improve. It can reliably diagnose injury to the spleen and liver and hemoperitoneum after abdominal trauma.[10] However, CT still remains suboptimal in diagnosing hollow viscus injury, specifically injuries of the bowel, pancreas, and diaphragm. In situations where US is not available, or where the presence of intra-abdominal injury remains a possibility after CT, there is a role for DPL. All three modalities offer high sensitivity and specificity for diagnosis of intra-abdominal injury, although the specificity for an operative lesion is lower in DPL and US.[11]

The utility of DPL in trauma is to identify intra-abdominal hemorrhage in the grossly unstable patient where US is unavailable or technically inadequate, and the patient is too unstable for CT scanning. Less commonly, it is used in the identification of hollow viscus or diaphragmatic injury in the hemodynamically stable patient with penetrating or blunt abdominal trauma.

Diagnostic peritoneal lavage has drawbacks, mainly its invasiveness compared to CT and US. Limitations of DPL include its inability to diagnose retroperitoneal injuries and its lack of sensitivity when diagnosing diaphragmatic, and intestinal injury. Diagnostic peritoneal lavage has a high false positive rate, ranging from 13% to 54%, resulting in non-therapeutic laparotomies.[4,10,12–16]

The only absolute contraindication to DPL is a patient who has a clear indication for immediate laparotomy. Patients with obvious peritoneal signs or unstable vitals after abdominal trauma should proceed directly to laparotomy.[17] Relative contraindications include prior abdominal surgery, obesity, coagulopathy, and second or third trimester pregnancy.

Box 34.2 Equipment for DPL

Equipment	Additional Information	Technique
Foley catheter	Not necessary if US shows empty bladder	Open, semi-open, closed
1% lidocaine for local anesthesia	Epinephrine preferred	Open, semi-open, closed
Nasogastric tube		Closed supraumbilical, possible open supraumbilical
Skin preparation materials (e.g., drapes, betadine)		Open, semi-open, closed
DPL catheter with a right angle adaptor, extension tubing set without a one-way valve and a non-Leur-lock syringe		Open, semi-open, closed
Warm saline	1 L in adult 15 ml/kg in children	Open, semi-open, closed
No. 11 scalpel		Closed and open
Trocar		Semi-open and closed
No. 10 blade		Open or semi-open
Flexible guidewire		Closed

589

Technique	Circumstance
Supraumbilical	Pregnancy; pelvic fracture with hematoma; or previous infraumbilical scar
Infraumbilical	Majority unless relative contraindications as described above
Open	Previous surgery with concern for adhesions; obesity; pregnancy
Semi-open	Similar in complications to closed, still preferred in some centers for increased visualization of peritoneum
Closed (Seldinger)	Generally similar to semi-open in complications, may be faster and performed without assistance

Procedure

Diagnostic peritoneal lavage can be performed by the open, semi-open, or closed techniques. It may also be performed in the supra- or infraumbilical position (Table 34.1).

A Foley catheter should be placed prior to any of these techniques. Optimally, a nasogastric tube should be placed for decompression of the stomach before a DPL with a supraumbilical approach is performed. The patient should be supine with the abdomen prepped and draped in standard sterile fashion. Local anesthesia with 1% lidocaine with epinephrine should be used. After an initial wheal is place in the supra- or infraumbilical area, the needle should be directed downward and perpendicular to the skin to provide deeper anesthesia to the peritoneum.

For the semi-open method, a 4–6 cm skin incision is made with a No. 10 scalpel in the infraumbilical ring in the midline. Blunt dissection with Army–Navy retractors and hemostats should proceed down to the fascial fibers of the linea alba. Next, a 2–3 mm incision is made in the linea alba with a No. 15 or 11 scalpel. Towel clips are placed in this small opening to grasp both sides of the rectus fascia and are lifted upwards. It is now safe to pass a catheter through the opening into the peritoneal cavity. The trocar and catheter are inserted at a 45–60° angle caudad. The trocar is advanced 0.5–1.0 cm, puncturing the peritoneum into the peritoneal cavity, and then is held as

the catheter is advanced another several centimeters. The trocar is then withdrawn.

The fully open technique is similar to the semi-open technique, except that the incision in the linea alba is extended to several centimeters to allow direct visualization of the peritoneal cavity. The peritoneum is grasped with a hemostat above and below, a nick is made in the peritoneum with a No. 11 or 15 blade and the catheter is passed through the opening. A purse string suture is made around the catheter through the peritoneum with an absorbable suture such as 3.0 Vicryl®, to prevent the fluid from leaking out. The full open technique may be safer, but takes longer and is more technically demanding (Figures 34.2 and 34.3).

The closed technique is performed in a percutaneous fashion with a catheter advanced over a wire (Seldinger technique). A small gauge (No. 18) needle at least 2.5 inches is inserted into the peritoneal cavity in the infraumbilical midline just below the umbilicus. The needle should be aimed slightly towards the patient's feet. A flexible J guidewire is then passed through the needle into the peritoneal cavity, aimed toward the right or left pelvic gutter. The needle is removed. A soft catheter is then passed over the guidewire into the peritoneal cavity using a twisting motion as the catheter is advanced. A small incision with a No. 11 scalpel at the site of entry through the skin may be necessary to pass the catheter. There are a variety of proprietary and hospital-designed kits to perform lavage. Some may have minor variation on the equipment above, such as an addition catheter to pass the wire through or a dilator (Figure 34.4).

Both techniques are comparably accurate and safe.[18,19] The closed technique takes less time but more often results in procedure failure. The time involved varies by study, with mean times ranging from 2 to 17.8 minutes for closed, and from 11 to 26.8 minutes for open.[19,20] Once the catheter has been passed into the peritoneal cavity, a right angle adapter, extension tubing, and a non-Leur-lock syringe are attached. Aspiration of 10 cc of gross blood or any bile or fecal material is considered a positive test and no lavage is necessary. If < 10 cc of gross blood is aspirated it is returned to the peritoneum, then the peritoneum is lavaged. No aspirated material should also result in proceeding to lavage. Lavage is accomplished by instilling 1000 cc in adults, or 15 mg/kg in children, of warm normal saline or lactated Ringer's solution. Just prior to complete emptying of the bag of fluid, the intravenous (IV)

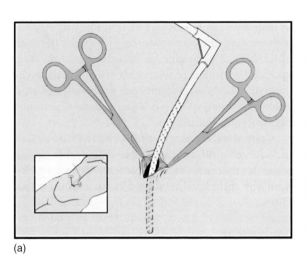

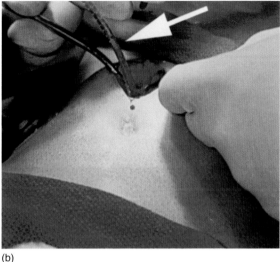

(a) (b)

Figure 34.2 (a) Illustration of open diagnostic peritoneal lavage (DPL) technique. (b) Photograph of the introduction of the DPL catheter under direct vision, using the open technique. (From Mandavia D, Newton E, Demetriades D. *Colour Atlas of Emergency Trauma*. Cambridge: Cambridge University Press, 2003.)

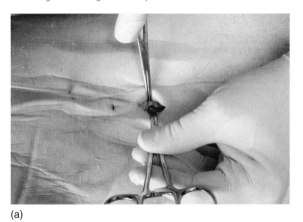

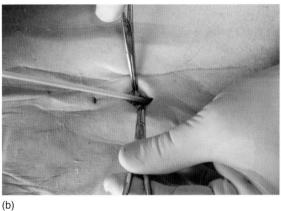

(a) (b)

Figure 34.3 Infraumbilical cadaveric model using open technique. In (a) the peritoneum is visualized, in (b) the catheter has been inserted. (Courtesy of Taku Taira, MD and the New York University School of Medicine.)

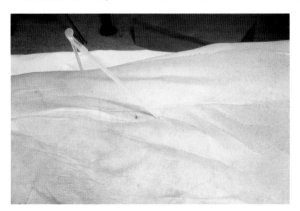

Figure 34.4 Cadaveric model with diagnostic peritoneal lavage (DPL) catheter inserted by closed technique.

bag is then placed below the patient and fluid is allowed to siphon back to the bag. While the absolute volume that needs to be returned is unclear, the smaller the volume returned, the less sensitive the test will be. The test characteristic probably plateau at about 600–750 cc returned with 1 L instilled.

The criteria for considering a DPL positive are free aspiration of 10 cc of gross blood, or analysis of DPL aspirate with $> 100\,000$ red blood cells (RBC)/mm^3, > 500 white blood cells (WBC)/mm^3, or amylase $> 175\,\text{IU}/100\,\text{ml}$. Patients with $> 100\,000\,\text{RBC}/\text{mm}^3$ should proceed to laparotomy. Patients with RBC counts between 10 000 and 100 000 should be admitted for observation and/or further testing, such as CT

591

Table 34.2 Diagnostic peritoneal lavage (DPL) fluid analysis

	Positive	Observation or further testing
Blood	10 cc gross blood or > 100 000 RBC/mm³	10 000–100 000 RBC/mm³ > 5000 RBC/mm³ in GSWs or low chest SWs (concern for diaphragmatic injury)
WBC	> 500 WBC/mm³	
Amylase	> 175 IU	
Other	Any bile, fecal material, or bowel contents	

GSWs, gunshot wounds; IU, international unit; RBC, red blood cells; SWs, stab wounds; WBC, white blood cells.

scanning. In patients with gunshot wounds, or lower chest stab wounds, a RBC/mm³ count of > 5000 is considered suspicious for injury and further study, exploration by laparoscopy or laparotomy, or observation is warranted (Table 34.2).

In patients with pelvic fracture, DPL should be performed though a supraumbilical incision to avoid passing the catheter through an anterior retroperitoneal hematoma.[11]

Complications

Complication rates are similar for all techniques.[11,19,21,22]

Arthrocentesis and arthrogram

Indications and contraindications

Arthrocentesis, the puncture and aspiration of a joint, and arthrogram, the injection of fluid into the joint, have many diagnostic roles in trauma. Indications for arthrocentesis in the setting of trauma includes: (1) diagnosis of injury to bony or ligamentous structures by confirming the presence of blood in the joint, i.e., hemarthrosis; (2) detection of an intra-articular fracture by aspiration of blood and fat globules from the joint space; and (3) determining if a laceration extends into a joint space by observing fluid instilled into a joint by arthrocentesis extravasate from the space into the laceration. Diagnostic reasons to perform arthrocentesis are rare but may be used to determine whether there is an occult fracture or

ligamentous/meniscal tear. This would be seen in the patient with severe pain and a negative radiograph or inability to ambulate with an effusion after trauma. A therapeutic role of arthrocentesis includes injection of lidocaine, bupivicaine, or morphine into the joint space, all of which provide pain relief. This may be done in patients with significant pain and large effusions after trauma. Often this can be done in conjunction with a diagnostic tap.

Contraindications to arthrocentesis in trauma include cellulitus overlying the area to be tapped, or in the trajectory of the needle. Relative contraindications include bleeding diathesis and prosthetic joints.

Equipment

Box 34.3   Equipment arthrocentesis
- 18-gauge needle for fluid aspiration
- 25–27-gauge needle for local anesthetic
- 10–20 cc syringe
- Local anesthetic (lidocaine or bupivicaine)
- Povidone–iodine solution for sterilizing the procedure site
- Alcohol 10% isopropryl wipe to cleanse the iodine solution
- Sterile gloves and drapes.

The equipment needed for arthrocentesis includes an 18-gauge needle for fluid aspiration, a 25–27-gauge needle for local anesthetic, a large 10–20 cc syringe, local anesthetic (lidocaine or bupivicaine), povidone–iodine solution for sterilizing the procedure site, alcohol 10% isopropryl wipe to cleanse the iodine solution, and sterile gloves and drapes. The procedure for traumatic arthrocentesis is similar to that for non-traumatic, although a lavender top for cell count analysis, a green top for crystal analysis, and a culture medium may also be sent.

Procedure

Sterile technique should be used. Landmarks should be clearly identified before attempting arthrocentesis. Alternatively, US may help identify the area of greatest effusion and maximize the likelihood of a successful tap. Once the area to be aspirated is identified, the area is widely cleansed with a povidone–iodine solution that is allowed to dry for several minutes to produce the desired antimicrobial effect.

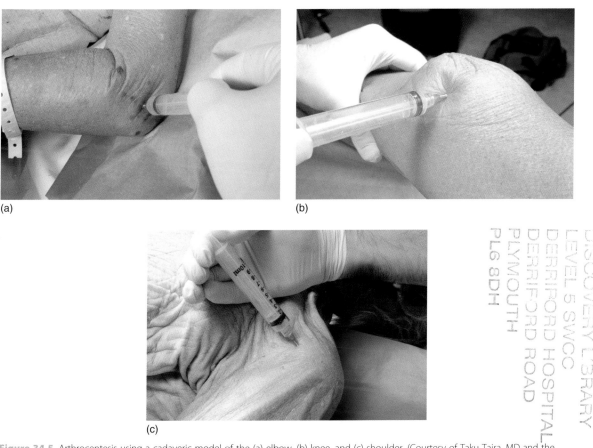

(a)

(b)

(c)

Figure 34.5 Arthrocentesis using a cadaveric model of the (a) elbow, (b) knee, and (c) shoulder. (Courtesy of Taku Taira, MD and the New York University School of Medicine.)

The area is then cleansed with alcohol to avoid introducing iodine into the joint space, causing local inflammation. Next, the area is draped in a sterile fashion and local anesthesia can be performed with 1% or 2% lidocaine given through a 25–27-gauge small bore needle. Skin, subcutaneous tissue, and the joint capsule itself should be anesthestized. Insertion of the arthrocentesis needle should be relatively painless if anesthetic has been given properly. When inserting the 18-gauge arthrocentesis needle, make sure not to "bounce" the needle off of the bone or cartilage, as this can damage these structures. Once synovial fluid begins to flow into the syringe, hold the needle steady and withdraw as much fluid as possible. Once fluid stops flowing, the joint is either dry or a clot has lodged in the needle. Try to withdraw or advance the needle slightly, reinject a small amount of aspirate and withdraw again to attempt to aspirate more fluid. If unable, withdraw the needle

completely and apply a dressing. In the setting of acute trauma, laboratory analysis of the synovial fluid adds little to the gross inspection for blood and fat globules (Figure 34.5).

Saline arthrogram

The approach to performing an arthrogram is the same as arthrocentesis. However, sterile saline is injected into the joint. The volume injected depends on the joint; it must be sufficient to distend the joint capsule and allow the fluid to extravasate through any communicating wound. In the knee, low volumes of fluid under low pressure may not be accurate. The sensitivity of the test is dependent on the size of the laceration, the rate of injection, and the amount of fluid. Recent data suggest that around 90–190 ml are required for a 95% sensitivity with 1.0–2.6 cm lacerations.[22,23] When the pressure in the joint capsule

593

Table 34.3 Synovial fluid analysis

	Color	WBC/µg	% PMN	Culture	Crystals
Normal	Clear	< 200	< 25	Negative	None
Non-inflammatory/ traumatic	Yellow or red	$< 200–2000$	< 25	Negative	None
Inflammatory	Yellow	$200–50\,000$	> 50	Negative	Uric acid or calcium pyrophosphate
Septic	Yellow	$> 50\,000$	> 50	$> 50\%$ positive	none
Fracture	Clear/ red May find fat globules	NA	NA	NA	none

NA, not applicable; PMN, polymorphonuclear leukocytes; WBC, white blood cells.

makes it difficult to instill further fluid, remove the needle. Once the needle is removed, the joint can be manipulated either by flexion and extension of the joint or by milking the fluid externally; however, manipulation may be contraindicated by the presenting trauma. If there is a communicating laceration, fluid should be seen draining from the laceration. If you do not get fluid, the joint should be re-tapped to remove the fluid. Consider installation of anesthesia into the joint at the end of the procedure.

Historically, methylene blue has been used and is described in several procedure manuals; it has never been shown to be better than saline alone and may be absorbed systemically.

Analysis of fluid

The full analysis of the fluid is described below (Table 34.3). However, when looking for a fracture or ligamentous injury the laboratory evaluation is of minimal assistance. The main question is, is there blood, blood and fat, or neither. Normal fluid is clear. Straw colored or red fluid is indicative of a traumatic injury. However, fluid from a traumatic injury can also appear yellow. Normal synovial fluid has < 200 WBC/ml and $< 25\%$ polymorphonuclear leukocytes (PMN). The differential for synovial fluid with < 2000 WBC/ml and $< 25\%$ PMN includes trauma, osteoarthritis, and other non-inflammatory conditions. The differential for synovial fluid with $200–50\,000$ WBC/ml and $> 50\%$ PMN includes the inflammatory arthropathies, such as gout, pseudogout, Lyme, lupus, and the spondyloarthropathies. Synovial

fluid with $> 50\,000$ WBC/ml and $> 50\%$ PMN indicates septic joint. The Gram stain of fluid from a septic joint will reveal organisms in $> 50\%$ of cases, whereas the Gram stain will be negative in all other cases.

Complications

Complications are uncommon but include infection, bleeding, and allergic reaction to local anesthetic. Infection, caused by skin bacteria being introduced into the joint space, occurs at a rate of 1 per 10 000 aspirations.[24] Bleeding into a joint space after arthrocentesis with resultant hemarthrosis generally occurs only when a patient is on anticoagulants or has a bleeding diathesis. Complications from arthrogram are the same with the addition of discomfort due to the expansion of the joint with extra fluid. This discomfort may last several days until the fluid reabsorbs but may be ameliorated by removing the fluid after the initial procedure.

Slit-lamp exam

Indications and contraindications

The slit-lamp exam, in conjunction with tonometry and the fluorescein exam, is used to diagnose corneal abrasions, foreign bodies, burns, and iritis after trauma to the eye. The slit lamp allows detailed evaluation of the external eye and the anterior chamber and is the instrument of choice in the ED for the diagnosis of anterior chamber hemorrhage and inflammation.

The slit-lamp exam is contraindicated in the unstable patient or those who are unable to sit up. Portable slit lamps, although uncommon in EDs, can be used in supine patients.

Equipment

> **Box 34.4 Slit-lamp examination equipment**
> - Functional slit lamp
> - Fluorescein strips
> - Anesthetic drops (proparicaine 0.5%)

The slit-lamp exam requires a functional slit lamp, fluorescein strips, and anesthetic drops, usually proparicaine 0.5% ophthalmic drops.

Sodium fluorescein is a water-soluble chemical that absorbs blue light and emits green light when exposed to an alkaline environment. The tear film over intact corneal epithelium is neutral, but the Bowman membrane, just under the corneal epithelium, is alkaline. When a corneal abrasion exposes the Bowman membrane and fluorescein is applied, the fluorescein will fluoresce, absorbing blue light and emitting green light.

Anesthetic ophthalmic drops are controversial because of the theoretical risk of punctuate keratitis that they can cause. However, they are usually required to perform an adequate examination of the eye.

Procedure

The slit-lamp exam can be divided into three parts: the general screening exam of the anterior segment of the eye; inspection with fluorescein for corneal abrasions; and examination of the anterior chamber looking for iritis or hemorrhage.

The first step looks at the anterior segment of the eye. Abnormalities discovered in this step include corneal perforation and foreign bodies (Table 34.4). For this step, the microscope should be directly in front of the patient's eye with the light source at a 45° angle. The slit beam is set to white light at minimum width and the power source is set at half power. One focuses the light beam on the cornea by moving the base of the slit lamp back and forth until the cornea comes into focus. Once the cornea is in focus, move the slit lamp back and forth to scan from side to side, searching the cornea and conjunctiva for foreign bodies or abrasions. Then, one pushes the slit lamp

Table 34.4 Foreign body patterns

Foreign bodies in the eyelids	Vertical and linear, and multiple
Embedded foreign body	Circular margin
Embedded metallic foreign bodies	Circular margin with surrounding rust circle
Burn injury	Diffuse punctate fluorescence

in slightly to focus on the iris. If the depth of the anterior chamber seems reduced, one must consider a corneal perforation. This set up can also be used to examine the inverted eyelids for retained foreign bodies.

The second step will identify cells and flare in the anterior chamber, suggestive of iritis. The beam width is narrowed as much as possible and the height is decreased to 3–4 mm. The light source is turned to high power. Looking through the eyepiece, the light source is focused on the middle of the cornea and then is advanced slightly to a focal point on the anterior surface of the lens. The light is then pulled back to the halfway point between the lens and the cornea and is now focused in the anterior chamber. Normal aqueous fluid in the anterior chamber is clear. Small particles floating in the aqueous fluid are cells; an aqueous that lights up indicates the protein "flare" of iritis. Traumatic iritis usually has an onset 1–4 days after an injury. This step is usually performed before fluorescein has been applied to the eye, because fluorescein can penetrate a damaged cornea, producing a false flare.

The third step of the slit-lamp exam inspects for corneal abrasions and is performed in a similar fashion to the first step, after fluorescein has been applied to the eye and the slit lamp is switched to the blue light. The slit-lamp beam should be widened to 3–4 mm and may be decreased to half power. A patient can tolerate a wider beam of blue light compared to white light. One applies fluorescein to the eye by holding the strip by the non-orange end, placing a single drop of sterile saline on the orange tip of the applicator, and touching the wet end gently inside the patient's lower lid. The strip is withdrawn and the patient is instructed to blink. Blinking spreads the fluorescein over the eye. One should be careful not to apply an excess of fluorescein as this will obscure the examination. A thin layer of fluorescein is preferred. Corneal defects are detected by scanning across the cornea looking for areas of fluorescein uptake (green). Corneal abrasions usually have sharp and linear margins.

The Seidel test may be performed to detect perforation of the globe. To perform the Seidel test, one applies a large amount of fluorescein by wetting the fluorescein strip with several drops of saline while holding the strip against the inner lower eyelid. Flooding the eye will result in a stream of fluorescein leaking from the ruptured globe that looks green under cobalt blue light or a Wood's lamp.

Tonometry may be performed to assess intraocular pressure. It is indicated in iritis, retrobulbar hemmorhage or suspicion of increased ocular pressure (e.g., acute angle-closure glaucoma in the post-traumatic setting). Most EDs will have a Tono-Pen® or Schiotz tonometer or applanation tonometer. If none of these are available, the physician can assess gross intraocular pressure by pressing gently on the closed eye with the index finger and comparing it to one's own eye firmness or the patient's other eye. High intraocular pressure causes a decrease in compressibility of the globe. Tonometry should not be performed when globe rupture is suspected as increasing the intraocular pressure by pressing on the eye can cause loss of vitreous humor to a ruptured globe.

Complications

Fluorescein will permanently stain contact lenses and should not be used when a patient is wearing them. The patient should not replace their lenses for several hours. Fluorescein solutions, but not drops, are associated with bacterial infection. The solution is rarely associated with vagal reactions and generalized convulsions, but the reactions are thought to be related to a compound in the solution other than fluorescein.[25,26] Paper strips impregnated with fluorescein are not associated with the same complication, are safe, and are widely used.

Conclusion

There are many diagnostic tests that emergency physicians are skilled at performing or interpreting that do not have a role in trauma. For example, lumbar puncture is utilized in the evaluation of atraumatic subarachnoid hemorrhage (SAH), but does not have a role in the evaluation of traumatic SAH. Similarly, paracentesis is useful in the evaluation of the cirrhotic patient to diagnose intraperitoneal infection, but does not have a role in the trauma room. In addition, advances in radiology have made some of the diagnostic procedures discussed in this chapter, such as DPL and blind pericardiocentesis, relatively uncommon in institutions where emergency US and high-definition CT scanning are readily available.

References

1. Shoemaker WC. Algorithm for early recognition and management of cardiac tamponade. *Crit Care Med* 1975;**3**(2):59–63.

2. Bolanowski PJ, Swaminathan AP, Neville WE. Aggressive surgical management of penetrating cardiac injuries. *J Thorac Cardiovasc Surg* 1973;**66**(1):52–7.

3. Salem K, Mulji A, Lonn E. Echocardiographically guided pericardiocentesis – the gold standard for the management of pericardial effusion and cardiac tamponade. *Can J Cardiol* 1999;**15**(11):1251–5.

4. Meredith JW, Ditesheim JA, Stonehouse S, Wolfman N. Computed tomography and diagnostic peritoneal lavage. Complementary roles in blunt trauma. *Am Surg* 1992;**58**(1):44–8.

5. Tsang TS, El-Najdawi EK, Seward JB, et al. Percutaneous echocardiographically guided pericardiocentesis in pediatric patients: evaluation of safety and efficacy. *J Am Soc Echocardiogr* 1998; **11**(11):1072–7.

6. Callahan JA, Seward JB, Tajik AJ. Cardiac tamponade: pericardiocentesis directed by two-dimensional echocardiography. *Mayo Clin Proc* 1985;**60**(5):344–7.

7. Clarke DP, Cosgrove DO. Real-time ultrasound scanning in the planning and guidance of pericardiocentesis. *Clin Radiol* 1987;**38**(2):119–22.

8. Hamaya Y, Dohi S, Ueda N, Akamatsu S. Severe circulatory collapse immediately after pericardiocentesis in a patient with chronic cardiac tamponade. *Anesth Analg* 1993;**77**(6):1278–81.

9. Mandavia DP, Hoffner RJ, Mahaney K, Henderson SO. Bedside echocardiography by emergency physicians. *Ann Emerg Med* 2001;**38**(4):377–82.

10. American College of Emergency Physicians, Clinical Policies Committee.Clinical policy: critical issues in the evaluation of adult patients presenting to the emergency department with acute blunt abdominal trauma. *Ann Emerg Med* 2004;**43**(2):278–90.

11. Liu M, Lee CH, P'Eng K. Prospective comparison of diagnostic peritoneal lavage, computed tomographic scanning, and ultrasonography for the diagnosis of blunt abdominal trauma. *J Trauma* 1993; **35**(2):267–70.

12. Bain IM, Kirby RM, Tiwari P, et al. Survey of abdominal ultrasound and diagnostic peritoneal lavage for suspected intra-abdominal injury following blunt trauma. *Injury* 1998;**29**(1):65–71.

13. Fryer JP, Graham TL, Fong HM, Burns CM. Diagnostic peritoneal lavage as an indicator for therapeutic surgery. *Can J Surg* 1991;**34**(5):471–6.

14. Henneman PL, Marx JA, Moore EE, Cantrill SV, Ammons LA. Diagnostic peritoneal lavage: accuracy in predicting necessary laparotomy following blunt and penetrating trauma. *J Trauma* 1990;**30**(11):1345–55.

15. Drost TF, Rosemurgy AS, Kearney RE, Roberts P. Diagnostic peritoneal lavage. Limited indications due to evolving concepts in trauma care. *Am Surg* 1991; **57**(2):126–8.

16. Sözüer EM, Akyürek N, Kafali ME, Yildirim C. Diagnostic peritoneal lavage in blunt abdominal trauma victims. *Eur J Emerg Med* 1998; **5**(2):231–4.

17. Cheng AB, Testa P, Legome E, Kaplan LJ. Penetrating abdominal trauma. *EMedicine.* Available from http://emedicine.medscape.com/.

18. Cué JI, Miller FB, Cryer HM, 3rd, et al. A prospective, randomized comparison between open and closed peritoneal lavage techniques. *J Trauma* 1990; **30**(7):880–3.

19. Hodgson NF, Stewart TC, Girotti MJ. Open or closed diagnostic peritoneal lavage for abdominal trauma? A meta-analysis. *J Trauma* 2000;**48**(6):1091–5.

20. Velmahos GC, Demetriades D, Stewart M, et al. Open versus closed diagnostic peritoneal lavage: a comparison on safety, rapidity, efficacy. *J R Coll Surg Edinb* 1998;**43**(4):235–8.

21. Davis JW, Hoyt DB, Mackersie RC, McArdle MS. Complications in evaluating abdominal trauma: diagnostic peritoneal lavage versus computerized axial tomography. *J Trauma* 1990;**30**(12):1506–9.

22. Nord RM, Quach T, Walsh M, Pereira D, Tejwani NC. Detection of traumatic arthrotomy of the knee using the saline solution load test. *J Bone Joint Surg Am* 2009;**91**(1):66–70.

23. Keese GR, Boody AR, Wongworawat MD, Jobe CM. The accuracy of the saline load test in the diagnosis of traumatic knee arthrotomies. *J Orthop Trauma* 2007;**21**(7):442–3.

24. Katz W. Diagnosis of monoarthritis, polyarthritis, and monoarticular rheumatic disorders. In Katz W (ed.), *Rheumatic Disorders: Diagnosis and Treatment.* Philadelphia, PA: JB Lippincott, 1977: pp. 192–7.

25. Cohn HC, Jocson VL. A unique case of grand mal seizures after fluress. *Ann Ophthalmol* 1981; **13**(12):1379–80.

26. Department of Opthalmology, University of Oregon Health Science Center. *National Registry of Drug-Induced Ocular Side Effects.* Portland, OR: University of Oregon Health Science Center, 1979: Case Reports 404a, 404b, and 421.

Trauma procedures II

Nancy Kwon, Sajan Patel, and Elizabeth L. Mitchell

Cricothyrotomy

Indications

Cricothyrotomy is indicated in establishing an emergent airway when orotracheal or nasotracheal intubation fails or is contraindicated, as in suspected cervical spine injury with airway compromise, upper airway hemorrhage, difficult patient anatomy due to congenital or traumatic distortions, massive emesis, or airway obstruction due to foreign body, trauma, or angioedema. It is estimated that between 1 and 3% of airways in the emergency department (ED) are managed by cricothyrotomy.[1,2] One study found that the rates of cricothyrotomies at one institution declined from 1.8% to 0.2% after the establishment of an emergency medicine residency.[3] The authors attributed this decline to increased faculty supervision, less cricothyrotomies being performed on patients with suspected cervical spine injury, and increased competency in endotracheal intubation.

Contraindications

Cricothyrotomy should not be performed in patients who can safely be intubated via nasotracheal or orotracheal intubation. It is contraindicated in patients with fracture or serious injury to the cricoid cartilage or larynx, who should instead be managed with tracheostomy. Needle cricothyrotomy is preferred in patients under the age of 12.

The following equipment is required to perform the cricothyrotomy: No. 11 blade scalpel, curved hemostat, Trousseau dilator, tracheal hook, and a tracheostomy tube (preferably 6 mm diameter, maximum 8 mm). A 6 mm endotracheal tube can be used temporarily; however, it is less desirable as its longer length makes it difficult to secure, increasing the risk

of dislodgment or mainstem bronchus intubation. Preparation for the procedure requires gloves, protective gown, face shield, chlorhexidine or povidone iodine, gauze pads, lidocaine, 10 ml syringe, tape, and suture or tying material. A bag-valve device and oxygen source should be available to ventilate the patient once an airway is established.

Box 35.1   Cricothyroidotomy equipment

Technique	Equipment
Standard	No. 11 blade scalpel
	Curved hemostat
	Trousseau dilator
	Tracheal hook
	Tracheostomy tube (preferably 6–8 mm diameter, maximum 8 mm)
	Gloves, protective gown, face shield, chlorhexidine or povidone iodine, gauze pads, lidocaine, 10 ml syringe, tape, and suture or tying material
Rapid four step	No. 20 blade scalpel, tracheal hook, cuffed tracheostomy tube, gloves, protective gown, face shield, chlorhexidine or povidone iodine, gauze pads, lidocaine, 10 ml syringe, tape, and suture or tying material
Seldinger	Commercial kit:
	Gloves, protective gown, face shield, chlorhexidine or povidone iodine, gauze pads, lidocaine, 10 ml syringe, tape, and suture or tying material

Trauma: A Comprehensive Emergency Medicine Approach, eds. Eric Legome and Lee W. Shockley. Published by Cambridge University Press. © Cambridge University Press 2011.

Procedure

There are three cricothryotomy techniques commonly utilized: standard, rapid four-step, and the Seldinger technique.

Standard technique

Cricothyrotomy is performed with the patient supine. If time permits, the area can be sterilized with chlorhexidine or iodine and infiltrated with lidocaine for the conscious patient.

The cricothyroid membrane can be identified by standing on the patient's side, stabilizing the larynx with the thumb and middle finger of the non-dominant hand, palpating the thyroid cartilage with the index finger and walking the finger inferiorly to palpate the cricothyroid membrane, which is the depression between the thyroid and cricoid cartilage. It can be estimated as one finger-breath below the laryngeal prominence ("Adam's apple"). It's important to keep the larynx immobilized with the non-dominant hand for the entire procedure.

A 2–3 cm vertical midline incision is made through the skin alone with the No. 11 blade scalpel. A vertical incision has two advantages over horizontal incision: it avoids injuring the recurrent laryngeal nerves and allows for extension of the incision if the membrane is missed. After initial skin incision, the curved hemostat is used to bluntly dissect the subcutaneous tissue down to the trachea. The cricothyroid membrane should be reidentified before proceeding. Next, a 1 cm horizontal incision through the cricothryoid membrane into the trachea is made. To prevent esophageal perforation, the scalpel should not go deeper than 1cm. To avoid injuring the cranially located vocal cords, the blade should be aimed in the caudad direction while cutting.

An audible pop or rush of air may be heard when the trachea is entered. After removing the blade from the incision, the index finger of the non-dominant hand is inserted to dilate and maintain the opening. A tracheal hook is then inserted under the thyroid cartilage and retracted upward (cephalad). Next, the curved hemostat or Trousseau dilator is inserted to open the membrane horizontally in the inferior portion of the cricothyroid membrane incision. The two legs of the dilator and the tracheal hook form a triangle, allowing room for the tracheostomy tube. The tracheostomy tube with the obturator in place is inserted into the trachea and the tracheal hook and dilator are removed. The obturator is removed from the inside of the tubing while the inner cannula is held in place and the adapter attached. The cuff of the tube is inflated with air from the 10 ml syringe. The tracheostomy tube can now be connected to a bag-valve device or mechanical ventilator and proper placement can be tested by observing symmetrical chest rise and by auscultating for breath sounds. Once proper placement is confirmed, the tube can be secured with a cloth tie around the neck or sutured in place.

A chest X-ray should be obtained to confirm proper placement of the tube. The cricothyrotomy can be used for 72 hours to manage the airway. If more time is needed, a surgical consult should be obtained to place a tracheostomy for long-term airway management.

Rapid four-step technique

Brofeldt et al. introduced their rapid four-step technique (RFST) as an alternative to the standard cricothryotomy.[4] The only equipment required is a No. 20 blade scalpel, tracheal hook, and cuffed tracheostomy tube. The physician stands at the patient's head as if performing endotracheal intubation. The cricothyroid membrane is palpated (step 1) and a horizontal stab incision is made through both skin and membrane (step 2). The larynx is stabilized by placing the tracheal hook under the cricoid cartilage in the inferior portion of the incision and retracted in a caudad direction (step 3). Of note, this differs from the standard technique where the hook is placed under the thyroid cartilage in the superior portion of the incision. The fourth and final step is placement of the tracheostomy tube into the trachea.

The RFST is reported to be three times faster than the standard technique.[5] Studies comparing the complication rates of RFST with the standard technique are conflicting, with some authors finding similar rates,[2,5] but more severe complications associated with RFST.[5] Others report significantly higher complication rates in RFST when performed on cadavers.[6] The provider must weigh the benefits of quick and simple airway access against a potentially higher complication rate when deciding between these two techniques.

The Seldinger technique

Commerical cricothyrotomy kits are available to perform the procedure using the Seldinger technique. Included in the kits are scalpel, syringe, needle with overlying catheter, guidewire, tissue dilator that fits inside the modified airway catheter, and tracheostomy tape or tie (Figure 35.1).

The cricothyroid membrane is palpated while the larynx is immobilized as described above. A small amount of water or saline is drawn into the syringe using the needle with overlying catheter. Negative pressure is applied to the syringe as the needle with catheter is inserted caudally into the cricothryoid membrane at a 45° angle. When bubbles appear, the syringe and then needle are removed, leaving the catheter in place. The guidewire is threaded through the catheter into the trachea. The catheter can now be removed by sliding it over the guidewire. Using the scalpel, a small incision is made at the entrance point of the guidewire. The tissue dilator–airway catheter unit is advanced over the guidewire through the skin incision, subcutaneous tissue, and into the trachea until the cuff and catheter abut the neck. Leaving the catheter in the trachea, the tissue dilator and guidewire unit are removed. The airway catheter is secured to the neck with tape or ties after proper placement is checked with auscultation (Figure 35.2).

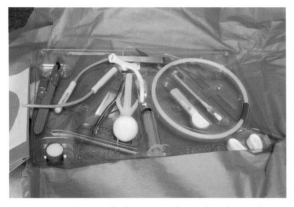

Figure 35.1 Photograph of commerical cricothyroidotomy kit.

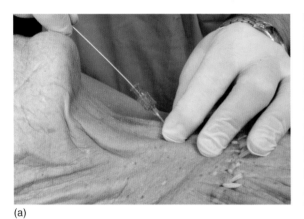

(a)

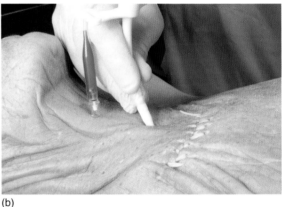

(b)

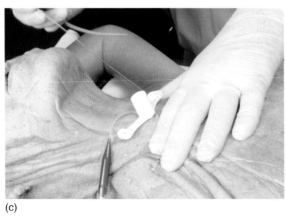

(c)

Figure 35.2 Cricothyroidotomy using Seldinger technique (cadaveric model). (a) A needle and wire is placed through the cricothyroid membrane. (b) After the hole is slightly widened with an introducer, the airway is placed. (c) The wire is removed from the tube and the balloon is inflated.

Complications

The overall complication rate of cricothyrotomies performed in the ED is estimated at 14–23%.[2,7] The major complications of cricothyrotomy are hypoxia due to prolonged time in securing the airway, malposition of the tracheostomy tube, esophageal perforation, subcutaneous emphysema, and hemorrhage. Adequate training and experience decreases cricothryotomy procedure time,[8] and subsequent risk of hypoxia. Malposition of the tracheostomy tube can be avoided by confirming placement by observing chest rise, auscultating the lungs for breath sounds, and a chest X-ray. To prevent esophageal perforation, precautions such as covering all but 1 cm of the blade can be taken when entering the trachea. Subcutaneous emphysema can be prevented by limiting the lateral incision to avoid gaps around the tracheostomy tube that can lead to subcutaneous air trapping. Excessive bleeding can be controlled with gauze and pressure. If a major artery or vein is cut, exploration and ligation may be necessary.

Tube thoracostomy

Indications

Chest tube insertion is indicated in trauma to drain blood or air from the pleural space (e.g., pneumothorax, hemothorax, or hemopneumothorax). It can be utilized emergently or non-emergently. Emergent tube thoracostomy is performed to relieve a pneumothorax that is large, recurrent or persistent, iatrogenic, under tension, in a patient on mechanical ventilation, or in a clinically unstable patient. Non-emergent indications include processes that are generally delayed complications from trauma such as empyemas or pleural effusions.

Contraindications

The only absolute contraindication to tube thoracostomy is if the lung is completely adherent to the chest wall. Relative contraindications include patients on anticoagulation therapy, patients with a bleeding diathesis, or patients with an expectation of receiving resuscitative thoracotomy. If time permits, the coagulopathy should be corrected before performing the thoracostomy.

The following equipment is used to perform a tube thoracostomy and is often included in a preassembled tray: scalpel with No. 11 blade, curved Kelly clamps, one small gauge (25) and one larger gauge (18) needle along with a 10 ml and 20 ml syringe for superficial and deep local anesthesia, 1% lidocaine, needle driver, silk or nylon size 1.0 or larger sutures, scissors, and appropriate chest tube. Sterile drapes, gown, gloves, chlorhexidine or povidone iodine, and a pleural draining system should be at hand.

Chest tube size should be chosen based on the indication. In general, a larger chest tube allows rapid evacuation of large pneumothoraces and fluid collections. A large pneumothorax in a stable patient can be evacuated with a 16–22-French (Fr) chest tube. If the patient is unstable or is receiving mechanical ventilation, a larger 24–28-Fr tube should be used. Pleural effusions can be drained with smaller bore 8- or 16-Fr catheters under ultrasound or computed tomography (CT) guidance using the Seldinger technique. Parapneumonic effusions and empyemas require 20-Fr or larger bore tubes. Hemothorax requires a large bore 32- or 40-Fr catheter to rapidly drain and tamponade the bleeding site.

Box 35.2 Thoracostomy equipment

- Scalpel with No. 11 blade
- Curved Kelly clamps
- One small gauge (25) and one larger gauge (18) needle along with a 10 ml and 20 ml syringe for superficial and deep local anesthesia
- 1% lidocaine (or bupivicaine)
- Needle driver
- Silk or nylon size 1.0 or larger sutures
- Scissors, and appropriate chest tube
- Sterile drapes, gown, gloves, chlorhexidine or povidone iodine, and a pleural draining system should be at hand

---

Box 35.3 General guidelines for chest tube size in trauma

Indication	Size
Large pneumothorax (stable patient)	16–22Fr
Large pneumothorax (unstable, ventilated)	24–28Fr
Hemothorax	32–40Fr

These chest tubes sizes are guidelines. Patient body habitus may alter the size of the tube used. For example, a 60kg teenager with a large hemothorax may not have adequate intercostal space to accommodate a 40-Fr tube.

Procedure

The incision site should be determined and marked before beginning the procedure. The most common site is the 4th or 5th intercostal space (about the level of the nipple in males) in the anterior axillary or mid-axillary line. The actual pleural insertion of the tube will occur one intercostal space above this site to prevent air entry after the chest tube is removed (Figure 35.3).

The patient should be supine with the ipsilateral arm placed over the patient's head. The area is sterilized with chlorhexidine or povidone iodine solution and draped with sterile towels. The incision site is infiltrated with 1% lidocaine using the 25-gauge needle. Next, the 18-gauge needle and 20ml syringe is used to infiltrate the subcutaneous tissue, intercostal muscles, and the periosteal surface of the rib below

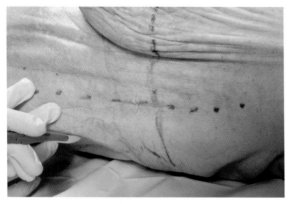

Figure 35.3 Incision site for thoracostomy tube placement (cadaver model). (Courtesy of Taku Taira, MD and the New York University School of Medicine.)

the insertion site with 10–20 ml of lidocaine. With negative pressure applied to the syringe, the needle is advanced until a flash of fluid or air enters the chamber, indicating entry into the pleural space. Lidocaine is injected to anesthetize the parietal pleura and the needle and syringe are withdrawn.

A 2–3cm skin incision is made parallel to and just above the rib to avoid injuring the neurovascular bundle. Kelly clamps are used to bluntly dissect the subcutaneous tissue in a cephalad direction towards the superior intercostal space (where the chest tube will be inserted). The intercostal muscles are dissected just above the inferior rib of this space. The Kelly clamp or index finger can be used to penetrate the parietal pleura and enter the pleural space (Figure 35.4). There should be a give when entering the pleural space and fluid or air may leak through the incision. The index finger should sweep the parietal pleura to ensure proper placement and that no adhesions between lung and pleura exist. Small adhesion may be broken up by the sweep of the finger.

The leading end of the chest tube should be clamped with the Kelly clamp and inserted through the incision site and directed cephalad through the wound track and into the pleura. The Kelly clamp is removed. General recommendations are that the chest tube is advanced cephalad and anterior if draining a pneumothorax, or inferiorly and posteriorly if draining fluid, although clinical situations (e.g., adhesions) may modify this. Proper placement is confirmed with the appearance of condensation or pleural fluid within the tube. The tube should be advanced until all holes are within the pleural space (Figure 35.5).

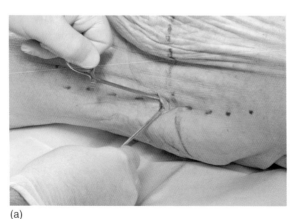

(a)

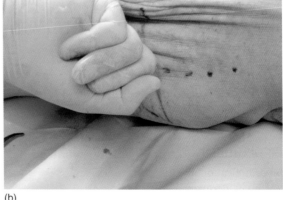

(b)

Figure 35.4 (a) Kelly clamp used to dissect and penetrate parietal pleura. (b) Index finger used to sweep the pleura.

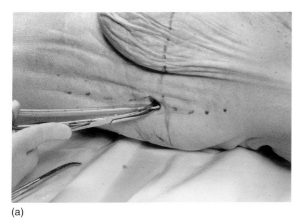
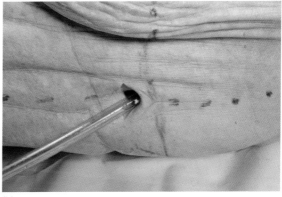

(a) (b)

Figure 35.5 (a) Chest tube inserted using clamp. (b) Photograph shows proximal hole of chest tube outside chest wall (must be inserted into pleural space).

The skin incision should be closed with mattress or interrupted sutures, with the loose ends of the sutures wrapped around and tied to the tube to anchor it. The tube should be taped to the patient's side and the site should be covered with sterile petrolatum gauze. The chest tube should be connected to a pleural drainage system, with a recommended initial setting of 20 cm of water. Bubbles will be seen in the chambers if a pneumothorax is being evacuated; fluid will collect if draining a hemothorax or pleural effusion.

A chest X-ray should be obtained to confirm placement. The gap in the radio-opaque lining of the chest tube represents the most proximal drainage hole and must be located within the pleural space to be functional.

The chest tube should be removed after the original indication has resolved. For pneumothorax, the chest tube can be removed after full re-expansion of the lung is seen on chest X-ray along with a trial of underwater seal to ensure the lung stays expanded without suction. If draining pleural fluid, the chest tube can be removed after lung expansion is seen on chest X-ray and fluid drainage is < 200ml per day. Some clinicians advocate clamping the chest tube 12–24 hours before removal to test for persistent air leak or fluid reaccumulation.[9]

Complications

The complication and adverse event rate of tube thoracostomies performed in the ED may be as high as 14–37%.[10–12] The most common complications are recurrent pneumothorax and tube malpositioning.[12]

Other complications include bleeding and hemothorax from intercostal artery laceration, lung parenchyma perforation, perforation of thoracic or intra-abdominal organs, subcutaneous placement, subcutaneous emphysema, re-expansion pulmonary edema, pneumonia, empyema, clotting, kinking or dislodgement of the chest tube, and infection. Antibiotic prophylaxis has been controversial in the setting of trauma. There may be a slight reduction in pneumonia and pneumonitis with the use of first generation cephalosporins for 24 hours, however the data is not strong.[9,13]

Intraosseus access

Indications

Intraosseus cannulation is utilized in the emergent setting when peripheral access for fluid resuscitation and medication is required and cannot be readily obtained. Although it can be used in any age group, it is primarily used in infants and children as it more typically provides faster access than central access.

The veins indirectly accessed via intraosseous cannulation drain the medullary sinus and are held open by the bony matrix. They do not collapse in hypovolemia, making them a reliable access point in the critically ill child. Intraosseous access is more difficult in older patients because of their thicker cortex and narrower bone marrow cavity.

Several studies have shown that intraosseous cannulation provides faster and more reliable access in children.[14–16] In their review of intraosseous cannulation, Buck et al. found that most providers could establish an intraosseous line within 1–2 minutes with a success rate of approximately 80%.[16] A randomized trial comparing intraosseous access and intravenous (IV) access for fluid resuscitation in 60 hypovolemic children found that within 5 minutes, intraosseous access was successful in 100% of the cases while IV access was successful in only 67% of the cases. Furthermore, the researchers reported that establishing intraosseous access was twice as fast as establishing IV access. Once established, both routes were equally as effective in rehydrating the patient.[15]

Contraindications

Intraosseous cannulation is absolutely contraindicated when there is a fracture near the insertion site as extravasation through a fracture may lead to a compartment syndrome. Relative contraindications include a previous attempt at intraosseous access at the same site, osteogenesis imperfecta, osteoporosis, and overlying burns or infection.

Equipment

Box 35.4 Equipment for intraosseous access
- Antiseptic cleanser
- 1% lidocaine with 25-gauge needle and syringe
- 5–10 ml syringe
- Intraosseous needle or system

The following equipment is used to establish intraosseous access: antiseptic cleanser, 1% lidocaine with 25-gauge needle and syringe, 5–10 ml syringe, and intraosseous needle or system. Several different intraosseous needles and systems are available. The intraosseous needles are manually placed while the newer Bone Injection Gun (BIG)® and E-Z IO® systems automatically penetrate the medulla using spring-loaded needles or drill handles (Figure 35.6). The manual needles contain a stylet to prevent occlusion of the needle with bone fragments or marrow.

Procedure

Intraosseous lines are most often placed in the anteromedial aspect of the tibia 1–2 cm distal to the tibial tuberosity. Alternative sites include the distal tibia 1–2 cm proximal to the medial maleolus, the anterior aspect of the distal femur, sternum,

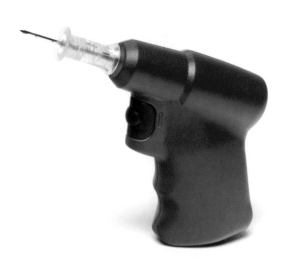

Figure 35.6 Photograph of EZ-IO® gun.

and the lateral aspect of the proximal humerus. Because of their relatively superficial location, large marrow cavity, and lack of intervening vessels and nerves, the proximal tibia and distal femur are preferred sites. The following procedure will be described with the proximal tibia as the insertion site (Figure 35.7).

The insertion site should be sterilized with povidone-iodine or chlorhexidine. If the patient is awake, lidocaine should be used to anesthetize the skin, subcutaneous tissue, and periosteum. The patient's leg can be placed on a rolled towel or sheet for stabilization. The patient's distal thigh and knee is held with the non-dominant hand while the dominant hand holds the intraosseous needle. The needle is inserted 1–2 cm distal to the tibial tuberosity on the anteromedial aspect of the tibia either perpendicular to the tibial surface or at a 60–75° angle caudad to avoid the growth plate. The needle is driven into the medullary cavity using significant force and a twisting, to-and-fro motion. A sudden decrease in resistance will be felt when the medullary cavity is reached. At this point, the stylet is removed and a 5–10 ml syringe is attached to the needle. Blood or marrow is aspirated to confirm placement in the medulla. Next, the needle is flushed with 5–10 ml of saline. Proper placement is confirmed if there is no resistance with the flush and if there are no signs of extravasation of the

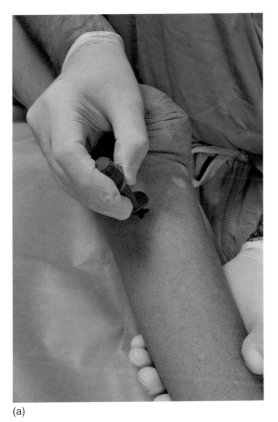

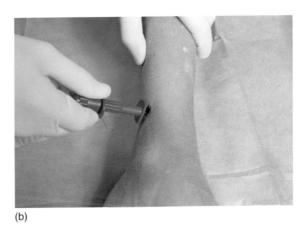

(a)

(b)

Figures 35.7 Manual intraosseous insertion (cadaveric model): (a) anteromedial tibia; (b) distal tibia.

saline into the leg. The needle should be flushed with saline, then connected to IV tubing and secured with tape and gauze dressing.

Any fluid required for resuscitation can be delivered safely through the intraosseous line. Various medications, including catecholamines, antibiotics, and blood products can also be infused (Table 35.1). Rapid volume repletion requires an infusion pump or pressure bag; if these are not available, manual push of the syringe may be necessary. The intraosseous line can also be used to draw various labs, including blood cultures, chemistries, blood gases, hematocrit, and type and screen. Complete blood count should not be drawn through the intraosseous line as the white cell count will be abnormal and spurious.

Table 35.1 shows common medications and fluids in trauma deliverable through an intraosseous line.[17] The intraosseous line should be replaced with an IV line as soon as possible. Long-term placement has been associated with higher risk of complications.[18]

Complications

A meta-analysis of 30 major studies of intraosseous infusion revealed a <1% rate of complications in over 4200 cases.[18] The most common complications include subcutaneous and subperiosteal infiltration of fluid, which carry the risk of causing compartment syndrome or skin necrosis. Although rare, serious complications include tibial fracture, growth plate injury, fat and marrow embolization, cellulitis, and osteomyelitis. Rosetti et al. found that only 27 (0.6%) of over 4000 intraosseous infusions were complicated by osteomyelitis, and these cases usually occurred in bacteremic patients or in patients whose intraosseous lines were left in place for prolonged periods of time.[18] The concern over the long-term effects of intraosseous placement on bone growth was addressed by Claudet et al., whose 29-month follow-up radiologic study revealed no significant difference in tibial growth in patients who had an intraosseous line.[19] Microscopic fat and marrow emboli were found to occur after all

605

Table 35.1 Medications and fluids that can be given through an intraosseous line

Medications and fluids

- Antibiotics
- Depolarizing and non-depolarizing paralytics
- Atropine
- Calcium gluconate and chloride
- Intravenous contrast media
- Dexamethasone
- Diazepam, lorazepam, midazolam
- Dopamine and dobutamine
- Epinephrine
- Norepinephrine
- Lidocaine
- Morphine, fentanyl, hydromorphone
- Naloxone
- Phenobarbital and phenytoin
- Blood products
- Intravenous resuscitation fluids (normal saline and Ringer's lactate)

intraosseous cannulations in one study, however they had no clinical significance.[20]

Genitourinary procedures in trauma patients

Indications

Injuries to the genitourinary (GU) system (Table 35.2[21]) are often secondary to other more life-threatening injuries to the chest, abdomen, and central nervous system; injuries such as renal vein lacerations or a fractured kidney can lead to rapid instability or mortality in the trauma patient.[22] Approximately 10% of multitrauma patients have GU involvement.[23]

Because of its less common occurrence and subtle presentation, GU injuries may be overlooked in the initial evaluation of the trauma victim. However, after the primary survey for life-threatening injuries, Foley catheter placement or evaluation of the spontaneously voided urine may disclose the signs of urinary tract injury.

The diagnostic evaluation of the GU tract is performed in a retrograde fashion. Genitourinary

Table 35.2 Anatomical concepts in genitourinary (GU) procedures[21]

- The main difference in the genitourinary tract anatomy of male and female patients is at the level of the lower tract
- The female urethra is shorter (4cm) than the male (20cm)
- The male urethra passes through the body of the prostate, the urogenital diaphragm and the penis
- The urogenital diaphragm anatomically divides the urethra into two portions: the anterior urethra, below the inferior aspect of the urogenital diaphragm, and the posterior urethra above the inferior aspect of the urogenital diaphragm
- The kidneys lie in the retroperitoneal space. They are surrounded by perinephric fat between the anterior and posterior layers of the renal fascia. The kidney is encapsulated by an adherent fibrous tissue known as the renal capsule. The renal capsule is adherent to the kidney; it may act to contain blood or urine from renal injuries
- The perinephric space lies between the anterior renal fascia (Gerota's) and the posterior renal fascia. It is closed superiorly, medially, and laterally but may open into the iliac fossa inferiorly, communicating with the anterior and posterior paranephric spaces. The normal perinephric space contains the kidney and fat but blood from renal trauma may collect in this space
- The ureter passes inferiorly and medially to connect the kidney with the bladder. Each ureter is approximately 30cm long with a lumen that is 2–4 mm in diameter
- The adult testis is approximately 3–5cm in length and 2–3cm in transverse diameter and depth. At the upper pole of the testes is the appendix of the testis which is a 3–5mm appendage to the testis
- The female urethra lies at the superior aspect of the vagina. The urethral meatus is occasionally not obvious. The urethral meatus is an anteroposterior slit with rather prominent margins that is situated directly superior to the opening of the vagina and approximately 2.5cm inferior to the glans clitoris. It is the first of three orifices encountered when examining any female genitalia cephalad to caudad in the lithotomy position

trauma is divided into lower tract injuries (i.e., bladder or urethral injury), upper tract injuries (i.e., renal or ureteral injury), and external genitalia injuries (i.e., penile, scrotal, and testicular injury). Injuries are also categorized based on blunt or penetrating mechanisms of injury. Generally, blood at the urethral meatus or gross hematuria will identify significant lower urinary tract injuries.[22] In the secondary exam, other noteworthy findings to look for include hematoma on the shaft of the penis, scrotum, or perineum, or blood at the vaginal introitus. A rectal exam may assist in determining bowel or bladder injuries, and may suggest a pelvic fracture. A high-riding prostate, which suggests pelvic fracture, is due to disruption of the puboprostatic ligaments and the prostatomembranous urethra causing retropubic venous bleeding. The resulting pelvic hematoma can displace the prostate superiorly, resulting in a boggy, ill-defined mass on rectal examination.[22] The actual incidence of this is unknown, but likely rare.

Urethral catherization

Indications

In the major trauma patient, indications for urethral catheterization are to relieve acute urinary retention due to neurologic injury or pain, assist the patient who has inability or significant difficulty in voiding due to painful injuries or medical treatments, and allow for rapid evaluation of the urine and provide ongoing monitoring of urine output. It may also be used for the urologic study of the lower urinary tract.[24]

While relatively simple to perform, it is not without morbidity, especially patient pain and discomfort and urinary tract infections. Urethral catheterization is performed differently in males, females, and children, and factors such as age, anatomy, and prior surgeries may make catheterization more difficult.

Contraindications

Initial placement of a Foley catheter via the penile urethra is generally contraindicated in patients with blood at the urethral meatus, boggy or "high-riding" prostate, or a perineal hematoma. This may worsen a possible urethral injury. Blood is seen in 37–93% of cases, and the amount of blood at the meatus does not appear to correlate with the severity of the injury.[25] A palpably distended bladder or inability to void, perineal bruising, and perineal ecchymosis are all suggestive of urethral disruption.[25] Rectal exam may reveal an elevated or displaced prostate gland in 34% of cases, but may not even be palpated because of

hematoma that surrounds the prostate in the setting of pelvic fracture.[26]

In addition, if difficulty is encountered that is felt potentially due to a urethral injury (not just prostatic hypertrophy) the placement should be delayed pending a urethrogram.

Box 35.5 Equipment for urethral catheterization (Foley catheterization)

- Foley catheter
- Lubricant (Surgilube®) or lidocaine gel (preferred)
- 10 cc syringe
- Collection (drainage) bag
- Tubing
- Sterile drapes, sterile gloves, sterile cleansing solution (povidone–iodine), sterile gauze and cotton balls, sterile specimen cup
- Forceps
- Benzoin
- Tape

Most catheterization kits have all of the standard equipment needed to perform urethral catheterization, although some leave out the Foley catheter and sterile gloves, which are obtained separately. In the average adult, an 18-Fr Foley is adequate, but one may need a smaller or larger catheter based on the patient's size, age, and whether they have complicating factors. A smaller catheter may be selected in patients with strictures, masses, or phimosis. A larger catheter may be selected in patients with benign prostatic hypertrophy. Other types of catheters include Coudé catheters to overcome prostatic hypertrophy or red-rubber catheters used for one time straight catheterization.

Male catheterization

In the male patient, the urethra is more easily evident. Although the urethra may be more easily identifiable, insertion of the catheter may be more difficult. The normal male urethra is much longer than the female urethra. It is approximately 20 cm long from the external urethral meatus to the bladder neck. The posterior prostatic urethra is approximately 3.5 cm long, and the contiguous external sphincter or urogenital diaphragm that encompasses the membranous urethra is 4 cm from the bladder neck.[24] In males, the catheter should be fully inserted to the balloon-inflating side-arm channel before it is safe to inflate the balloon. Urine may appear

607

in the Foley catheter prior to fully entering the bladder. Premature inflation of the catheter balloon prior to full insertion may result in urethral injury.

After sterile preparation and draping of a sterile field, the penis should be held by the clinician's non-dominant hand. The penis should be held upright during urethral catheterization in order to provide the most direct entry into the bladder.[24] If the patient is uncircmcumcised, the foreskin should be retracted while the penis is held upright, and the dominant hand should be used to sterilize the glans penis with povidone–iodine. An appropriate size catheter is then used after the tip of the catheter has been liberally coated with Surgilube®. In addition, if time permits, the distal part of the urethra should be slowly injected with 5–10cc of lidocaine gel (viscous lidocaine) in order to distend the urethra and to alleviate the discomfort that accompanies the procedure. This can be done through a syringe filled with gel or a commercially available Uro-Jet®. After injecting the gel, the meatus should be gently pinched and held for approximately 1.0–1.5 minutes to allow the gel to take effect.

In general, the catheter should pass relatively easily in most male patients. Once the catheter is advanced almost the length of the catheter to the hub for the balloon and urine flow is seen, the balloon should be slowly inflated with 10ml of water. If resistance or patient discomfort occurs during balloon inflation, the balloon should be deflated and catheter position should be re-evaluated.[24] Pain or resistance signifies that the catheter may still be positioned within the urethra.

Following successful catheter passage and balloon inflation, the catheter should be slowly withdrawn until the balloon abutting the bladder neck prevents further withdrawal.[24] The catheter is then connected to a sterile drainage bag.

Complications

Certain anatomical abnormalities may occur which may make catheterization in the male difficult. Some of these include urethral stricture, meatal stenosis, edema of the foreskin, phimosis, and prostatic enlargement.

Meatal stenosis: The urethral meatus may be narrowed either as a congenital condition or from scarring from infection or prior instrumentation. The stenosis may prevent catheterization of a normal-sized catheter, but may allow passage of a smaller catheter.

Urethral stricture: Inability to pass the catheter through the anterior or bulbous urethra is most often the result of urethral stricture disease; however, in the setting of acute trauma, it may also be from a partial or full urethral tear. If such resistance is met during catheterization, the catheter should never be forced. Forcing a catheter may cause perforation of the urethra and false passages, bleeding, and ultimately increased scarring.[24] Inability to negotiate a urethral stricture with a simple straight Foley catheter or Coudé catheter should lead to a urologic consultation for potential dilation.[24]

Edema of the foreskin: Patients with penile trauma, paraphimosis, anasarca, or lymphatic obstruction from disease processes may have marked edema of the foreskin. Such edema may make it difficult to visualize the urethral meatus and glans. The urethral meatus may be identified with gentle manipulation of the foreskin. Utilizing cold packs and direct pressure may also assist in reducing some of the swelling.

Prostate enlargement: Prostatic enlargement is frequently encountered during catheterization of older male patients. If urethral catheterization is unsuccessful or contraindicated, a larger catheter may be used. Even though this may seem counterintuitive, the larger catheter is stiffer and can overcome the obstruction, while a smaller one does not have the needed rigidity. Other options are a firm, angulated Coudé catheter or a suprapubic catheter.[27]

Phimosis: Phimosis exists when retraction of the foreskin proximally over the glans penis cannot occur due to recurrent inflammation or trauma which causes scarring.[24] In some instances, the phimotic opening becomes so small that the urethral meatus cannot be accessed. If the patient requires urgent catheterization the physician may need to perform a dorsal slit of the foreskin to expose the glans and urethral meatus or to dilate the phimotic opening sufficiently to identify the urethral meatus and catheterize the patient.[24]

Use of antibiotics in catheterization

The use of antibiotics before simple catheterization has not shown to be efficacious in preventing infection.[28,29] Furthermore, the most recent endocarditis guidelines from the American Heart Association do not recommend prophylactic antibiotics for patients with valvular heart disease or structural abnormalities undergoing simple catheterization.[30]

Table 35.3 Pediatric catheter size and type

Age	Catheter size and type
Infant	5–8 Fr feeding tube
1–3 years	8 Fr feeding tube
4–6 years	10 Fr feeding tube
7–12 years	10–12 Fr red-rubber catheter
>12 years	14 Fr red-rubber catheter

Female catheterization

In the supine position, the opening of the urethra is the most superior orifice and directly above the vaginal introitus, and below the glans clitoris. The clinician's non-dominant hand is used to separate the labia and expose the urethral meatus. Following sterile preparation and draping, the lubricated catheter is advanced. Once urine is freely flowing into the Foley catheter, and the resistance of the bladder wall is felt with advancement of the catheter, the balloon on the catheter can be safely inflated.

In some patients such as children, post-menopausal women, and patients who have had prior surgery the urethral meatus may not be obvious. In such patients, palpation may be necessary to aid in identification of the meatus. Occasionally, the urethral meatus recedes superiorly into the vagina and is not immediately visible. Anticipation of such cases will allow the examiner to gently advance an index finger into the vagina in the superior midline. The urethral meatus can usually be palpated and often visualized as a soft mound surrounded by a firmer ring of supporting periurethral tissue. Rarely, the meatus will have receded so far superiorly that it cannot be visualized at all, and catheterization must be carried out by palpation alone. From the meatus (if the patient assumes a supine position), the urethra proceeds straight back to slightly downward as it advances into the bladder just behind the symphysis pubis.[24]

Urethral catheterization in the pediatric population

The general procedure of urethral catheterization in the pediatric population is similar in terms of anatomy and procedure. Many considerations need to be taken into account for the pediatric population. Some of these include pain and anxiety. Patients may require sedation and restraint for the procedure, the anatomy may be more difficult to ascertain.

Equipment

Same as adult catheterization, except for actual catheter (Table 35.3).

Percutaneous suprapubic cystostomy

Percutaneous suprapubic cystostomy is utilized to access the bladder and allow for drainage when the urethra is inaccessible secondary to trauma or other causes such as stricture which prevents catheterization through the urethra.

Indications

In general, any patient who would require a urethral catheter but a catheter cannot be utilized through the urethra is a candidate for a suprapubic cystostomy tube. In the trauma patient, the most likely indication would be pelvic trauma with urethral disruption. Because trauma patients often need surgical intervention because of associated injuries, a large suprapubic catheter can be placed intraoperatively rather than at the bedside. If the patient does not require surgery, a percutaneously placed Foley catheter can be placed emergently and definitive urologic surgery can be done electively after the patient's condition has stabilized.[24]

Contraindications (including relative)

1. Patients without a definable bladder.
2. Patients in whom the bladder volume is so small that risk of penetration through and through the bladder or bowel exists.
3. Individuals who have a history of previous lower abdominal surgery, intraperitoneal surgery, or irradiation with extensive adhesions or adherence of the bowel to the anterior bladder wall.
4. Patients with clinically important bleeding diatheses or anticoagulation.

Box 35.6 Percutaneous suprapubic cystostomy equipment

- A kit with a guidewire Seldinger technique to gain bladder access and allow suprapubic access.
- An 8-Fr or 12-Fr trocar type cystostomy tube.
- Several common kits include the Cook Peel-Away® sheath unit and the Cystocath®.

Procedure

The following comments describe the placement of the Cook Peel-Away® sheath, a commonly used kit; however, other kits or hospital kits are fully appropriate. It would be helpful to use bedside ED ultrasound prior to the procedure to assure a full bladder and for improved localization.

Clinicians familiar with the Seldinger technique of vascular access should be able to readily place a suprapubic catheter using most of the commercially available kits. If available, ultrasound confirmation of a full bladder should be done prior to attempting to access the bladder.

Key points

- In awake patients, anesthetize the skin, the subcutaneous tissue and rectus abdominis muscle fascia with 1% lidocaine.
- Aim the introducer needle at a 10–20° angle toward the pelvis.
- Aspirate urine through the introducer needle and syringe to confirm bladder puncture.
- The Cook Peel-Away® sheath and indwelling fascial dilator are then passed together over the wire into the bladder. The guidewire and dilator are removed, leaving only the Peel-Away® sheath inside the bladder.
- A Foley balloon catheter is then passed through the indwelling intravesical sheath into the bladder. The balloon is inflated. The Peel-Away® sheath is withdrawn from the bladder and anterior abdominal wall and peeled away from the catheter leaving only the indwelling suprapubic Foley catheter.

Complications

Some of the complications include bowel perforation, extravasation into the intraperitoneal or extraperitoneal space, infection, bleeding, or displacement of the tube, or placement other than in the bladder.[24] Other complications include hernia through the incision site, kinking or blockage of the tube, and iatrogenic misplacement of the guidewire during the procedure.[24,31,32]

Genitourinary radiologic procedures in the trauma patient

In GU trauma, the lower urinary tract is evaluated before the upper urinary tract.[24] The exception is the blunt abdominal trauma patient with hematuria (gross or microscopic) and signs of shock, indicating a renal injury and need for immediate diagnosis and treatment.[33]

Retrograde urethrogram and cystogram (or CT cystogram) are the procedures of choice to diagnose and evaluate injury to the lower urinary tract, and are performed in that order.

Retrograde urethrogram

Indications

A retrograde urethrogram is indicated whenever there is uncertainty about the integrity of the urethra, such as when blood is found at the urethral meatus.

Contraindications

There are no absolute contraindications to a retrograde urethrogram.

A relative contraindication would be an unstable patient who requires other immediate first-aid.

Box 35.7 Equipment for retrograde urethrogram

- Foley catheter
- 60 ml Toomey syringe or Christmas tree syringe
- Water-soluble contrast medium diluted to 10% strength to prevent inflammation caused by extravasation. (This is controversial, some authors recommend half-strength or full-strength contrast.)

Contrast agents currently recommended include Renografin® or Hypaque®, diluted to a 1:10 ratio with normal saline.[24]

Procedure

A retrograde urethrogram is performed using 30ml of a solution of contrast medium which is administered through a Foley catheter.[34] The catheter is positioned in the very distal urethra and the balloon is inflated with 2ml of saline to hold it in place.[34] Another option is to use the Christmas tree syringe alone; inserting the tip into urethral meatus and injecting contrast. The contrast is then slowly injected into the urethra, taking precaution not to force the contrast material in, which will lead to filling of the venous plexus system and may obscure the study.

The study should optimally be conducted using fluoroscopy, however, as this is often not immediately available, it can be performed with a KUB taken

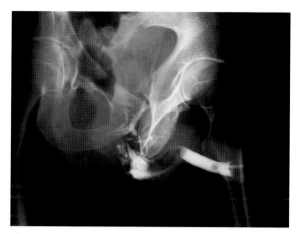

Figure 35.8 Retrograde urethrogarm with urethral tear. (Courtesy of David T. Schwartz, MD.)

during injection of the last 10 cc of contrast material. An oblique radiograph is obtained with the shaft of the penis perpendicular to the torso in order to visualize the full length of the urethra, and the nature of the injury will improve visualization, but may be difficult to perform with significant pelvic trauma.[34] Figure 35.8 shows a retrograde urethrogram with a urethral tear. This procedure is not performed in women; their shorter urethra are not prone to the same sheering forces and traumatic injuries.

A retrograde urethrogram will display a flame-like pattern of contrast outside of the urethra as displayed in the figure above if a urethral tear is present. Contrast material may be present in the bladder if the tear is partial, whereas a complete tear will reveal no contrast material in the bladder.[24]

One needs to be certain that the "extravasation" one is seeing is not filling of the venous plexus at the distal urethra. Repeating the KUB after the patient voids will show resolution of this finding in a non-injured urethra, whereas the finding will persist in a urethral tear.

Retrograde or CT cystogram

Indications

A retrograde cystogram is performed to rule out a bladder rupture. The indications are generally the same as for a retrograde urethrogram, however, there should be a mechanism of pelvic trauma, not just injury to the distal urethra.

Contraindications

There are no absolute contraindications to a retrograde urethrogram.

A relative contraindication would be an unstable patient who requires other immediate procedures first.

Procedure

A retrograde cystogram is performed similar to a retrograde urethrogram, except that for a cystogram the bladder should be distended by about 400 ml of contrast.[35] The central piston is removed from a 60 ml catheter tip syringe and the catheter tip is inserted into the Foley catheter. The syringe is held above bladder level and contrast material is poured into the open end of the syringe and the bladder is allowed to fill by gravity. In an adult or a child aged over 11 years, 400 cc of contrast needs to be instilled to completely fill the bladder. In a child under 11 years of age, the formula for determining the amount of contrast needed is (age+2)×30. Alternatively, one can fill the bladder with 100cc of contrast material and obtain a KUB looking for gross extravasation. If this is not observed, the remaining 300 cc of contrast needs to be instilled and the KUB retaken. If the patient has a bladder contraction before the full amount of contrast is instilled, one should instill an additional 50 cc of contrast and obtain the KUB. Volumes <400 cc in an adult, and less than the appropriate calculated amount in children under 11 years of age, can result in false-negative studies.[36]

Following the instillation of contrast material, a scout film, a filled film, and a postvoid film are performed.[35] With a CT cystogram, the Foley catheter is clamped while the CT abdomen/pelvis is performed with IV contrast. As the contrast-enhanced urine fills and distends the bladder, CT images are obtained.

A cystogram may reveal either an intraperitoneal tear or an extraperitoneal tear. An intraperitoneal tear is demonstrated when contrast extravasates outside the bladder and into the interperitoneal space. This will show on the film as contrast material accumulating either around the loops of bowel or in the dependent parts of the peritoneal cavity.[35] Figure 35.9 shows an intraperitoneal bladder tear. On the cystogram, extraperitoneal tears will show contrast leaking around the base of the bladder or in the prevesical space (Figure 35.10).[35] Figure 35.11 shows an extraperitoneal bladder rupture.

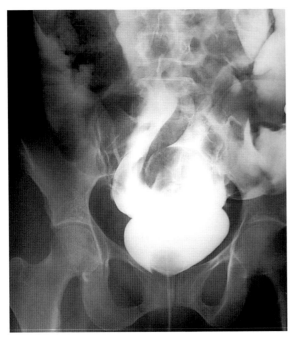

Figure 35.9 Intraperitoneal bladder tear. (Courtesy of David T. Schwartz, MD.)

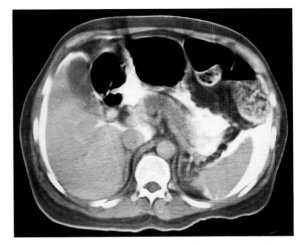

Figure 35.10 Computed tomography (CT) of intraperitoneal bladder rupture. The CT scan shows extravasated contrast throughout abdomen. (Courtesy of David T. Schwartz, MD.)

Complications

Complications from retrograde urethrogram and cystogram are rare. The rate of significant adverse reaction to contrast material is much lower than the estimated 1 in 1000 to 1 in 10000 cases from IV injection of contrast medium.[24]

Ultrasound in GU trauma

Indications

The main purpose of utilizing ultrasound in the trauma patient is to assess for traumatic hemoperitoneum. The focused abdominal sonography in trauma (FAST) study is insensitive for most renal injuries as they are retroperitoneal and the study does not look specifically for renal injury. Intraperitoneal bladder rupture leaves free fluid in the abdomen that may be indistinguishable from hemoperitoneum.

Testicular injuries are most often caused by a fall or kick and often occur in the setting of playing a sport.[22] Some of the more common injuries that result from direct trauma to the testes include testis rupture, tunica albuginea breach, testicular hematoma, testis avulsion, epididymis injuries, and hematocele.[37] Other injuries that can result are lacerations to the scrotum or other penetrating injuries. Common symptoms include severe pain, dizziness, nausea, vomiting, and urinary retention.[22] Examination may reveal tenderness, swelling, and hematoma. Ultrasound can be utilized as a bedside modality in order to diagnose some of these conditions in the ED. Testicular color Doppler ultrasonographic examination is the diagnostic procedure of choice to evaluate the testis.[22] The diagnosis of testicular rupture, which is based on an ultrasound finding of discontinuity of the echogenic tunica albuginea, can be important because early surgery results in salvage of the testis in 80–90% of rupture cases.[37]

Contraindications

There are no absolute contraindications; relative contraindications are the need for emergent life-saving procedures that take precedence.

Box 35.8 Equipment for testicular ultrasound

- A broadband linear ultrasound transducer capable of high-resolution imaging (up to 10 MHz) that can perform power and spectral Doppler ultrasonography.

A broadband linear ultrasound transducer capable of high-resolution imaging (up to 10MHz) that can perform power and spectral Doppler ultrasonography is needed.[38] Color Doppler is a

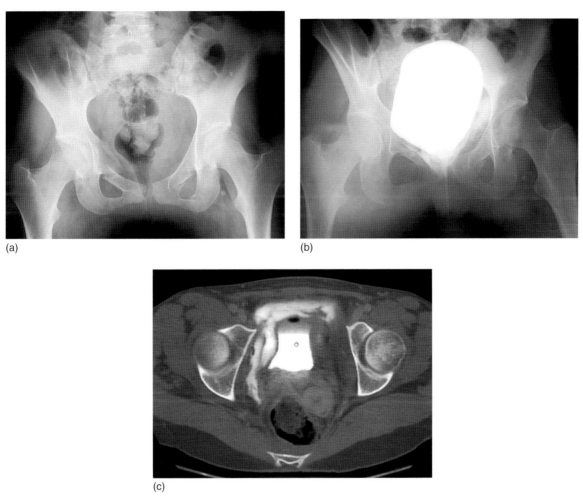

(a)

(b)

(c)

Figure 35.11 Extraperitoneal bladder rupture: (a) pelvic fractures (type IC2); with (b) cystogram; and (c) CT scan showing an extraperitoneal bladder rupture. This was a young woman who was a passenger in a motor vehicle collision. She was hemodynamically stable but had gross hematuria. No other injuries were found. (Courtesy of David T. Schwartz, MD.)

color-based display of blood flow in vessels of the scrotal contents and provides one color for flow towards the transducer and another for flow away from the transducer.[38] Power Doppler is not sensitive to direction, but possesses more likelihood that blood flow is registered.[38] The ability to measure the power of the Doppler signal rather than the Doppler frequency shift has been shown to enhance its sensitivity.[39]

Procedures

Ultrasound

Ultrasound is performed with a 5.0- or 7.5-MHz transducer.[34] An ultrasound examination positive for injury reveals loss of the normal homogeneous testicular pattern.[22] Typically, the unaffected hemiscrotum is scanned first to familiarize the patient with the process and decrease anxiety regarding discomfort. The scrotum should be scanned in at least two planes (short and long axes).[38] Using the highest resolution transducer, the scan is begun in a longitudinal axis to the testicle with the direction indicator toward the head, and is then repeated with the probe turned 90° toward the patient's right to obtain a short axis view.[38]

Power and spectral Doppler are utilized to assess blood flow in the patient with an acute scrotum secondary to trauma, and specifically helps to identify decreased or absent flow in testicular torsion, hemorrhage, hematoma, and rupture.[38] While power

613

Table 35.4 Testicular ultrasound patterns

Scrotal hematoma	A scrotal hematoma would appear as an echogenic collection between the tunica dartos and tunica vaginalis, or in the scrotal septum, and as time passes the hematoma would appear more sonolucent[34]
Hematocele	A hematocele is a complex collection seen between the leaves of the tunica vaginalis that can appear similar to testicular rupture[34]
Testicular rupture	Testicular rupture occurs when the tunica albuginea is disrupted with extrusion of the testicular parenchyma into the scrotal sac.[34] On ultrasound, the margins of the testis are poorly defined and the echogenicity of the testis is heterogeneous[34]
Hydrocele	A hydrocele is a serous collection between the layers of the tunica vaginalis which may also represent hematoma that has liquefied[34]
Testicular contusion	Testicular contusion is represented on ultrasound as a focal region of heterogeneity within the background uniform homogenous pattern of the testicular parenchyma.[34] Ultrasound appearance would show an echolucent fluid collection around the testis[34]
Testicular torsion	Testicular torsion is diagnosed when blood flow in the symptomatic testis is absent or markedly reduced compared with the normal side. The optimal Doppler settings should thus be set using the normal testis as a control[46]

Doppler allows for detection of blood flow within the testicle, the spectral or pulsed wave Doppler allows identification of the type of flow (venous or arterial).[38]

A simpler and easier test to assess for testicular perfusion than Doppler ultrasound is use of a Doppler stethoscope. Although this modality has not been well-studied with the advent of the Doppler ultrasound, its ease of use may be an adjunct to assessing blood flow to the testicle. Doppler stethoscope should never be utilized as the sole method in determining testicular perfusion as it is operator-dependent, and false negatives may occur secondary to hyperemia from inflammation.[40–45]

The stethoscope may be used as an adjunct for rapid assessment of blood flow when performing such procedures such as manual detorsion of the testicle, and also can be used in conjunction with the ultrasound to assess flow.[24]

The specific technique for testicular ultrasound is as follows: First the area of maximum testicular swelling is found and an aqueous transmission gel (Surgilube®) is placed over the scrotum. The testicle is held in one hand and the Doppler probe in the other and any overlying skin is displaced as much as possible. The Doppler probe is placed in the center of the testicle and pointing slightly caudally so that pulsations in the cord are not detected. The pulsation in the affected testicle is compared with the unaffected side. Decreased or absent flow to the affected testicle suggests torsion.[24] The funicular compression test should be performed to confirm that flow signals are related to perfusion to the testicle. If the increased signal lessens on compression of the patient's spermatic cord, then the signal is most probably coming from the patient's testicle and not from inflamed scrotal tissues. If there is no change in the signal on adequate cord compression, the increased flow may be originating in inflamed scrotal tissue, and torsion or testicular avulsion should be suspected (Table 35.4[34,46]).[24]

Complications

The complications are few and mainly related to pain and discomfort.

Spermatic cord anesthesia

Indications

During the assessment and treatment of patients with traumatic injuries to the scrotum and testicles, the examination and procedures could be uncomfortable and extremely painful. Local anesthesia of the spermatic cord can be performed to alleviate the pain from trauma and procedures such as ultrasound of the scrotum. Local anesthesia using plain lidocaine can be performed by injecting at the external inguinal ring.[24,47]

Contraindications

Absolute contraindications are severe allergy to anesthetic. Relative contraindications are the need for emergent life-saving procedures that take precedence.

Box 35.9 Equipment for spermatic cord anesthesia

- 10cc syringe
- 18-gauge needle or smaller
- Gauze
- Sterile gloves
- Povidone–iodine
- Sterile drapes

Procedure

First the overlying skin is sterilely prepped. The spermatic cord is grasped between the thumb and index finger. If the cord is swollen or difficult to grasp, the cord may be identified at the pubic tubercle. One percent plain lidocaine is directly injected into the cord (up to 10 cc) using a syringe and needle.[24]

Box 35.10 Procedures and skills in GU trauma – essential information

- Although GU trauma is often secondary to other more life-threatening injuries, a high suspicion and a careful examination are needed in order not to miss an injury.
- The presence of blood at the urethral meatus generally signifies a lower tract injury.
- Diagnostic evaluation of the GU tract is performed in a retrograde fashion. Evaluation of urethral injury precedes bladder injury which precedes ureteral or renal injury.
- Procedures such as urinary catheterization are important in the trauma patient, but numerous factors can make this straightforward procedure complicated. Ultrasound (FAST) is a bedside procedure that can easily be performed rapidly, but is relatively insensitive for GU injuries.
- Ultrasound can be rapidly diagnostic in the patient with scrotal trauma for injuries such as testicular rupture, hematoma, and torsion, but it is operator-dependent and absence of injury on examination does not necessarily rule-out injury. With high clinical suspicion, operative exploration may need to be undertaken.

References

1. McGill J, Clinton JE, Ruiz E. Cricothyrotomy in the emergency department. *Ann Emerg Med* 1982; **11**(7):361–4.

2. Bair AE, Panacek EA, Wisner DH, Bales R, Sakles JC. Cricothyrotomy: a 5-year experience at one institution. *J Emerg Med* 2003;**24**(2):151–6.

3. Chang RS, Hamilton RJ, Carter WA. Declining rate of cricothyrotomy in trauma patients with an emergency medicine residency: implications for skills training. *Acad Emerg Med* 1998;**5**(3):247–51.

4. Brofeldt BT, Panacek EA, Richards JR. An easy cricothyrotomy approach: the rapid four-step technique. *Acad Emerg Med* 1996;**3**(11):1060–3.

5. Holmes JF, Panacek EA, Sakles JC, Brofeldt BT. Comparison of two cricothyrotomy techniques: standard method versus rapid four-step technique. *Ann Emerg Med* 1998;**32**(4):442–6.

6. Davis DP, Bramwell KJ, Vilke GM, et al. Cricothyrotomy technique: standard versus the rapid four-step technique. *J Emerg Med* 1999;**17**(1):17–21.

7. Erlandson MJ, Clinton JE, Ruiz E, Cohen J. Cricothyrotomy in the emergency department revisited. *J Emerg Med* 1989;**7**(2):115–18.

8. Mutzbauer TS, Munz R, Helm M, Lampl LA, Herrmann M. Emergency cricothyrotomy–puncture or anatomical preparation? Peculiarities of two methods for emergency airway access demonstrated in a cadaver model. *Anaesthesist* 2003;**52**(4):304–10.

9. Miller KS, Sahn SA. Chest tubes. Indications, technique, management and complications. *Chest* 1987;**91**(2):258–64.

10. Helling TS, Gyles NR, 3rd, Eisenstein CL, Soracco CA. Complications following blunt and penetrating injuries in 216 victims of chest trauma requiring tube thoracostomy. *J Trauma* 1989;**29**(10):1367–70.

11. Chan L, Reilly KM, Henderson C, Kahn F, Salluzzo RF. Complication rates of tube thoracostomy. *Am J Emerg Med* 1997;**15**(4):368–70.

12. Sethuraman KN, Duong D, Mehta S, et al. Complications of tube thoracostomy placement in the emergency department. *J Emerg Med*, 2008 (Epub. ahead of print).

13. Maxwell RA, Campbell DJ, Fabian TC, et al. Use of presumptive antibiotics following tube thoracostomy for traumatic hemopneumothorax in the prevention of empyema and pneumonia–a multi-center trial. *J Trauma* 2004;**57**(4):742–8; discussion 8–9.

14. Fuchs S, LaCovey D, Paris P. A prehospital model of intraosseous infusion. *Ann Emerg Med* 1991; **20**(4):371–4.

15. Banerjee S, Singhi SC, Singh S, Singh M. The intraosseous route is a suitable alternative to intravenous route for fluid resuscitation in severely dehydrated children. *Indian Pediatr* 1994; **31**(12):1511–20.

16. Buck ML, Wiggins BS, Sesler JM. Intraosseous drug administration in children and adults during cardiopulmonary resuscitation. *Ann Pharmacother* 2007;**41**(10):1679–86.

17. Hoffman ME, Ma OJ. Intraosseous Infusion. In Reichman EF, Simon RR (eds), *Emergency Medicine Procedures*. New York: McGraw-Hill, 2004: pp. 383–90.

18. Rosetti VA, Thompson BM, Miller J, Mateer JR, Aprahamian C. Intraosseous infusion: an alternative route of pediatric intravascular access. *Ann Emerg Med* 1985;**14**(9):885–8.

19. Claudet I, Baunin C, Laporte-Turpin E, et al. Long-term effects on tibial growth after intraosseous infusion: a prospective, radiographic analysis. *Pediatr Emerg Care* 2003;**19**(6):397–401.

20. Orlowski JP, Julius CJ, Petras RE, Porembka DT, Gallagher JM. The safety of intraosseous infusions: risks of fat and bone marrow emboli to the lungs. *Ann Emerg Med* 1989;**18**(10):1062–7.

21. Cowan N. The genitourinary tract; techniques and anatomy. In Adam, A, Dixon AK (eds), *Grainger and Allison's Diagnostic Radiology*, 5th edn. Philadelphia, PA: Churchill Livingstone, 2008: pp. 813–32.

22. Schneider R. Genitourinary system. In Marx JA (ed.), *Rosen's Emergency Medicine: Concepts and Clinical Practice*. Philadelphia, PA: Mosby/Elsevier, 2006: pp. 524–36.

23. McAninch, J. Injuries to the genitourinary tract. In Tanagho EA, McAninch JW (eds), *Smith's General Urology*, 15th edn. New York: McGraw-Hill Co., 1999: pp. 330–49.

24. Schneider RE. Urologic procedures. In Roberts JR, Hedges JR (eds), *Clinical Procedures in Emergency Medicine*, 4th edn. Philadelphia, PA: WB Saunders, 2004: pp. 1098–100.

25. Colapinto V, McCallum RW. Injury to the male posterior urethra in fractured pelvis: a new classification. *J Urol* 1977;**118**(4):575–80.

26. Rosenstein DI, Alsikafi NF. Diagnosis and classification of urethral injuries. *Urol Clin North Am* 2006;**33**(1):73–85, vi–vii.

27. Selius BA, Subedi R. Urinary retention in adults: diagnosis and initial management. *Am Fam Physician* 2008;**77**(5):643–50.

28. Niel-Weise BS, van den Broek PJ. Antibiotic policies for short-term catheter bladder drainage in adults. *Cochrane Database Syst Rev* 2005;**3**:CD005428.

29. Warren JW. Catheter-associated urinary tract infections. *Infect Dis Clin North Am* 1997;**11**(3):609–22.

30. Nishimura RA, Carabello BA, Faxon DP, et al. ACC/AHA 2008 guideline update on valvular heart disease: focused update on infective endocarditis: a report of the American College of Cardiology/American Heart Association Task Force on Practice Guidelines: endorsed by the Society of Cardiovascular Anesthesiologists, Society for Cardiovascular Angiography and Interventions, and Society of Thoracic Surgeons. *Circulation* 2008;**118**(8):887–96.

31. Rao AR, Hanchanale VS, Sharma M, Gordon A, Motiwala H. Incisional hernia around the suprapubic catheter: an unusual complication. *Hernia* 2007; **11**(1):61–2.

32. Dogra PN, Goel R. Complication of percutaneous suprapubic cystostomy. *Int Urol Nephrol* 2004; **36**(3):343–4.

33. Nicolaisen GS, McAninch JW, Marshall GA, Bluth RF, Jr., Carroll PR. Renal trauma: re-evaluation of the indications for radiographic assessment. *J Urol* 1985;**133**(2):183–7.

34. Mirvis SE, Shanmuganathan K. Trauma to the genitourinary tract. In Adam, A, Dixon AK (eds), *Grainger and Allison's Diagnostic Radiology*, 5th edn. Philadelphia, PA: Churchill Livingstone, 2008: pp. 919–36.

35. Hustey F, Wilber LM. The pelvis. In Schwartz D, Reisdorff E (eds), *Emergency Radiology*. New York: McGraw-Hill, 2000: pp. 243–68.

36. Cass AS. False negative retrograde cystography with bladder rupture owing to external trauma. *J Trauma* 1984;**24**(2):168–9.

37. Guichard G, El Ammari J, Del Coro C, et al. Accuracy of ultrasonography in diagnosis of testicular rupture after blunt scrotal trauma. *Urology* 2008; **71**(1):52–6.

38. Blaivas M, Brannam L. Testicular ultrasound. *Emerg Med Clin North Am* 2004;**22**(3):723–48, ix.

39. Albrecht T, Lotzof K, Hussain HK, et al. Power Doppler US of the normal prepubertal testis: does it live up to its promises? *Radiology* 1997; **203**(1):227–31.

40. Valla JS, Kurzenne JY, Bastiani F, et al. Testicular exploration by Doppler ultrasonography in children. Importance, indications, limitations. Apropos of 90 cases. *Chir Pediatr* 1985;**26**(6):351–5.

41. Perri AJ, Rose J, Feldman AE, et al. An evaluation of the role of the Doppler stethoscope and the testicular scan in the diagnosis of torsion of the spermatic cord. *Invest Urol* 1978;**15**(4):275–7.

42. Perri AJ, Slachta GA, Feldman AE, Kendall AR, Karafin L. The Doppler stethoscope and the

diagnosis of the acute scrotum. *J Urol* 1976;
116(5):598–600.

43. Perri AJ, Morales JO, Feldman AE, Kendall AR, Karafin L. Necrotic testicle with increased blood flow on Doppler ultrasonic examination. *Urology* 1976;**8** (3):265–7.

44. Brereton RJ. Limitations of the Doppler flow meter in the diagnosis of the "acute scrotum" in boys. *Br J Urol* 1981;**53**(4):380–3.

45. Haynes BE. Doppler ultrasound failure in testicular torsion. *Ann Emerg Med* 1984; **13**(12):1103–7.

46. Akin EA, Khati NJ, Hill MC. Ultrasound of the scrotum. *Ultrasound Q* 2004;**20**(4):181–200.

47. Smith DE. Treatment of epididymitis by infiltration at spermatic cord with procaine hydrochloride. *J Urol* 1941;**46**:74–6.

Chapter 36

Wound management

Vincent J. Markovchick and Maria E. Moreira

Introduction

Wound management and wound closure are visible and important procedures that an emergency physician is frequently called upon to perform. The results of this procedure will be an observable reminder of the care rendered on that emergency department visit for the rest of that patient's life. Therefore, it is imperative that emergency physicians be well versed in wound management techniques in order to optimize the functional and cosmetic result.

Wound evaluation

History

It is important to determine whether the wound represents a cut or crush injury secondary to sharp or blunt trauma. In addition, the mechanism of wounding should be carefully ascertained to determine whether or not a high degree of bacterial inoculum was introduced into the wound at the time of injury (Table 36.1).

The exact time of injury will assist in determining the approach to closure. Significant comorbidities (diabetes, human immunodeficiency virus [HIV], malnourishment, etc.) of the patient should be elicited to help determine risk of infection or poor healing. Tetatus status should be checked and appropriate immunization provided.[1]

Physical examination

The precise anatomical location, length in centimeters and direction of the wound should be documented in the medical record either in text or by drawing. The additional physical examination documentation is dependent upon the underlying anatomy (e.g., ductal function, joint penetration, neurovascular injury).

Table 36.1 Examples of high-risk wounds

- Blunt force wounds with devitalized tissue
- Full thickness wounds from bites, including human bites
- Wounds exposed to fertile soil
- Wounds made while the body part is submerged in lakes, ponds, or streams
- Wounds in areas of the body in which there is a high degree of bacteria on the surface of the skin such as wounds in the perineum or axilla

Appropriate sensory and motor functions should be established before anesthetic infiltration. After the sensory examination is completed, local anesthetics may be administered, facilitating a complete examination of the wound. Wounds over tendons require direct visualization in a full range of motion This is important as the tendon could have been in a different position during injury and the site of injury can be missed if the tendon isn't placed through a full range of motion. Wounds over joints should be explored. If penetration is unclear, a common technique is injection of saline or dilute methylene blue to look for extravastion consistent with a violated joint space. If there is a possibility of an underlying fracture, X-rays should be obtained.

If the mechanism of injury is such that there may be a foreign body in the wound, obtain a radiograph. In the case where the wound can be absolutely and thoroughly explored and no foreign bodies are visible, radiographs may not be necessary. However, 0.6–4.3% of superficial wounds undergoing adequate exploration have been noted to have retained foreign bodies detected by radiography.[2] A study on cadavers showed a 90% sensitivity of X-rays for detecting

Trauma: A Comprehensive Emergency Medicine Approach, eds. Eric Legome and Lee W. Shockley. Published by Cambridge University Press. © Cambridge University Press 2011.

glass.[3] When looking at gravel detection, plain radiographs of chicken legs showed a sensitivity of < 75% for particles < 0.5 mm with a sensitivity of 97.7% for 2 mm and 1 mm particles.[4] Other modalities that are helpful in the evaluation of foreign bodies include computed tomography (CT), magnetic resonance (MR), and ultrasound. Ultrasound is easy and can be done at the bedside, but results are operator dependant. Computed tomography and MR are more expensive and the cost benefit needs to be analyzed. It is always reasonable to tell a patient that there may be a very small foreign body that is unvisualized or irretrievable. In wounds that overlie a duct such as the lacrimal ducts or Stensen's ducts, careful exploration and examination must be carried out to determine whether or not the integrity of these ducts is compromised. Examination should be carried out under sufficient lighting. Complete hemostasis should be obtained by the use of tourniquets on digits or extremities, and by the use of anesthetics with epinephrine in other very vascular areas such as the scalp and face. Although blind clamping of vessels is strongly discouraged, in some instances ligation of ongoing bleeding vessels may be appropriate. For example, if after injecting a facial laceration with lidocaine with epinephrine and applying pressure there is considerable bleeding with an identifiable vessel causing the bleeding, that vessel can be ligated.

In addition to looking in the wound, it should be palpated for foreign bodies and underlying fractures. Care must be taken to avoid laceration or penetrating injury to examine for sharp objects. Caution must be used when performing motor examination on the hand to determine the integrity of the tendon. Examination of a digit against resistance carries the risk of converting a partial tendon laceration with preserved function to a complete tendon laceration. The determination of whether or not there is a partial tendon laceration should be made by visual exploration while the patient and examiner carefully take the digit through its full range of motion without resistance.

Wound preparation

A critical factor in the prevention of infection from traumatic wounding is meticulous wound preparation. After adequate anesthesia the surrounding skin should be prepped with an antiseptic solution such as povidone–iodine. Solutions that should not be used in the wound include hydrogen peroxide, rubbing alcohol, and full strength betadine or scrub. Following the surrounding wound preparation, the wound should be irrigated. Many experts recommend at least 5–10 pounds of pressure per square inch based on physics, but no outcome data exists.[5–7] This pressure can be achieved by using a 30–60 ml syringe and a 19-gauge needle or splash shield.[8] Recent studies have shown that tap water is just as safe and efficacious as sterile saline solution.[9–12] Wounds, particularly those on the upper extremity, can be irrigated safely and adequately under a brisk flow from a faucet. Maintaining adequate pressure in wound irrigation is an important factor in reducing the bacterial count in traumatic wounds.[6,8] The amount of irrigant is probably important; the incidence of infection has been related inversely to the amount of irrigation.[13] Some wounds may not require irrigation. In a study done by Hollander et al., irrigation did not make a difference in clean, non-contaminated facial and scalp lacerations.[14] Following irrigation, the wound should be explored and any foreign body or devitalized tissue should be removed or debrided.

In abrasions in which there is ground-in dirt and debris, all of this material must be removed by mechanical scrubbing after obtaining local or topical anesthesia. If the area is widespread, procedural sedation may be necessary. If the dirt and debris are ground-in sufficiently deep into the layers of the dermis, a stiff bristle brush can assist in removing the foreign material. A new, stiff toothbrush is an ideal instrument to perform this function. Following removal with a brush, any additional material should be removed by sharp debridement. If foreign material is left in the dermis, this may result in permanent tattooing.

Tissue excision and foreign body removal

There are two schools of thought regarding tissue excision, particularly on wounds that have ragged edges. The first school of thought is to excise all ragged wounds in order to create a straight line in order to facilitate closure. However, excising a wound creates tension. This may necessitate undermining of the wound edge, which in turn can compromise circulation to the edges. Therefore, our recommendation is that wounds with viable skin edges should be meticulously closed without sharp excision. Tissue that is clearly non-viable at the wound edges or on the tips of flaps should be sharply excised. The

619

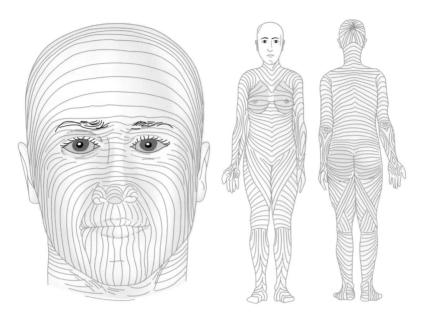

Figure 36.1 The natural lines of tension are perpendicular to the longitudinal orientation of the underlying muscles. Wounds occurring along these lines generally have a more favorable cosmetic outcome. (From Mahadevan S, Garmel G. *An Introduction to Clinical Emergency Medicine.* Cambridge: Cambridge University Press, 2005.)

amount of excision should be the minimum necessary to remove devitalized tissue.

The wound should be visually explored after obtaining hemostasis, and all foreign bodies should be removed. Particular care must be taken with proximally based flaps, since large amounts of debris can be imbedded very high up under the flap into the subcutaneous tissue. These wounds should be meticulously and extensively explored. If there is any question of retained foreign body, radiographs should be obtained.

Wounds made by broken glass that extend through subcutaneous tissue should be X-rayed in order to rule out foreign body in muscle tissue. Alternatively, ultrasound may be considered. Foreign body should generally be removed; however, occasionally it is prudent to leave them embedded when the removal is expected to be prolonged, difficult, and traumatic. The patient must be informed that the foreign body is being left in the wound and the reason why. Follow up with a surgeon is appropriate to consider removal under ultrasound or fluoroscopy.

Wound closure

At the extremes there are two basic types of wound closure with very different goals, i.e., functional and cosmetic closures. In reality, closure is usually some combination of both. The goal of a functional wound closure is to return the injured part to full function as soon as possible. It should be considered for all wounds over large joints and on extremities. Cosmetic closure is closure of a wound in a manner such that it results in the least visible scarring. All wounds of the face and, in certain individuals, wounds of the torso and extremities except the hands and feet should have a cosmetic closure.

Cosmetic closures

There are several factors that contribute to more visible scarring: (1) wounds perpendicular or oblique to lines of dynamic and static skin tension; (2) wounds under significant amounts of tension; (3) inversion of wound edges; (4) uneven wound edges; (5) delayed sutured removal; (6) tissue necrosis; (7) sunlight exposure.

An example of a wound that is perpendicular or oblique to the normal lines of skin tensions is a vertical laceration of the forehead that is perpendicular to the normal lines of skin tension. One must be particularly cognizant of these tension lines when excising the wound or making an elective incision. If at all possible, such incisions should be made parallel to the lines of skin tension (Figure 36.1).

Wounds that are under significant amounts of tension may ultimately heal with a wider scar if they are closed in a single layer. If the sutures are removed in 1 week, depending on the area of the body, the wound may have only 5% of its ultimate tensile strength.[15] Significant tension on the wound may cause the scar to widen slightly over time. In order

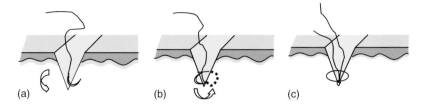

(a)　　　　　　　(b)　　　　　　　(c)

Figure 36.2 Placing intradermal sutures increases the risk of infection in a wound. However, deep sutures can remove "potential" spaces where fluid collection may distort tissue anatomy and/or predispose to infection. In addition, deep sutures facilitate closure of wounds which are widely open at the surface. This sequence (a–c) demonstrates burying the knot. (From Mahadevan S, Garmel G. *An Introduction to Clinical Emergency Medicine.* Cambridge: Cambridge University Press, 2005.)

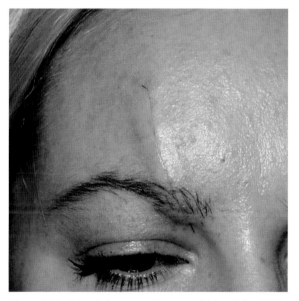

Figure 36.3 Subcuticular suture. (Courtesy of Adam Kolker, MD.)

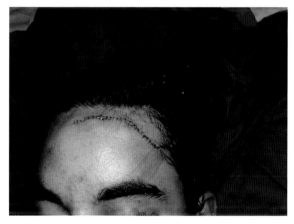

Figure 36.4 Layered closure with simple interrupted sutures. (Courtesy of Adam Kolker, MD.)

to prevent this, close wounds with significant tension in layers with either running subcuticular or interrupted subcuticular absorbable sutures will minimize this possibility. Meticulous technique should be exercised when placing these deep sutures. They should be synthetic, absorbable material that will stay in place for 3–4 weeks before dissolving such as polyglycolic acid sutures, e.g., Vicryl® or Dexon®. When placing deep sutures, care must be used in order to perfectly align the tissue planes and bury the knot by starting at the deepest point of the wound (Figure 36.2). Running subcuticular sutures can be placed either in a completely buried fashion or, if non-absorbable suture is used, by one percutaneous needle stick at each end of the wound (Figure 36.3). After the deep sutures, the skin is closed in a surface layer using a non-absorbable 5–0 or 6–0 suture. If necessary, the wound edges can be optimally approximated by careful placement of skin

sutures at appropriate depths. Surface sutures for linear lacerations can be a simple running (Figure 36.4), a running suture, or a running locked suture. For wounds that are stellate or have multiple components to them, the top layer suture should be interrupted non-absorbable sutures (Figure 36.5).

Wound edges invert due to incorrect technique in the placement of suture or tissue adhesive. This inversion of the wound edges results in a depression in the scar and increases its visibility due to shadowing (Figure 36.6). In the correct technique, the suture is passed perpindicular through both sides of the wound. Placement of the sutures in this manner will most often result in slight eversion of the wound edges, which gives the best long-term cosmesis. The horizontal mattress suture, a naturally everting suture, may be the best choice in wounds that tend to invert. Horizontal mattress can be either an interrupted or a running horizontal mattress.

Uneven wound edges result in more visible scarring. If one edge is higher than the other, particularly if it is horizontal on the face, the ultimate scar will

621

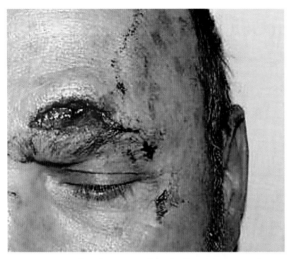

Figure 36.5 Stellate laceration of the forehead. (Courtesy of Adam Kolker, MD.)

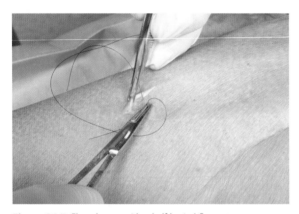

Figure 36.7 Flap closure with a half-buried flap suture.

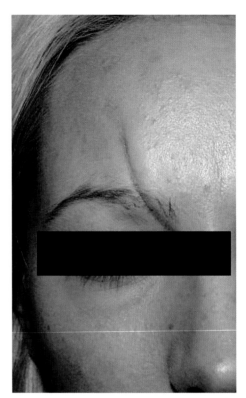

Figure 36.6 Depressed wound requiring revision. (Courtesy of Adam Kolker, MD.)

cast a shadow in normal lighting and magnify the scar. Care must particularly be taken in a wound made by blunt trauma in which there may be differential swelling of the wound edges over time, i.e., the lower edge will tend to drain its edema where the upper edge will maintain it, and over time an uneven wound edge may result. Therefore, proper placement of the surface sutures should minimize or prevent this occurrence.

Permanent suture marks may occur if percutaneous surface sutures are left in a wound for > 7 days. Therefore, surface sutures should optimally be removed within this period of time and, if necessary, the wound reinforced with Steri-Strips® or tissue adhesive.

Tissue necrosis, particularly when it involves a distally based flap, will result in more noticeable scarring. This can be minimized by careful debridement of non-viable edges and meticulous placement of the suture. Suture placed at the tip of the flap may compromise the venous or lymphatic return, with resultant necrosis These flap sutures may be placed as a buried absorbable subcutaneous suture, intradermal suture, or as a half-buried flap suture on the surface (Figure 36.7). Stellate lacerations, especially on the extremities or body, with multiple component parts may be best closed via an absorbable purse string suture that is carefully placed. In areas of the body with less robust blood supply such as the pretibial area, a flap may be closed using an advancement flap (e.g., V–Y closure) with less tension.

If the vermillion border of the lip is malaligned by > 1 ml, it will result in a noticeable scar. Therefore, meticulous care must be taken to align the vermillion border and to obtain a watertight mucosal closure in order to get the optimal cosmetic result. If the laceration results in an irregular vermillion margin, a full thickness wedge of lip tissue can be removed to produce a single linear scar with an intact vermillion. A significant amount of the lip (in some cases up to a third) can be removed without appreciable distortion in the symmetry of the lip.

Research on wounds exposed to ultraviolet light within 6 months following the injury revealed that traumatic wounds exposed to ultraviolet light showed greater scarring and worse cosmetic outcome at 2–3 months.[16] Therefore, it is recommended that sunscreen with a sun protection factor (SPF) of 15 or greater be applied every day for at least 6 months to a maturing scar that will be exposed to sunlight.

Basic and advanced techniques

Basic techniques

There are three types of closure options available in traumatic wounds: primary closure; delayed primary closure; and healing by secondary intention. Basic techniques include simple interrupted sutures, simple running sutures, and mattress sutures.

Primary closure

Primary closure is closure of a wound shortly after the time of wounding. In general, the acceptable time frame for safely performing primary closure is up to 24 hours for wounds of the face or scalp and up to 8 hours for wounds in other areas of the body. The type of closure and choice of material will depend upon the type of wound, area of the body, and whether one is performing a cosmetic or functional closure.

Delayed primary closure

Delayed primary closure is defined as closure of a wound using the same techniques as one would use with a primary closure, but this is performed 4–5 days following the wounding with the ideal time period of approximately 96 hours after wounding. This method of closure is most often used for wounds that are contaminated by virtue of being "old" or having a mechanism in which there was a high degree of bacterial inoculum at the time of wounding. Examples of these wounds are full-thickness mammalian bites, lacerations suffered in lakes, streams, ponds, or fertile soil, and wounds on body areas with a high degree of bacterial contamination such as the perineum or axilla. When delayed primary closure is indicated, the wound should receive meticulous wound preparation and irrigation, bleeding should be controlled, a fine, dry mesh gauze should be placed inside the wound, the wound should be dressed, and the patient should be instructed to return in 4–5 days for delayed primary closure. If, when the patient returns, there is no visible infection, i.e., purulence or cellulitis surrounding the wound edges, the wound should be anesthetized, reirrigated and closed using whatever technique is indicated to obtain the optimal functional or cosmetic closure. Even though some practitioners administer antibiotics, there is no evidence to support the practice. Outside of immuncompromised patients or patients with a very high degree of contamination, we do not recommend prophylactic antibiotics.

Healing by secondary intention

For wounds such as small, deep stab wounds or puncture wounds, this is the method of choice in which the wound is decontaminated as best possible and then allowed to heal by secondary intention, which is healing by granulation tissue. That is, not closing the wound, but allowing it to fill in with scar tissue and naturally contract.

Simple interrupted sutures

Simple interrupted sutures are adequate for many functional closures (Figure 36.8). Care must be taken to meticulously place these sutures the same distance on either side of the wound and in a perpendicular or hourglass fashion so as to avoid uneven or inversion of the wound edges. Historically, the least reactive, non-absorbable material has been used on external structures; however, some newer data suggests that, at least in children, absorbable gut is probably appropriate on the face.

Simple running sutures

Simple running sutures are adequate for small linear lacerations in which the wound is under minimal or very little tension or as the top layer in a cosmetic closure. Running sutures may be simple running or running locked (Figure 36.9) sutures. Running locked are probably best for non-cosmetic areas under greater tension in which hemostasis may be an issue. The advantage from running sutures are they are faster to perform than interrupted and their tension is self adjusting. (Each suture will achieve the same-tension.) The disadvantage is that it does not work well on stellate, curved, or complex lacerations and if it breaks it compromises the entire repair (Table 36.2).

623

Table 36.2 Properties of running and locked sutures

Advantages of running suture	Advantages of locked suture
• Faster	• Able to close wounds with greater tension
• Self-adjusting for equal tension	• Potentially stronger
Disadvantage of running suture	**Disadvantage of locked suture**
• Works well only on straight lacerations	• Takes longer
• If disrupted or broken while placing, must be restarted	• Greater scarring potential
• If broken after placement, may open wound	

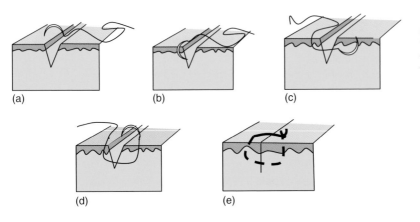

(a)   (b)   (c)

(d)   (e)

Figure 36.8 Sequence illustrating the placement of a simple interrupted suture (a–e). (From Mahadevan S, Garmel G. *An Introduction to Clinical Emergency Medicine.* Cambridge: Cambridge University Press, 2005.)

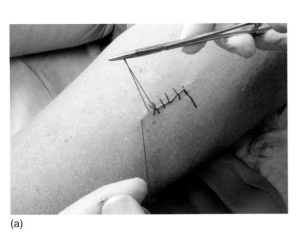

(a)

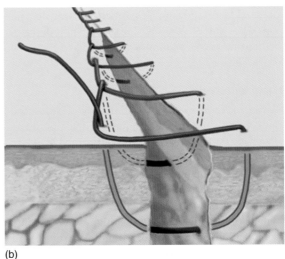

(b)

Figure 36.9 (a) Photograph of running locked suture. (Courtesy of Taku Taira, MD and the New York University School of Medicine.) (b) Running locked suture technique.

Mattress sutures

The two choices for basic wound closure in which wounds are under significant tension are vertical or horizontal mattress sutures. Vertical mattress sutures are preferred by some and the placement of these sutures are so that the tension is taken primarily by the far suture and the wound edge is everted by the near suture (Figure 36.10). The theoretical

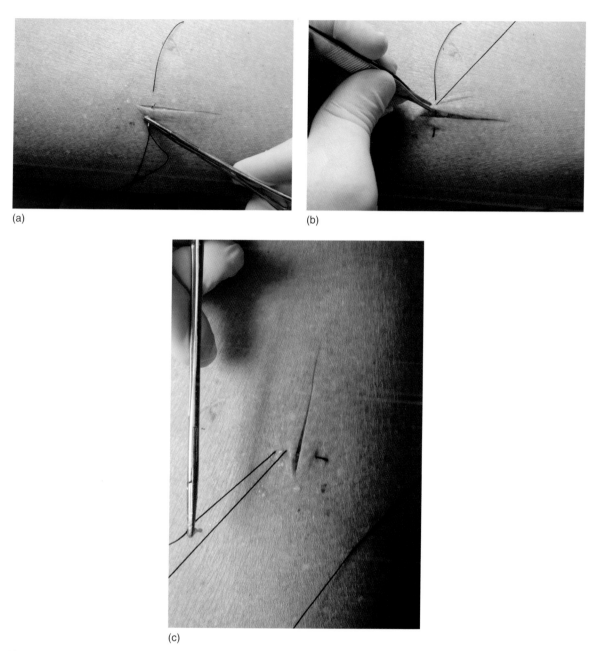

(a)

(b)

(c)

Figure 36.10 Vertical mattress sutures being placed (a–c).

disadvantage of this suture is that the near suture, if improperly placed, may cause necrosis of the wound edges. The other alternative for mattress sutures is the horizontal mattress suture, which is placed in a rectangular fashion (Figure 36.11). The advantage of this suture is that it is extremely strong; it will not pull through, even in areas in which the skin is delicate and thin such as the fingertips, and is a naturally everting suture. Care must be taken to ensure proper tension when tying to avoid excessive eversion of the wound edges. This type of suture is ideal in areas of tension, such as over joints, in which movement of the joint will create strain on the wound edges. Horizontal mattress sutures may also be placed as a running suture which is advantageous when the wound edges are tending to invert or possibly overlap.

625

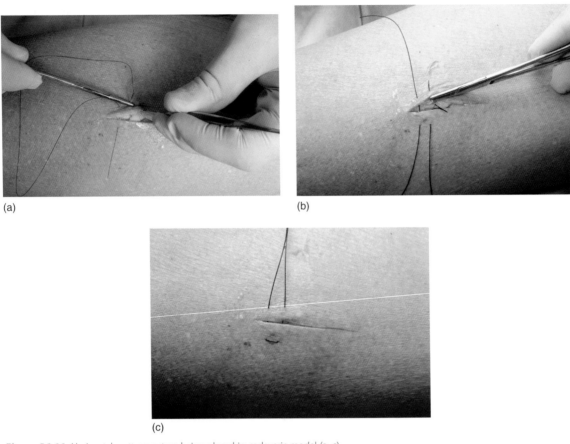

Figure 36.11 Horizontal mattress suture being placed in cadaveric model (a–c).

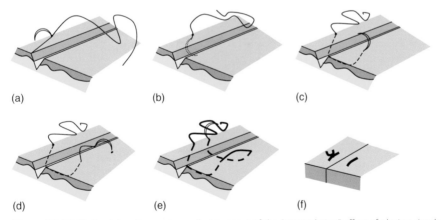

Figure 36.12 Horizontal mattress sutures alleviate some of the "strangulation" effect of placing simple interrupted sutures along the margin of a wound under high tension (a–f). (From Mahadevan S, Garmel G. *An Introduction to Clinical Emergency Medicine*. Cambridge: Cambridge University Press, 2005.)

Horizontal mattress sutures can be used in areas in which the skin is extremely thin, such as the eyelids, to ensure the optimal cosmetic closure (Figure 36.12).

Another technique for one-layer wound closure is that of the running subcuticular suture. Technically this is a somewhat more difficult suture to master, since care must be taken to pass the needle perfectly

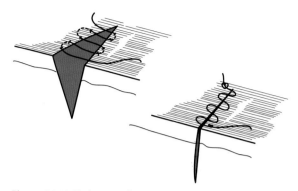

Figure 36.13 Technique of subcuticular suture placement.

horizontal and at the same distance from the surface with the in-and-out pass (Figure 36.13). In addition, each subsequent pass on the opposite side of the wound edge should be slightly behind where one came out on the opposite side. These sutures may be absorbable or non-absorbable sutures. With non-absorbable, an entry and exit on either end of the wound can be used and the tension on this suture can be adjusted over time. It may be left in place for several weeks and then removed.

Advanced techniques

Advanced suture techniques involve deep layer closures of wounds. This is usually done when an optimal cosmetic result is important. The ideal suture for this is a synthetic, polyglycolic acid absorbable suture (e.g., Dexon® or Vicryl®) since it will remain in place for 3–4 weeks before it is fully absorbed, at which time the wound will have adequate tensile strength so as not to separate or widen over time. The technique of placing these sutures involves starting and ending subdermally and making the pass at the same vertical depth and directly opposite on the other side. This suture is normally placed in a vertical fashion, but in wounds with minimal room for maneuvering, it can be placed in a tangential fashion. If the exit and entrance back into the dermis is not the same depth on both sides, this will result in uneven wound edges.

Flap closure

Care must be taken when closing flaps so as not to compromise the venous or lymphatic return from the tip of the flap. This is particularly important in distally based flaps. A suture or a combination of sutures that result in compromising the circulation to the tip of the flap must be avoided. Flaps may be closed with

a half-buried horizontal mattress suture from the surface (Figure 36.14) or with a completely buried absorbable suture in which the knot is placed intradermally.

If the flap has non-viable edges and is in an area of the body in which the circulation is somewhat compromised, such as the anterior pretibial area, the non-viable flap edges may be excised. However, if this would result in an inability to pull the flap back into place without putting an inordinate amount of tension on the wound, a V–Y closure is recommended (Figure 36.15).

Stellate lacerations

Stellate lacerations, a series of small flap lacerations in a circular pattern, most commonly occur in areas such as the scalp but may be encountered on the face or extremities. The ideal method of bringing these small flaps together is to do a purse string suture with absorbable material followed by either a single- or double-layered closure of the remainder of the laceration. Care should be taken not to place the sutures too close to the tip of the small flap that has been closed with the purse string suture (Figure 36.16).

Nailbed lacerations

In lacerations involving the nail bed in which the nail is avulsed or loose, the nail should be trimmed back to give exposure to the lacerated nail bed. It should be closed very carefully with an absorbable suture so as to evenly approximate the lacerated nail bed. For wounds through the nail that penetrate the nail bed where the nail is adherent on both sides, one method of closure is to use an adhesive glue on the surface of the nail bringing it directly together; in turn it will bring the lacerated nail bed in good anatomical position for healing. If the nail bed is allowed to heal unevenly, this may result in a permanent deformity of the nail. Following closure of the nail bed, if the nail has been avulsed, it should be cleansed and irrigated and used as a stint dressing on top of the exposed nail bed. The nail can be sutured in place with a horizontal mattress suture through the area of the cuticle with the nail in position under the cuticle so as to prevent adhesions between the germinal matrix and cuticle. Other methods described to replace the nail plate include tissue adhesives or chloramphenicol ointment.[17,18] With these techniques, the nail plate will work itself loose on its own. When a patient presents with an isolated subungal hematoma, nailbed removal

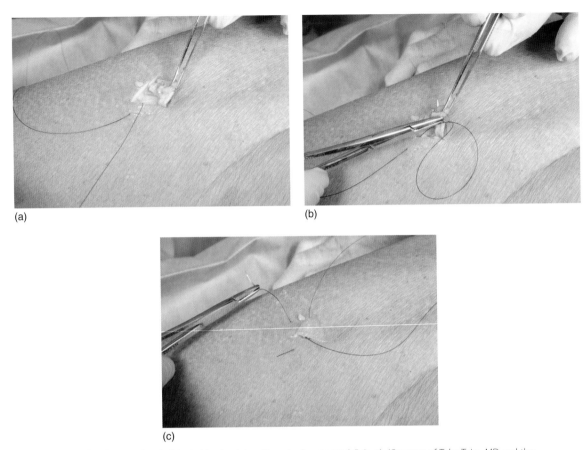

(a)

(b)

(c)

Figure 36.14 Flap closure using half-buried horizontal mattress (cadaveric model) (a–c). (Courtesy of Taku Taira, MD and the New York University School of Medicine.)

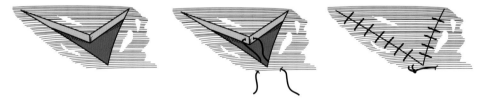

Figure 36.15 Drawing of flap closure.

is not required. If the nail is adherent to the nail bed, removal to suture the nailbed laceration confers no outcome improvement over simple trephination. This is regardless of the size of the hematoma.[19]

Extensor tendon repair

Tendons should be repaired with non-absorbable sutures, such as nylon or Prolene®, and a modified Kessler suture is an acceptable method for tendon repair. Following the repair of a tendon, the digit or joint should be immobilized in a splint for at least 2 weeks. Flexor tendons, due to their fine mechanism and need for perfect alignment, should be repaired in an operating room with proper equipment and conditions.

Special considerations

Scalp

Wounds of the scalp may produce significant ongoing hemorrhage. Although uncommon, they, may result in hypovolemic shock if the bleeding is not adequately controlled.[20,21]

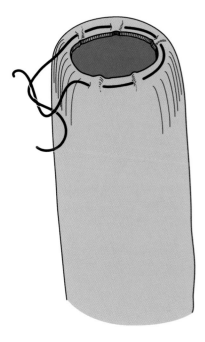

Figure 36.16
Purse string suture technique.

Initial methods for control of the bleeding include direct pressure on the wound edges, liberal injection of Xylocaine with epinephrine, and placing Raney clips or a temporary tight closure with a running, locked, non-absorbable suture that will later be removed in order to adequately irrigate the wound and perform a proper closure. If the scalp wound causes a large rent in the galea, it may be closed with the surface suture extending down through the galea or in an additional layer with either 3–0 or 4–0 suture. All scalp lacerations should be visually and palpably inspected for foreign bodies or fractures. One other method that has been proven efficient and fully appropriate to close scalp wounds is simple staples. They may, in most circumstances, be considered the treatment of choice in the emergency department. In addition, the hair apposition technique (HAT), although not widely used in emergency departments, seems to be an effective, inexpensive, and relatively simple method for closing minor scalp wounds.[22–27]

Face

All full-thickness wounds of the face, with the exception of the eyelids, are candidates for layered closure in order to obtain the optimal cosmetic results. Recent evidence suggests, however, that single-layer closure of non-gaping simple facial wounds < 3 m produces comparable results to double-layer closure and can be accomplished more rapidly.[28] It is important to determine what the underlying anatomy is, particularly the nerves and ducts, in order to adequately explore for injury of these deep structures. Wounds of the eyelid margin that include the tarsal plate require special techniques of repair, and if one is unskilled in closing the tarsal plate, it should be referred to the appropriate specialist. Wounds involving the lower lacrimal duct apparatus on the medial aspect of the inferior eyelid should be referred to an ophthalmologist for microscopic operative repair over stents. Wounds over the parotid gland should be carefully inspected for penetration into the parotid gland, and if the parotid gland appears to be penetrated, determination should be made as to whether or not Stensen's duct has been violated. Exploration of the orifice of Stensen's duct opposite the upper 2nd molar should be done, and if there is bleeding from the duct, it should be presumed that the duct is violated. Another technique would be to place a solution of dilute methylene blue into the wound and examine the mouth for the appearance of the blue dye at Stensen's duct intraorally. Alternatively, fluorescein and an ultraviolet light can be used in a similar fashion. Full-thickness, through-and-through lacerations of the lips should be repaired in three layers in which the first layer would be absorbable suture intraorally with a water-tight closure tested by reirrigating the wound from the outside. Following the secondary irrigation, the lip should be closed with the second layer using absorbable 4.0 or 5.0 deep sutures, and the last or top layer using non-absorbable sutures to the vermillion border with absorbable sutures of 5.0 in the vermillion. The key suture here is careful and perfect approximation of the vermillion border. Wounds of the eyelids should be carefully inspected and the eyelids should be everted, and if there is a through-and-through laceration or penetration of the eyelid, very careful exam of the globe should be performed to exclude globe injury or penetration.

Pinna

Wounds of the pinna that violate the cartilage generally can be repaired by approximating the skin overlying the cartilage, placing it back into its proper anatomical position. If the wound is large and under any tension involving the cartilage, the cartilage may be closed with an absorbable suture. It is important

Table 36.3 Brief review of sutures[1]

Suture	Characteristics
Absorbable vs. non-absorbable	Major division. If they lose tensile strength within 60 days considered absorbable. Non-absorbable generally below skin
Tensile strength	Highly dependent on material and size. Larger the first number, thinner the suture
Ease of handling/security	Depends on memory (ability to return to original position), pliability and coefficent of friction
Multifilament vs. monofilament	Multifilament handle easier and tie better, but may be more prone to infection, avoid with higher risk wound. Monofilament may have lower infection risk, but are more difficult to handle and tie
Tissue reactivity	Higher with natural products (silk and gut) lower with synthetics
Specific types: absorbable	
Chromic gut	Good for about 10–14 days, high tissue reactivity, most common for mucosal surfaces
Fast absorbing gut	Used when wound has low tension and removal may be difficult
Polyglactin 910 (Vicryl®) or (Polysorb®)	Synthetic, low reactivity, handles well, common in subcuticular or dermal sutures. Completely breaks down in about 3 months. Fascial wounds
Poliglecaprone 25 (Monocryl®)	Similar to Vicryl® but less reactivity, good handling, use where minimal tissue reaction is needed
Polydioxanone (PDS II)	Monofilament polymer with excellent strength and long lasting. Good for high tension or contaminated areas. Low reactivity. Consider with cartilage
Polytrimethylene carbonate (Maxon®)	Monofilament that is strong and handles very well. Long lasting with minimal tissue reaction
Specific types-non-absorbable	
Nylon (Ethilon®)	Common removables, monofilament, good strength, fair handling, less expensive than Dermalon® and Surgilon® which handle somewhat easier
Polybuster (Novafil®)	Monofilament, good elasticity, good for subcuticular
Polypropolene (Prolene®)	Monofilament, good plasticity, but somewhat difficult to handle and expensive, poor knot security. Good for subcuticular
Polyester(Dacron®), (Ethibond®)	Multifilament with low reactivity, good strength, and handling good for mucosa

following closure of lacerations of the pinna that a stent dressing with cotton behind and in the ear, followed by a comfortable compression dressing, be placed so as to prevent hematoma formation between skin and cartilage.

Intraoral lacerations

Lacerations of the oral mucosa should be closed if they are gaping, will catch food particles or teeth, or have ongoing hemorrhage. Lacerations of the tongue should be closed if they are gaping, have ongoing

hemorrhage, or are vertical through the anterior surface of the tongue.[29,30] This should be accomplished using absorbable suture in a simple interrupted or horizontal mattress fashion to control ongoing hemorrhage and to prevent continued contamination of the wound with saliva.

Hands and feet

Failure to appreciate the underlying anatomy and adequately examine for injuries to nerves, bones, joints, and tendons may result in increased morbidity.

Table 36.4 Overview of specific wound management

Wound	Management	Pitfalls	Suture	Other
Lip	Vermillion border first (6–0 NA), then inside-out closure, approximate wet dry border, then orbicularis oris (absorbable), then close skin.	Vemillion border needs perfect closure Explore for foreign body Watertight closure	Mucosal gut or Vicryl® intraoral/deep, polyester or nylon for outside surface	Consult if significant avulsion or tissue loss
Ear	Debride cartilage only if devitalized, can lose up to 5 mm and retain shape Close posterior to anterior, suture cartilage only if defect	Cartilage is avascular, requires coverage, critical to prevent hematoma	Consider PDS II for cartilage if needed Close surface with nylon or other monofilament	Consult for tissue loss, unable to cover cartilage
Eyelid	Repair with 6–0 or 7–0, consider horizontal mattress stitch for fine skin. May leave small superficial approximated defects	Exclude puncta/lacrimal laceration, instill fluorescein if unsure, consult for medial lacerations, marginal lacerations, tarsal plate through and through	Superficial non-absorbable, nylon (Ethilon®) most common, consider Dermalon® or Surgilon® for handling	Consult freely if any concerns of duct or muscle, margin injury
Intraoral	Repair if > 2 cm, gaping, or likely to trap food, or occlusive surface of teeth	Make sure to explore if there's missing teeth Use of antibiotics unclear	Can use absorbables, polyester sutures probably best, chromic gut and silk still common	
Limb	May need to undermine as a large amount of tension, use deep sutures, consider mattress sutures		Can use larger sutures, leave in longer, 4–0 or 5–0, 3–0 or 4–0 deep Vicryl® most common deep, consider PDS II if tension and not clean for deep	
Tongue[30,32]	Repair if > 1 cm in length that extends into the muscular layers or through and through. Deep lateral border lacerations. Bisecting lacerations should be sewn Lacerations that bisect the tongue		Chromic or gut most common Silk easy to use and soft, but higher reactivity	Consult for significant tissue loss, hemorrhage, or partial amputations

Placing the sutures too close to the wound edges can lead to closure failure if subsequent swelling causes the sutures to pull through. Wounds of the hands and feet should be closed with the minimum number of sutures placed at least 3–4 mm from the wound edges. In areas of very high tension, horizontal mattress sutures are ideal. Hand lacerations < 2 cm may heal without suturing with the same cosmetic result.[31]

The choice of suture material is outlined in Table 36.3. Aftercare instructions should include the signs and symptoms of infection, the timing of the suture removal, and instructions on how to care for the wounds. Wounds closed over joints should be splinted for at least 7 days and, if wounds are closed properly, they should have a watertight seal. In about 24 hours, the patient may shower but should not submerge the injured part under water until removal of the sutures.

See Table 36.4 for an overview of specific wound management.[30,32]

Controversies

Antibiotics

Antibiotics are commonly used with the intent to "prevent infections." However, there is a paucity of randomized, controlled clinical trials with adequate numbers to scientifically support the common practice of administering prophylactic antibiotics. Studies have also been inconsistent in the definition of infection and in wound-surveillance protocols. A meta-analysis of randomized trials looking at use of prophylactic antibiotics in simple non-bite wounds showed lack of evidence for protection against infection.[33]

In a study looking at clean, incised hand wounds with the inclusion of trauma to the skin, tendon, and nerves, there were no statistically significant differences in infection rates between the groups treated with antibiotics and those that were not.[34] It is unclear from this study if antibiotics would benefit a certain subgroup of patients that is at higher risk for infection at baseline (i.e., diabetics).

Evidence exists for the use of antibiotics in hand injuries involving fractures, contaminated wounds, crush injuries, animal bites, and human bites. However, not all hand injuries with fractures require antibiotics. For example, antibiotics do not provide added benefit over thorough wound preparation and careful soft tissue repair in the case of open fractures of the distal phalanx.[35]

Debridement is more effective in reducing infection than antibiotics in the setting of dog-bite wounds. However, when a wound cannot be thoroughly irrigated, as occurs with puncture wounds, the infection rate increases. Therefore, antibiotics may not be necessary in deep, open dog-bite wounds that can be well irrigated. They are warranted for dog-bite wounds on the hand or those presenting as puncture wounds that cannot be adequately irrigated or debrided.[36]

In conclusion, antibiotics should be considered in patients with higher risk of infection, secondary to other underlying medical conditions or state of the wound at presentation. Antibiotics are also generally recommended for highly contaminated wounds or wounds that cannot be adequately irrigated or debrided. If antibiotics are to be used, they should be selected based upon the most likely bacterial, etiologic agent and they should be generic, inexpensive, and broad spectrum. In general, coverage for skin flora with a first-generation cephalosporin or semi-synthetic penicillin is appropriate. An example would be cephalexin or dicoxicillin. For those with diabetes or an immunocompromised state, more broad spectrum is reasonable, such as amoxicillin–clavulanate, a penicillinase-resistant penicillin. There is no good reason to prescribe expensive antibiotics when the scientific basis for their use is marginal at best.

Saline vs. tap water

Recent studies have shown that tap water is safe and efficacious and does not result in any increased risk of infection compared to sterile saline. This irrigation can be accomplished on extremity wounds by holding them under a vigorous stream of tap water.[10]

Sterile gloves vs. exam gloves

A prospective multicenter trial has shown that there is no increased risk of infection using standard exam gloves vs. sterile gloves in accomplishing wound repair.[37] Other studies in surgical and dental patients support this data.[38]

High pressure vs. low pressure irrigation

There is *in vitro* scientific basis for the use of high pressure irrigation in that studies have shown that the level of bacteria from a contaminated wound is significantly decreased with irrigating pressures of at least 8 psi.[5–7] Low pressure irrigation is unlikely to accomplish the same ends. On the other hand, there is no evidence that in a simple clean wound, high pressure irrigation makes a difference in outcome.[14]

Complications and adverse outcomes

All patients should be informed that even "clean" wounds have up to a 5% incidence of infection. Contaminated wounds, such as bites of the hand, have a higher incidence of infection, as do wounds in the elderly and in immunocompromised patients. Retention of foreign body in wounds will result in inflammatory reactions and possibly infection.[39] Therefore, foreign bodies should always be removed when possible, and if a decision is made to leave a foreign body in the wound, the patient should be informed as to why this decision is being made, i.e., the morbidity of attempting to remove it is far greater than the risk of leaving it in. Any foreign body that may cause an inflammatory response or may cause long-term discomfort should be referred for removal.

References

1. Singer AJ, Dagum AB. Current management of acute cutaneous wounds. *N Engl J Med* 2008;**359** (10):1037–46.

2. Weinberger LN, Chen EH, Mills AM. Is screening radiography necessary to detect retained foreign bodies in adequately explored superficial glass-caused wounds? *Ann Emerg Med* 2008;**51**(5):666–7.

3. Arbona N, Jedrzynski M, Frankfather R, et al. Is glass visible on plain radiographs? A cadaver study. *J Foot Ankle Surg* 1999;**38**(4):264–70.

4. Chisholm CD, Wood CO, Chua G, Cordell WH, Nelson DR. Radiographic detection of gravel in soft tissue. *Ann Emerg Med* 1997;**29**(6):725–30.

5. Edlich RF, Rodeheaver GT, Morgan RF, Berman DE, Thacker JG. Principles of emergency wound management. *Ann Emerg Med* 1988;**17**(12):1284–302.

6. Hollander JE, Singer AJ. Laceration management. *Ann Emerg Med* 1999;**34**(3):356–67.

7. Singer AJ, Hollander JE, Quinn JV. Evaluation and management of traumatic lacerations. *N Engl J Med* 1997;**337**(16):1142–8.

8. Stevenson TR, Thacker JG, Rodeheaver GT, et al. Cleansing the traumatic wound by high pressure syringe irrigation. *JACEP* 1976;**5**(1):17–21.

9. O'Neill D. Can tap water be used to irrigate wounds in A&E? *Nurs Times* 2002;**98**(14):56–9.

10. Moscati RM, Mayrose J, Reardon RF, Janicke DM, Jehle DV. A multicenter comparison of tap water versus sterile saline for wound irrigation. *Acad Emerg Med* 2007;**14**(5):404–9.

11. Bansal BC, Wiebe RA, Perkins SD, Abramo TJ. Tap water for irrigation of lacerations. *Am J Emerg Med* 2002;**20**(5):469–72.

12. Valente JH, Forti RJ, Freundlich LF, Zandieh SO, Crain EF. Wound irrigation in children: saline solution or tap water? *Ann Emerg Med* 2003;**41**(5):609–16.

13. Peterson L. Prophylaxis of wound infection. *Arch Surgery* 1945;**50**(4):177–83.

14. Hollander JE, Richman PB, Werblud M, et al. Irrigation in facial and scalp lacerations: does it alter outcome? *Ann Emerg Med* 1998;**31**(1):73–7.

15. Trott A. Surface injury and wound healing. In Trott A (ed.), *Wounds and Lacerations Emergency Care and Closure*. Saint Louis, MO: Mosby, 1991: pp. 12–23.

16. Due E, Rossen K, Sorensen LT, et al. Effect of UV irradiation on cutaneous cicatrices: a randomized, controlled trial with clinical, skin reflectance, histological, immunohistochemical and biochemical evaluations. *Acta Derm Venereol* 2007;**87** (1):27–32.

17. Pasapula C, Strick M. The use of chloramphenicol ointment as an adhesive for replacement of the nail plate after simple nail bed repairs. *J Hand Surg Br* 2004;**29**(6):634–5.

18. Richards AM, Crick A, Cole RP. A novel method of securing the nail following nail bed repair. *Plast Reconstr Surg* 1999;**103**(7):1983–5.

19. Roser SE, Gellman H. Comparison of nail bed repair versus nail trephination for subungual hematomas in children. *J Hand Surg Am* 1999;**24**(6):1166–70.

20. Lemos MJ, Clark DE. Scalp lacerations resulting in hemorrhagic shock: case reports and recommended management. *J Emerg Med* 1988;**6**(5):377–9.

21. Turnage B, Maull KI. Scalp laceration: an obvious 'occult' cause of shock. *South Med J* 2000; **93**(3):265–6.

22. Hock MO, Ooi SB, Saw SM, Lim SH. A randomized controlled trial comparing the hair apposition technique with tissue glue to standard suturing in scalp lacerations (HAT study). *Ann Emerg Med* 2002;**40** (1):19–26.

23. Hogg K, Carley S. Towards evidence based emergency medicine: best BETs from the Manchester Royal Infirmary. Staples or sutures in children with scalp lacerations. *Emerg Med J* 2002;**19**(4):328–9.

24. Hogg K, Carley S. Towards evidence based emergency medicine: best BETs from the Manchester Royal Infirmary. Staples or sutures for repair of scalp laceration in adults. *Emerg Med J* 2002;**19**(4):327–8.

25. Ong ME, Chan YH, Teo J, et al. Hair apposition technique for scalp laceration repair: a randomized controlled trial comparing physicians and nurses (HAT 2 study). *Am J Emerg Med* 2008;**26**(4):433–8.

26. Ong ME, Coyle D, Lim SH, Stiell I. Cost-effectiveness of hair apposition technique compared with standard suturing in scalp lacerations. *Ann Emerg Med* 2005;**46** (3):237–42.

27. Weick R, Stevermer JJ. Hair apposition technique is better than suturing scalp lacerations. *J Fam Pract* 2002;**51**(10):818.

28. Singer AJ, Gulla J, Hein M, et al. Single-layer versus double-layer closure of facial lacerations: a randomized controlled trial. *Plast Reconstr Surg* 2005;**116**(2):363–8; discussion 69–70.

29. Brown DJ, Jaffe JE, Henson JK. Advanced laceration management. *Emerg Med Clin North Am* 2007;**25** (1):83–99.

30. Ud-din Z, Aslam M, Gull S. Towards evidence based emergency medicine: best BETs from the Manchester Royal Infirmary. Should minor mucosal tongue lacerations be sutured in children? *Emerg Med J* 2007;**24**(2):123–4.

633

31. Quinn J, Cummings S, Callaham M, Sellers K. Suturing versus conservative management of lacerations of the hand: randomised controlled trial. *BMJ* 2002;**325**(7359):299.

32. Patel A. Tongue lacerations. *Br Dent J* 2008;**204**(7):355.

33. Cummings P, Del Beccaro MA. Antibiotics to prevent infection of simple wounds: a meta-analysis of randomized studies. *Am J Emerg Med* 1995;**13**(4): 396–400.

34. Whittaker JP, Nancarrow JD, Sterne GD. The role of antibiotic prophylaxis in clean incised hand injuries: a prospective randomized placebo controlled double blind trial. *J Hand Surg Br* 2005;**30**(2):162–7.

35. Stevenson J, McNaughton G, Riley J. The use of prophylactic flucloxacillin in treatment of open fractures of the distal phalanx within an accident and emergency department: a double-blind randomized

36. Callaham M. Prophylactic antibiotics in common dog bite wounds: a controlled study. *Ann Emerg Med* 1980;**9**(8):410–14.

37. Perelman VS, Francis GJ, Rutledge T, et al. Sterile versus nonsterile gloves for repair of uncomplicated lacerations in the emergency department: a randomized controlled trial. *Ann Emerg Med* 2004;**43** (3):362–70.

38. Rhinehart MB, Murphy MM, Farley MF, Albertini JG. Sterile versus nonsterile gloves during Mohs micrographic surgery: infection rate is not affected. *Dermatol Surg* 2006;**32**(2):170–6.

39. Hollander JE, Singer AJ, Valentine SM, Shofer FS. Risk factors for infection in patients with traumatic lacerations. *Acad Emerg Med* 2001;**8**(7):716–20.

placebo-controlled trial. *J Hand Surg Br* 2003;**28** (5):388–94.

37

Universal/standard precautions

David Peak

Introduction

In 1987 and 1988, the Centers for Disease Control and Prevention (CDC) published documents designed to protect healthcare workers (HCW) from transmission of blood-borne pathogens under the name of universal precautions (UP) which recommended blood and body fluid precautions be consistently used for all patients regardless of their infectious status. This represented a fundamental change from the previous 1983 document that recommended precautions only when a patient was known or suspected to be infected with blood-borne pathogens.[1,2] In 1996, UP and body substance isolation protocols were incorporated into a strategy called standard precautions (SP).[3] Standard precautions combine the major features of UP and body substance isolation into a single set of precautions used for the care of all patients in hospitals and are based on the principle that all blood, body fluids, secretions and excretions (except sweat), as well as non-intact skin and mucous membranes may contain transmissible infectious agents. Standard precautions constitute the primary strategy of the prevention of healthcare-associated transmission of infectious agents among patients and healthcare personnel.

General principles

Standard precautions are recommended for the care of all hospital patients. Standard precautions apply to blood and body fluids, non-intact skin, mucous membranes and secretions/excretions (except sweat), and entail proper hand hygiene, the use of personal protective equipment (PPE), as well as safe disposal of sharp instruments and proper decontamination techniques.[4]

Fundamental components necessary to prevent transmission of infectious agents in the healthcare setting include healthcare system components, surveillance of healthcare-associated infections, education of HCW, patients, and visitors, hand hygiene and PPE, safe work practices, appropriate placement of patients within the hospital, and environmental issues of decontamination. While some of these issues may not seem important to the emergency physicians, all are important as a breakdown in any area will affect the entire system.

Healthcare organizations can demonstrate a commitment to the prevention of infectious agent transmission by incorporating infection control into the organization's overall objectives. Since multiple federal bodies have explicit goals in this regard, it is imperative that healthcare organizations commit an infrastructure to support and monitor adherence to standard and transmission-based precautions. Healthcare organizations must provide fiscal and human resources to establish and maintain infectious control programs that fit the specific organizational requirements. The positive influence of institutional leadership has repeatedly been demonstrated to increase adherence to recommended practices.[5–12]

Specific components to enhance infection control include dedicated infection prevention and control professionals, appropriate staffing levels, clinical microbiology support, adequate supplies and equipment including ventilation systems, monitoring (including assessment and correction of system failures), and a feedback mechanism for HCW and administrators.[13–20] An institutional culture of safety is the shared commitment of the administration and HCW to ensure the safety of the work environment.[21,22]

Trauma: A Comprehensive Emergency Medicine Approach, eds. Eric Legome and Lee W. Shockley. Published by Cambridge University Press. © Cambridge University Press 2011.

A culture of safety encourages every individual to project a level of awareness and accountability for safety. The culture of safety has a direct bearing on the adherence to recommendations for transmission prevention and, in turn, adherence decreases transmission of infectious agents in healthcare settings.[21–26]

Box 37.1 Essentials of standard precautions

- Standard precautions are recommended for the care of all hospital patients.
- Standard precautions apply to blood and body fluids, non-intact skin, mucus membranes, and secretions and excretions (except sweat).
- Standard precautions entail proper hand hygiene, the use of PPE, and safe disposal of sharp instruments and proper decontamination techniques.

Infection transmission prevention: specific principles

There are two tiers of precautions to prevent transmission of infectious agents according to the CDC Healthcare Infection Control Practices Advisory Committee: (1) SP; and (2) transmission-based precautions (TBP).[27] Barrier protection devices such as gloves, gowns, masks, and eye protectants may be used for both SP as well as TBP.

Gloves

Gloves should be worn when there is a risk for direct contact with blood or body fluids, mucous membranes, non-intact skin, or other potentially infectious material, as well as when having direct contact with patients who are colonized or infected with pathogens transmitted via the contact route. Gloves manufactured for healthcare purposes are subject to the US Food and Drug Administration (FDA) evaluation and clearance.[28] Gloves should never be reused and must be changed between patients. Hand hygiene following glove use is recommended.

Gowns

Isolation gowns are used to protect the healthcare provider and their clothing from becoming contaminated with infectious material. Gowns should also be worn as part of contact precautions when the presence of excessive wound drainage, fecal incontinence, or the presence of other bodily fluids suggest an increased potential for contamination and transmission. Isolation gowns should be worn when exposure to blood and body fluids is likely, such as with trauma patients as part of SP.

Masks/eye protection

Exposure of mucous membranes of the eyes, nose, and mouth to blood and body fluids has been associated with the transmission of infectious agents to healthcare personnel.[29–32] The prevention of mucous membrane exposure to infectious agents by using personal protection equipment is part of SP for routine care of the major trauma patient.

Masks are used for three primary purposes in the healthcare setting: (1) to protect HCW from contact with infectious materials from patients such as respiratory secretions and sprayed blood or body fluids; (2) to protect patients during procedures requiring sterile technique from infectious agents possibly contained in the mouth or nose of a HCW; (3) placed on coughing patients to limit potential dissemination of infectious secretions as part of respiratory hygiene/cough etiquette. The routine surgical mask, while not adequate for some infectious airborne particles (e.g., N-95 is used for tuberculosis [TB] transmission), is appropriate for the major

---

Box 37.2 Barrier protection

Barrier	Common uses
Eye shields or goggles	Goggles and face shields add additional protection to the eyes from splashes, sprays, and respiratory droplets.
Gloves	Used when there is a risk for direct contact with blood or body fluids, mucus membranes, non-intact skin, or other potentially infectious material.
Masks	Used to protect from contact with infectious materials such as respiratory secretions and sprayed blood or body fluid, and to protect patients during procedures requiring sterile technique.
Gowns	Used to protect the healthcare provider and their clothing from becoming contaminated with infectious material.

trauma patient. Masks should not be confused with particulate respirators that are used to prevent inhalation of small particles that may contain infectious agents transmitted via the airborne route.

Goggles and face shields add additional protection to the eyes from splashes, sprays, and respiratory droplets. Personal eyeglasses without sideguards and contact lens are not considered adequate protection.

Standard precautions

Standard precautions should be applied to the care of all patients in all healthcare settings. Standard precautions also represent the primary strategy for the prevention of healthcare-associated transmission of infectious agents among patients and HCW. Implementation of SP includes hand washing before and after every patient contact, use of barrier precautions such as gloves, gowns, and masks/eye protection for patients with potential ability to cause contamination, safe handling of sharp instruments, and proper cleaning/disinfection and disposal of equipment or linens that have likely been contaminated. All spills of blood and blood-contaminated body fluids should be promptly cleaned by a person wearing gloves and using an Environmental Protection Agency-approved disinfectant or a 1 : 10 to 1 : 100 solution of household bleach. Visible material should first be removed with disposable towels or other means to prevent direct contact. The area should then be decontaminated with an appropriate disinfectant. Since 1991, training and implementation of UP as well as monitoring of compliance of PPE to prevent mucocutaneous exposures has been legally mandated by the Occupational Safety and Health Administration and by CMS.[33] Policies issued by the American College of Emergency Physicians and the American College of Surgeons Committee on Trauma endorse current CDC recommendations for SP.

Transmission-based precautions

Transmission-based precautions are used in addition to SP for patients who are known or suspected to be infected or colonized with infectious agents and which require additional control measures to effectively prevent transmission. Transmission-based precautions are used when the routes of transmission are not completely interrupted by SP and are divided into three categories: (1) contact precautions; (2) droplet precautions; and (3) airborne precautions. For some infectious agents, multiple routes of transmission are possible.

Contact transmission

Contact transmission (CT) is the most common mode of transmission and is divided into two groups: direct and indirect contact. Direct transmission occurs when microorganisms are transferred from one infected individual to another without a contaminated intermediate person or object. Indirect transmission involves the transfer of microorganisms through a contaminated person (e.g., HCW) or object. Contact precautions are intended to prevent transmission of infectious agents transmitted by direct or indirect contact.

Contaminated hands of HCW are important contributors of indirect infection transmission. Other examples include contaminated patient-care devices, shared clothing or toys, and components of PPE including laboratory coats, gowns, and uniforms. Hand hygiene is considered the single most important practice to reduce the transmission of infectious agents in healthcare settings. Its effectiveness has been demonstrated in multiple studies.[10,34,35] Hand washing should be considered essential when delivering care to the trauma patient.[22,36–39]

In the absence of visibly soiled hands, alcohol-based products for hand disinfection are preferred over soap and water because of their superior microbiocidal activity, convenience, and reduced drying of skin.[10] Easily accessible alcohol-based waterless hand disinfection agents have also been shown to improve hand washing compliance.[40,41]

Barrier protection with gloves, isolation gowns, and mucous membrane protectants are also an important component of contact precautions when there is concern for exposure to a microorganism potentially transmitted by HCW. Wearing gown and gloves prior to room entry and discarding before exiting should be done to contain pathogens. Barrier devices should also be worn as part of contact precautions when the presence of excessive wound drainage, fecal incontinence, or the presence of other bodily fluids suggests an increased potential for contamination and transmission such as the major trauma patient.

Respiratory transmission

Respiratory agents that emergency providers must consider include traditional and emerging respiratory pathogens including highly virulent and resistant strains as well as bioterrorism-related agents.[42]

637

Implementation of proper protocols can minimize infection transmission to hospital personnel and other patients (e.g., immunocompromised patients). The increasingly crowded nature of emergency departments (EDs) further elevates the risk of contagion. Healthcare facilities should have policies/procedures in place for respiratory control with operational plans for handling individual patients as well as large outbreaks.[43] While this is not generally a concern in the individual trauma, it may be reasonable to consider with bioterrorism or major disasters. Both the World Health Organization and the CDC provide general recommendations for handling of patients with suspected respiratory infections including proper hand hygiene and wearing face masks and eye protection.[41,43] The CDC recommends that tissues and masks as well as access to sinks or hand washing stations should be made readily available for all symptomatic patients who enter the ED. Respiratory transmission is generally divided into two groups: droplet transmission or airborne transmission.

Droplet transmission

Droplet transmission is technically a form of CT and some infectious agents that are transmitted via droplet transmission may also be transmitted via direct or indirect contact. Examples of infectious agents that are transmitted via the droplet route include *Bordetella pertussis*, influenza virus, adenovirus, rhinovirus, *Mycoplasma pneumoniae*, SARS-associated coronavirus, group A streptococcus, and *Neisseriea meningitides*.[44–49] Respiratory droplet transmission occurs when infectious agents travel directly from the respiratory tract of an infectious individual to susceptible mucosal surfaces of the recipient over short distances and can be generated when an infected individual coughs, sneezes, or talks as well as during procedures such as suctioning, endotracheal intubation, chest physiotherapy, and cardiopulmonary resuscitation.[50–56] Large particle droplets have traditionally been defined as being > 5 μm in size and are generally thought not to remain infective over long distances and, therefore, do not require special air handling and ventilation. Historically the area of defined risk has been a distance of ≤ 3 ft and is based on epidemiologic and simulated studies of selected infectious agents.[57,58] Experimental studies with smallpox and investigations during the 2003 global

SARS outbreaks suggest that droplets with these two infections could reach persons located six or more feet from the source patient.[59–61] It may be prudent to wear a mask when within 6–10 ft of suspected patients to ensure adequate protection.

Airborne transmission

Airborne transmission occurs by dissemination of small particles or droplet nuclei containing infectious agents capable of remaining infective over longer distances and times. Infectious agents in this category include Aspergillus species, *Mycobacterium tuberculosis*, rubeola virus, and varicella virus.[62–64]

Preventing the spread of pathogens that are transmitted via airborne transmission requires the use of special air handling and ventilation techniques to contain and safely remove the infectious agents with monitored negative air pressure.[65,66] Negative pressure isolation systems prevent contaminated air from traveling to other areas of the hospital, which is the most efficient method for containment of airborne respiratory pathogens. When the organism load is high, negative pressure rooms may not remove all pathogens and may need to be augmented by high efficiency particulate air (HEPA) filtration systems and/or ultraviolet lights. The performance of procedures that can generate small particle aerosols such as endotracheal intubation, bronchoscopy, and open suctioning of the respiratory tract has been associated with transmission of infectious agents to healthcare personnel. Use of a particulate respirator is recommended during aerosol-generating procedures and in general contact with patients suspected of *M. tuberculosis*, SARS, or avian or pandemic influenza viruses. Healthcare workers exposed to suspect individuals should wear CDC and Occupational Safety and Health Administration (OSHA) approved NIOSH certified N-95 or powered air-purifying respirators. These precautions generally do not apply to the trauma patient but should be kept in mind when treating a patient felt to be at higher risk, either by demographics or findings on examination or studies.

Blood-borne

Blood-borne exposures occur through needlesticks or other sharp instruments, or through contact of mucous membranes or non-intact skin with an affected patient's blood or blood containing bodily fluids. Healthcare workers delivering emergency care face a higher risk of exposure to blood-borne pathogens than in many other clinical settings. Surgeons and emergency providers in training incur a higher risk when considering the numerous encounters and propensity for error while learning new technical skills.[67-69] Patients seen in hospital EDs are, in general, at higher risk of being infected with a transmissible pathogen than the general population and HCW are often unaware of the patient's infectious disease serostatus.[70-73] Uncooperative and agitated patients secondary to injury, shock, or intoxication further increase the risk. The risk of blood-borne transmission of an infectious agent is dependent upon the frequency of important exposures, the prevalence of disease in the patient population, the concentration of the infectious pathogen in the implicated body fluid, the volume of infective material transferred, the route of inoculation, and the effectiveness of post-exposure treatment.[74]

Prevention of blood exposure through safe practices, barrier precautions, safe needle devices, and other innovations is the best way to prevent transmission of blood-borne pathogen transmission.[75] The Federal Needlestick Safety and Prevention Act, requiring the use of safer devices, became law in November 2000.[76] An 11-step process for the selection of sharps injury prevention devices is available from http://www.cdc.gov/sharpssafety/wk_operational_selection.html. A significant and sustained decrease in percutaneous injuries (up to 60%) has been associated with adoption and education of SP.[77-79]

Percutaneous injuries

Up to 800 000 needlestick and other percutaneous injuries are reported annually among US HCW.[80,81] According to one study, more than half of HCW have experienced percutaneous exposures to blood and body fluids.[82] The majority of these exposures are with hollow-bore needles. Infectious exposures can result in substantial health consequences and psychological stress for providers and their families and friends.[83] Injuries due to needles and other sharp instruments have been associated with transmission of at least 20 different blood-borne pathogens including hepatitis B virus (HBV), hepatitis C virus (HCV), and human immunodeficiency virus (HIV) to healthcare personnel.[32,75,84]

Hepatitis B

Hepatitis B is present in high titers in blood and serous fluids (up to 10^9 virons per milliliter), whereas the titer in semen, saliva, and vaginal secretions is generally 1000–10 000 times lower and very low in urine and feces uncontaminated with blood.[85-104] There is no known risk for HBV infection from exposure to intact skin. While HIV and HCV are susceptible to a variety of disinfectants and drying, HBV is resistant to drying, ambient temperatures, simple detergents, and alcohol and has been found to be stable on environmental surfaces for at least 7 days.[92-95] Since its availability in 1981, hepatitis B vaccine has been recommended to HCW with anticipated exposure to blood and/or body fluids. In 1991, OSHA issued a standard that required employers to offer the hepatitis B vaccine at no cost to employees with anticipated contact with blood or other infectious materials.[96] The rate of HBV transmission to susceptible HCW ranges from 6% to 30% after a single needlestick exposure, with the greatest risk when a source patient is HbeAg positive.[97] Hepatitis B transmission to HCW declined approximately 95% secondary to widespread immunization of HCW and the use of SP.[98] Post-exposure prophylaxis (PEP) with hepatitis B immune globulin and initiation of hepatitis B vaccine is more than 90% effective in preventing HBV infection. The incubation period for acute hepatitis B ranges from 45 to 160 days, with an average of 120 days.[99] Approximately one-third to one-half of persons with acute HBV virus develop symptoms of hepatitis including fever, nausea, abdominal pain, and jaundice. Most infections resolve, but approximately 5–10% of patients develop chronic infection that carries a 20% lifetime risk of dying from cirrhosis and a 6% risk of dying of liver cancer.[100]

Hepatitis C

Hepatitis C is the most common chronic blood-borne infection in the United States, affecting approximately 4 million people.[101] The seroprevalence rates in the general population are estimated to be 1.8% but higher numbers (2–18%) are estimated among hospitalized, emergency, and trauma patients, and as much as 20% among dialysis patients and 60–90% among hemophilia patients.[102-107] The rate of HCV seroconversion to HCW through a needlestick injury is 1.8% (range 0–10%) per injury based on prospective studies.[108] The risk of transmission following needle-stick exposure that contains HCV antibodies but not HCV RNA is close to zero. Hepatitis C risk after mucous membrane exposure is believed to be very small. There is no known risk with exposure to intact skin. The incubation period for acute hepatitis C infection ranges from 2 to 24 weeks, with an average of 6–7 weeks.[109] Hepatitis C often occurs with little or only mild symptoms, but active liver disease occurs in 70% of patients and chronic infection develops in 75–85% of patients. Of the patients with active liver disease, 10–20% develop cirrhosis and 1–5% develop liver cancer. Hepatitis C's RNA is a direct indicator of infection and can be detected in as little as 10 days after exposure.[110,111] Hepatitis C antibodies are detected within 6 months of most persons who become infected.[112] Testing for HCV antibodies and alanine aminotranferase (ALT) levels should be done in follow up within several days post-exposure and again at 4–6 months for HCW with percutaneous, mucosal, or non-intact skin exposure to blood or body fluids from a patient with HCV antibodies and/or HCV RNA. Although there is no PEP regimen for HCV, post-exposure testing of both the source patient, if known, and HCW can help guide further care. Interferon therapy may prevent chronic HCV infection when administered to patients with acute HCV infection.[113,114] In settings in which a more rapid detection may change clinical care, HCV RNA testing may be performed earlier than the usual 4–6 week post-exposure interval.

Human immunodeficiency virus

The percentage of HIV-positive patients in EDs and trauma centers based on studies from the late 1980s through 1993 range from 2.1% to 7.2%, with the highest seroprevalence rates in urban, inner-city populations.[115–119] Percutaneous injury, usually with a hollow-bore needle, is the most common mechanism for occupational HIV transmission.[120] The estimated rate of HIV transmission with a percutaneous injury is 0.3% (3/1000; 95% confidence interval [CI] 0.2–0.5%).[120–122] Findings in a case-control study of needlestick injuries suggest the risk of transmission likely exceeds 0.3% for percutaneous injuries involving a larger volume of blood and higher titers of HIV.[123] The risk after mucus membrane exposure is approximately 0.09% (95% CI 0.006–0.5%).[124] There are no reports of seroconversion with isolated intact skin exposure. There is no evidence that HIV can be transmitted via aerosolized particles. An exposure is defined as a percutaneous injury or contact of mucus membrane or non-intact skin with blood, tissue, or other potentially infectious body fluids including cerebrospinal fluid, synovial fluid, pleural fluid, peritoneal fluid, pericardial fluid, and amniotic fluid. Feces, nasal secretions, saliva, sputum, sweat, tears, urine, and vomitus are not considered infectious unless they are visibly bloody.

Management of HCW soon after exposure to blood or body fluid from HIV-infected patients is important in reducing the likelihood of infection. All institutions should have a readily available policy for managing exposures that should comply with the regulations of OSHA. Exposed HCW should have HIV antibody testing to determine baseline status. If possible, depending on ability, consent, and local legal considerations, the source patient should be tested as soon as practical. When considering PEP, the provider must consider the risk of infection with the risk of toxicity, inconvenience, and side effects of PEP therapy. Injuries may be classified as high-risk injuries if percutaneous injuries occur with a hollow-bore needle, injuries from a hollow-bore needle with visible blood on the device, or exposure to a needle that was in an artery or a vein of the source patient. Lower risk injuries are defined by exposure with a solid needle, superficial appearing, and occuring from a low-risk source patient such as a patient with an HIV viral load of < 1500 copies/ml. Mucocutaneous exposures are considered very low risk except if from large volumes of blood from an HIV-positive patient with a high viral load (> 1500 copies/ml).

Adherence to prevention standards

Despite the fact that prevention recommendations work, multiple studies have shown limited adherence to recommended practices and higher self-reported adherence than observed adherence. Observed adherence to SP have ranged from 43% to 89%.[125–132] The degree of adherence depends both on individual factors (knowledge, past experience, perception of risk) and institutional factors (safety climate, policies/procedures, education, and training). Adherence improvement requires the institution to incorporate infection control practices into the organization's safety culture and overall objectives. Reasons for individual HCW lack of adherence to precaution guidelines include the perception of a low-risk procedure or patient, time factors, interference with dexterity, and equipment not being readily available.[133] Non-adherence among HCW has also been associated with inadequate knowledge, forgetfulness, workload, workplace safety climate, and the perception that colleagues also failed to adhere.[134–140]

Multidrug resistant organisms

Multidrug resistant organisms (MDROs) are defined as microorganisms that are resistant to one or more classes of commercially available antimicrobial agents.[141] Multidrug resistant organisms include methicillin resistant *Staphylococcus aureus* (MRSA), vancomycin resistant enterococcus (VRE), multidrug resistant *Streptococcus pneumoniae* (MDRSP), multidrug resistant gram-negative bacilli (MDR-GNB), and vancomycin resistant *S. aureus* (VRSA).

Multidrug resistant organisms are transmitted by the same routes as antimicrobial sensitive infectious agents. Patient-to-patient transmission via hand carriage by HCW has been a major factor accounting for the increase in incidence and prevalence.[142–144] During the last several decades, the prevalence of MDROs in US hospitals and medical centers has increased steadily.[145] Multidrug resistant organisms have been associated with increased lengths of stay, costs, and mortality.[146] Once MDROs are introduced into a healthcare setting, transmission and persistence of the resistant strain is determined by the availability of vulnerable patients, selective pressure exerted by antimicrobial use, increased potential for transmission from larger numbers of colonized or infected patients, and the impact of implementation and adherence to prevention efforts.[147] There is epidemiologic evidence to suggest that MDROs are often transmitted via the hands of HCW.[148] Hands are easily contaminated during the process of caregiving or from contact with environmental surfaces in proximity to infected or colonized patients.[149]

Certain organisms are considered to be of special epidemiological importance. These organisms are characterized by the following: a propensity for transmission within healthcare facilities; resistance to first-line therapies; and an association with serious clinical disease. These organisms are of special concern because the mode of transmission is often suspected to be patient to patient via staff. Examples include *C. difficile*, norovirus, respiratory syncytial virus,

influenza, rotavirus, Enterobacter species, Serratia species, group A streptococcus, MRSA, and VRE.

Clostridium difficile is a spore forming gram-positive anaerobic bacillus that is the most common microbial causative agent of antibiotic associated diarrhea and pseudomembranous colitis. *Clostridium difficile* has been responsible for many large, difficult to control outbreaks in healthcare settings. Factors lending to outbreaks include environmental contamination, persistence of spores for a long period, resistance of spores to commonly used disinfectants and antiseptics, exposure of patients to courses of antimicrobial agents, and hand carriage by HCW to other patients.[150]

Prevention of transmission relies on accurate identification of patients, rigorous adherence to contact precautions with environmental cleaning using a bleach containing disinfectant (5000 ppm) and hand hygiene with soap and water rather than alcohol-based hand cleaners when applicable. In the trauma patient, this means that the usual SP should be followed and that prophylactic antibiotics without a clear basis, i.e., lacerations, should not be given.

Vancomycin-resistant Enterococcus (VRE) has emerged the past 10–15 years to become endemic in many healthcare facilities in the United States.[151] The bacteria usually reside in the intestine or genital tracts and are transmitted by HCW via CT with contaminated blood, urine, or feces of affected patients.[152] In 1995, the CDC published recommendations to prevent transmission of VRE including surveillance for identification, isolation of affected patients, hand washing by HCW, and environmental disinfection.[153]

Methicillin-resistant *Staphylococcus aureus* was first identified in 1961 and now accounts for over half of hospital-associated staphylococcal infections in intensive care units and over half of soft tissue and skin infections. Almost 1% of the US population is colonized with MRSA. Transmission may occur via direct contact or indirect contact (e.g., toys, towels, etc.). It can be divided into hospital-acquired MRSA and community-acquired MRSA, each with very distinct genetic elements leading to distinct resistance patterns. Hospital-acquired MRSA is resistant to multiple antibiotics and has been associated with greater hospital length of stays as well as increased mortality compared to MSRA.[154,155] Community-acquired MRSA is primarily important for skin and soft tissue infections that present in outpatient settings.

Post-exposure evaluation

Although prevention is the best strategy for protecting HCW from occupation transmission of infectious agents, exposures will occur. Institutions must have in place a protocol for evaluation, counseling, treatment, and follow up of occupational exposures as well as OSHA-compliant incident reporting and exposure control measures.[156,157] Access to clinicians who can provide post-exposure care should be available during all work hours. Prompt reporting is important, not only for management of the post-exposure HCW, but also to identify workplace hazards and to evaluate preventive measures.[158] Healthcare workers' orientation and education should include measures to prevent exposures, personal risk of occupational pathogen exposure, and the principles of post-exposure management including early reporting.[159] When reporting, the HCW should be evaluated and counseled regarding the risk of transmission, the potential usefulness of PEP for HIV and HBV, the need for follow-up evaluation, and precautions for secondary transmission during the follow-up period.[160] Cutaneous injuries should be washed with soap and water. Eyes and affected mucus membranes should be copiously irrigated. Local treatment with antiseptics, bleach, or other agents is not recommended.[161] Next, efforts to identify, evaluate, and test the source patient for evidence of HIV, HBV, and HCV should be undertaken. Finally, the circumstances of the exposure should be recorded including date, time, job duty, type of exposure including amount and type of fluid involved, type of device used, and severity of exposure.

Timely reporting of blood-borne pathogen exposure is required to ensure adequate counseling, prophylactic treatment, and establish legal prerequisites for workers' compensation.[162] The HIV, HBV, and HCV infections have implications for personal health, relationships, and insurance coverage.[163] Failure to report an occupational exposure could lead to the denial of subsequent insurance claims.[164] Counseling may also alleviate the anxiety associated with such exposures.[165]

A significant proportion (up to 60%) of percutaneous injuries are not reported.[166–170] Reasons cited for not reporting percutaneous exposures include time and inconvenience, the perception of no utility in reporting, and ignorance of to whom to report the incident.[152,171] Additional factors associated with under-reporting include exposures to physicians, mucocutaneous exposures, and a higher number of injuries.[172]

Post-exposure prophylaxis

If a needlestick exposure occurs the affected area should be washed with soap and water. If a mucous membrane was exposed it should be irrigated with clean water, saline, or sterile irrigants. No evidence suggests that washing with an antiseptic or squeezing the wound will reduce transmission. After the affected area has been washed or irrigated, the HCW should report to the department responsible for managing exposures.

Exposure to HBV poses a high risk for infection that can be somewhat ameliorated by vaccination and PEP. Recommendations for HBV post-exposure management include initiation of the hepatitis B vaccine series to any susceptible, unvaccinated person who sustains blood- or body-fluid exposure. Initiation of hepatitis B immune globulin depends on the source patient's hepatitis B surface antigen status and the antibody response of the affected HCW previously vaccinated with the hepatitis B vaccine series. A multiple dose regimen of HBIG in the occupational setting within 1 week of percutaneous exposure afforded an estimated 75% protection from HBV infection.[173] A combination of hepatitis B vaccination initiation and HBIG therapy after birth in perinatal exposure is 85–95% effective in preventing transmission.[174–175] Hepatitis B vaccine may be safely administered to infants, children, and adults. Common side effects include pain at the injection site and fever. Anaphylaxis is rare but may occur.

If post-exposure HIV prophylaxis treatment is recommended, baseline laboratory studies are drawn, although this can be done in early follow up. Deciding which agents and how many agents to use for PEP is primarily empiric and may be affected by known or suspected resistance of the source virus to particular antiviral agents. Post-exposure prophylaxis has been demonstrated to reduce risk of HIV transmission by approximately 80%, although the numbers of patients who seroconverted are small and the confidence intervals are wide.[176] The ideal HIV post-exposure prophylactic drug would have a high activity against the offending virus and a rapid onset of action. The selection of a drug regimen for HIV PEP must balance the risk of infection against the potential toxicities of the agents used. Because PEP therapy is potentially toxic, its use is not justified for exposures thought to pose a negligible risk of transmission. Most institutions have a pre-existing protocol for treatment. However, if the case is particularly complex, consultation with an infectious disease consultant or another healthcare provider with experience with antiretroviral agents is recommended. Post-exposure prophylaxis should be initiated when indicated as soon as possible, preferably within hours after exposure. While early treatment seems to lead to better outcomes, the absolute time that makes a difference is unclear. A general recommendation is to attempt to start treatment within 2 hours but continue to initiate treatment up to 36 hours after exposure. Some providers will treat up to 72 hours for very high-risk exposures. Rapid HIV testing of the source patient can facilitate making timely decisions regarding use of HIV PEP after occupational exposures to source patients with unknown HIV status.

Current CDC recommendations call for two or more drug PEP regimens based on the level of risk of HIV transmission represented by the type of exposure. Many institutions have a policy or recommendations to ensure proper risk assessment, prophylaxis regimen, and follow up. Persons receiving PEP should complete a full 4-week regimen unless the source patient can be tested and is negative. A reasonable current recommendation would be to use two-drug regimen and to add an additional drug for higher risk exposures, although some recommend a three-drug regimen for all patients. For *source patients with known HIV infection and if information regarding previous anti-retroviral therapy, current level of viral suppression, genotypic or phenotypic resistance profile is known*, standard PEP regimens may be inappropriate and expertise *in providing an unique PEP regimen* should be sought. In the US, assistance with choosing a drug regimen can be obtained by calling the National Clinician's Post-Exposure Prophylaxis Hotline at 888–448–4911. A substantial proportion (one third to one half) of persons taking PEP after occupational exposures to HIV-positive sources do not complete the full 4-week regimen because of side effects. Most side effects are mild and include nausea, fatigue, diarrhea, headache, and vomiting but serious side effects may occur which mandate reliable follow up. Human immunodeficiency virus serology should

be performed at baseline, 6 weeks, 12 weeks, 6 months, and 12 months post-exposure.[177] In patients who seroconvert after HIV exposure, the median time to the development of detectable antibody is 2.4 months with 95% of infected individuals developing detectable antibody within 6 months.[178] Patients receiving PEP should be monitored for drug toxicity with complete blood count including differential, hepatic, and renal function tests at baseline and 2 and 4 weeks after initiation of treatment. *These tests do not have to be done prior to first dose unless clinically indicated.* No work restrictions apply while taking PEP but medical attention should be sought for viral syndrome symptoms. Persons exposed to HIV should be urged to prevent secondary transmission by refraining from donating blood products, semen, tissue, or organs, to avoid pregnancy, refrain from breast feeding if possible, and to abstain from or use condoms during sexual intercourse, especially during the first 6–12 weeks when seroconversion is most likely.[179]

Vaccination and chemoprophylaxis for respiratory pathogens

The CDC currently recommends *annual* influenza vaccinations for HCW.[180] Research has demonstrated that influenza vaccination of HCW leads to decreased in-patient mortality. The US government has developed interim plans adopted by many institutions for vaccination plans for certain respiratory pathogens (e.g., anthrax and smallpox).

Under-appreciation of the risk of exposure is commonly reported as a contributor to exposure to infectious material. Standard precautions including gloves, gowns, and mucous membrane protection should be commonly worn when taking care of patients in whom there is a risk of exposure to blood or bodily fluids such as victims of trauma. Masks should be worn during endotracheal intubation, suctioning, bronchoscopy, and cardiopulmonary resuscitation as part of droplet precautions/standard precautions. The use of masks and gowns is also recommended during sterile procedures to protect patients. The US Department of Health and Human Services recommends that in outbreak settings for respiratory pathogens, aerosol-generating procedures and treatments, including nebulized medications, use of bilevel positive air pressure be avoided when possible.[181] When essential for patient care, HCW

643

Table 37.1 Overview of barrier protection recomendations in trauma

	Hand hygiene	Gloves	Gown	Mask	Eye protection	Respirator
All pts	X					
All trauma pts	X	X	X			
All penetrating trauma pts	X	X	X	X	X	
Intubation	X	X	X	X	X	X*
Central line†	X	X	X	X	X	
Chest tube†	X	X	X	X	X	
Suturing	X	X	X	X	X	

*Respirator indicated when suspicion for respiratory pathogen capable of airborne transmission.
†Optimally central lines and chest tubes should be done under sterile conditions, although immediacy of patient's condition may not allow this.
pts, patients

should use N-95 or powered air-purifying respirators as part of TBP during suspected respiratory pathogen outbreaks.

Special populations

Providers must ensure protection of themselves and their staff to ensure their own health and to ensure that further patient care can be provided. The lessons of the 2003 SARS outbreak highlighted this rule. It is tempting to treat unstable patients *without* SP for fear that the delay in therapy will impact the outcome. The amount of time taken to employ appropriate precautions is trivial in the overall scale of treatment delivery. Administrators and educators must enforce this message to care providers.

Pregnant patients and women who are breast feeding can receive the hepatitis B vaccine and immunoglobulin. Pregnancy should not rule out the use of PEP for HIV when indicated. Antiviral agents have been linked to fetal carcinogenicity, mutagenicity, neurologic abnormalities, and early death as well as lactic acidosis of pregnant women. Pregnant females should not receive efavirenz and tenofovir disoproxil fumarate. A negative pregnancy test or a signed consent form may be required in some institutions prior to initiating PEP in women of childbearing age. Ideally, an expert in HIV treatment or a high-risk obstetrician should help make PEP recommendations for pregnant females.[182]

Healthcare personnel and facilities confront a different set of issues when dealing with a HazMat or bioterrorism event. Providing medical care for patients potentially contaminated with hazardous material presents a complex situation. There are OSHA guidelines for HCW who may care for patients from HazMat incidents, including availability of protective equipment. The CDC has designated anthrax, smallpox, plague, tularemia, viral hemorrhagic fever, and botulism as high priority agents owing to their properties of ease of dissemination, transmission, and high risk of significant morbidity and mortality. Infection control issues in bioterrorism events include: identifying persons exposed/infected, preventing transmission, providing treatment, protecting the healthcare environment, providing adequate supplies of PPE, and allocating staff to care for potentially infectious patients. The CDC and the Association of Professionals in Infection Control and Epidemiology have published plans for bioterrorism events.[182] Federal agencies, state, and county health departments can also be consulted for the most current information.

Biological foreign body implantation

Physicians involved in the management of victims of blast injuries or explosions should be aware of the possibility of biological foreign bodies capable of transmitting of infection agents.[183] Such foreign bodies (e.g., bone fragments from suicide bombers) must be considered in the treatment of the victims. Care should also be taken to prevent exposure of this material to HCW during evaluation and treatment of wounds. Post-exposure prophylaxis against hepatitis B and HIV should be considered when treating patients with allogenic biological foreign bodies.[184]

References

1. Centers for Disease Control and Prevention. Recommendation for prevention of HIV transmission in health-care settings. *MMWR* 1987;**36**(2S):1S–18S.

2. Garner JS, Simmons BP. Guideline for isolation precautions in hospitals. *Infect Control* 1983;**4**:245–325.

3. Garner JS. Guideline for isolation precautions in hospitals. *Infect Control Hosp Epidemiol* 1996;**17**:53–80.

4. Centers for Disease Control and Prevention. Update: universal precautions for prevention of transmission of human immunodeficiency virus, hepatitis B virus, and other bloodborne pathogens in health-care settings. *MMWR* 1988;**37**:377–88.

5. IOM. Antimicrobial Resistance: Issues and Options. Workshop report. In: Harrison PF, Lederberg J, eds. Washington, DC: National Academy Press; 1998:8–74.

6. Shlaes DM, Gerding DN, John JF, Jr., et al. Society for Healthcare Epidemiology of America and Infectious Diseases Society of America Joint Committee on the Prevention of Antimicrobial Resistance: guidelines for the prevention of antimicrobial resistance in hospitals. *Infect Control Hosp Epidemiol* 1997;**18**(4):275–91.

7. Friedman C, Barnette M, Buck AS, et al. Requirements for infrastructure and essential activities of infection control and epidemiology in out-of hospital settings: a consensus panel report. Association for Professionals in Infection Control and Epidemiology and Society for Healthcare Epidemiology of America. *Infect Control Hosp Epidemiol* 1999;**20**(10):695–705.

8. Goldmann DA, Weinstein RA, Wenzel RP, et al. Strategies to prevent and control the emergence and spread of antimicrobial-resistant 178 microorganisms in hospitals. A challenge to hospital leadership. *JAMA* 1996;**275**(3):234–40.

9. Scheckler WE, Brimhall D, Buck AS, et al. Requirements for infrastructure and essential activities of infection control and epidemiology in hospitals: a consensus panel report. Society for Healthcare Epidemiology of America. *Infect Control Hosp Epidemiol* 1998;**19**(2):114–24.

10. Centers for Disease Control and Prevention. Guideline for hand hygiene in health-care settings: recommendations of the Healthcare Infection Control Practices Advisory Committee and the HICPAC/SHEA/APIC/IDSA Hand Hygiene Task Force. *MMWR* 2002;**51**(16)(RR-16):1–44.

11. Larson EL, Early E, Cloonan P, Sugrue S, Parides M. An organizational climate intervention associated with increased handwashing and decreased nosocomial infections. *Behav Med* 2000;**26**(1):14–22.

12. Pittet D, Hugonnet S, Harbarth S, et al. Effectiveness of a hospital-wide programme to improve compliance with hand hygiene. Infection Control Programme. *Lancet* 2000;**356**(9238):1307–12.

13. Jackson M, Chiarello LA, Gaynes RP, Gerberding JL. Nurse staffing and health care-associated infections: proceedings from a working group meeting. *Am J Infect Control* 2002;**30**(4):199–206.

14. O'Boyle C, Jackson M, Henly SJ. Staffing requirements for infection control programs in US health care facilities: delphi project. *Am J Infect Control* 2002;**30**(6):321–33.

15. Peterson LR, Hamilton JD, Baron EJ, et al. Role of clinical microbiology laboratories in the management and control of infectious diseases and the delivery of health care. *Clin Infect Dis* 2001;**32**(4):605–11.

16. McGowan JE, Jr., Tenover FC. Confronting bacterial resistance in healthcare settings: a crucial role for microbiologists. *Nat Rev Microbiol* 2004;**2**(3):251–8.

17. Curtis JR, Cook DJ, Wall RJ, et al. Intensive care unit quality improvement: a "how-to" guide for the interdisciplinary team. *Crit Care Med* 2006;**34**(1):211–18.

18. Pronovost PJ, Nolan T, Zeger S, Miller M, Rubin H. How can clinicians measure safety and quality in acute care? *Lancet* 2004;**363**(9414):1061–7.

19. Goldrick BA, Dingle DA, Gilmore GK, et al. Practice analysis for infection control and epidemiology in the new millennium. *Am J Infect Control* 2002;**30**(8):437–48.

20. Lundstrom T, Pugliese G, Bartley J, Cox J, Guither C. Organizational and environmental factors that affect worker health and safety and patient outcomes. *Am J Infect Control* 2002;**30**(2):93–106.

21. Moore D, Gamage B, Bryce E, Copes R, Yassi A. Protecting health careworkers from SARS and other respiratory pathogens: organizational and individual factors that affect adherence to infection control guidelines. *Am J Infect Control* 2005;**33**(2):88–96.

22. Tokars JI, McKinley GF, Otten J, et al. Use and efficacy of tuberculosis infection control practices at hospitals with previous outbreaks of multidrug-resistant tuberculosis. *Infect Control Hosp Epidemiol* 2001;**22**(7):449–55.

23. LeClair JM, Freeman J, Sullivan BF, Crowley CM, Goldmann DA. Prevention of nosocomial respiratory syncytial virus infections through compliance with glove and gown isolation precautions. *N Engl J Med* 1987;**317**(6):329–34.

24. Maloney SA, Pearson ML, Gordon MT, et al. Efficacy of control measures in preventing nosocomial

transmission of multidrug-resistant tuberculosis to patients and health care workers. *Ann Intern Med* 1995;**122**(2):90–5.

25. Montecalvo MA, Jarvis WR, Uman J, et al. Infection-control measures reduce transmission of vancomycin-resistant enterococci in an endemic setting. *Ann Intern Med* 1999;**131**(4):269–72.

26. Lynch P, Cummings MJ, Roberts PL, et al. Implementing and evaluating a system of generic infection precautions: body substance isolation. *Am J Infect Control* 1990;**18**(1):1–12.

27. Siegel JD, Rhinehart E, Jackson M, Chiarello L, Healthcare Infection Control Practices Advisory Committee. *Guideline for Isolation Precautions: Preventing Transmission of Infectious Agents in Healthcare Settings*. Available from http://www.cdc.gov/ncidod/dhqp/pdf/isolation2007/pdf.

28. Food and Drug Administration. *Medical Glove Guidance Manual*. Available from http://www.fda.gov/cdrh/dsma/gloveman/gloveman99.pdf.

29. Rosen HR. Acquisition of hepatitis C by a conjunctival splash. *Am J Infect Control* 1997;**25**(3):242–7.

30. Hosoglu S, Celen MK, Akalin S, et al. Transmission of hepatitis C by blood splash into conjunctiva in a nurse. *Am J Infect Control* 2003;**31**(8):502–4.

31. Keijman J, Tjhie J, Olde Damink S, Alink M. Unusual nosocomial transmission of *Mycobacterium tuberculosis*. *Eur J Clin Microbiol Infect Dis* 2001;**20**(11):808–9.

32. Do AN, Ciesielski CA, Metler RP, et al. Occupationally acquired human immunodeficiency virus (HIV) infection: national case surveillance data during 20 years of the HIV epidemic in the United States. *Infect Control Hosp Epidemiol* 2003;**24**(2):86–96.

33. Office of Occupational Health and Safety. Occupational exposures to bloodborne pathogens: final rule. *Federal Regist 1991; 29 CFR, part* 1910.**1030**:64004–64182.

34. Jarvis WR. Handwashing – the Semmelweis lesson forgotten? *Lancet* 1994;**344**(8933):1311–12.

35. Daniels IR, Rees BI. Handwashing: simple, but effective. *Ann R Coll Surg Engl* 1999;**81**:117–18.

36. Doebbeling BN, Stanley GL, Sheertz CT, et al. Comparative efficacy of alternative hand-washing agents in reducing nosocomial infections in intensive care units. *N Engl J Med* 1992;**327**:88–93.

37. Conly JM, Hill S, Ross J, Lertzman J, Louis TJ. Handwashing practices in an intensive care unit: the effects of an educational program and its relationship to infection rates. *Am J Infect Control* 1989;**17**:330–9.

38. Goldman DA, Freeman J, Durbin WA, Jr. Nosocomial infection and death in a neonatal intensive care unit. *J Infect Dis* 1983;**147**:635–41.

39. Bauer TM, Ofner E, Just HM, Just H, Daschner FD. An epidemiological study assessing the relative importance of airborne and direct contact transmission of microorganisms in a medical intensive care unit. *J Hosp Infect* 1990;**15**:301–9.

40. Bischoff WE, Reynolds TM, Sessler CN, et al. Handwashing compliance by health care workers. *Arch Intern Med* 2000;**160**:1017–21.

41. World Health Organization. *Hospital Infection Control Guidance for Severe Acute Respiratory Syndrome (SARS)*. Available from http://www.who.int/csr/sars/infectioncontrol/en.

42. Rothman RE, Irvin CB, Moran GJ, et al. Respiratory hygiene in the emergency department. *Ann Emerg Med* 2006;**48**:570–82.

43. Centers for Disease Control and Prevention. *Public Health Guidance for Community-Level Preparedness and Response to Severe Acute Respiratory Syndrome (SARS), Version 2, Supplement I, Section III: Infection Control In Healthcare Facilities*. Available from http://www.cdc.gov/ncidod/sars/guidance/I/healthcare.htm.

44. Musher DM. How contagious are common respiratory tract infections? *N Engl J Med* 2003;**348**(13):1256–66.

45. Steinberg P, White RJ, Fuld SL, et al. Ecology of *Mycoplasma pneumoniae* infections in marine recruits at Parris Island, South Carolina. *Am J Epidemiol* 1969;**89**(1):62–73.

46. Dick EC, Jennings LC, Mink KA, Wartgow CD, Inhorn SL. Aerosol transmission of rhinovirus colds. *J Infect Dis* 1987;**156**(3):442–8.

47. Scales D, Green K, Chan AK, et al. Illness in intensive-care staff after brief exposure to severe acute respiratory syndrome. *Emerg Infect Dis* 2003;**9**(10):1205–10.

48. Varia M, Wilson S, Sarwal S, et al. Investigation of a nosocomial outbreak of severe acute respiratory syndrome (SARS) in Toronto, *Canada*. *CMAJ* 2003;**169**(4):285–92.

49. Bridges CB, Kuehnert MJ, Hall CB. Transmission of influenza: implications for control in health care settings. *Clin Infect Dis* 2003;**37**(8):1094–101.

50. Papineni RS, Rosenthal FS. The size distribution of droplets in the exhaled breath of healthy human subjects. *J Aerosol Med* 1997;**10**(2):105–16.

51. Loeb M, McGeer A, Henry B, et al. SARS among critical care nurses, *Toronto*. *Emerg Infect Dis* 2004;**10**(2):251–5.

52. Fowler RA, Guest CB, Lapinsky SE, et al. Transmission of severe acute respiratory syndrome during

intubation and mechanical ventilation. *Am J Respir Crit Care Med* 2004;**169**(11):1198–202.

53. Gehanno JF, Kohen-Couderc L, Lemeland JF, Leroy J. Nosocomial meningococcemia in a physician. *Infect Control Hosp Epidemiol* 1999;**20**(8):564–5.

54. Ensor E, Humphreys H, Peckham D, Webster C, Knox AJ. Is *Burkholderia (Pseudomonas) cepacia* disseminated from cystic fibrosis patients during physiotherapy? *J Hosp Infect* 1996;**32**(1):9–15.

55. Christian MD, Loutfy M, McDonald LC, et al. Possible SARS coronavirus transmission during cardiopulmonary resuscitation. *Emerg Infect Dis* 2004;**10**(2):287–93.

56. Valenzuela TD, Hooton TM, Kaplan EL, Schlievert P. Transmission of "toxic strep" syndrome from an infected child to a firefighter during CPR. *Ann Emerg Med* 1991;**20**(1):90–2.

57. Feigin RD, Baker CJ, Herwaldt LA, et al. Epidemic meningococcal disease in an elementary-school classroom. *N Engl J Med* 1982;**307**(20):1255–7.

58. Dick EC, Jennings LC, Mink KA, Wartgow CD, Inhorn SL. Aerosol transmission of rhinovirus colds. *J Infect Dis* 1987;**156**(3):442–8.

59. Downie AW, Meiklejohn M, St Vincent L, et al. The recovery of smallpox virus from patients and their environment in a smallpox hospital. *Bull World Health Organ* 1965;**33**(5):615–22.

60. Fenner F, Henderson DA, Arita I, Jezek Z, Ladnyi ID. The epidemiology of smallpox. In Fenner F, Henderson DA, Arita I, Jezek Z, Ladnyi ID (eds), *Smallpox and Its Eradication*. Geneva, Switzerland: World Health Organization, 1988: pp. 169–209.

61. Wong TW, Lee CK, Tam W, et al. Cluster of SARS among medical students exposed to single patient, Hong Kong. *Emerg Infect Dis* 2004;**10**(2):269–76.

62. Bloch AB, Orenstein WA, Ewing WM, et al. Measles outbreak in a pediatric practice: airborne transmission in an office setting. *Pediatrics* 1985;**75**(4):676–83.

63. LeClair JM, Zaia JA, Levin MJ, Congdon RG, Goldmann DA. Airborne transmission of chickenpox in a hospital. *N Engl J Med* 1980;**302**(8):4503.

64. Riley RL, Mills CC, Nyka W, et al. Aerial dissemination of pulmonary tuberculosis. A two-year study of contagion in a tuberculosis ward. *Am J Hyg* 1959;**70**:185–96.

65. Centers for Disease Control and Prevention. Guidelines for environmental infection control in health-care facilities. Recommendations of CDC and the Healthcare Infection Control Practices Advisory Committee (HICPAC). *MMWR* 2003;**52**(RR10);1–42.

66. Centers for Disease Control and Prevention. Guidelines for preventing the transmission of *Mycobacterium tuberculosis* in health-care settings, 2005. *MMWR Recomm Rep* 2005;**54**(17):1–141.

67. Jagger J, Bentley M, Tereskerz P. A study of patterns and prevention of blood exposures in OR personnel. *AORN J* 1998;**67**:978–81.

68. Babcock HM, Fraser V. Differences in percutaneous injury patterns in a multi-hospital system. *Infect Control Hosp Epidemiol* 2003;**24**:731–3.

69. Tokars JI, Bell DM, Culver DH, et al. Percutaneous injuries during surgical procedures. *JAMA* 1992;**267**:2899.

70. Caplan ES, Preas MA, Kerns T, et al. Seroprevalence of human immunodeficiency virus, hepatitis B virus, hepatitis C virus, and rapid plasma regain in a trauma population. *J Trauma* 1995;**39**:533–7.

71. Kelen GD, Fritz S, Oaqish BF, et al. Unrecognized human immunodeficiency virus infection in emergency department patients. *N Eng J Med* 1988;**318**:1645–50.

72. Kelen GD, Green GB, Purcell RH, et al. Hepatitis B and hepatitis C in emergency department patients. *N Engl J Med* 1992;**326**:1399–404.

73. Schoenbaum EE, Webber MP. The underrecognition of HIV infection in women in an inner-city emergency room. *Am J Public Health* 1993;**83**:363–8.

74. Xeroulis G, Inaba, K, Stewart TC, et al. Human immunodeficiency virus, hepatitis B and hepatitis C seroprevalence in a Canadian trauma population. *J Trauma* 2005;**59**(1):105–8.

75. Centers for Disease Control and Prevention. Updated US Public Health Service guidelines for the management of occupational exposures to HBV, HCV, and HIV and recommendations for postexposure prophylaxis. *MMWR* 2001;**50**(RR-11):1–52.

76. Needlestick Safety and Prevention Act of 2000, Pub. L. No. 106–430, 114 Stat. 1901, *November 6, 2000*.

77. Beekman SE, Vlahow D, Koziol DE, et al. Temporal association between implementation of universal precautions and a sustained, progressive decrease in percutanous exposures to blood. *Clin Infect Dis* 1994;**18**:562–9.

78. Fahey BJ, Koziol DE, Banks SM. Frequency of nonparental occupational exposures to blood and body fluids before and after universal precautions training. *Am J Med* 1991;**90**:145–53.

79. Haiduven DJ, Demaio TM, Stevens DA. A five-year study of needlestick injuries: significant reduction associated with communication, education, and convenient placement of sharps containers. *Infect Control Hosp Epidemiol* 1992;**13**:265–71.

80. Occupational safety: selected cost and benefit implications of needlestick prevention devices for

647

hospitals. Washington, DC: General Accounting Office, November 17, 2000 (GAO–01–60R).

81. NIOSH Alert: preventing needlestick injuries in health care settings. Washington, DC: National Institute for Occupational Safety and Health, 1999; 2000–108.

82. Hersey JC, Martin LS. Use of infection control guidelines by workers in healthcare facilities to prevent occupational transmission of HBV and HIV: results from a national survey. *Infect Control Hosp Epidemiol* 1994;**15**:243–52.

83. Worthington MG, Ross JJ, Bereron EK. Posttraumatic stress disorder after occupational HIV exposure: two cases and a literature review. *Infect Control Hosp Epidemiol* 2006; **27**:215–17.

84. Collins CH, Kennedy DA. Microbiological hazards of occupational needlestick and 'sharps' injuries. *J Appl Bacteriol* 1987;**62**:385–402.

85. Hoffnagle JH. Hepatitis B. In Haubrich WS, Schaffner F, Berk JE (eds), *Gastroenterology*, 5th edn. Philadelphia, PA: WB Saunders, 1994: pp. 2062–3.

86. Jenison SA, Lemon SM, Baker LN, et al. Quantitative analysis of hepatitis B virus DNA in saliva and semen of chronically infected homosexual men. *J Infect Dis* 1987;**156**:299–307.

87. Centers for Disease Control. Lack of transmission of hepatitis B to humans after oral exposure to hepatitis B surface antigen-positive saliva. *MMWR* 1978;**27**:247–8.

88. Villarejos VM, Visona KA, Guitierrez A. Role of saliva, urine and feces in the transmission of type B hepatitis. *N Engl J Med* 1974;**291**:1374–8.

89. Di Bisceglie AM, Dusheiko GM, Kew MC. Detection of markers of hepatitis B virus infection in urine of chronic carriers. *J Med Virol* 1985;**16**:337–41.

90. Feinman SV, Berris B, Rebane A, et al. Failue to detect hepatitis B surface antigen (HbsAG) in feces of HbsAg-positive persons. *J Infect Dis* 1979:**140**:407–10.

91. Irwin GR, Allen AM, Bancroft WH, et al. Hepatitis B antigen in saliva, urine and stool. *Infect Immun* 1975;**11**:142–5.

92. Sattar SA, Springthorpe VS. Survival and disinfectant inactivation of the human immunodeficiency virus. *Rev Infect Dis* 1991;**13**:430–47.

93. Van Bueren J, Simpson RA, Jacobs P, et al. Survival of human immunodeficiency virus in suspension and dried onto surfaces. *J Clin Microbiol* 1994;**32**:571–4.

94. Cuypers HTM, Bresters D, Winkel IN, et al. Storage conditions of blood samples and primer selection affect yield of cDNA polymerase chain reaction products of hepatitis C virus. *J Clin Microbiol* 1992;**30**:3320–4.

95. Pattison CP, Boyer KM, Maynard JE, et al. Epidemic hepatitis in a clinical laboratory: possible association with computer card handling. *JAMA* 1974;**230**:854–7.

96. US Department of Labor Occupation Safety and Health Administration. 29 CFR part 1910.1030. Occupational exposure to bloodborne pathogens: final rule. *Fed Regist* 1991;**56**:64004–182.

97. Centers for Disease Control and Prevention. Immunization of health care workers: recommendations of the Advisory Committee on Immunization Practices and the Hospital Infection Control Practices Advisory Committee. *MMWR* 1997;**46** (RR-18):1–42.

98. Occupational Safety and Health Administration. Preamble-bloodborne pathogens (**29** CFR 1910.1030).

99. Beltrami EM, Williams IT, Shapiro CN, Chamberland ME. Risk and management of blood-bourne infections in health care workers. *Clin Micribiol Rev* 2000;**13**:385–407.

100. Shapiro CN. Occupational risks of infection with hepatitis B and hepatitis C virus. *Surg Clin North Am* 1995;**75**;1047–56.

101. CDC Recommendations for prevention and control of hepatitis C virus infection and HCV-related chronic disease. *MMWR* 1998:**47**(RR-19):1–39.

102. Alter MJ, Kruszon-Moran D, Nainan DV, et al. The prevalence of hepatitis C virus infection in the United States, 1988 through 1994. *N Engl J Med* 1999;**341**:556–61.

103. Kelen GD, Green GB, Purcell RH, et al. Hepatitis B and hepatitis C in emergency department patients. *N Engl J Med* 1992;**326**:1399–404.

104. Henein M, Lloyd L. HIV, hepatitis B, hepatitis C in the code one trauma population. *Am Surg* 1997;**63**:657–8.

105. Louie M, Low DE, Feinman SV. Prevalence of bloodborne infective agents among people admitted to a Canadian hospital. *Can Med Assoc J* 1992;**146**:1331–4.

106. Alter MF, Mast EE. The epidemiology of viral hepatitis in the United States. *Gastroenterol Clin N Am* 1994;**23**:437–55.

107. Kaplan AJ, Zone-Smith LK, Hannegan C, Norcross ED. The prevalence of hepatitis C in a regional Level I trauma center population. *J Trauma* 1992;**33**:126–9.

108. Sulkowski MS, Ray SC, Thomas DL. Needlestick transmission of hepatitis C. *JAMA* 2002;**287**:2406–13.

109. Koretz RL, Brezina M, Polito AJ, et al. Non-A, non-B posttransfusion hepatitis: comparing C and non-C hepatitis. *Hepatology* 1993;**17**:361–5.

110. Farci P, Alter HJ, Wong D, et al. A long-term study of hepatitis C virus replication in non-A, non-B hepatitis. *N Eng J Med* 1991;**325**:98–104.

111. Prince AM, Brotman B, Inchauspe G, et al. Patters and prevalence of hepatitis C virus infection in posttransfusion non-A, non-B hepatitis. *J Infect Dis* 1993;**167**(6):1296–1301.

112. Villano SA, Vlahov D, Nelson NE, et al. Persistence of viremia and the importance of long-term follow-up after acute hepatitis C infection. *Hepatology* 1999;**29**:908–14.

113. Jaeckel E, Cornberg M, Wedemeyer H, et al. Treatment of acute hepatitis C with interferon alfa-2b. *N Engl J Med* 2001;**345**:1452–7.

114. Lampertico P, Rumi M, Romeo R, et al. A multi-center randomized controlled trial of recombinant interferon-alpha2b in patients with acute transfusion-associated hepatitis C. *Hepatology* 1994;**19**:19–22.

115. Tardiff K, Marzuk PM, Leon AC, et al. Human immunodeficiency virus among trauma patients in New York City. *Ann Emerg Med* 1998;**32**:151–4.

116. Kelen D, DiGiovanna T, Bisson L, et al. Human immunodeficiency virus infection in emergency department patients. *JAMA* 1989;**262**:516–22.

117. Orr MD, Hoos A, Reister DE, et al. HIV-1 infection in patients with penetrating trauma in San Antonio, Texas. *JAMA* 1989;**262**:1629.

118. Baker JL, Gabor KD Sivertson KT, et al. Unsuspected human immunodeficiency virus in critically ill emergency patients. *JAMA* 1987;**257**:2609.

119. Nagachinta T, Gold CR, Cheng F, et al. Unrecognized HIV-1 infection in inner-city emergency department patients. *Infect Control Hosp Epidemiol* 1996;**17**:174–7.

120. Gerberding JL. Occupational exposure to HIV in health care settings. *N Engl J Med* 2003;**348**:826–33.

121. Bell DM. Occupational risk of human immunodeficiency virus infection in healthcare workers: an overview. *Am J Med* 1991;**102**(Suppl. 5B):9–14.

122. Ippolito G, Puro V, Heptonstall J, et al. Occupational human immunodeficiency virus infection in health care workers: worldwide cases through September 1997. *Clin Infect Dis* 1999;**28**:365–83.

123. Cardo DM, Culver DH, Ciesielski CA, et al. A case control study of HIV seroconversion in health care workers after percutaneous exposure. *N Eng J Med* 1997;**337**:1485.

124. Ippolito G, Puro V, De Carli G, et al. The risk of occupational human immunodeficiency virus infections in health care workers. *Arch Intern Med* 1993;**153**:1451–8.

125. Kelen GD, Green GB, Hexter DA, et al. Substantial improvement of compliance with universal precautions in an emergency department following institution of policy. *Arch Intern Med* 1991;**151**:2051–6.

126. Kelen GD, DiGiovanna TA, Celentano DD, et al. Adherence to Universal (barrier) Precautions during interventions on critically ill and injured emergency department patients. *J Acquir Immune Defic Syndr* 1990;**3**(10):987–94.

127. Huff JS, Basal M. Universal precautions in emergency medicine residencies. *Ann Emerg Med* 1989;**18**:798.

128. Baraf LJ, Talan DA. Compliance with universal precautions in a university hospital emergency department. *Ann Emerg Med* 1989;**18**:654–7.

129. Courington KR, Patterson SL, Howard RJ. Universal precautions are not universally followed. *Arch Surg* 1991;**126**(1):93–6.

130. DiGiacomo JC, Hoff WS, Rotondo MF, et al. Barrier precautions in trauma resuscitation: real-time analysis utilizing videotape review. *Am J Emerg Med* 1997;**15**(1):34–9.

131. Helfgott AW, Taylor-Burton J, Garcini FJ, Eriksen NL, Grimes R. Compliance with universal precautions: knowledge and behavior of residents and students in a department of obstetrics and gynecology. *Infect Dis Obstet Gynecol* 1998;**6**(3):123–8.

132. Moore S, Goodwin H, Grossberg R, Toltzis P. Compliance with universal precautions among pediatric residents. *Arch Pediatr Adolesc Med* 1998;**152**(6):554–7.

133. Henry K, Campbell S, Maki M. A comparison of observed and self-reported compliance with universal precautions among emergency department personnel at a Minnesota public teaching hospital. *Ann Emerg Med* 1992;**21**:940–6.

134. Becker MH, Janz NK, Band J, et al. Nonadherence with universal precautions: why do physicians and nurses recap needles? *Am J Infect Control* 1990;**18**:232–9.

135. Diekema DJ, Albanese MA, Schuldt SS, Doebbeling BN. Blood and body fluid exposures during clinical training: relation to universal precautions knowledge. *J Gen Intern Med* 1996;**11**:109–11.

136. Evanoff B, Kim L, Murtha S, et al. Adherence with universal precautions among emergency department personnel caring for trauma patients. *Ann Emerg Med* 1999;**33**:160–5.

137. Gershon RR, Karkashian CD, Grosch JW, Murphy LR. Hospital safety climate and its relationship with safe work practices and workplace exposure incidents. *Am J Infect Control* 2000;**28**:211–21.

138. Michalsen A, Delclos GL, Felknor SA, et al. Adherence with universal precautions among physicians. *J Occup Environ Med* 1997;**39**:130–7.

139. Dejoy DM, Searcy CA, Murphy LR, Gershon RR. Behavioral diagnostic analysis of adherence with

universal precautions among nurses. *J Occup Health Psychol* 2000;5:127–41.

140. Ferguson KJ, Waitzkin H, Beekman SE, Doebbeling BN. Critical incidents of nonadherence with standard precautions guidelines among community hospital-based health care workers. *J Gen Intern Med* 2004;**19**:726–31.

141. Institutes of Medicine. Antimicrobial resistance: issues and options. Workshop report. In Harrison PF, Lederberg J (eds), *Forum on Emerging Infections*. Washington, DC: National Academy Press, 1998: pp. 8–74.

142. Blok HE, Troelstra A, Kamp-Hopmans TE, et al. Role of healthcare workers in outbreaks of methicillin-resistant *Staphylococcus aureus*: a 10 year evaluation from a Dutch university hospital. *Infect Control Hosp Epidemiol* 2003;**24**(9):679–85.

143. Muto CA, Jernigan JA, Ostrowsky BE, et al. SHEA guideline for preventing nosocomial transmission of multidrug-resistant strains of Staphylococcus aureus and enterococcus. *Infect Control Hosp Epidemiol* 2003;**24**(5):362–86.

144. Tammelin A, Klotz F, Hambraeus A, Stahle E, Ransjo U. Nasal and hand carriage of *Staphylococcus aureus* in staff at a department for thoracic and cardiovascular surgery: endogenous or exogenous source? *Infect Control Hosp Epidemiol* 2003;**24**(9):686–9.

145. Klevens RM, Edwards JR, Tenover FC, et al. Changes in the epidemiology of methicillin-resistant *Staphylococcus aureus* in intensive care units in US hospitals, 1992–2003. *Clin Infect Dis* 2006;**43**(3):387–8.

146. Song X, Srinivasan A, Plaut D, Perl TM. Effect of nosocomial vancomycin-resistant enterococcal bacteremia on mortality, length of stay, and costs. *Infect Control Hosp Epidemiol* 2003;**24**(4):251–6.

147. Siegel JD, Rhinehart E, Jackson M, et al. *Management of Multidrug-resistant Organisms in Healthcare Settings*, 2006. Available from http://www.cdc.gov/ncidod/dhqp/pdf/ar/MDROGuideline2006.pdf.

148. Duckro AN, Blom DW, Lyle EA, et al. Transfer of vancomycin-resistant enterococci via health care worker hands. *Arch Intern Med* 2005;**165**:302–7.

149. Bhalla A, Pultz NJ, Gries DM, et al. Acquisition of nosocomial pathogens on hands after contact with environmental surfaces near hospitalized patients. *Infect Control Hosp Epidemiol* 2004;**25**:164–7.

150. McFarland LV, Mulligan ME, Kwok RY, Stamm WE. Nosocomial acquisition of *Clostridium difficile* infection. *N Engl J Med* 1989;**320**(4):204–10.

151. Centers for Disease Control and Prevention. Nosocomial enterococci resistance to vancomycin – United States, 1989–1993. *MMWR* 1993;**42**:597–9.

152. Rosenthal E, Pradier C, Keita-Perse O, et al. Needlestick injuries among French medical students. *JAMA* 1999; **281**:1660.

153. Hospital Infection Control Practices Advisory Committee. Recommendations for preventing the spread of vancomycin resistance: recommendations of the Hospital Infection Control Practices Advisory Committee (HICPAC). *MMWR* 1995;**44**(RR–12):1–13.

154. Noskin GA, Rubin RJ, Schentag JJ, et al. The burden of *Staphylococcus aureus* infections on hospitals in the United States: an analysis of the 2000 and 2001 Nationwide Inpatient Sample Database. *Arch Intern Med* 2005;**165**:1756–61.

155. Cosgrove SE, Qi Y, Kaye KS, et al. The impact of methicillin resistance in *Staphylococcus aureus* bacteremia on patient outcomes: mortality, length of stay, and hospital charges. *Infect Control Hosp Epidemiol* 2005;**26**:166–74.

156. U.S Department of Labor Occupation Safety and Health Administration. 29 CFR Part 1901.1030. Occupational exposure to blood borne pathogens: final rule. *Red Regist* 1991; **56**:64004–182.

157. Centers for Disease Control and Prevention. Public Health Service statement on management of occupational exposure to human immunodeficiency virus, including considerations regarding zidovudine postexposure use. *MMWR* 1990;**39**(RR-1):1–14.

158. Beltrami EM, Williams IT, Shapiro CN, et al. Risk and management of blood-borne infections in health care workers. *Clin Microbiol Rev* 2000;**13**:385–407.

159. Gerberding JL. Management of occupational exposures to bloodborne viruses. *N Engl J Med* 1995;**332**:444–51.

160. Centers for Disease Control and Prevention. Public Health Service statement on management of occupational exposure to human immunodeficiency virus, including considerations regarding zidovudine postexposure use. *MMWR* 1990;**39**(RR-1):1–14.

161. Cardo DM, Castro KG, Polder JA, et al. Management of occupational exposures to HIV. In Schochetman G, George JR (eds), *AIDS Testing: A Comprehensive Guide to Technical, Medical, Social, Legal, and Management Issues*, 2nd edn. New York: Springer-Verlag, 1994: pp. 361–75.

162. Osborn EH, Papadakis MA, Gerberding JL. Occupational exposures to body fluids among medical students: a 17-year longitudinal study. *Ann Intern Med* 1999;**130**:45–51.

163. Perry J, Jagger J. Lessons from an HCV-infected surgeon. *Bull Am Coll Surg* 2002;**87**:8–13.

164. Tereskerz PM, Jagger J. Occupationally acquired HIV: the vulnerability of health care workers under

workers' compensation laws. *Am J Public Health* 1997;**87**:1558–62.

165. Sohn JW, Kim SH, Han C. Mental health of healthcare workers who experience needlestick and sharps injuries. *J Occup Health* 2006;**48**:474–9.

166. Centers for Disease Control and Prevention. Evaluation of safety devices for preventing percutaneous injuries among health-care workers during phlebotomy procedures-Minneapolis-St. Paul, New York City, and San Francisco, 1993–1995. *MMWR* 1997;**46**:20–5.

167. Hamory BH. Underreporting of needlestick injuries in a university hospital. *Am J Infect Control* 1983;**11**:174–7.

168. Mangione CM, Gerberding JL, Cumings SR. Occupational exposure to HIV: frequency and rates of underreporting of percutaneous and mucocutaneous exposures by medical housestaff. *Am J Med* 1991;**90**:85–90.

169. McGeer A, Simor AE, Low DE. Epidemiology of needlestick injuries in house officers. *J Infect Dis* 1990;**162**:961–4.

170. O'Neil TM, Abbott AV, Radecki SE. Risk of needlesticks and occupational exposures among residents and medical students. *Arch Intern Med* 1992;**152**:1451–6.

171. Makary MM, Al-Attar A, Holzmueller CG, et al. Needlestick injuries among surgeons in training. *N Engl J Med* 2007;**356**:2693–9.

172. Doebbeling BN, Vaughn TE, McCoy KD, et al. Percuteous injury, blood exposure, and adherence to standard precautions: are hospital-based health care providers still at risk? *Clin Infect Dis* 2003;**15**:1006–13.

173. Grady GF, Lee VA, Prince AM, et al. Hepatitis B immune globulin for accidental exposures among medical personnel: final report of a multicenter controlled trial. *J Infect Dis* 1978;**138**:625–38.

174. Beasley RP, Hwang L-Y, Lee GC-Y, et al. Prevention of perinatally transmitted hepatitis B virus infections with hepatitis B immune globulin and hepatitis B vaccine. *Lancet* 1983;**2**:1099–102.

175. Stevens CE, Toy PT, Tong MJ, et al. Perinatal hepatitis B virus transmission in the United States: prevention by passive-active immunization. *JAMA* 1985;**253**:1740–5.

176. Cardo DM, Culver DH, Ciesielski CA, et al. A case-control study of HIV seroconversion in health care workers after percutaneous exposure. *N Engl J Med* 1997;**337**:1485–90.

177. Panililio AL, Cardo DM, Grohskopf LA, et al. Updated US Public Health Service guidelines for the management of occupational exposures to HIV and recommendations for postexposure prophylaxis. *MMWR Recomm Rep* 2005;**54**:1.

178. Busch MP, Satten GA. Time course of viremia and antibody seroconversion following human immunodeficiency virus exposure. *Am J Med* 1997;**102** (Suppl. 5B):117–24.

179. Centers for Disease Control and Prevention. Public Health Service guidelines for the management of health-care worker exposures to HIV and recommendations for postexposure prophylaxis. *MMWR* 1998;**47**(RR-7):1–34.

180. Centers for Disease Control and Prevention. *Updated Interim Influenza Vaccination Recommendations: 2004–2005 Influenza Season.* Available from http://www.cdc.gov/flu/protect/whoshouldget.htm.

181. US Department of Health and Human Services. *HHS Pandemic Influenza Plan: Supplement 4: Infection Control: Personal Protective Equipment For Special Circumstances.* Available from http://www.hhs.gov/pandemicflu/plan/sup4.html.

182. Association of Professionals in Infection Control Bioterrorism Task Force. Bioterrorism readiness plan: a template for health care facilities. *Surg Serv Manage* 1999;**5**:43–54.

183. Wong JM, Marsh D, Abu-Sitta G, et al. Biological foreign body implantation in victims of the London July 7th suicide bombings. *J Trauma* 2006;**60**:402–4.

184. Health Protection Agency. *Post Exposure Prophylaxis Against Hepatitis B for Bomb Victims and Immediate Care Providers. Considerations of Other Blood Borne Viruses (Hepatitis C and HIV).* Available from http://hpa.org.uk/explosions/BBV.htm.

38

Prehospital care

Aaron Eberhardt and Christopher B. Colwell

Introduction

From an historical prospective, the prehospital administration of medical care is a relatively new concept. While most emergency practitioners believe that the delivery of medical care in the prehospital setting has led to increased survival for patients, the practice of Emergency Medical Services (EMS) remains controversial. Core EMS practices such as airway management and trauma care are being questioned and continually refined. Emergency Medical Services is entering a time of self-assessment and paradigm shift never before seen its history.

The mix of tradition and progress in EMS has led to ever-increasing complexity in the medical administration and management of prehospital medical care. Perhaps even more challenging then the medical issues currently facing prehospital care is the overwhelming complexity of personnel management, politics, and funding that affect the delivery of evidence-based, outcome-oriented prehospital medical care.

Prehospital trauma systems

The delivery of prehospital medical care to the trauma patient is one component of the trauma care systems within the United States.[1] The development of trauma care systems has led to the need for developing appropriate trauma destination policies and optimal ambulance staffing.

The development of trauma care systems has led to trauma center categorization. The American College of Surgeons Committee on Trauma periodically publishes criteria guidelines for the categorization of levels of trauma care (Table 38.1). Based on hospitals' availability of resources, staffing, and research commitment they are categorized from Level I (providing

Table 38.1 American College of Surgeons trauma center levels: general overview of criteria

Level	General principles
I	Regional resource trauma center. Should be able to provide for all aspects of care. In addition should have a teaching, research, and community outreach component. Usually have medical education component associated
II	Can provide initial definitive care, regardless of severity of injury. Can be located in suburban or urban area. May provide leadership when Level I center unavailable
III	Serves communities that do not have immediate access to higher level care. Can provide prompt assessment, resuscitation, and possible transfer. Have general surgeons available along with transfer and resuscitation protocols
IV	Provide advance level trauma support in rural or remote areas prior to transport. May be a clinic. Physicians may not be available at all times

the most comprehensive care) to Level IV (providing the least comprehensive care). Depending on the size of the community, all or none of these types of hospitals may be available. Destination policies and protocols are therefore extremely varied depending on the availability of local hospital resources and the ability to transfer to a more definitive care facility.

In systems with only one hospital within a reasonable transport distance the destination for trauma victims is straightforward. Systems in which there are multiple levels of care possible need to develop more complex destination protocols to guide prehospital personnel in the transport of the trauma patient. The development of destination protocols involves a number of considerations including patient condition, the potential for injury based on mechanism, and the options for trauma care within the system. Factors considered in destination policies include anatomic considerations, physiologic factors, mechanism of injuries, combinations thereof, and high-risk modifying conditions such as extremes of age and advanced pregnancy. In 2005, the Centers for Disease Control and Prevention (CDC) put together a National Expert Panel on Field Triage (NEPFT) which made recommendations on determining the most appropriate destination facility within a trauma care system. These were evidence-based recommendations that updated those initially made by the American College of Surgeons in 1986. In January of 2009 the CDC published these guidelines for the field triage of trauma patients. These guidelines help to clarify which patients should be transported to a Level I facility and which patients can be safely triaged to facilities with a lower designation.[2] Most destination protocols for trauma patients will be some variation on this algorithm. Their recommendations are summarized in Table 38.2.[2]

Given the great diversity of practice environments and constraints on each individual EMS system the optimal ambulance staffing will also vary greatly from one EMS system to the next. Large urban EMS systems will have very different staffing needs than smaller rural-based systems. Emergency Medical Technicians (EMTs) are largely credentialed to one of three levels. EMT-Basic (EMT-B) undergo over 120 hours of training that generally focuses on basic life support (BLS) treatment and intervention including cardiopulmonary resuscitation (CPR), non-invasive airway support such as bag-valve-mask, hemorrhage control, and immobilization. Obtaining EMT-B certification is a prerequisite for becoming an Emergency Medical Technician-Intermediate or Paramedic (EMT-I and EMT-P).

The next level of EMT provider is EMT-I. The training is approximately 300–500 hours more then EMT-B. An EMT-I will have all of the EMT-B skills as well as a list of more advanced skills and knowledge that are largely dictated by local protocol. The EMT-I will usually be trained in endotracheal intubation and intravenous (IV) line placement. An EMT-I will have a number of medications that are available to him or her; however, the list will not be nearly as comprehensive as the list of medications that a full EMT-P has available.[3]

Paramedics (EMT-P) complete between 750 and 1500 hours of training above EMT-B level. Paramedics have extensive training in advanced skills including patient assessment and management, pharmacology, and advanced airway interventions. The exact nature of the scope of practice for each level will be determined by local and state regulations.

The overall staffing pattern of a premedical system is based on few parameters. First, the type of providers on each ambulance should be considered. This will largely be determined by the availability of providers and the needs within an individual system. For instance, training and retaining a paramedic can be expensive and smaller agencies may not have the funding to employ a large number of paramedics. In this instance it may make sense to mix crews (one EMT-P with one EMT-B or I) or to have increased numbers of EMT-B and EMT-I providers. Second, consideration needs to be given to the number of each type of provider practicing within the system in order to maintain a certain baseline proficiency in the provider's skill sets. Evidence suggests that systems with too many paramedics may have worse outcomes in cardiac arrest.[4] This may be due to the fact that the paramedics in some systems are not seeing enough cases to maintain good practical skills since the fixed number of encounters is spread over larger numbers of providers.

Western Europe has a number of well-developed EMS systems, the large majority of which are not associated with fire services. Traditionally, many of these countries have relied on physicians to provide prehospital care, although many are now moving to tiered response schemes that involve greater use of non-physician medical providers. Many dispatch systems in Western Europe also use more aggressive screening methods and prioritization of calls that might direct some patients away from ambulance transport and towards alternative sites for care.

Non-ambulance transport

The air medical transport system involves the use of aircraft to transport and care for patients. Air medical transport is a well-established part of the modern trauma system. While early literature described a benefit in patient outcomes by using helicopters to transport trauma patients,[5–7] more recent literature has called this benefit into question.[8–10]

Table 38.2 Criteria established by the National Expert Panel on Field Triage for transport by Emergency Medical Services (EMS) directly to a trauma center when available[2]

Physiologic criteria	Glasgow Coma Scale score < 14
	Systolic blood pressure < 90 mmHg
	Respiratory rate of < 10 of > 29 breaths/min in adults or < 20 in children < 1 year of age
Anatomic criteria	All penetrating injuries to the head, neck, torso, and extremities proximal to the elbow and knee
	Flail chest
	Two or more proximal long bone fractures
	Crushed, degloved, or mangled extremity
	Amputation proximal to the wrist or ankle
	Pelvic fractures
	Open or depressed skull fractures
	Paralysis
Mechanism criteria	Falls
	1. Adults: > 20 ft
	2. Children (< 15 years old): > 10 ft or 2–3 times the child's height
	Auto accidents
	1. Intrusion > 12 inches to the occupant site of > 18 inches anywhere
	2. Ejection (partial or complete)
	3. Death in the same passenger compartment
	Auto–pedestrian or auto–bike accidents where the victim is thrown, run-over, or there is significant impact (> 20 mph) Motorcycle accidents involving speeds of > 20 mph
Special considerations	Age > 55 or < 15 years
	Anticoagulation and bleeding disorders
	Burns
	1. Without other trauma: to a burn center
	2. With other trauma: to a trauma center
	Time sensitive extremity injury
	End-stage renal disease requiring dialysis
	Pregnancy > 20 weeks or
	EMS provider judgment

The American College of Emergency Physicians publication *Principles of EMS Systems* summarizes the goal of air medical transport. An air medical system should "provide critical care medical transport that results in similar or better patient outcome over a larger geographic area than can be achieved by ground transport during the same elapsed time."[3] In order to achieve this goal it is imperative that the physician and EMS personnel understand the capabilities and limitations of the EMS and air medical system in which they operate. An understanding of the available services that the air medical transport team can provide, the time in which they can provide these services, and the limits on both care and transport need to be appreciated.

The use of air medical transport of the trauma patient largely falls into two categories: interfacility transfer and the transport of patients from the scene to a trauma center. Interfacility air medical transport is an integral part of regionalized trauma care. Fixed-wing and helicopter transfer of patients has made specialty trauma services available to a wider range of patients within a region. The benefit of air medical transfer is to extend the trauma management of patients over longer distances or to areas that are inaccessible by ground.[3]

Rural EMS systems have a number of unique aspects that make helicopter transport from the scene potentially advantageous. Rural systems may have fewer hospitals with fewer resources covering a wide geographical region. This leads to prolonged travel distance and therefore prolonged time to reach a definitive care site. Air medical transport provides a solution to these constraints. In these situations, helicopters may allow for trauma patients to reach a hospital more quickly than is possible by ground transport.

Helicopter transport within urban or suburban EMS systems is more controversial. The main issue facing urban EMS helicopter use is the proper utilization of the service. Numerous guidelines exist that attempt to establish the criteria needed to activate a helicopter response.[11,12] Several studies indicate that helicopter transport within urban systems is largely over-utilized for the transport of non-critical patients.[10,13] While a certain amount of "overtriage" may be acceptable in the prehospital setting, this can lead to increased cost of medical care and risk to patients and providers that may not be necessary. Bledsoe et al. performed an observational meta-analysis of peer-reviewed literature regarding helicopter transport of trauma patients.[13] By analyzing studies that used validated criteria for identifying non-critical patients they showed that approximately 60–69% of patients transported by helicopter had relatively minor injuries. Additionally they found that approximately one in four patients transported by helicopter did not require hospital admission.[13] Eckstein et al. came to a similar conclusion for children and adolescents.[10]

An important consideration in the over-utilization of helicopter transport is the concern about safety. Baker et al. reviewed EMS helicopter crashes over a 22-year period and found a 39% fatality rate during these accidents.[14] A more disturbing finding is that the fatality rate appears to be getting worse.[14] These studies call into question how to appropriately use helicopters for the treatment and transport of trauma patients within an urban EMS system. The issue is compounded by the fact that helicopter transport is significantly more expensive than ground transport. The identification of the subset of patients that would benefit from helicopter transport should remain the focus of further research. The EMS system personnel and medical directors must work to develop protocols and guidelines that emphasize the appropriate use of helicopter transport.

Box 38.1 Essential literature in helicopter transport

- Ringburg AN, deRonde G, Thomas SH, et al. Validity of helicopter Emergency Medical Services dispatch criteria for traumatic injuries: a systemic review. *Prehosp Emerg Care* 2009;**13**:28–36.
- Eckstein M, JantosT, Kelly N, et al. Helicopter transport of pediatric trauma patients in an urban Emergency Medical Services system: a critical analysis. *J Trauma* 2002;**53**:340–4.
- Bledsoe BE, Wesley, KA, Eckstein M, et al. Helicopter scene transport of trauma patients with non-life-threatening injuries: a meta-analysis. *J Trauma* 2006;**60**:1257–66.
- Baker SP, Grabowski JG, Dodd RS, et al. EMS helicopter crashes: what influences fatal outcome? *Ann Emerg Med* 2006;**47**:351–6.

Direct patient care

Historically ambulances were largely transportation vehicles that brought injured patients from the accident scene or battlefield to hospitals or other healthcare facilities. Little actual medical care took place in the ambulance. Over the past few decades the practice of prehospital medicine has evolved considerably. Now paramedics can provide a variety of medical interventions in the field. In the prehospital management of the trauma patient, there are multiple interventions that fall within the scopes of practice of the EMT and paramedic. As the practice of prehospital medical care continues to evolve, the utility of these interventions should be analyzed and refined to improve patient outcomes. A complete review of all the possible interventions for the trauma patient is beyond the scope of this chapter; however, airway management, cervical spine immobilization, IV access, splinting, and pain control are among the most commonly performed prehospital interventions.

Airway management of the trauma patient

Airway management of a trauma patient is an important skill for all prehospital providers. The prehospital provider must be adept at a number of different ways of managing the airway that are commensurate with the provider's level of training. Airway management can range from simple maneuvers such as repositioning the airway (chin lift) and applying oxygen, to non-invasive assisted ventilation or airway adjuncts, to the definitive management of the airway with endotracheal intubation or surgical cricothyroidotomy.

The appropriate manner in which to manage the airway of a trauma patient can be a difficult decision. The provider needs to understand his or her own skill level, the patient's needs given the level of physiological distress, and the appropriate airway intervention for that patient in the prehospital setting. In general, the least invasive method should be employed that yields adequate oxygenation and ventilation.

Traditionally, paramedics have performed out-of-hospital endotracheal intubation as the airway of choice for definitive airway management in the trauma patient. A majority of the historical data on the benefits and side effects largely rely on paramedic self-reporting of their field experience. More recent literature has called this practice into question. In 2000, Gausche et al. reported the effect of out-of-hospital pediatric intubation on critically injured children.[15] This article showed that the addition of out-of-hospital endotracheal intubation to a paramedic scope of practice that already includes the bag-valve-mask did not improve survival to discharge or neurological status at discharge. Subgroup analysis further showed an increase in mortality of patients in respiratory arrest and victims of non-accidental trauma as well as worse neurological outcome in patients suffering from foreign body aspiration. Some research involving adult patients has raised concerns as well. In a study published in 2007 by Cudnick et al., prehospital intubation was associated with increased mortality among trauma victims at all distances from the hospital.[16] In the San Diego Paramedic Rapid Sequence Intubation Trial, paramedic rapid sequence intubation (RSI) in severely head injured patients was associated with increased mortality and decreased "good" outcomes.[17] This was compared to historical controls within the same system.

A number of studies have also documented a significant number of complications with out-of-hospital endotracheal intubation. In 2001 Katz et al.

documented that 25% of the patients evaluated had improperly placed endotracheal tubes, of which 67% were in the esophagus.[18] In 2003, Dunford et al. used recording oximeters throughout the course of prehospital rapid sequence intubation attempts.[19] In this evaluation, 57% of trauma victims receiving RSI endotracheal intubation demonstrated desaturation. The median time of desaturation in these patients was 2 minutes and 40 seconds with a mean decrease in saturation of 22% from baseline.

Although there are studies that have found better rates of successful intubation in the field, no definitive research has found endotracheal intubation by field providers to improve outcomes. With this in mind, medical directors and EMS systems should carefully evaluate the use of prehospital intubation in trauma patients. Prolonging scene times and engaging in multiple attempts to accomplish this procedure may well be harmful. It is possible that there is a subset of trauma patients that benefit from out-of-hospital endotracheal intubation, especially those with prolonged transport times.

Cervical spine immobilization

Cervical spine immobilization is one of the most frequently utilized prehospital interventions performed on trauma patients. This is despite a lack of Class I or II medical evidence to support the use of cervical spine immobilization in patients following trauma.[20] While ethical constraints will likely never allow rigorous clinical trials to establish Class I or II evidence, it is generally accepted that patients with known cervical injury or a mechanism with the potential for cervical injury should receive spinal immobilization. While spinal immobilization is very common it does carry some risks to the patient. Immobilization causes back and head pain, can cause skin breakdown on pressure points if a patient is immobilized for prolonged periods, and can limit effective breathing. As with all medical decisions, a risk–benefit analysis should be done when considering spinal immobilization. The primary concern is for the pathological movement of the spinal cord during the prehospital evaluation and transport of a patient. This is exemplified historically by the significant percentage of spinal cord injuries that are estimated to occur after the initial injury either during the transport of the patient or early in the patient's evaluation.[21–25] There are a number of case series that chronicle the poor outcomes of mishandled cervical spine injuries.[24–27] With these considerations in mind, there are a few aspects of spinal immobilization that need to be considered including the indications to immobilize the cervical spine in the prehospital setting and the most appropriate method of performing this procedure.

No universal indications for prehospital cervical spinal immobilization currently exist. The EMS agencies will generally have their own established protocols that range from complete immobilization of all trauma victims with a potential of cervical spine injury, to the EMS provider evaluating certain clinical parameters and making a decision in the field about the necessity of cervical spine immobilization (also called selective immobilization). Domeier et al. reported on a protocol for selective spine immobilization by EMS personnel based on five clinical assessment parameters.[28] By applying this protocol, they reported 91% sensitivity with a 40% specificity to detect spinal column or cord injuries.[28] While this study provided reasonable evidence that prehospital evaluation for cervical spine injury is feasible with a reasonable degree of certainty, it should be stressed that it was not 100% sensitive and there were a number of patients that did not receive cervical spine assessment when indicated. This exemplifies the fact that it is difficult to get strict compliance to a protocol. Given the high medicolegal risk of a missed cervical spine injury, a conservative policy is advocated.

There have been numerous studies performed looking at the best way to immobilize the spine. The historical practice of immobilizing the cervical spine with sandbags and tape alone may not be effective. A combination of a rigid cervical collar, supportive blocks on each side of the head, and a rigid backboard with straps for securing the patient is the most effective means of limiting spinal movement after a traumatic injury.[29]

Intravenous access

Traditionally prehospital personnel have started IVs in the upper limbs or external jugular vein (if authorized) as a peripheral line site. While no good patient outcome data exists to support this practice, it is generally accepted that the trauma patient should receive at least one (and in many cases two) large bore peripheral IV line in a timely manner. This should be balanced by the potential for prolonging transport times and the questionable efficacy and necessity of prehospital fluid resuscitation. Risks of line placement include infection, infiltration, and pain resulting from placement attempts. Having early IV access can be valuable in the resuscitation of the trauma patient, especially in the case of developing hemorrhagic shock when severe vasoconstriction can make the procedure much more difficult and time consuming. Guisto and Iserson have demonstrated that paramedics can place a 12-gauge IV line approximately 84% of the time.[30]

Splinting

Although orthopedic extremity injuries are commonly encountered in the prehospital setting, there is little Class I evidence to support the use of splinting in the field. On the other hand, splinting of traumatic orthopedic injuries is generally believed to provide a number of benefits: decreased pain, tissue damage, blood loss, and possibly fatty embolism.

In the case of open fractures, splinting may be further advantageous. By applying gentle traction and placement of a splint, the ellipse created by an opening in the skin from a fracture will become more linear. This will have the effect of providing less room for bleeding to occur and may lead to faster tamponade of the bleeding site. This measure may have a significant impact if bleeding is potentially severe, such as with femur fractures.

Pelvic fracture can lead to life-threatening hemorrhage in the trauma patient. Historically, military anti-shock trousers (MASTs)/pneumatic anti-shock garments (PASGs) immobilization devices were used in an attempt to stabilize the fractured pelvic ring and tamponade and reduce associated bleeding. Now it is generally advocated that unstable pelvic fractures in the trauma patient may be secured with sheet immobilization or pelvic binders in order to reduce the potential of life-threatening bleeding.

Pain control

A number of studies suggest that emergency physicians as well as prehospital personnel fail to adequately assess and treat pain.[31] Both the Joint Commission and the American College of Emergency Physicians have clearly identified the assessment and treatment of pain as a major priority.[32,33] The National Association of EMS Physicians (NAEMSP) have extended this priority into the prehospital setting, stating in a 2003 policy statement that "the relief of pain and suffering of patients must be a priority of every emergency medical services (EMS) system."[34]

Given this extensive national attention, it is important for protocols to be in place that address the treatment of pain in the prehospital trauma patient. The NAEMSP policy statement outlines a number of aspects of protocol development felt necessary when considering the development of a pain protocol.[34]

Box 38.2 NAEMSP recommended aspects of a pain protocol

- Presence and severity of pain
- Use of a reliable tool for this assessment
- Indications and contraindications for pain management
- Non-pharmacological interventions
- Pharmacological interventions
- Patient monitoring
- Communication of appropriate information to receiving medical personnel
- Quality improvement measures

Non-pharmacological management of pain in the prehospital setting is fairly limited; however, there are some simple interventions that can be employed. Methods include therapeutic communication, splinting, elevation of injured limbs, and applications of cryotherapy to painful musculoskeletal injuries.

Pharmacological management of pain in the prehospital setting is more complex. The guidelines listed above indicate that, after the recognition of pain, a reliable tool should be employed to measure the pain level and to follow the effect of the pain medication. The three most widely described tools to assess pain are the Visual Analog Scale (VAS), the Numeric Rating Scale (NRS), and the Verbal or Adjective Rating Scale. Several sources endorse the NRS for use in the prehospital setting.[31,34]

The ideal agent for pain control in the prehospital setting is unclear. A number of narcotic and non-narcotic agents have been used. For the trauma patient with significant pain, opiates have emerged as a safe and effective means of managing pain. Limited data exists for the prehospital administration of opiates for trauma patients. Morphine has many advantages for the prehospital setting. It can be used IV or intramuscularly (IM). When used IV it has a

relatively quick onset of action and a half-life of 2–3 hours.[31] An added benefit to the use of morphine is the ability to reverse unwanted respiratory depression side effects with the use of naloxone if necessary. Historically there has been reluctance to use morphine secondary to fears of respiratory depression and hypotension.[34] With more experience, morphine has been shown to be relatively safe. In 2007 a randomized, double-blinded study with 106 patients compared low dose to higher dose morphine for the treatment of pain. The dose of 0.1 mg/kg IV followed by 0.05 mg/kg every 5 minutes showed better pain control at 10 minutes than the lower dose of 0.05 mg/kg morphine then 0.025 mg/kg every 5 minutes.[35] At 30 minutes the pain control was similar. Given the results of this study, if pain control is desired during transport the higher dose may be given. This study also demonstrated relatively few side effects, concluding that this dosing regimen is "safe in the prehospital setting."[35]

Fentanyl is a synthetic opiate that has some significant advantages for use in the prehospital setting. Fentanyl is more potent, has a faster onset of action, and less histamine release than morphine. Like morphine, undesired respiratory depression can be reversed with naloxone. These features have a theoretical advantage for EMS use in which transport times are relatively short and fast pain control is desired. These advantages were evaluated in one study in which Fentanyl was compared with morphine for acute pain control in the prehospital setting.[36] This randomized, double-blinded trial failed to show a significant difference in pain control in transport times of < 30 minutes, stating that morphine and Fentanyl were "comparable" in treating acute pain. The most serious side effect that has been described with Fentanyl use is chest wall rigidity that requires paralysis in order to ventilate the patient.[31] This is exceedingly rare.

Multitrauma/incident command

All EMS systems should have plans that address the response to incidents that involve multiple patients; also referred to as Multiple Casualty Incidents (MCIs). This may or may not be considered a "disaster." A disaster is defined as any situation that overwhelms a system's resources to respond to that situation and therefore a disaster for one system (eight victims of a motor vehicle accident in a rural area with a single hospital not resourced to take eight patients at once), might not qualify as a disaster in another (urban area with multiple trauma centers). Initial evaluation of the scene is important. An accurate initial assessment will mobilize appropriate resources without overcommitting assets that could risk response to other areas or responsibilities. A good initial assessment will determine the nature of the incident, extent of the damage that occurred, approximate number of victims and types of injuries involved, any hazards rescuers face, and best access to the scene. Once this assessment is performed, this information will need to be communicated to a centralized communication center or regional trauma center.

The next priority for those responding first to an incident will be the organization of a command post. The Incident Command System (ICS) is a standard emergency management system and a very effective way of establishing operational control and a coordinated response to a multiple casualty incident. It is adaptable to all types of incidents that may involve multi-agency or multi-jurisdictional response. There are five sections of the ICS structure: incident command, operations, planning, logistics, and finance.

Once the command post has been established, triage can begin. Triage is the process of sorting and classifying patients based upon the severity of their injuries and the likelihood of survival. The goal of triage is to do the most good for the greatest number of patients. If the potential exists for the incident to qualify as a disaster, responders must assume they will not have enough resources to provide standard care for all victims, and therefore the triage process will help determine priority for treatment and transport from the scene. Although the triage process may occur at or near the scene of an incident, in some situations the scene may be too dangerous and it is best performed some distance from the scene and maybe even at a hospital.

Triage categories generally include red (critical), who receive the highest priority for treatment and transport, yellow (moderate), who are treated and transported after all patients designated as red have been cared for, and green (walking wounded), who are treated after reds and yellows have been managed. There is also a black (expectant) category that may be appropriate in some situations, which includes patients who are either dead or are not expected to survive their injuries. Lessons learned from responses to MCIs have included the importance of performing triage of all patients before initiating treatment, insuring all responders understand the incident command structure, communication from the scene, and the importance of appropriate use of resources, staging of vehicles, and identification of responders. A well-identified and recognized command presence at a scene, and at the hospital as well, will help to ensure a coordinated and cooperative response that will promote effective management.

Protocol development

The development of a set of written protocols is one of the core responsibilities of a medical director and can be very challenging. Because EMTs are certified and not licensed, they must operate under the oversight of a licensed medical provider. Protocols establish the standards EMTs are expected to meet and provide under specific circumstances, and generally focus on direct patient care, while policies and procedures tend to address operational and other nonclinical situations. Protocols have been developed to address most any situation, although the nature of emergency care is such that, as complete as a set of protocols may be, situations will arise where actions that fall outside of the protocols will need to be considered. This is where on-line medical direction can play an important role. Protocols will typically have a set of standing orders that specify specific actions, treatments, or other approaches providers may take without making direct contact with a physician. They will also typically specify what can be done in addition to the standing orders with a direct order from on-line medical control. Although some protocols can be written based on guidelines established by national experts (Advanced Cardiovascular Life Support [ACLS] is an example of this), others will be more system specific or may have little in terms of evidence to base them on. Protocols for an EMS system should be written by medical directors that are knowledgeable on best evidence-based practices but also on system-specific as well as area-specific issues and challenges. For example, protocols that address destination decisions based on specialized services provided by some hospitals (such as trauma centers) are very appropriate for urban systems that transport to a number of different facilities, but don't have much of a role in rural areas which may only have a single hospital available to transport to.

Writing a protocol is only one step in the process of implementing a new protocol. Critical to successful implementation is providers understanding why a protocol is written and what the intended goal is. Communication and education are key steps in the process. A good protocol will need to be flexible and be able to adapt to changing needs in a system.

Conclusions

Prehospital care of the trauma patient continues to be a process in evolution. Prehospital care plays an important role in the overall care of the trauma patient, and quality assurance systems with input from all involved will help to ensure optimal outcomes. Research is continuing to refine the role of prehospital interventions in the care of the trauma patient, and EMS leaders will need to stay current on this literature to ensure their practice is leading to better outcomes in their patients.

References

1. Peterson TD, Mello MJ, Broderick C, et al. *ACEP White Paper – Trauma Care Systems*. Dallas, TX: American College of Emergency Physicians, 2003.

2. Centers for Disease Control and Prevention. Trauma triage guidelines. *MMWR* 2009;**58**:1–35.

3. Brennan JA. *Principles of EMS Systems*. Boston, MA: Jones and Bartlett, 2006.

4. *Acad Emerg Med* 2006 **13**(5):Supplement 1.

5. Crowely RA, Hudson F, Scala E, et al. An economical and proved helicopter program for transporting the emergency critically-ill and injured patient in Maryland. *J Trauma* 1973;**13**:1029–38.

6. Baxt WG, Moody P. The impact of rotorcraft aeromedical emergency care service on trauma mortality. *JAMA* 1983;**249**:3047–51.

7. Baxt WG, Moody P, Cleveland HC, et al. Hospital-based rotorcraft aeromedical emergency care services and trauma mortality: a multicenter study. *Ann Emerg Med* 1985;**14**:859–64.

8. Cunningham P, Rutledge R, Baker CC, et al. A comparison of the association of helicopter and ground ambulance transport with the outcome of injury in trauma patients transported from the scene. *J Trauma* 1997;**43**:940–6.

9. Shatney CH, Homan SJ, Shreck JP, Ho CC. The utility of helicopter transport of trauma patients from the injury scene in an urban trauma system. *J Trauma* 2002;**53**:817–22.

10. Eckstein M, Jantos T, Kelly N, et al. Helicopter transport of pediatric trauma patients in an urban emergency medical services system: a critical analysis. *J Trauma* 2002;**53**:340–4.

11. Association of Air Medical Services. Position paper on the appropriate use of emergency air medical services. *J Air Med Transp* 1990;**9**(9):29–30, 32–3.

12. Air Medical Physicians Association. Medical condition list and appropriate use of air medical transport. *Prehosp Emerg Care* 2002;**6**:464–70.

13. Bledsoe BE, Wesley KA, Eckstein M, et al. Helicopter scene transport of trauma patients with nonlife-threatening injuries: a meta-analysis. *J Trauma* 2006;**60**:1257–66.

14. Baker SP, Grabowski JG, Dodd RS, et al. EMS helicopter crashes: what influences fatal outcome? *Ann Emerg Med* 2006;**47**:351–6.

15. Gausche M, Lewis RJ, Stratton SJ, et al. Effect of out-of-hospital pediatric intubation on survival and neurological outcome: a controlled clinical trial. *JAMA* 2000;**283**(6):783–90.

16. Cudnik MT, Newgard CG, Wang H, et al. Distance impacts mortality in trauma patients with an intubation attempt. *Prehosp Emerg Med* 2006;**12**(4):459–66.

17. Davis DP, Hoyt DB, Ochs M, et al. The effect of paramedic rapid-sequence intubation on outcome in patients with severe traumatic brain injury. *J Trauma* 2003;**54**:444–53.

18. Katz SH, Falk JL. Misplaced endotracheal tubes by paramedics in an urban emergency medical services system. *Ann Emerg Med* 2001;**37**(1):32–7.

19. Dunford JV, Davis DP, Ochs M, et al. Incidence of transient hypoxia and pulse rate reactivity during paramedic rapid-sequence intubation. *Ann Emerg Med* 2003;**42**:721–8.

20. Hadley MN, Walters BC, Grabb PA, et al. Guidelines for the management of acute cervical spine and spinal cord injuries. *Clin Neurosurg* 2002;**49**:407–98.

21. Brunette D, Rockswold G. Neurological recovery following rapid spinal realignment for complete cervical spinal cord injury. *J Trauma* 1987;**27**:445–7.

22. Burney RE, Waggoner R, Maynard FM. Stabilization of spinal injury for early transfer. *J Trauma* 1989;**29**:1497–9.

23. Geisler W, Wynne-Jones M, Jousse AT. Early management of the patient with trauma to the spinal cord. *Med Serv J Can* 1966;**22**:512–23.

24. Prasad VS, Schwartz A, et al. Characteristics of injuries to the cervical spine and spinal cord in the polytrauma patient population: experience from a regional trauma unit. *Spinal Cord* 1999;**37**:560–8.

25. Totten VY, Sugarman DB. Respiratory effects of spinal immobilization. *Prehosp Emerg Care* 1999;3:347–52.

26. Bohlman HH. Acute fractures and dislocations of the cervical spine: an analysis of three hundred hospitalized patients and review of the literature. *J Bone Joint Surg Am* 1979;**61**:1119–42.

27. Jeanneret B, Magerl F. Over distraction: a hazard of skull traction in the management of acute injuries of the cervical spine. *Arch Orthop Trauma Surg* 1991;**110**:242–5.

28. Domeier RM, Frederiksen SM, Welch, K. Prospective performance assessment of out-of-hospital protocol for selective spine immobilization using clinical spine clearance criteria. *Ann Emerg Med* 2005; **46**(2):123–31.

29. American College of Surgeons Committee on Trauma. *Advanced Trauma Life Support for Doctors: ATLS®️ Manual*, 7th edn. Chicago, Il: American College of Surgeons, 2004.

30. Guisto JA, Iserson KV. The feasibility of 12-gauge intravenous catheter use in the prehospital setting. *J Emerg Med* 1990;**8**(2):173–6.

31. McManus JG, Jr., Sallee DR, Jr. Pain management in the prehospital environment. *Emerg Med Clin N Am* 2005;**23**:415–31.

32. Joint Commission on Accreditation of Healthcare Organizations. *Comprehensive Accreditation Manual for Hospital, the Official Handbook*. Chicago, IL: JCAHO, 1998.

33. American College of Emergency Physicians. Clinical policy for procedural sedation and analgesia in the emergency department. *Ann Emerg Med* 1998;**31**:663–77.

34. Alonso-Serra HM, Wesley K, for the National Association of EMS Physicians Standards and Clinical Practices Committee. Position paper: prehospital pain management. *Prehosp Emerg Care* 2003; 7(4):482–8.

35. Bounes V, Charpentier S, Houze-Cefron CH, et al. Is there an ideal morphine dose for prehospital treatment of acute severe pain? A randomized, double-blind comparison of two doses. *Am J Emerg Med* 2008;**26**:148–54.

36. Galinski M, Dolveck F, Borron SW, et al. A randomized double-blind study comparing morphine with fentanyl in prehospital analgesia. *Am J Emerg Med* 2005;**23**:114–19.

Professionalism

Erica Kreisman and Lewis Goldfrank

Professionalism

The scope of professionalism is a broad one, encompassing that which guides us as human beings and governs us as physicians. Plato described the virtues of fortitude, temperance, justice, and wisdom. Aristotle related these virtues to the art of medicine stating that we must not only know virtue but we must also be good and do good. Edmund Pellegrino, a physician–ethicist stated that:

> The special claim of professionhood, of "learned professions". . . lies in their dedication to something other than self-interest while providing their services. That something else is a certain degree of altruism or suppression of self-interest when the welfare of those they serve requires it. This is the distinguishing feature of medicine, ministry, law and teaching that sets them apart. They are in this sense "professed," i.e., publicly committed to the welfare of those who seek their help. They thereby become ethical enterprises.[1]

And therein lies the crux of professionalism; a synthesis of knowledge, understanding of good, commitment to the public, and willingness for self-sacrifice.

Prehospital

In the the United States, at this time, there exists in excess of 45 million uninsured persons.[2] In 1986 Congress mandated access to emergency care when it passed the Emergency Medicine Treatment and Labor Act (EMTALA). This legislation was passed to prevent the unethical denial of emergency care based solely on an inability to pay. By passing this law, Congress, in effect, established a safety-net for our millions of uninsured, presumably made necessary because of "unethical" behavior of healthcare providers and the lack of organization of a universal healthcare system. While EMTALA addresses the fundamental behavior and interventions of physicians once a patient arrives in the Emergency Department (ED), the patient's relationship with the healthcare system begins in prehospital interaction. There is a limited amount of literature describing the nuances of the ethics of ambulance destination practices and the impact of a patient's insurance status on those decisions. Yet, anecdotally, it seems that many providers feel that there is a relationship between socioeconomic status and hospital destination. It is widely known which hospitals in an area are welcoming of the uninsured and as a result these facilities are given the greatest responsibility for this segment of the population. Emergency departments are open for care 24 hours a day, 7 days a week. The staff of these departments must be available to all, independent of class, color, religion, insurance, and any other potentially confounding factors; this is true for ambulatory or ambulance arrivals as well as patient transfers. Our duty is to care for any and all patients. This mandate is not primarily a legal one (although it is supported by our legal system) but rather stems from an ethical obligation articulated at the origin of the profession. The Hippocratic oath states: "I will remember that I remain a member of society, with special obligations to all my fellow human beings, those sound of mind and body as well as to the infirm."

Moral conflicts may arise when compassion for fellow human beings runs counter to external legal mandates or financial interests. Instead of looking to the law for guidance we should remain loyal to our patients' fiduciary interests. If we fail, not only do our patients suffer, but so too does the integrity of the medical profession.

Trauma: A Comprehensive Emergency Medicine Approach, eds. Eric Legome and Lee W. Shockley. Published by Cambridge University Press. © Cambridge University Press 2011.

- While EMTALA addresses the fundamental behavior and interventions of physicians once a patient arrives in the ED, the patient's relationship with the healthcare system begins in pre-hospital interaction.
- Our duty is to care for any and all patients.
- This stems from an ethical obligation articulated at the origin of the profession. The Hippocratic oath states: "I will remember that I remain a member of society, with special obligations to all my fellow human beings, those sound of mind and body as well as to the infirm."
- Moral conflicts may arise when compassion for fellow human beings runs counter to external legal mandates or financial interests.
- We should remain loyal to our patients' fiduciary interests.

Role of blood ethanol levels

The intoxicated patient presents a unique set of ethical dilemmas. The most general or overlying one is simple consent to, or refusal of, care. The Western model of medicine is now heavily reliant upon the principle of autonomy. Whereas in the past, the model was significantly more paternalistic, we practice now under a framework of shared responsibility; treatment is a collaborative relationship of both the physician and the patient. In the ED we often must care for a patient unable or unwilling to consent to care. As Beauchamp and Childress note, "Virtually all theories of autonomy agree that two conditions are essential for autonomy: 1. liberty (independence from controlling influences) and 2. agency (capacity for intentional action)."[3] It can be argued that neither of these requisite criteria are present in the intoxicated patient. In this instance, as in many others, we rely both upon the standard of implied consent which stipulates that emergent treatment should be provided, as well as a reasonable person standard which presumes that we will act in accordance with that which the ordinary citizen would desire. The law in New York, for example, defines an emergency situation as one that "Includes both the immediate endangerment of life or health or the need for the immediate alleviation of pain."[4] We are bound by a duty to treat in instances of imminent danger, life-threatening conditions, or the potential for permanent disability.

The question of drawing a blood alcohol level (BAL) arises often in the ED, yet we must remember that intoxication is a clinical diagnosis. We ought not to be lulled into complacency simply because a level is elevated while missing a more critical underlying etiology or explanation for the presence of slurred speech or lethargy. There is no example of this more illustrative than in the trauma patient. While a BAL can be used to guide therapy, it should do nothing more than raise suspicion for more significant injuries. As clinicians we tend to rely heavily on our physical examination, trusting the patient to tell us if something hurts or feels abnormal. This guidepost is often lost when a patient is intoxicated. There is little utility to routinely drawing alcohol levels; they may have a role in the care of the acutely traumatically injured as another piece of information in the context of other data.

The ethical debate becomes more complex when it is not the physician who is caring for the patient who requests the BAL, but rather when the medical team is asked to draw the blood sample by accompanying police officers. This situation may arise when a patient is brought in to the ED after a motor vehicle collision or other trauma by officers who believe that alcohol may have played a role in the traumatic event. Under these circumstances the providers must assess their goals and objectives. If an alcohol level is indicated in the care of the patient, if it would have been drawn under any circumstance then one ought to proceed in standard fashion. However, if the medical team would not have drawn the level, legal interventions and evidence collection are best left to the police department and investigators whereas the treating team must focus on treating the patient. Some police departments and precincts have medical personnel on staff whose job it is to collect data and this type of forensic evidence. Once the physician begins to move away from patient care, he or she runs the risk of losing sight of the primary objective, which is simply the care of the patient.

The broader social perspective may view driving while intoxicated as a public hazard and thusly argue for independent reporting or even mere complicity with police department staff. Medical academic bodies are divided in their opinions of this: Whereas the American College of Emergency Physicians (ACEP) does not support mandated reporting by healthcare providers (they do strongly advocate for mandatory testing by law enforcement officials), the American Academy of Emergency Medicine (AAEM) supports permissive reporting. This dichotomy is illustrative of the widely varying stances of many providers in this debate.

Family presence during resuscitation

Family presence during trauma resuscitations has received increasing support. While not many institutions have rules or standards that preclude family presence at the bedside, rarely is this offered. This absence of the family is usually attributable to physician discomfort or habit. Recent studies have shown that family presence may reduce anxiety and fear, while giving the family members a sense of closure should death occur.[5] Resuscitation staff fears that the public is not adequately prepared for participation in resuscitations, that care will be compromised or diverted, or concerns regarding potential litigation have not been substantiated. Family presence during resuscitation has also received recent publicity in the lay press which means that we, as providers of care, can expect increased interest and awareness in our patients.

It is difficult to make a sweeping recommendation regarding protocol and policy on an issue as emotional and contentious as this one. Lack of consistency in the available surveys on this issue limits the validity of conclusions.[6] Each case ought to be individually evaluated as many factors must be acknowledged and accounted for including availability of family support staff, hospital policy, provider comfort, and, perhaps most importantly, the actual logistics of making it possible. Family presence during resuscitation seems to help meet the emotional and spiritual needs of a patient's family while assisting the family to understand the severity of the patient's condition. Some have argued that family presence during resuscitation violates confidentiality and a patient's right to privacy.[5] While this concept is of concern, in many resuscitations there comes a point when the needs of the family take on mounting importance and their grieving process can and should be effectively integrated into our care. In many circumstances a tipping point is reached where the probability of survival is far less than the potential benefit to assist in the family grieving process, that family presence seems most appropriate. While perhaps more visually jarring, presence at trauma resuscitations may in fact mitigate a

Table 39.1 Best practices in delivering bad news or death notification

Preparation	A dedicated telephone for family use
	Ask if you can call anyone
	Be aware and respectful of religious differences and requirements
Language	Be direct and clear. Use simple terms
Culture	Be sensitive
Space	Private space – allow the family/survivors to stay
	Some will leave immediately, others will stay for a prolonged time
Contact	Physical contact is not always welcome. If in doubt, refrain

family's appreciation of the severity of injury, that, in addition to the immense investment of staff energy and resources, may ease understanding. The situation is best if resources allow for someone dedicated to the survivor's family. A staff member to answer questions, intervene if necessary or offer brief explanations may be invaluable. Chairs set off to the side may also be helpful. As younger physicians become more accustomed to family presence at the bedside during resuscitation and as more data emerges regarding both provider and family perspectives, it is possible that this approach will, at minimum, be an option increasingly available, perhaps even encouraged, in our hospitals and EDs.

Discussion of death

No one enjoys the telling of bad news. Yet, even though it is an essential professional skill, little time has been allocated for it in physician education. Many graduating students and residents feel unprepared to address the needs of patients and families at the end of life. It is our obligation to ensure that these skills are taught and modeled so that the next generation of physicians does not feel similarly ill-equipped or unqualified. Since traumatic death is often in the young and is unexpected, many families will have no forewarning of the discussion that will ensue in the ED. It is our duty and obligation to ensure that the truth is appropriately and honestly discussed in the most culturally sensitive and professional manner (Table 39.1). While a significant amount of literature exists regarding the telling of bad news or effective truth telling in palliative care, oncology, and pediatric literature, information is limited in trauma and emergency settings. Survivors of family catastrophes state that "A caring attitude of a well informed, sympathetic caregiver who gives families a clear message and is able to answer their questions"[7] is most comforting. The rank and attire of the truth teller seemed to matter little in this study. A general approach must assure that the member of the team whose task it is to tell the news has both the time and knowledge to answer the essential questions that will typically arise. A private space should be created, ideally with access to a phone so that calls can be made to other family or friends. While it is rarely possible for a physician or nurse involved in the resuscitation to stay with the family for a prolonged period of time, a social worker or member of the clergy (if requested) may be an appropriate replacement. Direct, clear language that is sensitive to the family's English proficiency and health literacy is essential. Euphemisms such as "He didn't make it," "He passed away," or "He is no longer with us" are vague and should be avoided. A debate exists with regard to the appropriateness of physical contact between the care provider and the family. Although some believe that touching a shoulder or hand can provide comfort or additional support, studies indicate that it may not always be welcome.[7] Recommendations cannot be made and individual decisions must be based on the provider's understanding of individual and cultural needs with any uncertainty leading to limiting physical contact.

Another complex professional exchange occurs when the family is not already aware of the situation and a telephone call must be placed to the family requesting them to come to the ED. Informing families of bad news is best done in person. If travel time makes this impractical, it may need to be done by telephone. Under these circumstances, establishing legitimacy, authority, and rapport in clear and simple language are of paramount importance. Early in the conversation, the physician should provide their name, the institution's name, and contact information so that the family can verify the information or obtain additional information. The Health Insurance Portability and Accountability Act (HIPAA) of 1996 created a heightened awareness of patient privacy and legality surrounding these issues, but a logical balance must be struck between providing comfort and information to the family while respecting a patient's privacy. The difficulty of discussing grave matters with previously unknown individuals over the telephone forces one to reflect as to whether a patient retains the right to privacy once dead. It is a good idea to determine if there is anyone with the person receiving the call, or if perhaps someone can be called to provide comfort and a safe environment. An attempt should be made for avoidance of driving and assistance should be offered to facilitate safer arrangements with a friend or family.

At the end of life the emergency physician must address not only the question of when not to resuscitate, but if withdrawal of the acute care that has already been initiated is appropriate. Advance directives refer to a spectrum of documentation enabling patients to specify instructions pertaining to healthcare decisions should they become incapacitated. A living will is a legal document that addresses the types of medical treatments desired, often related to specific circumstances and conditions. A Health Care Proxy designates a specific person to be responsible for making medical decisions should the patient become incapacitated. This person has essentially (with a few variations from state to state) the same right to request and refuse treatment that the patient would have if he or she had capacity. Durable Power of Attorney designates another person legally able to make decisions, enact bank transactions, and pay bills. With increasing understanding in the general population of advanced directives and their implementation becoming more widespread, emergency physicians must become comfortable with withdrawing care as patient preferences are elucidated. By the nature of emergency care, procedures and interventions are commonly initiated before the treating team has all of the relevant information about a patient's desires and wishes as well as prognosis. This approach to attempt to save the patient's life is clearly the proper course of action and it is defended by multiple ethical principles (beneficence, non-maleficence, presumed/implied consent) yet once the patient's desires are known there is an absolute obligation to respect and implement them. Withdrawal of treatment in concordance with a patient's advance directives is also consistent with ethical thinking and is felt to respect the patient's legal and moral right to self-determination and autonomy.[8]

Box 39.2   Essentials of advance directives

Living will	Legal document that addresses the types of medical treatments desired, often related to specific circumstances and conditions.
Health Care Proxy	Designates a specific person to be responsible for making medical decisions should the patient become incapacitated.
Durable Power of Attorney	Designates another person legally able to make decisions, enact bank transactions, and pay bills.

Although many providers feel uneasy about the withdrawal of care, most Western bioethicists believe that there is no ethical distinction between withholding or withdrawing care felt to be non-beneficial or unwanted.[2] Once the patient's wishes are determined, if care continues despite the clear expression of personal wishes to the contrary, the physician's actions can be considered "battery," which is defined legally as "unconsented bodily contact."[9] Compliance with Advance Directives is mandatory, not optional, in all 50 states.[10] Despite this standard, a survey of internists in 2004 found that 65% would not necessarily accept the directives of a living will if its instructions were in conflict with the physician's personal perspective of the patient's prognosis.[11] This is even more complex in trauma, where the prognosis is often unclear in the initial evaluation. Physicians providing trauma care must be knowledgeable and comfortable with end-of-life issues. In the case of trauma it is especially important to be sensitive and aware of options for organ donation. The legal next of kin, when they assume responsibility with regard to the body, will also assume a role regarding disposition of organs. Whereas some patients will have previously discussed wishes with family and friends, and some may have advance directives, many will not.

Resource allocation

Trauma can be considered a pandemic with over 400 deaths per day and nearly 150 000 deaths per year in the United States.[12] The care of these patients raises serious ethical questions. Many of these questions relate to resuscitation procedures (Who should perform them; the one who needs the experience or the one most experienced?). In addition there are questions regarding the treatment and sanctity of the newly dead. For years it was tacitly understood that procedures were performed on the newly dead, but as public awareness has increased and as physicians turn a critical eye on these practices they are less easily justified. Many professional groups have taken a position and consider practice on the newly dead unfavorable unless consent is obtained from the family.[13] The discussion of heroic interventions unlikely to change outcome can also fall within the purview of resource allocation. A classic example being resuscitative thoracotomy, where the risk to the care provider is real and the likely benefit to the patient is low. In blunt trauma with loss of vital signs, a meta-analysis of the literature shows survival rates of $< 1.5\%$.[14] When the risk of provider injury is factored into the equation, such dismal survival outcomes need to be considered before performing a thoracotomy despite being technically useful for learning. Prior to committing the team to performing a thoracotomy, the risks and survival benefits need to be carefully weighed. Many ethicists would consider it unjustified purely for learning.

Finding a balance between learning technical skills, acceptable risk to the healthcare provider, and proficiency with regards to aggressive resuscitation has forced new methods of teaching and skill development such as the use of medical simulators. Whereas earlier an argument was put forth regarding the importance of self-sacrifice and caring for the patient lying before us, it is also imperative that we are able to recognize the limitations of our own knowledge and skills to heal.

The immediate focus of medicine also shifts from being centered on the individual patient to the good of the group in circumstances of disaster and mass casualty. Triage and disaster medicine are commonly addressed in society, not solely in relation to possible terrorist attacks but also in our approach to preparing for natural disasters and pandemic illness. A classic example is influenza. With a recent outbreak of avian flu, many inadequacies of the current healthcare system became apparent. Calculated resource gaps demonstrate that there may be a time when not everything can be done and standards must be changed. A recurring question is the allocation of valuable and limited resources. Recurring shortage of blood products has led some to argue that resource allocation ought to factor into our daily algorithm and not solely be reserved for disaster situations. Yet the inevitable question is whether we, as healthcare providers, should be responsible for determining that allocation. Currently, there exist no guidelines for allocation of these limited resources, in contradistinction to our nation-wide organ shortage which is based on rules and lists. Perhaps this codification is the direction in which we are headed.

Triage standards, motivated primarily by the events of September 11, 2001 and the ensuing anthrax attacks, are being proposed in the critical care and emergency fields.[15–17] Although our primary obligation in day-to-day care is to the individual patient, the generally accepted goal of treatment during a mass casualty event is to save as many lives as possible.[17] It does not matter what the patient's individual belief systems are or were, if they are at odds with our own, or if they will require 2 or 20 units of blood, the physician is not in a position to pass judgment in the first critical moments. While resources should not be utilized indiscriminately, currently we act as physicians not epidemiologists? whereas inevitable disasters force us to create new organized standards for resource allocation that will result in life and death decisions.

The impact of the profession on our work

Day after day, trauma care takes its toll. We see the best of society, the occasional kindnesses and gratitude, but we are also frequently faced with society's worst events and behavior. The violence we do unto to each other, intentional and not, the unanticipated losses and those moments at life's end are exceptionally demanding. Many among us, who have lost sleep to images of our day, wished we had done something differently, said something kinder, or just taken the time to sit when company might have been needed. It is not easy to find the time amidst our demanding profession to care for ourselves, yet it is something that we must do.

Job satisfaction and fulfillment is impacted by a multitude of factors both personal as well as professional. A physician's self-reported satisfaction has been strongly linked to patient satisfaction, yet very little time is spent during our years in school and training on how to look after ourselves, deal with stress in a healthy, productive way and remain fulfilled, contented people. In addition to a positive impact on patients, physician satisfaction has also been linked to health and wellness of the physicians themselves, whereas increased dissatisfaction has conversely been linked to increasing burnout as well as

health problems among the physicians surveyed.[18,19] We must have the skills to cope with the inevitable day-to-day burdens of this profession. We must impart unto those in training the ability to not only care for others but to care for themselves. Self care is dependent on the recognition of signs of stress and the toll that it can take at work (lowering of mood, isolation, irritability, decreased quality of care),[19] and the ability to deal with it in a healthy, realistic manner.

Conclusion

Medicine is continually changing. Technology and the mores of society impact on our practice in both perceptible and imperceptible ways. As professionals and humanists we struggle with questions of death and dying, the impact of technology, the importance of autonomy, and clashes of ideology. The spectrum of trauma will challenge us with these issues. We must, however, as healthcare providers, primarily be advocates for our patients. We must strive to be true professionals: to achieve and maintain knowledge, understand good and commit to the public with willingness to self sacrifice.

References

1. Pellegrino, E. Professionalism,profession and the virtues of the good physician. *Mt Sinai J Med* 2002; **69**(6):378–84.

2. *US Census Bureau: Income, Poverty, and Health Insurance Coverage in the United States:2003.* Washington, DC: Government Printing Office, 2004.

3. Beauchamp TL, Childress JF. *Principles of Biomedical Ethics*, 3rd edn. New York: Oxford University Press,1989.

4. Kirrane BM, Drukteinis DA. Risk management and legal principles. In Flomenaum NE, Hoffman RS, Goldfrank LR, et al. (eds), *Goldfranks's Toxicologic Emergencies*, 8th edn. New York: McGraw-Hill, 2006: pp. 1879–85.

5. Mangurten J, Scott S, Guzzetta C, et al. Effects of family presence during resuscitation and invasive procedures in a pediatric emergency department. *J Emerg Nurs* 2006;**32**(3):225–33.

6. Halm MA. Family presence during resuscitation: a critical review of the literature. *Am J Crit Care* 2005; **14**(6):494–511.

7. Jurkovich GJ, Pierce B, Pananen L, Rivara FP. Giving bad news: the family perspective. *J Trauma* 2000; **48**(5):865–70; discussion 70–3.

8. Bookman K, Abbott J. Ethics seminars: withdrawal of treatment in the emergency department – when and how? *Acad Emerg Med* 2006;**13**(12):1328–32.

9. Iserson K, Sanders A, Mathieu D, eds. *Ethics in Emergency Medicine*, 2nd edn. Tucson, AZ: Galen Press, 1995.

10. Gillick M. Advance care planning. *N Engl J Med* 2004;**350**:7–8.

11. Hardin SB, Yusufaly YA. Difficult end-of-life treatment decisions: do other factors trump advance directives? *Arch Intern Med* 2004;**164**:1531–3.

12. Mackenzie E, Fowler C. Epidemiology in trauma. In Moore E, Feliciano, D, Mattox K (eds), *Trauma*, 5th edn. Norwalk, CT: McGraw-Hill, 2003: pp. 21–37.

13. Schmidt TA, Abbott JT, Geiderman JM, et al. Ethics seminars: The ethical debate on practicing procedures on the newly dead. *Acad Emerg Med* 2004;**11**(9): 962–6.

14. Eckstein M, Henderson S. Thoracic Trauma. In Marx J, Walls R, Hockberger R (eds), *Rosen's Emergency Medicine: Concepts and Clinical Practice*, 6th edn. Philadephia, PA: Mosby, 2006: pp. 453–88.

15. Hick JL, O'Laughlin DT. Concept of operations for triage of mechanical ventilation in an epidemic. *Acad Emerg Med* 2006;**13**:223–9.

16. Rubinson L, Nuzzo JB, Talmor DS, et al. Augmentation of hospital critical care capacity after bioterrorist attacks or epidemics: Recommendations of the Working Group on Emergency Mass Critical Care. *Crit Care Med* 2005;**33**:2393–403.

17. Agency for Healthcare Research and Quality. *Bioterrorism and Other Public Health Emergencies: Altered Standards of Care in Mass Casualty Events.* AHRQ Publication No. 05–0043. Washington, DC: AHRQ, 2005.

18. Brown S, Gunderman R. Viewpoint: enhancing the professional fulfillment of physicians. *Acad Med* 2006;**81**(6):577–82.

19. Hughes G. Professional issues in emergency medicine: UK perspective. *Emerg Med Australas* 2004;**16**(7):5–6, 422–8.

Chapter 40

Communication and interpersonal issues in trauma

Matthew R. Levine

Introduction

Trauma teams come together when summoned to care for the acutely injured patient. Teams are comprised of individuals from multiple disciplines such as emergency medicine, surgery, nursing, radiology, and others. Team membership may change based on the month, week, day, or time of day. The size may also vary significantly based on type of injury or patient hemodynamics, institutional protocols or type of institution, i.e., teaching vs. community. There are structured routines with both the specialty derived guidelines of care (Advanced Trauma Life Support [ATLS®]) institutional and that are clearer than most other medical specialty guidelines. There is clear and meaningful purpose – to treat patients and train novices.

Trauma teams face significant challenges. There may be limited information during the initial evaluation. There are rapid changes in patient status. Decisions are made under pressure. The environment is often noisy and emotional. There is a fluctuating incoming workload with task overload at times, and multitasking is essential. Membership frequently changes so team members may not be familiar with one another, which can impair effective communication. Communication may be challenged by interdepartmental rivalry or varying prioritizations. There may be multiple levels of decision-making authority. Members-in-training must receive mentorship and teaching while acute care proceeds smoothly.

Effective teams have core attributes: clear mission and focus, collective commitment, and standards of practice. They have formal structure and unambiguous roles and responsibilities. Leadership is dynamic. Communication is effective. There are processes for objective monitoring and feedback.[1,2]

Leadership

The team leader

The performance of trauma teams is dependent on an identified team leader.[3,4] The ATLS® teaches a "vertical" model of resuscitation, that is, tasks happen sequentially. However, in large hospitals and trauma centers, "horizontal" resuscitation, in which ATLS® tasks are performed simultaneously by multiple providers, is more efficient. Resuscitation time was reduced by 54% after implementing horizontal resuscitation with precise task allocation.[5] Proper horizontal resuscitation requires a more sophisticated level of organization, with preassigned roles and direction by a single individual.[4]

The leader's attention must focus on strategic direction, prioritization, and support. The leader must be prepared to adapt and make revisions when necessary. Effective leaders are involved, monitor performance, provide hands-on treatment when necessary, and are willing and able to teach. They establish norms and routines that are positive and safe.[6]

Multiple surveys and studies of videotaped trauma resuscitations reveal that many trauma team leaders but perform medical tasks well, tend to be deficient in communication and delegation.[7–11] Frequent deficiencies are failure to communicate clearly with other team members and not announcing the overall plan. A common mistake is to ask for something in a general manner without specifically asking one individual. In many cases leaders do not verbalize their thought process or assertively lead with clear verbal instructions.[9] A notable comment from a nursing journal highlights concerns by nurses when trauma team leader communication is ineffective:

> A vital part of the specific training of a trauma nurse is gathering the ability to rapidly identify who is in fact

Table 40.1 Recommended leadership style based on scenario

Team experience		Injury severity		Recommended leadership style	
High	Low	High	Low	Directive	Empowered
X		X		If unusual presentation	If common presentation
X			X		X
	X	X		X	
	X		X		X

leading the initial evaluation and resuscitation of the injured patient at any given moment, regardless of formal title or area of specialty.[12]

Early communication by the team leader is good practice.[3] Teams comprised of individuals who are familiar with each other work with greater efficiency than teams of strangers.[13,14] To help minimize effects of uncertainty and unfamiliarity, preassigned roles should be given to each team member and team orientation and introductions should be a priority.[4] When the leader initiates a structure, resuscitation teams are more dynamic, work more effectively, and are more likely to perform tasks correctly and at the right time.[15]

Leadership style

Team leadership style can be categorized by two broad terms: directive and empowered leadership.[16] Directive leadership is autocratic. Plans are developed without team consultation, the team is expected to carry out orders, and resuscitations are run by the leader without input from others. Team members have fewer opportunities to increase their expertise. When power and authority are used to limit others, barriers may be created within teams.[17]

In contrast, empowered leadership encourages team participation in decision making and task management, delegates responsibility and authority, and allows others to take initiative. Empowered leadership provides other team members opportunities to think, apply knowledge, and learn by doing. Empowered leadership also enhances group commitment. Increased participation leads to greater "buy-in" and motivation – people support what they help build.[18] Trauma teams are problem solving units, so knowledge within the group ultimately enhances its function.[19] These benefits of empowered leadership

are realized at a later point in time so they may not be immediately obvious.[18]

The proper leadership style for an individual scenario depends on two important situational elements: illness severity and team experience (Table 40.1). When illness severity is high, there is less time to diagnose, construct a plan, seek consensus, and implement treatment. A directive approach would be favored for critical trauma patients when the team is inexperienced. When the team is experienced and the patient is critical, other situational elements may be considered such as the novelty of the condition. A critical patient with a common condition and a highly skilled team can still be managed by empowered leadership. Empowered leadership can almost always be used when the patient is not critically ill, and usually when the team is experienced.

Therefore, the leader must maintain *situational awareness* – the ability to *diagnose the situation*[6,16] – in order to select the leadership style to best effect team outcome.

Positioning of the team leader

The trauma team leader can be positioned at the bedside close to the patient ("hands-on"), or away from the team ("hands-off").

During "horizontal" resuscitations many tasks occur simultaneously. Loss of situational awareness can occur if the leader focuses too much on one aspect. This is a particular risk when the leader becomes involved in a demanding procedure. Important information may not be recognized as important or properly integrated; conflicts of priorities may result. In arrest scenarios as part of ATLS® training, the leader is encouraged to stand back to enable delegation and monitoring of the process. This positioning clearly defines the leadership role and develops an empowering approach to team management. "Hands-off" positioning allows observation of all activity to provide direction to individual team members, while allowing the opportunity to maintain situational awareness. Resuscitation research shows the "hands-off" approach to be more effective for team dynamics and increases the level of task performance.[15]

The "hands-on" leader has been shown to be less likely to initiate a structure within the team and was less effective overall. The team was less dynamic, showing little interaction and cooperation. Many "hands-on" activities by the leader could have been delegated.

However, in situations with few or inexperienced team members, the "hands-on" style may be required to rapidly assess and treat the injured patient. So the ultimate decision for "hands on" or "hands off" positioning requires situational awareness.

Who should lead?

Evidence-based recommendations regarding who should lead the trauma team are scant. There is little difference demonstrated in the performance of emergency physicians vs. trauma surgeons as the team leader. The presence of an attending trauma surgeon was shown to decrease resuscitation time and time to the operating room without decreasing mortality.[20] Senior surgical residents performed similarly to trauma surgeons for the primary and secondary survey, but scored significantly lower than the trauma surgeon for items such as constructing a definitive plan.[4]

Generally, the leader should be *experienced* in trauma management from an emergency, intensive care unit (ICU), or surgical specialty, and have completed training in trauma care.[3] Experienced leaders were more likely to make their part in the team understood, plan the work to be done, and set expectations.[15] More experienced leaders were associated with decreased resuscitation times.[5] When determining who should lead, focus should be on team performance and patient welfare.

Leadership roles in trauma can change fluidly even within the same case.[6] This allows novices to practice and lead in a setting that provides protection and support. A common practice of this is found in teaching centers with senior emergency medicine or surgical residents. Shared leadership can create redundancy which enhances reliability. While leadership can be shared sequentially, it cannot be shared *simultaneously*.

Box 40.1 Trauma team leadership essential information

- The performance of a trauma team is dependent on its team leader.
- Communication is a common deficiency of trauma team leaders.
- The team leader should initiate a structure in the trauma room by introducing team members and assigning roles before patient arrival.
- The team leader must be able to diagnose the *situation* to choose the appropriate leadership style to optimize team function and learning.

- The team leader may assume a position away from the bedside to best observe and direct team activity whenever possible.
- Experience in trauma care is essential in selection of the team leader.
- The team leader must be able to manage conflicts without introducing barriers within the team while patient care continues.

Table 40.2 Means to settle conflicts

Accommodation	Concedes to other's position
Avoidance	Ignores, denies, or escapes
Collaboration	Assertively seeks win–win outcome
Competition	Interested only in winning
Compromise	Seeks to have a matter settled if not resolved

Conflict management and communication

When more than one individual is involved in a complex situation, conflict may occur. The means by which conflicts are settled are listed in Table 40.2.[21] Certain means are more constructive than others, such as collaboration and compromise. Use of power or authority may introduce team barriers,[17] as may avoidance. Use of this leadership style should be judicious and reserved for critical situations. When managing conflicts, many sources recommend learning one's own triggers to anger, the practice of active listening, and not blaming or personalizing conflicts.

Conflicts often result from unclear orders, missed input, or distractions. Optimal communication can help prevent conflicts. Communication is transmitted and received verbally (words and voice intonation) and non-verbally (facial expressions and gestures). The sender is responsible for conveying information accurately and concisely and verifying that important information was received. The receiver is responsible for actively listening, acting or answering the communication, or requesting clarification when the information is unclear.

The team leader has ultimate responsibility for the conduct of the resuscitation and must determine when to end or temporarily suspend the discussion to ensure treatment continues efficiently. Sometimes a final resolution may not occur but effective management of the conflict by the leader still promotes team success and mutual respect.

Teamwork

Teamwork does not come naturally. It does not result from simply working together. However, with appropriate team training, effective communication is increased.[22] Multidisciplinary medical teams have teamwork difficulties attributed to professional barriers, perceived inequity in status, and separate lines of management control and payment systems. These barriers perpetuate role rigidity, low morale, and outdated working practices.[23] Team members have different training backgrounds and disciplines and may not appreciate each other's strengths and weaknesses.[24]

Medical training traditionally emphasizes technical and clinical skills, not team skills. Physicians are taught to be self sufficient and individually responsible for the care they deliver. The ATLS® focuses more on clinical management than team leadership skills. Few trauma team members have had formal teamwork training. Superb individuals may not perform well in teams. A convenience sample of 54 malpractice incidents from 8 institutions from 1985 to 1996 found there were 8.8 teamwork failures per case and teamwork failures contributed to over half the deaths and disabilities.[25]

Box 40.2 Teamwork essential information

- Trauma teams face challenges beyond the application of medical skills. These are seldom formally taught in medical training.
- Teamwork is not a natural product of working together but can be taught.
- Team training has demonstrated effectiveness in analogous medical and non-medical teams, has been recommended by the Institute of Medicine, and may be a future endeavor to improve trauma care.
- Nurses and prehospital personnel are a vital part of the trauma team.

High reliability organizations

According to high reliability organization (HRO) theory, accidents occur because individuals are unable to sense and anticipate the myriad of problems generated by a complex system. Trauma teams have been compared to other HROs in nuclear power, aviation,

Table 40.3 Attributes of teams in high reliability organizations

Division of tasks

Shared responsibility

Trust and respect

Monitoring other team members

Broadcasting information to ensure team awareness

---

and aircraft carrier crews with respect to teamwork principles. All involve quick decision making despite incomplete data and effective coordination of team members to rapidly accomplish complex high stakes tasks. While patients are different and less predictable than machinery, there are still valuable team lessons from other HROs that are applicable to medical teams.[26] To achieve high performance, teams in HROs learn several attributes (Table 40.3).[19,27]

Team training and crew resource management

Team training in aviation has changed several problematic cultures that may also apply to medicine.[10] One includes steep hierarchies in which the senior is not open to input from the junior. Another is the denial of the effect of stress and fatigue on performance. The widespread application of teamwork training in aviation has changed the perception of the airline captain as the lone authority with the silent crew following orders, to a crew with all members encouraged to provide insights and input. Basic principles of team training are listed in Table 40.4.

The Institute of Medicine's landmark report *To Err is Human: Building a Safer Healthcare System* recommends that:

> Healthcare organizations should establish team training programs for personnel in critical care areas (e.g., the emergency department, intensive care unit, operating rooms) using proven methods such as the crew resource management techniques employed in aviation, including simulation.[24]

Crew Resource Management (CRM) was born in 1979 from a NASA workshop that examined the role that human error played in air crashes. The widespread implementation of CRM in aviation since then has led to reduction in aviation mishaps beyond those explained by improvements in equipment and technology. The core concept of CRM is to train teams to

Table 40.4 Basic principles of team training

Team communication and coordination are crucial

Attitudes and behaviors are malleable and predict performance. Personalities are not

Others besides the leader contribute to problem solving

Group knowledge decreases errors

Table 40.5 Crew Resource Management elements

Adaptability/flexibility

Assertiveness

Communication

Decision making

Leadership

Situational awareness

use all available information, insights, and input to achieve safe and efficient operations.[28] Team communication and coordination behaviors are identifiable, teachable, and applicable to high-stakes environments. These are not practiced reliably, regularly, or well unless established by specific training and reinforcement.[24,29] Crew Resource Management training achieves proficiency in the functions listed in Table 40.5. Team members are taught fine points of verbal and non-verbal communication, specific listening skills, and debriefing after work scenarios. These all build team knowledge and increase team performance.

Crew Resource Management training applied to medical teams increases team concepts and communication in the operating room and the emergency department.[3,30] There are barriers, however, to widespread implementation of team training for medical teams.[8] It requires resources and commitment. Teams must train together regularly to sustain benefits of team training. Coordination of training team members from different fields and levels of training is difficult. Whether CRM is the model to be adopted for future trauma team training, team training is proven effective, a specific Institute of Medicine recommendation, and may be a major endeavor to optimize trauma care. Simulators are often used in CRM and have become more prevalent in medical training and show promise in increasing trauma team effectiveness.

Prehospital trauma system

The pivotal events of trauma resuscitation link the prehospital phase of care to definitive management of the injured patient.[4] The goal of EMS and hospital team communication is the efficient transfer of important prehospital information to ensure team and hospital preparedness. Communication with EMS begins by radio or phone contact to aid prehospital medical and transport decisions. Contacts with EMS are often brief because many urban systems have short transport times and favor a "scoop and run" approach for trauma. Rural systems with longer transport times may have more involved communications. Whenever time permits, personnel receiving the call should try to obtain information that will help the team prepare for patient arrival, such as mechanism of injury, vital signs, and mental status. Prehospital personnel possess important information such as initial assessment, changes in patient status, mechanism of injury, scene description, and extrication details. This information should be obtained without delaying patient care. If not handled well, important information may be lost when prehospital providers depart.

Nursing participation in the trauma team

Nurses are a vital part of the trauma team. The presence of highly skilled, experienced, and empowered nurses provides additional redundancy, reducing error likelihood.[6] It is often the direct responsibility of the trauma nurse to ensure continuous effective monitoring and uninterrupted delivery of supportive care during the imaging procedures or intervention.[12]

Feedback and evaluation

Provision of feedback is a core attribute of effective medical teams.[2] Individuals are likely to perform better individually and within a group when they know they will be evaluated.[27] Evaluation helps prevent a natural tendency toward less motivation and effort when subjects work collectively rather than individually.[27]

Feedback can occur during trauma resuscitations, immediately afterwards, or at a later date. Anticipated briefings during and after care of the trauma patient provide opportunity for real time feedback and immediate learning. The concept of briefings is used in other analogous HROs. Morbidity and mortality conferences are a traditional educational setting. These should include multiple specialties, including non-physicians, and emphasize, in addition to clinical management and system factors, teamwork, collegiality, and respect for everyone's role and insight. The use of video recordings of trauma resuscitations has been found to improve education, feedback, compliance with protocols, identify errors in techniques, improve usage of time, identify equipment failures, and achieve quality control. However, due to numerous factors such as privacy, liability and logistical issues, the use of this is not universal.[4,7,9,31,32]

Interdepartmental and medical staff issues

Effective trauma care requires institutional leadership and commitment.[14] Trauma care is labor and resource intensive, which may make it seem unappealing to hospital administration. The benefits of a trauma service to an institution, however, are significant. Trauma care emphasizes that a hospital is a 24-hour tertiary care institution. A hospital that can handle trauma can likely handle diverse medical scenarios. Communities see trauma centers as "go-to" hospitals.[14]

Excellent trauma care requires establishment of a culture within the institution. Key tasks in establishing a culture are providing direction, aligning people, motivating people, planning, budgeting, organizing, staffing, controlling, and problem solving.[33] For a team to succeed over time it must function in a collaborative environment to achieve standards of excellence, receive external support, and have principled leadership and commitment.[2] Given the two major services involved in trauma are emergency medicine and surgery, it is imperative they are cooperative and collaborative. In addition to using the skill sets discussed above in daily interactions, other ways to work together include joint conferences, case reviews, research, protocol development quality management committees, and training excercises.

References

1. Katzenbach JR, Smith DK. *The Wisdom of Teams: Creating the High Performance Organization.* New York: Harper Collins, 1994.

2. Larson CE, LaFasto FM. *Teamwork: What Must Go Right/What Can Go Wrong.* Newbury Park, CA: Sage Publications, 1989.

3. Cole E, Crichton N. The culture of a trauma team in relation to human factors. *J Clin Nurs* 2006;**15**:1257–66.

4. Hoff WS, Reilly PM, Rotundo MF, DiGiacomo JC, Scwab CW. The importance of the command-physician in trauma resuscitation. *J Trauma* 1997;**43**:772–7.

5. Driscol PA, Vincent CA. Organizing an efficient trauma team. *Injury* 1992;**23**:107–10.

6. Klein KJ, Zieger JC, Knight AP, Xiao Y. *A Leadership System for Emergency Action Teams: Rigid Hierarchy and Dynamic Flexibility.* Available from http://knowledge.wharton.upenn.edu/papers/1282.pdf.

7. Bergs EAG, Rutten FLPA, Tadros T, Krijnen P, Schipper IB. Communication during trauma resuscitation: do we know what is happening? *Injury* 2005;**36**:905–11.

8. Helmreich RL. On error management: lessons from aviation. *BMJ* 2000;**320**:781–5.

9. Ritchie PD, Cameron PA. An evaluation of trauma team leader performance by video recording. *Aust NZ J Surg* 1999;**69**:183–6.

10. Sexton JB, Thomas EJ, Helmreich RL. Error, stress, and teamwork in medicine and aviation: cross sectional surveys. *BMJ* 2000;**320**:745–9.

11. Sugrue M, Seger M, Kerridge R, Sloane D, Deane S. A prospective study of the trauma team leader. *J Trauma* 1995;**38**:79–82.

12. Hertz D, Ben Ezer Y. Pitfalls in trauma team work. *Aust Emerg Nurs J* 1997;**1**:30–1.

13. Guzzo RA, Dickson MW. Teams in organizations: recent research on performance and effectiveness. *Ann Rev Psychology* 1996;**47**:307–38.

14. Harris BH, Butler LJ. Teamwork in pediatric trauma centers. *Sem Ped Surg* 2001;**10**:35–7.

15. Cooper S, Wakelam A. Leadership of resuscitation teams: 'lighthouse leadership'. *Resuscitation* 1999;**42**:27–45.

16. Yun S, Faraj S, Sims HP, Jr. Contingent leadership and effectiveness of trauma resuscitation teams. *J App Psych* 2005;**90**:1288–96.

17. Christie J. Collaborative practice. In Langstaff D, Christie J (eds), *Trauma Care: A Team Approach.* Oxford: Butterworth Heinemann, 2000: pp. 310–22.

18. Vroom VH. Leadership and the decision making process. *Organ Dyn* 2000;**28**:82–94.

19. Xiao Y, Moss JA. Practice of high reliability teams: observations in trauma resuscitation. Human Factors and Ergonomics 44th Annual Meeting. Minneapolis/St. Paul, MN, 2001.

20. Khetarpal S, Steinbrunn BS, McGonigal MD, et al. Trauma faculty and trauma team activation: impact on

trauma system and patient outcome. *J Trauma* 1999;**47**:576–81.

21. Masters MF, Albright RR. *The Complete Guide to Conflict Resolution in the Workplace*. New York: American Management Association, 2002.

22. Awad SS, Fagan SP, Bellows C, et al. Bridging the communication gap in the operating room with medical team training. *Am J Surg* 2005;**190**:770–4.

23. Millward LJ, Jeffries N. The team survey: a tool for health team development. *J Adv Nurs* 2001;**35**:276–87.

24. Kohn LT, Corrigan JM, Donaldson MS (eds). *To Err is Human: Building a Safer Healthcare System*. Washington, DC: National Academy Press, 2000.

25. Risser DT, Rice MM, Salisbury ML, et al. The MedTeams Research Consortium: the potential for improved teamwork to reduce medical errors in the emergency department. *Ann Emerg Med* 1999;**34**:373–83.

26. Ruchlin HS, Dubbs NL, Callahan MA. The role of leadership in instilling a culture of safety: lessons from the literature. *J Healthcare Management* 2004;**49**:47–58.

27. Xiao Y, Plasters C, Seagull FL, Moss JA. Cultural and institutional conditions for high reliability teams.

IEEE International Conference on Systems. *Man and Cybernetics* 2004;**3**:2580–5.

28. Lauber JK. Cockpit resource management: background and overview. In Orlady HW, Foushee HC (eds), *Cockpit Resource Management Training: Proceedings of the NASA/MAC Workshop*. Moffett Field, CA: NASA, 1987: Pub. no. 2455.

29. Musson DM, Helmreich RL. Team training and resource management in healthcare: current issues and future directions. *Harvard Health Policy Rev* 2004;**5**:25–35.

30. Morey JC, Simon R, Jay JD. Error reduction and performance improvement in the emergency department through formal teamwork training: evaluation results of the MedTeams project. *HSR* 2002;**37**:1553–81.

31. Michaelson M, Levi L. Videotaping in the admitting area: a most useful tool for quality improvement of the trauma center. *Eur J Emerg Med* 1997;**4**:94–6.

32. Santora TA, Trooskin SZ, Blank CA, Clark JR, Schinco MA. Video assessment of trauma response: adherence to ATLS® protocols. *Am J Emerg Med* 1996;**14**:564–9.

33. Kotter JP. *A Force for Change: How Leadership Differs from Management*. New York: The Free Press, 1990.

Trauma research

Jason S. Haukoos and Debra Houry

Introduction

Research is a process that begins with a well-developed question. A study is then designed in an effort to answer this question. The study is implemented and data are collected, compiled, and analyzed. Results are critically interpreted and incorporated into a manuscript, which after standing-up to rigorous peer-review, ends up in-press and contributing to the fund of knowledge (Figure 41.1).

This approach to scientific discovery spans all aspects of research, including basic science, clinical research, outcomes or health services research, and translation between each of these areas. Trauma-related research is no exception to this process.

Traumatic injuries have a wide physical, psychological, and financial impact on society.[1] While it is often predictable and preventable, substantial effort is still required to reduce trauma-related morbidity and mortality. Investigators continue to evaluate injury patterns and therapeutic approaches from the bench, to the bedside, to populations.[2–6]

Objectives

This chapter will not detail specific aspects of developing a study question, designing research protocols, performing data management or statistical analyses, or reporting results. There are a substantial number of resources to provide more detail in these areas.[7–9] This chapter, however, will: (1) provide a general overview of basic research methodologies and their relative strengths and weaknesses; (2) provide an overview of data sources available for trauma research, including de novo data, local trauma registries, and publicly-available national databases, and describe aspects of their validity and generalizability; (3) discuss trauma scoring systems, why they are important, and how to use them; and (4) describe

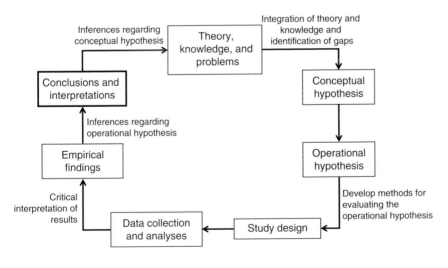

Figure 41.1 Conceptual framework for conducting research.

Trauma: A Comprehensive Emergency Medicine Approach, eds. Eric Legome and Lee W. Shockley. Published by Cambridge University Press. © Cambridge University Press 2011.

Table 41.1 Strengths and weaknesses of different basic study designs

Study design	Strengths	Weaknesses
Experimental	• Directly evaluates an intervention	• Limited generalizability
	• Well-defined study population	• Difficult to perform and time-consuming
	• Randomization balances study groups	• Expensive
	• Comparison group provides control (e.g., placebo or active control)	• Often funded by industry, which dictates study design and methodology
	• Prospective data collection	
	• Takes advantage of blinding	
Quasi-experimental	• Directly evaluates an intervention	• Pseudo-randomization
	• Comparison group provides control	• Study population may be less well defined
	• Prospective data collection	• Retrospective data collection (e.g., historical controls)
	• More generalizable	• Greater likelihood for introduced bias
	• Best approach when randomization is unethical	
Observational	• Often most generalizable	• Study groups seldom similar
	• Relatively easy to perform	• No direct control over intervention or use of other study design components (e.g., blinding)
	• Inexpensive	• Requires more sophisticated analytic methods to control for differences between study groups
	• Prospective data collection (e.g., prospective cohort study)	• Retrospective data collection (e.g., retrospective cohort or case-control study)
		• Typically unable to control for all confounding

controversies and difficulties of doing research with critically-ill trauma patients.

Basic research methodology

Study design is generally divided into the following three fundamental categories: experimental designs, quasi-experimental designs, and observational designs (Table 41.1).[7] Within each of these three categories, numerous design strategies influence how patients will be included and data collected.

Experimental designs are defined by the use of an intervention and true randomization (i.e., having equal probability of being assigned to one of two or more study arms). This generates two (or more) study groups that theoretically only vary by the intervention provided, and therefore provides the investigator with the opportunity to evaluate the true effect of the intervention.[9–11] These studies are considered to be the strongest in terms of evidence that contributes to the general knowledge base and therefore carry the most weight in terms of impacting future medical care. Of course, such studies may suffer from the same limitations as other designs, including selection biases, imbalanced patient assignment, recording or measurement biases, confounding, or other limitations.[7]

Quasi-experimental designs are defined by the use of an intervention with pseudo-randomization (e.g., using odd or even days to guide enrollment into specific arms of the trial).[9] Because true randomization does not occur in these settings, the two study groups often are not comparable. However, this study design does afford the investigator the opportunity to introduce an intervention and to evaluate its effect, recognizing the potential need for more complex analyses to control for variation among the two study groups.

Observational designs are often subcategorized into cohort, cross-sectional, or case-control designs, and include a relatively large number of potential design features, including various study sample selection and data collection methods.[7] While observational designs often have the most generalizability (because inclusion and exclusion criteria are not as limited as those for experimental or quasi-experimental designs), they also are often more limited by introduced bias or lack of control for confounding. Significant effort must be made to either control for these potential limitations in the study design, in obtaining or analyzing the data, or interpreting the results of the study.[11–20] It is important to recognize that study designs and other methods of conducting research are not, in general, specific to content areas. These methods, although briefly described, are the cornerstone of conducting sound research, including trauma-related research.

Trauma-related data sources

De novo data sources

Much of trauma research includes de novo data, or new data collected for the primary purpose of the study.[5] In this form of data collection, also called *primary data collection*, one can acquire data prospectively or retrospectively. The advantages of de novo data collection primarily stem from the fact that data are collected for the sole purpose of research. As such, investigators are able to specifically define each variable *a priori* and attempt to anticipate any problems with how they will be ascertained or defined during the performance of the study. Data collection in this fashion allows investigators to control several aspects of how their study will be carried out, including how data will be defined, what their forms will be (e.g., continuous vs. categorical), and what additional data will be required (e.g., confounders) that otherwise may not have been collected or easily obtained. Disadvantages of de novo data collection include having to acquire data that do not already exist and are limited by specific methodologies related to whether they are collected prospectively or retrospectively.

Data collected prospectively are typically considered the most valid because it allows for consistent and real-time oversight in order to minimize bias or missing data. This method is used exclusively in experimental research (from basic science to clinical to outcomes research), and commonly in quasi-experimental or observational research. Of course,

the quality of the final dataset will strongly depend on acquiring data in a valid and consistent fashion. Strategies to maximize prospectively-collected data include explicitly defining all variables, using standardized closed-response data collection instruments, and using consistent methodology to transfer data into electronic forms (if data collection includes paper-based data collection instruments).

Retrospective data collection, on the other hand, uses extraction of existing data (commonly from medical records) for the primary purpose of the study. Although this data collection method is more limited, in that data are gathered from records that were not recorded for research purposes, explicit methodology has been described to maximize the validity of data collected in this manner.[12] Retrospective data collection, however, limits which data may be obtained or how they were defined when they were documented because it relies on data that were (or were not) recorded for other purposes.

Existing data sources

Alternative methods of trauma research include the use of existing data sources. Such data may or may not have been primarily collected for research purposes. If the existing data were collected for research purposes and are now being used for other research, this form of evaluation is referred to as *secondary data collection* or a secondary analysis of an existing dataset.[21] The advantages of using an existing dataset that was primarily collected for other research is that those data already exist (thus removing the need to collect de novo data), and were specifically collected for research, thus theoretically conforming to the advantages of these types of data. Disadvantages, however, include the fact that the investigators have no control over how the data were originally collected or how the individual variables were defined.

Institutional and state trauma registries

Institutional and state trauma registries also provide sources of data for trauma-related research.[22,23] As of 2006, 32 states maintained centralized registries and countless more individual hospitals maintain their own trauma registries. Although the American College of Surgeons Committee on Trauma (ACSCOT) has attempted to help standardize which data are included in these registries, there still remains substantial variability in their composition and content.[24,25]

As with most registries, trauma registries have certain strengths and weaknesses. Advantages of these types of registries include their large numbers of patients and variables, which provide some of the best sources of information about severe injuries. Data collected for these types of registries are also often done using systematic data collection procedures, have strict inclusion and exclusion criteria, and are rigorously maintained and easily accessible. Unfortunately, trauma registries also have a number of weaknesses that limit their use in trauma research. In almost all cases, data included in trauma registries are not population-based and are therefore restricted to numerator data, thus preventing investigators from accurately calculating incidence or prevalence measures. For example, it would be impossible to use a trauma registry to define the incidence of bicycle crashes in a community since only a proportion of all patients who experience a bicycle crash are included in the registry. In addition, registries commonly include older and more medically impaired patients than injury victims in surrounding communities due to the fact that registries usually are maintained at trauma referral centers. Registry patients also tend to have higher Injury Severity Scores (ISS) and more head, spine, and thoracic (and fewer orthopedic) injuries than at community facilities.[26,27]

National Trauma Data Bank®

The National Trauma Data Bank® (NTDB), developed by the ACSCOT is the largest aggregation of trauma registry data ever assembled, containing over two million records from trauma centers throughout the United States.[28] This database is primarily supported by the Health Resources and Services Administration (HRSA), the National Highway Traffic Safety Administration (NHTSA), and the Centers for Disease Control and Prevention (CDC). This database includes individual level demographic, injury, prehospital, emergency department, procedural, diagnostic, and outcome data from over 700 hospitals nationwide and across all trauma-center designation levels.

Similar to individual hospital trauma registries, the NTDB suffers from selected, or convenience, sampling. The NTDB National Sample Project was thus created to serve as a unique patient database from a nationally representative sample of trauma hospitals in order to allow statistically valid inferences about national injury incidence and prevalence. This database is not a subset of the NTDB database, but includes variables similar to those collected for the NTDB. The NTDB National Sample Project was developed in an effort to create national baseline estimates of variables and indices associated with traumatic injuries and can be used to provide nationally representative estimates of trauma mortality, ISS, length of stay (LOS), and patient demographics.

National Automotive Sampling System and the Fatality Analysis Reporting System

The National Automotive Sampling System (NASS), created in 1979, is sponsored by the US Department of Transportation, and operated by the National Center for Statistics and Analysis (NCSA) of the NHTSA.[29] It is primarily aimed at reducing motor vehicle crashes, injuries, and deaths nationwide. Two components of the NASS include the Crashworthiness Data System (CDS) and the General Estimates System (GES), both of which randomly select police crash reports from representative geographical areas of the United States. Crashworthiness Data System data are collected from field researchers who carefully study and record aspects of selected motor vehicle crashes, including exterior and interior vehicle damage, occupant injury, crash scene investigation, and environmental conditions, among others. General Estimates System data, on the other hand, comes from a larger sample of crashes, but only includes basic information from police accident reports. A number of clinical investigations have published results using these datasets.[30–34]

The Fatality Analysis Reporting System (FARS) was created in 1975 by the NCSA to assist in identifying traffic safety problems and to evaluate motor vehicle safety standards and highway safety initiatives. Fatality data include motor vehicle traffic crashes that result in the death of an occupant of a vehicle or a non-motorist, and includes data from all 50 states, the District of Columbia, and Puerto Rico.[35] The focus of these data are only those crashes in which a fatality occurred.

Trauma scoring systems

Historically, investigators have relied on standardized injury severity assessments to stratify groups of trauma patients, to control for severity when evaluating predictors of outcomes, or in evaluating trauma care and their systems. Trauma outcomes are fundamentally multivariate problems. Researchers, therefore, use multiple variables (e.g., age, comorbidities, injury severity, etc.) to predict these outcomes (e.g., survival), and statistical techniques such as multivariable logistic regression are often the cornerstone of such analyses.[36]

Examples of most of the trauma-related scoring systems are categorized into: (1) anatomical scoring systems(e.g., the Abbreviated Injury Scale [AIS], the Injury Severity Score [ISS], or the Anatomic Profile [AP]); (2) physiological scoring systems (e.g., the Glasgow Coma Scale [GCS] score, the Revised Trauma Score [RTS], or the Acute Physiology and Chronic Health Evaluation [APACHE]); or (3) combined scoring systems (e.g., the Trauma and Injury Severity Score [TRISS] or the A Severity of Characterization of Trauma [ASCOT]). They have existed for decades and have provided clinical investigators with the ability to control for variation among patients within trauma populations or to predict expected outcomes.[37]

Abbreviated Injury Scale and the Injury Severity Score

The AIS is an anatomical scoring system first introduced nearly 40 years ago, although revised since.[38] The AIS differs slightly from the Organ Injury Scale, which uses the same scoring system to categorize injuries across organ systems (Table 41.2).[39] The AIS is a consensus-derived, anatomical injury grading system that ranges from 1 (minor injury) to 6 (non-survivable injury).

The AIS does not reflect the combined effects of multiple injuries, but forms the foundation of the ISS, which does.[40] Historically, the ISS has been used to predict mortality and multiple organ failure. It is defined as the sum of squares of the highest AIS in the three most severely injured body regions. Six body regions are defined, and include the head and neck, face, thorax, abdomen and visceral pelvis, bony pelvis, and extremities and external structures. To calculate the ISS, only the most severe injury per body region is allowed, and the ISS ranges from 1 to 75, with 75 being assigned to anyone with an AIS of 6. For example, a patient with a small subdural hematoma (head AIS = 4), a parietal lobe contusion (head AIS = 3), a major liver laceration (abdominal AIS = 4), and a displaced tibial fracture (extremity AIS = 3), would have an ISS of 41 (i.e., $4^2 + 4^2 + 3^2$).

Table 41.2 Abbreviated Injury Scale (AIS) and Organ Injury Scale (OIS)

AIS	OIS	Injury
1	1	Minor
2	2	Moderate
3	3	Serious
4	4	Severe
5	5	Critical
6	6	Non-survivable

The ISS has several limitations, including the inability to account for multiple injuries to the same body region. It also limits the total number of contributing injuries to three, thus possibly limiting its utility, especially among patients with penetrating injuries where multiple injuries are common. The ISS also equally weights injuries across body regions, ignoring the differential associations between injuries and mortality (e.g., head injuries are more strongly associated with mortality than extremity injuries). In addition, mortality is not a linear function of the ISS. In fact, it is possible to have a higher mortality with a lower ISS, depending on the different combinations of AIS scores. Finally, many ISS values (between 1 and 75) do not exist due solely to how the score is calculated, and the same ISS values can result from multiple different AIS combinations or injury patterns. Overall, this makes the ISS heterogeneous with limited predictive value, particularly in the acute setting, in patients with penetrating trauma, and in patients at the extremes of age.

More recently, a modified, or new ISS (NISS) was reported.[41] This score is based on the three most severe injuries regardless of body region. The NISS has been demonstrated to be a more accurate predictor of trauma mortality than the ISS, especially among those with penetrating trauma and is increasingly being used.[36,42]

Anatomic Profile

The AP was developed in response to some of the limitations of the ISS.[37,43] It summarizes all serious injuries (defined by an AIS $\geq$ 3) into the three categories (A: head and spinal cord; B: thorax and anterior neck; and C: all remaining serious injuries) and all other non-serious injuries into their own

Table 41.3 Revised Trauma Score

Glasgow Coma Scale score	Systolic blood pressure (mmHg)	Respiratory rate (beats/ min)	Coded value
13–15	> 89	10–29	4
9–12	76–89	> 29	3
6–8	50–75	6–9	2
4–5	1–49	1–5	1
3	0	0	0

category (D). Each component is calculated as the square root of the sum of squares of the AISs for all serious injuries within each region. A region with no injury receives a score of zero. Probability of survival is calculated using logistic regression, and the AP performs somewhat better than the ISS although it is more complex.[44]

International Classification of Diseases

Another, more recent, method of scoring anatomic injury uses the *International Classification of Diseases, Ninth Edition* (ICD-9) codes.[45] This method, termed the ICD-9 Injury Severity Score (ICISS), uses the product of individual survival risk ratios calculated from each ICD-9 discharge diagnosis to estimate survival. This methodology provides a slightly better prediction of survival than the ISS and includes all injuries. It also does not require specialized coding as with the AIS. Although this methodology appears to be superior to the ISS, it is limited by in that not all injuries may be coded and that it still requires more thorough validation prior to widespread use.

Revised Trauma Score

The RTS is one of the more common physiologic scoring systems and was originally suggested and has been used primarily as a triage tool in the pre-hospital setting.[46] In fact, its efficiency is related both to the speed in which it can be applied and its objectivity. The RTS is a combination of three specific physiologic parameters, namely, the GCS score, systolic blood pressure, and respiratory rate. Each of these parameters is divided into five groups on a scale from 0 to 4, resulting in a score that ranges from 0 to 12 (Table 41.3).

An RTS < 11 is used to indicate the need for transport to a designated trauma center. The coded version of the RTS is used more frequently for quality assurance and outcome prediction, and is:

$$RTSc = [0.7326 \times SBPc] + [0.2908 \times RRc] + [0.9368 \times GCSc]$$

Although more complicated to calculate, the coded version of the RTS provides for a more precise prediction of outcome because each of its three components is weighted differently, with GCS having the greatest weight.

The RTS has several limitations. Its primary limitation is related to the GCS. As originally described, the GCS was intended to measure functional status of the central nervous system in trauma. Therefore, problems inherent in using the GCS (e.g., scoring intubated, pediatric patients, or intoxicated patients) are reflected in the RTS. Recent research has shown that the motor component alone is as predictive as the total GCS.[47] This may require revision of the RTS.

Acute Physiology and Chronic Health Evaluation

The APACHE was introduced in 1981 and a revision (i.e., the APACHE II) was introduced 4 years later.[48,49] It is one of several intensive care-based scoring systems, and is used widely for the assessment of illness severity, including in both medical and surgical patients. This scoring system incorporates the patient's age, previous health status, and 12 routine physiologic measurements (e.g., vital signs, results from arterial blood gases, serum chemistries and blood counts, and renal function) ranges from 0 to 71, and provides a general measure of illness severity. The score incorporates variables at admission and at 24 hours after admission to the intensive care unit in order to estimate mortality. Unfortunately, patients with trauma only compromised 8% of the study population used to develop APACHE II, and they had a relatively low mortality, although traumatic brain injury was heavily weighted in those who did die.[49]

In 1992, researchers demonstrated that APACHE II was inferior to the TRISS in predicting mortality in injured patients, and its poor performance was primarily related to the absence of an anatomic component in the APACHE system.[50] A method to calculate a more refined score (i.e., APACHE III) was therefore published in 1991 in an effort to address these issues.[51] This score has not been widely accepted, in part, because it is proprietary and it has not yet been convincingly validated in patients with trauma.

Trauma and Injury Severity Score

The TRISS is arguably the most widely recognized and used tool to predict mortality in patients with trauma.[52,53] It combines both anatomic and physiologic measures of injury severity (i.e., the ISS and RTS, respectively), and patient age and mechanism of injury (either blunt or penetrating). This score was also developed using multivariable logistic regression and quickly became the standard methodology for outcome assessment among trauma patients after standing-up to external validation in both adult and pediatric populations (Box 41.1).[53]

Box 41.1   Trauma and Injury Severity Score

Survival probability $= 1/(1 + e^{-b})$
where "b" is calculated as for patients with blunt mechanisms as:

$$b = -0.4499 + (0.8085 \times RTS) \\ - (0.0835 \times ISS) - (1.743 \times \text{Age Index})$$

or for patients with penetrating mechanisms as:

$$b = -2.5355 + (0.9934 \times RTS) \\ - (0.0651 \times ISS) - (1.136 \times \text{Age Index})$$

where age index is equal to 0 if the patient is younger than 54 years or equal to 1 if 55 years or older.

Its limitations have been widely noted and include its modest predictive ability, incorporation of the ISS with its inherent limitations (although incorporating the NISS improves the overall score) and the RTS with its inherent limitations, and the lack of incorporation of pre-existing conditions, which contribute to mortality.

A Severity Characterization Of Trauma

In an effort to improve TRISS, Champion et al. developed ASCOT.[54] This score uses the AP in place of the ISS and categorizes age into deciles. Additional

changes include the individual components of the coded RTS. Unfortunately, the predictive performance of ASCOT is only slightly better than the ISS, and this coupled with the complexity of the AP has dissuaded investigators from using it.

More recently, investigators have conducted more elaborate and computationally complex modeling to attempt to provide additional guidance for predicting survival following trauma and incorporating pre-existing conditions into such models.[36,42,55]

Controversies and difficulties of research with critical patients

One of the major difficulties conducting research with trauma patients is the inability to obtain consent from critically ill patients. In addition, patients may be in pain, or have impaired cognition because of injury or intoxication.[56]

In 1996, the "Final Rule" was codified into Federal Regulations.

This rule allows a limited category of research bearing more than minimal risk to go forward without informed consent. The Emergency Research Waiver Rule permits Institutional Review Boards to waive the requirement for informed consent when certain conditions are met, including: patients who are in a life-threatening situation that necessitates intervention; obtaining informed consent from a legally authorized representative (LAR) is not feasible within the time period necessary to initiate the experimental intervention; and available treatments are unproven or unsatisfactory.[58] In addition, researchers must consult with representatives of the communities in which the research will be carried out and publicly disclose the risks and benefits of the proposed research to those communities (see Box 41.2).

The first large multicenter clinical trial conducted under the Emergency Research Waiver Rule was a study of an oxygen-carrying blood substitute, Baxter Laboratories' HemAssist®.[59] This study was ended early after review of two adverse events found that the diaspirin cross-linked hemoglobin group had higher mortality rates than the control group. Lewis et al. examined the decision to terminate the study and concluded that the Data Monitoring Committee had appropriately allowed the study to begin and the committee monitored the study and protected patient interests in the absence of informed consent.[60]

Box 41.2 The Final Rule[57]

Section 50.24(a)
This rule describes the following criteria that must be met for a clinical investigation to be eligible for an exception from the informed consent requirements. The responsible Institutional Review Board must find and document the following:

- The human subjects are in a life-threatening situation and available treatments are unproven or unsatisfactory.
- Obtaining informed consent is not feasible because of the subjects' medical conditions and the intervention under investigation must be administered before consent can feasibly be obtained from the subjects' legally authorized representative.
- Participation in the research holds out the prospect of direct benefit to the subjects because evidence supports the potential of the intervention.
- The clinical investigation could not practicably be carried out without the exception from informed consent.
- The proposed investigational plan defines the length of the potential therapeutic window based on scientific evidence, and the investigator has committed to attempting to contact a legally authorized representative for each subject within that window of time.
- In addition, public disclosure to the community, consultations with the community, and establishment of an independent data monitoring committee are required.

Patients in this trial received the diaspirin treatment within 60 minutes of arrival to the emergency department. Because these were critically injured patients with hemorrhagic shock, prospective consent would be difficult to obtain for all patients. The investigators retrospectively reviewed the informed consent process and found that of 98 patients, prospective consent was obtained from only two patients, three family members, and one LAR (6%). In addition, consent to continue was requested for 89 patients (89%) and full participation was granted for 87 of these patients (98%).[59] This suggests that the Final Rule can be applied to emergency research and that patients and LARs agree to continue participation in most cases.

A more controversial use of the Final Rule was applied to a clinical trial for patients with hemorrhagic shock that compared Polyheme® (Northfield Laboratories Inc., Evanston, IL), an oxygen-carrying resuscitative fluid, to saline. This clinical trial was classified as a prehospital study, as patients were enrolled prior to their arrival at the emergency department. Because patients in hemorrhagic shock are critically ill, most are unable to consent to participation in a research study. In addition, the vast majority of paramedics do not give blood products in the prehospital setting so Polyheme® would be a treatment that patients would normally not be able to receive in the field.[58] Thus, from these criteria, the Polyheme® study qualified for waiver of consent. Once in the hospital, the control group received standard treatment including blood. However, patients in the experimental arm received up to 6 units of Polyheme® for up to 12 hours (and instead of blood transfusions).[58] From a consent perspective, it would still be difficult to obtain consent to continue from a LAR during this critical 12-hour time period, contributing to the rationale for using waiver of consent. The Final Rule allows patients to participate in research to obtain treatments they would not have access to otherwise. However, patients in hemorrhagic shock would have access to blood transfusions once in the hospital. A controversy arose with the Polyheme® trial due to the the consideration that patients randomized to the experimental arm would not have received the standard care. Holloway also wrote about concerns regarding community consultation for the study.[61] Of the four community information sessions conducted for the Duke University site, one was at a rotary club, two were at malls, and one was at a baseball game. He asserted that many urban, African-Americans were not engaged in these consultations to an appropriate extent. Use of emergency consent should be used cautiously with these concerns in mind and adequately addressed prior to initiating the study. Critics of the Final Rule state that meeting all the requirements lengthens the study approval process and increases the cost of conducting a trial. In these instances, consent by proxy may be an alternative for emergency research. Wright et al. utilized consent by proxy for a clinical trial of progesterone vs. placebo for traumatic brain injury.[62] The time to initiation of experimental treatment through proxy consent was approximately 379 minutes; the authors projected that this would have been reduced to approximately 92 minutes under the Final Rule. In addition, 25 patients were not enrolled because of failure to identify either the patient or a LAR in a

Box 41.3 Advanced trauma research example

A 40-year-old male presented after a motorcycle crash. Prehospital vitals include a blood pressure of 90/60 mmHg, a respiratory rate (RR) of 8 beats/min, a heart rate (HR) of 120 beats/min, and a Glasgow Coma Scale (GCS) score of 10. After thorough evaluation, he was found to have a subarachnoid hemorrhage and a Grade 3 liver laceration as well as an open femur fracture and a closed non-displaced tibial shaft fracture.

Revised Trauma Score (RTS)

Variable	Coded value
GCS = 10	3
Systolic blood pressure (SBP) = 90 mmHg	4
RR = 8 beats/min	2

RTS = [0.9368 GCS value] + [0.7326 SBP value] + [0.2908 RR value]
RTS = [0.9368 3] + [0.7326 4] + [0.2908 2]
RTS = [2.89] + [2.93] + [0.58]
RTS = 6.32
The RTS ranges from 0 to 7.84. An RTS of 6 predicts a survival probability of approximately 92% whereas an RTS of 7 predicts a survival probability of approximately 97%.

Abbreviated Injury Scale and the Injury Severity Score (AIS and ISS)

Region	Injury description	AIS	Top three squared
Head and neck	Subarachnoid hemorrhage	3	9
Face	No injury	0	
Chest	No injury	0	
Abdomen	Grade 3 liver laceration	4	16
Extremity	Open femur fracture	4	16
	Closed tibia fracture	2	
External	No injury	0	
	Injury Severity Score:		**41**

Trauma and Injury Severity Score [TRISS]

Survival probability = $1/(1 + e^{-(0.4499 + (0.8085\ RTS) - (0\ 0835\ ISS) - (1.743\ Age\ Index))})$
Survival probability = $1/(1 + e^{-(0.4499 + (0.8085\ 6322) - (0\ 0835\ 41) - (1743))})$
Survival probability = 77.5%

---

timely fashion. So despite the longer approval process and costs associated with the Final Rule, the authors concluded that because of these findings, investigators conducting time-critical studies should make efforts to comply with the Final Rule. Additionally, prehospital research is difficult to conduct because there is often little or no agreement on clear definitions, standard data elements, and validated severity scoring for traumatic conditions.[63] Also, the implementation of randomized controlled trials in the prehospital setting is often very difficult and

not always possible or suitable given the short treatment period and limited interventions available to Emergency Medical Services (EMS). A search of all the scientific studies in medicine from 1985 to the mid 1990s revealed 5842 publications on prehospital EMS, but only 54 were randomized trials and only one was a double blind randomized controlled trial that showed a positive outcome to a trial.[64] However, the prehospital setting is an important part of trauma treatment and studies should be conducted in this setting despite the limitations and difficulties

Table 41.4 Glossary of commonly used terms

Basic science research	Research conducted in a laboratory, typically using molecular, cellular, organs, or animals (exclusive of humans) as subjects
Clinical research	Research that involves humans as subjects in the study and typically involves inferences at the individual patient level
Health services (outcomes) research	Research that involves humans as subjects and typically involves inferences at the population level
Experimental study design	One of three main categories of research design. This includes an intervention (e.g., a new drug) and randomization, and is considered the most valid design available to researchers. A randomized, controlled, trial represents an experimental design
Quasi-experimental study design	This study design includes an intervention but uses quasi-randomization (e.g., randomizing by alternating days)
Observational study design	This study design includes no intervention and is typically subcategorized into: (1) cohort studies; (2) cross-sectional studies; or (3) case-control studies
Prospective data collection	Collecting data de novo and real-time
Retrospective data collection	Collecting data from existing data sources
Primary data analysis	Using data collected primarily for the current study
Secondary data analysis	Using data collected primarily for another purpose to conduct a study
Trauma registry	Centralized database, typically maintained by individual hospitals with trauma designations, of selected trauma patients and characteristics associated with the traumatic event, the care provided to the patient, and outcomes. National registries include the National Trauma Data Bank® (NTDB), the NTDB National Sample Project, and the National Automotive Sampling System and Fatality Analysis Reporting System
Trauma scoring systems	Standardized injury severity assessments used to stratify groups of trauma patients, to control for severity of injury when evaluating outcomes, or in evaluating trauma care and their systems
Anatomical scoring systems	Trauma scoring systems based on anatomical regions (e.g., Injury Severity Score)
Physiological scoring systems	Trauma scoring systems based on the patient's physiology (e.g., Glasgow Coma Scale score)
Combined scoring systems	Trauma scoring systems based on both anatomical and physiological components (e.g., Trauma and Injury Severity Score)
The Final Rule	Federal regulations that describe criteria that must be met for clinical investigation to be eligible for exception from the informed consent requirements

inherent with EMS research. This is reflected, in part, by the development of the Resuscitation Outcomes Consortium (ROC).[65] The ROC is primarily funded by the National Institutes of Health and includes multiple EMS systems across North America in an effort to conduct collaborative clinical trials of promising new treatments for cardiac arrest and severe traumatic injuries.

Conclusions

Trauma care is enhanced by our ability to understand trauma epidemiology, and diagnostic and therapeutic approaches. Research, spanning from the laboratory to populations, is critical for the continued advancement of how trauma patients are managed. The validity of such research is predicated on the questions posed, the methods used, and how the results are interpreted and incorporated into patient care. Although much progress has been made over the past several decades, there is still a significant need for well-trained clinician-scientists who will continue to advance trauma research (see Box 41.3 for an example, and Table 41.4 for a glossary of commonly used terms).

References

1. Centers for Disease Control and Prevention. *CDC Injury Fact Book*. Available from http://www.cdc.gov/ncipc/fact_book/Introduction-2006.pdf.

2. Stahel PF, Smith WR, Moore EE. Role of biological modifiers regulating the immune response after trauma. *Injury* 2007;**38**:1409–22.

3. Escobar GA, Cheng AM, Moore EE, et al. Stored packed red blood cell transfusion up-regulates inflammatory gene expression in circulating leukocytes. *Ann Surg* 2007;**246**:129–34.

4. Smith W, Williams A, Agudelo J, et al. Early predictors of mortality in hemodynamically unstable pelvis fractures. *J Orthop Trauma* 2007;**21**:31–7.

5. Murrell Z, Haukoos JS, Putnam B, et al. The effect of older blood on mortality, need for ICU care, and length of ICU stay after major trauma. *Am Surg* 2005;**71**:781–5.

6. Cothren CC, Moore EE, Hedegaard HB, et al. Epidemiology of urban trauma deaths: a comprehensive reassessment 10 years later. *World J Surg* 2007;**31**:1507–11.

7. Rothman KJ, Greenland S. *Modern Epidemiology*, 2nd edn. Philadelphia, PA: Lippincott, Williams and Wilkins, 1998.

8. Rivara FP, Cummings P, Koepsell TD, et al. *Injury Control: A Guide to Research and Program Evaluation*. New York: Cambridge University Press, 2001.

9. Campbell DT, Stanley JC. *Experimental and Quasi-Experimental Designs for Research*. Boston: Houghton Mifflin Company, 1963.

10. Krause MS, Howard KI. What random assignment does and does not do. *J Clin Psychol* 2003;**59**:751–66.

11. Lewis RJ. Modeling complex systems: gaining valid insights and avoiding mathematical delusions. *Acad Emerg Med* 2007;**19**:795–8.

12. Gilbert EH, Lowenstein SR, Koziol-McLain J, et al. Chart reviews in emergency medicine research: where are the methods? *Ann Emerg Med* 1996;**27**:305–8.

13. Worster A, Bledsoe RD, Cleve P, et al. Reassessing the methods of medical record review studies in emergency medicine research. *Ann Emerg Med* 2005;**45**:448–51.

14. Day S, Fayers P, Harvey D. Double data entry: what value, what price? *Controlled Clin Trials* 1998;**19**:15–24.

15. Harrell FE. *Regression Modeling Strategies: With Applications to Linear Models, Logistic Regression, and Survival Analysis*. New York: Springer-Verlag, 2001.

16. Hosmer DW, Lemeshow S. *Applied Logistic Regression*, 2nd edn. New Jersey: John Wiley and Sons, 2000.

17. Royston P. A strategy for modeling the effect of a continuous covariate in medicine and epidemiology. *Stat Med* 2000;**19**:1831–47.

18. Haukoos JS, Newgard CD. Advanced statistics: missing data in clinical research – part 1: an introduction and conceptual framework. *Acad Emerg Med* 2007;**14**:662–8.

19. Newgard CD, Haukoos JS. Advanced statistics: missing data in clinical research – part 2: multiple imputation. *Acad Emerg Med* 2007;**14**:669–78.

20. Newgard CD, Hedges JR, Arthur M, et al. Advanced statistics: the propensity score – a method for estimating treatment effect in observational research. *Acad Emerg Med* 2004;**11**:953–61.

21. Ungar TC, Wolf SJ, Haukoos JS, et al. Derivation of a clinical decision rule to exclude thoracic aortic imaging in patients with blunt chest trauma after motor vehicle collisions. *J Trauma* 2006;**61**:1150–5.

22. Haukoos JS, Gill MR, Rabon RE, et al. Validation of the Simplified Motor Score for the prediction of brain injury outcomes after trauma. *Ann Emerg Med* 2007;**50**:18–24.

23. Guice KS, Cassidy LD, Mann NC. State trauma registries: survey and update – 2004. *J Trauma* 2007;**62**:424–35.

24. Mann NC, Mullins RJ. Research recommendations and proposed action items to facilitate trauma system implementation and evaluation. *J Trauma* 1999;**47**:S75–8.

25. Mann NC, Guice K, Cassidy L, et al. Are statewide trauma registries comparable? Reaching for a national trauma dataset. *Acad Emerg Med* 2006;**13**:946–53.

26. Waller JA, Skelly JM, Davis JH. Trauma center-related biases in injury research. *J Trauma* 1995;**38**:325–9.

27. Lowenstein S. Trauma registries: tarnished gold. *Ann Emerg Med* 1996;**27**:389–91.

28. American College of Surgeons Committee on Trauma. *National Trauma Data Bank*. Available from http://www.facs.org/trauma/ntdb.html.

29. National Center for Statistics and Analysis of the National Highway Traffic Safety Administration.

National Automotive Sampling System. Available from http://www-nrd.nhtsa.dot.gov/departments/nrd-30/ncsa/NASS.html.

30. Newgard CD, Lewis RJ. Effects of child age and body size on serious injury from passenger air-bag presence in motor vehicle crashes. *Pediatrics* 2005;**115**:1579–85.

31. Wood DP, Veyrat N, Simms C, et al. Limits for survivability in frontal collisions: theory and real-life data combined. *Accid Anal Prev* 2007;**39**:679–87.

32. Jehle D, Kuebler J, Auinger P. Risk of injury and fatality in single vehicle rollover crashes: danger for the front seat occupant in the "outside arc." *Acad Emerg Med* 2007;**14**:899–902.

33. Cook A, Shackford S, Osler T, et al. Use of vena cava filters in pediatric trauma patients: data from the National Trauma Data Bank. *J Trauma* 2005;**59**:1114–20.

34. Millham FH, LaMorte WW. Factors associated with mortality in trauma: re-evaluation of the TRISS method using the National Trauma Data Bank. *J Trauma* 2004;**56**:1090–6.

35. National Center for Statistics and Analysis. *Fatality Analysis Reporting System: Fatal Crash Data Overview*. Available from http://www-nrd.nhtsa.dot.gov/pdf/nrd-30/NCSA/FARS/809–726/index.htm.

36. Haukoos JS. Advanced modeling strategies in emergency medicine research: is the pendulum swinging? *Ann Emerg Med* 2008;**52**(4):365–7.

37. Chawda MN, Hildebrand F, Pape HC, et al. Predicting outcome after multiple trauma: which scoring system? *Injury* 2004;**35**:347–58.

38. Kramer CF, Barancik JI, Thode HC. Improving the sensitivity and specificity of the abbreviated injury scale coding system. *Public Health Rep* 1990;**105**:334–40.

39. Moore EE, Shackford SR, Pachter HL, et al. Organ injury scaling – spleen, liver and kidney. *J Trauma* 1989;**29**:1664–6.

40. Baker SP, O'Neill B, Haddon W, et al. The injury severity score: a method for describing patients with multiple injuries and evaluating emergency care. *J Trauma* 1974;**14**:187–96.

41. Osler T, Baker SP, Long W. A modification of the injury severity score that both improves accuracy and simplifies scoring. *J Trauma* 1997;**43**:922–5.

42. Moore L, Lavoie A, Le Sage NL, et al. Using information on preexisting conditions to predict mortality from traumatic injury. *Ann Emerg Med* 2008;**52**(4):356–64.

43. Copes WS, Champion HR, Sacco WJ, et al. Progress in characterizing anatomic injury. *J Trauma* 1990;**30**:1200–7.

44. Frankema SP, Steyerberg EW, Edwards MJ, et al. Comparison of current injury scales for survival chance estimation: an evaluation comparing the predictive performance of the ISS, NISS, and AP scores in a Dutch local trauma registration. *J Trauma* 2005;**58**:596–604.

45. Osler T, Rutledge R, Deis J, et al. ICISS: an International Classification of Disease-9 Based Injury Severity Score. *J Trauma* 1996;**41**:380–6.

46. Champion HR, Sacco WJ, Copes WS, et al. A revision of the Trauma Score. *J Trauma* 1989;**29**:623–9.

47. Haukoos JS, Gill MR, Rabon RE, et al. Validation of the Simplified Motor Score for the prediction of brain injury outcomes after trauma. *Ann Emerg Med* 2007;**50**:18–24.

48. Knaus WA, Zimmerman JE, Wagner DP, et al. APACHE – Acute Physiology and Chronic Health Evaluation: a physiologically based classification system. *Crit Care Med* 1981;**9**:591–7.

49. Knaus WA, Draper EA, Wagner DP, et al. APACHE II: a severity of disease classification system. *Crit Care Med* 1985;**13**:818–29.

50. Vassar MJ, Wilkerson CL, Duran PJ, et al. Comparison of APACHE II, TRISS, and a proposed 24-hour ICU point system for prediction of outcome in ICU trauma patients. *J Trauma* 1992;**32**:490–9.

51. Knaus WA, Wagner DP, Draper EA, et al. The APACHE III prognostic system. Risk prediction of hospital mortality for critically ill hospitalized adults. *Chest* 1991;**100**:1619–39.

52. Boyd CR, Tolson MA, Copes WS. Evaluating trauma care: the TRISS method. Trauma Score and Injury Severity Score. *J Trauma* 1987;**27**:370–8.

53. Furnival RA, Schunk JE. ABCs of scoring systems for pediatric trauma. *Pediatr Emerg Care* 1999;**15**:215–23.

54. Champion HR, Copes WS, Sacco WJ, et al. Improved predictions from A Severity Characterization of Trauma (ASCOT) over Trauma and Injury Severity Score (TRISS): results of an independent evaluation. *J Trauma* 1996;**40**:42–8.

55. Bergeron E, Rossignol M, Osler T, et al. Improving the TRISS methodology by restructuring age categories and adding comorbidities. *J Trauma* 2004;**56**:760–7.

56. Nee PA, Griffiths RD. Ethical considerations in accident and emergency research. *Emerg Med J* 2002;**19**:423–7.

57. Offices of the Secretary, DHHS, FDA. Protection of humans subjects: informed consent and waiver of informed consent requirements in certain emergency research circumstances: Final Rule. *Fed Reg* 1996;**61**:51498–533.

58. Kipnis K, King N, Nelson RM. An open letter to institutional review boards considering Northfield laboratories Polyheme® trial. *Am J Bioethics* 2006;**6**:18–21.

59. Sloan EP, Koenigsberg M, Brunett PH, et al. Post hoc mortality analysis of the efficacy trial of diaspirin cross-linked hemoglobin in the treatment of severe traumatic hemorrhagic shock. *J Trauma* 2002;**52**:887–95.

60. Lewis RJ, Berry DA, Cryer H, et al. Monitoring a clinical trial conducted under the Food and Drug Administration regulations allowing a waiver of prospective informed consent: the diaspirin cross-linked hemoglobin traumatic hemorrhagic shock efficacy trial. *Ann Emerg Med* 2001; **38**:397–404.

61. Holloway KF. Accidental communities: race, emergency medicine, and the problem of Polyheme®. *Am J Bioeth* 2006;**6**(3):7–17.

62. Wright DW, Clark P, Pentz R, et al. Enrolling subjects by exception from consent versus proxy consent in trauma care research. *Ann Emerg Med* 2008;**51**(4):355–60.

63. Osterwalder JJ. Insufficient quality of research on prehospital medical emergency care – where are the problems and solutions? *Swiss Med Wkly* 2004;**134**:389–94.

64. Callaham M. Quantifying the scanty science of prehospital emergency care. *Ann Emerg Med* 1997;**30**:785–90.

65. National Institutes of Health. *Clinical Research Consortium to Improve Resuscitation Outcomes*. Available from http://www.nhlbi.nih.gov/funding/inits/resus_faq.htm#sci.

Chapter

42

Trauma nursing

Nancy Martin, Julie Mayglothling, and Marion Machado

Care of the injured patient has evolved greatly in the past two decades. With the development of rapid prehospital care and transport, severely injured patients who might have died at the scene are being brought to trauma centers alive. Because of the increased challenges of caring for this complex population, trauma nursing has developed into a highly specialized field. Coordinating care for the injured patient requires the nurse to have an understanding of both the immediate needs of the patient as well as the impact injuries will have on the patient's outcome. Detailed medical history is often not available, and there may be no time for diagnostic tests. The initial evaluation needs to be performed expeditiously; it is geared towards initiation of resuscitation and rapid diagnosis of all injuries with the intent to treat the greatest threat to life first.

It is difficult to provide firm recommendations as to the nurse staffing levels that are optimal or necessary in the trauma resuscitation area. The number of nurses necessary to provide the level of care is dependent upon the availability of other staff, such as medical technicians and assistants. At least two nurses with training in trauma should optimally be present for each resuscitation. In addition, each emergency department (ED) that treats victims of trauma should have a pre-defined plan as to how additional resources, including nurses, can be called upon in case of increased patient volume.

Initial trauma resuscitation is often a high-stress environment where a number of activities are carried out simultaneously or in rapid succession. This necessitates that the nurse be able to function effectively in demanding situations. Prior to caring for these critical trauma patients, the Emergency Nurses Association recommends nurses should have at least 6 months experience in an ED or a critical care setting.[1]

Additionally the nurse should be proctored by a more senior and experienced nurse prior to assuming the responsibility of trauma resuscitation. Educational preparation should include courses such as Trauma Nursing Core Course (TNCC), Advanced Trauma Care for Nurses (ATCN), Course in Advanced Trauma Nursing (CATN), and Emergency Nursing Pediatric Course (ENPC) (Table 42.1). It is recommended by the American College of Surgeons that nurses take at least one of these courses.[2] These courses are offered through national organizations such as the Society of Trauma Nurses and the Emergency Nurses Association. Some states have enacted programs certifying nurses to become Trauma Nurse Specialists (TNS). The purpose of the TNS program is to increase the competency of nurses in the delivery of care to critically injured patients. While obtaining certification through these various courses may be important, it is equally important to ensure maintenance of competencies. One common option is to perform routine evaluations to ensure that existing competencies are retained and new knowledge related to trauma care is incorporated into practice. The exact methodology utilized to maintain these competencies is often dictated by state or national verifying agencies.

The primary nurse's role in the trauma room is multifaceted and begins prior to the patient's arrival. Based on the prehospital report, the nurse should have the necessary equipment at the bedside, ready for use. Suggested equipment for the care of the injured patient can be found in the Advanced Trauma Life Support® (ATLS®) manual; however, many trauma centers will have their own specific preferences of what type and amount of equipment to utilize.[3] Having the appropriate equipment at the bedside reduces delay in therapy, which may have a

Table 42.1 Suggested qualifications and certifications of the resuscitation nurse

Qualifications	6–12 months experience in an emergency department/or critical care setting
Educational preparation	• Trauma Nursing Core Course (TNCC)
	• Advanced Trauma Care for Nurses (ATCN)
	• Course in Advanced Trauma Nursing (CATN)
	• Emergency Nursing Pediatric Course (ENPC)
	• Advanced Cardiac Life Support (ACLS)

direct effect on the patient's ultimate outcome. If the resuscitation nurse is the first person to receive prehospital communication regarding the patient, the other members of the team should be provided with a brief, concise report that should include: patient age, mechanism of injury, injuries (known and suspected), vital signs, and treatment rendered in the field. Equipment setup should also include provision of personal protective equipment for all members of the team that will be in direct contact with the patient.

Upon the patient's arrival the nurse is responsible for setting up the monitoring equipment, measuring vital signs, and assisting the physicians with emergency procedures such as endotracheal intubation, placement of chest tubes, etc. Hypothermia can be dangerous to a trauma patient; the nurse should obtain an initial core temperature and ensure that the patient does not unnecessarily lose body heat. This requires avoidance of exposure except when medically necessary, maintenance of environmental temperature, and provision of blankets, fluid warmers, and body warmers. Once the initial evaluation has been completed, and the patient stabilized as much as possible, the physician team leader will decide the next step. This may be transfer to another area within the hospital for definitive care, transport to the radiology suite for further tests, or transfer to a higher level of care at another hospital. The nurse should take reasonable steps to ensure that the patient's care will not deteriorate once they leave the ED. This entails ensuring adequate monitoring will take place, all essential lines and tubes are secured,

and any necessary drugs are available during transport. Lastly, the nurse is responsible for adequate documentation of the initial condition of the patient at arrival, the vital signs during the stay in the ED, and all procedures performed, including fluid resuscitation, transfusions, and medications administered. Any relevant history obtained from the patient or the prehospital providers should also be documented.

> **Box 42.1 Responsibilities of the resuscitation nurse(s)**
>
> • Assist with set up of equipment based on prehospital report.
> • Relay information from prehospital report to other providers.
> • Upon the patient's arrival, set up the monitoring equipment, measure vital signs, and assist as necessary with emergency procedures (including assisting with or primarily obtaining intravenous access).
> • Obtain an initial core temperature and ensure that the patient does not unnecessarily lose body heat.
> • Ensure that the patient's care will not deteriorate once they leave the ED.
> • This entails ensuring adequate monitoring will take place, essential lines and tubes are secured, and any necessary drugs are available during transport.
> • Adequately document the initial condition of the patient, the vital signs during the stay, and all procedures performed, including fluid resuscitation, transfusions, and medications administered.

While all of the above nursing procedures are to be performed during the initial evaluation, the specific member of the team who actually performs each task will vary based on the composition of the team. The team composition is influenced by the size of the hospital and whether the hospital has a teaching mission. There usually are more trained personnel available at designated trauma centers and at teaching hospitals. The nurse, along with the physician team leader, should define the roles of individual members of the team such as medical students, residents, student nurses, and medical assistants. In addition, the nurse plays a key role in coordinating care, including the timing of radiology, evaluation by consulting services, and social workers. Because of the size and composition of the team, communication plays a major role in prevention of errors and maintaining a controlled environment during the trauma resuscitation.

Trauma nurse coordinator/trauma program manager

Trauma has been a leader among medical specialties in critically evaluating care and patient outcomes. Modern trauma care is increasing in complexity and involves multiple specialties. This has led to the need for a person with a nursing background who can coordinate the care among specialties throughout the continuum. In the late 1970s, as trauma centers were developing, the role of the Trauma Coordinator or the Trauma Program Manager (TPM) was created. The TPM is usually a registered nurse who works in close collaboration with the Trauma Medical Director (TMD) to ensure the services and systems are in place to care for the injured patient. The American College of Surgeons Committee on Trauma *Resources for the Optimal Care of the Injured Patient 2006* provides details regarding the role and responsibility of the TPM.[3] The document describes the clinical aspects of the TPM as coordinating management across the continuum of care, the planning and implementation of clinical management guidelines, and the continuous monitoring of patient outcomes. The TPM is also responsible for development of trauma education programs, not only within the hospital, but for referral facilities, prehospital, and community prevention programs. Performance improvement (PI) is the backbone of any mature trauma program. The TPM is responsible for the maintenance of the trauma registry that provides the necessary information for an effective PI program. As an administrative position, the TPM is also responsible for ensuring compliance with the regulatory guidelines that are mandatory for trauma center verification. The TPM also has responsibility for managing the operational, personnel, and financial aspects of the trauma program.

The majority of trauma in the United States is initially evaluated in the EDs of hospitals that are not designated trauma centers. In these situations the trauma physician leader and the nurse together need to develop a plan as to whether the patient will stay at the receiving hospital or should be transferred to a designated trauma center for higher level of care. The key to this decision is the balance between the needs of the patient and the available resources at the receiving hospital. For some patients the decision is

straightforward. Such patients fall into two broad categories. The first consists of patients with derangements in physiology, usually from bleeding that requires surgical or radiological control not available at the receiving hospital. The second category consists of patients whose anatomic injury requires specialized care (i.e., severe single system injury requiring highly specialized care or injuries involving multiple body regions requiring coordinated care from multiple specialties). In some patients the decision is not straightforward and considerable judgment is required on the part of the physician and nurse. Once the decision is made to transfer the patient to a higher level of care, the physician and the nurse should directly speak to the receiving personnel at the other hospital to ensure that all pertinent information about the patient is accurately conveyed. The nurse should further ensure that proper monitoring will occur during transport and that all lines and tubes are adequately secured so that they are not dislodged during transport. Finally, the nurse should oversee the proper gathering of all documentation, including copies of all radiological and laboratory tests, to send to the other hospital.[4]

Death due to a traumatic event often poses challenges to all involved in the patient's care. It may be especially challenging for the resuscitation nurse involved in the care of the deceased patient. The nurse must assist with providing an environment of dignity for the patient and the family. Because many traumatic deaths occur in young, healthy adults, the family reaction to death is one of intense grief. Anger, immense sorrow, and disbelief are some of the reactions that can be anticipated in a traumatic death. A multidisciplinary approach should be taken by the nurse in dealing with issues surrounding traumatic death. The nurse may have involvement from the chaplain or social worker to assist the family, provide resources and assist in decision making. The nurse may activate agencies dealing with organ donation and or the medical examiner. The nurse works with the physician and acts as a liaison with these agencies, providing details of the event, injuries, and resuscitation efforts.

References

1. Emergency Nurses Association. *So You Want to be an Emergency Nurse*. Available from http://www.ena.org/careercenter/.

2. American College of Surgeons Committee on Trauma. *Advanced Trauma Life Support for Doctors: Instructors*

Course Manual. Chicago, IL: American College of Surgeons, 2008.

3. American College of Surgeons Committee on Trauma. *Resources for Optimal Care of the Injured Patient 2006*. Chicago, IL: American College of Surgeons, 2006.

4. Von Rueden KT, Hartsock RL. Nursing practice through the cycle of trauma. In McQuillan KA, Von Rueden KT, Hartsock RL, et al. (eds), *Trauma Nursing: From Resuscitation through Rehabilitation*, 3rd edn. Philadelphia, PA: WB Saunders, 2002: pp. 107–28.

Index